MOSBY'S
Family Practice Sourcebook

An Evidence-Based Approach to Care

Fourth Edition

MOSBY'S
Family Practice Sourcebook

An Evidence-Based Approach to Care

Fourth Edition

Michael Evans, M.D., CCFP

Director, The Health Knowledge Lab, Centre for Effective Practice
Associate Professor, Department of Family and Community Medicine
University of Toronto
Toronto, Ontario, Canada

ELSEVIER
MOSBY

Notice

Pharmacology is an ever-changing field. Standard safety precautions must be followed, but as new research and clinical experience broaden our knowledge, changes in treatment and drug therapy may become necessary or appropriate. Readers are advised to check the most current product information provided by the manufacturer of each drug to be administered to verify the recommended dose, the method and duration of administration, and contraindications. It is the responsibility of the licensed prescriber, relying on experience and knowledge of the patient, to determine dosages and the best treatment for each individual patient. Neither the Publisher nor the editor assume any liability for any injury and/or damage to persons or property arising from this publication.

Library and Archives Canada Cataloguing in Publication

Evans, Michael, 1964-
    Mosby's family practice sourcebook: an evidence-based approach to care / Michael Evans. – 4th ed.
Includes bibliographical references and index.
ISBN-13: 978-0-7796-9906-3   ISBN-10: 0-7796-9906-8
1. Family medicine—Textbooks. I. Title. II. Title: Family practice sourcebook.

RC55.E92 2005   610   C2005-905887-0

Publisher: Ann Millar
Managing Developmental Editor: Martina van de Velde
Developmental Editor: May Look
Projects Manager: Liz Radojkovic
Publishing Services Manager: Pat Joiner
Senior Book Designer: Kathi Gosche

Elsevier Canada
905 King Street West, 4th Floor, Toronto ON, Canada M6k 3G9
Phone: 1-866-896-3331
Fax: 1-866-359-9534
ISBN-13: 978-0-7796-9906-3
ISBN-10: 0-7796-9906-8

Printed in the United States of America.

2 3 4 5   10 09 08 07 06

Those of us who practice academic medicine receive praise for our academics, but rarely for our medicine. Our peers, the clinicians who "just see patients" but who make the whole system of care actually click—those who stop on the way home for a visit with an elderly patient or get up in the middle of the night to deliver a baby—practice in relative obscurity. It is our good fortune that many of the contributors to this book are these sorts of practitioners. They would argue that the smile of a kid or the hug of an elderly patient is more than enough recognition. We disagree, and dedicate this book to the "general practitioners" in the community.

ACKNOWLEDGEMENTS

Any act of scholarship is rarely the accomplishment of one individual, and this is especially true of *Mosby's Family Practice Sourcebook*. The process of becoming a better caregiver is, in many ways, the process of becoming a more reflective practitioner. We are starting to understand that reflection should not be limited to the clinic, but applied to life. How we understand and enjoy our lives seems a critical, but rarely acknowledged, attribute of thoughtful practice. Ken Marshall epitomizes this concept (see Preface). His ability to set aside the status quo and delineate the truth remains unparalleled. He set a very high standard for this edition to meet.

Our section editors were chosen essentially for their clinical expertise, but also most definitely for their ability to collaborate with colleagues and reflect their knowledge needs. Their hard work and attention to detail allowed us to successfully find and utilize the many talented clinicians who contributed to this work. Rita Shaughnessy, the librarian for our department, and Vivian Yee who worked with Rita, supported our many authors with the latest articles to inform best practice. Personal mentors, all black belts at reflective practice and working without a trace of ego, include Drs. Dave Davis, John Frank, Phil Ellison, and Louise Nasmith (for Michael Evans) and Drs. Kirk Lyon, Morris Rotbard, and John Stewart (for Jamie Meuser).

This book could not have happened but for the efforts of two people. Ann Millar, the acquisitions editor and prime mover from Elsevier Canada, worked with us all to realize a novel relationship between a publisher and an academic institution. It is always interesting to observe an individual who has the patience to watch us, her less experienced partners, make the necessary mistakes to move forward. Thank you, Ann, for your sagacity.

As the new edition had over 170 contributors, significant organizational and relationship management was key to the book's development, and there is always somebody who actually does the necessary day-to-day, behind-the-scenes activities to get this kind of work done. Solé Fernandez was that person for the *Sourcebook*. We all have a new and significant respect for her Chilean approach to life and the fundamental importance of complete but quiet competence and a sunny disposition.

Projects like this one focus on the big picture, covering all the important topics and making sure the information is accurate and helpful. However, to be delivered to the printer, the "devil is in the details." May Look, our developmental editor—working in conjunction with Martina van de Velde from Elsevier Canada—was critical to this process. It helped that she has an inspired sense of humour. We wondered if this was a job requirement. Mike would also like to acknowledge Kevin and the various forms of caffeine available at The Urban Annex Cafe, where most of the book was written.

Finally, we would like to thank our "den mother," Louise Nasmith. Louise is Chair of our department and has many laudable qualities, but chief among these is her ability to make us feel that we are special, and that if we veer off the beaten track, we are supported. Merci, Louise.

Mike Evans & Jamie Meuser

PREFACE

First things first. Without Ken Marshall and his passion for the right answers, none of this would be possible. The foundation of the book you now hold is based wholly on his efforts to create *Mosby's Family Practice Sourcebook* and its subsequent editions. I remember when Ken asked me to edit a section of a previous edition of this book on a topic I was purportedly quite knowledgeable about. I read his draft and made significant edits (thankfully in pencil). I then looked hard at the literature to support my changes. Of course, I ended up erasing most of my edits.

Unlike many of our brethren, Ken was able to look retirement in the eye and claim that his work was done, and asked me to take over as the new editor of the *Sourcebook* series. As I discussed this possibility with seasoned clinicians, residents, and academics, all were keen on a new edition as they found the *Sourcebook* incredibly useful at the bedside. "The perfect mix of the evidence and the practical," they said. With the many people who work closely with me reminding me of my limitations, we decided that I could not replicate Ken's task of editing another version solo. In consultation with James Meuser and Louise Nasmith, we hatched the idea of developing "panels" (see our list of section editors), with significant expertise in managing primary care problems at the bedside. These people are smart and exuberant and it was an honour to work with them. Our new model was to have one editor but also many contributors and section editors. The end result is that this book is truly the good work of over 170 contributors. Most book chapters are written solely by highly published authors. Although this is true of some of our own chapters, it was very rewarding for us to augment this method and synergize it with the experience of people who take care of patients most days. The process of community scholarship came to be the most rewarding part of this new edition.

By building on Ken's work and harnessing the many talents that reside within the Department of Family & Community Medicine at the University of Toronto, I think we have gained new chapters that are truly world class yet retained the spirit of why this book had become so very popular. Examples include more powerful sections on addictions, vascular risk reduction, and sexually transmitted infections. We have added a new section, "Approach to Common Problems," which has been very highly regarded by early reviewers. One rarely sees guidelines on the most common problems we see. Ken's evidence-based and practical approach remains a core attribute, and by unanimous vote of the panel, we have retained colourful features that likely only exist when there is a solo editor, such as the medical usefulness of wine corks and an overview of causative factors for farts.

Our new task will be to take all this useful content and put it into formats that are accessible at the point of curiosity and make it easier for you to manage knowledge. We think this will be an ongoing labour of love for the newly minted Centre for Effective Practice and any feedback and advice is most welcome.

Finally, and on a more personal note, Jamie Meuser is a good friend and the spirit behind the team-building exercise that made this book unique and possible. People do stuff for Jamie that they would not do for the rest of us—this is because they all like him. I am grateful for his partnership in this project.

Mike Evans
January, 2005

No family physician, no matter how competent and dedicated, can acquire or keep in his or her head the vast and changing body of medical data that is needed for adequate care of patients. My goal in writing this annual book is to supplement the already extensive knowledge and skills of practicing family physicians with an up-to-date database that can be accessed quickly and easily.

This book deals primarily with conditions seen and treated by family physicians in an outpatient setting. Some material on inpatient treatment is included, primarily so that office-based family physicians have information with which to counsel patients or their families. Community health issues are also part of the text because prevention of disease is an important part of our mandate.

The *Family Practice Sourcebook* is not a textbook, and only rarely is an attempt made to cover all aspects of any medical condition. Rather, this is an up-to-date, annual reference manual dealing with selected aspects of a wide variety of subjects chosen because of their usefulness or interest for family physicians. Many of the entries are practical therapeutic programs for disorders such as acne, Parkinson's disease, or sexually transmitted diseases, while others cover the background data required by family physicians for making rational decisions about controversial issues such as cholesterol or prostate-specific antigen screening. I hope this text will facilitate the practice of "evidence-based," or if that is not possible, at least "reference-based" office medicine. To help achieve this, almost all of the data in this text has been extracted from recent articles in the medical literature and in most cases the full citations appear at the end of each topic.

HOW TO USE THIS BOOK

Finding Your Way Around the Text

There are six ways of finding your way around the text:

1. Index. Using the index is the most efficient way of finding what you want quickly. Drugs are listed by both generic and trade names.
2. Table of Contents. The table of contents lists the major subject areas covered.
3. Inside front and back covers. A more detailed table of contents is given that corresponds to the outlines described below.
4. Outlines. At the beginning of each subject area listed in the table of contents is an outline of topics covered in that section.
5. Cross references. Related subjects are listed beneath the section and topic headings ("See also ...").
6. Random perusal. This is the most fun. It requires a bit of time and if possible a winter evening in front of a crackling fire.

Errors

I have tried to minimize errors in this volume, but I cannot guarantee that none are present. Therefore anyone using this book should verify the accuracy of the contents, particularly in terms of drugs and dosages, before basing patient treatment on them.

Kenneth G. Marshall, M.D.

PREFACE TO THE SECOND EDITION

In the second edition of *Mosby's Family Practice Sourcebook*, I have modified much of the text by integrating into it information and perspectives obtained from reviewing hundreds of articles from recent medical literature. The result is an up-to-date, succinct, and readable review of data that are relevant to office-based family practice.

An accessible overview such as this is particularly important in the era of proliferating clinical guidelines. Family physicians are overwhelmed by them, and all too often they provide little help: Have recent guidelines been published on this topic? If so, where? Did I receive them? If I did, where are they? Are there several guidelines on the same topic? If there are, which should I use? Which ones are evidence based? If I find the appropriate guideline, can I easily extract from it the information I need?

Hibble and associates collected all the guidelines that were available in 22 general practices in Great Britain. They ended up with 855, which formed a pile 68 cm (27 inches) high and weighing 28 kg (61 lb). Some of the guidelines were so detailed that they were presented in small book format. As Gray put it, "The present position is intolerable [and a major effort has to be directed into managing] knowledge and know how." Slawson and Shaugnessy's objective of "Patient Oriented Evidence that Matters (POEM)" seems to be the ideal one for busy primary care practitioners. My goal has been to make the book a "POEM."

Kenneth G. Marshall, M.D.

PREFACE TO THE THIRD EDITION

As in the two previous editions of *Mosby's Family Practice Sourcebook*, I have collected from the literature a vast amount of pertinent up-to-date information and have presented it in an easy-to-read integrated fashion. I have taken this approach because I think most of us absorb new information better when it is presented in context.

The third edition of the *Family Practice Sourcebook* has been extensively revised with new material culled from over 750 articles published in 1999 in 96 different medical journals. All told, the book contains more than 4000 references, the vast majority from articles published within the last 5 years. Although I have been responsible for most of this work, Dr. Michael Evans from the University of Toronto has used his expertise in critical appraisal to thoroughly revise the section on mood disorders.

Extensively updated topics include gastroesophageal reflux disease, Barrett's esophagus, and esophageal carcinoma; *Helicobacter pylori* and non-ulcer dyspepsia; beta-blockers and spironolactone for heart failure; homocysteine and coronary artery disease; chronic fatigue syndrome and fibromyalgia; hormone replacement therapy; surgical correction of refractive errors; male infertility; concussion in the athlete; screening for colon cancer, diabetes, and prostate cancer; causes of chronic cough; the circumcision controversy; new drugs for dementia, Parkinson's disease, diabetes, and obesity; shaken baby syndrome; urine testing for sexually transmitted diseases; chronic prostatitis; and screening of relatives of patients with subarachnoid hemorrhages for aneurysms.

The medical literature is full of "pearls," often embedded in pages and pages of turgid text. I pride myself in having become a fairly expert miner. I hope you enjoy the material I have extracted and compiled for you.

Kenneth G. Marshall, M.D.

Project Leader:
James Meuser, M.D., C.C.F.P., F.C.F.P.
Centre for Effective Practice
University of Toronto
Ontario, Canada

SECTION EDITORS AND CONTRIBUTORS:
(All Affiliated with the Department of Family &
Community Medicine, University of Toronto, Toronto,
Ontario, Canada)

Common Problems in Family Medicine
Section Editor: Michael Evans
Contributors:
Alison C. Bested
Mel Borins
Riina I. Bray
June Carroll
Michael Evans
Rick Glazier
Dawn Martin
Ross Upshur
Kingsley Watts
David Gordon White

Community Health: Prevention
Section Editors: James Meuser, Ross Upshur
Contributor:
Michael Evans

Community Health: Travel Health
Section Editors: James Meuser, Ross Upshur
Contributors:
Denise Chan
David Lawee
Andrea Somers

Immunizations
Section Editors: James Meuser, Ross Upshur
Contributors:
Eleanor Colledge
Benjamin Comeau
Dean Elterman
Lien Ngoc Luu
Dharini Mahendira
James Meuser
Jacqueline Sandoz
Jessica Tomlinson
Kathryn A. Towns
Sharonie Valin
Karen Weyman

Cardiovascular System
Section Editors: Frank Martino, Nicholas Pimlott
Contributors:
Zishan Allibhai
Sheldon Cheskes
Michael Evans
Karl R. Hartwick
Hashmat Khan
Noah Levine
George Porfiris

Central Nervous System
Section Editors: William J. Watson, Kingsley Watts
Contributors:
François-Gilles Boucher
Amita Dayal
Karl Iglar
Elaine Parker
William F. Sullivan
William J. Watson

Dentistry
Section Editors:
Risa Bordman, Roy Wyman
Contributor:
Barnett I. Giblon

Dermatology
Section Editors:
Risa Bordman, Roy Wyman
Contributors:
Risa Bordman
Russell Goldman
Angela Hwang
Chiu Lee
Dana McKay
James Meuser
Vsevolod Perelman
George Porfiris
David Wheler
Winnie Wong
Roy Wyman
Tanya Wyman

Gastroenterology

Section Editors: Frank Martino, Nicholas Pimlott
Contributors:
Sanjay Agarwal
Michael Evans
Michael Garay
Jeff Handler
Susan Hayward
Diane L. Kelsall
Judy Maynard
Louie Mavrogiannis
James Meuser
Jeffrey W. Sutherland
Shane Teper

Geriatrics

Section Editors: Frank Martino, Nicholas Pimlott
Contributors:
Teresa E. Killam
Robert Lam
Ken Marshall
Nicholas Pimlott

Hematology

Section Editors: Risa Bordman, Roy Wyman
Contributors:
Risa Bordman
Michael Evans
Jeff C. Kwong
Calvin Tai-Ien Lian
Elaine Parker
Lisa Salamon
Ken Uffen

Immunology

Section Editors: James Meuser, Ross Upshur
Contributors:
Gordie Arbess
Chris A. Cavacuiti
Brian M. Cornelson
Abbas Ghavam-Rassoul
Charlie B. Guiang
Ally Murji
Serena Verma
Shirin Yazdanian

Infectious Disease

Section Editors: James Meuser, Ross Upshur
Contributors:
Sean Caine
Eleanor Colledge
Michael Curry
Laurie Dunn
Dean Elterman
Michael Evans
Michael Humphreys
David W. Knox
Mark A. Mandell
James Meuser
David Rosenstein
Jacqueline Sandoz
Ross Upshur
Sharonie Valin
Erika Weir

Mental Health and Addictions: Addictions

Section Editors: William J. Watson, Kingsley Watts
Contributors:
Chris A. Cavacuiti
Meldon Kahan
Lisa Lefebvre
Peter Selby
Kay Shen
Kingsley Watts

Mental Health and Addictions: Mental Health

Section Editors: William J. Watson, Kingsley Watts
Contributors:
Jameet Bawa
Mel Borins
Amita Dayal
Melvin Goodman
Cynthia Nathanson
Elaine Parker
Giovanna Sirianni
Kingsley Watts
William J. Watson

Metabolic/Endocrine

Section Editors: Frank Martino, Nicholas Pimlott, James Meuser

Contributors:

Nalin Ahluwalia
Serena Beber
Carrie Bernard
Yemisi Bolaji
Riina I. Bray
Michael Evans
John Graham
Rahim Hirji
Lynn Margaret Marshall
Christine Papochek
Elaine Parker
John Stewart
Sharon Marie Thomson
Ingrid Tyler
Jessica J. Yu
Heather Zimcik

Nephrology

Section Editors: Frank Martino, Nicholas Pimlott

Contributors:

Sanjay Agarwal
Nalin Ahluwalia
Michael Evans
Sharon Marie Thomson

Ophthalmology

Section Editors: Risa Bordman, Roy Wyman

Contributors:

Rubi Alvi
Liane Bacal
Risa Bordman
Daniel M. Mandell
Mark A. Mandell
Ian Pun
Albert Yeung

Otolaryngology

Section Editors: Risa Bordman, Roy Wyman

Contributors:

Loredana Di Santo
Albert Flores
Kate Lazier
Jennifer Rotstein
Rebecca Stoller
Roy Wyman
Tanya Wyman

Pediatrics

Section Editors: Susan Edwards, Sheila Dunn

Contributors:

Katherine Bingham
Jeff A. Bloom
Sarah Bradford-Relyea
Julie A Brahm
David W. Cadotte
Melanie Campbell
Vicky Chan
Susan A. Deering
Susan Edwards
Michael Evans
Jonathan Gabor
R. Rishi Gupta
Amanda Chia-Ming Hu
Dirk Huyer
Andrea Iaboni
Maria N. Ivankovic
Mark S. Landis
Jennifer MacIsaac
Mark A. Mandell
Niraj D. Mistry
Sergio Muraca
Michelle S. Naimer
Karen A. Ng
Netee Papneja
Tripti Papneja
Jacqueline Poitras
Cara A. Polson
Jennifer Stulberg
Jeff Tanguay
Diana Toubassi
Ingrid Tyler
William J. Watson
Daphne Williams

Respirology

Section Editors: Frank Martino, Nicholas Pimlott
Section Reviewer: Alan G. Kaplan

Contributors:

Anthony D'urzo
Michael Evans
Alan G. Kaplan
Josiah Lowry
Lynn Margaret Marshall
John C. Rea
Vasant Solanki
Michael Varenbut

Rheumatology

Section Editors: Risa Bordman, Roy Wyman
Contributors:
Risa Bordman
Riina I. Bray
Richard Glazier
Lynn Margaret Marshall
Catherine Paris
Vsevolod Perelman
Joy C. Schuurman
Kevin Shi
Roy Wyman
Tanya Wyman

Sports Medicine, Exercise, and Injuries

Section Editors: Risa Bordman, Roy Wyman
Contributors:
Julia Alleyne
Risa Bordman
Tom Chan
Ian Cohen
Shafik Dharamshi
Michael Evans
Ian Finkelstein
Grant Lum
Natalie K. Mamen
Bruce Topp
Howard A. Winston
Roy Wyman

Urology

Section Editors: Risa Bordman, Roy Wyman
Contributors:
Risa Bordman
Michael Evans
Barnett I. Giblon
Paul Gragg
Michelle Greiver
Jonathan Kerr
Hashmat Khan
David MacPherson
Ron Phillipson
Jeff Weissberger

Women's Health: Breast Diseases

Section Editors: Sheila Dunn, Susan Edwards
Contributors:
Sheila Dunn
Michael Evans
Ruth Heisey
Sandra Messner

Women's Health: Gynecology

Section Editors: Sheila Dunn, Susan Edwards
Contributors:
Viola Antao
Sandra Chery
Sheila Dunn
Michael Evans
Kymm Feldman
Milena Forte
Batya Grundland
Hansa Meera Gupta
Jean Marmoreo
Sandra Messner
M. Claire Murphy
Pari Oza
Lea Rossiter
Nihad Abu Setteh
Christine Singh
Fay Sliwin
Rajani Vairavanathan
Sharonie Valin
Erica Weir
Karen Wong

Women's Health: Obstetrics

Section Editors: Susan Edwards, Sheila Dunn
Contributors:
Julia Alleyne
Ruth Brooks
Susan Edwards
Michael Evans
Karen Fleming
Difat Jakubovicz
Alice Ordean
Lisa Salamon
Rajani Vairavanathan
William J. Watson
Daphne Williams

CONTENTS

COMMON PROBLEMS IN FAMILY MEDICINE

KNOWLEDGE MANAGEMENT

Knowledge management in primary care is at an important crossroads. We spend considerable time and resources managing things like money, our offices, and people, yet we do little to manage perhaps our most important resource: knowledge.[1] When we consider evidence-based medicine (EBM), we must contextualize it within the larger background of knowledge management in the busy primary care clinic. Most likely, the practical evidence-based clinicians of the future will not just be those trained in critical appraisal but rather will also include those trained in using multiple high-quality knowledge products.[2] These products are certainly more reproducible and sustainable. Consider this textbook. Some will use it, with other textbooks, as their primary sources of information. Others will find a textbook too dated or not portable enough. Five years ago the publisher would simply have put it into circulation as a printed text, but now web, CD, and PDA versions need to be contemplated for use at the point of care.

Managing these knowledge products will likely depend largely on technology, but the uptake in practice will often depend on content. "eHealth" can only work if the provided content fits the question or need in practice and can save time. New trainees exemplify the use of current technology; they do not carry around the black books and textbooks that the older clinicians did, but instead house and access their knowledge in PDAs and on websites.

When examining how doctors answer questions, we see that most questions are not answered. The medical field still has considerable progress to make in creating knowledge resources that fit within the time constraints of a busy clinic.[3] Additionally, most practitioners have lacked a supportive environment for a complex and multifaceted decision-making process. We have all watched as the business of "summarizing" health data has slowly evolved. Initially every organization imaginable developed new guidelines. These were initially over 200 pages and only written by specialists. The guidelines have evolved and are now more succinct and have improved formatting with tables, algorithms, and in general, a more inclusive process. These have all showed little impact in changing physician behaviour but do represent an honest attempt to administer best evidence.[4] As with didactic lectures, what may make sense (knowing more leading to better practice) doesn't fully translate to optimizing practice.[5] The guidelines do, however, set the stage for more barrier-sensitive tools.

Currently the educational landscape is changing into a virtual cottage industry in summarizing services that synthesize the evidence and toolkits that make best practice easier. (See www.healthknowledgecentral.org to view a collection of resources.) These resources are being combined with multifaceted interventions such as small group learning, better formatting, patient versions, targeted communities of practice, and end-user involvement, thereby marking the evolution from a unifaceted knowledge source (a guideline) to multifaceted toolkits to enable best practice.[6] Although this model forces us to "trust" a resource, as efficiency is prioritized over validity, it works if this is understood and the clinician uses quality knowledge products. At this point in time our efforts are likely making a difference with the reflective practitioner, or the clinicians that are ready to make a change, but we need to create long-term knowledge management support if we want to affect the bulk of practitioners. Physicians are likely no different than the rest of the population when it comes to what typically changes behaviour: marketing, incentives, packaging, timing, and happiness of our "customers." These techniques need to be combined with the very best information if we are to achieve sustainable knowledge management.

_____ ◈ REFERENCES ◈ _____

1. Gray JA: Where's the chief knowledge officer? To manage the most precious resource of all (editorial), *BMJ* 317(7162):832-840, 26 September 1998.
2. Evans M, Creating knowledge management skills in primary care residents: a description of a new pathway to evidence-based practice, *ACP J Club* 135(2):A11-12, Sep-Oct 2001.
3. Ely JW, Osheroff JA, Ebell MH, et al: Obstacles to answering doctors' questions about patient care with evidence: qualitative study, *BMJ* 324(7339):710, Mar 23 2002.
4. Shaneyfelt TM, Mayo-Smith MF, Rothwangl J: Are guidelines following guidelines? The methodological quality of clinical practice guidelines in the peer-reviewed medical literature, *JAMA* 281(20): 1900–1905, 1999.
5. Davis DA, Thomson MA, Oxman AD, et al: Changing physician performance: a systematic review of the effect of continuing medical education strategies, *JAMA* 274(9): 700–705, 1995.

6. Davis D, Evans M: The professional development of the family physician: managing knowledge in primary care. In Jones R, Britten N, Culpepper L, et al, ed., *Oxford Textbook of Primary Medical Care,* Oxford ; New York, 2003: 3

EVIDENCE-BASED MEDICINE
(See also attitudes, physician; clinical practice guidelines; medical education; periodic health examination; screening)

Good physicians are skeptical about much of what they do and most of what they read, including this text. Being skeptical helps keep us attuned to new evidence and probably keeps us from harming our patients by either prematurely endorsing new investigative or therapeutic procedures or rigidly sticking to outmoded interventions. Skepticism is one of the driving forces behind "evidence-based medicine" and is well exemplified by the critical approach taken by the Canadian Task Force on Preventive Health Care[1] and the U.S. Preventive Services Task Force.[2] However, skepticism carried to extremes leads to diagnostic and therapeutic paralysis. This is captured in the phrase "evidence-based medicine is necessary but not sufficient." This is especially true in primary care, where the evidence often is either unavailable or needs to be extrapolated to a specific population or setting. Evidence-based data are only part of what physicians require to care adequately for their patients. They need easy access to accurate information that is relevant to everyday practice; as Slawson and Shaughnessy[3] put it, they are looking for "Patient Oriented Evidence that Matters (POEM)." Finding what we need among the 6 million medical articles that are published annually requires us all to develop some understanding of how to perform critical appraisals of the medical literature.[4]

Although randomized controlled trials are the gold standard for evidence-based medicine, they are not always applicable to the patients seen in family medicine. Controlled trials often enroll patients from referral centres, and women, elderly patients, and patients with comorbid illnesses are commonly excluded from such trials. Drug trials may give good information about when to start medications but no evidence-based data on when to stop them.[5]

Randomized controlled trials and critical appraisals apply to populations of patients, not to individual patients. To practice high-quality medicine, family physicians must use evidence-based guidelines but at the same time recognize the physical, psychological, ethical, spiritual, and social uniqueness of each patient. When patient individuality is incorporated into management decisions, "evidence-based" recommendations must often be abandoned.[6] Expert opinion, whether verbal or in the form of a review article, is a common but sometimes unreliable source of information for general practitioners. Antman and associates[7] compared current written reviews of "experts" in the specific content area of myocardial infarction with current meta-analyses on the same subject. The reviews of the "experts" often contained potentially harmful recommendations and omitted newer beneficial therapeutic modalities. (On the other hand, meta-analyses may lead to erroneous conclusions compared with large randomized controlled trials.[8-10]) Oxman and Guyatt[11] analyzed the methodological rigour of a number of review articles and concluded that the greater the expertise of the authors, the poorer the quality of the reviews. It may be that some "experts" are consciously or unconsciously biased because they have vested interests in certain viewpoints or,[11] to put it more bluntly, they value their personal experience more than randomized controlled trials.[3]

It has often been stated that only 10% to 20% of medical interventions are evidence based. When this hypothesis was tested on in-patients for general medical services in Oxford, England,[12] and Ottawa, Canada,[13] 82% of the decisions made in the English study and 84% of those in the Canadian study were evidence based. It is likely less in the community setting. Classification of categories of evidence and strength of recommendations is discussed in the section on clinical practice guidelines.

──────────── ◈ REFERENCES ◈ ────────────

1. Canadian Task Force on the Periodic Health Examination: *Canadian guide to clinical preventive health care,* Ottawa, 1994, Canada Communication Group.
2. U.S. Preventive Services Task Force: *Guide to clinical preventive services,* ed 2, Baltimore, 1996, Williams & Wilkins.
3. Slawson DC, Shaughnessy AF: Obtaining useful information from expert based sources, *BMJ* 314:947-949, 1997.
4. Miser WF: Critical appraisal of the literature, *J Am Board Fam Pract* 12:315-333, 1999.
5. Knottnerus JA, Dinant GJ: Medicine based evidence, a prerequisite for evidence based medicine: future research methods must find ways of accommodating clinical reality, not ignoring it (editorial), *BMJ* 315:1109-1110, 1997.
6. Tonelli MR: The philosophical limits of evidence-based medicine, *Acad Med* 73:1234-1240, 1998.
7. Antman EM, Lau J, Kupelnick B, et al: A comparison of results of meta-analyses of randomized control trials and recommendations of clinical experts: treatments for myocardial infarction, *JAMA* 268:240-248, 1992.
8. LeLorier J, Grégoire G, Benhaddad A, et al: Discrepancies between meta-analyses and subsequent large randomized, controlled trials, *N Engl J Med* 337:536-542, 1997.
9. Bailar JC III: The promise and problems of meta-analysis (editorial), *N Engl J Med* 337:559-561, 1997.
10. DerSimonian R, Levine RJ: Resolving discrepancies between a meta-analysis and a subsequent large controlled trial, *JAMA* 282:664-670, 1999.
11. Oxman AD, Guyatt GH: The science of reviewing research, *Ann NY Acad Sci* 703:125-133, 1993.

12. Ellis J, Mulligan I, Rowe J, Sackett DL (A-Team, Nuffield Department of Clinical Medicine): Inpatient general medicine is evidence based, *Lancet* 346:407-410, 1995.
13. Michaud G, McGown JL, van der Jagt R, et al: Are therapeutic decisions supported by evidence from health care research? *Arch Intern Med* 158:1665-1668, 1998.

UNCERTAINTY

(See also attitudes, physician; informed consent; investigations; positive predictive value; risk analysis; risk assessment in pregnancy; screening)

Uncertainty permeates clinical medicine and is likely ineradicable. Uncertainty stems from two primary sources:

1. Lack of knowledge to inform decisions because such knowledge does not exist, which is the reason for continued research;
2. Lack of knowledge to inform decisions because knowledge cannot be accessed; knowledge translation, evidence-based medicine, and lifelong learning are responses to this situation.

A third consideration is failure to access knowledge when knowledge exists; this is called ignorance.

Many persons believe that the greatest problem with uncertainty in medicine is the failure of physicians to discuss how pervasive it is.[1] Consequently, a detrimental way for health professionals to deal with uncertainty is to deny it. For example, breast surgeons may be quite certain that the treatment they recommend is correct even though no consensus exists in the literature. Baumann and associates[2] label this the "micro-certainty, macro-uncertainty" phenomenon.

Over a decade ago Biehn[3] from the University of Western Ontario wrote about some of the methods of dealing with uncertainty in family medicine. He pointed out that family physicians probably see more patients with undifferentiated diseases than do any other group of physicians and that this necessarily leads to uncertainty. (See discussion of physician attitudes.) Biehn suggested that one of the first ways of dealing with this issue is to ensure that the presenting complaint is the patient's real reason for coming to the office and not just a ticket of admission for a hidden agenda. If the patient has a hidden agenda and the physician brings it out and deals with it, the anxiety of both the patient and physician will drop dramatically, and the vague presenting complaint is likely to resolve spontaneously. Patients probably have even more difficulty living with uncertainty than do physicians.[4,5] As Wardle and Pope[4] point out, shades of grey and risk spectrum are not part of most people's conception of illness. Even evidence-based medicine leaves substantial grey areas of practice that cannot be easily eradicated.[6] Valerie Mike, a statistician, has articulated an ethics of evidence that consists of the following two postulates[7]:

1. The creation, dissemination and use of the best possible scientific evidence as a basis for every phase of medical decision making
2. The need to increase awareness of and come to terms with the extent and ultimately irreducible nature of uncertainty

The first imperative imposes on clinicians a duty to be aware of the best evidence; the second postulate applies equally to providers and patients.

❧ REFERENCES ❧

1. Chalmers I: Well informed uncertainties about the effects of treatments, *BMJ* 328:475-476, 2004.
2. Baumann AO, Deber RB, Thompson GG: Overconfidence among physicians and nurses: the "micro-certainty, macro-uncertainty" phenomenon, *Soc Sci Med* 32:167-174, 1991.
3. Biehn J: Managing uncertainty in family practice, *Can Med Assoc J* 126:915-917, 1982.
4. Wardle J, Pope R: The psychological costs of screening for cancer, *J Psychosom Res* 36:609-624, 1992.
5. Angell M: Shattuck Lecture–evaluating the health risks of breast implants: the interplay of medical science, the law, and public opinion, *N Engl J Med* 334:1513-1518, 1996.
6. Naylor CD: Grey zones of clinical practice: some limits to evidence-based medicine, *Lancet* 345(8953):840-842, 1995.
7. Mike V: Outcomes research and the quality of care: the beacon of an ethics of evidence, *Eval Health Prof* 22:3-32, 1999.
8. Gianakos D: Accepting limits (editorial), *Arch Intern Med* 158:1059-1061, 1998.
9. Kassirer JP: Our stubborn quest for diagnostic certainty: a cause of excessive testing, *N Engl J Med* 320:1489-1491, 1989.

A BRIEF PRIMARY CARE APPROACH TO DIZZINESS

Basics

One in four people experience severe dizziness over their lifetime, typically when they get older (50% of people >65).[1] Patients may become frustrated because a single cause with a cure is often not found. This is especially true in the elderly or people with prolonged symptoms. A study of general practice attendees found that one in five experienced recurrent and frequent dizziness, 15% of these were disabled by their symptoms, and 29% were more handicapped 18 months later.[2] The evidence base for dizziness is limited and tends to focus on the discrete diagnoses rather than the broad approach to "dizziness."

What is most common?

- Most community samples reveal Benign Positional Vertigo (BPV) and labrynthitis as the most common causes of dizziness for a patient presenting to the clinic.[3,4]
- This may not be true for the elderly, as reflected in one U.K. seniors study in which it was found that central vascular disease and spondylosis were the two most common diagnoses. (See geriatric syndrome below.)[5]

- Kroenke's review[6] cited the following causes (and prevalence): BPV (16%), psychiatric (16%), metabolic infections (16%), labrynthitis (9%), medication (5.9%), presyncope (arrhythmia, hypotension) (6%), cerebrovascular (6%), Meniere's disease (5%), stroke (2.9%), transient ischemic attack (TIA) (2.6%), central vestibular causes (multiple sclerosis, migraine, epilepsy) (1.2%), acoustic neuromas (0.7%), and "unknown" (13%).

How can I diagnose the cause?

There is no perfect diagnostic algorithm with high utility. The pearls below can help differentiate causes of disease.

Consider the Patient's Description[7]

1. *Presyncope: The feeling one is about to faint.* This condition can be accompanied by light-headedness, buzzing, "rubbery legs," visual field constriction, and diaphoresis. Presyncope is poorly studied, but the cause is typically vasovagal (patient often has a history of similar episodes when he or she becomes generally ill), or due to orthostatic hypotension (especially when symptoms are predictable after getting up suddenly). Etiology can be vasovagal (post-vomiting, micturation, defecation, coughing), vascular (hypotension, vertebrobasilar insufficiency, subclavian steal), cardiac (arrhythmia, valvular problems), or neurological (seizure, hydrocephalus). Cervical spondylosis can cause dizziness through neurological pathways by chronic degeneration of the cervical spine, which gradually compresses one or more of the nerve roots. This can exacerbate or cause dizziness. By age 60, 70% of women and 85% of men show changes consistent with cervical spondylosis on x-ray examination. Finally, it is important to consider a cardiac cause, especially when symptoms are accompanied by chest pain or arrhythmia.

2. *Dysequilibrium: A sensation of imbalance, usually accompanied by fear of falling.* This can be partly due to aging because the ability of the cerebellum to process sensory input slows. Common causes include peripheral neuropathies, deconditioning, Parkinson's disease, and use of certain medications.

3. *Vertigo: The illusion of false motion.* The patient has the sensation of the external environment moving, as opposed to the complaint of spinning within the head, which is typically functional or psychogenic in origin. One question has been validated in trials: "When you have dizzy spells do you feel light-headed or do you feel the world spin around you as if you have just gotten off a playground roundabout?"[8] The patient may have associated nausea, vomiting, diaphoresis, and nystagmus worsened by head movement. The body always adapts with neurochemical changes to make vertigo a temporary condition. Common etiologies include BPV, vestibular neuronitis, Meniere's disease, and migraines. Rare, but serious, causes include stroke

and acoustic neuromas, although the latter is often combined with unsteadiness.

Consider that Dizziness in the Elderly May Be More of a Syndrome Than a Symptom.[9] Dizziness in the elderly, while occasionally a precise diagnosis, typically finds its cause in multiple domains (cardiovascular, neurological, sensory, psychological, and medication-related), and dizziness may be a geriatric syndrome, similar to delirium and falling. If so, an impairment reduction strategy, proven effective for other geriatric syndromes, may be effective in reducing the symptoms and disabilities associated with dizziness.

Consideration of Precipitants:
Consideration of Associated Symptoms:
- Change in head position (BPV)
- After getting up (orthostatic hypotension) or with exertion (cardiac or vascular)
- With uneven ground or in the dark (disequilibrium)

Consideration of Associated Symptoms:
- Recent viral illness (vestibular neuronitis, labrynthitis, vasovagal response)
- Hearing loss, fullness in ear, tinnitus (Meniere's disease or acoustic neuroma, the latter typically with unsteadiness)
- Neurological deficit (stroke, TIA)
- Chest pain with activity or palpitations (cardiac)
- Panic (dizziness is one of the key symptoms of panic, and more than four out of five people with panic disorder report it.)[10]

Consideration of Duration:[11]
- Seconds = BPV
- Minutes = cerebrovascular ischemia
- Hours = Meniere's disease
- Days = viral labrynthitis
- Months = a central process

Consideration of Red Flags:
- Absence of vertigo, age >69, or presence of a neurological deficit.
- This is based on one trial done in the ER that followed 124 patients 1 month after discharge for serious causes of dizziness (TIA, stroke, arrhythmia, seizure, and medication toxicity). The follow-up was short, and this rule has not been validated in a separate population.[12]

Testing

General exam with a focus on the ear, nose, and throat (ENT) in vertigo and metabolic or cardiac systems for non-vertigo dizziness. The Dix-Hallpike manoeuvre is helpful for confirming the diagnosis of BPV.[13] The patient is positioned on the examining bed so that his or her head will drop below the top of the bed when he or she lies down. The clinician fully supports the head as it drops down below the level of the bed, and the head is rotated to one side. (It is recommended to have a bucket available!) Repeat and turn head the other way if necessary. If symptoms are reproduced, count the seconds to nystagmus (typically 3 to 40 seconds) where the slow phase of the nystagmus goes toward the affected ear. Symptoms typically resolve in 30 seconds. Magnetic resonance imaging (MRI) is the most precise test if central lesions are suspected.[14]

Management of Common Causes of Dizziness

Treatment is based on the individual cause(s) of dizziness. In general, antihistamines can help for short-term management of the most disturbing symptoms.

- Choices include meclizine (antivert 12.5 to 25 mg), dimenhydrinate (Gravol 12.5 to 25 mg), betahistine dihydrochloride (Serc 8 to 16 mg), diazepam, and prochlorperazine. These can all be quite sedating, so nighttime use and low dosing is recommended.
- Patients can be instructed to lie still, with eyes closed, in a darkened room during acute episodes to reduce vertigo and vomiting.
- Some patients, especially those with BPV, respond well to adaptation exercises (analogous to becoming used to motion on ships and reducing seasickness) such as the Cawthorne-Cooksey exercises.[15]
- If available, consideration of referral to a physiotherapist for head and neck exercises that rehabilitate the vestibular system may be helpful.[16]
- For elderly patients with multiple causes, consider a harm reduction strategy.
- **Labrynthitis:** Reassurance and management as above.
- **BPV:** This condition may result from free-floating debris in the endolymph of the posterior semicircular canal. This debris moves with position change, causing an abnormal perception of movement and classic symptoms of vertigo. A Cochrane review of treatments for BPV yielded 11 trials, 9 of which were excluded due to a high risk of bias.[17] The 2 remaining trials compared the Epley manoeuvre[18] with a sham procedure among 86 patients referred to specialty care and showed a benefit in conversion of the Dix-Hallpike test from positive to negative, as well as resolution of symptoms by patient report. Lorazepam and diazepam had no effect in 1 small randomized controlled trial.[19] The Epley procedure is done for left side-induced BPV by starting with the Dix-Hallpike manoeuvre to the right and holding until symptoms resolve, then having the patient roll slowly onto his or her right shoulder so the patient is facing down toward the floor for 10 to 20 seconds. The patient then sits up with his or her head still facing the right shoulder, then the head is faced forward and the chin is tilted down. Symptoms resolve more rapidly when the head is repeatedly put in the inciting position. Most patients are better within 3 months. Antihistamines may help.
- **Medication-induced:** Consider the cost/benefit of removing common culprits: the aminoglycosides, loop diuretics, salicylates, anticonvulsants, and psychotropics, especially TCA's, haloperidol, benzodiazepines, and lithium.

❧ REFERENCES ❧

1. Yardley L, Owen N, Nazareth I, et al: Prevalence and presentation of dizziness in a general practice community sample of working age people, *Br J Gen Pract* 48(429): 1131-1135, Apr 1998.
2. Nazareth I, Yardley L, Owen N, et al: Outcome of symptoms of dizziness in a general practice community sample, *Fam Pract* 16(6):616-618, Dec 1999.
3. Nazareth I, Yardley L, Owen N, Luxon L: Outcome of symptoms of dizziness in a general practice community sample, *Fam Pract* 16(6):616-618, Dec 1999.
4. Jayarajan V, Rajenderkumar DJ: A survey of dizziness management in General Practice, *Laryngol Otol* 117(8): 599-604, Aug 2003.
5. Colledge NR, Barr-Hamilton RM, Lewis SJ, et al: Evaluation of investigations to diagnose the cause of dizziness in elderly people: a community based controlled study, *BMJ* 313(7060):788-792, Sep 28 1996.
6. Kroenke K, Lucas C, Rosenberg ML, et al: One-year outcome for patients with a chief complaint of dizziness, *J Gen Intern Med* 9(12):684-689, Dec 1994.
7. Link N, Tanner M: *Bellevue guide to outpatient medicine: an evidence-based guide to primary Bellevue,* London, 2001, BMJ Publishing.
8. Evans JG: Transient neurological dysfunction and risk of stroke in an elderly English population: the different significance of vertigo and non-rotatory dizziness, *Age Ageing* 19:43-49, 1990.
9. Tinetti ME, Williams CS, Gill TM: Dizziness among older adults: a possible geriatric syndrome, *Ann Intern Med* 132(5):337-344, Mar 7, 2000.
10. Cox BJ, Hasey G, Swinson RP, et al: The symptom structure of panic attacks in depressed and anxious patients, *Can J Psychiatry* 38:181-184, 1993.
11. Byrne M: Assessment of the dizzy patient, *Aust Fam Phys* 31-38, Aug 2002.
12. Herr RD, Zun l, Matthews JJ: A directed approach to the dizzy patient, *Ann Emerg Med* 18:664-672, 1989.
13. Dix MR, Hallpike CS: Pathology, symptomatology and diagnosis of certain common disorders of the vestibular system, *Proc Roy Soc Med* 45:341–354, 1952.
14. Hasso AN, Drayer BP, Anderson RE, et al: Vertigo and hearing loss, American College of Radiology, ACR Appropriateness Criteria, *Radiology* 215(Suppl):471-478, Jun 2000.
15. See http://www.dizziness-and-balance.com/treatment/cawthorne.html last accessed May 11, 2004.
16. Yardley L, Beech S, Zander L, et al: A randomised controlled trial of exercise therapy for dizziness and vertigo in primary care, *Br J Gen Pract* 48:1136-1140, 1998.
17. Hilton M, Pinder D: The Epley (canalith repositioning) manoeuvre for benign paroxysmal positional vertigo (Cochrane Review). In: *The Cochrane Library,* Issue 3, 2003. Oxford: Update Software, last updated October 25, 2001.
18. Epley JM: The canalith repositioning procedure: for treatment of benign paroxysmal positional vertigo, *Otolaryngol Head Neck Surg* 107:399-404, 1992.
19. McClure JA, Willett JM: Lorazepam and diazepam in the treatment of benign paroxysmal vertigo, *J Otolaryngol* 9:472–477, 1980.

AN APPROACH TO COMPLEMENTARY AND ALTERNATIVE MEDICINE (CAM)

Complementary medicine is controversial. The number of patients who use complementary and alternative treatments has increased. Physicians are concerned that patients may delay seeking treatments that can be life-saving. Patients may be spending time and considerable money for approaches that are not effective and in fact are harmful. Often no scientific basis for many approaches exists, and there is lack of regulation and proper training of some alternative practitioners. Finally, patients tend to not tell their doctor they are using alternatives because of fear of being dismissed, ridiculed, or judged. One study found that half of patients in a family practice were using at least one alternative therapy, and only half of them had told their family physician.[1]

There are hundreds of different health practices including Craniosacral Therapy, Chelation, Massage Therapy, Orthomolecular Medicine, environmental medicine, nutritional therapy, Therapeutic Touch, Emotional Field Therapy, Shiatsu, Ayurvedic Medicine, and Chinese Traditional Medicine. Many of these are intertwined into specific cultures. Some physicians use relatively safe complementary modalities that have support in the scientific literature.

Common Therapies

Acupuncture

The literature on acupuncture has mixed reviews.[2-7] The National Institutes of Health, in their "non-advocate," multidisciplinary Consensus Conference in 1997, felt there was some evidence of effectiveness of acupuncture for post-operative and chemo-induced nausea and vomiting, certain pain syndromes, addiction, stroke rehabilitation, headache, dysmenorrhea, tennis elbow, carpel tunnel syndrome, and fibromyalgia.[8] A recent systematic review concluded that "acupuncture for acute low back pain has not been well studied and although 10 randomized controlled trials (RCTs) exist for chronic back pain, its value remains in question. Recent studies suggest that acupuncture is more effective than sham treatments and other questionable interventions (e.g. TENS or NSAIDs for chronic back pain) but it is less effective than massage."[9]

Side Effects. Occasionally, mild pain, minimal bleeding, or bruising can result from needle insertion. Infections like AIDS and hepatitis have been spread through improper sterilization. Most practitioners use disposable needles; others use expensive electrical and laser acupuncture, which avoids needles. Physicians should advise patients to be careful when choosing an acupuncturist and to select someone who uses disposable needles.

Certain acupuncture points are contraindicated during pregnancy because acupuncture can cause miscarriages.

Pneumothorax secondary to improper needling happens occasionally, and patients presenting with sudden onset of shortness of breath should be asked if they have had acupuncture recently.

Manipulation

Most patients seek manipulation for back pain. A 2003 systematic review looking at 38 RCTs, including 12 that looked at manipulation in combination with other therapies, concluded that it was superior to sham treatment but not superior to other standard treatments. Results were similar for both acute and chronic back pain.[10] Chiropractors spend a considerable part of their day treating low back pain and can develop expert multifaceted skills and good satisfaction ratings as compared with medical care.[11] At least two randomized studies show that chiropractic manipulations reduced migraine frequency and severity.[12,13]

Contraindications. Manipulation should not be performed on an infected joint; if there is bone or joint pathology; if a patient has a blood dyscrasia, or is on anticoagulant therapy; if there is a vertebral artery syndrome or an abdominal aorta with extensive atherosclerosis; if there is a neurological lesion involving the spinal cord, or there is a vertebra that is weakened by osteoporosis or the presence of a tumour or fracture. There is controversy over the relationship between neck manipulation and stroke.[14-16] The incidence of cerebrovascular accidents after neck manipulation has been estimated by various authors to range from 1 in 400,000 to between 3 and 6 per 10 million manipulations.[17] The exact mechanism and relationship remain unclear.

Herbs

Generalizing about herbal medicine can be difficult because different parts of the plant may have different effects, there are many genus of the same plant, and soil and climate conditions and storage affect potency. Although herbs have been used for centuries and are relatively safe, literature on toxicity and side effects of the use of plant products is growing. Toxic ingredients, pesticides, and non-declared drugs or added chemicals have contaminated some herbal preparations. Herbs can have anticholinergic, hallucinogenic, cathartic, irritative, carcinogenic, and allergic effects. Although efforts are being made to make the process more systematic, at this time the predictability of potency or active ingredient in over-the-counter herbals is not guaranteed, so it can be difficult to generalize from the trial literature.

RCT's have shown Gingko to slow the onset of Alzheimer's disease and intermittent claudication, although the clinical relevance is debated and Gingko increases the risk of bleeding; St. John's Wort to be effective for mild to moderate depression (but not severe depression and with considerable drug interactions) with possibly favourable tolerance when compared with tricyclics and SSRIs; saw palmetto may be used effectively for prostatism, and feverfew has been useful for migraine headaches. Echinacea may be helpful in the treatment of upper respiratory tract infections, but trial data are not fully convincing.[18]

Homeopathy

Homeopathy, a system of medicine first developed in the 19th century in Germany, works on the premise that the substance that causes symptoms in a healthy person can be used, if the substance is given in very small doses, to treat those same symptoms in a sick person. Homeopathic medications are extremely diluted and made from fresh plant, animal, or biological sources.

Negative Trials. Homeopathy has not been shown to be useful for regular headaches, migraines,[19] or chronic asthma.[20] Arnica, a popular remedy for trauma, has not been shown to be useful in a review of eight trials.[21] Ernest Ernst, likely the most published researcher in complementary medicine,[22] believes that there is no evidence that homeopathy is better than placebo.

Positive Trials. Meta-analysis by Kleijnen et al,[23] Linde et al,[24] and Cucherat[25] have reflected both the promise of homeopathy and the methodological flaws. Homeopathy appears to be fairly safe and rarely causes serious side effects. Homeopathy was shown to be useful in double-blind controlled trials in post-operative ileus,[26] the treatment of influenza-like syndromes,[27] perennial allergic rhinitis, children with diarrhea, hay fever,[28] vertigo, mild traumatic brain injury,[29] and acute otitis media.[30]

Communication Issues in CAM

Discussing CAM with patients should be no different than usual patient-centred care. Rather than attacking patient's beliefs, it is helpful to understand where they are coming from and how they developed these opinions and sometimes mistrust of modern medicine. Many patients do not see their views as a mistrust of biomedical medicine, but rather as complementary self-care. The care, time, and framework of understanding that many alternative medicine caregivers can provide can be truly helpful, especially if interwoven into the patient's culture.

Physicians cannot be expected to have expertise in every alternative treatment. However, it is important to become familiar with the expanding field of complementary medicine so we can help patients make informed decisions about choices for their care. This is especially true regarding drug interactions. Ask every patient if he or she is using herbs, vitamins, homeopathy, or seeking other alternative treatments.

❧ REFERENCES ❧

1. Elder NC, Gillcrist A, Minz R: Use of alternative health care by family practice patients, *Arch Fam Med* 6(2): 180-184, 1997.
2. Lewith GT, Machin D: On the evaluation of the clinical effects of acupuncture, *Pain* 16:111-127, 1983.
3. Richardson PH, Vincent CA: Acupuncture for the treatment of pain: a review of evaluative research, *Pain* 24:15-40, 1986.
4. Gunn CC, et al: Dry needling of muscle motor points for chronic low back pain, *Pain* 26:277-290, 1986.
5. Vickers AJ: A systemic review of acupuncture antiemesis trials, *J R Soc Med* 89(6):303-311, 1996.
6. Trinh K: An evidence-based review of acupuncture, *Can J of Diagnosis* 3:81-84, 2004.
7. Smith LA, Oldman AD, McQuay HJ, et al: Teasing apart the quality and validity in systematic reviews: an example of acupuncture in chronic neck and back pain, *Pain* 86: 119-132, 2000.
8. National Institute of Health (NIH): Acupuncture, *JAMA* 280(17):1518-1524, 1998.
9. Cherkin DC, Sherman KJ, Deyo RA, et al: A review of the evidence for the effectiveness, safety, and cost of acupuncture, massage therapy, and spinal manipulation for back pain, *Ann Intern Med* 138:898-906, 2003.
10. Assendelft WJ, Morton SC, Yu EI, et al: Spinal manipulative therapy for low back pain: meta-analysis of effectiveness relative to other therapies, *Ann Intern Med* 138:871-881, 2003.
11. Hertzman-Miller et al: Comparing the satisfaction of low back pain patients randomized to receive medical or chiropractic care: results from the UCLA low-back pain study, *Am J Pub Health* 92(10):1628-1633, 2002.
12. Parker GB, Tupling H, Pryor DS: A controlled trial of cervical manipulation of migraine, *Aust N Z J Med* 8:589-593, 1978.
13. Parker GB, Pryor DS, Tupling H: Why does migraine improve after a clinical trial? Further results from a trial of cervical manipulation of migraine, *Aust N Z J Med* 10: 193-194, 1980.
14. Williams LS, Biller J: Vertebrobasilar dissection and cervical spine manipulation: a complex pain in the neck, *Neurology* 60:1408-1409 2003.
15. Smith WS, Johnston SC, Skalabrin EJ, et al: Spinal manipulative therapy is an independent risk factor for vertebral artery dissection, *Neurology* 60:1424-1428, 2003.
16. Rothwell DM, Bondy SJ, Williams JI, et al: Chiropractic manipulation and stroke: a population-based case-control study (editorial), *Stroke* 32:1054-1060, 2001.
17. Meeker WC, Haldeman S: Chiropractic: a profession at the crossroads of mainstream and alternative medicine, *Ann Intern Med* 136: 216-227, 2002.
18. Ernst E: The risk-benefit profile of commonly used herbal therapies: Ginkgo, St. John's Wort, ginseng, echinacea, saw palmetto, and kava, *Ann Intern Med* 136(1):42-53, Jan 1 2002.
19. Ernst E: Homeopathic prophylaxis for headache and migraine? A systemic review, *J Pain Symptom Manage* 18:353-357, 1999.
20. Linde K, Jobst KA: Homeopathy for chronic asthma, *Cochrane Database Syst Rev* CD000353, 2000.

21. Ernst E: Efficacy of homeopathic arnica, *Arch Surg* 133:1187-1190, 1998.

22. Ernst E: A systemic review of systemic reviews of homeopathy, *Br J Clin Pharmacol* 54, 577-582, 2002.

23. Kleijnen J, Knipschild P, Riet G: Clinical trials of homeopathy, *BMJ* 302:316-323, 1991.

24. Linde K, et al: Are the clinical effects of homeopathy placebo effects? A meta-analysis of placebo-controlled trials, *Lancet* 350:834-843, 1997.

25. Cucherat M, Haugh MC, Gooch M, et al: Evidence of clinical homeopathy, *Eur J Clin Pharmacol* 56:27-33, 2000.

26. Barnes J, Resch K, Ernst E: Homeopathy for postoperative ileus? A meta-analysis, *J Clin Gastroenterol* 225(4):628-633, 1997.

27. Vickers AJ, Smith C: Homeopathic Oscillococcinum for preventing and treating influenza and influenza-like syndromes, *Cochrane Database Syst Rev* CD001957, 2000.

28. Reilly DT, et al: Is homeopathy a placebo response? Controlled trial of homeopathic potency, with pollen in hayfever as model, *Lancet* 881-886, Oct 18 1986.

29. Chapman EH, Weintraub RJ, Milburn MA, et al: Homeopathic treatment of mild traumatic brain injury: a randomized double-blind placebo-controlled trial, *J Head Trauma Rehabil* 14:521-542,1991.

30. Jacobs J, Springer DA, Crothers D: Homeopathic treatment of acute otitis media in children: a preliminary randomized placebo controlled trial, *Pediatr Infect Dis J* 20:177-183, 2001.

AN APPROACH TO ENHANCING MOTIVATION AND CHANGING BEHAVIOUR

(See also addictions)

Introduction

Several studies in various clinical settings have demonstrated the effectiveness of changing behaviour by using a method of structuring and conducting conversations known as *Motivational Interviewing* (MI). Developed by Miller and Rollnick in health promotion studies among heavy drinkers, most of the supporting evidence for MI is in the field of addiction.[1] More recently it has been applied to several areas of lifestyle change from changing water disinfection practices in Zambia,[2] to exercise prescriptions,[3] to improving nutritional practices.[4]

Motivational Interviewing was originally developed as an approach to facilitating change for addiction therapists, counsellors, and psychiatrists.[5] Proficiency at MI for the purposes of evaluation entailed structured training and skills beyond the reach of most primary care providers. Hence, until recently, there were few published studies using brief motivational interventions among family physicians. Over the past few years there have been several attempts to introduce MI interventions to brief office-based physician encounters. In particular *Health Behaviour Change*[6] (HBC) provides a brief, practical MI approach incorporating the patient-centred clinical method with elements of solution-focused therapy.[7]

Change

The physician's natural inclination as a problem solver is to fix things, provide advice, and argue for change. Patients who are not ready to make changes often respond with silence, anger, or avoidance. The physician's resulting frustration often increases his or her cynicism about health prevention and promotion. This may lead to either avoiding the issue entirely, or pushing patients harder to stimulate change. Ironically, these approaches are counterproductive, leading to a decrease in motivation in people who would otherwise benefit from making lifestyle changes.

Prochaska and DiClemente's transtheoretical stages of change (SOC) model[8] (see section on stages of change), now familiar to most health professionals, was helpful with providing a theoretical framework for understanding that patients may be at different places in terms of readiness to change. The SOC model encouraged primary care providers to alter their strategies for different patients, and thus reduce the discrepancy between the patient's lack of readiness to change and the physician's view that change was urgently necessary. Also, enabling a patient to move from one stage of change to the next is a more achievable and thus rewarding target for both the caregiver and patient.

However, this model also has limitations. For example, the stages are somewhat arbitrary and do not adequately capture the complexity of the process for all individuals. Additionally, the SOC model *does not* address the more central issue of *why* people are at different stages and what moves them forward or back.

Using the SOC model as a starting point, Miller and Rollnick's review of the literature on facilitating change revealed several conclusions.

1. Even very brief interventions increase the likelihood of change.
2. The longer that people remain engaged in treatment, the greater the likelihood of change.
3. Most of the change effect can be predicted after the first few sessions.
4. Counsellor characteristics affect outcomes.
5. Conversational style and direction affect outcomes.

That counsellor characteristics increase the likelihood of change is consistent with numerous studies of counselling outcomes; that is, approximately 40% of the effect of counselling can be attributed to the characteristics identified by Carl Rogers[9]—*accurate empathy* (skillful reflective listening with a non-judgemental attitude), *warmth*, and *genuineness.*[10]

More novel was the notion that, independent of the counsellor, conversations that included more talk about change and discussion of future goals and expressed optimism (*change talk*) were more likely to lead to change than conversations that involved argument, expressed pessimism, or included reasons for maintaining the status quo (*resistance talk*). In other words, when we "dance, and don't wrestle" we can improve outcomes.[11]

Motivation

Miller and Rollnick's observational work with patients who were considering change identified three recurring, interrelated themes.

1. The *importance* of changing for the patient
2. The patient's *confidence* in being able to make the change
3. The patient's *readiness* to make the change

In general, the more important the issue is to the patient and the more confident the patient is of succeeding, the more likely he or she will be to commit to making a change, and, hence, the more highly *motivated* the patient is.

Rather than being clearly structured methods, MI and HBC are ways of working with patients that emphasize collaboration over confrontation, eliciting intrinsic motivation over education, and patient autonomy over physician authority. This patient-centred approach makes it a natural fit with family medicine.

Using the HBC model to enhance motivation involves exploring the answers to the following questions[12]:

1. *"Why should I change?"* (Importance) Encourage patients to weigh competing values, benefits, and perceptions of risk.
2. *"How can I change?"* (Confidence) Explore issues of self-efficacy, past experience, and alternative solutions with the patient.
3. *"When shall I change?"* (Readiness) Allow the patient to weigh the competing priorities in their own lives with their assessment of their confidence.

Ambivalence

Answers to these questions inevitably involve some degree of uncertainty or *ambivalence* regarding making changes. Uncertainty is generally lowest when the patient is not at all interested in changing (precontemplation), or is clearly ready to make changes (action). During the process of considering change, of moving from low motivation to high motivation, the patient naturally experiences a rise in ambivalence. The contemplation stage corresponds to a point where ambivalence peaks, and is characterized by the phrases "I want to, *and* I don't want to," or "I know how, *and* I do not know how." Ambivalence regarding importance, confidence, and/or readiness is a natural part of the process of change. For the most part people resolve the ambivalent feelings or thoughts and either choose to change or remain where they are. When people get stuck in ambivalence, problems persist or get worse.[5]

In using HBC techniques, the practitioner seeks to initially enhance and then resolve ambivalence by exploring the patient's perspective and helping to clarify goals, values, and beliefs that support change. This is done in the context of a natural tendency for patients to resist change. This *resistance*, whether it be "yes, but . . ." statements, outright anger, or simply forgetting to make the changes, is simply seen as information that he or she is not ready, or that the process is moving too quickly. Resistance is an indication that the physician should slow down or back off.

Enhancing Motivation for Health Behaviour Change

Sources of individual motivation to change can be either extrinsic, involving external reasons such as rewards, parental approval, the law, or other, or intrinsic, arising from personal values, beliefs, self-image, or other.

Four General Principles that guide MI and HBC:

1. *Express Empathy.* As in all forms of "talk therapy," empathic listening is vital to joining and building the trust that opens up possibilities for change.
2. *Develop Discrepancy.* In general, change is motivated by a discrepancy between present behaviour and important personal goals, beliefs, and values. Drawing attention to these discrepancies and encouraging "change talk" may help resolve ambivalence.
3. *Roll with Resistance.* Avoid arguing for change, and other forms of "resistance talk" that tend to reduce motivation to change.
4. *Support Self-confidence.* Small successes and emotional support increase confidence. The patient is responsible for choosing and carrying out change.

The Spirit of the Method

Many types of questions can be used to propel a conversation that enhances motivation, but the most important characteristic on the physician's part is a genuine curiosity regarding what motivates and inhibits the individual's path to change.

Examples of HBC techniques:

1. Use a *decisional balance* in which the patient is asked to reflect on the relative merits and drawbacks of making the proposed change. For example, "What is the downside of continuing to smoke?"
2. Ask *open-ended questions that evoke change talk* such as "What worries you about your current lack of exercise?"
3. Use *scaling questions* to assess motivation and to help set small goals, such as "What would it take for your confidence to leave your husband to increase from a two to a three out of ten?"
4. *Reflect and elaborate on small goals* (e.g., "So you are interested in changing your eating habits some day. Is there anything you could do now that would be a start?")
5. *Provide information and elicit a response* such as, "Drinking more than two to three drinks per day is

often a cause of high blood pressure. What do you think about your own drinking pattern?"

6. *Back off to reduce resistance* (e.g., "It sounds as though you are not really interested in getting help at the moment.")

The aim of assessing and then exploring importance and confidence with respect to a specific change is to resolve the patient's ambivalence to the point at which he or she feels ready to make a change that is congruent with his/her goals. For example, "So it sounds like you are ready to give up the drug you have been doing. Would you be interested in starting to talk about this?" When the patient indicates he/she is willing to try, the process of enhancing motivation shifts to negotiating a change plan.

Negotiating a Change Plan:

1. *Establish the end point.* Clarify the patient's goals. In the case of drinking alcohol this may be abstinence, but it may be merely cutting down to four beers per day.

2. *Consider change options.* Discuss different ways of achieving the goal. Guide the conversation toward initial achievable, small goals that lead toward the big goal. This can be done by simply asking the patient, or by prompting with gentle suggestions such as, "As a first step, have you considered not smoking in your apartment any more?"

3. *Detail a plan.* Ideally, co-establish a clear, small, observable goal that is as specific and precise as possible. For example, in clarifying the discussion, you might say, "So we have been discussing losing weight, and you want to start exercising once a week by walking to the park and back every Saturday morning before breakfast. Is that right?"

4. *Elicit commitment.* It is crucial that the patient feels ready to commit to the plan, and that the patient sees it as achievable. Ask, "Are you sure that this is something that you can do every week?"

5. *Establish follow-up.* Ongoing support and problem solving is helpful to most patients.

This iterative method by which the physician moves the patient forward and then reassesses the patient's response is continued in subsequent sessions. Failure to complete the goal is seen as either a lack of readiness or as resistance. Either way, it suggests a need to reassess readiness and continue the process. Small successes are reinforced and built upon. The result is a gradual acquisition of new patterns of behaviour and thought and increased awareness of the process of change, coupled with a greater sense of self-efficacy—the feeling that one is capable of making changes in one's life.

_____ ❧ **INTERNET SOURCES** ❧ _____

www.motivationalinterview.org

_____ ❧ **REFERENCES** ❧ _____

1. Miller WR: Motivational interviewing with problem drinkers, *Behav Psychother* 11(2)147-172, 1983.

2. Thevos AK, Olsen SJ, Rangel JM, et al: Social marketing and motivational interviewing as community interventions for safe water behaviors: follow-up surveys in Zambia, *Int Q Community Health Educ* 21(1):51-65, 2002-2003.

3. Scales R, Miller JH: Motivational techniques for improving compliance with an exercise program: skills for primary care clinicians, *Curr Sports Med Rep* 2(3):166-172, Jun 2003.

4. Thorpe M: Motivational interviewing and dietary behavior change, *J Am Diet Assoc* 103(2):150-151, Feb 2003.

5. Miller WR, Rollnick: *Motivational interviewing: preparing people for change,* ed 2, New York, 2002, Guilford Press.

6. Rollnick S, Mason P, Butler C: *Health behavior change: a guide for practitioners,* New York, 1999, Churchill Livingstone.

7. O'Hanlon W, Weiner-Davis M: *In search of solutions: a new direction in psychotherapy,* New York, 1989, Norton.

8. Prochaska JO, DiClemente CC: *The transtheoretical approach: crossing the traditional boundaries of change,* Malabar, FL, 1984, Krieger.

9. Miller SD, et al: No more bells and whistles, *Fam Ther Networker* 53-63, Mar-Apr 1995.

10. Rogers C: *On becoming a person,* Boston, 1961, Houghton Mifflin.

11. Miller WR, Benefield RG, Tonigan JS: Enhancing motivation for change in problem drinking: a controlled comparison of two therapist styles, *J Consult Clin Psychol* 61:455-461, 1993.

12. Rollnick S, Mason P, Butler C: *Health behavior change: a guide for practitioners,* New York, 1999, Churchill Livingstone.

AN APPROACH TO FATIGUE

(See also chronic fatigue syndrome; multiple chemical sensitivities; infectious mononucleosis; benefits of exercise; fibromyalgia; functional somatics syndromes)

A review of the literature for fatigue reveals two major points.

1. Diagnosis is the challenge because fatigue is very common, often due to life imbalance and psychological causes, but can be the presenting complaint of a wide range of diseases.

2. The evidence base is very limited to inform a reasonable approach.

Investigations for undifferentiated fatigue can range from hemoglobin, fasting blood sugar, and thyroid stimulating hormone (TSH) to advanced testing for autoimmune disorders and chronic infections and are likely heavily influenced by the clinician-patient relationship.

Prevalence

The prevalence of clinically significant fatigue depends on the threshold chosen for severity (usually defined in terms of associated disability) and persistence. The frequency with which patients complain of fatigue in family practice is estimated to vary from 6% to 32% internationally.[1] Fatigue is twice as common in women as in men but is not strongly associated with age or occupation. It is one of the most common presenting symptoms in primary care, being the main complaint of 5% to 10% of patients and an important subsidiary symptom in a further 5% to 10%.[2] There is often a mismatch when fatigue presents in primary care because it can be disabling for the patient but is often a non-specific symptom for the clinician.[3]

What is the Likely Diagnoses?

Ebell and Belden attempted to answer this question by extrapolating from several series of patients presenting with fatigue. One series involved Risdale's analysis of 220 patients presenting to the general practitioner with fatigue. The patients received a thorough history and physical; had tests done for complete blood count, fasting blood glucose, electrolytes, sedimentation rate, TSH, and urea; and were tested for mononucleosis if younger than age 40. Only 19 (8%) were given a diagnosis based on the laboratory evaluation. Based on five series, if 100 patients present to a primary care physician with fatigue, approximately 25 will be depressed; 25 will have another psychiatric diagnosis, such as dysthymia or anxiety; 15 will have an infection (e.g., postviral, hepatitis, mononucleosis, etc.); 15 will have another physiological cause of fatigue, such as undiagnosed diabetes, anemia, or hypothyroidism; and 20 will remain undiagnosed.

This analysis did not capture some other more subtle, but likely common, contributing factors such as sleep problems, lack of adequate exercise, and life imbalance (too much work, stress, or busyness with inadequate play, replenishment, or spiritual reflection and renewal).[4,5]

A Five-step approach that seems reasonable is the following:

1. Consider red flags; that is, review recent personal events such as accident, overwork, viral episode, weight loss, new medication, occupational issues, more sedentary lifestyle, and fever, and the general history of the patient (risk for anemia, pregnancy, cardiac problems, hepatitis or other chronic infection, mononucleosis, other). It may be helpful to ask the patient whether the sensation is fatigue or "overwhelming weakness," because the latter may predict disorders[6] such as an electrolyte disorder, hypoglycemia, or neuromuscular disease.
2. Consider a mental health diagnosis such as depression, anxiety, and/or drug dependency. The Patient Health Questionnaire, which is a rapid inventory that the patient fills out, is a validated and time-efficient option.[7]
3. Take a sleep history for insomnia, apnea, and/or movement disorder.

4. Rule out chronic fatigue syndrome: >6 months of fatigue that cannot be explained by another medical or psychiatric cause, including a BMI .40. Chronic fatigue syndrome reduces function significantly and is accompanied by four or more of the following:
   - Impaired memory and/or concentration
   - Sore throat
   - Tender lymph nodes
   - Muscle tenderness
   - Multi-joint pain with no swelling or erythema
   - New onset headache pattern
   - Unrefreshing sleep
   - Postexertional malaise >24 hrs
5. Order tests for hemoglobin, TSH, creatinine, electrolytes, fasting blood sugar, alanine transaminase (ALT), and transferrin saturation (for hemochromatosis). This list may be augmented or reduced depending on the previous four questions.

How Should I Manage Fatigue?

- An obvious starting point is to rule out primary disease. It may be helpful at the outset to tell the patient that 8% to 25% of patients with significant fatigue find a previously undiscovered abnormality in their work-up, and at least 50% will have a mental health cause. The first step is to make sure that they are not part of that 8% to 25% and if they are not, to review the possibility of a mental health diagnosis or unexplained symptoms. The degree of investigation will likely depend on the personalities of the clinician and patient.
- Lessons learned from management of chronic fatigue can be very helpful:
   - Institute a graded exercise program.[8]
   - Change cognitive "automatic thoughts:" "I am so tired, they must be missing a terrible diagnosis" toward, "I am tired, but worrying about some unlikely terrible illness is not going to help. I've had all the appropriate investigations and I will do best if I remain positive."
   - Detect and treat mental illness. Also, consider the "balance" in the patient's life in terms of work, family life, activity, and self-renewal.
   - Employ a patient-centred clinical method[9]: Work together to understand the experience of fatigue for the person and jot down what is likely causing it. Find a common ground in terms of investigations and management, and be realistic.

─────────────── ⤝ **REFERENCES** ⤞ ───────────────

1. Godwin M, Delva D, Miller K, et al: Investigating fatigue of less than 6 months' duration: guidelines for family physicians, *Can Fam Phys* 45:373-379, 1999.
2. Kroenke K, Mangelsdorff D: Common symptoms in ambulatory care: incidence, evaluation, therapy and outcome, *Am J Med* 86:262-266, 1989.

3. Sharpe M, Wilks D: ABC of psychological medicine: fatigue, *BMJ* 325:480–483, 2002.
4. Ridsdale L, Evans A, Jerrett W, et al: Patients with fatigue in general practice: a prospective study, *BMJ* 307:103-106, 1993.
5. Ebell M, Belden JL: What is a reasonable initial approach to the patient with fatigue? [Putting research into practice: clinical inquiries: from the family practice inquiries network], *J Fam Pract* 50:1,16-17, 2001.
6. Chaudhuri A, Behan PO: Fatigue in neurological disorders, *Lancet* 363: 978-988, 2004.
7. The Patient health questionnaire, http://www.deployment health.mil/guidelines/downloads/appendix2.pdf
8. Ridsdale L, Darbishire L, Seed PT: Is graded exercise better than cognitive behaviour therapy for fatigue? A UK randomized trial in primary care, *Psychol Med* 34(1):37-49, Jan 2004.
9. Stewart M, Crown JB, Weston WW, et al: *Patient centred medicine: transforming the clinical method,* Oxford, Eng, 2003, Radcliffe Medical Press.

AN APPROACH TO GENETICS

The mapping of the human genome heralds a new era in medicine, in which genetic tests will become increasingly available. These tests will be used in diagnosis, prenatal care, and reproductive decision making. They will help to predict susceptibility to common diseases such as heart disease, diabetes, and cancer and to choose appropriate medications.[1] Media attention to genetic discoveries and direct marketing of genetic testing to health care providers and the public[2] will result in increased public interest in genetics.[3,4] The public will turn to primary care providers for the information needed to make informed decisions about genetic services. Both the increasing number of genetic tests for common disorders and the lack of genetics professionals and resources will result in primary care providers playing an increasingly important role in this area.[5,6]

Table 1 lists many of the possible roles for family physicians as they integrate genetics into their practices.

Additionally, family physicians will need to critically appraise new genetic tests as they become available, balancing their potential harm and benefits before offering referral for genetic testing.[5]

In the postgenome mapping era, health care providers increasingly will need to see patients through a genetic lens. A three-generation family history, including both sides of the family, will be required for every chart and with regular updating. Pay attention to the unusual, be it early age of onset, multiple affected relatives, or uncommon conditions or diseases.

Genetic causes are more likely when disorders in the family:
- Occur at a younger age than usual
- Are unusual or rare
- Occur in more than one relative on the same side of the family
- Occur in more than one generation

Or in situations of:
- Consanguinity
- Three or more miscarriages
- History of infertility
- Stillbirth or childhood death
- Family history of birth defects, mental disability

Table 1 Primary Care Providers' Roles in Genetics[6-8]

- Taking an adequate family history
- Assessing risk of hereditary disorders
- Recognizing common genetic conditions
- Offering referral to genetics resources when appropriate
- Offering genetic testing when appropriate
- Providing information needed for informed decision making including risks, benefits, and limitations of genetic testing
- Recognizing and providing emotional support to those in need as a result of a genetic diagnosis or test result
- Coordinating appropriate screening and preventive care appropriate to genetic risk

From Carroll JC, Blaine S, Ashbury FD. In Knoppers BM, Scrive C, eds: *Genomics, health and society: emerging issues for public policy,* Ottawa, Canada: Policy Research Initiative, 1993, 67-81; Emery J, Hayflick S: *BMJ* 322:1027-1030, 2001; and Carroll JC, Heisey RE, Warner E, et al: *Can Fam Physician* 45:126-132, 1999.

Table 2 Potential Consequences of Genetic Testing

Potentially Beneficial

Clear Positive Result
- Clinical interventions or surveillance may improve outcomes
- Positive health behaviour may improve outcomes
- Family members at risk can be identified
- Relief of uncertainty

Clear Negative Result
- Avoidance of unnecessary interventions
- Relief from worry

Potentially Harmful

Clear Positive Result
- Anxiety, depression
- Insurance/job discrimination
- Guilt regarding transmission to family
- Fatalistic attitude to health

Clear Negative Result
- Complacency regarding health behaviour and screening
- Survivor guilt

Inconclusive Results

- A variation in a gene may be identified but it may not yet be known whether it is disease-associated or a harmless variant
- A gene mutation may not be identified, but the family history may imply a genetic basis to the disease, suggesting that the mutation may not yet have been discovered

Local genetics clinics are resources for advice and referral. Additional web-based resources are listed below. In the references section, 8, 9 and 10, are articles worth reading on this subject.

Genetic testing for adult-onset diseases differs from traditional medical tests. Test results come with a great deal of uncertainty, such as the following:

- Will the condition develop?
- At what age?
- How severe?
- Will interventions make a difference?

In contrast to other tests, genetic test results have direct implications for family members and have ethical, legal, and social consequences. Family physicians have an important role in discussing the potential consequences of genetic testing with their patients to help them determine if genetic testing would make a difference to their health and make informed choices about referral and testing. Some of the benefits, risks, and limitations of genetic testing are listed in Table 2.[8]

❧ INTERNET SOURCES ❧

The Genetics File; an excellent Australian resource for family physicians describing genetic disorders
http://murdoch.rch.unimelb.edu.au/GF/pages/GeneticsFile.asp
For reviews of genetic disorders and tests available
www.geneclinics.org
Online Mendelian Inheritance in Man
www.ncbi.nlm.nih.gov/omim/
A description of genetic disorders and helpful links
www.mtsinai.on.ca/familymedicine/genetics

❧ REFERENCES ❧

1. Burke W, Emery J: Genetics education for primary-care providers, *Nat Rev Genet* 3:561-566, 2002.
2. Greendale K, Pyeritz RE: Empowering primary care health professionals in medical genetics: how soon? how fast? how far? *Am J Med Genet* 106(3):223-232, 2001.
3. Andrykowski MA, Munn RK, Studts JL: Interest in learning of personal genetic risk for cancer: a general population survey, *Prev Med* 25:527-536, 1996.
4. Graham ID, Logan DM, Hughes-Benzie R, et al: How interested is the public in genetic testing for colon cancer susceptibility? Report of a cross-sectional population survey, *Cancer Prev Control* 2:167-172, 1998.
5. Acheson L: Fostering applications of genetics in primary care: what will it take? *Genet Med* 5(2):63-65, 2003.
6. Carroll JC, Blaine S, Ashbury FD: Family physicians and genetic medicine: roles and challenges. In Knoppers BM, Scriver C, eds: *Genomics, health and society: emerging issues for public policy*, Ottawa, Canada: Policy Research Initiative, 1993, 67-81.
7. Emery J, Hayflick S: The challenge of integrating genetic medicine into primary care, *BMJ* 322:1027-1030, 2001.
8. Carroll JC, Heisey RE, Warner E, et al: Hereditary breast cancer: psychosocial issues and family physicians' role, *Can Fam Physician* 45:126-132, 1999.
9. Gilchrist DM: Medical genetics: 3. An approach to the adult with a genetic disorder, *CMAJ* 167(9):1021-1029, 2002.
10. Evans JP, Skrzynia C, Burke W: The complexities of predictive genetic testing, *BMJ* 322:1052-1056, 2001.

AN APPROACH TO OBESITY
The Epidemic

Nearly one third (30.5%) of adults in the United States are obese. When rates of "overweight" and "obesity" are combined, the estimated prevalence is 64.5%. Since 1960, the prevalence of obesity in American adults has increased by 17.5%.[1]

Reasons for this may be simple, such as less activity, and/or higher intake of food, or complex. Consider power windows and typewriters, video games, the current size of the common bagel or serving of fries, and culture-specific consumption patterns and what is considered attractive appearance. In the United States the age of the house a person lives in is the most sensitive predictor of activity; that is, a new house often has no sidewalk, whereas most old neighbourhoods were designed with walking in mind.[2]

The prevalence of overweight children and teens ages 6 to 19 in the United States has tripled between 1990 and 2000.[1] Rates of childhood obesity have increased similarly in Canada and the United Kingdom.[3,4]

How do I tell whether they are obese?
Option 1: BMI (Weight in kg Divided by Height in Metres^2)

- Offers the simplicity of plotting a person on a nomogram. A person is overweight if the BMI is ≥25, and is obese if the BMI is ≥30.
- This formula can have false positives (the muscular) and false negatives ("potato-on-toothpick" bodies).

To use this formula, persons who are metrically challenged can take weight in pounds, multiply it by 703, and divide it by the height in inches squared. Therefore, for a 180 lb. person who is 5 foot 5 inches tall (65 inches), $180 \times 703 = 126,540$, divided by 65×65 (4,225) = 29.9.

Options 2 & 3: Waist Circumference (WC) and the Waist/Hip Ratio (WHR)

- WC is measured at the end of normal expiration, while the person is standing with feet hip-width apart, midway between the lower costal margin and the iliac crest. Put another way, find the smallest measurement below the rib cage and above the belly button. For WHR then compare to the widest part around the hips.
- The WHO considers ≥102 cm (40 in) in men and ≥88 cm (35 in) in women to indicate a high risk for diabetes, hypertension, and coronary heart disease. The Nurses' Health Study reported that women with waist circumferences of 76.2 cm (30 in) or greater had over twice the risk for coronary artery disease compared with thinner women.
- According to the appropriately named Lean and associates, health risks are significant for waist/hip ratios of > 0.95 for men and 0.80 for women.[5]

- The Nurses' Health Study found that women with a waist/hip ratio greater than 0.75 had over twice the risk for coronary artery disease as those with a lower ratio.6

Which one is best?

All approaches mentioned above are good, so pick the one that works best for you. A recent study comparing waist circumference, waist-hip ratio and BMI in an Australian population concluded that WHR was most strongly correlated with cardiovascular disease (CVD) risk factors in the general population.[7] NIH guidelines suggest treatment of all individuals with BMI >30 and of individuals with BMI 25.0-29.9 or those with increased WC who have two or more risk factors.[2,3] The Canadian Task Force on Preventative Health Care gives a B recommendation for weight reduction therapy of obese adults with obesity-related diseases.[8,9]

Why bother?

- An analysis of the Framingham Heart Study data showed a 3- to 7-year decrease in life expectancy among obese individuals compared with persons of normal weight.[10]
- The Nurses' Health Study found sharp increases in total cohort mortality for BMI >27 and weight gain over 10 kg after age 18. Women with BMI of 24 to 25 have a five-fold increase of developing diabetes than women with a BMI <22. Those with BMI >35 have a 93-fold increase risk.[11]
- Although cardiovascular disease accounted for most of the excess mortality, cancers were also contributing factors.[12]
- Obesity increases the risk for all heart diseases, arthritis, sleep apnea, gallbladder disease, cough and wheezing, various cancers, fatty liver, low back pain, and emotional distress and stigmatization.

Why are some people obese and others not?

Following are common reasons for obesity.
- There has been a greater consumption of high energy or high calorie foods and less activity.
- Twin studies suggest that about 70% of the influence on body weight is genetic, while about 30% is environmental. Twins brought up in variable obesogenic environments have strikingly similar BMIs.
- Non-exercise Activity Thermogenesis (NEAT): Small studies that look at non-obese volunteers who were fed 1000 excess kcal/day for 8 weeks and whose volitional exercise was strictly controlled revealed that weight gain ranged from 1.4 to 7.2 kg, and there was a ten-fold variation between individuals in fat storage. There was little inter-individual variation in basal metabolic rate and postprandial thermogenesis, but wide variations in NEAT accounted for the striking differences in fat accumulation.[13]

- One fourth of United States children watch 4 or more hours of television daily, and two thirds watch at least 2 hours per day. These figures are exclusive of time spent playing video games, watching videos, or working or playing on the computer.[14]

What works?

Big Picture. Although not so helpful for the clinic, it is important to remember that education, income levels, urban design, and media culture are large drivers of the obesity epidemic. For example, the impact of the use of technology such as escalators/elevators, desktop computer, power windows and lawnmowers, food processors, dishwashers, and remote controls on weight gain reveals an excess of as much as 5 kg (11 lbs) per year.

Dieting
- U.S. studies have shown that at any one time, 40% of women and 20% of men are dieting. However, in most studies, one third to two thirds of any initial weight loss is regained within a year and almost all of it within 5 years.[15,16] There is an absence of well-done diet trials showing long-term weight reduction. Recent work has focused on low-calorie versus low-fat (LF) versus low-carbohydrate (LC) diets. In general, the LC diets show slightly better outcomes at the beginning, but these diets usually level out at 1 year.[17] Concerns remain regarding the adverse effect of LC diets on other parameters, such as cardiac outcomes.
- The Mediterranean Diet, which is high in fruits, vegetables, legumes, and whole grains, has been examined for its impact on health outcomes rather than weight loss. It includes fish, nuts, and low-fat dairy products and emphasizes the use of olive oil. A recent Greek study showed that every 2-point increase in the Mediterranean diet score was associated with a 25% reduction in the risk of death from any cause, a 33% reduction in the risk of death from coronary heart disease, and a 24% reduction in the risk of death from cancer. The benefit was greater in women, in persons older than 55 years, in never-smokers, in heavier persons, and in sedentary persons.[18]

Drugs
- A systematic review of long-term results with orlistat (Xenical 120 mg tid pc) treated patients showed that they lost an average of 2.7 kg, and patients on sibutramine (Meridia 10 to 15 mg od) experienced 4.3 kg greater weight loss compared with a placebo. The number of patients achieving 10% or greater weight loss was 12% higher with orlistat and 15% higher with sibutramine therapy. Weight loss maintenance results were similar. Orlistat, which works by reducing fat absorption with meals and thus has a behavioural effect, caused gastrointestinal side effects, and sibutramine, which inhibits norepinephrine and serotonin uptake and

works on the satiety centre, was associated with small increases in blood pressure and pulse rate. In most studies, weight gain occurs with the cessation of pharmacotherapy. Other studies have found that topiramate, metformin, and zonesamide have been of some value in select populations.[19]

Limiting "Passive Overconsumption of Foods". This is so common that it needs to be singled out. The passive overconsumption of foods occurs when the diet is high in energy-dense foods, which tend to be highly processed, micronutrient-poor, and high in fats, sugars, or starch. A meta-analysis of 16 trials of high-fat versus low-fat diet suggested that a reduction in fat content by 10% corresponds to a reduction in 3 kg of body weight.[20]

National Weight Control Registry (NWCR)[21]

- The NWCR is a longitudinal prospective study of individuals 18 years and older, who have successfully maintained a 14-kg (30-1b) weight loss for a minimum of 1 year. Currently, the registry includes nearly 3,000 individuals followed for a mean of 5.5 years. Data is collected annually on weight, eating habits, and exercise patterns.
- Registry members report that weight loss has led to significant improvements in self-confidence, mood, and physical health. Surprisingly, 42% of participants report that maintaining their weight loss is less difficult than initially losing the weight.
- Successful weight losers report making substantial changes in eating and exercise habits to lose weight and maintain the loss.
- Two-thirds of these successful weight losers were overweight as children, and 60% report a family history of obesity.
- Approximately 50% of participants lost weight on their own without any type of formal program or help.

How did they lose weight?

- Successful weight-loss strategies used by individuals were variable and could have included more than one of the following: 90% used diet *and* activity strategies, 88% restricted food intake, and 44% instituted portion control. Forty-four percent counted calories, 33% focused on a low fat diet, and 22% exchanged foods in their diet (e.g., Splenda for sugar).
- These individuals exhibited high levels of physical activity (2800 Cal/wk or 60 min/day), but simple walking was the most frequently cited physical activity.
- Most individuals had a feedback system; 75 % weighed themselves weekly.
- Ninety percent eat breakfast. Most ate regular meals, had less than three meals out and less than one fast food meal per week.

Practical pearls

- **All diets work**. Self-assessment, awareness, education, regular weighing and documentation, and adherence

to a protocol all seem to predict a reduction in weight. Readiness to change is a key variable.

- Any diet is likely effective; however, some have negative effects on certain groups of dieters, such as those with kidney or heart problems. Perhaps the key message is that **the concept of "diet" is a short-term one and longer term issues such as participation of the person's social network, eating less processed foods, care for depression and anxiety, and making activity a habit are key components in successful dieting.** Weight Watchers is a good choice if the individual is looking for a program.
- **Reduction in calorie intake is likely the area of greatest opportunity.** This being said, after 1 year there does not seem to be any difference between very low-calorie and regular low-calorie diets.[22]
- **Health improvement comes with a weight loss of 5% to 10%, whereas most patients target 2 to 3 times this amount.** Obese persons who lost 5% to 7% of their weight, reduced saturated fat intake, were active 25 minutes/day, and increased fibre intake, reduced progression to diabetes by over 50% compared with control diet groups.[23]
- Review what was successful for individuals in the NWCR outlined above. A reasonable approach seems to be as listed below:
  - **Assess readiness to change** and consider the patient's unique risk factors and situation. It may be helpful to focus on the unique problem (e.g., patient only eats at night or eats to relieve stress, patient finds activity painful, patient has limited awareness of caloric value of common foods). Helpful resources exist that enable patients to assess their readiness.[24,25]
  - If available, have the patient (and their partner, if applicable) **see a dietician** for an analysis and food diary. Most dieticians can personalize this to a variety of cultures and situations.
  - **Reduce caloric intake by 500 to 1000 kcal/day or 300 –to 500 kcal/day if they are just overweight.** This will typically lead to a weight loss of 2 to 4 kg/wk (1 to 2 lbs/wk). At 6 months most patients will have met the target of 10% weight loss, and a maintenance program can be developed.
  - Consider **simple behavioural problem solving.**
    - Encourage self-monitoring of weight, food intake, and physical activity. Consider various outcomes beyond weight (mood, body shape, waist circumference).
    - Encourage identification and control of stimuli that provoke overeating.
    - Encourage patient to build a supportive social network and environment.
    - Encourage patient to focus on two to three realistic objectives.
  - **Pharmacotherapy may be useful** in "kick-starting" the patient, but is expensive for some and is limited in the long term.

- **Tailor a simple activity program**. Some limited data shows support that weight or resistance training may be the most effective activity (by increasing lean muscle mass and therefore basal metabolic rate), but simply taking additional steps every day is likely more realistic. A pedometer is an excellent way to provide feedback.
- **Document progress** with regular visits in the acute 6-month period and regularly after that. Be realistic. (Maintain a 5% to 10% weight loss target as opposed to "wedding weight.") Document reasons for failure, since this is the norm, not the exception, and continue to assess motivation and confidence.

◢ REFERENCES ◣

1. Ogden CL, Carroll MD, Flegal KM: Epidemiologic trends in overweight and obesity, *Endocrinol Metab Clin North Am* 32(4):741-60, 2003.
2. Frank L, Engelke P: How land use and transportation systems impact public health: a literature review of the relationship between physical activity and built form, *CDC Working Papers*, http://www.cdc.gov/nccdphp/dnpa/pdf/aces-workingpaper1.pdf, Nov. 29, 2004.
3. Tremblay MS, Katzmarzyk PT, Willms JD: Temporal trends in overweight and obesity in Canada 1981-1996, *Int J Obesity* 26:538-543, 2002.
4. Ebbeling CB, Pawlak DB, Ludwig DS: Childhood obesity: public-health crisis, common sense cure, *Lancet* 360:473-82, 2002.
5. Lean ME, Han TS, Seidell JC: Impairment of health and quality of life in people with large waist circumference, *Lancet* 351:853-856, 1998.
6. Rexrode KM, Carey VJ, Hennekens CH, et al: Abdominal adiposity and coronary heart disease in women, *JAMA* 280:1843-1848, 1998.
7. Dalton M, Cameron AJ, Zimmet PZ, et al: Waist circumference, waist-hip ratio and body mass index and their correlation with cardiovascular disease risk factors in Australian adults, *J Int Med* 254:555-563, 2003.
8. Expert Panel on the Identification, Evaluation, and Treatment of Overweight and Obesity in Adults: executive summary of the clinical guidelines on the identification, evaluation, and treatment of overweight and obesity in adults, *Arch Intern Med* 158:1855-1867, 1998.
9. Douketis JD, Feightner JW, Attia J, et al: Periodic health examination, 1999 update. 1. Detection, prevention and treatment of obesity, *Can Med Assoc J* 160:513-525, 1999.
10. Shaper AG, Wannamethee G, Walker M: Body weight: implications for the prevention of coronary heart disease, stroke, and diabetes mellitus in a cohort study of middle aged men, *BMJ* 314:1311-1317, 1997.
11. Willett WC, Manson JE, Stampfer MJ, et al: Weight, weight change, and coronary heart disease in women: risk within the "normal" weight range, *JAMA* 273:461-465, 1995.
12. Ford ES: Body mass index and colon cancer in a national sample of adult US men and women, *Am J Epidemiol* 150:390-398, 1999.
13. Levine JA, Eberhardt NL, Jensen MD: Role of nonexercise activity thermogenesis in resistance to fat gain in humans, *Science* 283:212-214, 1999.
14. Andersen RE, Crespo CJ, Bartlett SJ, et al: Relationship of physical activity and television watching with body weight and level of fatness among children: results from the Third National Health and Nutrition Examination Survey, *JAMA* 279:938-942, 1998.
15. Serdula M, Collins ME, Williamson DF, et al: Weight control practices of U.S. adolescents and adults: Youth Risk Behavior Survey and Behavioral Risk Factor Surveillance System, *Ann Intern Med* 119:667-671, 1993.
16. Horm J, Anderson K: Who in America is trying to lose weight? *Ann Intern Med* 119:672-676, 1993.
17. Yancy WS, Olsen MK, Guyton JR, et al: A low-carbohydrate, ketogenic diet versus a low-fat diet to treat obesity and hyperlipidemia, *Ann Intern Med* 140:769-777, 2004.
18. Trichopoulou A, Costacou T, Bamia C, et al: Adherence to a Mediterranean diet and survival in a Greek population, *N Engl J Med* 348:2599-2608, 2003.
19. Padwal R, Li SK, Lau DCW: Long-term pharmacotherapy for obesity and overweight (Cochrane Review). In *The Cochrane Library*, ed 4, Chichester, UK, 2003, John Wiley & Sons, Ltd.
20. Astrup A, Grunwald GK, Melanson EL, et al: The role of low fat diets in body weight control: a meta-analysis of ad libitum dietary intervention studies, *Int J Obes Relat Metab Disord* 24(12):1545-1552, 2000.
21. Klem ML, Wing RR, McGuire MT, et al: A descriptive study of individuals successful at long-term maintenance of substantial weight loss, *Am J Clin Nutr* 66:239-246, 1997.
22. Serdula MK, Khan LK, Dietz WH: Contempo updates: weight loss counseling revisited, *JAMA* 289(14):1747-1750, 2003.
23. Tuomilehto J, et al: Prevention of type 2 diabetes mellitus by changes in lifestyle among subjects with impaired glucose tolerance, *N Engl J Med* 344:1343-1350, 2001.
24. Kushner RF, Kushner N, Vincent E: *Dr. Kushner's Personality Type Diet*, New York: St. Martin's Press, 2003.
25. The Partnership for Health Weight Management; http://www.consumer.gov/weightloss

AN APPROACH TO PATIENT-PHYSICIAN COMMUNICATION

Competent health care delivery in medicine is heavily influenced by the doctor-patient relationship. Overwhelming evidence suggests that a patient-centred approach to this relationship can significantly influence health care outcomes, including patient satisfaction.[1-3] This is of critical importance in the practice of primary care medicine, where relationships are developed and strengthened over time and physicians may see patients through many stages of the life cycle.[4,5] The patient-centred model is a conceptual framework based on six interconnected components: exploring both disease and the illness experience, understanding the whole person, finding common ground regarding management, incorporating prevention and health promotion, enhancing the doctor-patient relationship, and being realistic.[6]

The patient history is well documented as the most powerful diagnostic tool in medicine.[7-9] Considering most physicians conduct approximately 200,000 interviews in a career,[10] the quality of the clinical interview is critical to establishing effective and efficient doctor-patient relationships. Additionally, competent communication in the clinical interview can yield huge benefits, such as fewer patient complaints, fewer clinical errors and medical litigation, more accurate diagnosis and care, and a reduction in avoidable stress on both physician and patient.[11]

Martin's Map[12] (Figure 1) provides a realistic framework for flexibly organizing and integrating medical content with a patient-centred approach. Medical interviews do have structure and organization; they are not passive, haphazard events. The interview map was derived and substantiated through existing medical, teaching, and learning literature and research.[13-15] Martin's Map is meant to be a guide that presents an effective and efficient route to organizing a medical interview while still responding to individual patient differences.

The Beginning

The first part of the medical interview should elicit the patient's agenda, including expectations for the office visit. The physician should gain as comprehensive as possible understanding of the patient's reason for coming and his or her expectations. Avoid getting sidetracked by one issue, assuming either that it is the only concern or the most pressing concern. At the beginning of the interview, physicians often provide premature reassurance and health teaching without clearly understanding the patient's agenda. The medical literature is rich with examples of the fact that understanding the patient's perspective at the beginning contributes directly to better health care outcomes.[16,17] If it becomes evident there is not enough time allotted to attend to all expectations, stop, negotiate, and prioritize. Finding common ground begins at this point. Unlike other specialties, doctor-patient relationships in family medicine evolve through continuity of care, meaning multiple visits over time. It is not necessary to address and resolve every issue in one visit.

The interview should always begin with an open-ended question, allowing patients to verbalize in their own words what brought them in. Understanding the patient's agenda and expectations for the visit, as fully and as early as possible is the foundation of the patient-centred interview and critical to its outcome. Open-ended questions facilitate this foundation. More directed, close-ended questions about the presenting complaint illness begin only after the patient has had an opportunity to give his or her agenda. Documentation reveals that physicians often interrupt patients within seconds of the patient's initial statements, often prematurely directing the conversation.[18-20] Studies show that patients do not consume valuable time unnecessarily if allowed to talk. Most patients provide relevant information and conclude their list of complaints within 2 minutes.[21] Exploration of the patient's agenda and concerns includes both the exploration of the disease process and the illness experience. Questions relating to these should be interwoven throughout the interview, but initial understanding and exploration of the patient's agenda begins immediately through open-ended questioning. The physician should not move on to the middle of the interview until he or she has a clear, comprehensive understanding of the patient's agenda and expectations.[22] This includes both a beginning exploration of the patient's illness experience (ideas, feelings, expectations, effects on functioning) and an exploration of the history of presenting illness.

A free-flow exchange of information can make the "beginning" the most time-consuming part of the interview. However, the information acquired minimizes what you may need to explore in the "middle" of the interview and helps you tailor the rest of the interview efficiently. Additionally, you are building a relationship with the patient by joining and establishing rapport. If the patients begin repeating themselves and information becomes redundant, stop and summarize your understanding to regain control and refocus the interview.

When you feel you have a comfortable understanding of the patient's agenda, reflect this back for clarification and verification before continuing. You should include some reference to the patient's expectations regarding the outcome of the appointment and a further inquiry as to whether there are any additional concerns to discuss. Before moving on to the "middle" or "body" of the interview, use a transitional/bridging statement to signify a change in direction or tempo of the interview; that is, a statement of what you are doing and why you are doing it.

Middle

The purpose of the middle of the interview is twofold. First, continue to gather relevant information, both verbally and through the physical examination to either confirm or discount hypothesis related to the preliminary differential diagnosis. Second, increase your understanding of this patient's specific life context that may affect the treatment and management plan. If the beginning of an interview is considered the "patient's turn," the middle of the interview is the "physician's turn." Patients who feel that the physician is really listening during the beginning of the interview tend to stay focused during history taking and are more open to recommended treatment and management plans. Patients who do not feel they are being heard tend to interrupt more often until their feelings are acknowledged.[23,24]

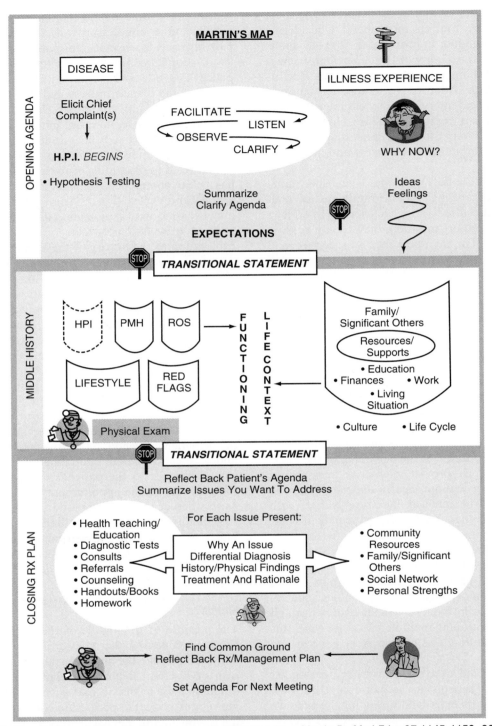

Figure 1 Martin's Map for Organizing a Medical Interview" (Modified from Martin D: *Med Educ* 37:1145-1153, 2003. Printed with permission from Dawn Martin, DFCM, St. Joseph's Health Centre, University of Toronto.)

One way to think of history taking is through the metaphor of *pockets* (Figure 2). A pocket is a specific piece of bounded history. Each pocket contains all the questions related to a distinct part of the history. Once the physician goes into a pocket, he or she should clean out the pocket by asking all *relevant* questions before moving to another pocket. This keeps both the physician and patient focused and organized. Interviews become disjointed and difficult for the patient to follow when the physician jumps back and forth between pockets without

WHAT'S IN A POCKET?

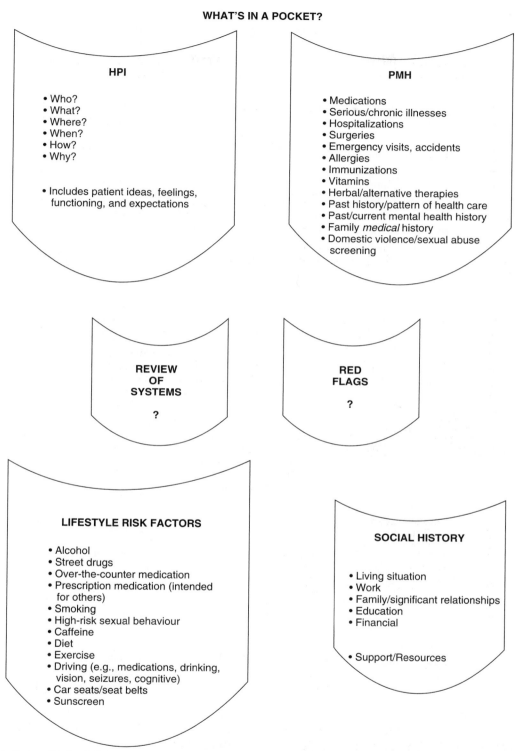

HPI

- Who?
- What?
- Where?
- When?
- How?
- Why?

- Includes patient ideas, feelings, functioning, and expectations

PMH

- Medications
- Serious/chronic illnesses
- Hospitalizations
- Surgeries
- Emergency visits, accidents
- Allergies
- Immunizations
- Vitamins
- Herbal/alternative therapies
- Past history/pattern of health care
- Past/current mental health history
- Family *medical* history
- Domestic violence/sexual abuse screening

REVIEW OF SYSTEMS

?

RED FLAGS

?

LIFESTYLE RISK FACTORS

- Alcohol
- Street drugs
- Over-the-counter medication
- Prescription medication (intended for others)
- Smoking
- High-risk sexual behaviour
- Caffeine
- Diet
- Exercise
- Driving (e.g., medications, drinking, vision, seizures, cognitive)
- Car seats/seat belts
- Sunscreen

SOCIAL HISTORY

- Living situation
- Work
- Family/significant relationships
- Education
- Financial

- Support/Resources

Figure 2   What's in a Pocket? (Reprinted with permission from Dawn Martin, DFCM, St. Joseph's Health Centre, University of Toronto.)

any apparent direction or link between questions. A disorganized history increases the risk of missing pertinent information and adds unnecessary time to an interview.

When a physician is finished asking the questions relevant to a specific pocket, he or she should signal the intention to move into another pocket by using signposts.

Signposts increase time efficiency by guiding patients through the interview and help the physician stay organized and focused. For example, "I think I have an understanding of your past medical history and care; now I want to ask you some specific questions about your headaches."

Not all questions in a pocket are relevant to every patient. The patient's chief complaint and expectations elicited at the beginning of the interview determine relevant questions. At this point, a comprehensive understanding of the patient's agenda and expectations for the visit helps the physician tailor the history-taking (the middle) part of the interview. The physician mentally scans the contents of the different pockets for the necessary questions.

There are a few general rules when asking questions within pockets. Whenever possible, questions should be asked from least sensitive to most sensitive and close-ended to open-ended. The former helps build rapport and the latter enhances efficiency. These rules extend to deciding which questions should be asked first. In most interviews, the retrieval of medical information is perceived as less sensitive than social history and subsequently acts to build rapport. Usually, patients are expecting to answer questions related to their medical health; therefore, medical data collection is a way of building rapport. There is a logical sequence to data collecting.

In most clinical encounters during history taking, *relevant* patient medical history (PMH) questions should be asked first. Information retrieved at this point may help to inform questions in other pockets. For instance, the use of medications often helps the physicians understand a patient's current and/or past medical conditions. The history of presenting illness (HPI) follows PMH and appears in the middle of the interview for the purpose of *completing* any unfinished HPI questions that were not presented or retrieved at the beginning of the interview. The scope of questions changes continually throughout the interview based on elicited information and physical findings. Because review of symptoms (ROS) follows later in the interview, much of the relevant information may be answered by the data obtained earlier. Red flag questions narrow the focus of inquiry by quickly ruling in or out low probability, but acute diagnosis. Red flags might also include the necessary screening questions that uncover potential risk factors for a proposed treatment, such as "Any history of blood clots?" "Any history of liver disease?" when trying to decide whether to prescribe birth control pills.

Lifestyle risk factors tend to be associated with patients' beliefs and values about their health, which may be at odds with medical recommendations. As a result, this inquiry can be very sensitive despite being a routine set of questions for physicians. Condensing risk factors into one pocket helps in recall and diminishes the patient's perception of judgment. Questions related to health pre-

vention have been included in this pocket because they are linked to lifestyle. Lifestyle questions follow the medical history but come before the social history because positive answers to lifestyle screening questions may influence questions related to social history.

A patient's social history should be explored after the medical history and inquiry into lifestyle risk factors, because the beginning of the interview and subsequent medical history lay the foundation for rapport building. The information gathered can help the physician more sensitively and accurately inquire about the patient's disease/illness experience and how it is affecting their ability to function.

No standardized set of questions is related to cultural determinants and life cycle stages, although these factors directly influence diagnostic treatment and management decisions. As a result, the questions appear on the interview map not as pockets, but reminders.

Closing

The purpose of the closing is to present the diagnosis, rationale, treatment, and management plan based on the history/physical/diagnostic tests. Treatment and management plans should not be presented as one "run-on" sentence. Issues should be presented one at a time with efforts made to address questions and find common ground before moving on to the next concern. Health teaching should fall under the closing phase of the interview, after relevant medical and social histories, so explanations can be tailored to the patient. The interview closes with a summary of the agreed upon plan[25] and recommendations, when relevant, for a return visit.

❧ REFERENCES ❧

1. Stewart M, Brown JB, Donner A, et al: The impact of patient-centered care on outcomes, *J Fam Pract* 49:796-804, 2002.
2. Mead N, Bower P: Patient-centered consultations and outcomes in primary care: a review of the literature, *Patient Educ Couns* 48:51-61, 2002.
3. Beckman H, Kaplan S, Frankel R: Outcome-based research on doctor-patient communication. In: Stewart M, Roter D, eds: *Communicating with medical patients,* Newbury Park, CA, 1989, Sage.
4. Parboosingh J: A catalyst for change in communication skills: the Canadian Breast Cancer Initiative, *Cancer Prev Control* 3:19-24, 1999.
5. Handfield-Jones R, Kocha W: The role of the medical organization in supporting doctor-patient communication, *Cancer Prev Control* 3:46-50, 1999.
6. Stewart M, Brown JB, Weston WW, et al: *Patient-centered medicine: transforming the clinical method,* ed 2, Oxford, Eng, 2003, Radcliffe Medical.
7. Platt R: Two essays on the practice of medicine: Manchester University, *Med School Gazette* 27:139-145, 1947.
8. Peterson MC, Holbrook JH, DeVon H, et al: Contributions of the history, physical examination and laboratory

investigation in making medical diagnoses, *West J Med* 156:163-165, 1992.

9. Hasnain M, Bordage G, Connell KJ, et al: History taking behaviors associated with diagnostic competence of clerks: an exploratory study, *Acad Med* 76:14-17, 1997.

10. Kurtz S, Silverman J, Draper J: *Teaching and learning communication skills in medicine,* Oxford, Eng, 1998, Radcliffe Medical.

11. Levinson W, Roter DL, Mullooly JP, et al: Physician-patient communication: the relationship with malpractice claims among primary care physicians and surgeons, *JAMA* 277:533-559, 1997.

12. Martin D: Martin's Map: a conceptual framework for teaching and learning the medical interview using a patient-centred approach, *Med Educ* 37:1145-1153, 2003.

13. Smith RC, Marshall-Dorsey AA, Osborn GG, et al: Evidence-based guidelines for teaching patient-centered interviewing, *Patient Educ Couns* 2000;39:270:36.

14. Mead N, Bower P: Patient-centred consultations and outcomes in primary care: a review of the literature, *Patient Educ Couns* 48:51-61, 2002.

15. Street RL Jr, Millay B: Analyzing patient participation in medical encounters, *Health Communication* 13(1):61-73, 2001.

16. Lang F, Floyd MR, Beine LB, et al: Sequenced questioning to elicit the patient's perspective on illness: effects on information disclosure, patient satisfaction and time expenditure, *Fam Med* 34:325-330, 2002.

17. Simpson M, Buckman R, Stewart M, et al: Doctor-patient communication: the Toronto consensus statement, *BMJ* 303:1385-1387, 1991.

18. Beckman HB, Frankel RM: The effect of physician behavior on the collection of data, *Ann Intern Med* 101:692-696, 1984.

19. Marvel MK, Epstein RM, Flowers K, et al: Soliciting the patients' agenda: have we improved? *JAMA* 281:283-7, 1999.

20. Blau JN: Time to let the patient speak, *BMJ* 298(6665):39, 1989.

21. Langewitz Wolf, Martin Denz, Keller Anne, et al: Spontaneous talking time at start of consultation in outpatient clinical cohort study, *B M J* 325(7366):682-683, 2002.

22. Martina B, Bacheli B, Stotz M, et al: First clinical judgement by primary car physicians distinguishes well between non-organic causes of abdominal or chest pain, *J Gen Intern Med* 12:459-465, 1997.

23. Levinson W, Gorawara-Bhast R, Lamb J: A study of patient clues and physician responses in primary care and surgical settings, *JAMA* 286:1021-1027.

24. Lang F, Floyd MR, Beine KL: Clues to patient's explanations and concerns about their illnesses, *Arch Fam Med* 9:222-227, 2000.

25. Starfield B, Wray C, Hess K, et al: The influence of patient-practitioner agreement on outcome of care, *Am J Public Health* 71:127-131, 1981.

AN APPROACH TO PREVENTING THE SPREAD OF INFECTION IN THE OFFICE

Introduction

The outbreak of Severe Acute Respiratory Syndrome (SARS) and its rapid worldwide spread in early 2003 served to remind health care practitioners of the importance of infection control. This section summarizes the necessary steps health care providers can take to minimize the risk of spreading infections in their work settings, with an emphasis on a typical physician's office.

In the past, guidelines for infection control were oriented toward the patient with a known or suspected specific infection. More recently in the wake of SARS, guidelines have addressed symptoms such as fever or new respiratory symptoms. This syndromic approach is far more compatible with primary care, because patients with undifferentiated problems must be assessed in a safe setting, long before a specific diagnosis is known.

Principles of Transmission of Micro-Organisms

Understanding how micro-organisms can be transmitted forms the basis for measures to counteract possible spread.

A. Contact transmission: this includes direct and indirect contact as well large droplet transmission.
   1. Direct and Indirect Contact
      - Direct contact transmission is the transfer of micro-organisms from direct physical contact between a colonized individual and a susceptible second person.
      - Indirect contact refers to the passive transfer of micro-organisms to a susceptible individual via an intermediate object such as contaminated hands or instruments.
   2. Droplet transmission refers to transmission of micro-organisms by large droplets (>5μm) and is associated with coughing and sneezing. It is the principle mechanism whereby respiratory infections are spread to a distance up to approximately 1 metre from the patient. It is also the mode of transmission during procedures that are likely to generate splashes of blood, body fluids, secretions, or excretions.

B. Airborne transmission occurs by dissemination of either airborne droplet nuclei or dust particles containing micro-organisms. These can remain suspended in the air for long periods and can be widely dispersed by air currents, and thus may be inhaled by persons who are a considerable distance from the source patient. Chicken pox and TB are examples of illnesses spread by airborne transmission.

   Aerosolization, the process of creating very small droplets of moisture, was recognized during SARS as a mechanism whereby certain procedures could convert droplet transmission into airborne transmission for brief periods, facilitating inhalation of micro-organisms.

C. Common vehicle transmission refers to a single contaminated source such as food, medication, or intravenous fluid or equipment, each of which can transmit infection to multiple hosts. This may result in an explosive outbreak.

D. Vector-borne transmission is a process in which another organism transmits the infectious micro-organism. For example, the mosquito is the vector for the West Nile Virus, transmitting it from infected birds to susceptible humans.

Guidelines for Health Care Practice

Routine infection prevention practices

"Routine practices" is the term Health Canada uses to describe a system of infection prevention recommended in Canada, applicable to all health care settings. These prevention strategies are used during all patient care. They include the following:

- Hand washing with soap and water or an alcohol-based sanitizer before and after any direct contact with a patient is the single most important measure to prevent transmitting infection.
- The use of additional barrier precautions helps to prevent contact with a patient's blood and body fluids, non-intact skin, or mucous membranes.
- Wearing surgical masks and eye protection or face shields when appropriate helps to protect mucous membranes of the eyes, nose, and mouth in patient care procedures that are likely to generate splashes or sprays of any body fluid or secretions.
- Gloves should be worn when there is a risk of body fluid contact with hands. Gloves are an additional measure and not a substitute for hand washing.
- Gowns should be worn during procedures that are likely to generate splashes or sprays of any body fluid or secretions that could contaminate clothing.

Preventing respiratory illnesses

All patients presenting for care should be screened for symptoms of a febrile respiratory illness (FRI). The goal is to identify patients who *may* have an infectious illness early in the encounter to minimize the risk of transmission to staff or other patients. The approach should be to err on the side of caution.

Screening can be done at the time of booking an appointment or through patient self-screening on arrival via signage asking if the patient has a new or worse cough, shortness of breath, or a fever. Patients with a positive response to any of the questions should be asked to wash hands and wear a mask while waiting. The signage, waterless hand wash, and surgical masks should be readily available to all patients as close to the entrance as practical. If possible, symptomatic patients should wait in a separate area or keep one meter away from others. Office personnel who provide care should initiate droplet precautions including hand hygiene, a mask, and eye protection. Routine care can be provided. The patient should be assessed for further risks of SARS or other severe res-

piratory illness with questions about recent travel (past 30 days), possible contact with another sick person who has travelled recently, and contact with others in their family and work or social setting, who may have similar symptoms. The responses to these questions and the clinical assessment will determine whether continued precautions are required. Patients with positive answers and an FRI should be advised to follow up with a primary care provider if there is no improvement within 72 hours.

Special office considerations for airborne infections

Patients with known or suspected infectious TB, measles, varicella, or disseminated herpes zoster require additional precautions to prevent spread to other susceptible patients or personnel. Such patients should be identified as early as possible in the booking process, and should not wait in the common waiting room but be placed directly in an examining room. If possible, the visit should be scheduled to minimize exposure of other patients, such as the beginning or end of the day. Ideally the patient should be seen in a negative pressure room with exhaust vented to the outside or filtered through a high efficiency filter, but this is not available in most settings; therefore, a designated room should be used and the door must remain closed. The patient should wear a surgical mask when not in a negative pressure room. Unless they have documented immunity to the suspected infection, health care workers (HCWs) who enter the room should wear an N-95 mask.[1]

For varicella, items and services that have been in contact with skin lesions should be cleaned before the next patient is admitted to the room. If possible, allow sufficient time for the air to be free of aerosolized droplets before using it for the next patient (in the case of TB) or for non-immune patients (in the case of measles or varicella).

Individuals susceptible to varicella, including staff, should not enter the room. For infectious TB, all staff should wear a mask.

Special office considerations for antibiotic-resistant organisms

Colonization or infection with bacteria that are resistant to many antibiotics is becoming an increasing problem in all health care settings. Patients are at the highest risk for acquiring an antibiotic resistant organism such as methicillin-resistant *Staphylococcus aureus* (MRSA) or vancomycin-resistant enterococci (VRE) when hospitalized. They may require subsequent care in the physician's office.

Family physicians should be specifically notified by the discharging institution if patients have MRSA or VRE. The charts of such patients should be flagged to facilitate recognition.

Both MRSA and VRE are spread by contact, usually from the hands of health care providers. In addition it is likely that VRE is spread by contaminated equipment or environmental surfaces. The following precautions are recommended for patients in the office with either MRSA or VRE; additional ones follow for managing patients with VRE.

1. Patient should be moved to an examining room as soon as possible.
2. The HCW should wear gloves when entering the room. For MRSA wear a mask as well to prevent nasal cell inoculation. For VRE a mask is not necessary, but a gown should be worn. Regular disposal of gloves, masks, or gowns is sufficient.
3. Wipe all equipment such as stethoscope, thermometers, and blood pressure cuffs with the disinfectant used in the office or with 70% alcohol.
4. Wash hands thoroughly before leaving the room and again outside the room as an added safety measure. Antimicrobial soap is recommended; an alcohol-based hand wash after regular soap is also effective.

The following additional steps are recommended when caring for VRE patients:

5. Cover surfaces that will not be touched or used in the examination to limit contact with environmental surfaces.
6. After the patient leaves, wash all environmental surfaces that were touched or exposed with office disinfectant (see below). The person cleaning the room should wear gloves and a gown. Be sure to note door handles, light fixtures, and surfaces that may be touched by the health care worker or patient.

Patients discharged from the hospital with MRSA are usually on eradication therapy. Contact the infection control practitioner or infectious diseases specialist if treatment or follow-up strategies have not been identified for the patient.

Immunization of medical office workers

All employees in a medical office should have documented, current immunization for communicable diseases that are preventable by vaccine. This includes poliomyelitis, pertussis, measles, rubella, influenza, hepatitis B, tetanus, and diphtheria toxoids. Varicella vaccine is recommended for susceptible HCWs unless they are immunocompromised or pregnant.

Tuberculosis skin testing with the two-step method is recommended for all HCWs at the beginning of employment. Routine follow-up skin testing is not recommended except for situations of exposure to a known case of TB, clinical symptoms suggesting active TB, or annually for HCWs at risk of contact with TB.

Pneumococcal vaccine is indicated for susceptible individuals regardless of occupation. This includes persons over the age of 65, and those with asplenia or splenic dysfunction, sickle cell disease, or the following chronic conditions: chronic respiratory disease, cirrhosis, alcoholism, chronic renal disease, diabetes mellitus, chronic cerebrospinal fluid (CSF) leaks, HIV, and other immune suppressive conditions.

Personnel health

The routine practices described above should minimize the risk of HCWs acquiring disease from patients. An HCW with dermatitis is at risk because of compromise of the skin as a protective barrier. Good preventative skin care is important, and any dermatitis should be covered with a bandage. Gloves should be worn if there is a potential exposure to blood or other body fluids.

All practices should educate individual health care providers about their personal responsibility in disease prevention and the steps they can take to minimize the spread of FRI, including the following:

- Having an annual influenza immunization
- Not working when ill
- Reporting any symptoms of an FRI to their supervisor
- Covering the mouth when coughing
- Washing hands frequently

Disinfection and Sterilization of Medical Instruments
General principles

A detailed discussion of disinfection and sterilization of medical instruments is beyond the scope of this article, but may be found in several of the references. (For example, see The College of Physicians & Surgeons of Ontario publication "Infection Control in the Physicians Office" [July 2004], available at the website indicated below.)

Medical instruments can be categorized according to how they are used to determine the level of cleaning and sterilization required (first proposed by Spaulding). In modified form, the classification is as follows:

- "Critical" instruments enter a sterile body site or vascular system and should be cleaned followed by sterilization.
- "Semi-critical" instruments come in contact with intact mucous membranes or non-intact skin and should be cleaned followed by high-level disinfection.
- "Non-critical" instruments come in contact with intact skin and should be cleaned followed by low- or intermediate-level disinfection.

Many offices choose to use disposable equipment such as vaginal specula or anoscopes rather than sterilization. Instruments should be cleaned of any organic material as soon as possible after use so that the material does not dry or interfere with the sterilization or disinfection process. Sterilization such as autoclaving completely kills all forms of microbial life.

Monitoring sterilization is important to ensure that the process has been accomplished. Monitoring includes manual indicators such as time, temperature, and pressure gauges, chemical indicators such as tape that changes colour, and biological indicators for weekly performance. The manufacturer instructions should be followed and regular maintenance checked and maintained.

A variety of packaging materials is available, many with convenient features such as self-sealing closures and chemical indicator strips. Wrapped packs should be stored in clean, dry areas such as closed shelves. Before use, packages should be checked to ensure that the seal is intact, there is no evidence of soiling, and the chemical indicators are the appropriate colour. With the integrity of the package maintained, sterilized equipment can be kept for long periods but should probably not exceed 1 year.

General housekeeping of the office

Medical offices should be cleaned at the end of the work day, with immediate attention for special situations such as spilled body fluids. Surfaces, toys, and objects should be cleaned with a low-level disinfective.

The following detergents are useful for daily cleaning of all surfaces in the office: phenolic, idophor, ammonia compounds, and sodium hypochloride (1:100 dilution of household bleach prepared weekly and stored at room temperature in an opaque container).

Spilled body fluids should be cleaned immediately. The person cleaning should wear household gloves, wipe up as much of the physical material as possible with disposable toweling, dispose in a covered garbage, and then clean the spill area with a prepared disinfective detergent and then rinse and dry with a disposable towel. Carpets are not an appropriate surface for patient care areas.

A refrigerator should be designated for medications or vaccines only; food and personal items should be stored in a separate refrigerator. Temperature monitors are available to ensure that the temperature of the medication or refrigerator is maintained between 2° and 8°. Manufacturer's instructions should be followed for vaccine handling and maintaining a basic cool chain.

Waste disposal

Most jurisdictions have specific legislation regarding biomedical waste. Anatomical waste consists of tissue, organs, and body parts, not including teeth, nails, and hair.

Non-anatomical waste consists of human liquid blood and blood products, items contaminated with blood that would release liquid or semi-liquid blood if compressed, and body fluids contaminated with blood excluding urine and feces. Sharps including needles and blades and broken glass and other materials capable of causing puncture or cuts that come into contact with human blood or body must also be handled carefully through disposable sharps containers with appropriate subsequent disposal.

For all types of waste, garbage containers should be waterproof and should have tight-fitting lids. Plastic bags should be used to line the containers.

Employee protocol following significant exposure to blood

Accidental exposure to blood or body fluids through needle stick injuries or splash accidents that contact mucous membranes should be addressed with prompt, organized action. Potential blood-borne infections include hepatitis B, hepatitis C, and HIV.

First aid includes encouraging bleeding after a sharp injury, then washing the area well with soap and warm water. For a splash accident infecting the eyes, the eyes should be flushed well for 10 minutes with cold water.

There are specific protocols for chemoprophylaxis following HIV and hepatitis B. Readers are referred to current sources. The risk of transmission of hepatitis C following subcutaneous exposure is about 3%. A health care worker who has been accidentally exposed should be monitored with a sense of testing and treatment should be started if infection is diagnosed.

NOTES

Surgical masks cover the nose and mouth of the wearer, providing a physical barrier to fluids, droplets, and particles. Along with eye protection, they are part of preventing droplet transmission. N-95 masks have a high degree of filtration and reduce the risk of inhaling airborne particles. Proper use of N-95 masks requires fit-testing to ensure a seal with the wearer's face. Details are available at http://www.osha-slc.gov.SLTC/etools/respiratory/index.html.

The primary sources and studies to support the infection control recommendations are voluminous and highly detailed. Following are references to authoritative sources readily available on the Internet, which form the basis of this summary.

http://www.cdc.gov/ncidod/hip/Guide/guide.htm

Routine Practices and Additional Precautions for Preventing the Transmission of Infection in Health Care http://www.hc-sc.gc.ca/pphb-dgspsp/publicat/ccdr-rmtc/99vol25/25s4/index.html

CPSO http://www.cpso.on.ca/publications/INF-CONTR.PDF

Guideline for Isolation Precautions in Hospitals CDC http://www.cdc.gov/ncidod/hip/ISOLAT/Isolat.htm

Public Health Guidance for Community-Level Preparedness and Response to Severe Acute Respiratory Syndrome (SARS) Version 2. Supplement I: Infection Control in Healthcare, Home, and Community Settings

Infection Control and Surveillance Standards Task Force of the Ontario Ministry of Health and Long-Term Care (MOHLTC): "Preventing Respiratory Illness in Community Settings: Recommendations for Infection

Control and Surveillance for Febrile Respiratory Illness (FRI) in Community Settings in Non-Outbreak Conditions" March 11, 2004, available at: www.health. gov.on.ca/english/providers/program/pubhealth/sars/sars mn.html

The full description of routine practices to prevent transmission of nosocomial pathogens can be found on the Health Canada website: http://www.hc-sc.gc.ca/ pphb-dgspsp/dpg_e.html#infection

http://www.hc-sc.gc.ca/pphb-dgspsp/dpg_e.html# infection

AN APPROACH TO SPECIAL POPULATIONS
Socio-Economic Status

Major differentials in socio-economic status (SES) persist in most societies and have major implications for health. Even among those with full-time employment, men in the lowest income grade have more than a three-fold increase in mortality compared with those in the highest grade.[1] This effect is not limited to those in the lowest SES groups, because even high SES groups have worse health than those with yet higher levels. If it was a disease, income-related excess mortality would be the second leading cause of potential years of life lost, following neoplasms.[2] The nature and direction of causative factors is complex and differs among groups because poor health can cause low SES, such as with severe and persistent mental illness; low SES can cause poor health, such as with inadequate income for a healthy diet; or a third factor can cause both low SES and ill health, such as in genetic factors. SES is also strongly implicated in health disparities involving ethnic and racial minorities and recent immigrants.

The challenge of low SES is often seen as one of financial access barriers to care, and this is a major concern in some settings. Even in countries with universal health care, however, low SES is associated with increased mortality, avoidable hospitalization, disability, higher health care costs, and lack of access to specialists and procedures.[2-7] Low SES is also associated with increased prevalence and severity of many chronic health conditions such as asthma and diabetes.[8,9] Reducing health care disparities has become a major policy focus in industrialized countries.[10-13]

What can family doctors do about this pervasive health issue? Advocacy for expanded access to care and for other appropriate public policies can occur at the level of the individual physician, through professional associations and other societal groups. There is evidence that directing attention to child poverty and early childhood development can be effective.[14,15] At the clinical interface, being aware of increased health needs and access barriers among patients with low SES is important for ensuring that patients get appropriate care. Health literacy, for example, is strongly associated with self-

management for chronic diseases and positive health outcomes, yet most health communication and written materials are at a high-literacy level.[16,17] Using plain language, employing low-literacy materials, correcting misconceptions, and ensuring appropriate referrals to medical specialists, non-medical health care providers, and community agencies and programs may help to reduce health care disparities.

✎ REFERENCES ✍

1. Marmot MG, Shipley MJ: Do socioeconomic differences in mortality persist after retirement? 25 year follow-up of civil servants from the first Whitehall study, *BMJ* 313: 1177-1180, 1996.
2. Wilkins R, Berthelot JM, Ng E: Trends in mortality by neighbourhood income in urban Canada from 1971-1996, *Health Rep* 13:S1-S28, 2002.
3. Pappas G, Hadden WC, Kozak LJ, et al: Potentially avoidable hospitalizations: inequities in rates between U.S. socioconomic groups, *Am J Public Health* 87:811-816, 1997.
4. Glazier RH, Badley EM, Gilbert JE, et al: The nature of increased hospital use in poor neighbourhoods: findings from a Canadian inner city, *Can J Public Health* 91: 268-273, 2000.
5. Alter DA, Iron K, Austin PC, et al: SESAMI Study Group: socioeconomic status, service patterns, and perceptions of care among survivors of acute myocardial infarction in Canada, *JAMA* 291:1100-1107, 2004.
6. Hawker GA, Wright JG, Glazier RH, et al: The effect of education and income on need and willingness to undergo total joint arthroplasty, *Arthritis Rheum* 46:3331-3339, 2002.
7. Roos NP, Mustard CA: Variation in health and health care use by socioeconomic status in Winnipeg, Canada: does the system work well? Yes and no, *Millbank Q* 75:89-111, 1997.
8. Mielck A, Reitmeir P, Wjst M: Severity of childhood asthma by socioeconomic status, *Int J Epidemiol* 25:388-393, 1996.
9. Brancati FL, Whelton PK, Kuller LH, et al: Diabetes mellitus, race, and socioeconomic status: a population-based study, *Ann Epidemiol* 6:67-73, 1996.
10. National Heathcare Disparities Report, http://www.ahcpr. gov/qual/nhdr03/nhdrsum03.htm, accessed April 14, 2004.
11. Health Canada, http://www.hc-sc.gc.ca/hppb/phdd/overview implications/01_overview.html, accessed April 14, 2004.
12. Health inequalities, *http://www.ohn.gov.uk/ohn/inequ.htm*, accessed April 14, 2004.
13. Health Inequalities Research Collaboration, http:// www.hirc.health.gov.au/, accessed April 14, 2004.
14. Devaney BL, Ellwood MR, Love JM: Programs that mitigate the effects of poverty on children, Future Child 7: 88-112, 1997.
15. Kangas O, Palme J: Does social policy matter? Poverty cycles in OECD countries, *Int J Health Serv* 30:335-352, 2000.
16. Gazmararian JA, Williams MV, Peel J, et al: Health literacy and knowledge of chronic disease, *Patient Educ* Counsel 51:267-275, 2003.

17. Williams MV, Davis T, Parker RM, et al: The role of health literacy in patient physician communication, *Fam Med* 34:383-389, 2002.

Gay and Lesbian Health Care

Current estimates indicate that 3% to 9% of men are gay or bisexual and 1% to 4% of women are lesbian or bisexual.[1] Negative experiences with health care providers are unfortunately very common among gay and lesbian patients.[2] Consequently, access to care is reduced for these groups due to concerns about disclosing sexual orientation that could engender homophobic responses. Lower income non-urban gay men are most likely to lack regular checkups and delay treatment.[3] Lesbian access to health care is also a concern. Basically cervical cancer is now seen as an STD secondary to transmission of human papilloma virus (HPV) or genital warts. Most of the evidence is penis to cervix but there is some emerging evidence that HPV can be transferred from woman to woman. Lesbians think they are protected, but they needed to be followed, especially if their is a history of sex with men.[4]

Compared with heterosexual women, health risks for lesbian women attending an STD clinic included a higher rate of bacterial vaginosis, a similar rate of abnormal cervical smears, and higher rates of hepatitis C due to contact with men who inject drugs.[3] Large national surveys show that lesbians and bisexual women have higher prevalence of obesity, alcohol use, and tobacco use and lower rates of parity and birth control pill use. They are also less likely to have health insurance coverage, pelvic examinations, or a mammogram.[5] Mental disorders appear to be higher in lesbians, gay men, and bisexuals, most likely as a result of responses to stigma, prejudice, and discrimination.[6] Gay men have higher risks of cardiovascular disease on the basis of increased rates of smoking and less access to preventive care.[7] Rates of HIV/AIDS, STDS, anal cancer, Hodgkin's disease, and hepatitis B are elevated in gay men.[8,9] The most effective interventions to reduce unprotected anal sex among gay men promote interpersonal skills, are delivered in community-level formats, and focus on younger populations or those at highest risk.[10]

Non-judgemental attitudes are essential in clinical care, as is willingness to routinely inquire about sexual orientation. Appropriate questions include asking if the patient is sexually active, who their partner(s) is/are, and whether they have sex with men, women, or both. As with all sexually active patients, physicians should be prepared to inquire in detail about sexual practices and be knowledgeable about risk behaviours. Gay and lesbian patients should be asked whether they wish their sexual orientation to be documented on their chart. Particular attention should be paid to establishing a welcoming environment and to ensuring routine preventive care.

A comprehensive guide to clinical care for gay and lesbian people has recently been published.[11]

❧ REFERENCES ❧

1. Friedman RC, Downey JI: Homosexuality, *N Engl J Med* 331:923-930, 1994.
2. Stevens PE, Hall JM: Stigma, health beliefs and experiences with health care in lesbian women, *Image J Nurs Sch* 20:69-73, 1988.
3. Fethers K, Marks C, Mindel A, et al: Sexually transmitted infections and risk behaviours in women who have sex with women, *Sex Transm Infect* 76:345-349, 2000.
4. Marrazzo JM: Genital human papillomavirus infection in women who have sex with women: a concern for patients and providers, *AIDS Patient Care Stds* 14:447-451, 2000.
5. Cochran SD, Mays VM, Bowen D, et al: Cancer-related risk indicators and preventive screening behaviors among lesbians and bisexual women, *Am J Public Health* 91:591-597, 2001.
6. Meyer IH: Prejudice, social stress, and mental health in lesbian, gay, and bisexual populations: conceptual issues and research evidence, *Psychol* Bull 129:674-97, 2003.
7. Jalbert Y: *Gay health: current knowledge and future actions*, Ottawa, 1999, Health Canada.
8. Koblin BA, Hessol NA, Zauber AG, et al: Increased incidence of cancer among homosexual men, New York City and San Francisco, 1978-1990, *Am J Epidemiol* 144:916-923, 1996.
9. Dean L, Meyer I, Robinson K, et al: *Lesbian, gay, bisexual, and transgender health: findings and concerns,* conference ed, New York, 2000, Columbia University.
10. Johnson WD, Hedges LV, Ramirez G, et al: HIV prevention research for men who have sex with men: a systematic review and meta-analysis, *J AIDS* 30 Suppl 1:S118-129, 2002.
11. Peterkin A, Risdon C: Caring for lesbian and gay people: a clinical guide, Toronto, 2003, University of Toronto.

The Homeless

Homeless and under-housed populations are growing in many urban areas. Although single men are the largest group, women and families with young children are often the fastest growing. Health risks are highly prevalent due to adverse environmental conditions, absolute poverty, exposure to physical, sexual, and psychological abuse, and lack of social support.[1] Mortality rates vary among countries but are consistently higher than among housed individuals of the same age and sex.[2] Highly prevalent conditions include mental health problems and respiratory and skin infections. Clinicians also need to be alert to risks for and occurrence of TB, HIV/AIDS, and hepatitis B and C. Commonly encountered mental health problems include depression, substance abuse, schizophrenia, and personality disorders. Special populations to be aware of include youth, pregnant women, and older adults. Street youth are often faced with challenges of abusive families of origin, exploitative relationships, psychological distress, violence, substance use, and sexually transmitted disease.[3,4] Young homeless women have a tenfold mortality risk and are particularly at risk from HIV, drug overdose, and suicide.[5]

Primary care physicians should be aware that homeless persons often have difficulty affording prescription medications, keeping them safe from loss or theft, and being able to adhere to medication regimes. They should also be aware of barriers to accessing a balanced diet, appropriate exercise, daily hygiene, logistics for chronic disease treatment and monitoring, and the ability to keep dressings clean and dry.[6] Outreach and case management programs for severe and persistent mental health problems and for substance use have demonstrated success in a variety of settings, as have programs to provide housing.[7] Referral to such programs and involvement of community agencies should be facilitated wherever possible.

❧ REFERENCES ❧

1. Martens WH: A review of physical and mental health in homeless persons, *Public Health Rev* 29:13-33, 2001.
2. Hwang SW: Mortality among men using homeless shelters in Toronto, Ontario, *JAMA* 283:2152-2157, 2000.
3. Walters AS: HIV prevention in street youth, *J Adolesc Health* 25:187-198, 1999.
4. Kamieniecki GW: Prevalence of psychological distress and psychiatric disorders among homeless youth in Australia: a comparative review, *Aust N Z J Psychiatry* 35:352-358, 2001.
5. Cheung AM, Hwang SW: Risk of death among homeless women: a cohort study and review of the literature, *Can Med Assoc J* 170:1243-1247, 2004.
6. Hwang SW, Bugeja AL: Barriers to appropriate diabetes management among homeless people in Toronto, *Can Med Assoc J* 163:161-165, 2000.
7. Rosenheck R, Kasprow W, Frisman L, et al: Cost-effectiveness of supported housing for homeless persons with mental illness, *Arch Gen Psychiatry* 60:940-951, 2003.

COMMUNITY HEALTH: PREVENTION

Topics covered in this section _____

Screening
Wellness
Preventable Risk Factors

_____

Before participating in a preventive program, patients and their physicians should be able to answer the following questions[1]:
1. Are there any proven benefits?
2. If so, how great are they?
3. Are there potential adverse effects?
4. If so, what are they, how serious are they, and how frequently do they occur?

Some preventive programs such as accident prevention, avoidance of high-risk behaviour, and selection of healthy lifestyle choices have virtually no adverse consequences. Even if the benefits have not been proved, there seems little harm in participating in such endeavors. On the other hand, preventive programs that involve screening for disease, classification of individuals into high- or low-risk categories for certain diseases, dietary interventions, or prophylactic drug regimens often have uncertain benefits and may have significant adverse consequences.[1]

In addition, the concept of selection bias is important in prevention. A specialist sees a select population for which the benefit of a screening program may seem intuitive, whereas the family doctor cares for a more general population for which the benefit is not as intuitive and the problems with "false-positives" are more pronounced. Also, patients strongly influence screening because they often perceive testing as black and white. Finally, associations and disease advocacy groups have incentives to push for their own disease but have less awareness of the multiple problems clinicians see and where their own silo fits into the priorities of the general population.

Methods for reporting the benefits of preventive programs may have a profound influence on whether the programs appear useful.[1] The standard reporting methods are as follows[1]:
1. Relative reduction of morbidity or mortality rates
2. Absolute reduction of morbidity or mortality rates
3. Number of patients who need to be treated to prevent one adverse event
4. Total cohort mortality rates

The essential clinical point of the reporting methods is that although few participants in any screening program benefit, the use of relative reduction greatly exaggerates the apparent benefits. Relative reduction rates should never be used to make decisions about the clinical usefulness of a program.[1]

The clinical significance of the benefits of preventive programs may be misconstrued in many other ways, including these:
- Surrogate rather than clinically significant outcomes are used. (For example, finding more "small" cancers is a surrogate outcome for decreased mortality rates.)[2]
- The risk level or disease prevalence of the population involved is not considered. (For example, lipid-lowering drugs are more effective for patients with proven coronary disease than for asymptomatic persons.)[2]
- The interval between the intervention and the benefit is not considered. (For example, if a decrease in prostate cancer death rates is ever proved to result from prostate-specific antigen (PSA) screening, this benefit will not be evident until 10 years after radical prostatectomy.)[2]
- The duration of the intervention required to achieve the benefit is not considered. (For example, hormone replacement therapy must be given for several decades to prevent hip fractures.)[2]
- One benefit may be overshadowed by another. (For example, the value of exercise in the prevention of coronary artery disease and fractures may be de-emphasized by the promotion of hormone replacement therapy for the same purpose.)[2]
- The observed benefit may be due to a "healthy user" effect rather than the intervention. (For example, women choosing hormone replacement therapy have a healthier lifestyle than those who choose not to take hormones.)[3-5]
- Benefits documented in clinical trials are assumed to occur in clinical practice. (This is often not the case because the populations are different or compliance is less stringent.)
- There is publication bias. (Positive results of preventive interventions are more often published than are negative results.)[2]
- Studies showing positive results are preferentially cited. (Authors may cite positive studies more often than negative ones.)[2]
- False-negative results are present. (If a study has inadequate power, a true beneficial result may not be shown–type II error.)[2]

All preventive screening or case-finding programs have the potential for causing harm. In general, the degree of harm increases with each level of the "screening cascade." Harm is least at the initial level, which is the screening process itself; intermediate at the second level, which is the investigation of abnormal screening results; and greatest at the third level, which is the treatment of identified disorders. Examples of physical harm are breast pain from compression during mammography or syncope from a venipuncture at level 1 of the screening cascade, urinary tract infection from prostate biopsy or perforated colon from colonoscopy at level 2, and impotence or death as a result of radical prostatectomy or the precipitation of an eating disorder as a result of dietary therapy at level 3.[6]

The psychological and social harm of preventive programs may be categorized as follows[6]:

1. Anticipated discomfort or perception of adverse effects resulting from preventive interventions
2. Unpleasant interactions with health care workers
3. Time required for preventive programs
4. Excessive overall awareness of health
5. Anxiety while anticipating the results of a screening test
6. Anxiety induced by a positive screening test result
7. Distress from being labelled as "sick" or at "high risk"
8. Psychopathological effects directly induced by a therapeutic program (such as strict dieting)
9. False assurance of disease-free status as a result of a negative screening test

Screening-induced psychological distress is discussed in more detail in the section on screening below, and harm to society as a whole is dealt with in the section on wellness.

Since few persons participating in preventive screening programs benefit and many are harmed, failure to obtain informed consent before participation is likely unethical.[7-9] Unfortunately, obtaining informed consent is difficult because of biased promotional literature,[10,11] physicians' lack of knowledge, patients' problems assimilating data, and lack of time for the process to unfold.[7] Suggested ways to facilitate informed consent are for physicians to base their recommendations, whenever possible, on evidence-based guidelines, such as those put forward by the Canadian Task Force on Preventive Health Care and the U.S. Preventive Services Task Force, and for physicians to refrain from promoting a preventive program on the basis of relative reduction of morbidity rates. Patient information material (decision aids) should be used whenever it is available in a balanced and easily understood form[7]; many brochures present a biased view that exaggerates benefits and glosses over adverse effects.[10,11]

The logistics of implementing systematic preventive programs in a physician's office are closely related to the organizational efficiency of the medical practice. McVea and associates[12] from the University of Nebraska surveyed eight midwestern practices that were interested enough in prevention to have requested "Put Prevention into Practice" (PPIP) kits from the American Academy of Family Practice. They found that even though all the clinicians were enthusiastic about prevention and reasonably knowledgeable about its benefits, none used the kits. Those offices that did not already have an organized system were unable to integrate the material into their routines, while well-organized offices had already made preventive interventions a part of their programs and had no need for the kits.

Specific aspects of prevention are covered in many sections of the text. Immediately following are the sections on screening, behavioural changes for prevention, and wellness.

❧ REFERENCES ❧

1. Marshall KG: Prevention. How much harm? How much benefit? 1. Influence of reporting methods on perception of benefits, *Can Med Assoc J* 154:1493-1499, 1996.
2. Marshall KG: Prevention. How much harm? How much benefit? 2. Ten potential pitfalls in determining the clinical significance of benefits, *Can Med Assoc J* 154:1837-1843, 1996.
3. Posthuma WF, Westendorp RG, Vandenbroucke JP: Cardioprotective effect of hormone replacement therapy in postmenopausal women: is the evidence biased? *BMJ* 308:1268-1269, 1994.
4. Rossouw JE: Estrogens for prevention of coronary heart disease: putting the brakes on the bandwagon, *Circulation* 94: 2982-2985, 1996.
5. Grover SA: Estrogen replacement for women with cardiovascular disease: why don't physicians and patients follow the guidelines? (editorial), *Can Med Assoc J* 161:42-43, 1999.
6. Marshall KG: Prevention. How much harm? How much benefit? 3. Physical, psychological and social harm, *Can Med Assoc J* 155:169-176, 1996.
7. Marshall KG: Prevention. How much harm? How much benefit? 4. The ethics of informed consent for preventive screening programs, *Can Med Assoc J* 155:377-383, 1996.
8. Foster P, Anderson CM: Reaching targets in the national cervical screening programme: are current practices unethical? *J Med Ethics* 24:151-157, 1998.
9. Austoker J: Gaining informed consent for screening: is difficult–but many misconceptions need to be undone (editorial), *BMJ* 319:722-723, 1999.
10. Welch HG: Finding and redefining disease (editorial), *Effect Clin Pract* 2:96-99, 1999.
11. Coulter A: Evidence based patient information is important, so there needs to be a national strategy to ensure it (editorial), *BMJ* 317:225-226, 1998.
12. McVea K, Crabtree BF, Medder JD, et al: An ounce of prevention? Evaluation of the "Put prevention into practice" program, *J Family Pract* 43:361-369, 1996.

SCREENING

(See also abdominal aortic aneurysm; alcohol abuse; attitudes, physician; breast cancer; cervical cancer; clinical practice guidelines; colon cancer; congenital anomalies; consensus conferences; glaucoma; group B streptococci; hemochromatosis; hypothyroidism; lipids; maternal serum screening; obesity; ovarian cancer; patient preferences; periodic health examination; pituitary incidentalomas; prevention; prostate cancer; testicular cancer; thyroid nodules; type 2 diabetes; urinalysis; wellness)

Screening is a public health program organized in such a way that an entire population is screened for a specified condition. Case finding is a program in which individual health care workers in practices and clinics screen their patients for one or more diseases.

Criteria Justifying a Screening Program

Criteria that should be met to justify a screening program include the following[1]:

1. The disease in question should be a serious health problem.
2. There should be a presymptomatic phase during which treatment can change the course of the disease more successfully than in the symptomatic phase.
3. The screening procedure and the ensuing treatment should be acceptable to the public.
4. The screening procedure should have acceptable sensitivity and specificity.
5. The screening procedure and ensuing treatment should be cost effective.

Effect of Screening on Apparent Prevalence Rates

Increased imaging resolution or other techniques that detect small lesions lead to an apparent increase in prevalence rates. For example, ultrasound increases the detection of abdominal aneurysms threefold, but most of the aneurysms are small. Computed tomography (CT) or magnetic resonance imaging (MRI) detects many prolapsed disks in asymptomatic persons.[2] The incidence of prostate cancer has been increasing rapidly over the past 2 decades, probably because of an increase in diagnoses resulting from increased numbers of transurethral prostatic resections for benign disease in the period 1973 to 1986[3] and the increased use of PSA testing thereafter.[4] Ultrasound screening of the thyroid gland in asymptomatic patients resulted in a "nodule" detection rate of 67%.[5]

A closely related issue is disease definition. If the threshold for diagnosing a condition is lowered, the prevalence of the disease will increase. The 1997 decision of the American Diabetes Association to lower the fasting glucose threshold for diabetes from 7.8 mmol/L (140 mg/dl) to 7.0 mmol/L (126 mg/dl) created 1.7 million new diabetics in the United States. If proposed new diagnostic thresholds for diabetes, hypertension, hypercholesterolemia, and obesity are all implemented, 75% of the U.S. adult population will be labelled as diseased.[6]

Clinical Significance of Detecting Small Lesions in a Screening Program

Autopsy studies have shown an extremely high prevalence rate of some cancers. In a 1985 autopsy study from Finland, 2.5-mm slices of thyroid were examined. At least one papillary carcinoma was found in 36% of cases. By extrapolation, if even thinner slices had been obtained, almost 100% of autopsy subjects would have had papillary carcinoma.[7] Ductal carcinoma in situ is found in 6% to 18% of autopsies of women who died of other diseases. How many of these would have progressed to clin-

ical cancer is unknown. This is an important issue because 30% to 40% of cancers diagnosed by mammography are ductal carcinomas in situ.[8]

Evidence that lowering diagnostic thresholds for diseases such as diabetes and hypercholesterolemia will decrease morbidity or mortality is absent or tenuous; in most instances guidelines are based on extrapolations from populations with more advanced disease. The certain result of lowering diagnostic thresholds will be an artifactual improvement in the outcomes of the identified diseases, since individuals with minimally elevated cholesterol, fasting glucose, or blood pressure will do better than those with more marked variations from the norm.[6] The harm of lowering thresholds is discussed below.

Lead Time Bias

Lead time bias is a failure to take into account the time of diagnosis of a disease.[2,9] For example, assume that a hypothetical cancer kills everyone affected by it 10 years after its onset, regardless of what treatment is offered. If one cohort of patients with this disease goes through a screening process that detects the lesions and leads to tumour resection 3 or 4 years before they become symptomatic, the 5-year survival rate will be much higher than in a control cohort in which resection takes place only when the tumour becomes symptomatic (i.e., 3 or 4 years later in the natural history of the disease). If the follow-up is longer, however, survival rates would equalize for the two groups; in this example, everyone would be dead by 10 years after onset.

Length Bias

Length bias refers to the fact that cancers having a slow rate of progression are more likely to be detected by screening techniques than are rapidly growing cancers. These are the tumours with the best prognosis, and therefore they would be expected to have a better prognosis whether or not early treatment is instituted.[2,9]

Overdiagnosis Bias

Overdiagnosis bias is the detection of a pseudodisease; that is, a subclinical disease that would not cause symptoms during the patient's life.[9] Detecting and treating such nonpathogenic conditions clearly results in excellent outcomes.

Efficacy of Screening

Although some screening or case-finding programs have led to decreased morbidity or mortality, such as with screening for phenylketonuria and thyroid-stimulating hormone in newborns, screening for bacteriuria in pregnant women, routine assessment of blood pressure, cervical cytology smears, and mammography in women between ages 50 and 69, other programs have not shown a benefit. For example, routine ultrasound screening of pregnant women at 15 to 22 weeks' gestation and 31 to 35 weeks' gestation has not improved perinatal outcome compared with control subjects who had ultrasound only if clinically indicated.[10] Other examples of screening or case-finding programs of no value, or unproved value, are digital rectal examination for the detection of prostate cancer, breast self-examination for the detection of breast cancer, examination of the skin for the detection of malignancy, examination of the testes for the detection of malignancy, periodic pelvic examinations for the detection of ovarian cancer, chest x-ray examination for the detection of lung cancer in smokers, sputum cytology for the detection of lung cancer in smokers, PSA screening for the detection of prostate cancer, measurement of blood cholesterol levels in asymptomatic average-risk children with the goal of decreasing cardiovascular mortality, assessment of blood glucose levels for the detection of diabetes mellitus in average-risk adults, and urine dipstick analysis for blood with the goal of detecting kidney, bladder, or ureteral malignancies. Most of the programs listed above are discussed and referenced elsewhere in the text, as well as in the reports of the U.S. Preventive Services Task Force[11] and the Canadian Task Force on Preventive Health Care.[12]

Adverse Effects of Screening

The adverse effects of screening are multiple, and many of these are discussed in the sections on prevention and wellness. The effect of screening programs on physicians and on patients' psychological states is dealt with here.

Effects of screening programs on physicians' practice patterns

Physicians are barraged with increasing numbers of guidelines recommending preventive screening interventions, and many are subject to audits assessing whether they comply adequately with these guidelines. There is concern that the increasing emphasis on prevention will take so much time and effort that physicians will be distracted from optimally diagnosing and treating the sick.[6,9]

Screening and psychological distress

Meador[13] points out that the search for disease may lead to the elimination of wellness, and Marteau[14] and Wardle and Pope[15] emphasize the degree of anxiety that screening procedures may invoke. Psychological distress may be manifested at several levels of screening programs. Some studies have found that in itself, publicity about screening programs may arouse concern about having serious disease,[16] whereas others have found no such association.[17] Patients often perceive recalls for further tests or the diagnosis of precancerous lesions such as cervical dysplasia or carcinoma in situ as a diagnosis of

cancer.[15] False-positive results of cancer screening may lead to devastating psychological effects that sometimes persist for prolonged periods even after thorough investigations have ruled out malignancy.[15,18,19] True-positive results not only engender distress because of the diagnosis (particularly if incurable cancer is detected[15]), but also may lead to disruption of family relationships, difficulty obtaining insurance, and job discrimination.[20]

Delay in receiving test results or failure to receive them may increase patient anxiety. Many physicians do not have reliable methods of determining whether the tests they have ordered are reported. Even if they get the results, many physicians do not pass this information on to their patients.[21]

Not all studies have found adverse psychological effects from screening. For example, a coronary risk factor and lifestyle intervention study led by nurses in a number of general practices in Great Britain found that if anything, the intervention group experienced less anxiety than the control group.[22]

Informed Consent for Screening

Informed consent is an important issue that is discussed in the earlier section on prevention.

Clinical Practice Guidelines for Screening

Different organizations often produce contradictory recommendations, which is a confusing aspect of clinical guidance. This occurs even though the evidence on which the recommendations are based is the same for all the organizations involved. The probable explanation is differing attitudes among the individuals who make up the issuing bodies. (See discussion of physician attitudes.)

Czaja and associates[23] point out that the recommendations of the Canadian Task Force on Preventive Health Care and the U.S. Preventive Services Task Force are more conservative than those of the National Cancer Institute and the American Cancer Society. The two task forces base their recommendations whenever possible on evidence from randomized controlled trials, whereas subspecialty groups such as the American Cancer Society more often accept "expert opinion."[24] Specialty societies are also more likely to emphasize the value of positive outcomes (such as finding "early" cancers) and to de-emphasize any detrimental effects that may result from false-positive results in persons without disease.[24]

A survey of American physicians found that the majority followed more interventionist guidelines, which were also the most heavily publicized ones. In terms of specialties, surgeons tended to favor more aggressive screening than did family physicians or internists, and gynecologists favored aggressive screening for cancers in women. Older physicians and those in solo practice were more conservative than younger physicians but were also more likely to favour outmoded screening procedures such as annual chest x-ray examinations.[23] Remarks by focus groups of family physicians and patients in the province of Quebec revealed that most patients and many physicians value early diagnosis regardless of whether this would improve the outcome, and that suspicion of "science" is common.[25] Goldbloom[26] suggests that part of the difficulty of giving up time-honoured practices even when evidence shows them to be useless is that such practices are comforting rituals that act as anxiolytics for both patients and doctors.

Sometimes physicians follow only selected recommendations of a guideline while ignoring others, a practice that may vitiate any possible benefit of the intervention. PSA screening for prostate cancer is an example. Although both the U.S. Preventive Services Task Force[11] and the Canadian Task Force on Preventive Health Care[12] give PSA screening a "D" recommendation (good evidence not to perform the test), other organizations such as the American Urological Association disagree. In 1992 the American Urological Association specifically recommended PSA screening for men between the ages of 50 and 70.[27] (This has subsequently been modified to recommend screening for men over the age of 50 who have at least a 10-year life expectancy.) The reason for the cut-off at 70 was that the life expectancy of most men over that age was considered too short for benefit to accrue from radical prostatectomy. In practice, primary care physicians avidly screened men for PSA but paid little or no attention to the upper age limit.[28] Almost certainly because of this, a third of all radical prostatectomies in the United States are performed on men over the age of 70.[29]

◿ REFERENCES ◿

1. Feldman W: How serious are the adverse effects of screening? *J Gen Intern Med* (Sept/Oct suppl 5):S50-S53, 1990.
2. Black WC, Welch HG: Advances in diagnostic imaging and overestimations of disease prevalence and the benefits of therapy, *N Engl J Med* 328:1237-1248, 1993.
3. Potosky AL, Kessler L, Gridley G, et al: Rise in prostatic cancer incidence associated with increased use of transurethral resection, *J Natl Cancer Inst* 82:1624-1628, 1990.
4. Potosky AL, Miller BA, Albertsen PC, et al: The role of increasing detection in the rising incidence of prostate cancer, *JAMA* 273:548-552, 1995.
5. Ezzat S, Sarti DA, Cain DR, et al: Thyroid incidentalomas: prevalence by palpation and ultrasonography, *Arch Intern Med* 154:1838-1840, 1994.
6. Schwartz LM, Woloshin S: Changing disease definitions: implications for disease prevalence: analysis of the Third National Health and Nutrition Examination Survey, 1988-1994, *Eff Clin Pract* 2:76-85, 1999.
7. Harach HR, Franssila KO, Wasenius VM: Occult papillary carcinoma of the thyroid: a "normal" finding in Finland; a systematic autopsy study, *Cancer* 56:531-538, 1985.
8. Ernster VL, Barclay J, Kerlikowske K, et al: Incidence of and treatment for ductal carcinoma in situ of the breast, *JAMA* 275:913-918, 1996.
9. Welch HG: Finding and redefining disease (editorial), *Eff Clin Pract* 2:96-99, 1999.
10. Ewigman BG, Crane JP, Frigoletto FD, et al: Effect of prenatal ultrasound screening on perinatal outcome: RADIUS Study Group, *N Engl J Med* 329:821-827, 1993.
11. U.S. Preventive Services Task Force: *Guide to clinical preventive services,* ed 2, Baltimore, 1996, Williams & Wilkins.
12. Canadian Task Force on the Periodic Health Examination: *Canadian guide to clinical preventive health care,* Ottawa, 1994, Canada Communication Group Publishing.
13. Meador CK: The last well person, *N Engl J Med* 330:440-441, 1994.
14. Marteau TM: Psychological costs of screening: may sometimes be bad enough to undermine the benefits of screening, *BMJ* 299:527, 1989.
15. Wardle J, Pope R: The psychological costs of screening for cancer, *J Psychosom Res* 36:609-624, 1992.
16. Kottke TE, Trapp MA, Fores MM, et al: Cancer screening behaviors and attitudes of women in Southeastern Minnesota, *JAMA* 273:1099-1105, 1995.
17. Wardle J, Taylor T, Sutton S, et al: Does publicity about cancer screening raise fear of cancer? Randomised trial of the psychological effect of information about cancer screening, *BMJ* 319:1037-1038, 1999.
18. Lerman C, Trock B, Rimer BK, et al: Psychological and behavioral implications of abnormal mammograms, *Ann Intern Med* 114:657-661, 1991.
19. Brett J, Austoker J, Ong G: Do women who undergo further investigation for breast screening suffer adverse psychological consequences? A multi-centre follow-up study comparing different breast screening result groups five months after their last breast screening appointment, *J Pub Health Med* 20:396-403, 1998.
20. Macdonald KG, Doan B, Kelner M, et al: A sociobehavioural perspective on genetic testing and counselling for heritable breast, ovarian and colon cancer, *Can Med Assoc J* 154:457-464, 1996.
21. Boohaker EA, Ward RE, Uman JE, et al: Patient notification and follow-up of abnormal test results: a physician survey, *Arch Intern Med* 156:327-331, 1996.
22. Marteau TM, Kinmonth AL, Thompson S, et al: The psychological impact of cardiovascular screening and intervention in primary care: a problem of false reassurance? *Br J Gen Pract* 46:577-582, 1996.
23. Czaja R, McFall SL, Warnecke RB, et al: Preferences of community physicians for cancer screening guidelines, *Ann Intern Med* 120:602-608, 1994.
24. Hayward RSA, Steinberg EP, Ford DE, et al: Preventive care guidelines: 1991, *Ann Intern Med* 114:L758-L783, 1991.
25. Beaulieu M-D, Hudon E, Roberge D, et al: Practice guidelines for clinical prevention: do patients, physicians and experts share common ground? *Can Med Assoc J* 161:519-523, 1999.
26. Goldbloom RB: Prisoners of ritual (editorial), *Can Med Assoc J* 161:528-529, 1999.

27. American Urological Association: Early detection of prostate cancer and use of transrectal ultrasound. In American Urological Association: *1992 Policy statement book,* vol 4, Baltimore, 1992, The Association, p 20.
28. Fowler FJ, Bin L, Collins MM, et al: Prostate cancer screening and beliefs about treatment efficacy: a national survey of primary care physicians and urologists, *Am J Med* 104: 526-532, 1998.
29. Murphy GP, Mettlin C, Menck H, et al: National patterns of prostate cancer treatment by radical prostatectomy: results of a survey by the American College of Surgeons Commission on Cancer, *J Urol* 152:1817-1819, 1994.

WELLNESS

"Wellness" or "health" is an evasive concept. In recent years, especially in North America, public concern about body functions and health has become an obsession.[1-8] Some phrases used to describe these attitudes include "death-denying culture,"[4] "an unhealthy obsession with health,"[5] "tyranny of health,"[6] "coercive healthism,"[7] "war on death,"[8] and "cultural imperialism."[9]

Meador[2] suggests that the search for disease may lead to the elimination of wellness. Barsky[1] points out that the health of Americans has increased immeasurably over the past few decades, but the subjective concept of being well has diminished.

Several reasons have been proposed for our concerns about health. A straightforward one is that increase in life expectancy has allowed more people to live long enough to acquire chronic diseases. More obvious is an epidemic of health awareness publicity. Diet programs, exercise programs, health spas, and publications on health proliferate without limit,[1] and almost a quarter of sites on the Internet are devoted to health.[10] Health is a huge commercial market that is exploited and expanded by advertising. If you have a cold and watch television, you may observe on commercials how a medication brings about instant health. If you then use the advertised medication and it fails to work for you, you feel not only cheated, but unhealthy. Because not everyone has a specific illness, the health promotion (and advertising) organizations delve into potential hidden disasters such as elevated cholesterol levels, prostate cancer, or skin cancer. Even normal anatomical or physiological traits such as baldness, wrinkles, and a touch of plumpness are targeted, since they become profitable if considered as treatable diseases.[1]

Førde suggests that the ever-increasing number of epidemiological reports on "risk" factors in daily life is promoting a lifestyle, the main focus of which is risk evasion. Since in his view acceptance of risk and uncertainty is necessary for self-realization and social functioning, a person obsessed with risk aversion is socially impaired. According to Førde, health promotion has become a form of "cultural imperialism"—that is, a moral crusade to change basic cultural norms with no assurance that the overall effect will not be deleterious.[9]

Another reason for our decreased sense of wellness is that greater availability of medical care and the growth of medical technology have paradoxically harmed us. In many parts of the Western world, people receive more medical care than ever before from an increasing variety of doctors who order escalating numbers of investigations. Investigations lead to more diagnoses and more treatments, but many of the detected "disorders,"—such as impaired glucose tolerance, mildly elevated lipid levels, ductal carcinoma in situ of the breast, small prostate cancers, or angiographically demonstrable coronary artery narrowing, may never cause clinically significant adverse effects and are best classified as "pseudodiseases." Unfortunately, once pseudodiseases are discovered, healthy persons are labelled as "sick" and subjected to medical or surgical interventions that offer questionable benefit and in many cases have serious adverse effects. Furthermore, current medical practice patterns have increased both the volume and the complexity of physicians' workloads. Physicians become distracted, which may be why many patients who have had myocardial infarctions (MIs) are not discharged on a regimen of aspirin or beta-blockers, or why patients often feel their doctors no longer listen to them.[11] A wonderful article illustrating the absurdities of excessive concern about health is "The Last Well Person" by Meador,[2] which appeared in the *New England Journal of Medicine* in 1994.

The perception of health as a precarious state besieged by a host of ailments destroys the concept of health as "physical, mental and social well-being,"[12] "something positive, a joyful attitude toward life,"[13] or "a buoyant life, full of zest."[14]

✑ REFERENCES ✍

1. Barsky AJ: The paradox of health, *N Engl J Med* 318: 414-418, 1988.
2. Meador CK: The last well person, *N Engl J Med* 330: 440-441, 1994.
3. Goodwin JS: Geriatrics and the limits of modern medicine, *N Engl J Med* 340:1283-1285, 1999.
4. Annas GJ: Reframing the debate on health care reform by replacing our metaphors, *N Engl J Med* 332:744-747, 1995.
5. Thomas L: Notes of a biology-watcher: the health-care system, *N Engl J Med* 293:1245-1246, 1975.
6. Fitzgerald FT: The tyranny of health, *N Engl J Med* 331: 196-198, 1994.
7. Scrabanek P: *The death of humane medicine and the rise of coercive healthism,* Bury Saint Edmunds, Eng, 1994, Crowley Esmonde, pp 37-41.
8. Herman J: The ethics of prevention: old twists and new, *Br J Gen Pract* 46:547-549, 1996.
9. Førde OH: Is imposing risk awareness cultural imperialism? *Soc Sci Med* 47:1155-1159, 1998.

10. Holmer AF: Direct-to-consumer prescription drug advertising builds bridges between patients and physicians, *JAMA* 281: 380-382, 1999.

11. Fisher ES, Welch HG: Avoiding the unintended consequences of growth in medical care: how might more be worse? *JAMA* 281:446-453, 1999.

12. World Health Organization: *Basic documents,* ed 35, Geneva, 1985, The Organization.

13. Sigerist HE: *The university at the crossroads: addresses and essays,* New York, 1946, Henry Schuman.

14. Breslow L: From disease prevention to health promotion, *JAMA* 281:1030-1033, 1999.

PREVENTABLE RISK FACTORS
Bicycle Helmets
(See also motor vehicle accidents)

Head injuries cause 75% of bicycle-related deaths.[1,2] Three case-control studies reported that bicycle helmets reduced the risk of head injury by 85%,[3] 69%,[4] and 63%.[5] In a Canadian study of deaths from bicycle-related injuries in Ontario between 1986 and 1991, 75% of the deaths were due to head injuries. Only 4% of those killed were wearing bicycle helmets.[2] In this study, 91% of deaths were the result of collisions with motor vehicles, males outnumbered females 3.5:1, and the risk of being killed was four times greater at night than during the day.[2] In Victoria, Australia, mandatory bicycle helmet use was associated with a 51% decrease in the number of cyclists killed or hospitalized with head injuries.[6] A case-control study has also shown that helmets protect against upper face and midface injuries.[7]

All types of helmets (soft shelled and hard shelled) are protective for all age groups.[5] Children under 6 years of age do not require a different type of helmet.[5]

An argument given against mandatory use of bicycle helmets is that fewer people might bicycle and therefore fewer people would gain the health benefits of that activity.[8] Several letters to the editor published in the *British Medical Journal*[9-11] and *JAMA*[12,13] suggest that this has happened in Australian states where such laws have been enacted. In fact, the decrease in bicycle use reported there was mainly in teenagers, while adult bicycling actually increased.[6,14] The peer-reviewed literature firmly supports the use of bicycle helmets as a protection against serious injury, and no solid evidence has been presented that mandatory helmet use decreases bicycle use.

❧ REFERENCES ☙

1. Friede AM, Azzara CV, Gallagher SS, et al: The epidemiology of injuries to bicycle riders, *Pediatr Clin North Am* 32:141-151, 1985.

2. Rowe BH, Rowe AM, Bota GW: Bicyclist and environmental factors associated with fatal bicycle-related trauma in Ontario, *Can Med Assoc J* 152:45-53, 1995.

3. Thompson RS, Rivara FP, Thompson DC: A case-control study of the effectiveness of bicycle safety helmets, *N Engl J Med* 320:1361-1367, 1989.

4. Thompson DC, Rivara FP, Thompson RS: Effectiveness of bicycle safety helmets in preventing head injuries: a case-control study, *JAMA* 276:1968-1973, 1996.

5. Thomas S, Acton C, Nixon J, et al: Effectiveness of bicycle helmets in preventing head injury in children: case-control study, *BMJ* 308:173-176, 1994.

6. Centers for Disease Control and Prevention: Mandatory bicycle helmet use–Victoria, Australia, *JAMA* 269(23):2967, 1993.

7. Thompson DC, Nunn ME, Thompson RS, et al: Effectiveness of bicycle safety helmets in preventing serious facial injury, *JAMA* 276:1974-1975, 1996.

8. DeMarco T: Helmet legislation could decrease cycling (letter), *Can Family Physician* 40:1703-1704, 1994.

9. Davis A: Cyclists should wear helmets: increasing the number of cyclists is more important (letter), *BMJ* 314:69, 1997.

10. Robinson DL: Cyclists should wear helmets: Australian laws making helmets compulsory deterred people from cycling (letter), *BMJ* 314:69-70, 1997.

11. Hillman M: Cyclists should wear helmets: health benefits of cycling greatly outweigh loss of life years from deaths (letter), *BMJ* 314:70, 1997.

12. Bayliss J: Do bicycle helmets protect, and should they be mandatory? (letter), *JAMA* 277:883, 1997.

13. Goldman D: Do bicycle helmets protect, and should they be mandatory? (letter), *JAMA* 277:883-884, 1997.

14. Thompson DC, Thompson RS: Do bicycle helmets protect, and should they be mandatory? (reply to letters), *JAMA* 277:884, 1997.

In-Line Skating

Elbow and wrist guards have been shown to decrease injuries to the elbows and wrists of in-line skaters. Data documenting the efficacy of helmets in this sport are not yet available.[1]

❧ REFERENCES ☙

1. Schieber RA, Branche-Dorsey CM, Ryan GW, et al: Risk factors for injuries from in-line skating and the effectiveness of safety gear, *N Engl J Med* 335:1630-1635, 1996.

Guns
(See also suicide)

In 1994 guns were owned by persons in 33% of urban, 39% of suburban, and 60% of rural U.S. households, and pistols made up more than 50% of the weapons in each category. Gun ownership is highest in southern and Rocky Mountain states. More men than women own guns, as well as more whites than blacks, Republicans than Democrats, and persons whose parents owned a gun than those whose parents did not.[1]

An analysis of the type of gun used in firearm-related homicides and suicides in Milwaukee, Wisconsin, between 1991 and 1994 found that handguns accounted for 89% of the homicides and 71% of the suicides.[2]

According to 1989 U.S. data, firearms accounted for 11% of childhood deaths, 17% of deaths among adolescents ages 15 to 19, and 41% of deaths of black males ages 15 to 19.[3] Many high school students take guns to school. Results of a Seattle survey found that 6% of the students had brought a handgun to school at least once,[4] and in Illinois, another survey revealed that a third of students had done so.[5] A survey of predominantly Hispanic adolescents in three New York City schools found that 21% carried a weapon to school and 42% reported having had a relative or close friend who was shot.[6] More recent data suggest some improvement. A survey of violence-related behaviour in U.S. high school students found that between 1991 and 1997, both fighting and the carrying of weapons, including guns, decreased.[7]

Adequate storage of guns in the home requires that they be unloaded and locked. A survey of parents of children in 29 urban, suburban, and rural pediatric practices from across the United States found that a third of families reported owning at least one gun. Of gun-owning families, 61% had at least one unlocked gun and 15% had at least one loaded gun. Only 30% kept all guns unloaded and locked.[8]

In 1998 an 11-year-old boy and a 13-year-old boy in Jonesboro, Arkansas, stole an arsenal of high-powered assault rifles from the grandfather of one of the boys and ambushed a public school, killing four children and one teacher and wounding many others. The editor of the *New England Journal of Medicine,* Dr. Jerome Kassirer, pointed out that almost all commentaries on this incident focused on the psychological or social circumstances that might have led these boys to commit such atrocities, while very few dealt with the fact that if the children had been unable to obtain weapons easily (i.e., if effective gun control laws had been in place), these deaths might not have occurred.[9]

In 1999 two adolescent boys killed a teacher, 13 fellow students, and themselves at Columbine High School in Littleton, Colorado. As in previous school shootings, much of the commentary focused on psychosocial issues, but one proposal that seemed to be gaining support was for personalized guns that could be fired only by the owners. Operating such guns would require either button codes or fingerprints, technologies that already exist.[10]

Accidental shootings, which are usually self-inflicted by young males, are reported to be a common sequel of gun ownership.[11] Six published case-control studies have reported that the relative risk of suicide among persons with access to guns in their homes varies from 1.4 to 4.8,[12] and a California population-based cohort study found that the risk of suicide in the first week after the purchase of a handgun was 57 times that of the general population.[13] Only two case-control trials have dealt with homicides and access to guns in the home; the relative risk for those with access to guns was 2.2 and 2.7.[12] In Washington State, 75% of the weapons used by children who shot themselves or others were stored in the home of the victim, a relative, or a friend.[14]

Statistics showing benefit from access to or use of guns usually come from questionnaires in which individuals are asked if they have successfully used guns to save lives or property.[12,15] Such case series carry little scientific weight.[12] Proponents of gun control interpret the literature as indicating that owning a gun increases a person's risk of death, whereas opponents claim that the medical literature on the topic is rife with publication and citation biases and that this is not a valid conclusion.[15]

Finally, a 2003 trial showed that brief counselling about firearm safety significantly increases the rate of safe storage. Most patients were not bothered by questioning about firearm use and safety. Further study is needed to determine whether counselling reduces the risk of injury or death.[16]

❧ REFERENCES ❧

1. Blendon RJ, Young JT, Hemenway D: The American public and the gun control debate, *JAMA* 275:1719-1722, 1996.
2. Hargarten SW, Karlson TA, O'Brien M, et al: Characteristics of firearms involved in fatalities, *JAMA* 275:42-45, 1996.
3. Fingerhut LA, Kleinman FC: *Firearm mortality among children and youth: advance data from Vital and Health Statistics No 178,* U.S. Dept of Health and Human Services, Pub No PHS 90-1250, Hyattsville, Md, 1989, National Center for Health Statistics.
4. Callahan CM, Rivara FP: Urban high school youth and handguns: a school-based survey, *JAMA* 267:3038-3042, 1992.
5. Koop CE, Lundberg GB: Violence in America: a public health emergency; time to bite the bullet back (editorial), *JAMA* 267:3075-3076, 1992. [Published errata appear in *JAMA* 268:3074, 1992, and 271:1404, 1994.]
6. Vaughan RD, McCarthy JF, Armstrong B, et al: Carrying and using weapons–a survey of minority junior high school students in New York City, *Am J Public Health* 86:568-572, 1996.
7. Brener ND, Simon TR, Krug EG, et al: Recent trends in violence-related behaviors among high school students in the United States, *JAMA* 282:440-446, 1999.
8. Senturia YD, Christoffel KK, Donovan M (Pediatric Practice Research Group): Gun storage patterns in U.S. homes with children, *Arch Pediatr Adolesc Med* 150: 265-269, 1996.
9. Kassirer JP: Private arsenals and public peril (editorial), *N Engl J Med* 338:1375-1376, 1998.
10. Teret SP, Webster DW: Reducing gun deaths in the United States: personalised guns would help–and would be achievable (editorial), *BMJ* 318:1160-1161, 1999.
11. Sinauer N, Annest JL, Mercy JA: Unintentional, nonfatal firearm-related injuries, *JAMA* 275:1740-1743, 1996.

12. Cummings P, Koepsell TD: Does owning a firearm increase or decrease the risk of death? *JAMA* 280:471-473, 1998.

13. Wintemute GJ, Parham CA, Beaumont JJ, et al: Mortality among recent purchasers of handguns, *N Engl J Med* 341: 1583-1589, 1999.

14. Grossman DC, Reay DT, Baker SA: Self-inflicted and unintentional firearm injuries among children and adolescents: the source of the firearm, *Arch Pediatr Adolesc Med* 153:875-878, 1999.

15. Kleck G: What are the risks and benefits of keeping a gun in the home? *JAMA* 280:473-475, 1998.

16. Albright TL, Burge SK: Improving firearm storage habits: impact of brief office counseling by family physicians, *J Am Board Fam Pract* 16:40-6, 2003.

Motor Vehicle Accidents

(See also alcohol; bicycle helmets; cocaine; exercise; post-traumatic stress disorder; prescriptions for elderly; sleep apnea; whiplash injury)

The last 75 years have seen a progressive decline in motor vehicle-related deaths per million vehicle miles travelled in the United States. In spite of this, motor vehicle accidents account for one third of injury-related deaths in the United States and are the leading cause of death among persons 1 to 24 years of age.[1]

Safety belts

Safety belt use is the single most effective method of reducing injuries and deaths in motor vehicle accidents. Seat belt use is higher in jurisdictions with safety belt laws. Young men are among those least likely to use safety belts.[2]

Air bags

The safety and efficacy of air bags have been well documented. However, a number of childhood fatalities have been reported to result from air bag deployment when the child was sitting in the front passenger seat, particularly if he or she was unrestrained or in a rear-facing child safety seat. Although deployment of the passenger-side air bag has reduced the overall risk of fatality for right front seat passengers by 18% in frontal crashes, the risk of death for children under age 10 in the right front passenger seat has increased by 34%.[3]

Protective measures for children in cars

The American Academy of Pediatrics and the Centers for Disease Control and Prevention have made a number of recommendations about infant and child car seats, booster seats, use of seat belts, and positioning of children in vehicles, including the following:

1. No matter what the age, rear seats are safer than front seats.[4-6]

2. All infants should be in a backward-facing seat strapped into the back seat until they are 1 year of age and weigh 9 kg (20 lb). Such seats should never be placed in the front passenger seat.[4,6] The shoulder straps in rear-facing seats should be in the lowest slots until the child's growth places the shoulders above that slot. If the tilt of the car seat causes the infant's head to flop forward, a rolled towel or newspaper should be placed under the depressed edge of the seat, raising it enough to keep the infant's head resting against the back of the seat.[4]

3. Children between 9 kg (20 lb) and 18 kg (40 lb) should be placed in a forward-facing child seat that is fastened into the back seat.[4,6]

4. Once the child surpasses 18 kg (40 lb), a belt-positioning booster with lap and shoulder belts may be used.[4,6]

5. Booster seats should be used until the child is 147 cm (58 in) tall, has a sitting height of 74 cm (29 in), and weighs 36 kg (80 lb). Without a booster seat the lap and seat belts are inadequately positioned and not only may not be protective but may be harmful. Most children outgrow booster seats by about age 10.[5]

6. Ideally a child who has outgrown a booster seat should be in the back seat, but if he or she is in the front passenger seat, the seat should be pushed as far back as possible to avoid injury if the air bag deploys.[4,6]

Non-use or misuse of restraint systems is responsible for numerous deaths and injuries. Children are twice as likely to be unrestrained if the driver is not using the seat belt system. Misuse of child safety seats is common; the most frequent errors are failure to attach the seat tightly to the vehicle and failure to adjust the harness so that the child is held snugly in place.[6]

Alcohol

In the United States, motor vehicle accidents are the leading cause of death among persons of all ages from 1 to 34 years, and slightly less than half of these fatal accidents are alcohol related. The cutoff point for blood alcohol levels in determining the above statistics is 0.1 g/dl (100 mg/dl). In the general population the risk of a motor vehicle accident has been shown to be much greater when this level is reached than at lower blood alcohol levels. However, lower levels are far from risk free. The risk begins to increase at levels of 0.02 g/dl (20 mg/dl), increases significantly at 0.05 g/dl (50 mg/dl), and increases rapidly at levels over 0.1 g/dl (100 mg/dl).[7] The risk of a fatal crash among drivers with blood alcohol levels of 0.05 to 0.09 g/dl is nine times greater than among those with no alcohol in the blood.[8]

Alcohol-impaired drivers are less likely to use seat belts than other drivers,[9] and children who are passengers in cars driven by drivers who have been drinking are less likely to be restrained.[10]

Evidence indicates that zero tolerance laws with respect to blood alcohol levels of drivers can dramatically decrease fatal motor vehicle accidents. This has been the case for drivers under the age of 21 in many U.S. states and for the entire population in Japan. In Maine a law that reduced the maximum allowable blood alcohol level to 0.05% for individuals with a previous conviction for driving while impaired cut the fatal accident rate for this population by 25%.[8]

Drivers 16 to 24 years of age are five times more likely to be involved in alcohol-related driving fatalities than drivers age 35 to 64, and in many instances this increased risk occurs with very low levels of blood alcohol. The reasons are uncertain, but the risk-taking behaviour of adolescents coupled with inexperience is most likely the major factor. It is also probable that less alcohol is required to impair adolescents than older drivers.[11] Although the frequency of driving after drinking has declined among U.S. high school seniors over the past 15 years, it is still a common occurrence.[12]

One of the medico-legal problems with the use of breathalyzers is that they require the person to blow into the device for a brief period. This has led to a number of court challenges in which individuals who had such conditions as asthma, chronic obstructive pulmonary disease, tracheostomy, or ankylosing spondylitis or who were experiencing severe emotional or physical distress were in some jurisdictions considered to have a reasonable excuse for not complying with police requests for breathalyzer tests.[13]

Seizures

The overall accident rate of drivers with controlled seizures is slightly increased and is comparable to the rates of patients with other significant medical disorders such as heart disease and diabetes. A short seizure-free period is the major risk factor for accidents in patients with seizure disorders; the risk is significantly reduced in those who have been seizure free for more than 6 to 12 months. The risk is also reduced in those who consistently have an aura before the onset of seizures.[14]

In the United States the seizure-free interval required to obtain a driver's license varies from 3 to 18 months depending on the state of residence. In practice this may have relatively little significance, since a high percentage of persons who have seizures never report their condition to the licensing authorities.[14]

Speed

Increasing the speed limit is associated with an increased mortality rate.[15] It has been estimated that an increase in impact speed of 10% results in approximately a 40% increase in mortality for both restrained and unrestrained occupants of a vehicle.[16]

Fog

Fog distorts drivers' perceptions of speed; they think they are going more slowly than they actually are and so tend to accelerate.[17] In foggy conditions the driver should check the speedometer frequently.

Sleep deprivation

Serious sleep deprivation is common among long-distance truck drivers, especially those who drive at night, and is responsible for numerous accidents.[18] Sleep apnea is also a risk factor for motor vehicle accidents.[19]

Geriatric drivers

Elderly people drive relatively few miles and tend to be law abiding. Therefore they account for a small proportion of total road accidents. On the other hand, on a per-mile-traveled basis, the accident rate is higher among elders than for younger individuals; by age 85 and over the accident rate is three times that of other drivers and is exceeded only by that of teenage drivers. Older drivers involved in accidents are more likely to be killed than are younger persons; those over age 85 have the highest death rate per accident of any group.[20] Use of long-acting benzodiazepines is associated with an increased rate of motor vehicle accidents in the elderly.[21]

Motorcycles

The death rate for motorcyclists is 35 times that of car occupants. Major injuries in motorcycle accidents are to the head and lower extremities. Helmets decrease fatal head injuries by 25%.[22]

Post-traumatic stress disorder and accidents

Post-traumatic stress disorder is a common sequel to motor vehicle accidents in both adults[23] and children.[24] In one study of children, post-traumatic stress disorder was identified in one third of those who were involved in vehicle accidents but in only 3% of those who sustained a sports injury. In spite of this high incidence the condition is rarely identified in daily clinical practice.[24]

✎ REFERENCES ✎

1. Centers for Disease Control and Prevention: Motor-vehicle safety: a 20th century public health achievement, *JAMA* 281: 2080-2082, 1999.
2. Nelson DE, Bolen J, Kresnow M-J: Trends in safety belt use by demographics and by type of state safety belt law, 1987 through 1993, *Am J Public Health* 88:245-249, 1998.
3. Braver ER, Ferguson SA, Greene MA, et al: Reductions in deaths in frontal crashes among right front passengers in vehicles equipped with passenger air bags, *JAMA* 278: 1437-1439, 1997.
4. Committee on Injury and Poison Prevention of the American Academy of Pediatrics: Selecting and using the most appro-

priate car safety seats for growing children: guidelines for counseling parents, *Pediatrics* 97:761-763, 1996.

5. Centers for Disease Control and Prevention: National child passenger safety week–February 14-20, 1999, *MMWR* 48: 83-84, 1999.

6. Winston FK, Durbin DR: Buckle up! is not enough: enhancing protection of the restrained child, *JAMA* 281:2070-2072, 1999.

7. Madden C, Cole TB: Emergency intervention to break the cycle of drunken driving and recurrent injury, *Ann Emerg Med* 26:177-179, 1995.

8. Hingson R, Heeren T, Winter M: Effects of Maine's 0.05% legal blood alcohol level for drivers with DWI convictions, *Public Health Rep* 113:440-446, 1998.

9. Foss RD, Beirness DJ, Sprattler K: Seat belt use among drinking drivers in Minnesota, *Am J Public Health* 84: 1732-1737, 1994.

10. Centers for Disease Control and Prevention: Alcohol-related traffic fatalities involving children–United States, 1985-96, *JAMA* 279:104-105, 1998.

11. Augustyn M, Simons-Morton BG: Adolescent drinking and driving: etiology and interpretation, *J Drug Educ* 25:41-59, 1995.

12. O'Malley PM, Johnston LD: Drinking and driving among U.S. high school seniors, 1984-1997, *Am J Public Health* 89:678-684, 1999.

13. Marks P: Drunk driving legislation: medicine and the law, *Medico-Legal J* 63:119-127, 1995.

14. Krauss GL, Krumholz A, Carter BA, et al: Risk factors for seizure-related motor vehicle crashes in patients with epilepsy, *Neurology* 52:1324-1329, 1999.

15. Rock SM: Impact of the 65 mph speed limit on accidents, deaths and injuries in Illinois, *Accid Anal Prevent* 27: 207-214, 1995.

16. Joksch HC: Velocity change and fatality risk in a crash– a rule of thumb, *Accid Anal Prevent* 25:103-104, 1993.

17. Snowden RJ, Stimpson N, Ruddle RA: Speed perception fogs up as visibility drops (letter), *Nature* 392:450, 1998.

18. Mitler MM, Miller JC, Lipsitz JJ, et al: The sleep of long-haul truck drivers, *N Engl J Med* 337:755-761, 1997.

19. Terán-Santos J, Jiménez-Gómez A, Cordero-Guevara J (Cooperative Group Burgos-Santander): The association between sleep apnea and the risk of traffic accidents, *JAMA* 340:847-851, 1999.

20. Martinez R: Older drivers and physicians (editorial), *JAMA* 274:1060, 1995.

21. Hemmelgarn B, Suissa S, Huang A, et al: Benzodiazepine use and the risk of motor vehicle crash in the elderly, *JAMA* 278: 27-31, 1997.

22. Rivara FP, Grossman DC, Cummins P: Injury prevention (first of two parts), *N Engl J Med* 337:543-548, 1997.

23. Blanchard EB, Hickling EJ, Vollmer AJ, et al: Short term follow up of post traumatic stress symptoms in motor accident vehicles, *Behav Res Ther* 33:369-377, 1995.

24. Stallard P, Velleman R, Baldwin S: Prospective study of post-traumatic stress disorder in children involved in road traffic accidents, *BMJ* 317:1619-1623, 1998.

Tap-Water Scalds

The risk of scalding from hot water depends on the water temperature and the duration of exposure. The usual home hot water heater is set at 60° C (140° F), and scalding at this temperature takes place in 5 to 6 seconds. Lowering the heater temperature to 49° C (120° F) will prevent many scalds in those most at risk (children under age 5, the disabled, and the elderly) because at this temperature, scalding occurs only after 9 minutes of exposure.[1]

─────────────── ◢ **REFERENCES** ◣ ───────────────

1. Huyer DW, Corkum SH: Reducing the incidence of tap-water scalds: strategies for physicians, *Can Med Assoc J* 156:841-844, 1997.

Topics covered in this section
Aviation Medicine
High-Altitude Medicine
Tropical / Travel Medicine

AVIATION MEDICINE
(See also cardiac arrest; insomnia; middle ear effusion)

Physiological Stresses of Air Travel
Commercial airplanes typically fly at altitudes of 1524 to 2438 m (5000 to 8000 ft) , resulting in decreased barometric pressures (565 mm Hg vs. 760 mm Hg at sea level). Consequently, PaO_2 also decreases while inflight, to approximately 55 mm Hg at 2438 m (8000 ft). This corresponds to a blood oxygen saturation level of 90% (when plotted on the oxyhemoglobin dissociation curve). Healthy individuals are able to tolerate this amount of hypoxia; however, passengers with pre-existing medical conditions may experience adverse effects. Other stresses include very low cabin humidity, cramped spaces, jet lag, carrying heavy belongings, and walking long distances through airport terminals. Major carriers assist passengers with special needs by pre-arranging special meals, wheelchair and trolley services, early boarding, and therapeutic oxygen.[1]

Flight Emergencies
Major medical emergencies aboard commercial aircraft are rare. A survey of nine U.S. airlines found that the rate was 1:58,000 passengers.[2] Studies report inflight death rates of 0.31 per million passengers.[1] Vasovagal episodes are the most common events, but cardiac, neurological, and respiratory problems make up the most serious events and account for the majority of instances in which an aircraft must be diverted.[3]

Before April 2004, the only medications mandated for inclusion in onboard emergency medical kits on U.S. airlines were 50% dextrose, nitroglycerin tablets, injectable diphenhydramine (Benadryl), and epinephrine 1:1000. The kits have now been expanded to include bronchodilator inhalers, oral antihistamines, non-narcotic analgesics, atropine, lidocaine, and nitroglycerin spray. Additionally, first-aid kits containing splints, bandages, and other such materials, and basic medical equipment such as stethoscopes, sphygmomanometers, oropharyngeal airways, and IV tubing are carried on board all U.S. air carriers.[1,3] Under a recent Federal Aviation Association (FAA) ruling, also effective as of April 2004, all commercial aircraft travelling with at least one flight attendant must carry automatic external defibrillators (AEDs). Evaluations of the use of AEDs during U.S. commercial air flights show survival rates ranging from 27% to 40%.[1,3]

According to an FAA study, physician travellers were available in 85% of reported inflight medical emergencies.[1,4] In the United States, Canada, and the United Kingdom, physicians do not have a legal duty to render assistance unless there is a pre-existing physician-patient relationship. However, many European countries and Australia do impose such legal obligations. By international law, the country in which the aircraft is registered has legal jurisdiction. The 1998 U.S. Aviation Medical Assistance Act provides limited "good Samaritan" protection to any medically qualified passenger who provides medical assistance aboard an aircraft. Many airlines augment voluntary assistance with inflight medical consultation by ground-based physicians. Volunteering health care professionals have several options for the management and stabilization of ill passengers: provision of supplemental oxygen, use of supplies in the emergency medical kit, ability to request the flight crew to lower the altitude of the aircraft to increase cabin pressure, consultation with ground-based medical support, or recommendation of diversion of the aircraft. Ultimately, the decision to divert the aircraft rests with the captain.[3]

Pre-existing Medical Conditions and Air Travel
Pregnancy and air travel
According to The American College of Obstetricians and Gynecologists, air travel is safe for most pregnant women up to 36 weeks' gestation. Most U.S. airlines allow pregnant women to fly up to 36 weeks' gestation on domestic flights. For international flights, 35 weeks' gestation is usually the limit. Women with multiple pregnancies, a history of preterm delivery, cervical incompetence, bleeding, or increased uterine activity that might result in early delivery should be encouraged to avoid air travel.[5] Because of the increased oxygen-carrying potential of fetal hemoglobin and increased fetal hematocrit, fetal PaO_2 changes very little at cabin altitudes under 2438 m (8000 ft).[1] Nevertheless, conditions that result in decreased placental oxygen reserve may be contraindications to flight or may necessitate medical oxygen therapy. These conditions include intrauterine growth restriction, post-maturity, pre-eclampsia, chronic hypertension, or placental infarction.[5]

Cardiac and pulmonary disease
Patients with stable pulmonary or cardiac disease may require supplemental oxygen during flight. The most practical means for assessing fitness to fly is to determine whether a patient can walk 46 m (50 yrds) at a normal pace or climb one flight of stairs without severe dyspnea.[1]

Cardiovascular contraindications to flight include the following: uncomplicated myocardial infarction (MI) within 2 to 3 weeks,[1] complicated MI within 6 weeks, unstable angina, severe congestive heart failure (CHF), uncontrolled hypertension, coronary artery bypass graft

(CABG) within 2 weeks, stroke within 2 weeks, uncontrolled ventricular or supraventricular tachycardia, Eisenmenger syndrome, and symptomatic valvular heart disease.[1]

Pneumothorax is strictly contraindicated for air travel since it may expand during flight and potentially progress to a tension pneumothorax. Safe travel may occur 2 to 3 weeks after radiological resolution.[1,6]

Diabetes mellitus

Persons with diabetes who require insulin will have to modify their doses if crossing several time zones. Travelling eastward means a short day and lower insulin doses, whereas travelling westward means a long day and larger doses. Frequent glucose self-monitoring is probably the easiest way of adjusting the doses.[1,7]

Recent surgery

Air travel should be discouraged for 1 to 2 weeks following open abdominal surgery. Ileus-associated gas volumes may expand by 25% at altitudes of 2438 m (8000 ft), and increased post-operative intra-abdominal pressures may result in complications such as wound dehiscence and hemorrhage. Laparoscopic abdominal surgical procedures are not as restrictive. Flight should also be avoided for 24 hours following colonoscopy because of residual intraluminal gas. Patients having undergone recent pneumonectomy or lobectomy have decreased pulmonary reserve and should be evaluated for fitness to travel as discussed above.[1] Recently applied casts should be bivalved.[7]

Conditions Associated with Air Travel

Aerotitis media

In a study of aerotitis media, 250 adult volunteers with a history of recurrent ear discomfort when flying were selected at random to receive 120 mg of oral pseudoephedrine (Sudafed) or placebo 30 minutes before departure. Ear discomfort was reported by 32% of those taking pseudoephedrine but 62% of those given placebo.[8] In contrast, a placebo-controlled double-blind trial of children ages 6 months to 6 years found no benefit from taking pseudoephedrine 30 to 60 minutes before flight departure.[9]

Infectious diseases on aircraft

One of the concerns about air travel is the possibility of increased risk of infection in the cabin environment. An evaluation of the concentration of organisms in the cabin air of domestic and international flights found the levels to be much lower than those in city locations such as bus and airline terminals or in shopping centers.[10]

The number of air exchanges per hour in an aircraft cabin varies with cruise conditions and ranges from 5 to 42. This compares favourably with the six air exchanges per hour recommended for hospital isolation rooms housing patients with active tuberculosis (TB).[11] A concern regarding air travel is organisms spread by tiny aerosol droplets, which in theory could circulate and recirculate in the cabin air for prolonged periods. Examples are measles, influenza, and TB.[12]

Studies of actual infection transmission in the aircraft cabin environment are few. One dramatic example was an outbreak of influenza affecting 59% of the occupants of an early model Boeing 737. The aircraft was delayed on the runway for 3 hours before takeoff, and the ventilation system was defective.[13]

Jet lag

Jet lag is a common result of crossing five or more time zones. Adjustment to a new time zone takes longer after an eastward than after a westward flight. Suggested preventive and management protocols are a good night's sleep before the flight, avoidance of alcohol during the flight, ingestion of plenty of fluids to avoid dehydration, and immediate adjustment to the time cycle of the destination. Exposure to several hours of bright outdoor light on arrival seems beneficial.[14,11] A recent Cochrane review found that melatonin, taken close to the target bedtime at the destination (10:00 P.M. to midnight), decreased jet lag from flights crossing 5 or more time zones in 8 of 10 trials. Daily doses of melatonin between 0.5 and 5 mg are similarly effective, except that people fall asleep faster and sleep better after 5 mg than 0.5 mg. One exception was a trial with 257 Norwegian physicians who had visited New York City for 5 days for a conference, which found no difference.[15] On balance and where available, melatonin can be recommended to adult passengers traveling across five or more time zones, particularly in an easterly direction.[16]

DVT and pulmonary embolism

The first case reports of deep vein thrombosis (DVT) associated with air travel were published in 1954, and the term "economy class syndrome" was coined by Symington and Stack in 1977. Recently, publicity has increased regarding the association of DVT and pulmonary embolism (PE) and long-haul flights. However, the majority of evidence is based on case reports and case-control and observational studies. According to WHO, there is insufficient data on which to base specific recommendations for prevention in the general public. General recommendations for passengers with no identifiable risk factors include frequent stretching and ambulation.[17-19] One recent randomized controlled trial (RCT) evaluated DVT prevention in high-risk subjects. Three hundred individuals were randomized to either no prophylaxis, aspirin use (400 mg for 3 days starting 12 hours before flight), and low-molecular-weight heparin (LMWH) (enoxaparine 1,000 IU SC 2 to 4 hours before flight). The incidence of thrombotic events was 4.8%, 3.6%, and 0.6% respectively, suggesting that LMWH may be indicated in high-risk patients.[20]

Scuba diving

Scuba divers who make only one dive on the day of or before a flight should wait 12 hours before flying; those who make several dives or who require decompression stops during ascent should wait 24 hours.[7] In general, physicians should encourage their patients to leave the last vacation day "dive-free."[1]

Mortality in general aviation accidents

Mortality rates of general aviation pilots involved in crash landings are lower among those who use both lap and shoulder restraints.[21]

Radiation exposure

Cosmic ray exposure is significantly increased at the altitudes flown by commercial jet aircraft. For occasional recreational travellers, the increased risk is minimal.[22]

―――――――――――― ◈ REFERENCES ◈ ――――――――――――

1. Aerospace Medical Association Medical Guidelines Task Force: Medical guidelines for airline travel, 2nd edition, *Aviat Space Environ Med* 74(5):A1-A19, 2003
2. Rayman RB: Aerospace medicine, *JAMA* 280:1777-1778, 1998.
3. Gendreau MA, DeJohn C: Responding to medical events during commercial airline flights, *NEJM* 346:1067-1073, 2002.
4. DeHart RL: Health issues of air travel, *Annu Rev Public Health* 24:133-151, 2003.
5. ACOG Committee on Obstetric Practice: Committee opinion: number 264, December 2001. Air travel during pregnancy, *Obstet Gynecol* 98:1187-1188, 2001.
6. Roby H, Lee A, Hopkins A: Safety of air travel following acute myocardial infarction, *Aviat Space Environ Med* 73:91-96, 2002.
7. Bettes TN, McKenas DK: Medical advice for commercial air travelers, *Am Fam Physician* 60:801-808, 1999.
8. Csortan E, Jones J, Haan M, et al: Efficacy of pseudoephedrine for the prevention of barotrauma during air travel, *Ann Emerg Med* 23:1324-1327, 1994.
9. Buchanan BJ, Hoagland J, Fischer PR: Pseudoephedrine and air travel–associated ear pain in children, *Arch Pediatr Adolesc Med* 153:466-468, 1999.
10. Wick RL Jr, Irvine LA: The microbiological composition of airliner cabin air, *Aviat Space Environ Med* 66:220-224, 1995.
11. Centers for Disease Control: Guidelines for preventing the transmission of tuberculosis in health-care settings with special focus on HIV-related issues, *MMWR* 39:1-29, 1990.
12. Wenzel RP: Airline travel and infection (editorial), *N Engl J Med* 334:981-982, 1996.
13. Moser MR, Bender TR, Margolis HS, et al: An outbreak of influenza aboard a commercial airliner, *Am J Epidemiol* 110:1-6, 1979.
14. Canada communicable disease report: travel statement on jet lag, *Can Med Assoc J* 155:61-63, 1996.
15. Spitzer RL, Terman M, Williams JBW, et al: Jet lag: clinical features, validation of a new syndrome-specific scale, and lack of response to melatonin in a randomized, double-blind trial, *Am J Psychiatry* 156:1392-1396, 1999.
16. Herxheimer A, Petrie KJ: (Cochrane Review) *Cochrane Database Syst Rev* (2):CD001520, 2002.
17. Mendis S, Yach D, Alwan A: Air travel and venous thromboembolism, *Bulletin of the World Health Organization* 80:403-406, 2002.
18. Lapostolle F, et al: Severe pulmonary embolism associated with air travel, *NEJM* 345:779-783, 2001.
19. Badrinath P: Air travel and venous thromboembolism: the jury is still out, *CMAJ*, 166:885, 2002.
20. Cesarone MR, et al: Venous thrombosis from air travel: the LONFLIT3 study – prevention with aspirin vs low-molecular-weight heparin in high-risk subjects: a randomized trial, *Angiology* 53:1-6, 2002.
21. Rostykus PS, Cummings P, Mueller BA: Risk factors for pilot fatalities in general aviation airplane crash landings, *JAMA* 280:997-999, 1998.
22. Barish RJ: In-flight radiation: counseling patients about risk, *J Am Board Fam Pract* 12:195-199, 1999.

HIGH-ALTITUDE MEDICINE   lm = 3.2ft

In susceptible individuals the hypoxia associated with high altitudes can induce a variety of symptoms. The most common and least serious, which affects one sixth to one third of recreational skiers in Colorado, is acute mountain sickness. Presenting complaints are headache plus at least one of the following: fatigue or weakness, gastrointestinal complaints, light-headedness or dizziness, and sleep disturbances.[1] Symptoms usually begin after 12 to 24 hours and peak on the second or third day.[2]

More serious are high-altitude pulmonary edema and high-altitude cerebral edema. These disorders are rare in individuals ascending less than 2500 m, but common in travellers ascending to 3500 m or more.[3] Symptoms of high-altitude pulmonary edema usually occur 2 to 3 days after arrival at altitude. Symptoms occur at night and include dyspnea with exercise, cough, weakness, and chest tightness. Signs include central cyanosis, rales, or wheezes (often over the right middle lobe), tachypnea, and tachycardia. High-altitude cerebral edema is manifested as mental changes and in many cases ataxia, which is a common early feature. Headache, nausea, vomiting, hallucination, disorientation, and confusion are often seen. The best way to prevent all these conditions is to ascend slowly, allowing time for acclimatization.

Optimal treatment of all these conditions is descent to lower altitudes, which is mandatory for patients with pulmonary or cerebral edema. Acetazolamide (Diamox) 250 to 500 mg twice a day has been used before ascent begins to prevent acute mountain sickness.[3] Dexamethasone (8 mg initially, then 4 mg every 6 hours) may also be used to reduce the incidence and severity of symptoms of acute mountain sickness, especially at altitudes above 4000 m.[4] It may be used when individuals must ascend rapidly or when they are intolerant of acetazolamide. Aspirin 325 mg taken 1 hour before ascent and repeated at 4 and 8 hours has been shown to prevent headaches caused by acute mountain sickness.[5] Nifedipine has been shown effective in the prevention and treatment of high-altitude pulmonary edema in susceptible individuals (given 10 mg orally initially, then 20 mg slow release preparation every 12 hours).[3]

─────────────── ✍ **REFERENCES** ✍ ───────────────

1. Harris MK, Terrio J, Miser WF, et al: High-altitude medicine, *Am Fam Physician* 57:1907-1914, 1998.
2. Peacock AJ: Oxygen at high altitude, *BMJ* 317:1063-1066, 1998.
3. Barry PW, Pollard AJ: Altitude illness, *BMJ* 326:915-919, 2003.
4. Dumont L, Mardirosoff C, Tramer MR: Efficacy and harm of pharmacological prevention of acute mountain sickness: quantitative systemic review, *BMJ* 321:267-272, 2000.
5. Burtscher M, Likar R, Nachbauer W, et al: Aspirin for prophylaxis against headache at high altitudes: randomised, double blind, placebo controlled trial, *BMJ* 316:1057-1058, 1998.

TROPICAL/TRAVEL MEDICINE
(See also high-altitude medicine, immunizations)

Approximately one billion passengers travel by air each year, and fifty million travellers from industrialized countries visit developing countries. Of this 50 million, 1% to 5% seek medical attention while travelling, 0.01% to 0.1 % require medical evacuation, and 1 in 100,000 dies.

To properly assess the geographical risk, the practitioner should inquire about the destination. The standard of public health services and availability of medical care is high and considered to be equivalent in North America, Western Europe, Israel, Australia and New Zealand, and Japan. Hence, travel to these destinations can be done with minimal preparation. In contrast, travel to Central and South America, the Middle East, the Indian subcontinent, Southeast Asia, and Africa may require significant preparation. The length of stay and the presence of specific epidemic/endemic issues such as malaria, yellow fever, dengue fever, meningococcal meningitis, or schistosomiasis require special consideration and often preventive intervention.

Affluent tourists need different preparation than, for example, those attending school as a student or teacher or staying with friends or relatives. Safari and rural travellers, travellers who are health care workers, veterinarians, animal handlers, and aid agency or missionary workers and volunteers all require detailed risk assessments..

The traveller's medical status must be taken into consideration. Diabetics and those who are on dialysis, who are immunocompromised (HIV, cancer, chemotherapy, etc.) and who have known allergies require additional preparation. Similarly, extremes of age, pregnancy, and even wearing contact lenses require targeted advice and preparation. In certain instances, preventive interventions may need to be influenced by a pre-existing condition. Glucose-6-phosphate dehydrogenase (G6PD) deficiency, for example, may complicate the recommendation for terminal treatment of malaria with primaquine (Table 3).

Sensible advice for travellers about immunization and other preventive interventions is based on risk assessment as outlined above. Children should have their core immunization updated-for dTaP (diphtheria-tetanus–acellular pertussis), Hib, Polio, and MMR (Measles, Mumps and Rubella). Immunization against hepatitis A and B, meningococcus, and varicella can also be considered.

Adult core immunization includes an update of TdP (tetanus-diphtheria-poliomyelitis toxoid) booster, a second dose of measles vaccine (alone or as MMR) for travel to areas with a high incidence of measles, and a single dose of rubella vaccine (alone or as MMR) for susceptible non-pregnant women of child-bearing age. The core immunization for seniors includes an update of influenza and pneumoncocal vaccines.

Twenty-one countries in Central, East, and West Africa and tropical South America south of the Panama Canal are located in the yellow fever endemic zone where the International Health Regulations defined by WHO apply. Furthermore, some 102 other countries not in yellow fever endemic zones require proof of vaccination from travellers who transit through an area infected with yellow fever. Yellow fever vaccination must be administered in travel clinics approved for that purpose.

When the administration of yellow fever vaccine is contraindicated, these clinics can issue an Exemption Certificate. Among those for whom an Exemption Certificate is recommended are infants less than 6 months, pregnant women, people with hypersensitivity to eggs, elderly people, and people with immunocompromise for any reason.

Cholera, or plague, vaccination is no longer required by any country. Selective immunization is based on the risks associated with any given itinerary.

Malaria

Malaria in humans is caused by one of four protozoan species of the genus *Plasmodium*: *P. falciparum*, *P. vivax*, *P. ovale*, or *P. malariae*. All species are transmitted by the bite of an infected female Anopheles mosquito, a species that habitually feeds from dusk to dawn. Occasionally, transmission occurs by blood transfusion or congenitally from mother to fetus. Although malaria can be a fatal disease, illness and death from malaria are largely preventable.

Yellow fever — Africa, central, S. America

Vaccine YF-VAX

~~Serious adverse~~ effects.

Table 3   Vaccines Against Common Infectious Agents for Travellers

Infection Agent (Vaccines)	Indications for Immunization Use
Hepatitis A (Avaxim, Havrix Vaqta)	Recommended for travel to developing countries, especially in rural areas or where the hygienic quality of the food and water supply is likely to be poor. Hepatitis A is endemic in Africa and Asia, South and Central America, and endemic areas of Russia and other countries that comprised the former Soviet Union. The vaccine is given in 2 doses, one before travel, the second dose within 6-12 months. While hepatitis A infection in children can be mild, children with this infection often act as a source of infection to others.
Hepatitis B (Recombivax HB Engerix B)	Recommended for travel for more than 6 months in areas with high levels of endemic hepatitis B, for those doing medical work, and those who are likely to have contact with blood or sexual contact with residents of such areas. The primary series consists of 3 injections given at 0, 30, and 180 days. Depending on the available time, the schedule can be accelerated: 0, 30, 60 days and 1 year OR 0, 7-10, 21 days, and 1 year.
Combined Hepatitis A and Hepatitis B (Twinrix) & (Twinrix Junior)	Given as 3 injections at 0, 30, and 180 days. An accelerated schedule for adults consists of 3 doses at 0, 7, 21 days, and 12 months.
Typhoid capsular polysaccharide (Typherix Typhim Vi) Oral attenuated Ty21a (Vivotef Berna Vivotef Berna L)	Recommended for travellers who will have prolonged exposure to contaminated food and water off the usual tourist itineraries. The primary series for the inactivated injectable vaccine is 1 injection. Booster is given every 3 years. The live-oral attenuated vaccine Ty21A provides protection for 7 years; it consists of 4 capsules taken every second day for 8 days for the Vivotef Berna and 3 doses of the Vivotef Berna L.
Traveller's diarrhea and cholera oral vaccine (Dukoral)	Indicated for the prevention of traveller's diarrhea and cholera in adults and children older than 2 years of age. The primary series consists of 2 oral doses at 1-week interval. The booster consists of 1 dose every 3 months. Traveller's diarrhea occurs during travel in an endemic area or 5-6 days after returning home from such areas. Traveller's diarrhea is a self-limited disorder and often resolves without specific treatment; however, oral rehydration is often beneficial to replace lost fluids and electrolytes. WHO's oral rehydration salts are widely available in developing countries. Simple diarrhea should be managed with over-the-counter antidiarrhoea medicine (Imodium, Pepto Bismal). Travelers who develop three or more loose stools in an 8-hour period–especially if associated with nausea, vomiting, abdominal cramps, fever, or blood in stools—may benefit from antimicrobial therapy. Antibiotics usually are given for 3-5 days. Currently, fluoroquinolones are the drugs of choice. Commonly prescribed regimens are 500 mg of ciprofloxacin twice a day or 400 mg of norfloxacin twice a day for 3-5 days.
Pre-exposure rabies (Imovax)	Immunization should be considered for persons intending to live or work in highly endemic areas, especially where rabies control programs for domestic animals are inadequate. The primary series consists of 3 intramuscular injections at 0, 7, and 21 or 28 days. Travellers should be warned that in the event of exposure to a rabid animal, thorough cleansing of the wound with soap and water is very important. Regardless of any previous immunization against rabies, persons exposed to rabies should receive 2 booster doses, one as soon as possible and a second booster in 3 days.
Japanese encephalitis (JE Vax)	A mosquito-borne viral encephalitis that occurs throughout most of East Asia from India east to Korea and Japan, in epidemics in late summer and early fall: Bangladesh, Burma, China, India, Japan, Kampuchea, Korea, Laos, Nepal; northern Thailand, northern Vietnam, eastern areas of the former Soviet Union, southern India, Indonesia, Malaysia, the Philippines, Sri Lanka, Taiwan, southern Thailand, and southern Vietnam. The primary series consists of 3 doses given 0, 7, and 21-28 days apart. Booster dose is given every 3 years. The vaccine is recommended for travel of more than 4 weeks in rural areas of endemic countries.
European tick-borne encephalitis	Transmitted by tick bite. The vaccine is recommended for long-term travellers to endemic areas of Russia and other countries that comprised the former Soviet Union and parts of Europe, from April through August. The vaccine is available in Austria and from travel clinics in London, England. In Canada, a physician may make a request for such a release to the Bureau of Biologics, Emergency Drug Release Program, Health Protection Branch.
Pre-travel Mantoux test	Recommended for medical personnel, missionaries, teachers, and children staying in endemic areas for prolonged periods of time. The Mantoux test could be repeated every 6 months or 6 weeks after return. Travellers who convert should be investigated for possible prophylactic treatment.

Continued

Table 3   Vaccines Against Common Infectious Agents for Travellers—cont'd

Infection Agent (Vaccines)	Indications for Immunization Use
Lyme disease (Lymrix)	Recommended for travellers to high-risk areas of the United States; available on the Internet at http://www.cdc.gov/ncidod/dvbid/lymeinfo.htm.
Meningococcal meningitis vaccine (Menoimune A/C/Y/W-135)	Recommended for travel into the sub-Saharan African meningitis belt: Chad, Ethiopia, Sudan, Niger, Nigeria, Ghana, Togo, and Burkina Faso and countries recognized as having an epidemic of meningococcal meningitis, especially during the dry season. The primary series consists of 1 injection that can be repeated every 5 years. Saudi Arabia requires evidence of immunization every 3 years for the purpose of Hajj and Umra.

Comments: 1. Most immunizing agents can be given simultaneously at different sites. 2. The efficacy of MMR may be impaired by the administration of immune serum globulin less than 2 weeks after the vaccine. If immune serum globulin is given first, an interval of 3 to 10 months may be required before giving MMR. 3. Concomitant use of Mefloquine may interfere with the response of the oral typhoid vaccine.

Many different species of mosquito exist, some of which carry some of the world's most common and most economically important infectious diseases. In addition to malaria and yellow fever, others include encephalitis (viral), dengue fever, West Nile virus, and leishmaniasis.

WHO and the CDC provide accurate and country-specific information on malaria risk and recommended chemoprophylaxis. However, many factors such as variations in local reporting rates and surveillance may significantly affect the reliability of these data.

The risk of transmission for malaria is variable and depends on the following factors:

- Increases in rural areas
- Varies seasonally in many locations; is highest at the end of the rainy season
- Proportional to the duration of an individual's exposure
- Decreases at altitudes above 2,000 m (6,500 ft)
- Decreases in tourist areas of Southeast Asia, Mexico, Central America, and South America
- Significant in urban travel in other malaria-endemic regions, such as sub-Saharan Africa, New Guinea, the Indian subcontinent, and the Amazon Basin

The spread of drug-resistant malaria and the prevalence of infection, especially with *P. falciparum,* have grown steadily. For example, malaria cases are at record levels on the Indian subcontinent, where an increasing proportion is due to drug-resistant *P. falciparum.* The malaria risk during a 1-month stay without chemoprophylaxis is estimated to be as follows:

- 1:30 or higher in Oceania (Papua New Guinea (PNG), Irian Jaya, Solomon Islands, and Vanuatu)
- 1:50 in sub-Saharan Africa
- 1:250 in Indian subcontinent
- 1:1,000 in Southeast Asia
- 1:2,500 in South America
- 1:10,000 in Central America

The prevention of malaria is an increasingly difficult problem because of the increase in multi–drug-resistant malaria strains. Hence, adopting the following personal protection measures against mosquito bites is essential.

- Remain in well-screened, air-conditioned areas from dusk to dawn.
- Apply non-aerosol mosquito repellent with concentration of DEET higher than 20% (Deep Woods Off, Muskol) to exposed areas at 4-hour intervals, especially from dusk to dawn (lower strengths of DEET shorten the time interval of effectiveness).
- Wear long-sleeved shirts and long pants tucked into boots or socks.
- Use permethrin-treated nylon mosquito bed nets (16X18 meshes).
- Take malaria prevention medication before, during, and after travel, as prescribed (Table 4).
- Pregnant women and children require special attention because of potential effects of malaria illness and the inability to use some drugs.

Symptoms of malaria may be very mild: fever, persistent headaches, muscular aching and weakness, vomiting, and/or diarrhea. The diagnosis of malaria is made by doing a malaria blood smear on one or more occasions. Since chloroquine-resistant malaria may be fatal, treatment should be prompt. Travellers should seek medical help as soon as possible. Self-treatment is advised only if prompt medical care is not available.

Travellers who elect not to take prophylaxis and plan to treat themselves only if they experience symptoms or who require or choose regimens that do not have optimal efficacy (for example, use of chloroquine for travel to areas with chloroquine-resistant *P. falciparum*), could be provided with a treatment dose of Fansidar or Malarone (Table 5). They should self-administer the prescribed dose if they develop a febrile illness during their travel and if professional medical care is not available within 24 hours. Self-treatment of a possible malarial infection

G6PD - avoid c̄ Primaquine, Chloroquine

Table 4 Malaria Prophylaxis

Drug	Adult Dosage	Pediatric Dosage
Chloroquine (Aralen) Only effective in central America, Haiti, Dominican Republic, and parts of the Middle East.	Two 250-mg tablets taken orally once a week starting 1 week before travel, once weekly during exposure, and once weekly for 4 weeks after leaving the malarious area.	Same weekly regimen as for adults but dosage is as follows: 5 mg per kg base (8.3 mg per kg salt), to a maximum of 300-mg base.
Mefloquine (Larium) May be used in second and third trimesters if use is warranted based on risk and the pregnant woman is unable to postpone travel plans. Avoid if there are seizure disorders, or a history of psychosis or cardiac conduction defects with arrhythmia.	One 250-mg tablet taken orally once a week starting 1 week before travel, once weekly during exposure, and once weekly for 4 weeks after leaving the malarious area.	Less than 15 kg (33 lb): 5 mg per kg. 15 to 19 kg (33 to 42 lb): one fourth of 250 mg. 20 to 30 kg (44 to 66 lb): one half of 250 mg. 31 to 45 kg (68 to 99 lb): three fourths of 250 mg.
Atovaquone250/Proguanil 100 (Malarone) Self-treatment ONLY if not taken for prophylaxis.	One adult tablet taken orally once a day starting 1 day before travel, once a day during exposure, and continuing daily for 7 days after leaving the malarious area.	11–20 kg (24–45 lb): 1 pediatric tablet. 21–30 kg (46–67 lb): 2 pediatric tablets. 31–40 kg (68–88 lb): 3 pediatric tablets. > 40 kg (> 88 lb): 1 adult tablet.
Doxycycline (Vibramycin) Alternative to Mefloquine in areas with resistant Plasmodium strains or when mefloquine is contraindicated. Side effects: photosensitivity, nausea, esophagitis, and monilial vaginitis.	One tablet 100 mg per day during exposure and for 4 weeks after return home.	Contraindicated in children less than 9 years old.

Thailand, Vietnam, Myanmar - Chloroquine & mefloquine resistance.

Table 5 Prophylaxis for Self-Treatment of Possible Malarial Infection

Self Treatment for Presumptive Diagnosis of Malaria		
Pyrimethamine-sulfadoxine (Fansidar) If in remote setting and medical care is not available or if on inadequate prophylaxis. Not in first or third pregnancy trimesters.	5 to 10 kg (11 to 22 lb): one-half tablet. 11 to 20 kg (24 to 44 lb): 1 tablet. 21 to 30 kg (46 to 66 lb): 1 and one-half tablets. 31 to 45 kg (68 to 99 lb): 2 tablets. > 45 kg: 3 tablets as a single dose.	
Malarone If not on Malarone prophylaxis.	11–20 kg: 1 adult tablet daily for 3 consecutive days. 21–30 kg: 2 adult tablets (as a single dose) daily for 3 consecutive days. 31–40 kg: 3 adult tablets (as a single dose) daily for 3 consecutive days. > 40 kg: 4 adult tablets (as a single dose) daily for 3 consecutive days.	
Terminal Prophylaxis		
Primaquine If at risk for relapsing type of malaria or for elimination of Plasmodium species in persons who travel for more than 2 months in a high-risk area. Contraindicated in pregnancy. Screen for G6PD.	15-mg base (26.3-mg salt) per day for 14 days before return home.	0.3 mg per kg base (0.5 mg per kg salt) per day for 14 days.

should be considered a temporary measure. Prompt medical evaluation is imperative.

Several new agents are under investigation. Azithromycin (Zithromax) is being evaluated as a potential suppressive agent with low toxicity. Some of the most interesting new antimalarial agents are derived from sweet wormwood *(Artemisia annua)*, known in China as "qinghaosu." Artemisinin (the plant's active component) and its synthetic derivatives have proved to be very effective treatments in persons infected with otherwise resistant Plasmodium strains, and they may have additional potential as prophylactic agents. Their chief disadvantage is a short half-life, which necessitates frequent dosing.

Acute Traveller's Diarrhea

Acute traveller's diarrhea occurs in 60% of travellers; 20% are bedridden for part of their trip. Fifty to 75% of cases are caused by *Escherichia coli*. Other pathogenic agents such as *Campylobacter jejuni,* shigella, salmonella, viruses, and parasites are rare.

The signs and symptoms consist of watery bowel movements with or without fever, blood in the stool, and abdominal cramps lasting 4 to 5 days. Complications may include reactive arthritis, post-infectious enteropathy, and Guillain-Barré syndrome.

Symptomatic treatment is often sufficient to control the illness. It includes rehydration (fluid, sugar, and salt replacement) with or without the use of antimotility agents. The use of antibiotics (fluoroquinolone) is reserved for severe cases. Pregnant women, children, seniors and the immunocompromised require special consideration.

Dengue Fever

Dengue fever is a viral illness transmitted by the Aedes aegypti, a domestic, day-biting mosquito that prefers to feed on humans. The spectrum of clinical illness ranges from a non-specific viral syndrome to severe and sometimes fatal hemorrhagic disease (DHF). The strain and serotype of the virus (DEN-1, DEN-2, DEN-3, and DEN-4), the age, the immune status, and genetic predisposition of the patient are important risk factors. There is no vaccine to prevent the disease.

Sexually Transmitted Diseases

Twenty-five infectious organisms can be transmitted through sexual activity. Hepatitis B is the only STD for which a vaccine is available. Travellers should practice safe sex and seek early diagnosis and treatment.

Bathing: Fresh water

In the tropics, watercourses, canals, lakes, and other water areas may be infested with larvae that can penetrate the skin and cause schistosomiasis (bilharziasis). Bathing and washing in waters likely to be infested with the snail host of this parasite or contaminated with human and animal excreta should be avoided. Only adequately chlorinated water may be considered safe for bathing. Swimming, fishing, and walking barefoot in rivers or watery rice paddies or on muddy land may expose travellers to leptospirosis infections, especially in Southeast Asia and the western Pacific regions. A wide range of trematodes causes swimmer's itch (cercarial dermatitis). It may be acquired in freshwater bodies of both temperate and tropical zones. These cercariae penetrate the skin and die, causing a localized or extended cutaneous allergic reaction. Treatment is symptomatic.

Bathing in unpolluted seawater does not in principle involve any risk of communicable disease. Travellers are nevertheless recommended to ascertain from local sources whether bathing is permitted and presents any hazards for health. Jellyfish stings may cause severe pain and skin irritation. In some areas, bathers should wear shoes as a protection against biting and stinging fish, coral dermatitis, and poisonous fish, shellfish, and sea anemones.

Traffic Accidents

Traffic accidents are a leading cause of death among travellers. A traffic accident in an area that is not well served medically is more likely to be fatal. Travellers should verify vehicle maintenance, state of the roads, and the possibilities of fuel supply, and should check carefully the insurance policy, the state of the tires, safety belts, spare wheel, lights, brakes, etc.

─────────────── ◢ INTERNET SOURCES ◣ ───────────────

The following on-line resources were used in the preparation of this section, and can serve as useful current information sources for clinicians and their patients:

Canada

http://www.voyage.gc.ca/main/sos/ci/all-en.asp
http://www.voyage.gc.ca/consular_home-en.asp
http://www.hc-sc.gc.ca/hpb/lcdc/osh/prof_e.html
http://www.hc-sc.gc.ca/hpb/lcdc/hp_eng.html

USA

http://www2.ncid.cdc.gov/travel/yb/utils/ybDynamic.asp
http://www.cdc.gov/health/diseases.htm
http://www.cdc.gov/travel/destinat.htm
http://www.cdc.gov/travel/yb/toc.htm

UK

http://www.fco.gov.uk/travel/countryadvice.asp

WHO

http://www.who.int/ith/

PAHO

http://www.paho.org

Global Weather

http://www.intellicast.com

IMMUNIZATIONS

Topics covered in this section

Storage and Shipping of Vaccines
Immunization Schedules for Children
Hemophilus B Immunization
Hepatitis B Immunization
Influenza Prevention
Measles-Mumps-Rubella and Rubella Immunization
Meningococcal Immunization
Pertussis Immunization
Pneumococcal Immunization
Polio Immunization
Rabies Immunization
Tetanus Immunization
Varicella Immunization

STORAGE AND SHIPPING OF VACCINES

Many vaccines are inactivated if they are exposed to high temperatures or if they are frozen. Vaccine inactivation through improper storage and handling probably occurs frequently in physicians' offices and may also occur during shipping, especially to remote regions.

Vaccines that do not need to be kept frozen should be stored between 2° and 8° C. Refrigerators containing vaccines should have temperature monitors that should be assessed frequently (optimally twice daily). Only vaccines should be kept in the refrigerator; food should be in another refrigerator to avoid temperature variations from frequent door opening and closing. Vaccines should not be kept in the refrigerator door and should be returned to the refrigerator immediately after use.[1-3]

❧ REFERENCES ❧

1. Health Canada: National guidelines for vaccine storage and transportation, *Can Comm Dis Report* 21-11:93-97, 1995.
2. http://www.who.int/vaccines-access/procurement/ PDF_Proc_Manual/18-9848.pdf (accessed 4 May/04).
3. http://www.cdc.gov/nip/publications/pink/Appendices/ appdx-full-d.pdf (accessed 4 May/04).

IMMUNIZATION SCHEDULES FOR CHILDREN

(See also Hemophilus B immunization; hepatitis immunization; measles-mumps-rubella immunization; pertussis immunization; polio immunization; rabies immunization; tetanus immunization; varicella immunization; pneumococcal immunization; meningococcal vaccine)

The recommended immunization schedules for children in Canada and the United States differ in only a few details. A comparison table is shown below.

HEMOPHILUS B IMMUNIZATION

(See also immunization schedules for children)

Until the introduction of immunization programs, *Haemophilus influenzae* type B (Hib) was the most common cause of bacterial meningitis in infants and young children. The case fatality rate for Hib meningitis was about 5%. Severe neurological sequelae occurred in 10% to 15% of survivors and deafness in 15% to 20%. Other diseases caused by Hib are acute epiglottitis, pneumonia, bacteremia, cellulitis, and septic arthritis.[1]

A variety of conjugate Hib vaccine formulations is available for infants and children, either as single entity vaccines or combined with other active immunizing agents.[2,3] Because of concern about decreased immune response to the Hib component of combined Hib/DTaP vaccines, such combinations are not recommended in the United States for the 2-, 4-, and 6-month vaccinations.[4] Across Canada, Pentacel (Act-Hib in combination DTaP and Polio) is now given. Several studies have shown that the Hib immune response was not reduced with Pentacel and that fewer postimmunization Hib infections occurred with its use.[5]

The recommended Hib immunization schedules vary based on age at first dose and vaccine used. The standard dosing schedule for an age of first dose of less than 6 months is 2, 4, and 6 months, with a booster dose at 15 to 18 months. Recent data from the United Kingdom indicate that vaccine efficacy remains high without a booster dose, even though declining antibody titres are seen. Therefore, a booster dose may not be necessary if a high uptake of primary immunization continues.[1] If Hib conjugate vaccine (PRP-OMP) (PedvaxHIB or ComVax) is given at ages 2 and 4 months, a booster dose at 6 months is not required.[4] Between 12 months and 5 years of age, nonimmunized children require only one dose of Hib vaccine for adequate protection.[1] Children older than 5 years do not require immunization.[1]

Rifampin prophylaxis is not required for Hib infection contacts who are over the age of 5 years or for those under 5 if they have been adequately immunized for their age. If one or more contacts under the age of 5 have not been adequately immunized for age or are immunocompromised, rifampin prophylaxis is usually indicated not only for the children who have not been immunized but also for those who have, since vaccinated children may still be carriers of the organism. In situations of this nature, consultation with local public health units is advisable.[1]

The usual rifampin regimen for prophylaxis against Hib infections is a 4-day course of 600 mg every 12 hours for adults, 20 mg/kg/day in 2 divided doses for children over the age of 1 month, and 10 mg/kg/day in 2 divided doses for children under the age of 1 month.

❧ REFERENCES ❧

1. *Canadian immunization guide,* ed 6. Ottawa, Canadian Medical Association, 2002. Accessed at http://www.phac-aspc.gc.ca/publicat/cig-gci/.
2. Supplementary statement on newly licensed *Haemophilus influenzae* type B (HIB) conjugated vaccines in combination with other vaccines recommended for infants. From: *Canada*

Table 6   Vaccination Schedule[1,2]

Vaccine		Birth	1mo.	2mo.	4mo.	6mo.	12mo.	15mo.	18mo.	24 mo.	4-6yr.	11-12yr.	14-16yr.
Hepatitis B	USA	X	X or	X or	X	X or	X or	X or	X				
	Can[3]	X			or							X	
DTaP	USA			X	X	X		X or	X		X	Td	
	Can.[4]			X	X	X			X		X		Td or dTaP[5]
IPV	USA			X	X	X or	X or	X or	X		X		
	Can.			X	X	(X)[6]			X		X		
Hib	USA[7]			X	X	X[8]	X or	X					
	Can.[9]			X	X	X			X				
MMR	USA						X				X		
	Can.						X	(X)[10]			X		
Varicella[11]	USA						X						
	Can.						X						
Pneumococcal[12]	USA			X	X	X	X or	X					
	Can.			X	X	X	X or	X					
Conjugate meningococcal	USA[13]												
	Can.[14]			X	X	X			OR				X
Influenza[15]	USA[16]					X →							
	Can.[17]					X →							
Hepatitis A	USA[18]									Hep A →			
	Can.[19]												

1. Adapted from Canadian Immunization Guide, ed 6, Ottawa, Canadian Medical Association, 2002. Accessed at http://www.phac-aspc.gc.ca/publicat/cig-gci/.
2. Adapted from CDC – MMWR: Recommended childhood and immunization schedule, USA, Jan-June 2004.
3. In Canada, routine hepatitis B immunization is often delayed until age 11 to 13 because of concerns about level and duration of protection when given in infancy.
4. In Canada this is usually a component of a combination vaccine (Pentacel, Quadricel).
5. In Canada it is now recommended that a booster of acellular pertussis be given at age 14 to 16.
6. This is an uneccessary dose but is often included for convenience.
7. In the USA, Hib is given on its own due to concerns about a lower immune response when it is given as a combination vaccine.
8. A 6-month dose is not necessary if the PRP-OMP vaccine is used.
9. In Canada, Hib is usually given in a combination vaccine because no decreased Hib response has been observed with Pentacel. If it is given separately as PRP-OMP, no 6-month dose is necessary.
10. A second dose of MMR at least 1 month after the first dose provides better measles protection. It can be given at 18 months or 4 to 6 years.
11. For persons ≥13 years old, two doses of varicella given at least 4 weeks apart should be given.
12. The number of doses of pneumococcal vaccine required depends on the age at which it is started.
13. In the USA the conjugate meningococcal vaccine is not yet available.
14. The number of doses of meningococcal vaccine required depends on the age at which it is started.
15. For children ≤ 9 years (Can.) or ≤ 8 years (USA), two doses of influenza vaccine at least 4 weeks apart are required when receiving the vaccine for the first time.
16. In the USA, influenza vaccine is recommended for persons ≥ 6 months with risk factors and household members of persons in groups at high risk. It is also encouraged for the 6- to 23-month age group because of an increased risk of infection–related hospitalization in this group. For healthy persons ages 5 to 49 years, the intranasal vaccine is an acceptable alternative to the intramuscular form.
17. In Canada the influenza vaccine is recommended annually for all persons ≥ 6 months of age.
18. In the USA, hepatitis A vaccine is recommended in certain regions and states.
19. In Canada, hepatitis A vaccine is not part of the recommended routine immunization schedule.

Communicable Disease Report 20:157-160, 1994, *Can Med Assoc J* 152:527-529, 1995.
3. Centers for Disease Control and Prevention: FDA approval for infants of a *Haemophilus influenzae* type b conjugate and hepatitis B (recombinant) combined vaccine, *JAMA* 277:620-621, 1997.
4. Zimmerman RK: The 2000 harmonized immunization schedule, *Am Fam Physician* 61:232-239, 2000.
5. Canada Communicable Disease Report: *Haemophilus Influenzae* type B disease control ssing Pentacel®, Canada, 1998-1999; 26(1), 2000.

HEPATITIS B IMMUNIZATION

(See also hepatitis; immunization schedules for children)

Primary Immunization

Hepatitis B vaccination is safe, and its use is cost effective. Two recombinant DNA hepatitis B vaccines are available in Canada and the United States (Recombivax HB and Engerix-B). These two vaccines can be used interchangeably. A combined hepatitis A/hepatitis B vaccine (Twinrix) is also available.[1]

The U.S. Centers for Disease Control (CDC) recommend primary hepatitis B immunization for the following[2]:

- All babies, at birth or within 2 months of delivery
- Children 0 to18 years old who have not been vaccinated
- Injection drug users
- Sexually active heterosexuals (more than one partner in prior 6 months or recently acquired STD)
- Men who have sex with men
- Household contacts and sexual partners of people with chronic hepatitis B
- People with jobs involving contact with human blood
- Patients on dialysis, or receiving regular blood products or with early renal failure
- Families of children adopted from areas with high rates of HBV infection (Southeast Asia, Africa, Amazon Basin, Pacific Islands, Middle East) with evidence of past infection
- Those travelling internationally for > 6 months in areas with high or intermediate HBV infection rates
- Inmates of correctional facilities
- Staff of institutions for developmentally disabled

Following the primary dose, boosters should be given after 1 and 6 months. If the vaccination series is interrupted, the second dose should be administered as soon as possible. The second and third doses should be separated by an interval of at least 2 months. If only the third dose is delayed, it should be administered when convenient.[3]

Vaccine dosage varies with age and should be checked for each product. Injections are given intramuscularly into the deltoid of adults and into the anterolateral thigh of children. Gluteal injections should be avoided because in this location the vaccine may be inadvertently deposited in the fat, resulting in lower effectiveness.[1]

After routine vaccination, post-vaccination testing for adequate antibody response is unnecessary. Post-vaccination testing IS recommended for persons whose medical management depends on knowledge of their immune status, such as immunocompromised patients, infants born to HbsAg-positive mothers, and health care workers and sex partners of persons with chronic hepatitis B infection. Post-vaccination testing should be completed 1 to 2 months after the third vaccine dose for results to be meaningful. A protective antibody response is 10 or more IU/mL.[3]

Response rates to hepatitis B immunization vary with age. For those under 2 years it is 95%; for those 2 to 19 years the rate is 99%; and for those over the age of 60 it is 50% to 70%.[1] Protection against both clinical disease and the carrier state has been documented to persist for 15 years,[4] but whether immunity will persist for longer periods is unknown at present. Response rates are lower in immunocompromised persons, and booster doses may be indicated. However, the timing and frequency of such boosters have not been established.[1]

Post-Exposure Prophylaxis for Hepatitis B

Hepatitis B immunoglobulin (HBIG, HyperHep) should be considered for post-exposure (within 7 to 14 days) prophylaxis of an infant born to an HBsAg-positive mother, for percutaneous or mucosal exposure to HBsAg positive blood, after sexual exposure to an HbsAg-positive person, or for household exposure of an infant under 1 year of age to a primary caregiver who has acute hepatitis B. In all cases, hepatitis B vaccine should be given at the same time but at a different site.[2]

All pregnant women should be screened for HBsAg. If a pregnant woman is HbsAg-negative but is at high risk of acquiring hepatitis B, she should be immunized. Infants born to HbsAg-positive mothers should receive 0.5 ml hepatitis B immunoglobulin at birth.[1]

Sexual contacts of a person with acute hepatitis B should receive active immunization. If prophylaxis can be started within 14 days of the contact, a single dose of HBIG should also be given. Household contacts need not be immunized except for infants under 1 year of age when the index case is the caretaker. HBIG is given in doses of 0.06 ml/kg.[2]

All health care workers should receive a primary hepatitis B immunization series and document their postimmunization antibody levels. If the levels are above 10 IU/L, long-term protection is likely even if the levels subsequently fall below 10 IU/L. If a health care worker is subject to percutaneous or mucosal exposure to blood or other body fluids, the risk level for hepatitis B and the HBsAg status of the source should be determined, as well as the anti-hepatitis B surface antigen (anti-HBs) level of the exposed health care worker. If the source is HbsAg-negative or is known to be at negligible risk, the only treatment for the health care worker is completion of regular primary immunizations if this has not already been done. If the HBsAg status of the source is unknown, management depends on the vaccination and immune status of the health care worker. If the health care worker has been fully immunized and has had protective levels of antibodies documented, no further action is required. If the health care worker has had two or more doses of vaccine but the worker's anti-HBs status is unknown, status should be determined as soon as possible. If the risk of exposure was high, the worker should receive one vaccination dose immediately. If it was low, the worker may wait for the results of the anti-HBs status determination and then receive vaccination only if it is negative. HBIG is indicated only if the health care worker has not been vaccinated, has received only one dose, or has not developed antibodies from a full vaccination course. HBIG should be given at once concomitantly with a full course of immunization.[2]

─────────── ✍ **REFERENCES** ✍ ───────────

1. *Canadian immunization guide,* ed 6. Ottawa, Canadian Medical Association, 2002. Accessed at http://www.phac-aspc.gc.ca/publicat/cig-gci/.
2. Centers for Disease Control and Prevention (CDC): *Vaccines to prevent hepatitis A and hepatitis B,* September 2002.
3. *Canadian immunization guide,* ed 6. Ottawa, Canadian Medical Association, 2002. Accessed at http://www.phac-aspc.gc.ca/publicat/cig-gci/.
4. Centers for Disease Control and Prevention (CDC): *Hepatitis B vaccine fact sheet,* August, 2002.
5. Koff RS: Hepatitis vaccines: recent advances, *Int J Parasitol* 33(5-6):517-523, May 2003.

INFLUENZA PREVENTION

Influenza virus infections rank as one of the most common infectious diseases in humankind. Approximately 21 million persons died worldwide in the 1918-1919 influenza pandemic, with 549,000 deaths in the United States. Today, in a typical season the acute febrile illness of influenza, with variable degrees of systemic symptoms, contributes to significant loss of work days, human suffering, mortality, and excess morbidity.[1] Rates of infection are highest among children, but serious illness and death are far more likely in the elderly and individuals with underlying medical conditions. Influenza affects 10% to 20% of the general population in the United States each year, accounting for 11,000 hospitalizations and 10,000 to 40,000 deaths annually.[2] Although rapid diagnostic tests on nasal secretions have become available, with respectable positive and negative predictive values in moderately high prevalence settings,[3] diagnosis is usually made on clinical grounds. Influenza outbreaks in temperate areas occur during the winter months, while in the Caribbean and other tropical regions, outbreaks occur throughout the year.

Vaccines

Influenza immunization decreases the incidence of pneumonia, hospitalization, and all cause mortality in both high- and low-risk individuals who are 65 years of age or older.[5] It also decreases both clinical and serologically confirmed influenza in those immunized, and leads to a modest decline in lost work time. The number needed to treat (NNT) ranges from 65 to 115 in the elderly to 13 in young, healthy adults.[2] Protection from the vaccine begins 1 to 2 weeks after injection and generally lasts 6 months. Protection may last for shorter periods in some elderly patients. Because of this short duration of protection, and the season-to-season variations in the prevalent circulating virus subtype, influenza vaccine must be given annually.

Two general types of vaccine are available, both with demonstrated efficacy in adults and children.[6] Inactivated intramuscular (whole or split virus) vaccine is the most widely available type worldwide. The split virus vaccine has fewer side effects and should be used for children 13

years of age or younger. Doses of whole and split viruses are 0.5 ml intramuscularly except for children between the ages of 35 months and 6 years, who should receive 0.25 ml. Children under age 9 years receiving influenza vaccine for the first time should be given two shots separated by at least 1 month. Vaccination of pregnant women in the second and third trimesters is safe and clearly indicated, since influenza complications are increased both in late pregnancy and the perinatal period. A randomized placebo-controlled study of healthy working adults found that the only adverse effect occurring more frequently in the cohort receiving the flu vaccine was arm soreness.[9] The only contraindication to flu vaccination is demonstrated anaphylactic reaction to egg or other vaccine components.[10]

An intranasal live virus vaccine is also available. It may be a more acceptable way to deliver vaccine protection to children and therefore has been promoted as an alternative to increase coverage in this group. Its higher cost, and concern over the potential for gene assortment between the live virus vaccine and non-human influenza viruses, may limit its usefulness. Although the intranasal vaccine is effective, a higher rate of rhinnorhea and pharyngitis were found in the intervention group.[12] Also, although it appears to induce excellent mucosal immunity, it has not yet been shown to be protective in immunocompromised individuals.[3]

Targeting the following groups for influenza immunization has been recommended[10]:

- *People at high risk of influenza-related complications:* Age over 65 years, chronic health conditions or immunosuppression (all ages), residents of nursing homes or chronic care facilities, children or adolescents on chronic ASA treatment.
- *People capable of transmission of influenza to those at high risk of complications:* Health care workers, household contacts (including children) of those at high risk.

Health policy and funding bodies are increasingly promoting influenza immunization for healthy adults and children. In the context of availability of inexpensive, safe, effective vaccines, this achieves a reduction in the reservoir of disease exposure for the vulnerable, decreases in loss of productivity due to illness in individuals and families, and enhanced protection for those (primarily in the 50- to 65-year age group) with undiagnosed chronic illness.[10] Advice from health care practitioners is among the most powerful positive influences on individuals' vaccination decision-making.[10] The area of public perception of influenza vaccine is of interest. For example, many patients perceive that the injection of the dead virus gives them the flu.

Antiviral Drugs

Prophylaxis against influenza with amantadine is 70% to 90% effective against influenza A (but ineffective against influenza B) when started before exposure. It is recommended for all patients in nursing homes during outbreaks of influenza A in the institution, whether or not they have been vaccinated. It can also be used for unimmunized health care workers and unimmunized household contacts of high-risk individuals during influenza A outbreaks. For adults the usual dosage for prophylaxis is 200 mg/day as a single dose or 100 mg twice a day.[10]

Neuraminidase inhibitors zanamivir (Relenza) and oseltamivir (Tamiflu) are effective against both influenza A and influenza B. Oseltamivir has been approved for prophylactic use in the United States, and is given orally at a dose of 75 to 150 mg once daily.

⋑ REFERENCES ⋐

1. Belshe RB, Mendelman PM, Treanor J, et al: The efficacy of live attenuated, cold-adapted, trivalent, intranasal influenza virus vaccine in children, *N Engl J Med* 338(20):1405-1412, May 14 1998.
2. Cifu A, Levinson W: Influenza: contempo updates, *JAMA* 284(22):2847-2849, 2000.
3. Bridges CB, Harper SA, Fukuda K, et al: Prevention and control of influenza—recommendations of the advisory committee on immunization practices (ACIP), *MMWR* 52(RR08):1-36, 2003.
4. Henley E: Prevention and treatment of influenza, *J Fam Prac* 52(11):883-886, 2003.
5. Nichol KL, Wuorenma J, von Sternberg T: Benefits of influenza vaccination for low-, intermediate-, and high-risk senior citizens, *Arch Intern Med* 158:1769-1776, 1998.
6. Dimicheli V, Rivetti D, Deeks JJ, et al: Vaccines for preventing influenza in healthy adults, *Cochrane Database Syst Rev* (4):CD001269, updated 2001.
7. Zangwill KM, Belshe RB: Safety and efficacy of trivalent inactivated influenza vaccine in young children: a summary for the new era of routine immunization, *Paed Infec Dis J* 23(3):189-197, 2004.
8. England JA: Maternal immunization with inactivated influenza vaccine: rationale and experience, *Vaccine* 21(24):3460-3464, 2003.
9. Nichol KL, Margolis KL, Lind A, et al: Side effects associated with influenza vaccination in healthy working adults: a randomized, placebo-controlled trial, *Arch Intern Med* 156:1546-1550, 1996.
10. National Advisory Committee on Immunization (NACI): Statement on influenza vaccination for the 2003-2004 season, *Can Comm Dis Rep* 29:1-20, 15 August, 2003.
11. Beyer WE, Palache AM, deJong JC, et al: Cold-adapted live influenza virus vaccine versus inactivated vaccine: systemic vaccine reactions, local and systemic antibody response, and vaccine efficacy. A meta-analysis, *Vaccine* 20(9-10):1340-1353, 2002.
12. Nichol KL, Mendelman PM, Mallon KP, et al: Effectiveness of live, attenuated intranasal influenza virus vaccine in healthy, working adults, *JAMA* 282:137-144, 1999.

MEASLES-MUMPS-RUBELLA AND RUBELLA IMMUNIZATION
(See also immunization schedules for children)

Large case series have demonstrated that administration of MMR vaccine is safe in children with egg allergy. However, precautions are needed: observation for 2 hours and appropriate treatment, if there is a history of active asthma or cardio-respiratory distress after egg ingestion.[1] In 1996 a combined attenuated measles-rubella vaccine free of egg protein (MoRu-Viraten) became available.

To eliminate measles from the population, more than a single early childhood vaccination is necessary. Two-dose measles vaccination is associated with a higher level of humoral immunity and clinical protection than a single dose. Maximum antibody levels are obtained if the initial immunizations are not given before 1 year of age, and if booster doses are given before entry to elementary school (ages 4 to 6) rather than before entry to middle school (ages 11 to 12).[2]

Acute arthralgias occur in about one fourth of women receiving rubella vaccination.[3] Current evidence suggests that a significant association exists between adult rubella vaccine and chronic arthritis in women.[4]

⋑ REFERENCES ⋐

1. Khakoo GA, Lack G: Recommendations for using MMR vaccine in children allergic to eggs, *BMJ* 320:929-932, 2000.
2. Hutchins SS, Dezayas A, Le Blond K, et al: Evaluation of an early two-dose measles vaccination schedule, *Am J Epi* 154(11):1064-1071, 2001.
3. Ray P, Black S, Shinefield H, et al: Risk of chronic arthropathy among women after rubella vaccination, *JAMA* 278:551-556, 1997.
4. Geier D, and Geier M: A one year follow-up of chronic arthritis following rubella and hepatitis B vaccination based upon analysis of the Vaccine Adverse Events Reporting System (VAERS) database, *Clin Exp Rheumatol* 20(6):767-771, 2002.

MENINGOCOCCAL IMMUNIZATION
(See also meningitis, immunization schedules for children)

Two types of meningococcal vaccines are available; polysaccharide vaccines (Men-Ps), and protein-polysaccharide conjugate vaccines (Men-C). Age-specific incidence rates (per 100,000 population per year and from 1985 to 2000 data) were 14.8 (less than 1 year old), 4.2 (1 to 4 years old), and 2.3 (15 to 19 years old). The overall case fatality rate ranged from 9% to 12% depending on the strain.[1]

Meningococcal Polysaccharide Vaccines
The Men-Ps are available as bivalent MenAC-Ps (active against serotypes A and C), and quadrivalent MenACYW-Ps (active against serotypes A,C,Y, and W-135) vaccines. There is no vaccine against serotype B disease. These vaccines are not recommended for routine

immunization in the general population because they induce a T-cell independent immune response that results in poor immunogenicity and protection in early childhood and a short duration of protection. In fact, studies have shown that in children under age 2 years, these vaccines are at best very poorly protective.[2]

Routine immunization

Routine immunization with MenACYW-Ps is recommended only in high-risk groups such as patients with immunodeficiencies and asplenia. It is also recommended for military recruits and should be offered to lab personnel who are routinely exposed to *Neisseria meningitides.* Immunization against serotype A is also recommended for travellers to the sub-Saharan belt of Africa. The effectiveness of, and need for, re-immunization is not well understood and should be considered only for those patients continuously exposed to serotype A disease or those with immunodeficiencies. The interval between boosters depends on the patient's age.[1]

Menactra.

Immunoprophylaxis

Polysaccharide vaccines should be given to unimmunized close contacts of known cases of serogroup A, Y, and W-135 disease, as well as in outbreak situations. In older children and adults these vaccines are known to provide a 1-year period of increased protection. For serogroup A disease, Men AC-Ps or MenACYW-Ps is recommended as a single dose for children over 18 months and adults, with 2 doses necessary for children ages 3 to 17 months. For serogroup Y or W-135 disease, one dose of MenACYW-P is recommended for people over 2 years. For serogroup C disease the conjugate vaccine is preferred, although Men AC-P or MenACYW-P may be given.[1]

Meningococcal Protein-Polysaccharide (Conjugate) Vaccines

Menjugate usu at 12 mo @, can be given .2,4,6 mo.

Early immunogenicity data on Men-C conjugate vaccine suggest it induces a high level of protection in infants as young as 2 months (greater than 95% with the three-dose, primary series). Immunological memory, and thus presumed protection, has been demonstrated at least 5 years after immunization. Because long-term data are not yet available, it is not known whether or not a booster will be needed to provide protection through adolescence. In addition, no data are available on Men-C use in outbreak control, immunodeficient patients, adults greater than 65 years, and pregnant or lactating women. Three conjugate vaccines are currently available that differ primarily in the protein that is used for conjugation.

Safety data on Men-C are mostly from the United Kingdom, where it has been used routinely for several years. In 12 million doses given between 1999 and 2000, the commonly seen side effects in infants were mild local reactions and irritability. In addition, fever over 38° C was seen in 9% of infants when other vaccines were administered at the same time, and headache and malaise occurred in up to 10% of older children and adults. Severe reactions were very uncommon (less than 0.01%), and no deaths were attributed to the vaccine. One U.K study found no significant differences in adverse reactions among the three different conjugate vaccine products.[1]

Routine immunization

Although recommended by most immunization organizations, the vaccine is often not covered by formularies because of its expense and limited effectiveness data. Informing the parent or individual of the current data is important. It is unknown if the meningococcal C vaccine can prevent disease, but in the United Kingdom there were decreased reports of group C disease following the national vaccination program.[3] One estimate is that if all 1.7 million children in Canada less than 5 years of age were vaccinated, then 22 cases and two deaths would be prevented in the first year.[4] This translates to having to vaccinate approximately 77,000 children to prevent one case, and 850,000 to prevent one death. It is a recommended vaccine for high-risk children, such as those with asplenia, or immunodeficiencies, in combination with the polysaccharide vaccine. Consideration should also be given to students living in university residences, due to a higher risk of serogroup C infection in this environment. Schedules differ depending on age. Men-C conjugate can be administered at the same time as DaPTP and Hib or MMR.[1]

Immunoprophylaxis

Men-C is recommended for all contacts over 2 months old of known serogroup C disease or in serogroup C outbreaks.[1]

◄ REFERENCES ►

1. *Canadian Immunization Guide,* ed 6,, Ottawa, Canadian Medical Association, 2002. Accessed at http://www.phac-aspc.gc.ca/publicat/cig-gci/. 151-165.
2. Canadian Communicable Disease Report, vol 27, ACS-6, Oct 2001.
3. MacLennan J: Meningococcal group C conjugate vaccines, *Arch Dis Child* 84:383-386, 2001.
4. Canada Health and Welfare Canada: *Statement on recommended use of meningococcal vaccines,* Canada Communicable Disease Report, ACS-5, 6, 2001,1-36.

PERTUSSIS IMMUNIZATION
(See also pertussis)

Almost all cases of pertussis are caused by *Bordetella pertussis,* and antigens from the bacteria and its toxin are administered in the acellular pertussis vaccination. Acellular pertussis vaccines are at least as effective as whole-cell vaccines and have fewer side effects, both in infants and adults.[1]

Immunization of infants against pertussis produces immunity in 80% to 90% of recipients. However, the acquired immunity wanes in time. Loss of protection begins within 3 to 5 years, and no antibodies are detectable after 10 to 12 years. Because of increasing rates of pertussis in adolescents and adults, and the low likelihood of side effects for the acellular vaccine, public health bodies are recommending dTap instead of Td for the routine adolescent booster.[2]

◢ REFERENCES ◣

1. Halperin SA, Scheifele D, Mills E, et al: Nature, evolution, and appraisal of adverse events and antibody response associated with the fifth consecutive dose of a five-component acellular pertussis-based combination vaccine, *Vaccine* 21(19-20):2298-2306, 2003.
2. National Advisory Committee on Immunization: Pertussis vaccine. In: *Canadian immunization guide,* ed 6, Ottawa, Canadian Medical Association, 2002. 169-176. Accessed at http://www.phac-aspc.gc.ca/publicat/cig-gci/.

PNEUMOCOCCAL IMMUNIZATION
(See also immunization schedules for infants and children)

Streptococcus pneumoniae (pneumococcus) is the leading cause of invasive bacterial infections, meningitis, bacterial pneumonia, and acute otitis media in children. Invasive disease is most common in the very young, the elderly, and high-risk groups (see below). Each year in Canada, there are approximately 65 cases of meningitis, 700 cases of bacteremia, 2200 cases of pneumonia requiring hospitalization and 9000 cases not requiring hospitalization, and an average of 15 deaths per year due to *S. pneumoniae* in children under 5 years of age.[1] Two pneumococcal vaccines are available in Canada.

Polysaccharide Vaccine

This preparation has been available since 1983 and immunizes against 23 types of pneumococci. Ninety percent of pneumoccocal bacteremia and meningitis are caused by these 23 serotypes. Available 23-valent vaccines are Pneumovax 23, Pnemo 23, Pnu-Immune. Epidemiological evidence suggests that pneumococcal vaccination is effective in preventing pneumococcal bacteremia.[2] The response of children less than 2 years of age to the polysaccharide vaccine is irregular; therefore, the vaccine is not recommended for this group.[3] Children from 24 to 59 months of age may receive the polysaccharide vaccine, but the conjugate vaccine is preferred. Antibody levels decline after 5 to 10 years. The duration of effective immunity is unknown.[2]

A single dose of polysaccharide pneumococcal vaccine should be given to the following groups:[1]
1) All persons 65 years and older. It can be given with the influenza vaccination at a different site. If immunization history is unknown, the vaccine should be given.
2) Individuals over 5 years of age with asplenia, splenic dysfunction, or sickle cell disease if not previously immunized.
3) Individuals over 5 years of age with the following conditions: chronic cardiorespiratory disease, cirrhosis, alcoholism, chronic renal disease, nephrotic syndrome, diabetes, chronic CSF leak, HIV, and other immunosuppresive conditions. The efficacy of the vaccine may be less than in immunocompetent persons, but benefits are still achieved.

Conjugate Vaccine

Pneumococcal conjugate vaccine (Prevnar™) immunizes against seven *S. pneumoniae* serotypes. It contains no thimerosal. Approximately 97% of infants achieve protective antibody titres after the primary series, with an observed protective efficacy of 89% to 97%.[2] Satisfactory safety and immunogenicity have been seen in HIV and sickle cell disease. Effectiveness in preventing otitis media is controversial. The vaccine does reduce the number of episodes caused by serotypes in the vaccine, but is accompanied by an increase in the number of infections caused by other serotypes and *H. influenzae.*[4,5] The long-term efficacy of the conjugate vaccine is not known.[3] In the short term, a recent review of a CDC program that monitors invasive pneumococcal infections in a population of 16 million in seven locations around the United States compared the rates of invasive pneumococcal disease before and after the introduction, in 2000, of the polyvalent pneumococcal vaccine for use in all children younger than 2 years and in high-risk children between the ages of 2 and 4 years. They found that the rate remained steady for older children (ages 3 and 4 years), declined a bit for 2-year-olds, and decreased significantly for children 1 year and younger. Among children 2 years and younger, the rate declined 69%, from 188 to 59 cases per 100,000. This translates to a NNT of 775. Interestingly, the rate of invasive disease also declined in older patients, even in adults. In all age groups, the benefit was largely from serotypes included in the vaccine. This is not a RCT and whether these results can be applied to other populations is yet to be seen.[6]

The conjugate pneumococcal vaccine is recommended by immunization authorities for all children 23 months and younger. Some parents may decide not to have their children vaccinated, given the cost and relative rarity of serious pneumococcal infection. It is also recommended for all children 24 to 59 months who are at risk for invasive pneumococcal infections, including children with sickle-cell disease, asplenia, HIV, immunocompromising conditions, and chronic medical conditions. It should also be considered in children of this age group who attend day care and aboriginal children living in isolated communities.[1]

Booster Doses and Re-immunization

Results from serologic and case studies indicate that polysaccharide vaccine-induced immunity decreases over time. Data are not yet available concerning persistence of immunity following the use of conjugate pneumococcal vaccine in infancy.

At present, routine re-immunization is not recommended but should be considered for those of any age at highest risk of invasive infection. People for whom re-immunization should be considered include those with functional or anatomic asplenia or sickle-cell disease; hepatic cirrhosis; chronic renal failure or nephrotic syndrome; HIV infection; and immunosuppression related to disease or therapy. A single re-immunization is recommended after 5 years in those over 10 years of age and after 3 years in those 10 years old or younger. Either conjugate vaccine or polysaccharide vaccine may be used for re-immunization. Any need for further subsequent re-immunization remains to be determined.[2]

Adverse reactions with both the conjugate and polysaccharide vaccines are mild and self-limiting.

—— ✒ REFERENCES ✑ ——

1. Canadian Immunization Guide, ed 6. Ottawa, Canadian Medical Association, 2002. Accessed at http://www.phac-aspc.gc.ca/publicat/cig-gci/.
2. Health Canada -Population and Public Health Branch Division of Immunization and Respiratory Diseases: Vaccine Preventable Diseases, Pneumococcal, April 2004 http://www.hc-sc.gc.ca/pphb-dgspsp/dird-dimr/vpd-mev/pneumococcal_e.html
3. National Advisory Committee on Immunization (NACI). Statement on recommended use of pneumococcal conjugate vaccine. CCDR 2002; 28 (ACS-2): 1-32.
4. Eskola J, Kilpi T, Palmu A, et al. Efficacy of a pneumococcal conjugate vaccine against acute otitis media. *N Engl J Med* 344:403-409, 2001.
5. Straetemans M, Sanders EAM, Veenhoven RH, et al: Pneumococcal vaccines for preventing otitis media (Cochrane Review). In: *The Cochrane Library*, Issue 4, 2003.
6. Whitney CG, Farley MM, Hadler J, et al. Decline in invasive pneumococcal disease after the introduction of protein-polysaccharide conjugate vaccine. *N Engl J Med* 348: 1737-1746, 2003.

POLIO IMMUNIZATION

(See also immunization schedules for children; polio)

One of the fears concerning poliomyelitis (polio) immunization is that the live virus vaccine may itself cause paralytic polio. The reason appears to be intramuscular injections of other drugs, usually antibiotics, within 30 days of receiving oral live polio vaccine.[1,2] This phenomenon was also noted in the prepolio vaccine era, when it was observed that polio developing in a child after tonsillectomy and adenoidectomy was likely to be bulbar, whereas polio striking a child who had had intra-muscular injections was likely to cause paralysis of the limb in which the injection was given.[2]

In 1999, to eliminate the risk for vaccine-associated paralytic polio, exclusive use of IPV (inactivated polio vaccine) was recommended for routine vaccination in countries where polio has been eradicated, and OPV (oral polio vaccine) subsequently became unavailable for routine use. However, because of superior ability to induce intestinal immunity and to prevent spread among close contacts, OPV remains the vaccine of choice for areas where wild poliovirus is still present. Until worldwide eradication of poliovirus is accomplished, continued vaccination of the North American population against poliovirus is necessary.[3]

Polio vaccines have been extraordinarily effective in eradicating the disease. The WHO target date for worldwide eradication of polio is 2005. To date, the Region of the Americas (36 countries), the Western Pacific Region (37 countries and areas including China), and the WHO European Region (51 countries) have been certified polio-free. Acute poliomyelitis is now found only in parts of Africa and South Asia. Six countries in the world were polio-endemic at the end of 2003, the lowest number ever.[4,5]

—— ✒ REFERENCES ✑ ——

1. Strebel PM, Ion-Nedelcu N, Baughman AL, et al: Intramuscular injections within 30 days of immunization with oral poliovirus vaccine–a risk factor for vaccine-associated paralytic poliomyelitis, *N Engl J Med* 332:500-506, 1995.
2. Wright PF, Karzon DT: Minimizing the risks associated with the prevention of poliomyelitis (editorial), *N Engl J Med* 332:528-529, 1995.
3. General Recommendations on Immunization, Recommendations of the Advisory Committee on Immunization Practices (ACIP) and the American Academy of Family Physicians (AAFP). (Accessed April 24, 2004, at http://www.cdc.gov/mmwr/preview/mmwrhtml/rr5102a1.htm).
4. W.H.O. Global Polio Eradication Initiative (Accessed April 24, 2004, at http://www.polioeradication.org/vaccines/polio-eradication/all/global/default.asp).
5. World Health Organization: Immunization, vaccines and biologicals. W.H.O Global Polio Eradication Initiative (Accessed April24, 2004, at http://www.who.int/vaccines-polio/all/news/files/pdf/news_20040420_global.pdf.
6. Centers for Disease Control and Prevention: Revised recommendations for routine poliomyelitis vaccination, *JAMA* 282:522, 1999.

RABIES IMMUNIZATION

(See also immunization schedules for children)

Epidemiology

Almost all cases of human rabies acquired from animals in North America result from bites of dogs, skunks, or foxes or from contact with bats. Rabies can also be transmitted by wolves, bobcats, bears, and groundhogs. Rabies can infect raccoons in the eastern United States and Canada as well as (rarely) cows, sheep, and horses; there are, however, no reports of transmission of the disease to humans from any of these sources.[1] Bites from squirrels, chipmunks, rabbits, hares, rats, mice, hamsters, guinea pigs, and gerbils rarely require post-exposure prophylaxis. However, the local medical officer of health or government veterinarian should be consulted.[2]

Rabies can be acquired only if a person has direct contact with saliva through a bite or scratch or through mucous membrane contact. With the exception of bats (see below), almost all reported cases are from bites. The risk of contracting the disease after a bite is 50 to 100 times greater than after a scratch.[1] The virus cannot be transmitted by petting a rabid animal, through contact with its blood, urine, or feces, or through being sprayed by a skunk.[2]

Since 1980, 58% of the cases of human rabies in the United States have been a result of contact with a rabid bat.[2] Even casual contact with bat variants of rabies may lead to infection, and therefore post-exposure immunization should be considered for all bat contacts unless the bat is collected safely and proved to be rabies free. Such contacts include individuals sleeping in a room where a bat is discovered, since a bite may neither be felt nor leave a mark.[2]

Post-Exposure Management

Immediate management of a bite from a potentially rabid animal includes thorough washing with copious amounts of soap, water, and a virucidal agent (such as a povidone-iodine solution), a process that markedly reduces the risk of infection.[2,3] Suturing of the wound should be avoided and, if required, antibiotics and tetanus prophylaxis should be given.[2] If a domestic dog, cat, or ferret is responsible for the bite and has rabies, it will become ill within 10 days. If a veterinarian believes that the animal appears healthy, it should be confined and watched for this period, but if it is behaving in an erratic fashion, it should be killed and its brain evaluated for rabies.[3] Post-exposure prophylaxis (PEP) should begin immediately if the animal is suspected or known to be rabid or if the animal develops rabies during confinement.[2] The immunization status of the animal is not a determining factor, since the degree of protection offered by animal rabies vaccines is less than that given by human vaccines.[1]

Three rabies vaccines are available in the United States: human diploid cell vaccine (HDCV; Imovax), rabies vaccine adsorbed (RVA), and purified chick embryo cell vaccine (PCECV). Only HDCV is available in Canada.[2] Standard injection technique is intramuscularly in the deltoid in adults or the upper anterolateral thigh in children. The vaccine should never be injected in the gluteal region.[2] Post-exposure vaccination in nonimmunized individuals consists of five 1-ml injections given on days 0, 3, 7, 14, and 28. In addition, human rabies immune globulin (HRIG;

Imogam Rabies-HT; BayRab) should be given at a dose of 20 IU/kg.[2-4] The U.S. Advisory Committee for Immunization Practices (ACIP) advises injecting as much of the HRIG as possible in and around the wound and then injecting any residual volume intramuscularly at a different site.[3] Post-exposure immunization of previously immunized individuals consists of two doses of rabies vaccine on days 0 and 3, without HRIG.[2] If PEP is begun in a patient and the animal is subsequently found to be rabies-free, the treatment can be discontinued.[4]

Pre-Exposure Management

Pre-exposure vaccination is given to high-risk individuals as a series of three shots on days 0, 7, and 21.[2] Individuals at risk include veterinarians and other animal handlers, spelunkers, and individuals travelling to regions where rabies is endemic (Asia, Africa, and Latin America) if they are unlikely to receive adequate medical care and PEP within 2 days of exposure to a possibly rabid animal.[1] Persons who have been immunized and are at continued high risk should either have their titres checked or receive a booster dose every 2 years.[2-4]

❧ REFERENCES ❧

1. Basgoz N: Case records of the Massachusetts General Hospital, Case 21-1998, *N Engl J Med* 339:105-112, 1998.
2. Canadian Immunization Guide. Ottawa, Canadian Medical Association, 2002: part 3 Active immunizing agents—Rabies vaccine. Health Canada. Population and Public Health Branch, 2002. Accessed at http://www. phac-aspc.gc.ca/publicat/cig-gci/.
3. Human rabies prevention–United States, 1999: recommendations of the Advisory Committee on Immunization Practices (ACIP), *MMWR* 48(RR-1):1-21, 1999.
4. A new rabies vaccine, *Med Lett* 40:64-65, 1998.

TETANUS IMMUNIZATION
(See also immunization schedules for children)

Assuming adequate childhood immunization, boosters of Td (combined tetanus and diphtheria toxoid) should continue to be offered at 10-year intervals after the age of 7 years.[1,2]

For persons that sustain a wound that is at risk of a tetanus infection (contaminated, for example, by soil or fecal matter), and whose previous immunization history is unknown or uncertain, both tetanus immune globulin and Td toxoid should be administered.[3]

❧ REFERENCES ❧

1. Zimmerman RK, Middleton DB, Burns IL, et al: Routine vaccines across the life span, 2003, *J Fam Pract* 52(1 suppl): S1-21, Jan 2003.
2. *Canadian Immunization Guide,* ed 6, Ottawa, Canadian Medical Association, 2002. Health Canada: (Accessed at http://www.phac-aspc.gc.ca/publicat/cig-gci/.

3. *Epidemiology and Prevention of Vaccine-Preventable Diseases–The Pink Book,* ed 8, February 2004: United States Department of Health and Human Services Centre for Disease Control and Prevention. (Accessed April 15, 2004, art http://www.cdc.gov/nip/publications/pink/).

VARICELLA IMMUNIZATION
(See also immunization schedules for children; infectious diseases in pregnancy; varicella; varicella in children)

Varicella zoster vaccine (Varivax) is a live attenuated vaccine constituted with the Oka strain of Varicella antigen. Although Varivax must be stored at −15° C, newer vaccines, such as Varivax II and Varilrix can be stored at 2° to 8°C for up to 90 days.[1]

Efficacy
Since its licensure in the United States in 1995, the incidence of varicella and related hospitalizations in the United States has fallen by 76% to 86% in 2001.[2] Postlicensure studies demonstrate that the vaccine provides 70% to 90% protection against varicella infection for 7 to 10 years and 95% protection against severe varicella for 7 to 10 years. Efficacy in immunocompromised individuals may not be as good.[1]

Breakthrough infections occur in 1% of vaccinated individuals per year. These infections are milder, briefer, and less likely to be complicated than usual varicella. An important risk factor for breakthrough varicella infection is administration of varicella vaccine less than 28 days after MMR immunization (2.5 times higher likelihood of breakthrough). Time since vaccination does not seem to be a risk factor.[2]

Cases of herpes zoster (HZ) associated with varicella immunization have been reported. However, these cases are mild and the risk of HZ following vaccination is less than the risk following wild-type varicella infection.

Recommendations and Dosing Schedule
In 2001, the Canadian Task Force on Preventive Health Care recommended immunization of all children 12 to 15 months and catch-up immunization for children up to 12 years of age (grade A). Susceptible adolescents and adults should also be immunized (grade B).[3] The same recommendations are made by the American Academy of Pediatrics (AAP),[4] the Advisory Committee on Immunization Practices (ACIP),[5] and the National Advisory Committee on Immunization (NACI).[6]

Susceptible individuals are those who have never been infected with varicella or those who have never been immunized. Routine serologic testing to assess immune status is not cost effective; a reliable history of chickenpox is considered sufficient evidence for immunity.[2]

Other populations in whom vaccination is recommended include: susceptible health care workers, susceptible women of childbearing age who are not pregnant, susceptible household contacts of immunocompromised people, and new immigrants from tropical climates (since they are more likely to be susceptible). Finally, children or adolescents on chronic salicylate therapy should be immunized due to the risk of Reye's Syndrome.[3-6]

Children under age 13 years require one dose (0.5 ml subcutaneously), while children older than 13 and adults require two doses given 4 to 8 weeks apart. Varivax can be administered simultaneously with MMR and other scheduled immunizations. If not given at the same time, there should be a minimum 28-day interval between giving any live-attenuated vaccines such as MMR and Varivax. The need for booster dosing is undetermined. Studies have shown protection lasting 11 to 20 years.[1-5]

Contraindications
Varivax should not be administered to those with a gelatin or neomycin allergy. The vaccine does not contain egg products, thimerosal, or aluminum. Individuals with cell-mediated (versus isolated humoral) immunodeficiency should not receive Varivax. Consultation should be obtained for HIV patients. The effects of Varivax in pregnancy are not known and therefore the vaccine should not be given. The American Academy of Pediatrics and ACIP recommend that pregnancy be avoided for 1 month after vaccination.

Safety and Precautions:
Adverse effects of Varivax include mild fever (10% to 15%), injection site reactions (20% to 24%), and maculopapular rash after the second dose (1% to 6%).[1-5]

Postexposure prophylaxis
If given within 3 to 5 days of exposure to an index case, varicella vaccine can prevent or reduce the severity of chickenpox in the exposed individual.[1]

Varicella zoster immune globulin (VZIG)
If administered within 96 hours of exposure, VZIG can modify or prevent varicella and prevent complications or death. The exposed individual's susceptibility status, exposure risk, and risk of complications of varicella will determine whether VZIG is indicated. It should be strongly considered in immunocompromised patients, newborns of mothers with onset of varicella from 5 days before to 48 hours postdelivery, and premature infants with postnatal exposure.[1,2]

_____ ◢ REFERENCES ◤ _____

1. *Canadian Immunization Guide,* ed 6, Ottawa, 2002, Canadian Medical Association, 223-232. Accessed at http://www.phac-aspc.gc.ca/publicat/cig-gci/.
2. *Epidemiology and Prevention of Vaccine Preventable Diseases— The Pink Book,* ed 8, 2004, National Immunization

Program CDC and Prevention, ch 13, Washington, DC, 2004, US Department of Health and Human Services.

3. Canadian Task Force on Preventive Health Care: www.ctfphc.org/Tables/Varicella_2001_tab.htm.

4. American Academy of Pediatrics: www.aap.org.

5. Adisory Committee on Immunization Practices: www.immunize.org/acip .

6. National Advisory Committee on Immunization: www.hc-sc.gc.ca/pphb-dgspsp/naci-ccni.

CARDIOVASCULAR SYSTEM

ABDOMINAL AORTIC ANEURYSM

Smoking is a major risk factor for the development of abdominal aortic aneurysms.[1]

The rate of rupture increases significantly for aneurysms greater than 5 cm in diameter. In a Mayo Clinic population study of the yearly rate of rupture based on the size of aneurysm as determined by the last ultrasound, no ruptures occurred in those less than 4 cm, and the rates were 1% for those 4 to 4.99 cm and 11% for those 5 to 5.99 cm. Rates of growth varied widely among individuals and from one period to another in the same individual. The authors recommended serial ultrasound examinations at annual intervals for aneurysms less than 4 cm in diameter and every 6 months for those between 4 and 5 cm. They also advised elective surgery once the aneurysm reached a diameter of 5 cm.[2] Although this is reasonable advice, Mason and associates[3] estimated that 72% of patients with untreated abdominal aortic aneurysms die of other causes and that operating on three individuals electively would be necessary to prevent one rupture.

The overall mortality rate for ruptured aortic aneurysms is about 80%. Two thirds of patients die before reaching the hospital, and of those who undergo surgery, more than one third die within 30 days.[4] In contrast, the operative mortality for elective resection of aneurysms is 5% to 6%.[5] A randomized controlled trial in the United Kingdom, in which open surgery was compared with ultrasonographic surveillance for aneurysms 4 to 5.5 cm in diameter, found no long-term benefit from surgery but a short-term survival disadvantage in that the 30-day mortality rate for the surgical patients was 5.8%.[5]

Endovascular grafting, which is being developed in a number of specialized centres, is a new method of controlling abdominal aortic aneurysms. In this procedure a graft is inserted via the femoral artery and is held in place by expandable stents. Only about half the patients with abdominal aortic aneurysms are suitable candidates for this procedure. Short- and medium-term results are comparable to those of open surgical repairs, but long-term results have not yet been reported.[6]

Although a number of vascular surgeons have advocated abdominal ultrasound screening, evidence supporting this is controversial. Mason and associates[3] recommend against it, not only because of the physical morbidity and mortality of surgery, but also because of the possible psychological harm to patients who are told they have an aneurysm, even if it is too small to warrant surgery at the time of diagnosis.

Recently from the United Kingdom there is emerging evidence from prospective, randomized trials that screening for abdominal aortic aneurysms may be cost effective in men over the age of 65.[7,8] However at the moment both the Canadian Task Force on Preventive Health Care[9] and the U.S. Preventive Services Task Force[10] give both screening by abdominal palpation and with abdominal ultrasound a "C" recommendation.

❧ REFERENCES ❧

1. Lederle FA, Johnson GR, Wilson SE, et al: Prevalence and associations of abdominal aortic aneurysm detected through screening, *Ann Intern Med* 126:441-449, 1997.
2. Reed WW, Hallett JW Jr, Damiano MA, et al: Learning from the last ultrasound: a population-based study of patients with abdominal aortic aneurysm, *Arch Intern Med* 157:2064-2068, 1997.
3. Mason JM, Wakeman AP, Drummond MF, et al: Population screening for abdominal aortic aneurysm: do the benefits outweigh the costs? *J Public Health Med* 15:154-160, 1993.
4. Norman PE, Semmens JB, Lawrence-Brown MM, et al: Long term relative survival after surgery for abdominal aortic aneurysm in Western Australia: population based study, *BMJ* 317:852-856, 1998.
5. UK Small Aneurysm Trial Participants: Mortality results for randomised controlled trial of early elective surgery or ultrasonographic surveillance for small abdominal aortic aneurysms, *Lancet* 352:1649-1655, 1998.
6. D'Ayala M, Hollier LH, Marin ML: Endovascular grafting for abdominal aortic aneurysms, *Surg Clin North Am* 78:845-862, 1998.
7. Multicentre Aneurysm Screening Study Group: Multicentre aneurysm screening study (MASS): cost effectiveness analysis of screening for abdominal aortic aneurysms based on four year results from randomized controlled trial, *BMJ* 325:1135-1142, 2002.
8. Earnshaw JJ, Shaw E, Whyman MR, et al: Screening for abdominal aortic aneurysms in men, *BMJ* 328:1122-1124, 2004.
9. Canadian Task Force on the Periodic Health Examination: *Canadian guide to clinical preventive health care,* Ottawa, 1994, Canada Communication Group—Publishing, 672-678.
10. U.S. Preventive Services Task Force: *Guide to clinical preventive services,* ed 2, Baltimore, 1996, Williams & Wilkins, 67-72.

ARRHYTHMIAS

Atrial Fibrillation

(See also anticoagulants; subclinical hyperthyroidism; transient ischemic attacks)

Epidemiology and complications

The prevalence of atrial fibrillation (AF) in developed countries increases with age. Between 60 and 69 years of age the prevalence is 3% to 4%, whereas for those over 70 it is estimated to be 9%.[1] Most patients have underlying heart disease, such as coronary artery disease, valvular disease, or cardiomyopathy, or systemic disorders, such as excessive use of alcohol or alcohol withdrawal, hyperthyroidism, cocaine or amphetamine intoxication, electrolyte imbalance, or the post-operative state.

The major complication of AF is stroke. In the pooled data of five randomized trials of patients with AF, the annual risk of stroke in patients younger than 65 with no risk factors was 1%, whereas it was 8.1% in patients older than 75 with one or more risk factors. The risk was the same whether AF was constant or paroxysmal. Risk factors include prosthetic valves, previous strokes or transient ischemic attacks, diabetes, hypertension, and coronary artery disease.[2] The risk of stroke in patients with lone AF is very low.

A small pilot case-control study of patients who had non-valvular AF and were not taking anticoagulants found that those with fibrillation performed less well on a battery of neuropsychological tests than did control subjects with no fibrillation. The authors postulated that this may have been due to small subclinical cerebral infarcts in the group experiencing fibrillation.[3]

─────────── ❧ REFERENCES ❧ ───────────

1. Ezekowitz MD, Levine JA: Preventing stroke in patients with atrial fibrillation, *JAMA* 281:1830-1835, 1999.
2. Atrial Fibrillation Investigators: Risk factors for stroke and efficacy of antithrombotic therapy in atrial fibrillation: analysis of pooled data from five randomized controlled trials, *Arch Intern Med* 154:1449-1457, 1994.
3. O'Connell JE, Gray CS, French JM, et al: Atrial fibrillation and cognitive function: case-control study, *J Neurol Neurosurg Psychiatry* 65:386-389, 1998.

Rate control and cardioversion

The rapid rate that often occurs with AF can be controlled with pharmacological or electrical conversion to sinus rhythm, often with maintenance pharmacotherapy, or by rate control alone without attempting to convert to sinus rhythm. Although conversion to sinus rhythm might seem the optimal approach, this has not been proved to decrease morbidity or mortality. Furthermore, any antiarrhythmic drug may be toxic. Recent studies have shown little difference between a rate-control strategy and a strategy to restore sinus rhythm in patients with persistent AF.[1] The large and well-done AFFIRM trial showed that there was no significant difference between rate control and rhythm control of AF with respect to overall mortality when 4060 patients were randomized to one or the other. In general, patients taking antiarrhythmic medications had more adverse effects than those who were not. Risk for stroke was similar in both rate- and rhythm-control groups and was related to absence of adequate anticoagulation. It might now be preferable to manage AF with rate control and anticoagulation.[2]

If cardioversion is planned for new-onset AF, up to half the patients will revert to sinus rhythm spontaneously. The success of cardioversion by whatever means necessary is better if the arrhythmia is treated within 24 to 48 hours of onset.[3,4] A variety of pharmacological agents are effective for restoring sinus rhythm; all are potentially toxic. Examples are class IA agents such as quinidine or procainamide (Pronestyl), class IC agents such as flecainide (Tambocor) or propafenone (Rythmol), and the class III agent ibutilide (Corvert). Amiodarone (Cordarone) and sotalol (Betapace, Sotacor), which are also class III agents, do not appear to be effective in converting recent-onset AF. Digoxin (Lanoxin) is also ineffective for this purpose.[1] An alternative to pharmacological cardioversion is electrical rhythm reversion, which is effective in up to 90% of patients.[3]

Since one of the major complications of cardioversion by any method is systemic embolization, current guidelines advise anticoagulation before and after the procedure, even though scant evidence supports or refutes this approach.[4] The American College of Chest Physicians recommends that patients who have had fibrillation for more than 24 to 48 hours and who do not require emergency cardioversion be given anticoagulants for 3 weeks before cardioversion is undertaken and for 4 weeks after it has been accomplished.[5]

The value of attempting to maintain sinus rhythm with pharmacological agents is controversial. Without treatment, only about one fourth of patients who have successfully undergone cardioversion will remain in sinus rhythm after 1 year, whereas with maintenance antiarrhythmic drugs, about half will still be in sinus rhythm after 1 year.[3] Quinidine has been associated with an increased death rate and is no longer used for maintenance purposes. Unfortunately, all the other drugs also have adverse effects, and whether it is better to use maintenance pharmacotherapy or simply to control the rate and give anticoagulants is unknown.[3,4]

If anticoagulation and rate control are the goals of therapy, the drug of choice is a beta blocker or either of the calcium channel blockers verapamil (Isoptin, Calan) or diltiazem (Cardizem). Amiodarone also controls the AF rate in maintenance doses of about 200 mg/day, but it is not widely used because of potential adverse effects, especially pulmonary toxicity.[6] Digoxin is not a good drug for rate control; although it controls resting rate, it does not control the rate when sympathetic tone is increased, such as during acute illness, thyrotoxicosis, or exercise. For patients whose rate cannot be adequately controlled with medications, radio-frequency energy applied to the atrio-ventricular node via an intra-cardiac catheter may modify the node sufficiently to control the ventricular rate in 75% of cases; in the remainder, complete atrioventricular block results and a permanent pacemaker is required.[7]

─────────────── ◢ REFERENCES ◣ ───────────────

1. Van Gelder IC, et al: A comparison of rate control and rhythm control in patients with recurrent persistent atrial fibrillation, *N Engl J Med* 347(23):1834, Dec 5, 2002.
2. Wyse DG, Waldo AL, DiMarco JP, et al: the Atrial Fibrillation Follow-up Investigation of Rhythm Management (AFFIRM) Investigators: a comparison of rate control and rhythm control in patients with atrial fibrillation, *N Engl J Med* 347(23):1825-1833, 2002.
3. Masoudi FA, Goldschlager N: The medical management of atrial fibrillation, *Cardiol Clin* 15:689-719, 1997.
4. Jung F, DiMarco JP: Antiarrhythmic drug therapy in the treatment of atrial fibrillation, *Cardiol Clin* 14:507-520, 1996.
5. Laupacis A, Albers G, Dalen J, et al: Antithrombotic therapy in atrial fibrillation, *Chest* 108(suppl 4):352S-359S, 1995.
6. Antman EM: Maintaining sinus rhythm with antifibrillatory drugs in atrial fibrillation, *Am J Cardiol* 78(suppl 4):67-72, 1996.
7. Morady F: Radio-frequency ablation as treatment for cardiac arrhythmias, *N Engl J Med* 340:534-544, 1999.

Anticoagulation and Aspirin
(See also anticoagulants)

Numerous clinical trials have conclusively shown that warfarin (Coumadin) in doses adjusted to maintain the international normalized ratio (INR) between 2 and 3 helps to prevent stroke in patients with AF. Fixed low-dose warfarin that maintains INR levels below 2 is not effective, nor are combinations of fixed low-dose warfarin and Aspirin.[1]

The greatest risk with warfarin therapy is major hemorrhage, and this increases with age and INR levels above 3. In the Stroke Prevention in Atrial Fibrillation (SPAF) II trial the incidence of intracerebral hemorrhage was nearly high enough to offset the benefits, particularly in those over the age of 75, but in almost all cases where this occurred the INR was above 3.[2] A Danish study found that among patients receiving adjusted-dose warfarin aimed at maintaining the INR between 2 and 3, the annual rate of major bleeding was 1.1%, which was not significantly different from the rate in patients treated only with Aspirin. In this study, age was not a risk factor for major bleeding in patients taking warfarin.[3] Aside from INR above 3, recognized risk factors for hemorrhage are a past history of serious gastrointestinal bleed-

ing, alcoholism, use of NSAIDs, and poor compliance with medications. Risk of falling has often been seen as a contraindication to anticoagulation. According to one decision analysis, if possible falling is the only contraindication, the benefits of warfarin far outweigh the risks, even in those over 75 years of age.[4]

In general, an INR of 2 is equivalent to a prothrombin time (PT) of 1.3, an INR of 3 to a PT of 1.5, and an INR of 4 to a PT of 2.

An overview of studies that evaluated the role of Aspirin in preventing stroke in patients with AF concluded that although less effective than warfarin, Aspirin reduced the risk of stroke by about 21%, with no clear relationship to dose.[5] A 1999 meta-analysis of the Cochrane database came to similar conclusions about Aspirin but noted that it primarily prevented non-disabling strokes; benefits from warfarin were much greater than those achieved with Aspirin and were particularly marked in patients who had experienced a previous stroke or transient ischemic attack.[6]

The risk of stroke in patients with AF increases greatly if the patient is older than 75 years or has comorbid conditions such as a previous stroke or transient ischemic attack, coronary artery disease, heart failure, previous hypertension, diabetes, mitral stenosis, prosthetic heart valves, or thyrotoxicosis. The risk is particularly high if the patient has several of these comorbid conditions. Unless warfarin is strictly contraindicated, it should be given to patients with comorbid conditions.[1]

Patients with no risk factors and who are less than 75 years of age should be on ECASA 325 mg OD. Patients who are over 75 or have any of the following risk factors should be on warfarin to maintain INR between 2-3: congestive heart failure (CHF), left ventricular hypertrophy (LVH), hypertension, diabetes, previous stroke or embolism, or mitral valve disease.

─────────────── ◢ REFERENCES ◣ ───────────────

1. Albers GW: Choice of antithrombotic therapy for stroke prevention in atrial fibrillation: warfarin, aspirin, or both? *Arch Intern Med* 158:1487-1491, 1998.
2. Stroke Prevention in Atrial Fibrillation Investigators: Warfarin versus aspirin for prevention of thromboembolism in atrial fibrillation: Stroke Prevention in Atrial Fibrillation II Study, *Lancet* 343:687-691, 1994.
3. Gulløv AL, Koefoed BG, Petersen P: Bleeding during warfarin and aspirin therapy in patients with atrial fibrillation: the AFASAK 2 study, *Arch Intern Med* 159:1322-1328, 1999.
4. Man-Son-Hing M, Nichol G, Lau A, et al: Choosing antithrombotic therapy for elderly patients with atrial fibrillation who are at risk for falls, *Arch Intern Med* 159: 677-685, 1999.
5. Atrial Fibrillation Investigators: The efficacy of aspirin in patients with atrial fibrillation, *Arch Intern Med* 157: 1237-1240, 1997.

6. Hart RG, Benavente O, McBride R, et al: Antithrombotic therapy to prevent stroke in patients with atrial fibrillation: a meta-analysis, *Ann Intern Med* 131:492-501, 1999.
7. Kopecky SL, Gersh BJ, McGoon MD, et al: Lone atrial fibrillation in elderly persons: a marker for cardiovascular risk, *Arch Intern Med* 159:1118-1122, 1999.
8. Hellemons BS, Langenberg M, Lodder J, et al: Primary prevention of arterial thromboembolism in non-rheumatic atrial fibrillation in primary care: randomised controlled trial comparing two intensities of coumarin with aspirin, *BMJ* 319:958-964, 1999.
9. Ackermann RJ: Anticoagulant therapy in patients aged 80 years or more with atrial fibrillation: more caution is needed (editorial), *Arch Fam Med* 6:105-110, 1997.
10. English KM, Channer KS: Managing atrial fibrillation in elderly people (editorial), *BMJ* 318:1088-1089, 1999.

Paroxysmal Atrial Fibrillation

Paroxysmal AF makes up over 40% of cases of fibrillation, but it has not been as well studied as persistent AF. The evidence available indicates that it is prudent to treat paroxysmal AF in a manner identical to persistent AF.[1] Sotalol has generally been considered the drug of choice for paroxysmal AF, but a comparative crossover study of sotalol 80 mg twice a day and atenolol 50 mg once daily found that they were equally effective in diminishing the number and frequency of episodes of fibrillation.[2] Digoxin should not be used for patients with paroxysmal AF, since it does not reduce the frequency of episodes or control the heart rate during attacks. Digoxin is contraindicated in patients with Wolff-Parkinson-White syndrome.[3]

❧ REFERENCES ❧

1. Aboaf AP, Wolf PS: Paroxysmal atrial fibrillation: a common but neglected entity, *Arch Intern Med* 156:362-367, 1996.
2. Steeds RP, Birchall AS, Smith M, et al: An open label, randomised, crossover study comparing sotalol and atenolol in the treatment of symptomatic paroxysmal atrial fibrillation, *Heart* 82:170-175, 1999.
3. Masoudi FA, Goldschlager N: The medical management of atrial fibrillation, *Cardiol Clin* 15:689-719, 1997.

Supraventricular Arrhythmias
(See also palpitations)

Two thirds of cases of paroxysmal supraventricular tachycardia are atrioventricular nodal re-entrant tachycardias, and most of the remainder are due to an accessory atrioventricular pathway. Radio-frequency ablation under fluoroscopic control is effective and has few adverse effects in the vast majority of cases.[1,2] Radio-frequency ablation is also effective in patients with Wolff-Parkinson-White syndrome and in many cases of atrial flutter.[1]

❧ REFERENCES ❧

1. Morady F: Radio-frequency ablation as treatment for cardiac arrhythmias, *N Engl J Med* 340:534-544, 1999.
2. Calkins H, Yong P, Miller JM, et al: Catheter ablation of accessory pathways, atrioventricular nodal reentrant tachycardia, and the atrioventricular junction: final results of a prospective, multicentre clinical trial, *Circulation* 99:262-270, 1999.

Pacemakers and Implantable Defibrillators
(See also cardiac arrest)

Rapid advances in technology have led to the development of single-lead cardioverter-defibrillators. The generator for these devices is usually implanted in the left pectoral area, and access to the heart is obtained via the left subclavian vein. Cardioverter-defibrillators are used primarily for patients with life-threatening ventricular arrhythmias. The apparatus can sense heart rates and institute a variety of remedial manoeuvres. It can provide demand ventricular pacing in cases of bradycardia; when tachycardia is detected, it can institute competitive rapid pacing to interrupt the re-entry circuit, or if that fails, it can defibrillate the heart.[1] Comparative studies have shown that cardioverter-defibrillators are more effective than antiarrhythmic drugs.[1,2]

Patients with cardioverter-defibrillators are usually examined every 3 to 4 months in a cardiac electrophysiology laboratory where the device is "interrogated" by means of a wand placed over the generator.

Patients may detect shocks from the device. In general an isolated shock can be assessed electively in the cardiac laboratory, but repetitive shocks require emergency assessment.[1]

Most household electromagnetic devices such as microwave ovens do not adversely affect cardioverter-defibrillators, but large industrial motors and arc welding equipment may do so.[1] Cellular telephones can interfere with implanted pacemaker functions when held over the pacemaker, but holding the phone over the ear does not cause problems.[3]

Patients with implantable defibrillators have reportedly suffered syncope and shocks as a result of standing for a while close to electronic surveillance equipment in stores. Simply walking by the equipment seems to be safe.[4]

❧ REFERENCES ❧

1. Groh WJ, Foreman LD, Zipes D: Advances in the treatment of arrhythmias: implantable cardioverter-defibrillators, *Am Fam Physician* 57:297-307, 1998.
2. Antiarrhythmics Versus Implantable Defibrillators (AVID) Investigators: A comparison of antiarrhythmic drug therapy with implantable defibrillators in patients resuscitated from near-fatal ventricular arrhythmias, *N Engl J Med* 337:1576-1583, 1997.
3. Hayes DL, Wang PJ, Reynolds DW, et al: Interference with cardiac pacemakers by cellular telephones, *N Engl J Med* 336:1473-1479, 1997.

4. Santucci PA, Haw J, Trohman RG, et al: Interference with an implantable defibrillator by an electronic antitheft-surveillance device, *N Engl J Med* 339:1371-1374, 1998.

Palpitations

Palpitations are common presenting complaints in primary care; in one general medical outpatient clinic they were noted in 16% of patients.[1] In a Harvard study of 130 patients who were referred for Holter monitoring because of palpitations, the group had a 28% lifetime prevalence of panic disorder, which was six times the rate in control subjects.[2]

Although anxiety disorders may cause palpitations, paroxysmal supraventricular tachycardia may mimic the symptoms of panic disorder.[3] In one study of patients with confirmed supraventricular tachycardia, two thirds of the patients met the criteria for panic disorder given in the *Diagnostic and Statistical Manual of Mental Disorders*, edition 4 (*DSM-IV*). Frequent symptoms included dizziness, shortness of breath, sweating, chest pain, fear of dying, flushing, tremulousness, and numbness. After definitive therapy, usually radio-frequency ablation, only 11% of patients whose symptoms had originally fulfilled the diagnostic criteria of panic disorder continued to experience such symptoms.[3]

The diagnosis of paroxysmal supraventricular tachycardia is usually easy if an electrocardiogram (ECG) can be obtained during an episode; otherwise it is difficult. The resting ECG of some patients may exhibit the delta wave typical of Wolff-Parkinson-White syndrome, but this is relatively uncommon. Holter monitoring, which records and saves all data over a 24-hour period, detects only a few cases because most patients do not have episodes of tachycardia during the monitoring period.[3] An alternative is the continuous-loop recorder, which the patient wears for up to 2 weeks. Data are monitored continuously but are saved for later analysis only if the patient manually activates the system when symptoms occur.[4]

Most ambulatory patients investigated for palpitations are found to have either normal sinus rhythm or benign atrial or ventricular ectopy. The treatment of choice for these conditions is reassurance; in a few instances beta blockers are needed. A CBC and sTSH should be done on all patients to rule out secondary causes of palpitations. Consider testing for pheochromocytoma. If the patient is on diuretics or ACE inhibitors, check the serum potassium. Most cases of supraventricular tachycardia and several variants of ventricular tachycardia are curable with radiofrequency ablation.[4]

—————————— ❧ **REFERENCES** ❧ ——————————

1. Kroenke K, Arrington ME, Mangelsdorff AD: The prevalence of symptoms in medical outpatients and the adequacy of therapy, *Arch Intern Med* 150:1685-1689, 1990.

2. Barsky AJ, Cleary PD, Coeytaux RR, et al: The clinical course of palpitations in medical outpatients, *Arch Intern Med* 155:1782-1788, 1995.

3. Lessmeier TJ, Gamperling D, Johnson V, et al: Unrecognized paroxysmal supraventricular tachycardia: potential for misdiagnosis as panic disorder, *Arch Intern Med* 157:537-543, 1997.

4. Zimetbaum P, Josephson ME: Evaluation of patients with palpitations, *N Engl J Med* 338:1369-1373, 1998.

ASPIRIN

(See also anemia; angina; asthma; asthma in children; atrial fibrillation; colon cancer; coronary artery disease; gout; migraines; myocardial infarction; niacin; non-steroidal anti-inflammatory drugs; peptic ulcer; thrombophlebitis; transient ischaemic attacks)

Aspirin has multiple reputed and proven benefits. It is also well known to have adverse effects on the gastrointestinal tract and to precipitate asthma in susceptible persons. Only a few of these topics are discussed here; others can be found elsewhere in the text.

Prevention of Neoplasms

Evidence is mixed that regular Aspirin use decreases the risk of several types of cancer. The most striking initially was colon cancer. However, a larger Physicians Health Study showed no advantage after 5 years of regular use,[1] but a more recent trial showed benefit for patients with a history of colorectal cancer and possibly adenomas. Use of Aspirin by patients without a history of adenomas or colorectal cancer solely to prevent colorectal cancer is not supported by the data, given the risks of major gastrointestinal hemorrhage (number needed to harm [NNH] = 300 to 800) or stroke (NNH = 800) with 5 years of Aspirin use. If a patient is already taking Aspirin to reduce the risk of cardiovascular disease (CVD), though, this study provides some proof of added benefit.[2]

Other cancer sites where regular Aspirin use is said to reduce risk are the esophagus, stomach, rectum, lung, and breast.[3,4] The absolute reduction rates are low, and whether potential benefits outweigh risks has not been established.

Pathophysiology of Antithrombotic Effect

Aspirin acetylates platelet prostaglandin G/H synthase, causing an irreversible loss of its cyclooxygenase activity. Cyclooxygenase is necessary for the formation of thromboxane A_2, which in turn causes platelet aggregation. This effect is produced within 1 hour by the oral ingestion of 100 mg of Aspirin. However, Aspirin also reversibly inhibits endothelial cell prostacyclin, a potent inhibitor of platelet aggregation. Some workers have hypothesized that lower doses of acetylsalicylic acid given at longer intervals may be the most effective prophylactic program against thromboembolic phenomena because they will cause less inhibition of endothelial prostacyclin.[5]

Gastrointestinal Bleeding

One of the major adverse effects of Aspirin is an increased incidence of gastrointestinal bleeding. An increased incidence of clinically significant bleeding episodes has been documented even with daily doses as low as 75[6] or 100 mg.[7] The 100-mg study emanating from Australia enrolled 400 men and women with an age range of 70 to 90 years.[5] Over a 1-year period the total percentage of overt bleeding episodes was 3% in treated patients versus none in the control group. In addition, the hemoglobin concentration of the treated group dropped by a mean of 0.33 g/dl (33 g/L), which was statistically significant, but more important, 17.4% of the Aspirin-treated group had a reduction of 1 g/dl (100 g/L) or more compared with 9.3% of the control subjects. The mean corpuscular volume increased in the treated group compared with the placebo group, perhaps because of an increase in reticulocytes. Gastrointestinal symptoms were reported by 18% of those taking Aspirin and by 12.5% of those given placebo.[7] Similar results have been reported in a Canadian study.[8]

In a British case-controlled study, the odds ratio for bleeding peptic ulcer disease in patients taking regular doses of Aspirin was 2.3 for 75 mg/day, 3.2 for 150 mg/day, and 3.9 for 300 mg/day. For enteric-coated Aspirin it was only 1.1.[9]

Hemorrhagic Stroke

A 1998 meta-analysis found that Aspirin was associated with an absolute increase in hemorrhagic strokes of 12:10,000 users.[10] In view of this it seems prudent to use Aspirin prophylactically for individuals at high risk of CVD but to refrain from using it as a primary preventive measure for those at low risk.[11]

Aspirin Sensitivity

Aspirin sensitivity with bronchospasm that is not allergic or IgE-mediated occurs in about 20% of persons with asthma.[12]

─────────────── ◢ **REFERENCES** ◣ ───────────────

1. Sturmer T, Glynn RJ, Lee IM, et al: Aspirin use and colorectal cancer: post-trial follow-up data from the physicians' health study, *Ann Intern Med* 1998:128:713-720.
2. Baron JA, Cole BF, Sandler RS, et al: A randomized trial of aspirin to prevent colorectal adenomas, *N Engl J Med* 348:891-899, 2003.
3. Thun MJ, Namboodiri MM, Calle EE, et al: Aspirin use and risk of fatal cancer, *Cancer Res* 53:60-74, 1993.
4. Schreinemachers DM, Everson RB: Aspirin use and lung, colon, and breast cancer incidence in a prospective study, *Epidemiology* 5:138-146, 1994.
5. Patrono C: Aspirin as an antiplatelet drug, *N Engl J Med* 330:1287-1294, 1994.
6. SALT Collaborative Group: Swedish aspirin low-dose trial (SALT) of 75 mg aspirin as secondary prophylaxis after cerebrovascular ischaemic events, *Lancet* 338:1345-1349, 1991.
7. Silagy CA, McNeil JJ, Donnan GA, et al: Adverse effects of low-dose aspirin in a healthy elderly population, *Clin Pharmacol Ther* 54:84-89, 1993.
8. Leibovici A, Lavi N, Wainstok S, et al: Low-dose acetylsalicylic acid use and hemoglobin levels: effects in a primary care population, *Can Fam Physician* 41:64-68, 1995.
9. Weil J, Colinjones D, Langman M, et al: Prophylactic aspirin and risk of peptic ulcer bleeding, *BMJ* 310:827-830, 1995.
10. He J, Whelton PK, Vu B, et al: Aspirin and risk of hemorrhagic stroke: a meta-analysis of randomized controlled trials, *JAMA* 280:1930-1935, 1998.
11. Boissel J-P: Individualizing aspirin therapy for prevention of cardiovascular events (editorial), *JAMA* 280:1949-1950, 1998.
12. Manning ME, Stevenson DD: Aspirin sensitivity: a distressing reaction that is now often treatable, *Postgrad Med* 90:227-233, 1991.

CARDIAC ARREST

(See also aviation medicine; exercise; heart failure; informed consent; pacemakers and implantable defibrillators; sports medicine; sudden infant death syndrome)

Sudden cardiac arrest claims 350,000 to 450,000 lives per year in the United States alone and is responsible for more than half of all deaths that are due to CVD. Our ability to recognize patients who are at high risk for cardiac arrest has improved, but 90% of cases of sudden death from cardiac causes occur in patients without identified risk factors. Although the majority of these cases of sudden death involve patients with pre-existing coronary heart disease, cardiac arrest is the first manifestation of this underlying problem in 50% of patients.[1] Ventricular arrhythmia resulting from coronary artery disease causes 80% of sudden cardiac deaths. Beta blockers have a significant protective effect against this event in both hypertensive and post-myocardial infarction (MI) patients.[2] Beta blockers are also protective against sudden cardiac death in patients with CHF.[3] For patients with previous documented Brugada syndrome, ventricular tachycardia, or ventricular fibrillation, an implantable cardioverter-defibrillator is generally the treatment of choice.[3]

Patients with hereditary or acquired Long Q-T syndrome as well as patients with re-entry arrhythmias such as Wolff-Parkinson-White (WPW) syndrome should be identified and treated to avoid sudden cardiac death in the otherwise young and healthy patient.[4] Numerous cohort studies have examined the relationship of fish consumption and sudden cardiac death. Most have shown a decrease in sudden cardiac deaths among those who ate fish as infrequently as once a week or even once a month, but no decrease in non-fatal cardiac events. A plausible explanation is that n-3 polyunsaturated fatty acids or some other component of fish is antiarrhythmic.

On the basis of this evidence it seems reasonable to recommend that everyone eat fish once a week and that patients with cardiac disease have two helpings of fish a week.[4] Moderate leisure activity such as walking or gardening has also been shown to decrease the risk of primary cardiac arrest.[5]

Hospitalized elderly patients with acute medical problems have a 10% to 17% chance of surviving to discharge after a cardiopulmonary resuscitation (CPR), although if they have chronic illnesses associated with a life expectancy of less than 1 year, their chance is less than 5%.[6] Some studies have found that even after a successful resuscitation, close to half the survivors have significant residual functional deficits,[7] whereas other studies report that 75% of survivors are able to live independently.[8]

Patients grossly overestimate their chances of recovery; in requesting advance directives, physicians and hospitals must give them accurate data so that they can give reasonable informed consent.[6] A factor contributing to their overly optimistic expectations of CPR may be the messages received from U.S. television programs such as *ER, Chicago Hope,* and *Rescue 911,* which portray an inordinately high success rate for resuscitation.[9] The major British medical television dramas *Casualty, Cardiac Arrest,* and *Medics* seem to give a more realistic perspective on the outcomes of this intervention.[10]

The results of resuscitation in nursing homes are abysmal, with virtually no long-term survivors. For the very few who survive to discharge, quality of life is awful.[11]

Reported overall survival rates after cardiac arrests outside of hospitals vary from 1.4% to 18%.[12] Results are slightly better if a bystander has initiated CPR[12,13] but markedly better if the arrest was witnessed by paramedics equipped with defibrillators.[13] A Scottish study found that about 40% of patients who had been successfully resuscitated away from a hospital were discharged without significant neurological sequelae.[14] Current evidence suggests that although both ventilation and external chest compression should be given in cases of arrest outside the hospital, chest compression alone can give good results.[12]

The automatic external defibrillator is a recent advance in CPR. This device, which is applied to a patient with no clinically detected pulse, senses cardiac rhythm and, if it detects a rapid ventricular tachycardia or ventricular fibrillation, automatically delivers a countershock.[12] A 2004 study found that citizens knowing CPR was the most helpful intervention, and rapid-defibrillation responses are a second priority for the resources of emergency-medical-services systems.[1]

A study from the Hospital for Sick Children in Toronto found that only 15% of children with out-of-hospital cardiac or respiratory arrests who were resuscitated in the emergency room survived to discharge and that all of the survivors were left with neurological deficits. The authors concluded that except for cases of severe hypothermia or episodes of recurrent (as opposed to persistent) arrest, continuation of resuscitation for out-of-hospital cardiac arrests is futile after 20 minutes or after the two doses of epinephrine have been administered.[15]

Most advance directives made by ambulatory patients are inaccessible to the health care team when a patient is transferred to a hospital and are therefore not used.[16]

❧ REFERENCES ❧

1. Stiel AG, Wells GA, et al: Advanced cardiac life support in out-of-hospital cardiac arrest, *N Engl J Med* 351:7, 647-656, 2004.
2. Kendall MJ, Lynch KP, Hjalmarson A, et al: Beta-blockers and sudden cardiac death, *Ann Intern Med* 123:358-367, 1995.
3. Goldberger JJ: Treatment and prevention of sudden cardiac death: effect of recent clinical trials, *Arch Intern Med* 159: 1281-1287, 1999.
4. Walker B: Congenital and acquired LQTS, *Can J Cardiol* 19:76-87, 2003.
5. Kromhout D: Fish consumption and sudden cardiac death (editorial), *JAMA* 279:65-66, 1998.
6. Lemaitre RN, Siscovick DS, Raghunathan TE, et al: Leisure-time physical activity and the risk of primary cardiac arrest, *Arch Intern Med* 159:686-690, 1999.
7. Murphy DJ, Burrows D, Santilli S, et al: The influence of the probability of survival on patients' preferences regarding cardiopulmonary resuscitation, *N Engl J Med* 330:545-549, 1994.
8. FitzGerald JD, Wenger NS, Califf RM, et al: Functional status among survivors of in-hospital cardiopulmonary resuscitation, *Arch Intern Med* 156:72-76, 1996.
9. de Vos R, de Haes HC, Koster RW, et al: Quality of survival after cardiopulmonary resuscitation, *Arch Intern Med* 159:249-254, 1999.
10. Diem SJ, Lantos JD, Tulsky JA: Cardiopulmonary resuscitation on television: miracles and misinformation, *N Engl J Med* 334:1578-1582, 1996.
11. Gordon PN, Williamson S, Lawler PG: As seen on TV: observational study of cardiopulmonary resuscitation in British television medical dramas, *BMJ* 317:780-783, 1998.
12. Awoke S, Mouton CP, Parrott M: Outcomes of skilled cardiopulmonary resuscitation in a long-term-care facility: futile therapy? *J Am Geriatr Soc* 40:593-595, 1992.
13. Ballew KA: Cardiopulmonary resuscitation, *BMJ* 324:1462-1465, 1997.
14. Norris RM (United Kingdom Heart Attack Study Collaborative Group): Fatality outside hospital from acute coronary events in three British health districts, 1994-5, *BMJ* 316:1065-1070, 1998.
15. Cobbe SM, Dalziel K, Ford I, et al: Survival of 1476 patients initially resuscitated from out of hospital cardiac arrest, *BMJ* 312:1633-1637, 1996.
16. Schindler MB, Bohn D, Cox PN, et al: Outcome of out-of-hospital cardiac or respiratory arrest in children, *N Engl J Med* 335:1473-1479, 1996.

17. Morrison RS, Olson E, Mertz KR, et al: The inaccessibility of advance directives on transfer from ambulatory to acute care settings, *JAMA* 274:478-482, 1995.

CARDIOMYOPATHY

Cardiomyopathies are diseases of the myocardium associated with cardiac dysfunction.[1,2] They can be divided into the following categories: dilated, hypertrophic, restrictive, right ventricular, and unclassified.[2] Dilated and hypertrophic cardiomyopathies will be discussed in this section.

Hypertrophic Cardiomyopathy

Hypertrophic cardiomyopathy is a genetic disorder characterized by disproportionate hypertrophy of the left ventricle, and occasionally the right ventricle. Cardiac hypertrophy with resulting ventricular dysfunction can also be acquired, with hypertension and aortic stenosis being the most common etiologies.[1,2]

In recent years, the diagnosis of asymptomatic hypertrophic cardiomyopathy through molecular genetic assays has become possible. As a result of such studies, it is clear that the disorder is more common (1:500) than was previously thought and that most patients have no or only mild symptoms.[3]

Hypertrophic cardiomyopathy is not always a progressive disease, and in some patients the symptoms abate over time. Prognostic indicators of a more severe course are advanced symptoms at the time of diagnosis, AF, basal outflow obstruction, severe ventricular hypertrophy, non-sustained ventricular tachycardia on Holter monitoring, family history of premature deaths from this disorder, and prior cardiac arrest.[3]

The drugs of choice for patients with hypertrophic cardiomyopathy who are in heart failure are beta blockers or verapamil. Both slow the heart, and the prolonged diastole allows increased filling of the ventricles. However, these drugs do not protect patients against sudden death.[4] Prophylactic drugs have not shown value in asymptomatic or mildly symptomatic patients. These patients should be encouraged to lead normal lives, but intense physical training or competitive athletics should probably be discouraged.[4] A few patients appear to benefit from antiarrhythmic agents such as amiodarone implantable cardioverter-defibrillators, or heart transplants.[3]

Dilated Cardiomyopathy

Dilated cardiomyopathies involve dilatation of one or both ventricles, along with impaired contraction. Physiologic compensation for the dilatation is invariably accompanied with ventricular hypertrophy. Patients affected with this condition have impaired systolic function and may present with overt heart failure, arrhythmias, or even sudden death.[2] Upon clinical presentation, heart failure is usually advanced.[5]

Idiopathic dilated cardiomyopathy is the major indication for heart transplantation in both adults and children. The condition is 2.5 times as common in males as in females, and 2.5 times as common in African-Americans as in whites. The disorder may develop in children or the elderly, but most patients are between 20 and 50 years of age.[6]

The prognosis of dilated cardiomyopathy is variable. Some patients remain stable for years, and others have a progressive downhill course. The average 5-year mortality is about 20%.[5] An observational cohort study found that adding metoprolol to the usual treatment with angiotensin-converting enzyme (ACE) inhibitors and diuretics reduced mortality and the need for cardiac transplantation.[7]

─────────── ❧ REFERENCES ❧ ───────────

1. Richardson P, Chairman: Report of the 1995 World Health Organization/International Society and Federation of Cardiology Task Force on the Definition and Classificatino of the Cardiomyopathies, *Circulation* 93:841, 1996.
2. Cooper LT: Definition and classification of the cardiomyopathies. In Rose BD, ed: *UpToDate,* Wellesley, MA, 2004.
3. Maron BJ, Casey SA, Poliac LC, et al: Clinical course of hypertrophic cardiomyopathy in a regional United States cohort, *JAMA* 281:650-655, 1999.
4. Spirito P, Seidman CE, McKenna WJ, et al: The management of hypertrophic cardiomyopathy, *N Engl J Med* 336:775-785, 1997.
5. Dec GW, Fuster V: Idiopathic dilated cardiomyopathy, *N Engl J Med* 331:1564-1575, 1994.
6. Barbaro G, Di Lorenzo G, Grisorio B, et al: Incidence of dilated cardiomyopathy and detection of HIV in myocardial cells of HIV-positive patients, *N Engl J Med* 339:1093-1099, 1998.
7. Di Lenarda A, Gavazzi MA, Gregori D, et al: Long term survival effect of metoprolol in dilated cardiomyopathy, *Heart* 79:337-344, 1998.

CONGENITAL HEART DISEASE
(See also pediatric heart murmur)

Epidemiology

The incidence of moderate and severe congenital heart disease (CHD) is about 6/1,000 live births. If minor cardiac lesions such as tiny muscular ventricular septal defects (VSDs) are included, the incidence is 75/1,000 live births.[1]

Risk factors include[2]:
- Chromosomal defects. Some are associated with severe congenital heart disease (e.g., trisomy 13 or 18), while others tend to cause more mild defects (e.g., Turner's syndrome and trisomy 21).
- Maternal illness (e.g., diabetes mellitus, systemic lupus erythematosus (SLE), rubella).
- Environmental exposure (e.g., to thalidomide, isotretinoin, or alcohol [fetal alcohol syndrome]).

The most common forms are[2]:
- Atrial septal defect (6% to 10% of CHD)
- Ventricular septal defect (0.5% of CHD)
- Atrioventricular canal defect (5% of CHD)
- Tetralogy of Fallot
- Transposition of the great arteries (5% to 7% of CHD)
- Patent ductus arteriosus
- Coarctation of the aorta (7% to 8% of CHD)

Atrial Septal Defect

Atrial septal defect (ASD) presents in children as a systolic flow murmur with splitting of S2, with typical onset after 1 year of age. Presentation in adults may include dyspnea on exertion, supraventricular arrthythmias, and right-sided heart failure.

Treatment is expectant for small defects, but closure of the defect is the treatment of choice for hemodynamically significant defects or in the presence of pulmonary hypertension.[3] Closure may include surgical repair or use of a patch (either from the patient's own pericardium or a synthetic patch). Family physicians should note that closure of the defect, especially later in life, does not necessarily prevent arrhythmia or stroke.

Ventricular Septal Defect

Small VSDs present with loud pansystolic murmurs early in infancy. Larger VSDs may not present until later, when there is more significant left-to-right shunting, and heart failure may occur. Heart failure is controlled medically to allow time for the VSD to close spontaneously. Surgical treatment is indicated for VSDs that fail to close or if refractory heart failure or other significant complications exist. Endocarditis prophylaxis is important.

Tetralogy of Fallot

The tetralogy of Fallot includes right-ventricular outflow-tract obstruction with ventricular septal defect. This allows unoxygenated blood to pass into the left ventricle. Treatment is surgical repair in early infancy, which often leads to significant pulmonary regurgitation (which may in turn lead to right-ventricular failure and an increased risk of atrial or ventricular tachycardia later in life). Often, pulmonary valve replacement is necessary, and some patients require ablation of abnormal electrical foci related to sugical scars.[4]

Transposition of the Great Arteries

An infant with this condition presents early after birth with severe cyanosis. Surgical treatment until the last decade mostly involved an atrial switch, where pulmonary venous return is diverted into the right ventricle and systemic venous return is diverted into the left ventricle.[4] Because the right ventricle must handle the systemic circulation, long-term sequelae (in adults) may include right-ventricular dysfunction and tricuspid regurgitation.[5] Damage to the sinus node may lead to atrial flutter.[5] Some patients may require heart transplantation. More recently, surgical repair has involved transposing back the great arteries.[4] Long-term outcomes from this procedure are not yet known.

Patent Ductus Arteriosus

Patent ductus arteriosus (PDA) is most common in premature infants, but it may also be diagnosed in full-term babies after 1 to 2 months, when it typically presents with a continuous murmur at the left sternal border.[2] Treatment in early childhood includes indomethacin and/or surgical ligation; surgery is necessary if manifestations of heart failure are present.[2]

PDA may not present until later in life. A small PDA may cause only a faint murmur, but may still increase the risk of endocarditis. Larger lesions, with more extensive left-to-right shunting, may lead to left ventricular dilatation, AF, and eventually, to pulmonary hypertension. Treatment in adults generally involves a transcatheter device, which significantly reduces the risk of endocarditis.[7] Surgery is required for ducts greater than 8 mm. Following treatment, patients should have periodic echocardiograms (ECGs) to monitor for reopening of the PDA.[4]

Coarctation of the Aorta

Coarctation of the aorta may present with sudden heart failure in infants when the ductus closes after birth. In older children and adults, presentation involves hypertension in the upper extremities with a bruit in the pulmonic area.

Treatment involves balloon dilatation with stenting, or surgical repair. Family physicians should be aware that even with repair, hypertension and even recurrence of the coarctation or aneurysm at the repair site may occur.[8] Ongoing monitoring should include monitoring for hypertension and periodic imaging to look for local complications.

◢ REFERENCES ◣

1. Hoffman JI, Kaplan S: The incidence of congenital heart disease, *J Am Coll Cardiol* 39(12):1890-1900, Jun 19 2002.
2. Congenital Heart Disease. In: Beers MH, Berkow R, eds: *The Merck manual of diagnosis and therapy,* ed 17, Whitehouse Station, 1999, Merck Research Laboratories, 2198.
3. Konstantinides S, Geibel A, Olschewski M, et al: A comparison of surgical and medical therapy for atrial septal defect in adults, *N Engl J Med* 333: 469-473, 1995.
4. Therrien J, Webb G: Clinical update on adults with congenital heart disease, *Lancet* 362: 1305-1313, 2003.
5. Wilson NJ, Clarkson PM, Barratt-Boyes BG, et al: Long term outcome after the Mustard repair for simple transposition of the great arteries: 28 year followup, *J Am Coll Cardiol* 32(3):758-765, 998.

6. Gelatt M, Hamilton RM, McCrindle BW, et al: Arrhythmia and mortality after the Mustard procedure: a 30 year single centre experience, *J Am Coll Cardiol* 29: 194-201, 1997.

7. Landzberg MJ, Bridges ND, Perry SB, et al: Transcatheter occlusion: the treatment of choice for the adult with a patent ductus arteriosus, *Circulation* 84 (suppl 2): 67, 1999.

8. Therrien J, Gatzoulis M, Graham T, et al: Canadian Cardiovascular Society: CCS Consensus Conference 2001 Update – recommendations for the management of adults with congenital heart disease (part 2), *Can J Cardiol* 18: 1029-1050, 2001.

CORONARY ARTERY DISEASE

(See also cardiac arrest; gastroesophageal reflux)

Overall Vascular Risk Reduction

When this chapter was first written, separation of the cardiac conditions was becoming increasingly important because each had different therapeutic modalities. However, while this is true, the current paradigm is switching to one of overall "vascular risk reduction." For example, with diabetes, previously physicians and patients spent considerable time focusing on lowering blood sugar. However, recent trials have shown that blood pressure and cholesterol are actually more important from an outcomes perspective, and that perhaps we shouldn't think of one as more important than the other, but rather that we have to target all three. The same is true in the prevention of diabetes; the key interventions are losing 5% to 7% of weight, reducing fat intake, increasing fibre, and being more active. This is clearly the same advice you would offer almost any patient with heart disease.

Over the last three decades the mortality rate from coronary artery disease (CAD) has decreased by 2% to 4% per year in the United States. About one fourth of the decline can be attributed to primary prevention and three fourths to secondary prevention and improved treatment.[1]

------------------------ ◙ **REFERENCES** ◙ ------------------------

1. Huang ES, Meigs JB, Singer DE: The effects of interventions to prevent cardiovascular disease in patients with type 2 diabetes mellitus, *Am J Med* 111:663-642, 2001.

2. Tuomilehto J, et al: Prevention of type 2 diabetes mellitus by changes in lifestyle among subjects with impaired glucose tolerance, *N Engl J Med* 344:1343-1350, 2001.

3. Hunink MG, Goldman L, Tosteson AN, et al: The recent decline in mortality from coronary heart disease, 1980-1990: the effect of secular trends in risk factors and treatment, *JAMA* 277:535-542, 1997.

Risk Factors for Coronary Artery Disease

(See also cardiac arrest; exercise; gastroesophageal reflux; hypertension; lipids; menopause; myocardial infarction; obesity; polycystic ovarian syndrome; poverty; smoking; vitamins)

The single biggest risk for coronary artery disease is being human. As Rose[1] pointed out, the most common cause of death in men with no apparent risk factors for coronary artery disease is coronary artery disease, and coronary artery disease is also the leading cause of death among U.S. women. Women tend to acquire coronary artery disease 10 years later than men, but once women have had an MI, their overall prognosis is worse than that of men. Female diabetics are more prone to coronary artery disease than are male diabetics, and women smokers have a higher risk of coronary artery disease than do men smokers.[2-4]

Another important risk factor is poverty and work status. Epidemiological evidence also suggests that diets low in fish or fibre (fruits, vegetables, and particularly cereals) and the presence of peripheral vascular disease are risk factors.[5-7] Children with homocystinuria have marked elevations of plasma homocysteine and suffer from premature vascular disease.[8]

Emerging Markers of Heart Disease Risk

Increasing evidence indicates that inflammation plays an important role in the development of atherosclerosis, and some studies have suggested that infection with *Chlamydia pneumoniae,* cytomegalovirus, or *Helicobacter pylori* may be the etiological factor responsible for such inflammation.[9] We still await patient-oriented evidence to support the use of these inflammatory markers in practice but the fact that at least 50% of emergency patients having MIs demonstrate normal cholesterol and/or triglyceride levels has raised interest in other possible markers of CAD. These include the following[10]:

Apolipoprotein A-I/II: found in high-density lipoprotein (HDL); play major roles in the removal of excess cholesterol from the tissues. The Apolipoprotein A's are useful in characterizing patients with genetic disorders that lead to low HDL levels.

Apolipoprotein B: the most abundant protein in low-density lipoprotein (LDL). Elevated levels of Apolipoprotein B have long been associated with increased risk for CAD, even in the presence of normal cholesterol levels. Apolipoprotein B analysis may be especially useful in assessing the number and size of LDL particles and provides more information than total LDL analysis in the prediction and risk of Ischemic Heart Disease (IHD).

High-sensitivity C-reactive protein: With respect to CVD risk prediction, individuals should be divided into the following risk categories:

- Less than 1 mg/L Low Risk
- 1 to 3 mg/L Average Risk
- Over 3 mg/L High Risk

Subjects with intermediate risk; that is, 10% to 20% 10-year CHD risk may benefit from CRP measurement, in that values over 3 mg/L might be used to increase intensity of evaluation and management. Those with over 20% 10-year CHD risk already qualify for intensive management.[11]

A number of epidemiological studies have documented an association between elevated plasma homocysteine levels (normal fasting levels are 5 to 15 µmol/L) and CAD, cerebrovascular accidents, and peripheral vascular disease. However, we await good evidence (apparently the trials are ongoing) that treating a high homocysteine, typically with folic acid, makes a difference in the patient's cardiac outcomes. Some clinicians do the test on patients with premature CAD and those with a very strong family history. The initial recommendation to treat elevated homocysteine levels is a diet rich in folic acid and vitamins B_6 and B_{12}. If that is ineffective, multivitamins containing 400 µg of folic acid, 2 mg of vitamin B_6, and 6 mg of vitamin B_{12} are prescribed.[12]

Psychosocial factors may alter risk factors for CAD by affecting health-related behaviours such as smoking and exercise, which in most studies are considered to be confounding variables, through direct pathophysiological changes, or by altering access to and quality of medical care. A systematic review of prospective cohort studies suggests that type A personality, hostility, depression, anxiety, work stress, and poor social supports are associated with increased risk of CAD. Among patients with known CAD, all these factors except type A personality are associated with a worse prognosis.[13]

Detection of Risk

Many available risk calculators typically utilize some component of the data from the Framingham study.[8] However, a recent European version based on a different population points out the limitations of the Framingham, in that it over-predicts in some populations (e.g., Europeans with low or medium levels of disease incidence) and can under-predict in others (e.g,. Southeast Asians). Additionally, it likely underestimates the importance of diabetes, raised triglyceride levels, and individuals with a family history of premature CAD or hyperlipidemia. Social factors such as poverty and job control and responsibility are hard to model.[14]

A risk analysis is helpful and contextualizes care. (See www.cebm.net/prognosis.asp, http://www.escardio.org, or www.riskscore.org.uk.) Questions remain about how patients perceive analyses or use them as motivation to improve self-management.[15]

Primary Prevention of Coronary Artery Disease

(See also alcohol; Aspirin; cardiac arrest; exercise; hormone replacement therapy; hypertension; lipids; obesity; relative risk reduction; risk factors for coronary artery disease; smoking; vitamin E)

Standard recommendations for the prevention of CAD depend on risk, and targets vary slightly depending on the country. Recent guidelines (PRODIGY 2003 guidelines for managing and detecting coronary artery

disease risk. Accessed at www.prodigy.nhs.uk August 4, 2003) suggest the following:

For people with diagnosed CHD, stroke, transient ischemic attacks, or peripheral vascular disease:

- Advice about how to stop smoking, including advice on the use of nicotine replacement therapy, and bupropion.
- Information about other modifiable risk factors and personalized advice about how they can be reduced, including advice about physical activity, diet, alcohol consumption, weight, and diabetes.
- Advice and treatment to maintain blood pressure (BP) below 140/85 mm Hg. People with diabetes should maintain their BP below 130/85 mm Hg, or below 135/75 mm Hg in the presence of microalbuminuria or proteinuria.
- Low-dose Aspirin. This can be the typical dose of 375 mg daily. For those who do not tolerate this dose the evidence is just as powerful for lower doses (75 or 81 mg daily). Other antiplatelet therapy is warranted if patient is hypersensitive to aspirin.
- Statins and dietary advice to lower serum total cholesterol by 20% to 25% or to reduce it below 5.0 mmol/L, whichever would result in the lower level. (Serum LDL cholesterol should be lowered by 30% or reduced to below 3.0 mmol/L, whichever would result in the lower level.)
- ACE inhibitors for people who also have left ventricular dysfunction. Note that beta blockers and spironolactone may also be added to therapy. Angiotensin 2 receptor antagonists are an alternative in people who are intolerant of ACE inhibitors.
- Beta blockers and ACE inhibitors for people who have had an MI.
- Warfarin or Aspirin for people over 60 years old who have AF. Note that the final choice depends on the individual's overall risk of stroke.
- Meticulous control of BP, cholesterol, and glucose in people who also have diabetes.

People with a 10-year CHD risk of more than 30% but who do not have CHD:

- Advice about how to stop smoking, including advice on the use of nicotine replacement therapy and bupropion.
- Information about other modifiable risk factors and personalized advice about how they can be reduced, including advice about physical activity, diet, alcohol consumption, weight, and diabetes.
- Advice and treatment to maintain blood pressure (BP) below 140/85 mm Hg. People with diabetes should maintain their BP below 140/80 mm Hg, or below 135/75 mm Hg in the presence of microalbuminuria or proteinuria.
- Low-dose Aspirin (75 mg daily) for those aged 50 years or over with a 10-year CHD risk greater than 15%, or people with diabetes, or people with target

organ damage.[15a] Note: only use other antiplatelet therapy if the individual is hypersensitive to aspirin.

- Statins and dietary advice to lower serum total cholesterol by 20% to 25% or to reduce it to below 5.0 mmol/L, whichever would result in the lower level. (Lower the serum LDL cholesterol by 30% or reduce to below 3.0 mmol/L, whichever would result in the lower level.)
- Meticulous control of BP and glucose in people who also have diabetes.

People with a calculated CHD risk of 15% to 30% over 10 years should receive:

- Advice about how to stop smoking, including advice on the use of nicotine replacement therapy and bupropion.
- Information about other modifiable risk factors and personalized advice about how they can be reduced, including advice about physical activity, diet, alcohol consumption, weight, and diabetes.
- Advice and treatment to maintain blood pressure (BP) below 140/90 mm Hg. People with diabetes should maintain their BP below 135/80 mm Hg, or below 135/75 mm Hg in the presence of microalbuminuria or proteinuria.
- Low-dose Aspirin (325 mg, 81 mg, or 75 mg daily) for those aged 50 years or over with a 10-year CHD risk greater than 15%, or for people with diabetes, or those with target organ. Note: only use other antiplatelet therapy if the individual is hypersensitive to Aspirin.
- Statins and dietary advice to lower serum total cholesterol below 5.0 mmol/L should be offered to people with diabetes, and people with a familial dyslipidaemia. Otherwise, offer diet and lifestyle advice, and follow-up every 3 to 5 years. (Consider the possibility of familial dyslipidemia if total cholesterol is greater than 7.8 mmol/L.

For those with 10-year CHD risk of less than 15%:

- Most of these people will not require treatment. They should be reassured and offered diet and lifestyle advice, including smoking cessation, to prevent coronary heart disease (CHD). Their 10-year risk of CHD should be reassessed after 3 to 5 years.
- People with BP above the usual treatment thresholds for hypertension should be offered advice and treatment, and people with a familial dyslipidemia should also be offered treatment.

Eating to Prevent Heart Disease

Much of the evidence showing that specific lifestyle measures reduce cardiovascular (CV) risk comes from observational studies rather than randomized controlled trials (RCTs). At least three dietary strategies are likely to be effective in preventing CHD[16]:

- Replace saturated and *trans*-fats with unsaturated fats (especially monounsaturated and nonhydrogenated polyunsaturated fat).

- Increase consumption of omega-3 fatty acids from fish oil or plant sources.
- Consume a diet high in fruits, vegetables, nuts, and whole grains and low in refined grains.

A Mediterranean diet contains many of the dietary elements that may be protective in CHD. (The data is largely from people with established CAD.) An examination of adherence to the Mediterranean diet and outcomes was assessed in 22,000 Greek adults aged 20 to 86 years. A two-point increment in the Mediterranean diet score reduced the risk of death by about 25%. Effects were important for older people, those taking less exercise, and any level of BMI, as well as cause of death or CHD or cancer.[17]

- Replace butter with olive oil and monounsaturated margarine (e.g., rapeseed- or olive oil-based).
- Eat less red meat. (Replace beef, lamb, and pork with poultry.) If eating red meat, use lean cuts. Remove the skin from poultry.
- Eat more fish, including at least one portion of oily fish per week (e.g., mackerel, herring, kipper, pilchard, sardine, salmon, or trout).
- Eat more bread, especially whole grain bread.
- Eat more root vegetables and green vegetables.
- Also encourage people to eat fewer commercial bakery and deep-fried foods, which contain high levels of *trans*-fats and sugar.
- People should aim to eat five portions of fruit and vegetables every day.

Reduced salt intake is recommended to reduce BP, especially in the elderly and those with higher initial BP levels. A systematic review found that reducing sodium intake by 6.7g per day for 28 days in people with hypertension reduced systolic BP by about 3.9/1.9 mm Hg.[9] Dietary supplements of antioxidants are not protective; the Heart Protection Study found that antioxidants such as beta carotene, vitamin C, vitamin E, copper, zinc, manganese, and flavonoids, given as dietary supplements, are of no benefit in the prevention of CHD.[18] Also, concerns have been raised about the safety of beta carotene supplements.[18]

Men should limit their alcohol consumption to a maximum of 21 units per week (i.e., a maximum of 3 units per day). For women, the maximum is 14 units per week (i.e., a maximum of 2 units per day).[19]

─────────── ≋ REFERENCES ≋ ───────────

1. Rose G: High-risk and population strategies of prevention: ethical considerations, *Ann Med* 21:409-413, 1989.
2. Mosca L, Grundy SM, Judelson D, et al: Guide to preventive cardiology for women, *Circulation* 99:2480-2484, 1999.
3. Thomas JL, Braus PA: Coronary artery disease in women: a historical perspective, *Arch Intern Med* 158:333-337, 1998.
4. Hoeg JM: Evaluating coronary heart disease risk: tiles in the mosaic, *JAMA* 277:1387-1390, 1997.

5. Morrison C, Woodward M, Leslie W, et al: Effect of socioeconomic group on incidence of, management of, and survival after myocardial infarction and coronary death: analysis of community coronary event register, *BMJ* 314:541-546, 1997.

6. Daviglus ML, Stamler J, Orencia A, et al: Fish consumption and the 30-year risk of fatal myocardial infarction, *N Engl J Med* 336:1046-1053, 1997.

7. Rimm EB, Ascherio A, Giovannucci E, et al: Vegetable, fruit, and cereal fiber intake and risk of coronary heart disease among men, *JAMA* 275:447-451, 1996.

8. Lloyd-Jones DM, Larson MG, Beiser A, et al: Lifetime risk of developing coronary heart disease, *Lancet* 353:89-92, 1999.

9. Graudal NA, Galloe AM, Garred P: Effects of sodium restriction on blood pressure, renin, aldosterone, catecholamines, cholesterols, and triglycerides, *JAMA* 279(17), 1383-1391, 1998.

10. Genest et al: Recommendations for the management of dyslipidemia and the prevention of cardiovascular disease: summary of the 2003 update, *CMAJ* 169(9):921-924, 2003.

11. Ridker P, Rifai N, Rose L, et al: Comparison of C-Reactive Protein and low-density lipoprotein cholesterol levels in the prediction of first cardiovascular events, *N Engl J Med* 347: 1557-1565, 2002.

12. Ridker PM, Manson JE, Buring JE, et al: Homocysteine and risk of cardiovascular disease among postmenopausal women, *JAMA* 281:1817-1821, 1999.

13. Hemingway H, Marmot M: Psychosocial factors in the aetiology and prognosis of coronary heart disease: systematic review of prospective cohort studies, *BMJ* 318:1460-1467, 1999.

14. Conroy et al: Estimation of ten-year risk of fatal cardiovascular disease in Europe: the SCORE project, *Eur Heart J* 24:987-1003, 2003.

15. British Heart Foundation (2002b) *How to use the coronary risk prediction charts for primary prevention.* Factfile 1/2002. British Heart Foundation. www.bhf.org.uk [Accessed: 5-8-2004].

15a. Ramsay L, Williams B, Johnston G, et al. Guidelines for management of hypertension: report of the third working party of The British Hypertension Society, *J Hum Hypertens* 13(9): 569-592, 1999.

16. Hu FB, Willett WC: Optimal diets for prevention of coronary heart disease, *JAMA* 288(20):2569-2578, 2002.

17. Trichopoulou A, et al: Adherence to a Mediterranean diet and survival in a Greek population, *N Engl J Med* 348:2599-2608, 2003.

18. Heart Protection Study Collaborative Group (2002a): MRC/BHF heart protection study of antioxidant vitamin supplementation in 20,536 high-risk individuals: a randomised placebo-controlled trial, *Lancet* 360:23-33, 2002.

19. Marmot MG: Alcohol and coronary heart disease, *Int J Epidemiol* 30(4), 724-729, 2001.

Angina

(See also coronary artery bypass grafting, angioplasty, and stenting)

Stable angina

All patients with angina should be taking Aspirin and beta-blockers (unless strictly contraindicated) because these two drugs are cardioprotective. (See earlier discussion of primary prevention ofCAD.) If Aspirin cannot be used, clopidogrel (Plavix) should be prescribed. Associated risk factors such as smoking, elevated lipid levels, diabetes, obesity, and a sedentary lifestyle should be aggressively treated.[1]

In patients with stable angina, proper use of nitroglycerin improves quality of life through symptom control. Short-acting nitroglycerin products may be given as sublingual tablets (Nitrostat) or sprays (Nitrolingual) to treat individual anginal attacks or they can be taken prophylactically before an activity known to induce angina. Isosorbide dinitrate (Isordil) comes in both oral and sublingual formulations; its rate of onset of action is slower than nitroglycerin, but its duration of action is up to 1 hour, so it is particularly useful as a prophylactic agent before activity. Long-acting nitrates include transdermal patches (Transderm-Nitro, Minitran), sustained-release isosorbide dinitrate (Isordil Tembids), standard-formulation isosorbide mononitrate (ISMO, Monoket), and sustained-release isosorbide mononitrate (Imdur). Because of nitrate tolerance, daily drug-free periods are required. Sustained-release isosorbide mononitrate is given once a day. Standard-formulation isosorbide mononitrate or sustained-release isosorbide dinitrate may be given twice a day provided that no more than 7 hours elapses between doses. Patches should be removed after 12 to 14 hours.[2] Patients taking nitrates must not use sildenafil (Viagra).

Beta blockers are excellent drugs for controlling angina, but if they are contraindicated, calcium channel blockers might be considered because they increase coronary blood flow and are effective in the symptomatic management of angina. However, because some of the shorter acting formulations have been associated with an increased incidence of MI, calcium channel blockers are no longer considered first-line agents for the treatment of either angina or hypertension. (See discussion of calcium channel blockers in the section on hypertension.) If calcium channel antagonists are needed, a long-acting nondihydropyridine drug should be chosen and short-acting dihydropyridine derivatives should be avoided.[1]

The role of bypass surgery or angioplasty in the management of angina is discussed in the section on coronary artery bypass grafting, angioplasty, and stenting.

Unstable angina

Braunwald[3] classifies unstable angina as follows:
- Class I. New-onset severe or accelerated angina developing within the past 2 months. Frequency of anginal episodes three or more per day. For patients who had stable angina, the episodes have become more frequent, last longer, are more severe, or are brought on by lesser degrees of exercise. No rest pain.
- Class II. Angina at rest within the last month but not the past 48 hours (angina at rest subacute).

- Class III. Angina at rest within the last 48 hours (angina at rest acute).

Current U.S. guidelines[4] suggest that for unstable angina and non-ST-segment elevation, MI patients should receive anti-ischemic therapy (oxygen, beta blockers, nitrates), antiplatelet therapy (aspirin, clopidrogel, Platelet glyco-protein IIb/IIIa inhibitors) and antithrombotic therapy (LMW heparin). They should be discharged on aspirin (75 to 325 mg per day) and clopidrogel (Plavix) 75 mg per day for those who cannot tolerate Aspirin or in addition to Aspirin for 1 to 9 months. Beta blockers should be started in all patients who do not have contraindications. Lipid lowering (statin) and diet therapy in patients with an LDL cholesterol level above 3.40 mmol/L (130 mg per dL), or in patients with an LDL cholesterol level higher than 2.60 mmol/L (100 mg per dL) after diet therapy. ACE-I is a recommended inhibitor in patients with CHF, left ventricular dysfunction (ejection fraction below 40%), hypertension, or diabetes mellitus.

One of the major changes in the care of patients with UA/NSTEMI has been the ACC/AHA class I indication for use of clopidogrel in addition to Aspirin in patients with acute coronary syndromes. Because of its safety profile (compared with ticlopidine [Ticlid]), clopidogrel currently is the preferred thienopyridine. This change occurred because of the findings of recent major clinical trials. The Clopidogrel in Unstable Angina to Prevent Recurrent Ischaemic Events (CURE) trial randomized more than 12,000 patients with UA/NSTEMI to receive clopidogrel or placebo in addition to Aspirin. Patients were followed for 3 to 12 months. In the CURE trial, death, MI, or stroke occurred in 9.3% of the patients treated with clopidogrel, compared with 11.5% of those who received placebo. The improvement occurred at the cost of a small, but significant increase in bleeding (relative risk: 27%), especially in patients who underwent coronary artery bypass grafting within 5 days of discontinuing clopidogrel therapy.

In an analysis of patients undergoing percutaneous coronary intervention (PCI-CURE study), patients were treated with clopidogrel or placebo for a median of 10 days before the intervention (all patients also received Aspirin). After the intervention, patients in the PCI-CURE study received open-label clopidogrel or ticlopidine for 4 weeks, followed by the initial study drug (clopidogrel or placebo) for an average of 8 months. The clopidogrel-treated patients had fewer early (30-day) and long-term CV events. It should be remembered that Aspirin is still the cornerstone of therapy.[5-7]

"Small molecule" glycoprotein IIb/IIIa inhibitors of platelet aggregation is an emerging therapy that is administered intravenously and may prove useful in the hospital setting.

The addition of unfractionated heparin (regular IV heparin) or low-molecular-weight heparin[8] to Aspirin for patients with unstable angina decreases both MI and death rates. Current data suggest that low-molecular-weight heparin (e.g., enoxaparin) is superior to unfractionated heparin for this purpose and that it should be given for at least 1 month to patients who have not had invasive therapy (angioplasty or coronary artery bypass surgery). Compared with unfractionated heparin, the LMW heparins are relatively more potent inhibitors of factor Xa. LMW heparins also have a more predictable pharmacology, which means that laboratory monitoring of anticoagulation status is not needed. Recent trial data have shown superior results with the use of enoxaparin compared with unfractionated heparin in patients with UA/NSTEMI.[9,10]

Beta blockers should be given to all patients with unstable angina, and nitrates are probably beneficial. Thrombolytic therapy is contraindicated for patients with unstable angina.[11]

Coronary Artery Bypass Grafting, Angioplasty, and Stenting

(See also anesthesia; informed consent; investigations; myocardial infarction; performance reports; practice patterns)

The number of invasive cardiac procedures performed varies widely among geographical regions. This is discussed under variations in medical care in the section on practice patterns.

Coronary artery bypass grafting (CABG) has been clearly shown to decrease mortality in patients with the following[1]:

A 2004 review concluded that:

- Coronary artery bypass grafting (CABG) is recommended for patients with left main CAD(ACC/AHA class I).
- CABG also is recommended for patients with three-vessel CAD or with two-vessel disease, including proximal left anterior descending coronary involvement with either decreased left ventricular function or diabetes mellitus (ACC/AHA class I).
- Percutaneous coronary intervention is recommended for other patients with multivessel CAD who have suitable anatomy for this technique and do not have depressed ventricular function or diabetes mellitus (ACC/AHA class I).
- Either percutaneous coronary intervention or CABG is considered suitable in patients with one- or two-vessel disease and none of the features mentioned above.
- As surgical procedures (e.g., minimally invasive surgery) and interventional procedures (e.g., drug-coated stents) improve, recommendations are likely to evolve.[12]

—————————— ❧ REFERENCES ❧ ——————————

1. Gibbons RJ, Chatterjee K, Daley J: ACC/AHA/ACP-ASIM guidelines for the management of patients with chronic stable angina: executive summary and recommendations: a

report of the American College of Cardiology/American Heart Association Task Force on Practice Guidelines (Committee on Management of Patients With Chronic Stable Angina), *Circulation* 99:2829-2848, 1999.

2. Parker JD, Parker JO: Nitrate therapy for stable angina pectoris, *N Engl J Med* 338:520-531, 1998.

3. Braunwald E: Unstable angina: a classification, *Circulation* 80:410-414, 1989.

4. ACC/AHA 2002 guideline update for the management of patients with unstable angina and non-ST-segment elevation myocardial infarction. A report of the American College of Cardiology/American Heart Association Task Force on Practice Guidelines (Committee on the Management of Patients with Unstable Angina). Accessed online July 11, 2004, at: http://www.americanheart.org/presenter.jhtml? identifier=3001260.)

5. Yusuf S, Zhao F, Mehta SR, et al: Effects of clopidogrel in addition to aspirin in patients with acute coronary syndromes without ST-segment elevation [published corrections appear in *N Engl J Med* 345:1716, 2001 and *N Engl J Med* 345:1506, 2001], *N Engl J Med* 345:494-502, 2001.

6. Mehta SR, Yusuf S, Peters RJ, et al: Effects of pretreatment with clopidogrel and aspirin followed by long-term therapy in patients undergoing percutaneous coronary intervention: the PCI-CURE study, *Lancet* 358:527-533, 2001.

7. Wiviott S, Braunwald E: Unstable angina and non–ST-segment elevation myocardial infarction: part I. Initial evaluation and management, and hospital care, *Am Fam Phys* 70(3):525-532, 2004.

8. Zed PJ, Tisdale JE, Borzak S: Low-molecular-weight heparin in the management of acute coronary syndromes, *Arch Intern Med* 159:1849-1857, 1999.

9. Magee KD, Sevcik W, Moher D, Rowe BH: Low molecular weight heparins versus unfractionated heparin for acute coronary syndromes, *Cochrane Database Syst Rev* (2): CD002132, 2004.

10. Antman EM, Cohen M, Radley D, et al: Assessment of the treatment effect of enoxaparin for unstable angina/non-Q-wave myocardial infarction. TIMI 11B-ESSENCE meta-analysis, *Circulation* 100:1602-1608, 1999.

11. Yeghiazarians Y, Braunstein JB, Askari A, et al: Unstable angina pectoris, *N Engl J med* 342:101-114, 2000.

12. Wiviott S, Braunwald E, Unstable Angina and Non–ST-Segment Elevation Myocardial Infarction: Part I. Initial Evaluation and Management, and Hospital Care, American Family Physician. *70-3. August 1, 2004*

Myocardial Infarction

(See also cardiac arrest; coronary artery bypass grafting and angioplasty; practice patterns; risks of exercise; smoking)

Panic disorder presenting as possible myocardial infarction

A series of 441 consecutive consenting patients with chest pain seen in the emergency room of a major Montreal teaching hospital specializing in heart disease was evaluated as to etiology and underlying psychiatric disorders. One fourth of these patients met the criteria for panic attacks in the *Diagnostic and Statistical Manual of Mental Disorders*, edition 3 revised *(DSM-III-R)*, and

of this group one fourth had suicidal thoughts in the week before being seen in the emergency room. In addition, close to 60% of patients with panic disorder had other Axis I psychiatric diagnoses, mainly generalized anxiety disorder, agoraphobia, major depression, and dysthymia. In only 2% of cases was the panic disorder recognized by the attending staff cardiologists in the emergency room. Seventy-five percent of the patients with panic disorder were discharged from the emergency room with the diagnosis "noncardiac chest pain."[1]

≈ REFERENCES ≥

1. Fleet RP, Dupuis G, Marchand A, et al: Panic disorder in emergency department chest pain patients–prevalence, comorbidity, suicidal ideation, and physician recognition, *Am J Med* 101:371-380, 1996.

Office or home management of suspected acute myocardial infarction

In cases of suspected MI, rapid transfer to an emergency facility for consideration of thrombolytic therapy is paramount. (In general, thrombolytic therapy is not given if symptoms have persisted for more than 12 hours.) If time permits, an immediate ECG should be obtained and sent with the patient along with previous ECGs if available, because changing electrocardiographic patterns, especially ST segment changes or new-onset left bundle-branch block, support the diagnosis of MI and determine whether thrombolytic therapy is indicated. (Enzyme changes are often not seen for at least 3 to 4 hours.)[1]

Aspirin has been shown to reduce mortality, so a half to one Aspirin should be given immediately.[2] Chewing and swallowing Aspirin results in a more rapid antiplatelet effect than occurs from swallowing intact tablets.[2] Aspirin should not be omitted because of a vague history of allergy or a remote history of gastrointestinal bleeding. The administration of aspirin does not interfere with subsequent thrombolytic therapy.[1]

A randomized double-blind study from Scotland showed a significant decrease in death rate measured at 30 months among patients with suspected acute MIs who received intravenous thrombolytic therapy with 30 units of anistreplase (Eminase) at home from their general practitioners compared with patients who received similar therapy only after arrival at the hospital.[3]

≈ REFERENCES ≥

1. Collins R, Peto R, Baigent C, et al: Aspirin, heparin, and fibrinolytic therapy in suspected acute myocardial infarction, *N Engl J Med* 336:847-860, 1997.

2. Feldman M, Cryer B: Aspirin absorption rates and platelet inhibition times with 325-mg buffered aspirin tablets (chewed or swallowed intact) and with buffered aspirin solution, *Am J Cardiol* 84:404-409, 1999.

3. Rawles J: Magnitude of benefit from earlier thrombolytic treatment in acute myocardial infarction: new evidence from Grampian Region Early Anistreplase Trial (GREAT), *BMJ* 312:212-215, 1996.

Secondary prevention of myocardial infarction
(See also exercise; hypertension; lipids; practice patterns; smoking)

Risk Stratification. For optimal provision of secondary prevention measures, patients who have had an MI should be stratified according to their degree of risk for further coronary events. This is best performed by testing left ventricular function with echocardiography and assessing ischemia with exercise testing.[1]

The first-year mortality rate after an MI is zero to 2% if the post-myocardial infarction exercise stress test is negative, but if it is positive, the total cardiac event rate is about 25%. In recent years the interval between MI and exercise testing has been decreasing, and in some centres, symptom-limited testing is being done as early as 4 to 7 days after the cardiac event. Usually one of two protocols is recommended: submaximal testing at 4 to 7 days followed by symptom-limited testing at 3 to 6 weeks, or symptom-limited testing at 2 to 3 weeks. Patients who have contraindications to exercise stress testing have a much higher mortality rate than those who are able to undergo the test.

Left ventricular function as determined by echocardiography is the single most important determinant of risk after MI. The 1-year mortality rate varies from 3% when the ejection fraction is greater than 50% to more than 40% when the ejection fraction is less than 30%.

_____ ❧ REFERENCES ❧ _____

1. Zellweger MJ, Lewin HC, Lai S, et al: When to stress patients after coronary artery bypass surgery? Risk stratification in patients early and late post-CABG using stress myocardial perfusion SPECT: implications of appropriate clinical strategies, *J Am Coll Cardiol* 37:144-152, 2001.

ELECTROCARDIOGRAMS

A long tradition in primary care holds that routine ECGs are a valuable part of the periodic health examination of middle-age or elderly patients. This is a myth.[1] The cardiogram has poor sensitivity and specificity for Q-wave MI in asymptomatic individuals, and the positive predictive value for this entity for 60-year-old men is calculated to be only 3%.[1] T-wave and ST segment changes are so common and so non-specific that they do not help identify patients at risk of CAD. The U.S. Preventive Services Task Force gives screening ECGs for middle-age and elderly men and women a "C" recommendation. They give a "D" recommendation for routine periodic health visits or routine pre-sports participation examinations in adolescents or young adults.[2]

A common argument for performing electrocardiography is to have ECGs available as a baseline in case cardiac symptoms develop in the future. The assumption is that the ECG will be relatively recent and rapidly accessible at whatever emergency room the patient goes to when symptoms of CAD develop. If the ECG is available, it will probably be helpful, but if cardiograms are going to be taken for this reason, the possible benefits for the very few must be weighed against the significant number of false-positive findings that would inevitably lead to unwarranted investigations for many patients.

_____ ❧ REFERENCES ❧ _____

1. Health Services Utilization and Research Commission: Anatomy of a practice guideline: tradition, science, and consensus on using electrocardiograms in Saskatchewan, *Can Fam Physician* 41:37-48, 1995.
2. U.S. Preventive Services Task Force: *Guide to clinical preventive services,* ed 2, Baltimore, 1996, Williams & Wilkins, 3-14.

HEART FAILURE

Congestive Heart Failure has an incidence approaching 10 per 1000 population among persons older than 65 years of age. Heart failure is the reason for at least 20% of all hospital admissions among persons older than 65.[1]

Definition of Heart Failure

Heart failure (HF) is defined by symptoms that are suggestive of cardiac dysfunction and objective evidence of cardiac dysfunction. In cases of doubt, response to a therapeutic trial may increase the diagnostic accuracy.

- *Systolic heart failure* is the presence of signs and symptoms of HF with an ejection fraction of less than 40%.
- *Diastolic heart failure* is the presence of signs and symptoms of HF in the absence of systolic dysfunction (left ventricular ejection fraction [LVEF] over 40%).

It is important to differentiate systolic from diastolic HF because research evidence for treatment is best established for systolic HF and for predicting prognosis, which is worse for systolic than for diastolic HF.[2-4]

The following is the New York Heart Association classification of CHF:

Class I	Symptoms with unusual activity (manual labour)
Class II	Symptoms with usual activity (light yardwork, sexual intercourse)
Class III	Symptoms with self-care activity (dressing, making bed)
Class IV	Symptoms at rest and worse with activity

A new classification system has recently been introduced that emphasizes the evolution and progression of HF and that will be clinically useful because it emphasizes that established risk factors and structural abnormalities are necessary for the development of HF, recognizes its progressive nature, and superimposes treatment strategies on the fundamentals of preventive efforts. This classification system is outlined below for reference but it has not as yet been widely adopted in clinical practice.[1]

Stage A: High risk for HF but no structural abnormality of the heart
Stage B: Structural abnormality but never had symptomatic HF
Stage C: Structural abnormality and current or previous symptoms of HF
Stage D: End-stage symptoms of HF that are refractory to standard treatment

Prognosis

The overall 5-year survival rate of patients with CHF is poor. Among U.S. Medicare patients in HF who were 67 years or older, 19% of black men, 16% of white men, 25% of black women, and 23% of white women survived 6 years from diagnosis.[5] The annual death rates for various degrees of HF based on the New York Heart Association classifications are estimated as follows[6]:

Class II   5% to 10% per year
Class III   10% to 20% per year
Class IV   20% to 50% per year

About half of the deaths from cardiac causes are sudden, and one fourth of these occur without prior worsening of HF.[6]

────── ❧ **REFERENCES** ❧ ──────

1. Jessup M, Brozena S: Medical progress: heart failure, *NEJM* 348:2007-2018, 2003.
2. Gomberg-Maitland M, Baran D, Foster V: Treatment of congestive heart failure. Guidelines for the primary care physician and the heart failure specialist, *Arch Intern Med* 161:342-352, 2001.
3. Hunt SA, Baker DW, Chin MH, et al: ACC/AHA guidelines for the evaluation and management of chronic heart failure in the adult, American College of Cardiology Web site. Available at: http://www.acc.org/clinical/guidelines/failure/hf_index.htm
4. Liu P: The 2001 Canadian cardiovascular society consensus guideline update for the management and prevention of heart failure, *Can J Cardiol* 17(Suppl E): 5E-24E, 2001.
5. Croft JB, Giles WH, Pollard RA, et al: Heart failure survival among older adults in the United States: a poor prognosis for an emerging epidemic in the Medicare population, *Arch Intern Med* 159:505-510, 1999.
6. Dracup K, Baker DW, Dubar SB, et al: Management of heart failure. II. Counseling, education, and lifestyle modifications, *JAMA* 272:1442-1446, 1994.

Systolic and Diastolic Heart Failure

Systolic HF is caused by a decreased contractility of the heart and is associated with dilation, which is often seen as an enlarged heart on a chest X-ray. Most people are familiar with systolic failure, which is much more common than diastolic failure. In systolic failure the LVEF is usually less than 40%.[1]

Diastolic HF is the inability of the heart to relax properly. Decreased cardiac compliance leads to inadequate filling of the ventricles during diastole. The chest X-ray may show no increase in heart size, and the LVEF is often greater than 40%. In fact, pure diastolic dysfunction may be defined as an elevated end-diastolic pressure without chamber enlargement.[1] Some of the causes of diastolic failure are hypertrophic cardiomyopathy, aortic stenosis, hypertension, and conditions such as cardiac amyloidosis and extensive scarring from CAD in which cardiac interstitial tissue is increased.[2] If a patient has evidence of systemic or pulmonary venous congestion in the absence of left ventricular enlargement, the odds are high that diastolic failure is a major component of the failure.[1] Treatment of diastolic failure is an area of growing research, but the key message is treating the underlying condition.

Many patients have a combination of systolic and diastolic failure. Physicians should not rule out HF in a patient with dyspnea on effort, orthopnea, and decreased energy just because the heart size is normal.[1]

Evaluation for HF includes a history and physical including assessment of a patient's mobility, ability to solve problems and perform routine and desired activities of self-management and daily living, assessment of volume status, CBC, urinalysis, serum electrolytes, blood urea, serum creatinine/calculated glomerular filtration rate, fasting blood glucose, aspartate transaminase, albumin, thyroid-stimulating hormone, ECG, chest X-ray, and two-dimensional echocardiography with Doppler to assess cardiac function (preferred) or radionuclide ventriculography. Brain natriuretic peptide (BNP) is an emerging test that has shown a high diagnostic predictive value for both systolic and diastolic HF but is not yet available in many settings.[3]

────── ❧ **REFERENCES** ❧ ──────

1. Cohn JN: The management of chronic heart failure, *N Engl J Med* 335:490-498, 1996.
2. Heart Failure Guideline Panel: Heart failure: management of patients with left ventricular systolic dysfunction, *Am Fam Physician* 50:603-616, 1994.
3. Congestive Heart Failure Guidelines 2003, Guidelines and Protocols Advisory Committee, British Columbia Ministry of Health. Accessed at www.healthservices.gov.bc.ca/msp August 1, 2004

Diet and Exercise
(See also exercise; nutrition)

Except in severe failure the maximum daily salt intake should be 3 g, which can be achieved by avoiding salty food and by not adding salt to food after it has been cooked. Patients with severe failure (e.g., those requiring at least 80 mg of furosemide per day) should limit their salt intake to 2 g per day. This involves avoiding milk products, prepared foods, and canned foods and is unpalatable for most patients.[1]

Data on alcohol in CHF are inconclusive. Alcohol is obviously contraindicated in alcoholic cardiomyopathy. In other cases expert opinion is that patients should not have more than one drink per day.[1]

Patients with stable HF should be encouraged to exercise regularly by walking or bicycling on flat terrain.[1,2] A 1999 randomized controlled trial of patients with stable HF found that in addition to improving quality of life, exercise decreased mortality rates.[3]

⚓ REFERENCES ⚓

---

1. Dracup K, Baker DW, Dubar SB, et al: Management of heart failure. II. Counseling, education, and lifestyle modifications, *JAMA* 272:1442-1446, 1994.
2. Willenheimer R, Erhardt L, Cline C, et al: Exercise training in heart failure improves quality of life and exercise capacity, *Eur Heart J* 19:774-781, 1998.
3. Belardinelli R, Georgiou D, Cianci G, et al: Randomized, controlled trial of long-term moderate exercise training in chronic heart failure, *Circulation* 99:1173-1182, 1999.

Pharmacotherapy

Patients with systolic HF should be on ACE inhibitor and beta blockers unless contraindications are present (angiotensin II antagonists (ARBs) can substitute if there is intolerance to these drug classes; i.e., ARBs can be used in combination with ACE inhibitors or with beta blockers). ACE inhibitors slow disease progression, improve exercise capacity, and decrease hospitalization and mortality. Beta blockers slow disease progression, decrease hospitalization and mortality, and improve quality of life but have little or no effect on objective measures of exercise duration. Both these medications can be titrated up slowly. Beta blockers should not be used in patients with asthma but can be used in patients with chronic obstructive pulmonary disease (COPD). Diuretics are used to control fluid, but the goal is always to stop the diuretic or use the most minimal dose once the patient is symptomatic. This is more often achieved after ACE inhibitors and beta blockers have been started and titrated to target doses, and then the diuretic can be stopped or used at minimum doses. Digoxin improves symptoms, exercise tolerance, and quality of life. Digoxin therapy has recently been associated with an increased risk of death from any cause among women (but not men) with HF and decreased LVEF. Therefore, digoxin (0.125-0.25 mg/day) should be used with caution in this group, and consideration should be given to obtaining a digoxin level when toxicity is suspected.[4] For moderate to severe heart failure, spironolactone at 25 mg per day

decreases mortality and hospitalization and improves symptoms. The publication of randomized Aldactone evaluation study (RALES)[5] proved this effect but was also associated with abrupt increases in the rate of prescriptions for spironolactone and in hyperkalemia-associated morbidity and mortality. Closer laboratory monitoring and more judicious use of spironolactone may reduce the occurrence of this complication.[6]

Table 7   ACE Inhibitors

Drug	Usual dose
Benazepril (Lotensin)	10-20 mg/day as a single dose
Captopril (Capoten)	25-50 mg bid or tid
Cilazapril (Inhibace)	2.5-5 mg/day as a single dose
Enalapril (Vasotec)	5-40 mg/day as a single dose or bid
Fosinopril (Monopril)	20 mg as a single daily dose
Lisinopril (Zestril, Prinivil)	10-40 mg/day as a single dose
Moexipril (Univasc)	7.5-30 mg/day in 1 or 2 divided doses
Perindopril (Coversyl)	4-8 mg/day as a single dose
Quinapril HCl (Accupril)	10-20 mg/day as a single dose
Ramipril (Altace)	2.5-10 mg/day as a single dose
Trandolapril (Mavik)	2-4 mg/day as a single dose

Table 8   Angiotensin II Antagonists

Drug	Usual dose
Candesartan Cilexetil (Atacand)	8-32 mg/day as a single daily dose
Eprosartan (Teveten)	400-800 mg/day as a single dose or bid
Irbesartan (Avapro)	150-300 mg/day as a single daily dose
Losartan (Cozaar)	25-100 mg/day as a single daily dose
Telmisartan (Micardis)	40-80 mg/day as a single daily dose
Valsartan (Diovan)	80-320 mg/day as a single daily dose

⚓ REFERENCES ⚓

---

1. Heart Failure Guideline Panel, Rockville, Maryland: Heart failure: management of patients with left ventricular systolic dysfunction, *Am Fam Physician* 50:603-616, 1994.
2. Pepper GS, Lee RW: Sympathetic activation in heart failure and its treatment with β-blockade, *Arch Intern Med* 159: 225-234, 1999.
3. Cleland JG, McGowan J, Clark A: The evidence for β blockers in heart failure: equals or surpasses that for angiotensin converting enzyme inhibitors (editorial), *BMJ* 318:824-825, 1999.
4. Congestive Heart Failure Guidelines 2003, Guidelines and Protocols Advisory Committee, British Columbia Ministry of Health. Accessed at www.healthservices.gov.bc.ca/msp August 1, 2004
5. Juurlink DN, Mamdani MM, Lee DS, et al: Rates of hyperkalemia after publication of the Randomized Aldactone Evaluation Study, *N Engl J Med* 351(6):543-51, Aug 5 2004.
6. Pitt B, Zannad F, Remme WJ, et al: The effect of spironolactone on morbidity and mortality in patients with severe heart failure, *N Engl J Med* 341:709-717, 1999.

HYPERTENSION

(See also hypertensive disorders of pregnancy)

Diagnosis

Definition and epidemiology

The definitions of hypertension according to the *Seventh Report of the Joint National Committee on Detection, Evaluation, and Treatment of High Blood Pressure (JNC VII)* are recorded in Table 9. Blood pressure should be recorded with the patient in the sitting position with the arm at heart level, and the mean of two readings taken 2 minutes apart should be used. The patient should have been resting for at least 5 minutes and have abstained from caffeine or smoking for at least 30 minutes. Normal readings are under 120/80 mm Hg.[1]

Patients with initial readings over 140/90 mm Hg should have at least 2 additional readings taken that visit. They should be scheduled for follow-up to further assess their blood pressure and search for evidence of target organ damage and associated risk factors by history, physical, and appropriate laboratory investigation.

For patients with BPs over 160/100 mm Hg, a diagnosis of hypertension can be made after three visits. Patients with BPs between 140-159/90-99 mm Hg should be reassessed over at least five visits in the ensuing 6-month period. This approach is based on a lower risk of complications in these patients. However, patients with target organ damage (Table 10) may be diagnosed as hypertensive after three visits.[2]

The category of prehypertension (120-139/80-89) deserves special consideration. The relationship between hypertension and CVD is linear across all levels of BPs greater than 115/75 mm Hg .[3] It is appropriate to stress lifestyle modifications in this group of patients as well to reduce overall CVD risk and prevent progression to sustained hypertension.[1] Those patients at the upper end of this range (greater than 135/85 mm Hg) have a relatively high risk of progression to sustained hypertension; as high as 25% for patients younger than 60 years old and 50% for those older than 60 over a 4-year follow-up period.[4]

Table 9   Definition of Hypertension

Blood pressure	Systolic (mm Hg)	Diastolic (mm Hg)
Normal	<120	<80
Prehypertension	130-139	80-89
Hypertension	>140	>90
Stage 1	140-159	90-99
Stage 2	>160	>100

Adapted from US Department of Health and Human Services, National Institutes of Health (NIH), National Heart, Lung and Blood Institute (NHLBI), and National High Blood Pressure Education Program (NHBEP): The Seventh Report of the Joint National Committee on Preventation, Detection, Evaluation, and Treatment of High Blood Pressure, August 2004, NIH Publication No. 04-5230: P.12 (Table 3).

Table 10   Target Organ Damage

Coronary artery disease
Left ventricular Hypertrophy
Stroke, including transient ischemic attacks and vascular dementia
Aortic and peripheral arterial disease
Hypertensive nephropathy (creatinine clearance < 1mL/sec)
Hypertensive retinopathy (eg. retinal arteriosclerosis)
Other asymptomatic atherosclerotic disease

Adapted from Hemmelgarn BR, et al, *Can J Cardiol* 20(1):31-40, 2004.

Laboratory Investigations

The usual laboratory investigations for patients with hypertension are aimed at assessing target organ damage and other risk factors for CAD. These are urinalysis; complete blood cell count; measurement of electrolytes, calcium, creatinine, and fasting glucose; lipid profile; and 12-lead ECG. Other investigations are optional and directed by the clinical findings.[1,2]

✎ REFERENCES ✐

1. Chobanian AV, Bakris GL, Black HR, et al: The Seventh Report of the Joint National Committee on Prevention, Detection, Evaluation, and Treatment of High Blood Pressure: The JNC 7 Report, *JAMA* 289:2560-2571, 2003. Developed by the National Heart, Lung, and Blood Institute and the National High Blood Pressure Education Program.
2. Hemmelgarn BR, Zarnke KB, Campbell NC, et al: The 2004 Canadian Hypertension Education Program recommendations for the management of hypertension: Part I-Blood pressure measurement, diagnosis and assessment of risk, *Can J Cardiol* 20(1):31-40, Jan 2004.
3. Lewington S, Clarke R, Qizilbash N, et al: Age-specfic relevance of usual blood pressure to vascular mortality: a meta-analysis of individual data for one million adults in 61 prospective studies, *Lancet* 360:1903-1913, 2002.
4. Vasan RS, Larson MG, Leip EP, et al: Assessment of frequency of progression to hypertension in non-hypertensive participants in the Framingham Heart Study: a cohort study, *Lancet* 139:272-281, 2001.

Secondary Hypertension

Except among persons who drink alcohol to excess, secondary hypertension is rare. Investigations for secondary hypertension are necessary only when it is clinically suspected. The following are important causes of the condition[1-4]:

- Alcohol
- Medications (e.g., oral contraceptives, NSAIDs, sympathomimetics such as appetite suppressants and decongestants)
- Renal parenchymal disease
- Renovascular disease
- Coarctation of the aorta

- Cushing's syndrome
- Primary hyperaldosteronism
- Pheochromocytoma
- Thyroid dysfunction (hyperthyroidism or hypothyroidism)
- Obstructive sleep apnea

Secondary hypertension may be suspected on the basis of the history, physical examination, or basic hypertensive investigations. It should be seriously considered in young patients or those with onset after the age of 55 years. Alcohol and drug use should be determined for all patients, as should the presence or absence of physical stigmata of Cushing's disease. The femoral artery pulsations and leg blood pressure should be checked as a screen for coarctation of the aorta in all young hypertensive patients. An abnormal urinalysis may point to renal disease, hypokalemia to primary hyperaldosteronism, and an abnormal thyroid-stimulating hormone level to thyroid disease.[1,4]

The following are other clues to secondary hypertension[1]:

- Abrupt onset of hypertension
- Severe hypertension (diastolic $\geq$110 mm Hg)
- Rapid worsening of hypertension
- Hypertension resistant to treatment

⬩ REFERENCES ⬩

1. Adcock BB, Ireland RB Jr: Secondary hypertension: a practical diagnostic approach, *Am Fam Physician* 55:1263-1270, 1997.
2. Silverberg DS, Oksenberg A: Essential and secondary hypertension and sleep-disordered breathing: a unifying hypothesis [Review] [207 refs], *J Hum Hypertens* 10(6):353-363, June 1996.
3. Dosh SA: The diagnosis of essential and secondary hypertension in adults, *J Fam Pract* 50(8):707-712, Aug 2001.
4. Hemmelgarn BR, Zarnke KB, Campbell NC, et al: The 2004 Canadian Hypertension Education Program recommendations for the management of hypertension: Part I-Blood pressure measurement, diagnosis and assessment of risk, *Can J Cardiol* 20(1): 31-40, Jan 2004.

White Coat Hypertension: Ambulatory Blood Pressure Monitoring (ABPM) and Self-Measurement of Blood Pressure (SMBP)

"White coat" hypertension presents a unique challenge in the evidence-based management of hypertension.

Approximately 20% to 25% of hypertensive patients have elevated office BPs and normal ambulatory or home BPs.[1,2]

When white coat hypertension is suspected based on self-measurement of blood pressure (SMBP) or other information from history, it should be further assessed by 24-hour ambulatory blood pressure measurement (ABPM). Den Hond and colleagues showed in a study of 257 hypertensive patients that SMBP was specific (89%) but not sensitive (68%) in its ability to detect white coat syndrome.[3] Physicians should use ABPM devices that have been validated independently.

Normal values for ABPM over 24 hours are less than 134/78 mm Hg, with daytime values less than 136/87mm Hg for men and less than 131/86 mm Hg for women. Blood pressure decreases by 10% to 20% overnight, so-called nocturnal "dipping" and individuals without this reduction are at increased CV risk.[4,5] Normal values for SMBP are less than 136/83 mm Hg. Values above this are associated with CV risk similar to office values greater than 140/90 mm Hg.[5]

Considerable controversy exists regarding the management of patients with AMBP and SMBP values below the levels stated above who have office values greater than 140/90 mm Hg; that is, white coat hypertension.[1,6,7] It is probable that their overall risk lies somewhere between "true" normotensive and sustained hypertensive. However, no long-term prospective trials exist to guide management.[1]

The family physician confronted with the patient in whom white coat hypertension has been documented could consider the following as a reasonably prudent approach based on expert opinion although not consensus.
1. Patients with risk factors such as diabetes mellitus, a history of CVD, or hyperlipidemia or stage 2 hypertension (greater than 160/100 mm Hg) should be treated to targets based on office BPs. This is based on the fact that in all large scale trials showing the benefit of treatment, outcomes were based on office BPs.[1]
2. Patients without risk factors and stage 1 office hypertension less than 159/99 mm Hg could be followed over time (3 to 6 months) with lifestyle modifications. Approximately 12% of patients followed over 3 to 6 months become normotensive.[1]
3. If office BPs do not become less than 140/90 mm Hg over time, the patient may be offered treatment with medication after a discussion of risks and cost (which in the case of thiazides is small). They should be advised that evidence for benefit is not as clear as it is for sustained hypertensive medications.[1]

ABPM has also been found useful in evaluating resistance to medication, possible hypotensive side effects from treatment, episodic hypertension, and autonomic dysfunction.[4,5]

⬩ REFERENCES ⬩

1. Moser M: White-coat hypertension—to treat or not to treat: a clinical dilemma (editorial), *Arch Intern Med* 161(22): 2655-2656, Dec 2001.
2. Grandi AM, Broggi R, Colombo S, et al: Left ventricular changes in isolated office hypertension: a blood pressure–matched comparison with normotension and sustained hypertension, *Arch Intern Med* 161:2677-2681, 2001.

3. Den Hond E, Celis H, Fagard R, et al: Self-measured versus ambulatory blood pressure in the diagnosis of hypertension, *J Hypertens* 21:717-722, 2003.
4. Chobanian AV, Bakris GL, Black HR, et al: The Seventh Report of the Joint National Committee on Prevention, Detection, Evaluation, and Treatment of High Blood Pressure: The JNC 7 Report, *JAMA* 289:2560-2571, 2003. Developed by the National Heart, Lung, and Blood Institute and the National High Blood Pressure Education Program.
5. Hemmelgarn BR, Zarnke KB, Campbell NC, et al: The 2004 Canadian Hypertension Education Program recommendations for the management of hypertension: Part I—Blood pressure measurement, diagnosis and assessment of risk, *Can J Cardiol* 20(1):31-40, Jan 2004.
6. Owens P, Atkins N, O'Brien E: Diagnosis of white coat hypertension by ambulatory blood pressure monitoring, *Hypertension* 34(2):267-272, Aug 1999.
7. Spence JD: Withholding treatment in white coat hypertension: wishful thinking (editorial), *Can Med Assoc J* 161: 275-276 1999.

Pseudohypertension

Pseudohypertension is found in 2% to 5% of elderly patients and may raise both the systolic and diastolic readings by as much as 20 to 30 mm Hg.[1] The diagnosis may be suspected in patients with very high readings and no signs of end organ damage, in patients who do not respond to intensive pharmacological therapy, and in those who have postural hypotension after minimal therapy.[2] The traditional confirmatory test on physical examination is Osler's manoeuvre, which consists of inflating the blood pressure cuff above the systolic reading while palpating the radial or brachial artery. If the artery can still be felt as a non-pulsatile cord when the cuff is inflated above the systolic reading, Osler's manoeuvre is positive and the patient probably has pseudohypertension.[1] Not all health care workers agree that this is a sensitive or specific test; Belmin and associates[3] found it insensitive and also found that a significant number of normotensive patients were Osler-test positive.

REFERENCES

1. Messerli FH, Ventura HO, Amodeo C: Osler's maneuver and pseudohypertension, *N Engl J Med* 312:1548-1551, 1985.
2. Fifth report of the Joint National Committee on Detection, Evaluation, and Treatment of High Blood Pressure (JNC V), *Arch Intern Med* 153:154-183, 1993.
3. Belmin J, Visintin J-M, Salvatore R, et al: Osler's maneuver: absence of usefulness for the detection of pseudohypertension in an elderly population, *Am J Med* 98:42-49, 1995.

Abdominal Bruits and Renovascular Hypertension

Between 7% and 31% of young individuals have abdominal bruits. Screening for such bruits in normotensive individuals is not indicated. However, about 80% of patients with angiographically documented renal artery stenosis have bruits; the specificity is particularly high if there is a systolic-diastolic bruit. The absence of a bruit does not rule out renovascular hypertension.[1]

REFERENCES

1. Turnbull JM: Is listening for abdominal bruits useful in the evaluation of hypertension? *JAMA* 274:1299-1301, 1995.

Treatment of Hypertension

Evidence for efficacy

Lowering BP decreases the incidence of CAD, stroke, CHF, and all-cause mortality.[1] It also decreases the rate of progression of renal failure[1] and the risk for left ventricular hypertrophy.[2]

Treatment of hypertension lowers the risk of CVD by 25% to 30% overall.[3] Antihypertensive therapy in clinical trials has been associated with reduction in incidence of stroke averaging 35% to 40%; in MI 20% to 25%; and in heart failure 50%.[1]

In patients with stage 1 hypertension (systolic BP 140-159 mm Hg and/or diastolic BP 90-99 mm Hg) and 1 or more CV risk factors, achieving a sustained reduction of 12 mm Hg in systolic BP over 10 years prevents one death for every 16 patients treated. In patients with CVD or target organ damage, such systolic BP reduction requires a number of only 9 to treat for 10 years.[4]

Treatment of isolated systolic hypertension in the elderly reduces the incidence of stroke and CAD.[4-6]

The results of the ongoing isolated systolic HYpertension in the Very Elderly Trial (HYVET) should guide clinical decisions around initiating treatment when hypertension is first diagnosed after age 80. However, therapy should be continued in previously treated patients who reach 80.[3]

REFERENCES

1. Chobanian AV, Bakris GL, Black HR, et al: The Seventh Report of the Joint National Committee on Prevention, Detection, Evaluation, and Treatment of High Blood Pressure: The JNC 7 Report, *JAMA* 289:2560-2571, 2003. Developed by the National Heart, Lung, and Blood Institute and the National High Blood Pressure Education Program.
2. Moser M, Hebert PR: Prevention of disease progression, left ventricular hypertrophy and congestive heart failure in hypertension treatment trials, *J Am Coll Cardiol* 27: 1214-1218, 1996.
3. Khan NA, McAlister FA, Campbell NR, et al: The 2004 Canadian recommendations for the management of hypertension: Part II – therapy, *Can J Cardiol* (20): 41-54, 2004.
4. Ogden LG, He J, Lydick E, et al: Long term absolute benefit of lowering blood pressure in hypertensive patients according to the JNC VI risk stratification, *Hypertension* 35:539-543, 2000.

5. Systolic Hypertension in the Elderly Program Cooperative Research Group: Prevention of stroke by antihypertensive drug treatment in older persons with isolated systolic hypertension: final results of the Systolic Hypertension in the Elderly Program (SHEP), *JAMA* 265:3255-3264, 1991.
6. Staessen JA, Fagard R, Thijs L, et al (Systolic Hypertension in Europe [Syst-Eur] Trial Investigators): Randomised double-blind comparison of placebo and active treatment for older patients with isolated systolic hypertension, *Lancet* 350:757-764, 1997.

Principles of management

1. Lifestyle modifications and pharmacotherapy. An important concept in the management of hypertension that is emphasized by both U.S. and Canadian guidelines is risk stratification of patients.[1,2] Characteristics of hypertensive patients at increased risk for complications include:

1. Male gender
2. Over 55 years of age
3. Smoker
4. Coronary Artery Disease
5. Left Ventricular Hypertrophy
6. Congestive Heart Failure
7. Peripheral Vascular Disease
8. Nephropathy
9. Retinopathy
10. Diabetes
11. Dyslipidemia
12. Positive family history for cardiovascular disease

Evidence-based guidelines recommend lifestyle modifications for all hypertensive patients. Those whose pressures are less than 160 mm Hg systolic or 100 mm Hg diastolic and who do not have target organ damage, clinical CVD, or diabetes may be given an initial 6- to 12-month trial of lifestyle modifications without drugs. Pharmacotherapy should be instituted in those with pressures greater than or equal to 160 mm Hg systolic or 100 mm Hg diastolic and in those with lower readings who have target organ damage, clinical CVD, renal failure, or diabetes[1,2]

Reducing hypertension-related complications in the general hypertensive population depends more on the extent of achieved BP lowering than on the choice of any specific first-line drug, although the evidence favouring thiazides is persuasive when combined with their low cost and high tolerability.[2] (See further discussion of thiazides in the section on drug choice.)

2. Overall vascular protection. The overall vascular protection strategy for patients with hypertension should include consideration of both statins and low-dose acetylsalicylic acid (ASA) in selected patients.[2]

2.1 Statins. Recent trials that included a large number of hypertensive patients with lipid levels that would not be considered elevated in the past have supported statin therapy for hypertensive patients at high risk for CVD (equal to or greater than three of the risk factors in Table 11).

In the ASCOT-LLA trial 10,305 individuals with hypertension and at least three other risk factors and a total cholesterol of 6.5 mmol/L or lower were randomly assigned to atorvastatin 10 MG OD or placebo (mean blood pressure at baseline was 164/95). Patients with known coronary disease or recent stroke or those selected for lipid-lowering treatment by their primary care physicians were excluded. The incidence of fatal and nonfatal MI was significantly reduced with atorvastatin (hazard ratio [HR] 0.64 95% CI 0.50 to 0.83). Relative benefits were consistent irrespective of baseline cholesterol levels. Stroke and total CV events were also significantly reduced with atorvastatin.[3]

The ALLHAT-LLT, PROSPER and HPS trials, all large prospective studies, also supported this approach.[4-6] Although the benefits of statins appear to be independent of baseline cholesterol levels, the trials to date have only included patients with normal or high-normal cholesterol levels. Further studies are needed to clarify if there is a cholesterol level below which statin therapy would not confer benefit.

2.2 ASA. Low-dose ASA therapy has been recommended for hypertensive patients over 50 years of age, providing their BP is well controlled.[2]

The Hypertension Optimal Treatment (HOT) trial of 18,790 hypertensive individuals age 50 to 80 years showed a significant reduction in major CV events, particularly MI, in those taking ASA 75 mg OD versus placebo. However, further analysis showed a trend toward increased life-threatening bleeding in those whose BP was not well controlled.[7]

3. Treatment targets. When treating hypertension, what level of BP readings should one aim for? Is there a J-curve; that is, does morbidity or mortality increase if target blood pressures are maintained below a certain level? The HOT randomized trial (which excluded patients with

---

Table 11   Cardiovascular Risk Factors for Consideration of Statin Therapy in Nonhyperlipidemic Patients with Hypertension

Characteristic:

Male

Age 55 or older

Left ventricular Hypertrophy

Other ECG abnormalities:
   Left bundle branch block, left ventricular strain pattern, abnormal Q waves or ST-T changes compatible with ischemic heart disease

Peripheral arterial disease

Previous stroke or transient ischemic attack

Microalbuminuria

Diabetes Mellitus

Smoking

Family History of premature CVD

Total cholesterol to HDL ratio greater than or equal to 6

Adapted from Sever PS, et al, for the ASCOT Investigators. *Lancet* 361: 1149-1158, 2003. Reprinted with permission from Elsevier.

isolated systolic hypertension) found no evidence of a J-curve and concluded that if 1000 patients achieved a pressure of 140/90 mm Hg, 5 to 10 CV events would be prevented per year. Lower levels gave only slight additional benefit but were not harmful.[7] In contrast, the Systolic Hypertension in the Elderly Program (SHEP) found a slight increase in CV events in patients whose diastolic pressure was lowered below 70 mm Hg and a more marked increase in those whose diastolic level reached 60 mm Hg or less.[8]

According to the Joint National Committee on the Detection, Evaluation and Treatment of High Blood Pressure, current evidence favours lowering pressures to levels achieved in clinical trials (usually below 140 mm Hg systolic and 90 mm Hg diastolic) for most patients and to below 130/80 mm Hg for diabetic patients and those with renal disease.[1] Some health care workers recommend target levels of 120/75 mm Hg for black patients and those patients with renal disease and protein excretion greater than 1 g/day.[8]

◢ REFERENCES ◤

1. Chobanian AV, Bakris GL, Black HR, et al: The Seventh Report of the Joint National Committee on Prevention, Detection, Evaluation, and Treatment of High Blood Pressure: The JNC 7 Report, *JAMA* 289:2560-2571. Developed by the National Heart, Lung, and Blood Institute and the National High Blood Pressure Education Program.
2. Khan NA, McAlister FA, Campbell NR, et al: The 2004 Canadian recommendations for the management of hypertension: Part II – therapy, *Can J Cardiol* (20):41-54, 2004.
3. Sever PS, Dahlof B, Poulter NR, et al (for the ASCOT Investigators): Prevention of coronary and stroke events with atorvastatin in hypertensive patients with average or lower than average cholesterol concentrations, in the Anglo-Scandanavian Cardiac Outcomes Trial-Lipid lowering arm (ASCOT-LLA): A multicentre randomized controlled trial, *Lancet* 361:1149-1158, 2003.
4. ALLHAT Officers and Coordinators for the ALLHAT Collaborative Research Group: Major outcomes in high-risk hypertensive patients randomized to angiotensin-converting enzyme inhibitor or calcium channel blocker vs diuretic: The Antihypertensive and Lipid-Lowering Treatment to Prevent Heart Attack Trial (ALLHAT), *JAMA* 288:2981-2997, 2002.
5. Shepherd J, Blau GJ, Murphy MB, et al (for the PROSPER study group): PROspective Study of Pravastatin in the Elderly at Risk. Pravastatin in elderly individuals at risk of vascular disease (PROSPER): a randomized controlled trial, *Lancet* 360:1623-1630, 2002.
6. Heart Protection Study Collaborative Group. MRC/BHF Heart Protection Study of cholesterol lowering with simvastatin in 20,536 high risk individuals: a randomized placebo controlled trial, *Lancet* 360:7-22, 2002
7. Hansson L, Zanchetti A, Carruthers SG, et al: Effects of intensive blood-pressure lowering and low-dose aspirin in patients with hypertension: principal results of the Hypertension Optimal Treatment (HOT) randomized trial. HOT Study Group, *Lancet* 351:1755-1762, 1998.
8. Somes GW, Pahor M, Shorr RI, et al: The role of diastolic blood pressure when treating isolated systolic hypertension, *Arch Intern Med* 159:2004-2009, 1999.
9. Moore MA, Epstein M, Agodoa L, et al: Current strategies for management of hypertensive renal disease, *Arch Intern Med* 159:23-28, 1999.

Lifestyle Modifications

(See also alcohol; exercise; NSAIDs; obesity)

Following are some of the non-pharmacological treatment modalities for hypertension. Many of these are discussed more fully in the ensuing paragraphs.
- Discontinue smoking
- Lose weight
- Exercise
- Discontinue or diminish alcohol consumption
- Discontinue NSAIDs; if possible, change diet

Smoking cessation

Smoking is not a risk factor for hypertension as such, but because it is a major CV risk factor, quitting is particularly important for hypertensive patients.[1]

Weight reduction

Weight reduction has been shown to lower BP independent of changes in diet and salt intake. Blood pressure is reduced approximately 2/1 mm Hg for each kilogram of weight loss.[2]

Exercise

Regular aerobic exercise such as 3 hours of brisk walking per week has been shown to reduce both the systolic and diastolic blood pressure in mild, moderate, and severe hypertension.[3] A study of Japanese men found that those who walked to work had a decreased risk of hypertension.[4]

Table 12 Lifestyle Interventions and Their Effect on Hypertension

Intervention	Targeted Change	SBP/DBP
Sodium reduction	100 mmol/day	-5.8 / -2.5
Weight loss	-4.5 kg	-7.2 / -5.9
Alcohol reduction	-2.7 drinks/day	-4.6 / -2.3
Exercise	3 times/week	-10.3 / -7.5
Dietary patterns	DASH diet	-11.4 / -5.5

From Campbell N, on behalf of the Canadian Hypertension Program: 2004 CHEP hypertension recommendations: What's new, what's old but still important in 2004. *Perspectives in Cardiology* 20(4):26, 2004. (Table 1). Available from: http://www.canadianstrokenetwork.ca/research/projects/downloads/hypertension2003.recommendations.pdf (accessed Jan. 6, 2005).

Thirty to 45 minutes of moderate exercise 3 to 5 times a week will result in an approximate reduction of systolic blood pressure of 4 to 9 mm Hg.[1]

Reduction in alcohol intake

Individuals who have less than three drinks per day did not show any elevation of BP. However, drinking more than that, even if in the form of binge drinking, caused a rise in BP.[5]

A reduction in alcohol intake to no more than two standard drinks per day for men and one standard drink per day for women can result in a reduction in BP of 2 to 4 mm Hg.[1]

Non-steroidal anti-inflammatory drugs

A large number of elderly patients with hypertension may have the disorder simply because they are taking, or have recently taken, NSAIDs. In one study 41% of elderly patients with hypertension had used NSAIDs in the previous year as compared with 26% of younger control subjects. The higher the dosage of NSAIDs, the more likely that the patients were started on antihypertensive therapy.[6] In a meta-analysis of a number of studies, an Australian group found that on average, NSAIDs elevated supine mean BP by 5 mm Hg. Furthermore, NSAIDs antagonized the BP-lowering effect of antihypertensive drugs, particularly beta blockers. Diuretics and vasodilators were less affected.[7]

Dietary changes

The Dietary Approaches to Stop Hypertension (DASH)[8] diet has been shown beneficial for both hypertension and for the prevention of hypertension. The efficacy of this diet is distinct from any benefits in weight reduction. It is a "feeding study" that lasted for 8 weeks, so is not necessarily reproducible in primary care; however, it emphasizes that these dietary changes make a difference. The DASH diet, which is high in fresh fruit and vegetables, nuts, legumes, and low-fat dairy products, but low in saturated fats, reduced BP by 7.2 mm Hg overall and by 11.4 mm Hg systolic. Interestingly, it also reduced headaches (36% vs. 47%).[2]

Sacks et al showed that a reduction in sodium intake to levels below 100 mmol/day and the DASH diet both lower BP substantially, with a greater effect in combination than singly. Long-term benefits depend on long-term compliance to diet changes and increased commercial availability of low-salt foods.[9]

The approximate reduction in systolic BP is 8 to 14 mm Hg for the DASH diet and 2 to 8 mm Hg for salt restriction.

A 1999 meta-analysis found that calcium supplementation or diets high in calcium resulted in a statistically significant[10] but clinically insignificant[11] reduction of both systolic and diastolic pressures. Caffeine can raise the blood pressure acutely but is not a cause of persistently elevated levels.[1] Excessive licorice ingestion may induce a hyperaldosterone-like syndrome with hypertension and a hypokalemic metabolic alkalosis.[12]

◈ REFERENCES ◈

1. Chobanian AV, Bakris GL, Black HR, et al. The Seventh Report of the Joint National Committee on Prevention, Detection, Evaluation, and Treatment of High Blood Pressure: The JNC 7 Report, *JAMA* 289:2560-2571, 2003. Developed by the National Heart, Lung, and Blood Institute and the National High Blood Pressure Education Program.
2. Khan NA, McAlister FA, Campbell NR, et al: The 2004 Canadian recommendations for the management of hypertension: Part II – therapy, *Can J Cardiol* (20):55-59, 2004.
3. Cléroux J, Feldman RD, Petrella RJ: Lifestyle modifications to prevent and control hypertension. 4. Recommendations on physical exercise training, *Can Med Assoc J* 160(suppl 9): S21-S28, 1999.
4. Hayashi T, Tsumura K, Suematsu C, et al: Walking to work and the risk for hypertension in men: the Osaka Health Survey, *Ann Intern Med* 130:21-26, 1999.
5. Marmot MG, Elliott P, Shipley MJ, et al: Alcohol and blood pressure: the INTERSALT study, *BMJ* 308:1263-1267, 1994.
6. Gurwitz FH, Avorn J, Bohn RL, et al: Initiation of antihypertensive treatment during nonsteroidal anti-inflammatory drug therapy, *JAMA* 272:781-786, 1994.
7. Johnson AG, Nguyen TV, Day RO: Do nonsteroidal anti-inflammatory drugs affect blood pressure? A meta-analysis, *Ann Intern Med* 121:289-300, 1994.
8. National Heart, Lung and Blood Institute Accessed April 8th 2004 http://www.nhlbi.nih.gov/health/public/heart/hbp/dash/index.htm
9. Sacks FM, Svetky LP, Vollmer WM, et al: Effects on blood pressure of reduced dietary sodium and the dietary approaches to stop hypertension (DASH) diet. DASH-Sodium Collaborative research Group, *N Engl J Med* 344:3-10, 2001.
10. Griffith LE, Guyatt GH, Cook RJ, et al: The influence of dietary and nondietary calcium supplementation on blood pressure: an updated metaanalysis of randomized controlled trials, *Am J Hypertens* 12:84-92, 1999.
11. Cappuccio FP: The "calcium antihypertension theory" (editorial), *Am J Hypertens* 12:93-95, 1999.
12. Heikens J, Fliers E, Endert E, et al: Liquorice-induced hypertension–a new understanding of an old disease: case report and brief review, *Netherlands J Med* 47:230-234, 1995.

Initiating Pharmacotherapy

Several drugs are supported by evidence as initial therapy. In general, one should start with a low dose and gradually increase as needed over several weeks. In most cases a thiazide diuretic (up to 25 mg) represents a good choice, but see Table 13 for compelling indications. A second drug from a different class (preferably a thiazide if it has not been used initially) should be added when a single drug in adequate doses fails to achieve BP goals.

If the patient experiences significant side effects while receiving the original drug, that drug should be discontinued and an antihypertensive from another class substituted.

Most patients should return for follow-up and adjustment of medications approximately monthly until target BP is reached. More frequent visits are indicated for patients with stage 2 hypertension (see Table 9) or with complicating co-morbid conditions.

Serum potassium should be monitored in the first 2 months of therapy, and creatinine should be monitored at least 1 to 2 times per year and more frequently with drugs affecting renal function, such as angiotensin converting enzyme inhibitors (ACEIs), angiotensin II antagonists (ARBs) and thiazides). After BP is stable at goal levels, follow-up visits are usually at 3- to 6-month intervals.[1]

More than one medication is usually needed for most patients. In the ALLHAT trial at the end of the 5-year follow-up, 63% of patients were on at least two antihypertensive agents.[2] Evidence supports the concept that combination therapy should be used if the response to standard monotherapy is only partial. Blood pressure reduction with combination drug therapy is usually additive, but adverse effects are not.[3] Non-compliance probably accounts for nearly half of all failures in the treatment of hypertension.[4]

❧ REFERENCES ❧

1. Chobanian AV, Bakris GL, Black HR, et al: The Seventh Report of the Joint National Committee on Prevention, Detection, Evaluation, and Treatment of High Blood Pressure: The JNC 7 Report. *JAMA* 289:2560-2571, 2003. Developed by the National Heart, Lung, and Blood Institute and the National High Blood Pressure Education Program.
2. ALLHAT Officers and Coordinators for the ALLHAT Collaborative Research Group: Major outcomes in high-risk hypertensive patients randomized to angiotensin-converting enzyme inhibitor or calcium channel blocker vs diuretic: the Antihypertensive and Lipid-Lowering Treatment to Prevent Heart Attack Trial (ALLHAT), *JAMA* 288:2981-2997, 2002.
3. Khan NA, McAlister FA, Campbell NR, et al: The 2004 Canadian recommendations for the management of hypertension: Part II – therapy, *Can J Cardiol* (20):55-59, 2004.
4. Stephenson J: Noncompliance may cause half of antihypertensive drug "failures," *JAMA* 228:313-314, 1999.

Factors influencing the choice of drugs

Patients without compelling indications. "Hypertension without compelling indications" refers to patients with high BP who do not have associated co-morbidities such as diabetes mellitus or ischemic heart disease.

Recent Canadian and American guidelines highlight the evidence supporting thiazides as "first among equals" as initial therapy in this group.[1,2]

The ALLHAT study, a double-blind trial of 42,418 patients randomly assigned to chlorthalidone, amlodipine, lisinopril, or doxazosin-based treatment found no difference between these four regimens in fatal and non-fatal MI or all-cause mortality. The chlorthalidone group had a statistically lower incidence of stroke than the groups taking doxazosin and lisinopril. The incidence of heart failure was also lower in the chlorthalidone group than the other three treatment groups.[3]

Support for using thiazides as first-line drugs also comes from a 1999 systematic review in which low-dose diuretics were found to reduce the risk of death, stroke, CAD, and CV events, whereas high-dose thiazide therapy, beta blocker therapy, and calcium channel blocker therapy did not decrease the risk of death or CAD. (ACE inhibitors were not assessed.)[3]

Alpha blockers are not recommended as first-line therapy for hypertension.[2]

Patients with Compelling Indications. Table 13 indicates the use of certain drugs for compelling indications. These selections are based on positive results from clinical studies. Combination therapy is often indicated or required and the information in Table 13 serves only as a starting point. Further therapy requires consideration of concurrent medications, tolerability, and BP targets.

Ischemic heart disease. Beta blockers are the preferred antihypertensive therapy for patients with stable angina. Long-acting calcium channel blockers may also be used if beta blockers are contraindicated such as for patients with asthma, or if BP does not reach target levels. Recent guidelines also recommend ACE inhibitors for all patients with documented CAD even if their BP is controlled. Evidence from several studies supports this, particularly the Heart Outcomes Prevention Evaluation (HOPE) trial and the EURopean trial On reduction of cardiac events with Perindopril in stable coronary Artery diease (EUROPA).[1,2,4,5]

Heart failure. ACE inhibitors are the drugs of first choice in hypertensive patients with HF.

Beta blockers and aldosterone antagonists (the latter for patients with New York Heart Association class III or IV symptoms or post MI) are also indicated and need careful titration, particularly beta blockers.[1,2]

ARBs are recommended if ACE inhibitors are not tolerated. The recommendation regarding ARBs is based on reduced mortality and rate of hospitalization vs placebo shown in the CHARM-ALTERNATIVE trial (relative reduction 23% 95% CI 11% to 33%). This benefit of ARBs in hypertension in HF patients was suggested earlier in a subgroup analysis from the Valsarten Heart Failure (ValHeFT) trial.[6,7]

An ACE inhibitor can be combined with an ARB if BP is not controlled.[2]

Diabetes mellitus. Because of the very high risk of cardiovascular and renal disease in patients with both diabetes

Table 13   Considerations in the Individualization of Antihypertensive Therapy

Initial therapy	Second-line therapy	Notes and/or cautions	
Hypertension without compelling indications for other medications	Thiazide diuretics, beta blockers, ACE inhibitors, ARBs, or long-acting dihydropyridine calcium channel blockers (CCBs)	Combinations of first-line drugs	Alpha blockers are not recommended as initial monotherapy. Beta blockers are not recommended as initial monotherapy in those over 60 years of age. Hypokalemia should be avoided in those who take prescribed diuretics. ACE inhibitors are not recommended as initial monotherapy in African Americans.
Isolated systolic hypertension without other compelling indications	Thiazide diuretics, ARBs, or long-acting dihydropyridine CCBs	Combinations of first-line drugs	Hypokalemia should be avoided in people who take prescribed diuretics
Diabetes mellitus with nephropathy	ACE inhibitors or ARBs	Addition of one or more of thiazide diuretics, cardioselective beta blockers, long-acting CCBs, or use of an ARB/ACE inhibitor combination	
Diabetes mellitus without nephropathy	ACE inhibitors, ARBs, or thiazide diuretics	Combination of first-line drugs or addition of cardioselective beta blockers and/or long-acting CCBs	If the serum creatinine level is greater than 150 mmol/L, a loop diuretic should be used as a replacement for low-dose thiazide diuretics if volume control is required
Angina	Beta blockers (strongly consider adding ACE inhibitors)	Long-acting CCBs	Avoid short-acting nifedipine
Prior MI	Beta blockers and ACE inhibitors	Combinations of additional agents	Avoid nondihydropyridine CCBs (diltiazem, verapamil)
Heart failure	ACE inhibitors, beta blockers, and spironolactone (ARBs if ACE-inhibitor intolerant)	Hydralazine/isosorbide dinitrate; thiazide or loop diuretics as additive therapy	
Past cerebrovascular accident or TIA	ACE inhibitor/diuretic combinations		BP reduction reduces recurrent cerebrovascular events
Renal disease	ACE inhibitors (diuretics as additive therapy)	Combinations of additional agents (ARBs if ACE-inhibitor intolerant)	Avoid ACE inhibitors if bilateral renal artery stenosis exists
Left ventricular hypertrophy	ACE inhibitors, ARBs, dihydropyridine CCBs, thiazide diuretics (beta blockers for patients under 55 years of age)		Avoid hydralazine and minoxidil

*Short-acting calcium channel blockers (CCBs) are not recommended in the treatment of hypertension. ACE: Angiotensin-converting enzyme; ARB: Angiotensin II receptor blocker; TIA: Transient ischemic attack.
This information was originally published in *Can J Cardiol* 20(1):41–54, 2004. Reprinted with permission.

and hypertension, the recommended target blood pressure for such individuals is 130/80 mm Hg.[1,2] Support for tight control comes from a United Kingdom Prospective Diabetes Study Group (UKPDS) report of hypertensive patients with type 2 diabetes who were treated with either a beta blocker or an ACE inhibitor as first-line therapy. (Other drug classes were added if necessary.) Mean blood pressures obtained were 144/82 mm Hg, and the incidence of macrovascular events, diabetes-related mortality, and visual loss was significantly lower than in the control group, who had a mean pressure of 154/87 mm Hg.[8]

For patients with diabetes and normal urinary albumin excretion (less than 30 mg/day), thiazides and ARBs have been added to ACE inhibitors as first-line therapy.[2] (ARBs were added on the basis of the LIFE trial, which showed a 39% reduction in all-cause mortality with Losarten in 1195 patients with mostly type 2 diabetes mellitus.[9] Thiazides were added following a subgroup analysis of the ALLHAT sudy, which showed no appreciable differences between thiazides and ACE inhibitors for all-cause mortality in patients with diabetes and hypertension.[3]

Antihypertensive medications may decrease glucose tolerance, and thiazide diuretics are commonly considered the worst offenders. They are not. All classes of antihypertensives decrease glucose tolerance over the short term, and multiple-drug regimens are more likely to do so than single-drug treatments.[10] However, the decreased glucose tolerance of thiazides seems to be self-limited and disappears with time.[11] Therefore, low-dose thiazides are acceptable treatment for diabetic patients provided that glucose levels are carefully monitored.[12] ACE inhibitors or ARBs are recommended as initial treatment for hypertensive (greater than 130/80 mm Hg) diabetics with albuminuria. If BP levels remain greater than 130/80 mm Hg, thiazides or long-acting calcium channel blockers may be added or the ACE inhibitor combined with an ARB.[2]

Alpha blockers are not recommended as initial therapy in hypertensive patients with diabetes.[2]

Chronic renal failure. The most important goal in the treatment of hypertension in patients with renal failure is to achieve good BP control (≤130/80 mm Hg) by whatever means are effective, and this often means using multiple drugs. For patients with proteinuria greater than 1 G/day, target BP should be less than 125/75 mm Hg.[2] Whenever possible, ACE inhibitors should be used because they have documented renal protective effects beyond that of BP control. In most cases diuretics are needed because of the salt and water retention that is usually part of renal failure. In renal failure brought about by severe BP failure, thiazides are ineffective and loop diuretics are required.[13]

If a patient has a creatinine level above 250 mmol/L (30 mg/dl), ACE inhibitors should be started at low doses and the creatinine level monitored closely. ACE inhibitors should not be used if the potassium is 5.5 mmol/L or greater.[14]

Cerebrovascular disease. In acute stroke, lowering the BP is controversial and caution is advised. After the acute phase, BP should be controlled, aiming for a target less than 140/90 mm Hg. A combination of thiazides and ACE inhibitors is recommended.[2]

Other considerations in choice of therapy

Reduction of left ventricular hypertrophy. Left ventricular hypertrophy (LVH) is an independent risk factor for CVD. Reduction of LVH is important because it is associated with improved prognosis. No evidence has shown that any one class of antihypertensives is superior to another in reducingLVH.[2,15]

Quality of life. No one class of antihypertensive agents is clearly superior to another in terms of quality of life. A 4-year follow-up of patients with mild hypertension taking a placebo or low doses of one of five classes of drugs (beta blockers [acebutolol], calcium channel blockers [amlodipine], diuretics [chlorthalidone], alpha₁ blockers [doxazosin], ACE inhibitors [enalapril]) found that quality of life improved in all groups, including those taking placebo.[16]

Cost. Antihypertensive drugs vary greatly in cost. The least expensive in most cases is a generic diuretic or beta blocker.

Age of patient. Hypertension affects two thirds of the population over age 65; in fact, this is the population with the poorest rates of BP control.[1] The recommendations for treatment of hypertension in the elderly, including isolated systolic hypertension, generally adhere to the same guidelines as younger patients. Side effects may be avoided by using lower initial dosages.[1]

However, current guidelines advise against the use of beta blockers as first-line agents, although they may play a role in combination therapy or in certain co-morbidities such as angina.[2] Messerli and colleagues in a meta-analysis of 10 trials involving 16,164 elderly patients found that diuretics were superior to beta blockers in all endpoints including stroke, CHD, CV mortality, and all-cause mortality. Beta blockers only reduced the odds for mortality from stroke.[17]

Race. African Americans may not respond as well to beta-adrenergic blockers or ACE inhibitors.[18]

ACE-inhibitor angioedema occurs 2 to 4 times more often in African American patients than in other patient groups,[3] and ACE inhibitors are not recommended as first-line therapy in this group.[2]

Arthritis. Arthritis is often treated with NSAIDs, but they tend either to cause hypertension or to counter the therapeutic effect of many antihypertensive drugs.

Hyperlipidemias. No good evidence supports that specific classes of antihypertensive drugs increase the risk of CV complications. The choice of antihypertensive drugs for hypertensive patients with hyperlipidemia should be the same as for hypertensive patients with normal lipid profiles.[19]

Peripheral vascular disease. Peripheral vascular disease is a marker for widespread atherosclerosis and equivalent in risk to ischemic heart disease. In most cases any class of antihypertensive may be used, including beta blockers, although beta blockers should be avoided in severe peripheral vascular disease. Aggressive management of other risk factors is important, as is the use of ASA therapy.[1,2]

Depression. Beta blockers are commonly believed to cause or aggravate depression; however, several studies have failed to show such a correlation.[20,21]

Potential favourable effects. Thiazide diuretics are useful in slowing demineralization in osteoporosis. Beta blockers can be used in the treatment of atrial tachyarrhythmias/fibrillation, migraine prophylaxis, thyrotoxicosis (short term), essential tremor, or perioperative hypertension. Calcium channel blockers may be useful in Raynaud's syndrome and certain arrhythmias. Alpha blockers have a role in the treatment of prostatism.[1]

Potential unfavourable effects. In patients who have a history of gout or hyponatremia, thiazides should be used with caution. Beta blockers should not be used in patients who have asthma, reactive airway disease, or second- or third-degree heart block. ACE inhibitors and ARBS are contraindicated in pregnancy and should be avoided in those who are likely to become pregnant. ACE inhibitors should not be used in patients with a history of angioedema. Aldosterone antagonists and potassium-sparing diuretics should generally be avoided in patients who have baseline (before drug therapy) serum potassium values above 5.0 MEQ/L.[1]

———————— ✍ REFERENCES ✍ ————————

1. Chobanian AV, Bakris GL, Black HR, et al: The Seventh Report of the Joint National Committee on Prevention, Detection, Evaluation, and Treatment of High Blood Pressure: The JNC 7 Report, *JAMA* 289:2560-71, 2003. Developed by the National Heart, Lung, and Blood Institute and the National High Blood Pressure Education Program.
2. Khan NA, McAlister FA, Campbell NR, et al: The 2004 Canadian recommendations for the management of hypertension: Part II – therapy, *Can J Cardiol* (20):55-59, 2004.
3. ALLHAT Officers and Coordinators for the ALLHAT Collaborative Research Group: Major outcomes in high-risk hypertensive patients randomized to angiotensin-converting enzyme inhibitor or calcium channel blocker vs diuretic: the Antihypertensive and Lipid-Lowering Treatment to Prevent Heart Attack Trial (ALLHAT), *JAMA* 288:2981-2997, 2002.
4. The Heart Outcomes Prevention Evaluation Study Investigators. Effects of an angiotensin converting enzyme inhibitor, ramipril, on cardiovascular events in high risk patients, *N Engl J Med* 342:1351-1357, 2000.
5. Fox KM (for the EURopean trial On reduction of cardiac events with Perindropil in stable coronary Artery disease Investigators): Efficacy of perindopril in reduction of cardiovascular events among patients with stable coronary artery disease: randomized double-blind, placebo-controlled, multicentre trial (the EUROPA study), *Lancet* 362:782-788, 2003.
6. Granger CB, McMurray JJ, Yusuf S, et al: The CHARM-Alternative trial, *Lancet* 362(9386):772-776, 2003.
7. Maggioni AP, Anand I, Gottlieb SO, et al: Effects of valsartan on morbidity and mortality in patients with heart failure not receiving angiotensin-converting enzyme inhibitors, *J Am Coll Cardiol;*40(8): 1414-1421, 2002.
8. UK Prospective Diabetes Study Group: Tight blood pressure control and risk of macrovascular and microvascular complications in type 2 diabetes: UKPDS 38, *BMJ* 317:703-713, 1998.
9. Dahlof B, Devereux RB, Kjeldsen SE, et al: Cardiovascular morbidity and mortality in the Losarten Intervention For Endpoint reduction in hypertension study (LIFE): a randomized trial against atenolol, *Lancet* 359:995-1003, 2002.
10. Gurwitz JH, Bohn RL, Glynn RJ, et al: Antihypertensive drug therapy and the initiation of treatment for diabetes mellitus, *Ann Intern Med* 118:273-278, 1993.
11. Freis ED: The efficacy and safety of diuretics in treating hypertension, *Ann Intern Med* 122:223-226, 1995.
12. Moser M: Management of hypertension, part I, *Am Fam Physician* 53:2295-2302, 1996.
13. Moore MA, Epstein M, Agodoa L, et al: Current strategies for management of hypertensive renal disease, *Arch Intern Med* 159:23-28, 1999.
14. Baker DW, Konstam MA, Bottoriff M, et al: Management of heart failure. I. Pharmacologic treatment, *JAMA* 272:1361-1366, 1994.
15. Dunn FG, Pfeffer MA: Left ventricular hypertrophy in hypertension (editorial), *N Engl J Med* 340:1279-1280, 1999.
16. Grimm RH Jr, Grandits GA, Cutler FA, et al: Relationships of quality-of-life measures to long-term lifestyle and drug treatment in the treatment of mild hypertension study, *Arch Intern Med* 157:638-648, 1997.
17. Messerli FH, Grossman E, Goldbourt U: Are beta blockers efficacious as first-line therapy for hypertension in the elderly? A systematic review, *JAMA* 279:1903-1907, 1998.
18. Hall WD, Reed JW, Flack JM, et al: Comparison of the efficacy of dihydropyridine calcium channel blockers in African American patients with hypertension, *Arch Intern Med* 158:2029-2034, 1998.
19. Feldman RD, Campbell N, Larochelle P, et al: 1999 Canadian recommendations for the management of hypertension, *Can Med Assoc J 161* (suppl 12):S1-S22, 1999.
20. Wurzelmann J, Frishman WH, Aronson M, et al: Neuropsychological effects of antihypertensive drugs, *Cardiol Clin* 4:689-701, 1987.
21. Prisant LM, Spruill WJ, Fincham JE, et al: Depression associated with antihypertensive drugs, *J Fam Pract* 33:481-485, 1991.

Step-Down Therapy

As many as one third of patients whose hypertension has been well controlled for at least 1 year may be able to decrease or even discontinue their medications.[1] No recent guidelines for this have been published. It is generally agreed that such an undertaking should be implemented gradually, close follow-up is indicated after medications are stopped, and success is most likely in patients who have made significant lifestyle improvements.[1,2] One suggested protocol from 1987 is that if patients who are taking more than one antihypertensive drug are normotensive for 6 to 12 months, all but one drug may be gradually withdrawn. A patient who remains normotensive for 6 to 12 months while taking one medication and whose pre-treatment pressure was only mildly elevated may have all medications discontinued.[3]

———————— ✍ REFERENCES ✍ ————————

1. Froom J, Trilling JS, Yeh S-S, et al: Withdrawal of antihypertensive medications, *J Am Board Fam Pract* 10:249-258, 1997.
2. Joint National Committee on Prevention, Detection, Evaluation and Treatment of High Blood Pressure: Sixth

report of the Joint National Committee on the Prevention, Detection, Evaluation and Treatment of High Blood Pressure, *Arch Intern Med* 157:2413-2446, 1997.

3. Dannenberg AL, Kannel WB: Remission of hypertension: the "natural" history of blood pressure treatment in the Framingham Study, *JAMA* 257:1477-1483, 1987.

Specific Antihypertensive Drugs

(See also benign prostatic hyperplasia; detrusor overactivity; heart failure; stress incontinence; urticaria and angioedema)

Diuretics and diuretics combined with potassium-sparing agents

Hypokalemia secondary to thiazide drugs is dose dependent[1] and is not usually a problem with doses less than 25 mg/day. One reason for treating even mild hypokalemia is that low potassium levels are associated with BP elevations.[2] Although oral supplements of potassium chloride are traditionally given to counter hypokalemia, the use of a potassium-sparing agent such as amiloride, triamterene, or spironolactone in conjunction with a thiazide should be considered for hydrochlorothiazide doses of 25 mg per day or more. There is evidence that this decreases the risk of primary cardiac arrest compared with control patients receiving equivalent doses of thiazides with or without potassium supplementation.[3] Some of the available combined products are Dyazide, Moduretic or Moduret, and Aldactazide (Table 14).

Thiazides are often combined with ACE inhibitors and ARBs, which both tend to conserve potassium so that supplementation is less likely to be necessary. However, creatinine and potassium levels still need to be closely monitored.

Other reputed adverse effects of thiazides are elevated cholesterol and glucose levels. When low doses are used, both of these effects tend to be short lived and either disappear with long-term therapy[4] or at least tend not to be progressive.[5] In the Systolic Hypertension in the Elderly Program (SHEP) program, in which chlorthalidone (Hygroton) in doses of 12.5 to 25 mg per day was the primary therapeutic agent, diabetic patients had as great a decrease in cerebrovascular events as did nondiabetic patients.[5]

Potassium supplementation

If hypokalemia is induced by diuretics, prescribing a combination of a thiazide and a potassium-sparing diuretic is often best. (See earlier discussion of diuretics.) Foods high in potassium include milk products, fruits, meat, and vegetables. A large number of commercial potassium supplements are available; the usual dose for oral replacement is about 20 mEq per day.

Calcium channel blockers

Traditional calcium channel blockers that block the L-channels are divided into three classes (Table 15). All calcium channel blockers increase coronary artery flow and are therefore antianginal agents. Verapamil has the most marked negative inotropic effect of all these agents. Verapamil and to a lesser extent diltiazem decrease atrioventricular node conduction and are therefore useful in patients with paroxysmal supraventricular tachycardia or AF with a rapid ventricular response.[6] Both verapamil and diltiazem may be used in patients with angina who are taking nitrates, because these agents do not tend to cause reflex tachycardia.

Calcium channel blockers have been known for some time to have no cardioprotective effect after MI.[6] Of more concern are reports of an association between both short-acting[7] and long-acting[8] calcium channel blockers and MI, but the true significance of this is uncertain, because other reports have not shown such a correlation.[9] Other reports suggest that these agents may lead to increased perioperative bleeding.[10] Some reports have claimed an association between calcium channel blockers and gastrointestinal hemorrhages,[11] but others have failed to confirm this finding.[12] Although some studies have found an increased risk of cancer in patients taking calcium channel blockers,[13] others report no such association, in particular the ALLHAT study.[14] An increased risk of suicide has been reported among patients taking these drugs.[15]

Beta blockers

Beta blockers decrease heart rate, systolic BP, myocardial contractility, and myocardial oxygen demand. Beta blockers without intrinsic sympathomimetic activity (ISA) are the only antihypertensive drugs shown to be cardioprotective; they reduce mortality after infarction, limit infarct size, and decrease arrhythmias and sudden death. Beta blockers may mask some of the symptoms of hypoglycemia in diabetic patients taking hypoglycemic

---

Table 14   Diuretics and Diuretics Combined with Potassium-Sparing Agents

Drug	Usual dose
Diuretics	
Hydrochlorothiazide (Hydrodiuril, Esidrix, HCTZ)	12.5-25 mg qam
Chlorthalidone (Hygroton)	25 mg qam
Indapamide (Lozide)	1.25-2.5 mg qam
Spironolactone (Aldactone)	25-100 mg qam
Diuretics Plus K+ Sparing Agents	
Hydrochlorothiazide 50 mg plus amiloride 5 mg (Moduretic, Moduret)	1/2 tablet qam
Hydrochlorothiazide 25 mg plus triamterene 50 mg (Dyazide)	1/2 tablet qam
Spironolactone 25 mg plus hydrochlorothiazide 25 mg (Aldactazide)	1 tablet qam

Table 15 Calcium Channel Blockers

Drug	Usual dose
Benzothiazepine Derivatives	
Diltiazem (Cardizem, Tiazac)	30-60 mg tid-qid for short acting; 60-180 mg bid for SR; 180-360 mg as a single dose for controlled delivery
Papaverine-Like Compounds	
Verapamil (Isoptin, Calan, Covera-HS)	80 tid for short acting; 180-240 mg as single dose for extended-release tablets
Dihydropyridine Derivatives	
Amlodipine besylate (Norvasc)	5-10 mg/day as a single dose
Felodipine (Renedil, Plendil)	2.5-10 mg/day as a single dose
Isradipine (DynaCirc)	2.5-5 mg bid for short acting; 5-10 mg/day as single dose for extended release
Nicardipine (Cardene)	20-40 mg tid for short acting; 30-60 mg bid for extended release
Nifedipine (Adalat, Procardia)	10-20 mg bid for short acting; 30-90 mg/day as a single dose for extended release
Nisoldipine (Sular)	20-40 mg/day as a single dose

Table 16 Beta Blockers

Drug	Usual dose
Non-selective, Without ISA	
Nadolol (Corgard)	80-240 mg/day as a single dose
Propranolol (Inderal)	40-160 mg bid for short acting; 80-320 mg once a day for extended release
Timolol (Blocadren)	5-30 mg bid
Selective, Without ISA	
Atenolol (Tenormin)	50-100 mg/day as a single dose
Metoprolol (Lopresor, Toprol-XL)	50-100 mg bid for short acting; 100 mg/day as a single dose for extended release
Non-selective, with ISA	
Pindolol (Visken)	5-15 mg bid
Selective, with ISA	
Acebutolol (Sectral)	100-400 mg bid
Beta-Adrenergic and Alpha₁ blocking Agents	
Labetalol (Trandate)	200-400 mg bid
Carvedilol (Coreg)	12.5 mg bid

ISA, Intrinsic sympathomimetic activity.

medications, but except for patients with recurrent hypoglycemic episodes, this is not a contraindication to using these agents, since the cardioprotective benefits far outweigh this adverse effect. Although beta blockers without intrinsic ISA may cause a slight lowering of HDL cholesterol and some elevation of triglycerides, the clinical significance of these changes is unknown; no human or animal data show that beta blockers promote atherogenesis. Beta blockers with intrinsic ISA activity do not adversely affect lipid profiles, but since they are not a good choice for cardioprotection, they have little role in the treatment of hypertension.

Beta blockers may lead to or aggravate urinary incontinence because of detrusor overactivity. This is because beta-adrenergic stimulation normally inhibits the detrusor muscle.[16]

Sotalol is not indicated for the treatment of hypertension.

ACE inhibitors and angiotensin II–blocking agents

ACE inhibitors (see Table 7) may cause disorders of taste, cough in up to 25% of patients, and rarely angioedema. An alternative for patients unable to tolerate ACE inhibitors is to try an angiotensin II–blocking agent (see Table 8). A more complete discussion of ACE inhibitors may be found in the section on heart failure.

With angiotensin II receptor antagonists, the incidence of cough is no greater than placebo. They rarely cause angioedema and occasionally cause hyperkalemia.[17-19]

Table 17 Alpha₁-Adrenergic Blocking Agents

Drug	Usual dose
Terazosin (Hytrin)	1-5 mg/day as a single dose
Prazosin (Minipress)	2-5 mg tid
Doxazosin (Cardura)	1-8 mg/day as a single dose

Alpha₁-adrenergic blocking agents

Reflex tachycardia often occurs in patients treated with alpha₁-blocking agents who are not also taking beta blockers. Alpha₁ blockers inhibit the alpha-adrenergic receptors of the internal bladder sphincter and may lead to incontinence. On the other hand, they may relieve the symptoms of benign prostatic hyperplasia.

⬿ INTERNET RESOURCES ⬾

National Heart Lung and Blood Institute: accessed April 12 2004 http://www.nhlbi.nih.gov/index.htm
Canadian Hypertension Society: accessed April 12 2004 http://www.chs.md
GAC Guidelines Advisory Committee : accessed April 12 2004 http://gacguidelines.ca/

⬿ REFERENCES ⬾

1. Knauf H: The role of low-dose diuretics in essential hypertension, *J Cardiovasc Pharmacol* 22(suppl 6):S1-S7, 1993.

2. Whelton PK, He J, Cutler JA, et al: Effects of oral potassium on blood pressure: meta-analysis of randomized controlled clinical trials, *JAMA* 277:1624-1632, 1997.

3. Siscovick DS, Raghunathan TE, Psaty BM, et al: Diuretic therapy for hypertension and the risk of primary cardiac arrest, *N Engl J Med* 330:1852-1857, 1994.

4. Freis ED: The efficacy and safety of diuretics in treating hypertension, *Ann Intern Med* 122:223-226, 1995.

5. Savage PJ, Pressel SL, Curb JD, et al: Influence of long-term, low-dose, diuretic-based, antihypertensive therapy on glucose, lipid, uric acid, and potassium levels in older men and women with isolated systolic hypertension: the Systolic Hypertension in the Elderly Program, *Arch Intern Med* 158:741-751, 1998.

6. Raspa RF, Wilson CC: Calcium channel blockers in the treatment of hypertension, *Am Fam Physician* 48:461-470, 1993.

7. Furberg CD, Psaty BM, Meyer JV: Nifedipine: dose-related increase in mortality in patients with coronary heart disease, *Circulation* 92:1326-1331, 1995.

8. Estacio RO, Jeffers BW, Hiatt W, et al: The effect of nisoldipine as compared with enalapril on cardiovascular outcomes in patients with non-insulin-dependent diabetes and hypertension, *N Engl J Med* 338:645-652, 1998.

9. Abascal VM, Larson MG, Evans JC, et al: Calcium antagonists and mortality risk in men and women with hypertension in the Framingham Heart Study, *Arch Intern Med* 158:1882-1886, 1998.

10. Zuccalà G, Pahor M, Landi F, et al: Use of calcium antagonists and need for perioperative transfusion in older patients with hip fracture: observational study, *BMJ* 314:643-644, 1997.

11. Pahor M, Guralnik JM, Furberg CD, et al: Risk of gastrointestinal hemorrhage with calcium antagonists in hypertensive patients over 67, *Lancet* 347:1061-1066, 1996.

12. Suissa S, Bourgault C, Barkun A, et al: Antihypertensive drugs and the risk of gastrointestinal bleeding, *Am J Med* 105:230-235, 1998.

13. Pahor M, Guralnik JM, Salive ME, et al: Do calcium channel blockers increase the risk of cancer? *Am J Hypertens* 9:695-699, 1996.

14. ALLHAT Officers and Coordinators for the ALLHAT Collaborative Research Group: Major outcomes in high-risk hypertensive patients randomized to angiotensin-converting enzyme inhibitor or calcium channel blocker vs diuretic: The Antihypertensive and Lipid-Lowering Treatment to Prevent Heart Attack Trial (ALLHAT), *JAMA* 288:2981-2997, 2002.

15. Lindberg G, Bingefors K, Ranstam J, et al: Use of calcium channel blockers and risk of suicide: ecological findings confirmed in population based cohort study, *BMJ* 316: 741-745, 1998.

16. Mold JW: Pharmacotherapy of urinary incontinence, *Am Fam Physician* 54:673-680, 1996.

17. Losartan for hypertension, *Med Lett* 37:57-58, 1995.

18. Gradman AH, Arcuri KE, Goldberg AI, et al: A randomized, placebo-controlled, double-blind, parallel study of various doses of losartan potassium compared with enalapril maleate in patients with essential hypertension, *Hypertension* 25:1345-1350, 1995.

19. Valsartan for hypertension, *Med Lett* 39:43-44, 1997.

VALVULAR HEART DISEASE

(See also anticoagulants; endocarditis prophylaxis; screening)

Heart Murmurs in Children

The ability of pediatric cardiologists to differentiate functional from organic murmurs in children by history and physical examination alone is excellent. Features suggesting organic disease include a pansystolic murmur, a murmur intensity of grade 3 or higher, and an abnormal second heart sound.[1]

Aortic Stenosis

The classic systolic ejection murmur of aortic stenosis is heard best over the base of the heart and is transmitted into the vessels of the neck. A long latent period occurs during the presymptomatic phase of aortic stenosis. Once symptoms such as angina, syncope, dyspnea, or HF occur, the mortality rate is very high over the ensuing 2 to 5 years. In general, surgery should be considered for all asymptomatic patients with declining left ventricular function as demonstrated by echo Doppler studies. It is also indicated for all symptomatic patients. Age is not a contraindication, and results are usually excellent.[2,3]

Aortic Insufficiency

The abnormal regurgitant flow of aortic insufficiency creates the decrescendo, blowing diastolic murmur, which is heard best along the left sternal border. In a 1994 study, nifedipine in doses of 20 mg twice a day was given to asymptomatic patients with aortic insufficiency who had normal left ventricular ejection fractions. This resulted in a significant delay in the need for valve replacement compared with the control group. The rationale for treatment with nifedipine is that arteriolar vasodilation increases forward flow and decreases the amount of aortic regurgitation, preventing left ventricular diastolic volume overload and subsequent dilation and hypertrophy.[4]

Mitral Stenosis

Mitral stenosis usually occurs due to progressive fibrosis, scarring, and calcification of the valve; however, rheumatic fever is still a common cause in underdeveloped countries. The typical murmur is a soft, low-pitched diastolic rumble best heard at the apex when the patient is in the left lateral decubitus position. Percutaneous balloon mitral commissurotomy appears to be the procedure of choice for most patients with mitral stenosis.[5]

Mitral Valve Prolapse

Mitral valve prolapse has a community prevalence rate of about 2.4% and is more common among women.[6] Two variants can be distinguished with two-dimensional echocardiography. The precision of this technique has evolved over the years and some have been falsely "labelled." In the common benign form, the valves are anatomically normal (normal variant mitral valve prolapse), and in a rare but serious variant, which is usually seen in older men or in patients with connective tissue diseases, they are deformed (primary mitral valve prolapse). Adverse sequelae such as cerebrovascular accidents, progressive severe mitral insufficiency, or endocarditis are generally limited to patients with primary mitral valve prolapse. Anxiety, atypical chest pain, and palpitations are not caused by mitral valve prolapse.[7]

Antibiotic prophylaxis against infective endocarditis is mandatory for patients with primary mitral valve prolapse, especially those with a systolic murmur. Prophylaxis for patients with normal variant mitral valve prolapse and no murmur is unnecessary.[7]

General Principles for Management of Valvular Heart Disease

Medical management is preferred in asymptomatic cases of valvular heart disease. Patients should be encouraged to avoid strenuous activity, and should be placed on diuretics and sodium restriction if CHF is present. Antibiotics are given in most cases for endocarditis prophylaxis for patients who are to undergo surgical or dental procedures. Echocardiography remains the gold standard for diagnosis and periodic assessment of patients with valvular heart disease. Surgery is recommended for most symptomatic patients or in cases where sudden decline of function has been demonstrated.[2]

Prosthetic Valves

The two major types of prosthetic valves are mechanical valves and tissue valves. Mechanical valves may be caged-ball (Starr-Edwards), single-tilting-disk (Medtronic-Hall, Bjork-Shiley), or bileaflet-tilting-disk (St. Jude). The most common tissue valve is the porcine heterograft valve. Porcine heterograft valves usually last 10 to 15 years and do not require long-term anticoagulation; mechanical valves last longer but require anticoagulation. Failure of porcine valves is usually gradual, so the replacement surgery can be elective.[8,9]

The surgical mortality of valve replacement depends largely on the patient's individual risk factors. Isolated aortic valve replacement in an otherwise healthy person has a 30-day mortality rate of 1% to 5%, while that for isolated mitral valve replacement is 2% to 8%.[8]

The risk of thrombosis depends on the type of mechanical valve; it is greatest for the caged-ball valves, least for the bileaflet-tilting-disk, and intermediate for the single-tilting-disk. One set of recommendations is that the INR should be maintained between 4 and 4.9 for patients with caged-ball valves or multiple prosthetic valves, between 3 and 3.9 for those with single-tilting-disk valves, and between 2.5 and 2.9 for those with bileaflet-tilting-disk valves. Patients with porcine heterografts may be given anticoagulants to achieve an INR between 2 and 3 for the first 3 months.

Modifications of these recommendations are required for patients at risk of bleeding, such as the very elderly.[9] The authors of a French study concluded that INR levels of 2 to 3 are acceptable for patients with single St. Jude bileaflet-tilting-disk valves implanted in the aortic or mitral regions.[10] Hirsh and associates[11] recommend INR levels of 2.5 to 3.5 for all mechanical prosthetic valves.

❧ REFERENCES ❧

1. McCrindle BW, Shaffer KM, Kan JS, et al: Cardinal clinical signs in the differentiation of heart murmurs in children, *Arch Pediatr Adolesc Med* 150:169-174, 1996.
2. Carabello BA, Crawford FA Jr: Valvular heart disease, *N Engl J Med* 337:32-41, 1997.
3. Otto CM: Timing of aortic valve surgery, *Heart* 84:211-219, 2000.
4. Scognamiglio R, Rahimtoola SH, Fasoli G, et al: Nifedipine in asymptomatic patients with severe aortic regurgitation and normal left ventricular function, *N Engl J Med* 331:689-694, 1994.
5. Farhat MB, Ayari M, Maatouk F, et al: Percutaneous balloon versus surgical closed and open mitral commissurotomy: seven-year follow-up results of a randomized trial, *Circulation* 97:245-250, 1998.
6. Freed LA, Levy D, Levine RA, et al: Prevalence and Clinical Outcomes of Mitral Valve Prolapse, *N Engl J Med* 341:1-7, 1999.
7. Nishimura RA, McGoon MD: Perspectives on mitral-valve prolapse, *N Engl J Med* 341:48-50, 1999.
8. Katz NM: Current surgical treatment of valvular heart disease, *Am Fam Physician* 52:559-568, 1995.
9. Vongpatanasin W, Hillis D, Lange RA: Prosthetic heart valves, *N Engl J Med* 335:407-416, 1996.
10. Acar J, Iung B, Boissel JP, et al: AREVA: multicentre randomized comparison of low-dose versus standard-dose anticoagulation in patients with mechanical prosthetic heart valves, *Circulation* 94:2107-2112, 1996.
11. Hirsh J, Dalen JE, Deykin D, et al: Oral anticoagulants: mechanism of action, clinical effectiveness, and optimal therapeutic range, *Chest* 108(suppl 4):231S-246S, 1995.

VASCULAR DISEASE

(See also transient ischemic attacks)

Arterial Disease

Peripheral vascular disease
(See also coronary artery disease)

In patients with claudication, the risk of death from all causes is 4 to 7 times greater and the risk of dying of CVD within 10 years is 15 times greater than the respective risks of patients who do not have claudication. The 5-year mortality rate for patients with claudication is 29%.[1] The mortality rate is particularly high in diabetic patients.[2] Claudication itself improves spontaneously in 40% of patients, and in only 7% does it progress to the point that amputation is required within the next 5 years.[3]

An objective measurement of peripheral vascular disease is the ankle-brachial index (ABI), which is determined by using Doppler probes to measure systolic pressures over the posterior tibial or dorsalis pedis arteries and comparing them with the branchial artery systolic pressure. Normally the ankle pressure is higher than the brachial pressure, so in normal individuals the index is greater than 1. Any value less than 1 is abnormal, and patients with rest pain usually have values less than 0.5. Diabetics tend toward lower ABI readings, which are measured via a toe systolic pressure index. Cases of peripheral vascular disease must be differentiated from spinal stenosis, neuropathy, arterial thrombois, and arterial embolism to ensure appropriate treatment. Risk factors such as hypertension, smoking, diabetes, obesity, and a sendentary lifestyle should be determined. Obtaining a medical history may also be problematic.[4] In one large study,[5] 83% of patients knew they had peripheral arterial disease yet only 49% of their physicians were aware of this history. Reliance on ABI may also be misleading because many patients with abnormal ABI do not have claudication symptoms by history.

First-line treatment for intermittent claudication is smoking cessation, correction of risk factors, and exercise.[3] In one study patients were instructed to walk for at least 30 minutes 3 times per week and continue walking to a point at which the claudication pain was near maximal. After 6 months the distance walked to onset and to maximal claudication pain increased by 120% to 180%.[6] Whether smoking cessation leads to improved walking distance is uncertain because of the poor quality of most studies,[3] but even if no improvement is achieved, smoking should be anathema to patients with claudication because of its adverse effect on CAD.

Pentoxifylline (Trental), usually given as 400 mg twice a day or three times a day, has increased pain-free walking distances. Because the quantitative effect is small, however, the drug's clinical usefulness for many patients is uncertain. Pentoxifylline is believed to decrease blood viscosity by making red blood cells more pliable.[3] One study found that verapamil (Isoptin, Calan, Covera-HS) in doses of 120 to 480 mg per day gave some symptomatic improvement.[7] Cilostazol (Pletal) has been recently approved by the U.S. Food and Drug Administration for the treatment of claudication (with a usual dosage of 100 mg twice a day). According to the *Medical Letter*, cilostazol has been shown to be moderately effective and may be worth trying in patients who cannot participate in exercise programs. This may be prescribed with an antiplatelet drug. There are concerns that it may prove cardiotoxic.[8]

Prophylactic Aspirin given over long periods to asymptomatic men is associated with a slight decrease in the need for vascular surgery.[8] Patients with peripheral vascular disease have a very high incidence of CAD, and prophylactic Aspirin is a reasonable option for this reason alone. Aspirin remains the best-tolerated and most cost-effective treatment for peripheral vascular disease. An alternative is clopidogrel (Plavix), which in doses of 75 mg per day has been shown to decrease the risk of MI, stroke, and vascular death in patients with peripheral vascular disease. Clopidogrel may be useful for patients who cannot tolerate aspirin, but it is more expensive than Aspirin.[10,11]

Another prophylactic drug that should probably be prescribed for all patients with peripheral vascular disease is the ACE inhibitor ramipril (Altace). In the HOPE study, patients treated with ramipril 10 mg per day had a decreased risk of coronary events, strokes, and total mortality.[11] Chelation therapy has no role in the treatment of peripheral vascular disease.[13]

---   ❧ REFERENCES ❧   ---

1. Criqui MG, Langoer RD, Fronek A, et al: Mortality over a period of 10 years in patients with peripheral arterial disease, *N Engl J Med* 326:381-386, 1992.
2. Barzilay JI, Kronmal RA, Bittner V, et al: Coronary artery disease in diabetic and nondiabetic patients with lower extremity arterial disease: a report from the Coronary Artery Surgery Study Registry, *Am Heart J* 135:1055-1062, 1998.
3. Girolami B, Bernardi E, Prins MH, et al: Treatment of intermittent claudication with physical training, smoking cessation, pentoxifylline or nafronyl, *Arch Intern Med* 159:337-345. 1999.
4. Ouriel K: Detection of peripheral arterial disease in primary care, *JAMA* 286:1380-1381, 2001.
5. Hirsch AT, Criqui MH, Treat-Jacobson D, et al: Peripheral arterial disease detection, awareness, and treatment in primary care, *JAMA* 286:1317-1324, 2001.
6. Gardner AW, Poehlman ET: Exercise rehabilitation programs for the treatment of claudication pain: a meta-analysis, *JAMA* 274:975-980, 1995.
7. Bagger JP, Helligsoe P, Randsbaek F, et al: Effect of verapamil in intermittent claudication: a randomized double-blind, placebo-controlled, cross-over study after individual dose-response assessment, *Circulation* 95:411-414, 1997.
8. Cilostazol for intermittent claudication, *Med Lett* 41:44-46, 1999.
9. Goldhaber SZ, Manson JE, Stampfer MJ, et al: Low-dose aspirin and subsequent peripheral arterial surgery in the Physicians' Health Study, *Lancet* 340:143-145, 1992.
10. CAPRIE Steering Committee: A randomised, blinded, trial of clopidogrel versus aspirin in patients at risk of ischaemic events (CAPRIE), *Lancet* 348:1329-1339, 1996.
11. Gorelick PB, Born GV, D'Agostino RB, et al: Therapeutic benefit: aspirin revisited in light of the introduction of clopidogrel, *Stroke* 30:1716-1721, 1999
12. Evaluation Study Investigators: Effects of an angiotensin-converting-enzyme inhibitor, ramipril, on cardiovascular events in high-risk patients, *N Engl J Med* 342:145-153, 2000.

13. van Rij AM, Solomon C, Packer SG, et al: Chelation therapy for intermittent claudication: a double-blind, randomized, controlled trial, *Circulation* 90:1194-1199, 1994.

Raynaud's phenomenon

Raynaud's phenomenon is a vasospastic disorder characterized by episodic ischemia of the digits of the hands and feet precipitated by cold exposure or emotional stress. Most cases of Raynaud's phenomenon are idiopathic and develop in women who are in their twenties and thirties. Underlying diseases to be ruled out include systemic lupus erythematosus, scleroderma and other types of vasculitis, myeloproliferative disorders, and cryoglobulinemia.[1] The risk that connective tissue disease will develop in patients with primary Raynaud's phenomenon is low, but the exact incidence is uncertain. In one meta-analysis, which included studies from rheumatology and immunology referral centres, the rate was a little more than 10%. This figure is certainly too high because of referral bias; many patients with Raynaud's phenomenon do not seek medical attention. Clinical predictors of progression included abnormalities of the nailfold capillaries, telangiectasia, puffy fingers, and sclerodactyly.[2] Symptomatic treatment involves keeping the patient warm, especially the extremities, and in some cases administering long-acting calcium channel blockers such as long-acting nifedipine (Adalat XL) or felodipine (Renedil, Plendil).[1] Direct vasodilators including nitroglycerin have been used topically in patients with Raynaud's phenomenon.

────────────────── **✍ REFERENCES ✍** ──────────────────

1. Keystone EC: Appropriate management of Raynaud's disease, *Patient Care Can* 7:14, 1996.
2. Spencer-Green G: Outcomes in primary Raynaud phenomenon: a meta-analysis of the frequency, rates, and predictors of transition to secondary diseases, *Arch Intern Med* 158:595-600, 1998.

Venous Disease

Thrombophlebitis
(See also anticoagulants; hormone replacement therapy; oral contraceptives; pulmonary embolism)

Difficulty making the clinical diagnosis. The clinical diagnosis of deep vein thrombosis (DVT) is notoriously difficult, and most patients have no suggestive signs or symptoms.[1] Among patients who do have symptoms or signs suggestive of phlebitis, only about one fourth actually have the condition. The accuracy of diagnosis among patients with symptoms can be greatly improved by using a clinical prediction guide. One point is given for each of the following factors[2]:

1. Active cancer
2. Paralysis or plaster immobilization of a lower limb

3. Recent confinement to bed for more than 3 days or recent major surgery
4. Localized tenderness along the deep venous system
5. Swelling of the entire leg
6. Calf swelling greater than 3 cm compared with the unaffected leg, as measured 10 cm below the tibial tuberosity
7. Pitting edema (greater than in the unaffected limb)
8. Superficial collateral veins

Two points are subtracted if an alternative diagnosis such as a Baker's cyst is highly suspected. The patient has a high probability of DVT with scores of 3 or higher, moderate probability if the score is 1 or 2, and low probability if it is zero or a negative number.[2] Differential diagnoses to consider include ruptured Baker's cyst, cellulitis, ruptured Achilles tendon, lymphedema, and superficial phlebitis. From a clinical viewpoint, all symptomatic patients should still be investigated. If a patient with a high or moderate probability of DVT has negative findings on ultrasonography, a venogram or serial testing is indicated. These options are also indicated if someone with a low probability has a positive ultrasonography result. On the other hand, ultrasonography negative for DVT in a patient with low probability of the condition does not require further investigation, whereas positive ultrasonography in patients with high or moderate probabilities is an indication for immediate treatment.[2]

Two practical, non-invasive procedures for assessing the presence of DVT are impedance plethysmography and compression ultrasonography. Neither is reliable for detecting isolated calf thrombophlebitis.[2] In most centres compression ultrasonography is now the procedure of choice.[3]

D-dimer testing. D-dimer is a fibrin degradation product that is usually increased in the presence of thromboembolic disease. D-dimer testing has come into vogue in the assessment of patients presenting with the potential for DVT. This test has a sensitivity for DVT of 80% but a specificity of only 30%. The negative predicative value exceeds 90% and rises to over 99% when combined with a negative Doppler test. Caveats to the use of d-dimer testing include the large number of conditions that will raise the d-dimer level, making its use in any decision tree problematic. Multiple studies have shown that a negative whole blood or ELISA d-dimer test in a patient with a low pre-test probability as defined by Wells criteria reliably excludes the diagnosis of DVT in a subgroup of patients with a less then 1% likelihood of DVT.[4-7] The d-dimer should not be used to exclude the diagnosis of DVT in any patients with a moderate- to high-pre-test probability of DVT.

Ultrasonography. Real-time ultrasonography processes the images rapidly enough to show the examiner what is going on at that instant. When used to diagnosis DVT, the probe is usually placed over the femoral vein in the groin and over the popliteal vein in the popliteal fossa. Each vein is compressed with the probe, and if the lumen is no longer visible, there is no contained thrombus.[3]

Proximal versus distal thrombosis. The distinction between proximal and distal (calf only) DVT is important because patients with thrombi limited to the calf rarely have pulmonary emboli, and if they do, the emboli are generally inconsequential. Neither impedance plethysmography nor ultrasound can rule out calf vein thrombosis, and since a certain percentage of calf vein thrombi propagate proximally, serial measurements are necessary to detect this eventuality. Various requirements for the number of repeat examinations have been published. One recent study evaluated patients with two ultrasound examinations 1 week apart; of all abnormal results, only 3% were found solely on the second visit. No treatment was given to patients with negative results on either the first or the second evaluation. After 6 months of follow-up, only 0.7% of patients who had negative results on the two initial evaluations showed clinical evidence of thromboembolic disease.[3]

Risk factors. Risk factors may be divided into those that are reversible and those that are permanent.[4] Reversible risk factors include trauma, surgery, temporary immobilization, travel, estrogen treatment, infection, Baker's cyst, and pregnancy.[8] Even "minor" surgery may be associated with a high incidence of thrombophlebitis; in one series of arthroscopies, calf or proximal deep vein thrombophlebitis developed in 18% of the patients as documented by venography.[9] One case-control study found that travel of 4 hours or more (mean 5.2) by plane, train, or car increased the odds ratio of thrombophlebitis fourfold.[10] Permanent risk factors include inherited disorders of coagulation, malignancy, permanent immobilization, and idiopathic recurrent-thromboembolic episodes.[4] Probable permanent risk factors are smoking and central abdominal obesity.[11]

Inherited disorders of coagulation. Some of the inherited disorders of coagulation inhibitors that predispose to thrombophlebitis are the thrombophilias, which include antithrombin III, protein C, and protein S deficiencies[12]; activated protein C resistance, which is usually caused by inheriting a mutation in factor V–factor V Leiden[12]; and G20210A prothrombin mutation.[13] Factor V Leiden is found in about 5% of individuals of European ancestry and between 11% and 21% of those with venous thromboembolism. Patients with factor V Leiden alone do not appear to be at major risk for recurrent thromboembolism, but if both G20210A prothrombin mutation and factor V Leiden are present, the risk is very high.[13] Whether women who want oral contraceptives should be screened for factor V Leiden is discussed in the section on oral contraceptives.

The antiphospholipid antibody syndrome consists of recurrent venous or arterial thrombosis; recurrent spon-taneous abortions, usually in the second trimester; and the presence of antiphospholipid antibodies (anticardiolipin antibodies or lupus anticoagulant). Testing for thrombophilias, particularly antithrombin III deficiency, protein C deficiency, protein S deficiency, and activated protein C resistance should occur before anticoagulation is begun or preferably after anticoagulation is stopped and the acute event is passed to provide the most accurate measures. Many cases are found in patients with systemic lupus erythematosus.[14] Stroke is one of the most serious complications of the antiphospholipid antibody syndrome. Treatment is lifelong use of warfarin (Coumadin)[14] except during pregnancy, at which time Aspirin, heparin, or a combination of the two is used.[15]

Cancer and thrombophlebitis. Although patients with cancer have long been known to have a higher risk of thromboembolic disease, extensive investigations looking for malignancy are not indicated for patients in whom thrombophlebitis develops.[16,17] A thorough history, a physical examination including a pelvic examination, a chest X-ray examination, and "routine" blood tests should suffice, because when cancer is related to a thrombotic event, the diagnosis of malignancy is often suspected at the time of initial presentation on the basis of clinical findings.[16,17] In cases with no clinical suggestion of malignancy, approximately 88 patients would have to be investigated to find one cancer, and many of the malignancies detected by this method would be incurable.[17]

Trauma and thrombophlebitis. A study from Sunnybrook Hospital in Toronto using serial impedance plethysmography and lower extremity contrast venography found that 58% of trauma patients had DVT, and in 18% of cases proximal DVT was present. Of 201 patients, only three (1.5%) had clinical symptoms or signs suggesting the disorder. None of the patients had received prophylaxis against thromboembolism at the time of the study.[18]

Prevention of thrombophlebitis. A variety of methods may prevent DVT in patients at risk. Physical measures include graduated compression stockings and intermittent-external pneumatic compression of the lower extremities. Commonly used drugs include warfarin, IV heparin, and low-molecular-weight heparin. Aspirin is not as effective as other modalities of prevention.[1]

Treatment of thrombophlebitis. The traditional initial treatment of thrombophlebitis is 5 days of IV (unfractionated) heparin followed by oral anticoagulation (warfarin) therapy for at least 3 months. Such therapy reduces the incidence of recurrent thrombosis from 25% to less than 4%. A simpler, more cost-effective method of initiating therapy is to use subcutaneous low-molecular-weight heparin (LMWH) or heparinoids administered on an outpatient basis (Table 18). Meta-analyses comparing LMWH with unfractionated heparin suggest that not only is LMWH more effective than unfractionated heparin, but it results in fewer major bleeding episodes.[19] Warfarin is contraindicated in pregnancy.

LMWH does not normally alter the partial thromboplastin time, so this is not monitored during therapy; INR is monitored in the usual way to control the level of concomitantly given warfarin. Heparin can cause thrombocytopenia through the development of heparin-dependent IgG antibodies, usually after 5 days of treatment. This complication appears to be less common in patients treated with LMWH than in those treated with unfractionated heparin.[20]

The optimal duration of therapy with anticoagulants is an area of controversy. The risk of recurrent thromboembolism is low in patients who have thrombosis limited to the calf veins and also in patients who have had a reversible risk factor such as surgery compared with those who have permanent risk factors such as cancer or those with idiopathic DVT. In the opinion of Hirsh, patients with a single episode of DVT associated with reversible risk factors that are no longer present should receive anticoagulants for 4 to 6 weeks if the thrombus is limited to the calf and for 12 weeks if proximal vein thrombosis is present.[8] The optimal duration of anticoagulation for patients without reversible risk factors who have had proximal venous thrombosis or pulmonary embolism is uncertain but is probably at least 6 months.[12] This view is substantiated by a 1999 report that studied patients with no known risk factors who experienced an initial episode of proximal venous thrombosis or pulmonary embolism. All patients were given anticoagulants for 3 months, and thereafter half were given placebo and half continued on warfarin. The study was terminated after only 10 months because the calculated annual recurrence rate in the placebo group was 27% compared with 1% in the anticoagulated group.[21]

If patients with a initial episode of thrombophlebitis are known to have a thrombophilia, longer periods of anticoagulation such as 1 to 3 years are probably indicated, but the optimal duration is unknown because the risk of hemorrhage may outweigh the benefits.[12] One decision analysis model of carriers of factor V Leiden who experienced a single thromboembolic event concluded that anticoagulation for periods of over 1 year would result in more major hemorrhages than pulmonary emboli prevented.[22]

The management of recurrent thrombophlebitis is also uncertain. A Swedish study found that after a second episode of thromboembolism, anticoagulation for a prolonged period resulted in fewer recurrences than occurred in those receiving anticoagulants for 6 months.[23] On an empirical basis, Ginsberg[24] recommended treating patients with two episodes of thromboembolism for 1 year and those with three or more episodes, for life. Bedridden cancer patients might require lifelong anticoagulation.[8]

Table 18   Low-Molecular-Weight Heparins and Heparinoids

Drug	Usual Dose for Postoperative Prophylaxis Against Deep Vein Thrombosis
Low-Molecular-Weight Heparins	
Ardeparin (Normiflo)	50 anti-Xa U/kg q12h
Dalteparin (Fragmin)	200 anti-Xa U/kg subcutaneously once daily
Enoxaparin (Lovenox)	40 mg subcutaneously once daily
Tinzaparin (Innohep)	175 anti-Xa U/kg once daily
Heparinoids	
Danaparoid (Orgaran)	750 anti-Xa U bid

Inferior vena cava filters can be placed through the transcutaneous route, which is being done more frequently.[25] Reputed indications are patients in whom anticoagulation is contraindicated and those with free-floating proximal-vein thrombi. The latter is a tenuous indication, since the risk of pulmonary embolism in patients taking anticoagulants is no higher in those with free-floating thrombi than in those with obstructing thrombi.[26] The efficacy of inferior vena cava filters has not been well studied. One 2-year randomized trial comparing inferior vena cava filters to 3 months of anticoagulation found no difference in mortality but an increased incidence of subsequent thrombophlebitis in the cohort with inferior vena cava filters.[25]

Post-thrombotic syndrome develops in an estimated 50% or more of patients with symptomatic DVT, usually within 2 years of the initial thrombotic episode. Wearing made-to-measure below-knee compression stockings during the day over a 2-year period (two new stockings every 6 months) decreases the risk by 50%.[27]

The management of excessively high INRs is discussed under anticoagulants in the hematology section.

------------------------------ **≈ REFERENCES ≈** ------------------------------

1. Weinmann EE, Salzman EW: Deep-vein thrombosis, *N Engl J Med* 331:1630-1641, 1994.
2. Anand SS, Wells PS, Hunt D, et al: Does this patient have deep vein thrombosis? *JAMA* 279:1094-1099, 1998.
3. Cogo A, Lensing AW, Koopman MM, et al: Compression ultrasonography for diagnostic management of patients with clinically suspected deep vein thrombosis: prospective cohort study, *BMJ* 316:17-20, 1998.
4. Moser KM, Fedullo PF, LittleJohn JK, et al: Frequent asymptomatic pulmonary embolism in patients with deep vein thrombosis, *JAMA* 271:223-225, 1994.
5. American College of Emergency Physicians: Clinical policy: critical issues in the evaluation and management of adult patients presenting with suspected pulmonary embolism, *Ann Emerg Med* 41:257-270, 2003.

6. American College of Emergency Physicians: Clinical policy to the initial approach to adults presenting with a chief complaint of chest pain, with no history of trauma, *Ann Emerg Med* 25:274-299, 1995.

7. American College of Emergency Physicians: Clinical policy: critical issues in the evaluation and management of adult patients presenting with acute myocardial infarction or unstable angina, *Ann Emerg Med* 35:521-544, 2000.

8. Hirsh J: The optimal duration of anticoagulant therapy for venous thrombosis (editorial), *N Engl J Med* 332: 1710-1711, 1995.

9. Demers C, Marcoux S, Ginsberg JS, et al: Incidence of venographically proved deep vein thrombosis after knee arthroscopy, *Arch Intern Med* 158:47-50, 1998.

10. Ferrari E, Chevallier T, Chapelier A, et al: Travel as a risk factor for venous thromboembolic disease: a case-control study, *Chest* 115:440-444, 1999.

11. Hansson P-O, Eriksson H, Wellin L, et al: Smoking and abdominal obesity: risk factors for venous thromboembolism among middle-aged men, *Arch Intern Med* 159:1886-1890, 1999.

12. Hirsh J: Duration of anticoagulant therapy after first episode of venous thrombosis in patients with inherited thrombophilia (editorial), *Arch Intern Med* 157:2174-2177, 1997.

13. De Stefano V, Martinelli I, Mannucci PM, et al: The risk of recurrent deep venous thrombosis among heterozygous carriers of both factor V Leiden and the G20210A prothrombin mutation, *N Engl J Med* 341:1801-1806, 1999.

14. Khamashta MA, Cuadrado MJ, Mujic F, et al: The management of thrombosis in the antiphospholipid-antibody syndrome, *N Engl J Med* 332:993-997, 1995.

15. Rai R, Cohen H, Dave M, et al: Randomised controlled trial of aspirin and aspirin plus heparin in pregnant women with recurrent miscarriage associated with phospholipid antibodies (or antiphospholipid antibodies), *BMJ* 314: 253-257, 1997.

16. Hettiarachchi RJ, Lok J, Prins MH, et al: Undiagnosed malignancy in patients with deep vein thrombosis, *Cancer* 83:180-185, 1998.

17. Sørensen HT, Mellemkjaer L, Steffensen FH, et al: The risk of a diagnosis of cancer after primary deep venous thrombosis or pulmonary embolism, *N Engl J Med* 338:1169-1173, 1998.

18. Geerts WH, Code KI, Jay RM, et al: A prospective study of venous thromboembolism after major trauma, *N Engl J Med* 331:1601-1606, 1994.

19. Siragusa S, Cosmi B, Piovella F, et al: Low-molecular-weight heparins and unfractionated heparin in the treatment of patients with acute venous thromboembolism: results of a meta-analysis, *Am J Med* 100:269-277, 1996.

20. Warkentin TE, Levine MN, Hirsh J, et al: Heparin-induced thrombocytopenia in patients treated with low-molecular-weight heparin or unfractionated heparin, *N Engl J Med* 332: 1330-1335, 1995.

21. Kearon C, Gent M, Hirsh J, et al: A comparison of three months of anticoagulation with extended anticoagulation for a first episode of idiopathic venous thromboembolism, *N Engl J Med* 340:901-907, 1999.

22. Sarasin FP, Bounameaux H: Decision analysis model of prolonged oral anticoagulant treatment in factor V Leiden carriers with first episode of deep vein thrombosis, *BMJ* 316:95-99, 1998.

23. Schulman S, Granqvist S, Holmström M, et al: The duration of oral anticoagulant therapy after a second episode of venous thromboembolism, *N Engl J Med* 336:393-398, 1997.

24. Ginsberg JS: Management of venous thromboembolism, *N Engl J Med* 335:1816-1828, 1996.

25. Decousus H, Leizorovicz, Parent F, et al: A clinical trial of vena caval filters in the prevention of pulmonary embolism in patients with proximal deep-vein thrombosis, *N Engl J Med* 338:409-415, 1998.

26. Pacouret G, Alison D, Pottier J-M, et al: Free-floating thrombus and embolic risk in patients with angiographically confirmed proximal deep venous thrombosis: a prospective study, *Arch Intern Med* 157:305-308, 1997.

27. Brandjes PM, Büller HR, Heijboer H, et al: Randomised trial of effect of compression stockings in patients with symptomatic proximal-vein thrombosis, *Lancet* 349: 759-762, 1997.

Pulmonary embolism
(See also thrombophlebitis)

The risk factors for pulmonary embolism are similar to those for thrombophlebitis and include trauma, surgery, HF, immobilization, cancer, and inherited disorders of coagulation. Important additional risk factors are obesity, smoking, and hypertension.[1]

Symptoms of pulmonary embolism include tachypnea and tachycardia, which are quite non-specific.[2] Blood gas concentrations are not sensitive enough to rule out pulmonary embolism. In one study 30% of patients with pulmonary emboli had a PaO_2 of more than 80 mm Hg,[3] while in another study between 8% and 23% had a normal A-a gradient.[4] In a third investigation 30% of patients with pulmonary embolism but no past history of cardiopulmonary disease had no diminution of the PaO_2 or the PCO_2 and also had normal A-a gradients.[5] Among patients with pulmonary emboli and a prior history of cardiopulmonary disease, 14% had all three values in the normal range.[5]

The standard investigative technique for suspected pulmonary embolism is a ventilation/perfusion (V/Q) lung scan.[2] This is a two-step procedure in which the pulmonary distribution of inhaled radioactive material (ventilation scan) is compared with the pulmonary distribution of intravenously injected radioactive material (technetium-99m). In a classic case of pulmonary embolism the ventilation scan is normal and the perfusion scan shows multiple perfusion defects. A "mismatch" occurs between the ventilation and perfusion scans.[2]

V/Q scans are reported as "normal," "low probability," "intermediate probability," and "high probability." In one study a pulmonary embolus was found in none of the patients with a "normal" scan, only 5% of those with a "low-probability" scan, 30% of those with "intermediate" results, and 90% of those with a "high-probability" scan.[6] Among those with "intermediate" results, 30% had a pulmonary embolism. Unfortunately, 50% to 70% of reports are in the intermediate range.[2] A suggested algorithm for this type of report, or for a low-probability report when the clinical probability of pulmonary embolism is high, is to perform duplex scanning of the leg veins; if this is negative and the patient's condition is stable, it is often safe simply to follow with serial duplex scanning or plethysmography of the leg veins because recurrent pulmonary embolism is extremely rare in the absence of proximal DVT.[2,7] A new technology that may be used for patients with "intermediate" V/Q scan results is helical computed tomography of the thorax. It has a sensitivity of 67% to 87% and a specificity of over 95%.[8]

Spiral CT scanning can demonstrate pulmonary emboli in the main, lobar, or segmental vessels with greater than 95% sensitivity and specificity. The modality is less sensitive for peripheral pulmonary emboli. It may also allow for the diagnosis of alternate conditions (i.e., tumour or pleural or pericardial disease). Subcutaneous low-molecular-weight heparin is reported to be as effective as IV-unfractionated heparin in the treatment of pulmonary embolism.[9,10]

────────────── ◢ **REFERENCES** ◣ ──────────────

1. Goldhaber SZ, Grodstein F, Stampfer MJ, et al: A prospective study of risk factors for pulmonary embolism in women, *JAMA* 277:642-645, 1997.
2. Bergus GU, Barloon TS, Kahn D: An approach to diagnostic imaging of suspected pulmonary embolism, *Am Fam Physician* 53:1259-1266, 1996.
3. Cvitanic O, Marino PL: Improved use of arterial blood gas analysis in suspected pulmonary embolism, *Chest* 95:48-51, 1989.
4. Stein PD, Goldhaber SZ, Henry JW: Alveolar-arterial oxygen gradient in the assessment of acute pulmonary embolism, *Chest* 107:139-143, 1995.
5. Stein PD, Goldhaber SZ, Henry JW, et al: Arterial blood gas analysis in the assessment of suspected acute pulmonary embolism, *Chest* 109:78-81, 1996.
6. Gottschalk A, Sostman HD, Coleman RE, et al: Ventilation-perfusion scintigraphy in the PIOPED study. II. Evaluation of the scintigraphic criteria and interpretations, *J Nucl Med* 34:1119-1126, 1993.
7. Hull RD, Raskob GE, Ginsberg JS, et al: A noninvasive strategy for the treatment of patients with suspected pulmonary embolism, *Arch Intern Med* 154:289-297, 1994.
8. Siegel MJ, Evens RG: Advances in the use of computed tomography, *JAMA* 281:1252-1254, 1999.
9. Büller HR, Gent M, Gallus AS, et al (Columbus Investigators): Low-molecular-weight heparin in the treatment of patients with venous thromboembolism, *N Engl J Med* 337:657-662, 1997.
10. Simmoneau G, Sors H, Charbonnier B, et al: A comparison of low-molecular-weight heparin with unfractionated heparin for acute pulmonary embolism, *N Engl J Med* 337:663-669, 1997.

Varicose veins

A variety of lower-leg symptoms such as heaviness, aching, swelling, cramps, restless legs, itch, and tingling have been attributed to varicose veins. A population survey in Edinburgh found a high incidence of such symptoms in individuals with and without varicose veins; the authors concluded that in only a small minority of patients, might surgery relieve these symptoms. Since previous studies have failed to show that early surgery prevents venous ulcers, improved cosmetic appearance remains one of the few specific indications for operative intervention.[1]

────────────── ◢ **REFERENCES** ◣ ──────────────

1. Bradbury A, Evans C, Allan P, et al: What are the symptoms of varicose veins? Edinburgh vein study cross sectional population survey, *BMJ* 318:353-356, 1999.

Venous ulcers
(See also ulcer, dermal)

Chronic venous ulcers result from dysfunction of the venous valves, which allows reflux of blood, increasing the pressure in the venous system. In some cases this is secondary to thrombophlebitis. If the valves of the perforating veins are also incompetent, the pressure is transmitted to the dermal capillaries with dilation of the capillaries and leakage of plasma and both red and white blood cells. Activation of the extruded white blood cells leads to the release of various toxic products that cause tissue destruction and ulceration.[1]

Venous ulcers are almost always located in an edematous limb in the region of the malleoli; the surrounding skin shows the typical pigmentation and induration of chronic venous insufficiency. Conservative treatment consists primarily of compression,[1,2] which may be accomplished with graded elastic compression stockings (with a 30- to 40-Torr gradient), elastic bandages, inelastic compression bands attached with Velcro (CircAid), or Unna gel paste gauze boots. Surgical interventions that can be used in selected cases consist of the stripping of superficial veins and at times the interruption of perforating veins; the latter can be performed through an endoscope, decreasing the degree of skin scarring.[1]

────────────── ◢ **REFERENCES** ◣ ──────────────

1. Angle N, Bergan JJ: Chronic venous ulcer, *BMJ* 314:1019-1022, 1997.
2. Fletcher A, Cullum N, Sheldon TA: A systematic review of compression treatment for venous leg ulcers, *BMJ* 315:576-580, 1997.

CENTRAL NERVOUS SYSTEM

Topics covered in this section

AMAUROSIS FUGAX

(See also cerebrovascular accidents)

The cardinal symptoms of amaurosis fugax include painless, transient, complete loss of vision that lasts only seconds to minutes and is often described as a sensation of a blind being pulled down over the eye. It is painless with sudden onset, and nearly always occurs in one eye. Vision is restored after each episode. About half of all cases of amaurosis fugax are caused by atherosclerosis, and in patients over 40 years of age it is the likely etiology. Spasm is a much more common cause in young individuals with no other evident disease or with a history of migraines; in these cases the course is usually benign. Lupus is a rare cause.[1,2] While there is no direct evidence for Aspirin use in amaurosis fugax, acetylsalicylic acid (ASA) has been shown to reduce the risk of stroke in patients with transient ischemic attacks (TIAs) and should therefore be of benefit in amaurosis fugax. Referral should be considered because a remedial cause can probably be found, such as carotid artery atherosclerosis. Surgery may be indicated in certain groups of patients to reduce the risk of future stroke. A thorough ophthalmological evaluation is necessary to rule out any abnormalities of the retina, optic nerve, visual fields, or other visual functions. A Cochrane review found that, for patients who presented with arterial vascular disease, there was no evidence that dipyridamole, in the presence or absence of another antiplatelet drug (chiefly aspirin), reduced the risk of vascular death, although it may reduce the risk of further vascular events. However, this benefit was found in only a single large trial and only in patients presenting after cerebral ischemia. No evidence showed that dipyridamole alone was more efficacious than aspirin.[3] Typical dosing of dipyridamole for amaurosis fugax caused by spasm is nifedipine 60 mg per day (20 mg of the regular formulations three times a day or Adalat XL 60 mg once daily).

◁ REFERENCES ▷

1. Winterkorn JMS, Kupersmith M, Wirtschafter JD, et al: Brief report: treatment of vasospastic amaurosis fugax with calcium-channel blockers, *N Engl J Med* 329:396-398, 1993.
2. Gautier JC: Amaurosis fugax (editorial), *N Engl J Med* 329:426-427, 1993.
3. De Schryver ELLM, Algra A, van Gijn J: Dipyridamole for preventing stroke and other vascular events in patients with vascular disease (Cochrane Review). In *The Cochrane Library,* issue 2, Chichester, UK, 2004, John Wiley.

AMYOTROPHIC LATERAL SCLEROSIS

Amyotrophic lateral sclerosis (ALS, motor neuron disease, Lou Gehrig's disease) is a neurodegenerative disease characterized by loss of upper and lower motor neurons. ALS usually affects middle-aged males and has a prevalence of 0.05/1000 in the population. Presently the United States has an estimated 20,000 to 30,000 cases. ALS is characterized by upper and lower motor neuron lesions, so patients tend to have weakness with fasciculations, muscle cramps, and signs of spasticity. The patient usually first notices clinical weakness in the hands or when climbing stairs because of weakness of the hip girdle. The diagnosis is made by clinical examination showing hyper-reflexia with pathological reflexes or corticospinal tract signs of abnormality, including ankle clonus and Babinski's sign. Confirmation of a lower motor neuron lesion is by electromyography. Both electrical and clinical sensory involvement is absent. Subjective and objective evaluations of pulmonary function should occur regularly. Subjective measures include assessing the strength of a cough or asking the patient to count as high as possible and comparing with prior visits. (With normal respiratory function one should be able to count up to 15.) Physicians should regularly obtain objective measures of forced vital capacity because respiratory failure and/or the development of pneumonia is the main cause of death.[1-5]

Most patients with ALS die within 5 years of diagnosis, but a few survive longer. The prognosis is worse for those with the bulbar form of the disease and for older patients. The cause of ALS is unknown, and no cure has been found. Riluzole (Rilutek) has been shown to slow the rate of progression of disease in a few patients but does not alter its natural history. Physical therapy (PT) and occupational therapy (OT) may aid with adaptation to weakness. Antisialorrhea agents are effective for the reduction of sialorrhea in most patients. Antidepressants are often required for the treatment of concomitant depression.[6] Amantadine or modafinil may alleviate fatigue, but their effectiveness is not universally accepted. Placement of tracheostomy and positive pressure ventilation is required for patients who elect to be on ventilator support. Placement of a percutaneous endoscopic gastrostomy (PEG) tube is required for selected patients when oral intake is no longer reliable. Supportive care is crucial for most patients. Although the medical options are limited, frequent clinic visits by the patient and a caring attitude on the part of the health care staff can be extremely helpful.

❧ REFERENCES ❧

1. Walling AD: Amyotrophic lateral sclerosis: Lou Gehrig's disease, *Am Fam Physician* 59:1489-1496, 1999.
2. Gaudette M, Saddique T: Amyotrophic lateral sclerosis overview. Available online: GeneReviews, update Feb 26, 2004-06-05.
3. Rowland LP, Shneider NA: Amyotrophic lateral sclerosis, *N Engl J Med* 344:1688-1700, 2001.
4. Daube J: Electrodiagnostic studies in amyotrophic lateral sclerosis and other motor neuron disorders, *Muscle Nerve* 23:1488-1502, 2000.
5. Saver DF, Scherger JE, Ferri FF, et al: Amyotrophic lateral sclerosis. In *First Consult,* Jan 9, 2004, www.firstconsult.com.
6. Lou JS, Reeves A, Benice T, et al: Fatigue and depression are associated with poor quality of life in ALS, *Neurology* 60:122-123, 2003.

BRAIN TUMOURS

The term *brain tumour* is used to refer to a variety of neoplastic processes of numerous histological types arising in or metastasizing to the brain. The clinical course involves a wide spectrum and expected prognoses of brain tumours. Some are histologically benign, such as most meningiomas and pituitary adenomas, for which surgical resection often is curative. At the other end of the spectrum are malignant primary brain tumours, such as glioblastoma multiforme, and most brain metastases that behave in an aggressive manner and are likely to end the patient's life within a year of diagnosis despite current multimodality therapies. Even slow-growing tumours, however, may significantly shorten a patient's life or cause debilitating symptoms, and low-grade tumours may evolve over time into malignant phenotypes.[1]

About 18,000 people are diagnosed annually with primary brain tumours in the United States, and about 13,000 people die as a result of progressive disease. Among adults with primary brain tumours, glioblastoma multiforme is the most aggressive and common. Metastatic brain cancers are more common than primary brain tumours, occurring with at least 10 times the frequency of primary brain tumours. Little is known about the exact cause of death of most patients with brain tumours; in most cases, death is assumed to be the direct result of tumour progression or the indirect consequence of an altered level of consciousness and being confined to bed. Many die at home with family and hospice caregivers.

Meningiomas are common intracranial neoplasms. Most are asymptomatic, and they either do not grow or grow very slowly. Optimal management of asymptomatic meningiomas is watchful waiting.[2]

An analysis of 19,000 patients with primary central nervous system neoplasms found that the overall 2- and 5-year survival rates were 36% and 28%, but prognosis varied greatly according to histological type and age (better for younger patients). For patients who survived 2 years, prognosis for survival was greatly improved, with an overall rate of 76%.[3]

The survival and life quality of patients with single brain metastases were no better after surgery plus radiation therapy than after radiation therapy alone.[4]

❧ REFERENCES ❧

1. Peterson K: Brain tumors, *Neurol Clin* 19(4):887-902, 2001.
2. Go RS, Taylor BV, Kimmel DW: The natural history of asymptomatic meningiomas in Olmsted County, Minnesota, *Neurology* 51:1718-1720, 1998.
3. Davis FG, McCarthy BJ, Freels S, et al: The conditional probability of survival of patients with primary malignant brain tumors: Surveillance, Epidemiology, and End Results (SEER) data, *Cancer* 85:485-491, 1999.
4. Mintz AH, Kestle J, Rathbone MP, et al: A randomized trial to assess the efficacy of surgery in addition to radiotherapy in patients with a single cerebral metastasis, *Cancer* 78:1470-1476, 1996.

CEREBRAL PALSY

Cerebral palsy (CP) refers to a wide range of conditions that affect posture and the control and coordination of movement. CP is usually diagnosed before age 2 based on maternal and infant history and signs of abnormal muscle tone and developmental delay. For differential diagnosis, degenerative central nervous system disorders must be ruled out. Although the underlying brain damage is not progressive, the signs of CP may become more or less noticeable over time. Improvements are possible with rehabilitation and proper management; therefore, early diagnosis and an individualized plan of management is important.[1] Attempts to identify CP in very young infants based on clinical examination, however, are unreliable. Observation of general movements may be an early, sensitive marker for CP.[2]

The incidence of CP is roughly 1 per 400 to 500 live births. The vast majority of children with CP (about 80%) are affected in utero, due to factors such as hypoxia or anoxia; brain malformation, which is sometimes caused by a genetic disorder; stroke; and exposure to maternal infection or toxins. A strong correlation has been shown between CP and extreme prematurity and/or low birth weight.[3] Whether perinatal factors and complications resulting in asphyxia also cause CP is still hotly debated.[4,5] The Society of Obstetricians and Gynaecologists of Canada has guidelines for fetal health surveillance to decrease the incidence of birth asphyxia.[6] Ten percent of children with CP acquire the condition from brain damage in the first few months or years of life.[7] In addition to clinical history and examination, neuroimaging, particularly MRI, can help to determine an etiology and timing of brain damage leading to CP. This information is often useful for prognosis and selecting approaches to management, and in some cases, can identify brain lesions or metabolic disorders that might be treatable.[8]

CP is classified according to clinical signs that suggest damage to different parts of the brain. Spastic CP, which is caused by impairment in the cortex, is most common (70% to 80% of patients) and is marked by stiff and permanently contracted limb muscles. Athetoid CP (10% to 20%), which is caused by damage to the basal ganglia, manifests itself in involuntary movements of the limbs and, in some cases, the face and tongue, resulting in grimacing or drooling. Ataxic CP (5% to 10%), which is caused by injury to the cerebellum, is characterized by difficulties in balance, depth perception, and coordination. Individuals often have a combination of these signs, particularly spasticity and dyskinesia.

Approximately 30% to 50% of individuals with CP have an intellectual disability, the vast majority in the mild-to-moderate range. Between 35% and 60% of children with CP develop epilepsy. Other challenges might include impaired vision and hearing, poor swallowing and hence nutrition, and speech and language disorders. Screening for and monitoring of these associated conditions is important. Little has been published on the physical effects of aging on adults with CP. Chronic back pain has been shown to be a problem in adulthood.[9] A recent study of older adults found a significant decline in the ability to walk and loss of some functions such as dressing over time.[10]

Management depends on the type and severity of CP and associated conditions present. Some form of PT to enhance and maintain motor skills and muscle strength and prevent contractures, and OT to help with activities of daily living, is generally needed.[11] Spasticity can also be addressed through medications like botulinum toxin type A and baclofen or through selective rhizotomy, but the long-term efficacy and complications arising from these interventions need to be studied further.[12,13] Speech-language therapy has been effective for individuals with CP, but there are not enough studies to show statistically that particular interventions lead to short- or long-term improvements in communication.[14] Mechanical devices may assist patients in sitting, walking, or communicating. Support to maintain oral feeding is often necessary because of oral motor delay and gastroesophageal reflux, which is associated with food refusal and dysphagia.[15] Behaviour therapy and counselling for children and young adults who have some form of CP can help to enhance self-image and coping and to avoid or reduce stereotyping, self-injury, or aggression that may arise from intellectual, emotional, and communicative difficulties. A holistic approach to management that optimizes the physical, affective, psychological, social, and spiritual well-being of people with CP and their caregivers is important. Family-centred care and enhancing participation in the community often improve the quality of function in individuals and satisfaction with services.[11,16]

❧ REFERENCES ❧

1. Scherzer AL, ed: *Early diagnosis and interventional therapy in cerebral palsy,* ed 3, New York, 2001, Marcel Dekker.
2. Ferrari F, Cioni G, Einspieler C, et al: Cramped synchronized general movements in preterm infants as an early marker for cerebral palsy, *Arch Pediatr Adolesc Med* 156:460, 2002.
3. Jarvis S, Glinianaia SV, Torrioli MG, et al: Cerebral palsy and intrauterine growth in single births: European collaborative study, *Lancet* 362:1106-1111, 2003.
4. MacLennan A: A template for defining a causal relationship between acute intrapartum events and cerebral palsy: international consensus statement, *Aust N Z J Obstet Gynaecol* 40:13-21, 2000.
5. Silvert M: Claim that events before birth cause cerebral palsy is disputed, *BMJ* 320:1626, 2000.
6. Liston R, Crane J, Hamilton E, et al (for the Society of Obstetricians and Gynaecologists of Canada and the Canadian Medical Protection Association): Fetal health surveillance in labour, *J Obstet Gynaecol Can* 24:250-276, 2002.
7. Cans C, McManus V, Crowley M, et al: Cerebral palsy of post-neonatal origin: characteristics and risk factors, *Paediatr Perinat Epidemiol* 18:214-220, 2004.
8. Ashwal S, Russman BS, Blasco PA, et al (for the Quality Standards Subcommittee of the American Academy of Neurology and the Practice Committee of the Child Neurology Society): Practice parameter: diagnostic assessment of the child with cerebral palsy, *Neurology* 62:851-863, 2004.
9. Jahnsen R, Villien L, Aamodt G, et al: Musculoskeletal pain in adults with cerebral palsy compared with the general population, *J Rehabil Med* 36:78-84, 2004.
10. Strauss D, Ojdana K, Shavelle R, et al: Decline in function and life expectancy of older persons with cerebral palsy, *Neurorehabil* 19:69-78, 2004.
11. Palisano RJ, Snider LM, Orlin MN: Recent advances in physical and occupational therapy for children with cerebral palsy, *Semin Pediatr Neurol* 11:66-77, 2004.
12. Tilton Ah, Maria BL: Consensus statement on pharmacotherapy for spasticity, *J Child Neurol* 16:66-67, 2001.

13. Boop FA, Woo R, Maria BL: Consensus statement on the surgical management of spasticity related to cerebral palsy, *J Child Neurol* 16:68-69, 2001.

14. Penningtoin L, Golbart J, Marshall J: Speech and language therapy to improve the communication skills of children with cerebral palsy, *Cochrane Database Syst Rev* 2004, 2:CD003466.

15. Field D, Garland M, Williams K: Correlates of specific childhood feeding problems, *J Paediatr Child Health* 39:299-304, 2003.

16. King S, Teplicky R, King G, et al: Family-centred service for children with cerebral palsy and their families: a review of the literature, *Semin Pediatr Neurol* 11:78-86, 2004.

CEREBROVASCULAR ACCIDENTS: STROKE

(See also amaurosis fugax; atrial fibrillation; subarachnoid hemorrhage; transient ischemic attacks; vertigo)

Stroke ranks second as the cause of mortality in Western countries, and is a major cause of disability.[1] More than 700,000 incidents of stroke are estimated to occur annually, and 4.4 million stroke survivors live with neurological sequelae of varying severity, rendering stroke the most frequent cause of acquired disability among adults and the cause of significant socio-economic effects. The economic burden of stroke, including both direct and indirect costs, was estimated by the American Heart Association to be $51 billion in 1999. The incidence of stroke increases exponentially with age. With the proportion of elderly people in the population rising, the overall incidence of stroke is likely to increase. Despite some advances in treatment of acute ischemic stroke, both primary and secondary prevention remain the cornerstone for management. A first-ever stroke significantly increases the likelihood of further events; about 33% of all strokes are estimated to be recurrent events. Thus, secondary prevention is of major importance.[2] Persons with a low level of risk factors have lifelong low levels of both heart disease and stroke. Stroke-prone individuals can be identified and targeted for specific interventions for modification of risk factors for ischemic stroke.

Classification

About 85% of strokes are ischemic strokes, while primary hemorrhages, either intracerebral or subarachnoid, constitute the remainder.[2] Transient ischemic attacks (TIAs) account for 15% to 20% of all cerebral ischaemic events, and about 15% of patients experiencing a stroke report a history of TIA. The retinal variant of TIA-transient monocular blindness (TMB) accounts for 25% of TIAs in the carotid territory. A recent study determined the risk of recurrent stroke to be 15% by 2 years post-initial stroke, which is over 15 times higher than the risk of stroke in the general population.

Risk Factors for Stroke

(See also lipids)

Non-modifiable risk factors

Age is the most important among these factors. Overall, the risk of stroke doubles in each successive decade after 55 years of age. After age 85, women have a slightly greater age-specific stroke incidence than men, and stroke-related case fatality rates are higher in women than men. In 1997, females accounted for 60.8% of stroke fatalities; overall, one in six women will die of stroke compared with one in 25 who will die of breast cancer. African Americans and Hispanic Americans have a higher stroke incidence and mortality rates adjusted for age and gender compared with whites. Some studies suggest that Chinese and Japanese populations generally have higher stroke rates as well.[3]

Lifestyle modifications

Smoking. Active smoking has long been recognized as a major risk factor for stroke. A meta-analysis of 22 studies suggested an approximate doubling of the relative risk of cerebral infarction among smokers versus non-smokers. The risk for stroke is not affected by a simple decrease in the number of cigarettes per day, stressing the necessity for complete cessation of smoking. The risk for vascular events might still be higher in former smokers, although the risk substantially decreases progressively after smoking cessation. The Framingham Heart Study found stroke risk to be at the level of nons-mokers at 5 years from cessation. However, an increased relative risk for stroke of 1.82 was found among non-smokers and long-term ex-smokers exposed to environmental tobacco smoke. Accordingly, current recommendations suggest complete cessation of smoking and avoidance of exposure to secondhand smoke.[3,4]

Physical activity. Regular physical activity has well-established benefits for reducing the risk of cardiovascular disease and stroke. Additional benefits are attained with intensive forms of physical activity compared with light-to-moderate activities and with increasing duration of exercise. These data are attributable particularly to relatively young patients. Guidelines endorsed by the Centers for Disease Control and Prevention and the National Institutes of Health recommend at least 30 minutes of moderate-intensity (40% to 60% of maximum capacity) physical activity on most (and preferably all) days of the week. The American Heart Association Guidelines for Primary Prevention of Cardiovascular Disease and Stroke 2002 suggest additional benefits are gained from vigorous-intensity activity (over 60% of maximum capacity) for 20 to 40 minutes, 3 to 5 days per week if there are no medical contraindications[4].

Weight management. Obesity, defined as a body mass index (BMI) greater than or equal to 30 kg/m^2, predisposes to cardiovascular disease in general and to stroke in particular. Obesity prevalence increases with advancing age, contributing to increased blood pressure, sugar, and lipids.[1] Several large studies, however, suggest abdominal obesity, rather than BMI or general obesity, is more closely related to stroke risk. Current recommendations consider maintaining BMI within 18.5 to 24.9 kg/m^2.

Dietary intake. Data regarding the effects of general nutritional status on stroke risk are limited. Evidence shows that a protective relationship may exist between stroke and consumption of fruits and vegetables, especially cruciferous and green leafy vegetables and citrus fruit and juice.[4] Current recommendations suggest an overall diet based on a healthy eating pattern with consumption of a variety of fruits, vegetables, grains, low-fat or nonfat dairy products, fish, legumes, poultry, and lean meats. This might require susceptible patients to modify food choices by reducing saturated fats.

Drug Treatment

Lipids management

Abnormalities of serum lipids (triglycerides, cholesterol, low-density lipoprotein [LDL], and high-density lipoprotein [HDL]) have traditionally been regarded as a risk factor for coronary artery disease (CAD). However, whether hyperlipidemia is a risk factor for stroke remains uncertain. A greater mortality from hemorrhagic stroke has been reported among those with serum cholesterol levels.

The exact mechanisms by which statins provide stroke protection are uncertain. Although some of the stroke reduction could be the result of lipoprotein alterations, statins may also act through mechanisms unrelated to their lipid-lowering properties, such as improved endothelial function, plaque stabilization, or antithrombotic, anti-inflammatory, and neuroprotective properties.[5] Recommendations of the American Heart Association for primary stroke prevention support the use of statins, especially in individuals with known coronary heart disease (CHD) and elevated LDL cholesterol levels.[4]

Antihypertensive therapy

Hypertension is the most important modifiable stroke risk factor, and its importance increases with age because the prevalence of hypertension and the average systolic blood pressure (BP) are higher in the elderly.[1] Even borderline hypertension or isolated systolic hypertension carries significant risk for stroke. Evidence of more than 30 years suggests that control of high BP contributes to the primary prevention of stroke as well as prevention of other target organ damage. Antihypertensive therapy can reduce relative risk for stroke by 35% to 45%. A similar reduction in stroke incidence can be obtained in elderly

patients with isolated systolic hypertension (relative risk reduction 30%), including those older than 80 years. A subset analysis of antihypertensive trials demonstrated that the more BP is lowered in a population, the greater the number of prevented strokes.[6] A systematic analysis of data obtained before 1997 confirms a 28% risk reduction for stroke recurrence with the institution of adequate antihypertensive therapy. The recent Perindopril Protection Against Recurrent Stroke Study (PROGRESS, n = 6105) further reinforces this, suggesting that a prevention of one stroke among every 14 patients treated for 5 years with a combination of perindopril (an angiotensin-converting enzyme [ACE] inhibitor) and indapamide (a diuretic).

Management of Diabetes

To date, good data do not exist to show that meticulous glycemic control will reduce the risk of stroke. However, case-control studies of stroke patients and prospective epidemiological studies have confirmed an independent effect of diabetes on ischemic stroke, with an increased relative risk in diabetics ranging from 1.8 to nearly sixfold. In the United States, a history of stroke was 2.5 to 4 times more common in diabetics than in persons with normal glucose tolerance.

Antithrombotic Therapy

Aspirin

Aspirin remains the cornerstone for primary prevention of myocardial infarction (MI); however, its role in primary stroke prevention is doubtful. At least eight trials included 59,977 patients analyzed for primary stroke prevention with different doses of Aspirin (75 to 990 mg per day). Three of the trials observed marginal increases of stroke risk, whereas others did not find significant reduction in stroke risk.[6] Meta-analysis of the six primary prevention stroke trials involving over 50,000 participants also showed the absence of risk reduction (odds ratio, 1.02). Moreover, Aspirin over a wide dose range (100 to 500 mg) did not affect severity of first-ever stroke. In secondary stroke prevention, Aspirin seems to be only moderately effective. Thus, a recent meta-analysis of 21 trials for stroke prevention suggests a 13% reduction in the relative risk for stroke; similar risk reduction within a 9% to 18% range was demonstrated in many other trials and meta-analyses.

The optimal Aspirin dose is still provoking heated debates. Some stroke experts favour higher doses of Aspirin (greater than or equal to 500 mg per day) for secondary stroke prevention. However, two trials directly comparing effects of Aspirin at low and high doses as well as six major meta-analyses did not demonstrate significant differences between stroke protection by Aspirin within the dose range of 50 to 1500 mg per day.[6-8] Thus, the protective effect of Aspirin appears to be comparable across all doses. Moreover, Aspirin-induced major gastrointestinal bleeding is also likely to be independent of aspirin dosage, although mild Aspirin-induced gastrointestinal toxicity appears to be dose-related in the range of 30 to 1300 mg per day. Accordingly, recent recommendations from several studies suggest using Aspirin in doses lower than 325 mg per day.

Thienopyridines

Combined analysis of four major trials for stroke prevention shows that thienopyridines (ticlopidine and clopidogrel) are modestly more effective (by 13%) than aspirin in secondary stroke prevention.[6] Currently, ticlopidine is only rarely used because of its relatively large incidence of a minor side effect (diarrhea) and less common serious side effects (neutropenia and thrombotic thrombocytopenic purpura [TTP]). The only large prospective trial assessing clopidogrel versus aspirin efficiency efficacy and safety that included a stroke population demonstrated roughly equivalent efficacy in stroke prevention for both medications. The clopidogrel group experienced slightly less gastric irritation and gastrointestinal bleeding but more rashes and diarrhea. Rare cases of TTP and one of hemolytic uremic syndrome have been recently reported in association with clopidogrel use.[7] No data exists regarding efficacy or safety of the combination of clopidogrel and Aspirin in secondary stroke prevention. The Clopidogrel in Unstable Angina to Prevent Recurrent Events (CURE) trial demonstrated significantly better prevention of the combined incidence of MI, stroke, and vascular death for the clopidogrel plus Aspirin combination versus Aspirin alone in patients with acute coronary syndrome without ST segment elevation. Major bleeding was significantly more common in the clopidogrel plus Aspirin group. The applicability of the CURE trial findings to a stroke population is questionable, however. This trial did not address the efficacy or safety of this combination in a stroke population. Overall, current recommendations consider clopidogrel to be an option for stroke prevention with greater applicability in cases of aspirin intolerance.[8]

Combination of Aspirin and dipyridamole

Although possible synergism of aspirin and dipyridamole in stroke prevention was first suggested years ago, meta-analyses of available data did not find that adding dipyridamole to Aspirin resulted in significant benefit over the use of Aspirin alone, until recently.[6] Currently, only one large randomized trial, The European Stroke Prevention Study-2 (ESPS-2, n = 6602, 2-year follow-up), demonstrated significant gain in stroke prevention using a combination of low-dose Aspirin (50 mg per day) with extended-release dipyridamole (ER-DP, 400 mg per day). Compared with placebo, Aspirin alone reduced the risk of stroke by 18%, dipyridamole

alone reduced it by 16%, and combination therapy reduced it by 37%. When compared with Aspirin alone, combination therapy had a relative risk reduction for stroke of 23% versus Aspirin alone. Presently, six major guidelines for stroke prevention consider a combination of Aspirin and ER-DP an option for initial therapy in stroke prevention.[8] This regimen, however, has the disadvantages of twice-daily dosing and an adverse effect profile that combines the effects of Aspirin and ER-DP.

Warfarin for non-cardiogenic stroke prevention

In contrast to cardiogenic stroke prevention, a dearth of evidence supports warfarin use in other clinical settings in symptomatic cerebrovascular disease. The Stroke Prevention in Reversible Ischemia Trial [SPIRIT]) using an international normalized ratio (INR) goal of 3 to 4.5 was stopped after only 14 months of average follow-up because of the high incidence of adverse effects of bleeding. The large Warfarin versus Aspirin Recurrent Stroke Study (WARSS, n = 2206, INR 1.4-2.8) demonstrated that warfarin is no more effective than Aspirin in prevention of stroke of presumably arterial origin, and no difference occurred in serious complications for these two agents. The subset analysis demonstrated that warfarin is not an option in cases of Aspirin failure for stroke protection. The recent recommendations of the American College of Chest Physicians[9] do not consider warfarin as an option for prevention of atherothrombotic stroke.

Carotid Endarterectomy

Symptomatic carotid stenosis

Three major trials (ECST, NASCET, and VA309) evaluated effects of carotid endarterectomy (CEA) for preventing stroke in patients with a recent TIA or ischemic stroke in the distribution of a proximal internal carotid artery stenosis. A recent report from the Carotid Endarterectomy Trialists' Collaboration[10] pooled all available data (n = 6092) with unification of measures of carotid stenosis to provide the most comprehensive evaluation of CEA-related stroke risk reduction in symptomatic carotid stenosis to date. CEA slightly increased the 5-year risk of ipsilateral ischemic stroke in patients with less than 30% stenosis, had no effect in patients with 30% to 49% stenosis, was of marginal benefit in those with 50% to 69% stenosis (absolute risk reduction 4.6%), and was highly beneficial in those with 70% stenosis or greater without near-occlusion or occlusion (absolute risk reduction 16.0%). No benefit occurred from surgery in patients with near-occlusion. These results draw attention to the necessity of accurate and reliable measurements of stenosis as the single most important indication for CEA. The beneficial effects of CEA are applicable only if the surgical complication rate is less than 7%.[10] The benefits of CEA are reduced by 20% for each 2% increase in the complication rate. Importantly, benefits of

CEA in the setting of symptomatic stenosis are likely to increase with age. The subset analysis of the NASCET trial demonstrated that the risk for stroke significantly increases with age in a medically treated group, whereas CEA-related stroke risk reduction (stenosis greater than 70%) is 28.9% for patients older than 75 years versus only 15.1% of risk reduction for patients age 65 to 74 years.[11] In patients older than 75 years, only three CEAs need to be performed to prevent one stroke within 2 years for stenosis greater than 70% and six CEAs when the stenosis is 50% to 69%.

Asymptomatic stenosis

Overall, the value of CEA for people with asymptomatic stenosis remains unclear. Results of several small trials were inconclusive, and only the Asymptomatic Carotid Atherosclerosis Study (ACAS; n = 1662; median follow-up, 2.7 years) found that statistically significant benefit of surgery for patients with high-grade stenosis was 60% to 99%. The aggregate rate of ipsilateral stroke, any perioperative stroke, or death in surgically treated patients was estimated at 5% over 5 years; in medically treated patients, the corresponding rate was 11% (53% relative risk reduction, 1% per year absolute risk reduction). There was no relationship between benefit and the degree of carotid artery stenosis above 60%. Women did not benefit from CEA, with 17% nonsignificant risk reduction in women versus 66% risk reduction in men, a difference ascribed in part to a higher rate of perioperative complications in women (3.6% vs. 1.7%). It must be noted that the study was not powered to detect differences between deciles of degree of stenosis or gender differences. Even more than for CEA of symptomatic stenosis, benefits of CEA in the setting of asymptomatic stenosis depend on surgical risk. The recommendation of the Stroke Council of the American Heart Association suggests consideration of performance of CEA for asymptomatic stenosis greater than 60% only by surgeons having individual rates of morbidity/mortality.

Managing Cardiac Risk Factors

Atrial fibrillation

The rate of ischemic stroke among patients with non-valvular atrial fibrillation (AF) not treated with antithrombotic therapy averages approximately 5% per year with wide, clinically important variation among subpopulations of AF patients. AF becomes an increasingly important cause of stroke with advancing age. In the Framingham Heart Study, the risk of stroke in AF patients rose from 1.5% in the 50- to 59-year age group to 23.5% in the 80- to 89-year age group.[12] More than 2 million adults in the United States have non-valvular AF, and approximately 36% of strokes in patients between the ages of 80 and 89 years are attributed to this condition. The risk is even higher for valvular AF, with an approximately 17-fold increase in stroke risk above that of age- and sex-matched control subjects. Although initial retrospective studies suggested that paroxysmal AF was associated with a lower stroke risk than chronic AF, analyses of recent trials data adjusted for confounding risk factors demonstrated similar stroke risk for both conditions.[6] Large prospective trials have established the benefits of antithrombotic therapy (warfarin, Aspirin) for stroke prevention, and this finding is reflected practically in all existing guidelines for stroke prevention.[8] Indications for using warfarin versus aspirin depend on stroke risk stratification. An analysis of five large randomized trials demonstrated that the relative risk for thromboembolic strokes for patients treated with warfarin was reduced by 68%.[1]

Antithrombotic therapy is not without risks for bleeding, including intracerebral hemorrhage. Taken together, primary prevention trials observed a rate of intracranial hemorrhages of only 0.3% per year among patients older than 75 years.[12] Some trials report a higher rate for this complication (up to 1.8% per year), usually associated with anticoagulation to a higher INR range used as a goal. The risk of intracranial hemorrhage rises dramatically at INR values over 4.0, stressing the necessity of meticulous control of INR during warfarin treatment. Many physicians are reluctant to prescribe warfarin to elderly patients with AF whom they deem at risk for falls. Given the significant stroke protection provided by warfarin, the risk of falls should not be overestimated. A recent study compared the benefits and risks of antithrombotic therapy in elderly persons with AF who were living in a community setting based on their risk of falls, and found that this factor was not important in determining their eligibility for treatment with oral anticoagulation.

Other cardiac risk factors

Several other potential cardiac risk sources for thromboembolic strokes theoretically might require long-term anticoagulation, including the following:

- Aortic arch atheroma, with increased risk for embolic strokes associated with plaques greater than 4 mm in thickness, ulcerated plaques, and those with mobile atheromatous components. In some reports, the annual stroke rate was up to 11.9% for these patients.
- Acute MI, following which there is a long-term risk of stroke of 1% to 2% per year. Stroke risk increases in the presence of akinetic or hypokinetic segments, ventricular aneurysms, and ischemic cardiomyopathy. (These patients are often placed on Aspirin therapy.)
- Left ventricular dysfunction with ejection fraction of < 35%
- Chronic left ventricular aneurysm when the risk of stroke is considered to be low, unless a thrombus that is mobile or pedunculated is present.
- Patent foramen ovale (PFO) is present in approximately 20% of normal individuals and in appro-

ximately 40% in patients with stroke. Among stroke patients with PFO, the risk of stroke recurrence is estimated to be only 1% to 2% per year; the risk might be substantially higher (up to 15%) in cases of complex PFOs (the combination of a large PFO and atrial septal aneurysm). Generally, PFO is considered a stroke risk factor in young patients with otherwise cryptogenic stroke.

- Prosthetic valve placement, which usually requires anticoagulation, unless the valve is porcine or fascia lata.
- Bacterial endocarditis is a stroke risk factor, but the value of anticoagulation in this condition is uncertain.

For each of these factors, the lack of controlled clinical trials and the heterogeneous nature of the potential cardiac sources of embolic stroke make it impossible to provide specific guidelines regarding the optimal long-term antithrombotic therapy for stroke prevention. In the absence of high-quality data for these conditions, either antiplatelet therapy or oral anticoagulation should be considered acceptable options. For prosthetic valves, lifetime anticoagulation is deemed appropriate, and the same approach might be reasonable for other cardiac diseases for which the risk of cerebral embolus is increased.

─────────────── ◢ **REFERENCES** ◣ ───────────────

1. Akopov S: Cohen S: Preventing stroke: a review of current guidelines, *J Am Med Dir Assoc* 4(5):S127-S132 (Suppl) September/October 2003.
2. Koennecke HC: 1 Secondary prevention of stroke: a practical guide to drug treatment, *CNS Drugs* 18(4):221-241, 2004.
3. Goldstein LB, Adams R, Becker K, et al: Primary prevention of ischemic stroke: a statement for healthcare professionals from the Stroke Council of the American Heart Association, *Stroke* 32:280-299, 2001.
4. Pearson TA, Blair SN, Daniels SR, et al: AHA guidelines for primary prevention of cardiovascular disease and stroke: 2002 update: consensus panel guide to comprehensive risk reduction for adult patients without coronary or other atherosclerotic vascular diseases, American Heart Association Science Advisory and Coordinating Committee, *Circulation* 106:388-391, 2002.
5. Gorelick PB: Stroke prevention therapy beyond antithrombotics: unifying mechanisms in ischemic stroke pathogenesis and implications for therapy: an invited review, *Stroke* 33:862-875, 2002.
6. Straus SE, Majumdar SR, McAlister FA: New evidence for stroke prevention, *JAMA* 288:1388-1395, 2002.
7. Cohen SN: Antiplatelet therapy to prevent ischemic stroke, *Fed Pract* 18:46-57, 2001.
8. Hart RG, Bailey RD: An assessment of guidelines for prevention of ischemic stroke, *Neurology* 59:977-982, 2002.
9. Gorelick PB, Sacco RL, Smith DB, et al: Prevention of a first stroke: a review of guidelines and a multidisciplinary consensus statement from the National Stroke Association, *JAMA* 281:1112-1120, 1999.
10. Chang CL, Donaghy M, Poulter N (World Health Organization Collaborative Study of Cardiovascular Disease and Steroid Hormone Contraception): Migraine and stroke in young women: case-control study, *BMJ* 318:13-18, 1999.
11. Schwartz SM, Petitti DB, Siscovick DS, et al: Stroke and use of low-dose oral contraceptives in young women: a pooled analysis of two U.S. studies, *Stroke* 29:2277-2284, 1998.
12. Finucane FF, Madans JH, Bush TL, et al: Decreased risk of stroke among postmenopausal hormone users, *Arch Intern Med* 153:73-79, 1993.
13. Faldeborn M, Persson I, Terent A, et al: Hormone replacement therapy and the risk of stroke: follow-up of a population-based cohort in Sweden, *Arch Intern Med* 153:1201-1209, 1993.
14. Petitti DB, Sidney S, Quesenberry C, et al: Stroke and cocaine or amphetamine use, *Epidemiology* 9:596-600, 1998.
15. Everson SA, Kaplan GA, Goldberg DE, et al: Anger expression and incident stroke: prospective evidence from the Kuopio Ischemic Heart Disease Study, *Stroke* 30:523-528, 1999.
16. McCormack JP, Levine M, Rangno RE: Primary prevention of heart disease and stroke: a simplified approach to estimating risk of events and making drug treatment decisions, *Can Med Assoc J* 157:422-428, 1997.
17. Howard G, Wagenknecht LE, Cai J, et al: Cigarette smoking and other risk factors for silent cerebral infarction in the general population, *Stroke* 29:913-917, 1998.

Management of Strokes

Both the American Heart Association and the American Academy of Neurology recommend the use of IV tissue plasminogen activator (t-PA) in selected patients when it can be administered within 3 hours of the onset of stroke symptoms. Selection criteria include absence of significant hypertension and use of computed tomography (CT) or magnetic resonance imaging (MRI) to rule out hemorrhage.[1,2] These recommendations were based on the National Institute of Neurological Disorders and Stroke (NINDS) trial, a randomized, placebo-controlled study that found a small but significant improvement in functional outcome at 3 months in patients receiving t-PA, but at the cost of an increase in intracerebral hemorrhage (6.4% versus less than 1%).[3] (When measured after 12 months, benefits in the NINDS trial were maintained; t-PA treatment of 100 patients prevented moderate to severe disability in 11 to 13 additional patients compared with those receiving placebo.[4]) A European trial of t-PA for stroke found no benefit and an intracerebral hemorrhage rate of 20%.[5] This discrepancy has been explained away on the grounds that the doses of t-PA were higher than those used in the NINDS study[6]; that the window of opportunity for administering the drug was up to 6 hours from the onset of symptoms, not 3 hours as in the NINDS trial[6]; and that numerous errors were made in the interpretation of the CT scans before treatment.[7] The last-mentioned phenomenon alone would appear to be a major obstacle to the widespread use of thrombolytic therapy; in one study of physician accuracy in interpreting CT scans in cases of suspected stroke, intracerebral hemorrhage was missed in 18% of cases.[8] Streptokinase trials to date have had an unacceptable rate of hemorrhage.[6]

How many patients suffering from strokes meet the inclusion criteria for t-PA therapy? In one Texas centre that strongly advocates the intervention, the reported rate was 6% to 7% of patients,[6] while in a Copenhagen series it was 5%.[9] However, since stroke patients who die or make a full recovery do not benefit from t-PA, the percentage of patients in the Copenhagen series who might have benefited from t-PA was calculated as only 0.4%.[9] Although some health care workers are enthusiastic proponents of t-PA use for strokes, others are skeptical, believing that more research is required before its widespread use is promoted.[9,10]

Two large multicentre studies have shown that daily Aspirin in doses of 160 mg[11] or 300 mg[12] given as soon as possible after an ischemic stroke resulted in slightly fewer deaths or recurrent strokes in the first weeks and in fewer deaths or dependent patients after several months.[12] According to 1998 guidelines from the United Kingdom, anyone who has had a stroke should take 75 mg of Aspirin daily for an indefinite period.[13]

The antithrombogenic agent clopidogrel (Plavix) given as a daily dose of 75 mg to patients with a history of stroke, MI, or peripheral vascular disease decreased the risk of further strokes, MIs, and vascular deaths. (See discussion of CAD.)[14]

Unfractionated heparin, which is frequently used for patients with ischemic strokes, is controversial in this case because of inconclusive proof of benefit and safety.[12,15] A trial of IV heparinoid showed benefits at 7 days, but by 3 months none was detectable.[15]

❧ REFERENCES ❧

1. Adams HP Jr, Brott TG, Furlan AJ, et al: Guidelines for thrombolytic therapy for acute stroke: a supplement to the guidelines for the management of patients with acute ischemic stroke; a statement for healthcare professionals from a special writing group of the Stroke Council, American Heart Association, *Stroke* 27:1711-1718, 1996.
2. Practice advisory: thrombolytic therapy for acute ischemic stroke–summary statement; report of the Quality Standards Subcommittee of the American Academy of Neurology, *Neurology* 47:836-839, 1996.
3. National Institute of Neurological Disorders and Stroke rt-PA Stroke Study Group: Tissue plasminogen activator for acute ischemic stroke, *N Engl J Med* 333:1581-1587, 1995.
4. Kwiatkowski TG, Libman RB, Frankel M, et al: Effects of tissue plasminogen activator for acute ischemic stroke at one year, *N Engl J Med* 340:1781-1787, 1999.
5. European Cooperative Acute Stroke Study (ECASS): Intravenous thrombolysis with recombinant tissue plasminogen activator for acute hemispheric stroke, *JAMA* 274:1017-1025, 1995.
6. Grotta J: t-PA: should thrombolytic therapy be the first-line treatment for acute ischemic stroke? The best current option for most patients, *N Engl J Med* 337:1310-1313, 1997.
7. Fisher M, Bogousslavsky J: Further evolution toward effective therapy for acute ischemic stroke, *JAMA* 279: 1298-1303, 1998.
8. Schriger DL, Kalafut M, Starkman S, et al: Cranial computed tomography interpretation in acute stroke: physician accuracy in determining eligibility for thrombolytic therapy, *JAMA* 279:1293-1297, 1998.
9. Jørgensen HS, Nakayama H, Kammersgaard LP, et al: Predicted impact of intravenous thrombolysis on prognosis of general population of stroke patients: simulation model, *BMJ* 319:288-289, 1999.
10. Caplan LR, Mohr JP, Kistler JP, et al: Should thrombolytic therapy be the first-line treatment for acute ischemic stroke? Thrombolysis–not a panacea for ischemic stroke, *N Engl J Med* 337:1309-1310, 1997.
11. CAST (Chinese Acute Stroke Trial) Collaborative Group: CAST: randomised placebo-controlled trial of early aspirin use in 20,000 patients with acute ischaemic stroke, *Lancet* 349:1641-1649, 1997.
12. International Stroke Trial Collaborative Group: The International Stroke Trial (IST): a randomised trial of aspirin, subcutaneous heparin, both, or neither among 19,435 patients with acute ischaemic stroke, *Lancet* 349:1569-1581, 1997.
13. Eccles M, Freemantle N, Mason J (North of England Aspirin Guideline Development Group): North of England evidence based guideline development project: guideline on the use of Aspirin as secondary prophylaxis for vascular disease in primary care, *BMJ* 316:1303-1309, 1998.
14. CAPRIE Steering Committee: A randomised, blinded trial of clopidogrel versus aspirin in patients at risk of ischaemic events (CAPRIE), *Lancet* 348:1329-1339, 1996.
15. Publications Committee for the Trial of ORG 10172 in Acute Stroke Treatment (TOAST) Investigators: Low molecular weight heparinoid, ORG 10172 (Danaparoid), and outcome after acute ischemic stroke, *JAMA* 279: 1265-1272, 1998.

Transient Ischemic Attacks
(See also anticoagulants; Aspirin; atrial fibrillation; transient global amnesia)

Measures to reduce stroke risk factors in patients who have had TIAs or previous strokes include discontinuing smoking, rigorously controlling blood pressure, losing weight if obese, increasing physical activity, and taking statins if lipid levels are elevated. Specific drugs for preventing future strokes are aspirin, ticlopidine (Ticlid), clopidogrel (Plavix), and anticoagulants (warfarin and heparin). Endarterectomy is beneficial for some patients.[1-5]

Aspirin

A collaborative overview of 145 randomized trials of antiplatelet therapy showed a relative reduction in strokes of 22% among patients with prior strokes or TIAs. This beneficial effect was noted among men, women, and the elderly with Aspirin doses that averaged 75 to 325 mg per day.[5] A 1999 metaregression analysis of the dose-response effect of Aspirin in patients who had suffered from TIAs found an overall reduction in strokes of 15%; doses of 50 mg per day were as effective as doses of 1500 mg per day.[6]

Ticlopidine and clopidogrel

Ticlopidine (Ticlid) has traditionally been prescribed for patients who cannot tolerate or do not respond to aspirin. Ticlopidine has many adverse side effects, some of which are fatal. There are few indications for its continued use, since the related drug clopidogrel (Plavix) is at least as effective as Aspirin and so far appears to be devoid of serious sequelae.[7]

Anticoagulants

Warfarin is the drug of choice for all patients with AF.[4] The role of warfarin for non-cardiac ischemic TIAs is uncertain; a number of clinicians use it for patients with TIAs that have not responded to aspirin or for patients with progressive strokes who are already receiving aspirin.[5] A European randomized trial comparing aspirin and the anticoagulant drug phenprocoumon (Marcoumar) was prematurely discontinued because of an excess of major hemorrhagic events (primarily intracerebral hemorrhages) in the arm of the study receiving anticoagulants. However, in this study the target INR was 3 to 4.5.[9]

Endarterectomy

The risk of stroke in patients who have had a TIA is 12% to 13% in the first year and 30% to 35% after 5 years. The risk of a subsequent stroke in a patient who has already had a stroke is between 25% and 45% after 5 years.[7] Published prospective studies report an absolute decrease in ipsilateral strokes of about 15% to 17% over 2 years in selected patients undergoing CEA compared with a medically treated control group. These patients had a carotid stenosis of greater than 70%; had experienced previous TIAs, amaurosis fugax, or a non-disabling stroke in the appropriate carotid territory; and were less than 80 years old. Surgery was most beneficial for those with a very tight stenosis (90% to 99%) and was considerably less valuable for those with a stenosis less than 70% (80% as measured in the European trial).[10,11]

Patients with a stenosis of 50% to 69% have only a moderate reduction in the risk of stroke, and this is eliminated if the combined risk of disabling stroke and death resulting from surgery exceeds 2%.[12] Surgery is riskier and less beneficial for women, who probably should not be treated operatively for stenosis less than 80% (90% as measured in the European trial).[13]

What is an acceptable morbidity and mortality rate for CEA in patients with TIAs? The consensus conference of the American Heart Association[14] and the guidelines of the Canadian Neurosurgical Society[15] put the upper limit for combined death and stroke from the operative procedure at 6% for patients who have had TIAs or mild strokes and at 3% for asymptomatic individuals. Since the overall death and stroke rate in the North American Symptomatic Carotid Endarterectomy Trial was 6.5%,[17] there must be few centres or surgeons meeting these standards. All candidates for CEA (and their family physicians) should become fully informed of the morbidity and mortality records of the surgeon and the centre where the operation would be performed.[17] (The role of endarterectomy is discussed in the earlier section on CEA.)

REFERENCES

1. Freestone B, Lip GYH, Rothwell P, et al: Stroke prevention: *Clinical Evidence* 10:246-272, 2003.
2. Alberts MJ (for the Publications committee of WALLSTENT): Results of a multicentre prospective randomised trial of carotid artery stenting vs carotid endarterectomy, *Stroke* 32:325, 2001.
3. Algra A, De Schryver EL, van Gijn J, et al: Oral anticoagulants versus antiplatelet therapy for preventing further vascular events after transient ischaemic attack or minor stroke of presumed arterial origin (Cochrane Review), In *The Cochrane Library*, issue 1, Chichester, UK, 2004, John Wiley.
4. Wolf PA, Clagett P, Easton D, et al: Preventing ischemic stroke in patients with prior stroke and transient ischemic attack: a statement for healthcare professionals from the Stroke Council of the American Heart Association, *Stroke* 30:1991-1994, 1999.
5. Antiplatelet Trialists' Collaboration: Collaborative overview of randomised trials of antiplatelet therapy. I. Prevention of death, myocardial infarction, and stroke by prolonged antiplatelet therapy in various categories of patients, *BMJ* 308:81-106, 1994.
6. Johnson ES, Lanes SF, Wentworth CE III, et al: A metaregression analysis of the dose-response effect of Aspirin on stroke, *Arch Intern Med* 159:1248-1253, 1999.
7. Gorelick PB, Born GV, D'Agostino RB, et al: Therapeutic benefit: Aspirin revisited in light of the introduction of clopidogrel, *Stroke* 30:1716-1721, 1999.
8. Brown J, Bernstein M: Antithrombotic therapy for patients with stroke symptoms, *Can Fam Physician* 42:1724-1730, 1996.
9. Stroke Prevention In Reversible Ischemia Trial (SPIRIT) Study Group: A randomized trial of anticoagulants versus

aspirin after cerebral ischemia of presumed arterial origin, *Ann Neurol* 42:857-865, 1997.

10. North American Symptomatic Carotid Endarterectomy Trial Collaborators: Beneficial effects of carotid endarterectomy in symptomatic patients with high-grade stenosis (NIH), *N Engl J Med* 325:445-453, 1991.

11. European Carotid Surgery Trialists' Collaborative Group: MRC European Carotid Surgery Trial: interim results for symptomatic patients with severe (70-99%) or with mild (0-29%) carotid stenosis, *Lancet* 337:1235-1243, 1991.

12. Barnett HJ, Taylor W, Eliasziw M, et al (North American Symptomatic Carotid Endarterectomy Trial Collaborators): Benefit of carotid endarterectomy in patients with symptomatic moderate or severe stenosis, *N Engl J Med* 339: 1415-1425, 1998.

13. European Carotid Surgery Trialists' Collaborative Group: Randomised trial of endarterectomy for recently symptomatic carotid stenosis: final results of the MRC European Carotid Surgery Trial (ECST), *Lancet* 351:1379-1387, 1998.

14. Moore WS, Barnett HJ, Beebe HG, et al: Guidelines for carotid endarterectomy: a multidisciplinary consensus statement from the Ad Hoc Committee, American Heart Association, *Circulation* 91:566-579, 1995.

15. Findlay JM, Tucker WS, Ferguson GG, et al: Guidelines for the use of carotid endarterectomy: current recommendations from the Canadian Neurosurgical Society, *Can Med Assoc J* 157:653-659, 1997.

16. Ferguson GG, Eliasziw M, Barr HW, et al: The North American Symptomatic Carotid Endarterectomy Trial: surgical results in 1415 patients, *Stroke* 30:1751-1758, 1999.

17. Gorelick PB: Carotid endarterectomy: where do we draw the line? *Stroke* 30:1745-1750, 1999.

CREUTZFELDT-JAKOB DISEASE AND BOVINE SPONGIFORM ENCEPHALOPATHY

(See also dementia; insomnia; transfusions)

Creutzfeldt-Jakob disease (CJD) is a rare and fatal human neurodegenerative disease characterized by a rapidly progressive dementia, myoclonus, and a periodic electroencephalogram (presence of periodic short wave complexes). CJD is classified as a *transmissible spongiform encephalopathy*, and is caused by the accumulation of an abnormal form of a normal cellular protein, the prion protein.[1] The annual worldwide incidence of CJD is 0.5 to 1 per million, affects both sexes equally, mainly in the 60- to 70-year age group,[2] and is the most common of the human prion diseases. (Others are kuru, familial Gerstmann-Sträussler-Scheinker syndrome, and fatal familial insomnia.) About 85% of CJD cases are sporadic; 10% to 15% are familial. In 1974, the first case of iatrogenic CJD was described, about 18 months after the insertion of a corneal graft; since then, about 300 cases of CJD have been linked to person-to-person transmission as a result of surgical or medical treatments; no cases have been linked to blood transfusions.[1] There is no effective treatment for CJD.

In 1996, a cluster of 10 cases in the United Kingdom affecting a much younger age group and presenting initially with psychiatric symptoms was termed "new variant Creutzfeldt-Jakob disease" (vCJD).[3] The cases were linked temporally and geographically to an outbreak of bovine spongiform encephalopathy (BSE), a prion disease affecting cattle; subsequent investigations have strengthened the belief that these cases were the result of transmission of the prion by ingestion of prion-infected beef. From October 1996 to November 2002, WHO recorded 129 cases in the United Kingdom, 6 in France and 1 each in Canada, Ireland, Italy, and the United States.[4] Intensive worldwide measures have been directed at identifying and preventing BSE in cattle, principally by banning the feeding of the protein.

──────── ❧ **REFERENCES** ❧ ────────

1. Knight RSG, Will RG: Prion diseases, *J Neurol Neurosurg Psychiatry* 75(Suppl I):i36-i42, 2004.
2. Stratton E: Surveillance for Creutzfeldt-Jakob disease in Canada, *Can Commun Dis Rep* 25(1):7-8, 1999.
3. Will RG, Ironside JW, Zeidler M, et al : A new variant of Creutzfeldt-Jakob disease in the UK, *Lancet* 347(9006): 921-925, 1996.
4. Variant Creutzfeldt-Jakob disease. *World Health Organization Fact Sheet N°180, revised* November 2002 (Accessed May 6, 2004 at http://www.who.int/mediacentre/factsheets/fs180/en/print.html).

HEADACHES

Investigations of Patients with Chronic Headaches

Headache investigation is really a two-step process:
1. Determining whether the headache is primary (not due to an underlying condition) or secondary (involving an underlying pathology and necessary investigations or referral).
2. Figuring out the cause of the primary headache (tension, migraine, and/or cluster) and the functional impact.[1]

Shown as follows, the SNOOP mnemonic can assist screening for secondary headaches.[2]

Systemic symptoms or signs (e.g., fever, myalgias, weight loss) or systemic disease (e.g., malignancy, AIDS)
Neurological symptoms or signs
Onset sudden (thunderclap headache)
Onset under age 5 or over 50 years of age
Pattern change
  • Progressive headache with loss of headache-free periods
  • Change in type of headache

Step 2 can be facilitated by understanding prevalence, pain, and disability. Tension-type headaches are experienced with mild-to-moderate pain and little disability by 38% of adults, whereas migraine affects approximately

12% of adults, is more severe, and can lead to moderate-to-high disability. Cluster headaches, which are experienced by 0.1% of adults, are severe and disabling. Additionally, duration can help differentiate headaches. Migraines typically last 5 to 72 hours, whereas cluster typically lasts less than 3 hours at the same time of day. Two other common scenarios are the "sinus headache," which is in fact migraine, and rebound headache caused by overuse of analgesic medications, and which occur more than 2 days a week or more than 10 days a month.[1]

No matter what the ultimate cause of the patient's headache, a longer differential diagnosis than primary headache disorder or neoplasm is vitally important to consider. A list of serious etiologies should be considered in the approach to the patient, including:

- Space-occupying lesion (tumour, abscess, hematoma, and so forth)
- Systemic infection such as meningitis or encephalitis
- Stroke (infarction, intracerebral bleed, and cerebral venous occlusion)
- Subarachnoid hemorrhage
- Systemic disorders such as thyroid disease, hypertension, pheochromocytoma, and so forth
- Temporal arteritis
- Traumatic head injuries
- Serious ophthalmological and otolaryngological causes of headache

Should patients with the clinical diagnosis of migraines or other types of benign chronic headaches have a CT or MRI scan? An evaluation of CT scans of 373 patients referred to a chronic headache clinic in a tertiary care centre in London, Ontario, found two osteomas, one low-grade glioma, and one aneurysm. The only lesion treated was the aneurysm. The authors state that this detection rate is the same as might be expected in the general population without headaches.[3] A study of imaging and headaches in children concluded that imaging was indicated only if neurological abnormalities were found on examination, a good history could not be obtained, or the child was very young.[4] If imaging is considered necessary, CT is usually the procedure of choice.[5]

REFERENCES

1. Taylor F, Hutchinson S, Graff-Redford S, et al: Diagnosis and management of migraine in family practice, *J Fam Pract* Jan;Suppl:S3-S24, 2004.
2. Dodick DW: Diagnosing headache: clinical clues and clinical rules, *Adv Stud Med* 3:87-92, 2003.
3. Dumas MD, Pexman JHW, Kreeft JH: Computed tomography evaluation of patients with chronic headache, *Can Med Assoc J* 151:1447-1452, 1994.
4. Maytal J, Bienkowski RS, Patel M, et al: The value of brain imaging in children with headaches, *Pediatrics* 96:413-416, 1995.
5. Goh RH, Somers S, Jurriaans E, et al: Magnetic resonance imaging: application to family practice, *Can Fam Physician* 45:2118-2132, 1999.

Psychiatric Disorders and Headaches

The overall prevalence of headaches in children 9 to 15 years of age is 10%. Children with psychiatric disorders have twice as high a prevalence rate of headaches as those without psychiatric disorders. The most frequently associated psychiatric disorders are depression and anxiety disorders among girls and conduct disorder among boys.[1]

REFERENCES

1. Egger HL, Angold A, Costello EJ: Headaches and psychopathology in children and adolescents, *J Am Acad Child Adolesc Psychiatry* 37:951-958, 1998.

Chronic Daily Headaches
(See also migraines)

The recently reported Landmark trial[1] reflected that many undiagnosed chronic headache sufferers actually have migraines. The trial looked at 1203 individuals with episodic headaches reporting to their general practitioners. The individuals in the trial then saw an expert panel unaware of their previous diagnosis; the expert panel showed that 94% of the individuals actually had a migraine. Many patients with migraines or other headaches are frequent users of analgesic drugs. This in itself can lead to withdrawal headaches, and a vicious circle of headaches–drugs–more headaches is established. Chronic tension headaches account for only a small proportion of chronic daily headaches. Patients with chronic daily headaches also frequently have anxiety or mood disorders.[2]

A useful trial to discuss with patients suffering from chronic tension-type headache is the 2001 trial by Holroyd that randomized patients with chronic headaches to an antidepressant (amitriptyline, up to 100 mg per day, or nortriptyline, up to 75 mg per day) versus a stress management program or both. Combined therapy was more likely to produce clinically significant (greater than or equal to 50%) reductions in headache index scores (64% of participants) than antidepressant medication (38% of participants), stress management therapy (35% of participants), or placebo (29%) used alone.[3] This data reflects that both medications and lifestyle strategies should be contemplated.

Overuse of analgesia (more than 2 days a week or more than 10 days a month) should be ruled out as a preventable cause. A population survey of patients with chronic daily headache reported that analgesic abuse existed in 17% of cases.[4] Almost any antimigraine drug, including Aspirin, NSAIDs, acetaminophen, codeine, ergotamine, and sumatriptan, may be responsible for analgesic overuse headache,[2] and this may lead to abuse of any of these drugs. For example, a Danish study of sumatriptan (Imatrex) use found that 5% of patients accounted for 40% of its total consumption.[5]

Clinical features of chronic headaches vary. Patients have daily or almost daily headaches with variable locations, and the headaches may be throbbing or steady. Patients often awaken with a headache. The headaches are often precipitated by physical exertion or intellectual effort, and the patient may have nausea, irritability, and difficulty concentrating.[2] Treatment of the disorder consists of withdrawal of the analgesics. This may be done rapidly or slowly, but if a barbiturate (e.g., Fiorinal) is involved, the withdrawal should be slow. Although many patients improve within 1 week, it may take up to 3 months for the maximal effect of analgesic withdrawal to be noted.[2]

▰ REFERENCES ▱

1. Tepper S, Newman L, Dowson A, et al: The prevalence and diagnosis of migraine in a primary care setting in the U.S.: insights from the Landmark Study. Poster presented at 44th Annual Scientific Meeting of the American Headache Society, June 21-23, 2002.
2. Mathew NT: Transformed migraine, analgesic rebound, and other chronic daily headaches, *Neurol Clin* 15:167-186, 1997.
3. Holroyd KA, O'Donnell FJ, Stensland M, et al: Management of chronic tension-type headache with tricyclic antidepressant medication, stress management therapy, and their combination: a randomized controlled trial, *JAMA* 286(16):1969-1970, 2001.
4. Castillo J, Munoz P, Guitera V, et al: Epidemiology of chronic daily headache in the general population, *Headache* 39:190-196, 1999.
5. Gaist D, Tsiropoulos I, Sindrup SH, et al: Inappropriate use of sumatriptan: population based register and interview study, *BMJ* 316:1352-1353, 1998.

Caffeine Withdrawal Headaches

The caffeine content of various beverages is as follows[1]:

6 ounces of brewed coffee	85-100 mg
6 ounces of instant coffee	65 mg
6 ounces of tea	40 mg
12 ounces of caffeinated soft drink	45 mg

Caffeine withdrawal symptoms usually begin within 12 to 24 hours of the last caffeine intake, reach their peak in 20 to 48 hours, and last for about a week.[2] In a Dutch study, individuals withdrawing from four to six cups of coffee per day had a high incidence of headaches beginning on day 1 and persisting as long as 6 days (mean 2.3 days).[3] A U.S. study found that even individuals taking an average of 2½ cups of coffee per day had withdrawal symptoms; 52% had moderate or severe headaches, and 8% to 11% had significant symptoms of anxiety or depression.[4]

▰ REFERENCES ▱

1. Hughes JR: Clinical importance of caffeine withdrawal, *N Engl J Med* 327:1160-1161, 1992.
2. Griffiths RR, Woodson PP: Caffeine physical dependence: a review of human and laboratory animal studies, *Psychopharmacology (Berl)* 94:437-451, 1988.
3. Van Dusseldorp M, Katan MB: Headache caused by caffeine withdrawal among moderate coffee drinkers switched from ordinary to decaffeinated coffee: a 12 week double blind trial, *BMJ* 300:1558-1559, 1990.
4. Silverman K, Evans SM, Strain EC, et al: Withdrawal syndrome after the double-blind cessation of caffeine consumption, *N Engl J Med* 327:1109-1114, 1992.

Cluster Headaches

Men are affected by cluster headache six times as frequently as women. Alcohol is a frequent triggering factor. The pain is unilateral and severe, is usually centred around the eye, comes on suddenly, and frequently awakens the patient from sleep. The usual attack lasts about 45 minutes.[1] In one study the most common behaviour observed during attacks of cluster headaches was walking with the trunk bent slightly forward while clutching the head, or sitting and rocking back and forth with the hands pressed over the painful area. Some patients banged their heads against a hard object, and others pressed a finger or thumb into the affected eye.[2]

Drugs used for treatment of the acute attack include Imitrex, dihydroergotamine (DHE, Migranal), ergotamine tartrate (Medihaler-ergotamine), ergotamine tablets or suppositories (Cafergot, Wigraine), inhaled oxygen at 8 L/min for 10 minutes, and 2% to 4% lidocaine (Xylocaine) by nasal instillation.[1] If lidocaine is used, it is administered by having the patient lie on the bed with the head hanging over the edge so the neck is extended 45 degrees and the head is rotated 30 to 40 degrees toward the side of the headache. The lidocaine is slowly dropped into the nostril ipsilateral to the pain. If the nostril is plugged, a topical decongestant is given.[1,3] More information on the usual dosages of these drugs may be found in Tables 19 and 20.

Lithium carbonate in doses of 300 mg twice a day to four times a day is often effective for the prophylaxis of cluster headaches. Serum lithium levels need be only between 0.4 and 0.8 mEq/L (0.4 to 0.8 mmol/L). Prednisone and methysergide (Sansert) are also effective prophylactic drugs. Prednisone is given in doses of 40 to 80 mg per day for 1 to 2 weeks and then tapered and discontinued over the following week, and methysergide is usually taken as 2 to 4 mg twice a day with meals. During cluster periods, ergotamine may be given at bedtime or on a regular basis twice a day to abort the headaches. For some patients, indomethacin (Indocin, Indocid) 25 to 50 mg three times a day prevents attacks.[1]

Table 19 Treatment of Acute Migraine Attacks

Drug	Usual dose
Simple analgesics	
Acetaminophen	650-1300 mg stat
Aspirin	650-1300 mg stat
Acetaminophen 500 mg + Aspirin 500 mg + caffeine 130 mg	A single dose stat
NSAIDs	
Diclofenac (Voltaren)	50-100 mg stat
Flurbiprofen (Ansaid, Froben)	100 mg stat
Ibuprofen (Motrin, Advil)	400-800 mg stat (10 mg/kg for children)
Indomethacin (Indocin, Indocid)	100 mg po or pr stat
Ketorolac (Toradol)	60 mg IM stat
Mefenamic acid (Ponstan)	500 mg stat
Naproxen (Anaprox)	550-825 mg stat
Serotonin agonists ("Triptans")	
Naratriptan (Amerge)	1-2.5 mg po
Rizatriptan (Maxalt)	5-10 mg po (tablet or wafer)
Sumatriptan (Imitrex)	25-100 mg po; 6 mg sc; 1 nasal insufflation
Zolmitriptan (Zomig)	2.5-5 mg po
Ergot derivatives	
Dihydroergotamine (Migranal)	1 spray (0.5 mg) each nostril; repeat once in 15 min prn
Dihydroergotamine (DHE)	1 mg IM stat; repeat q 1 hour X 2 prn
Ergotamine tartrate (Ergomar)	2 mg sl stat; repeat q 30 min X 2 prn
Ergotamine tartrate (Medihaler ergotamine)	1 inhalation of 360 µg stat; repeat q 5 min X 5 prn
Ergotamine caffeine (Cafergot)	2 tablets or 1 suppository stat; repeat with 1 tablet or 1/2 suppository q 30 min to maximum 6 tablets or 2 suppositories
Ergotamine-n-caffeine-n-belladonna alkaloids (Wigraine)	1-2 tablets or 1 suppository stat; repeat q 30 min to maximum 6 tablets or 2 suppositories
Drug combinations	
Butalbital-ASA-caffeine with or without codeine (Fiorinal)	Addictive; not recommended
Butalbital-acetaminophen-caffeine (Esgic Plus)	Addictive; not recommended
Narcotics—agonist-antagonist	
Butorphanol tartrate (Stadol)	1 spray in 1 nostril stat; repeat X 1 in 30-60 min prn
Topical nasal anesthetics	
Lidocaine (Xylocaine)	Nasal instillation of 0.5 ml of 4% solution
Antiemetics	
Metoclopramide (Maxeran)	10 mg po stat
Domperidone (Motilium)	10-20 mg po stat
Steroids	
Prednisone	Variable, e.g., 60 mg/day X 4 days with tapering over 10-14 days
Parenteral drugs in emergency room	
Chlorpromazine (Thorazine, Largactil)	12.5 mg IV as an initial dose repeated every 30 minutes to a maximum of 37.5 mg
Prochlorperazine (Compazine, Stemetil)	7-10 mg IV stat
Metoclopramide (Maxeran)	7-10 mg IV stat
Dexamethasone	20 mg IV with or without 3.5 mg of prochlorperazine
Ketorolac (Toradol)	60 mg IM

NSAIDs, Non-steroidal anti-inflammatory drugs.

Handwritten annotations:

Peds
· Ibuprofen
· Acetaminophen first line

- HA diary
- triptan off label for adolescents
- Ø proph. approved

C/I: Pregnancy, HTN, CVD, ✱ hepatic disease
- Constrict Cor. arteries

1, 2.5mg tablet (gentle, fewer SFx, adolescents)
tab: 25, 50, 100mg
Tablet + melt 2.5, 5mg, nasal spray 5mg
→ for N/V
; acute onset, works fast

SFx
Chest pain, jaw pain
→ muscular, esoph. spasm

Step up therapy
- NSAID/acetaminophen
- Triptans (5HT₁ agonists) Combo therapy of above
- important to determine when pt took tab if it didnt work

Triptans: Differential response to triptans so try all
· with an anti-emetic
- Early peak: 45min to onset
- Late peak: Amerge (1-2hour onset)
- Really quick → nasal spray
- lower adverse effects ā Amerge

For severe HA,
long HAs

Table 20 Prophylaxis of Migraines

Drug	Usual dose
Beta blockers	
Atenolol (Tenormin)	50-200 mg/day
Metoprolol (Lopressor)	100-200 mg/day
Nadolol (Corgard)	40-240 mg/day
Propranolol (Inderal)	40-320 mg/day
Calcium channel blockers	
Flunarizine (Sibelium)	5-10 mg qhs
Verapamil (Calan, Isoptin)	240-480 mg/day
Tricyclic antidepressants	
Amitriptyline (Elavil)	10-175 mg/day
Nortriptyline (Aventyl, Pamelor)	10-125 mg/day
Anticonvulsants	
Divalproex (Depakote)	250-1500 mg/day
Valproic acid (Depakene)	250-1500 mg/day
Non-steroidal anti-inflammatory drugs	
Naproxen sodium (Anaprox)	550 mg bid for 7 premenstrual days
Ergot derivatives	
Methysergide (Sansert)	2-6 mg/day (drug holiday 6 months)

Start low, go slow, build up gradually

Takes 4-6w to work
- Give 3 mo then grad. taper
- Can go back to Full dose

start 10 qhs

Topiramate
25-200 mg/d
Start 25 qhs

Look at Co-morbidities ie. Anx, depression, HTN, seizures, sleep

REFERENCES

1. Walling AD: Cluster headache, *Am Fam Physician* 47: 1457-1463, 1993.
2. Blau JN: Behaviour during a cluster headache, *Lancet* 342:723-725, 1993.
3. Kittrelle J, Grouse D, Seybold M: Cluster headache: local anesthetic abortive agents, *Arch Neurol* 42:496-498, 1985.

Migraines

(See also caffeine withdrawal headaches; chronic daily headaches; cluster headaches; investigations of patients with chronic headaches; risk factors for stroke)

In North America, approximately 18% of women and 6% of men suffer from migraines.[1] The association between migraines and stroke is equivocal. (See discussion of risk factors for stroke.) Many patients with migraines have superimposed withdrawal-type headaches from excessive use of medications to control the migraines (analgesic overuse headaches). Three fourths of women with migraines obtain relief with the onset of the menopausal period.[2]

The concept that migraine pain is directly caused by vascular hyper-reactivity with initial vasoconstriction followed by vasodilation is no longer tenable. It is now thought that dysfunction of the serotonergic system in the brainstem activates trigeminal nerve fibres that supply blood vessels of the pia and dura mater. This results in the release of vasoactive substances, causing inflammation and pain around the vessels. Vasoconstriction

and vasodilation are secondary phenomena. Serotonin is central to this process, which may explain the efficacy of dihydroergotamine and sumatriptan, agents that act on serotonin receptors.[3]

Migraines are divided into two main classes. Between 10% and 20% of patients have migraine with aura (classic migraine), and most of the remainder have migraine without aura (common migraine). A few patients have complicated migraines defined as neurological symptoms lasting for the duration of the headache and occasionally causing permanent sequelae. Well-known variants of this type are basilar, hemiplegic, and ophthalmoplegic migraines, the last usually occurring in children. Although migraines are classically unilateral and pulsatile, they are bilateral in 40% of cases and may be non-pulsatile. The criteria of the International Headache Society for making a diagnosis of migraine without aura state that nothing in the history or physical examination should suggest that the headaches are caused by another disease, that the patient must have had at least five attacks of headache lasting 4 to 72 hours, and that these must have had at least two of the following characteristics[2-4]:

- Unilateral
- Pulsatile
- Moderate-to-severe intensity
- Aggravated by physical activity such as walking upstairs

In addition, the patient should experience at least one of the following associated symptoms[3,4]:

- Nausea or vomiting
- Photophobia, phonophobia

One of the most important principles of the pharmacological treatment of acute migraine attacks is to initiate therapy early in the attack, using an effective dose of whatever drugs are chosen.[3] For anything but the mildest attack, the chosen antimigraine drug should be combined with an antiemetic such as metoclopramide (Maxeran) or domperidone (Motilium). Not only will metoclopramide or domperidone decrease the symptom of nausea, but it also facilitates the absorption of antimigraine drugs. Metoclopramide has the added advantage of providing specific antimigraine effects.[5]

The initial choice of an antimigraine drug should be acetaminophen,[2] Aspirin,[2] or a combination of these two agents plus caffeine.[6,7] Next on the list are NSAIDs, and if these fail, 5-HT$_1$ receptor agonists such as ergot derivatives or sumatriptan (Imitrex). Intense migraines persisting for many days may respond to a short course of oral steroids.[2] Very severe migraines usually respond to IV neuroleptics, dexamethasone, or metoclopramide.[3,4]

Acetaminophen or Aspirin should be given as soon as possible after the onset of the migraine with initial doses of 650 to 1000 mg[3] or 650 to 1300 mg.[4] Enteric-coated Aspirin should not be used because this formulation delays absorption.[3] The combination of acetaminophen

500 mg, aspirin 500 mg, and caffeine 130 mg as a single dose has been shown to control pain, nausea, photophobia, and phonophobia in adults with mild,[6] moderately severe,[6] and severe[7] migraines. A single oral dose of acetaminophen (15 mg/kg) is often effective in controlling migraines in children, but a single oral dose of ibuprofen (10 mg/kg) is said to be better.[8]

A variety of NSAIDs have proved beneficial (see Table 19).[3,4] Capobianco and associates[3] favour naproxen if oral medications are tolerated or indomethacin suppositories if nausea and vomiting occur.

Several 5-HT$_1$ receptor agonists, or "triptans," of which sumatriptan is the best known, are now available (see Table 19). The recurrence rate within 24 hours of successful treatment is 30% to 40%. A triptan should not be taken within 24 hours of using another triptan or an ergot derivative. A combination of triptans and selective serotonin reuptake inhibitors may induce the serotonin syndrome.[9] Triptans are often effective even if taken after the headache has been present for some time and is well established. → can use ē SSRI/TCA

Ergot is an agonist of 5-HT$_1$ receptors but is less selective than sumatriptan. Ergotamine derivatives should be given as soon as possible after the onset of the migraine. Oral absorption is relatively poor, so for some patients, rectal suppositories may be more effective. Because ergotamine derivatives may cause nausea and vomiting, the dose must be adjusted by cutting refrigerated suppositories in half or even quarters to prevent this reaction.[3] Ergotamine is available as tablets or suppositories combined with caffeine (Cafergot, Wigraine), as sublingual tablets (Ergomar), and as a metered-dose inhaler (Medihaler-ergotamine). The usual initial dose of tablets or suppositories is 1 to 2 mg, and these may be repeated every half hour to a maximum dosage of 6 mg. Dihydroergotamine (DHE) is available for IM injection and has recently been formulated as a nasal spray (Migranal). The usual initial dose is 1 to 3 mg intramuscularly or 1 spray of 0.5 mg in each nostril.

Drug combinations for migraines include acetaminophen or Aspirin with codeine and often caffeine; Aspirin, caffeine, and the barbiturate butalbital with or without codeine (Fiorinal) or acetaminophen; and caffeine and butalbital (Esgic and Esgic Plus). Evidence supporting the efficacy of these drug combinations is poor, they may lead to addiction, and they are thought to be a major cause of rebound headaches that lead to chronic daily headaches.[4] Because of the risk of severe dependence, their use should be discouraged.[10]

Butorphanol (Stadol) is a mixed narcotic agonist-antagonist, administered by nasal insufflation, that is marketed for migraine treatment. Each spray contains about 1 mg of butorphanol, which has the analgesic equivalency of 5 mg of parenterally administered morphine. The median duration of pain relief in migraine is

said to be 6 hours. A placebo-controlled study of 157 patients with migraines documented marked pain relief in 33% within 30 minutes, 47% within 1 hour, and 71% within 6 hours. Side effects, mainly dizziness, nausea, vomiting, and drowsiness, were prominent. Some patients also experienced confusion.[11] Butorphanol may be addictive and in some cases is sought by drug abusers.[12]

In a 1-month randomized placebo-controlled trial of ambulatory patients in a family medicine practice, a 4% solution of intranasal lidocaine relieved a little over one third of migraines within 15 minutes, with a relapse rate of 20% within 24 hours. In a 6-month follow-up open label trial, intranasal lidocaine relieved over 50% of migraines within 30 minutes, but as in the initial trial, the relapse rate was 20%. Severe headaches responded less well than moderate ones, and lidocaine retained its effectiveness over the 6-month period.[13]

Intranasal lidocaine is administered by having the patient lie on a bed with the shoulders overhanging the edge and the head hyperextended as far as possible and rotated 30 degrees toward the side of the headache. With a 1-ml syringe, 0.5 ml of a 4% solution of lidocaine is dripped over a 30-second period into the nostril on the side of the headache. When this is completed, the head is maintained in the same position for another 30 seconds. If the migraine is bilateral, the procedure is repeated with the head turned to the opposite side. The patient then moves back up the bed and lies supine (no pillow) for 2 to 3 minutes. If the patient responds to the initial dose but relapses, the lidocaine treatment may be repeated.[13]

When other medications fail and the patient has had headaches for several days, a short course of oral prednisone often breaks a migraine cycle.[3]

A variety of drugs given intravenously or intramuscularly in the emergency room have aborted migraines. These include chlorpromazine (Thorazine, Largactil) 12.5 mg intravenously as an initial dose repeated every 30 minutes to a maximum of 37.5 mg,[3] prochlorperazine (Compazine, Stemetil) 7 to 10 mg intravenously stat,[14] metoclopramide (Maxeran) 7 to 10 mg intravenously stat,[15] dexamethasone 20 mg intravenously with or without 3.5 mg of prochlorperazine,[16] and ketorolac (Toradol) 60 mg intramuscularly.[17] Akathisia is a common sequela of a single IV dose of prochlorperazine.[18]

Table 19 lists some drugs and usual doses used in the treatment of acute migraine attacks.

Few randomized trials of the non-pharmacological treatment of migraines have been published, and the magnitude of the placebo effect in most reports is uncertain. Almost all patients find some relief from retiring to a dark room and attempting to sleep. Cold compresses applied to the head are often useful.[19]

Measures to prevent migraines focus on lifestyle modifications and, if necessary, pharmacotherapy (see Table 20).

Menstrual migraine — most severe
— NSAID + triptan
— Pre-emptive if predictable (NSAID on day -1 for 5d,
— OCP / 3mo. cont. cycles   triptan)

The evidence that lifestyle factors contribute to migraines is largely anecdotal. Some of the more commonly accepted migraine triggers are bright or flickering lights, loud noises, strong odors, irregular sleeping patterns (sleeping in on weekends), missing meals, and specific dietary products, especially those containing nitrites, aspartame, or monosodium glutamate. Some of the foods that have been incriminated are alcohol, especially red wine; aged and processed cheese; aged, cured, or processed meats (hot dogs, bacon, smoked meat, many lunch meats); Chinese food (contains monosodium glutamate); chocolate; and caffeine-containing beverages. Biofeedback, relaxation therapy, and cognitive-behavioural therapy have reportedly decreased the frequency of migraines in some patients. Physiotherapy, osteopathy, chiropractic therapy, transcutaneous electrical stimulation, acupuncture, naturopathy, and homeopathy are of doubtful value.[19]

Indications for pharmacological prophylaxis of migraines include more than two or three migraines a month, attacks lasting longer than 48 hours, severe attacks, and non-response to therapy. Between 55% and 65% of patients respond to prophylactic therapy, but amelioration of symptoms may be delayed for 1 to 2 months. Starting with relatively low doses of prophylactic agents and raising them weekly if the response is inadequate is a wise approach.[3]

Beta blockers are the agents of first choice (see Table 20).[3] Beta blockers with intrinsic sympathomimetic activity such as pindolol (Visken) and acebutolol (Sectral) are ineffective.[4]

Most calcium channel blockers are of questionable value in the prophylaxis of migraines. Verapamil (Calan, Isoptin) seems to be marginally beneficial, the data for nifedipine are inconclusive, and diltiazem has not been adequately studied. If verapamil is used, the daily maintenance dose is 240 to 480 mg.[3] Flunarizine (Sibelium) has been effective at a usual maintenance dose of 5 to 10 mg qhs.[4]

Some patients respond well to tricyclic antidepressants such as amitriptyline (Elavil) with a usual daily maintenance dose of 10 to 175 mg or nortriptyline (Aventyl, Pamelor) in a daily maintenance dose of 10 to 125 mg.[3,4] An advantage of nortriptyline is that it has fewer anticholinergic side effects than amitriptyline.[4] Valproic acid (Depakene) and divalproex (Depakote) are effective prophylactic agents for migraines with a daily maintenance dose of 250 to 1500 mg.[3,4] For some patients, daily use of NSAIDs is an effective prophylactic regimen.[3] Naproxen sodium (Anaprox) 550 mg twice a day may be used for 1 week a month before the menstrual period as prophylaxis against premenstrual migraines.[4]

The semisynthetic ergot preparation methysergide (Sansert) is a serotonin antagonist and an effective prophylactic agent against migraines. The daily maintenance dose is 2 to 6 mg. The major problem with the drug is that it can induce retroperitoneal or pleuropulmonary fibrosis with continuous use in about 1 in 1500 patients. Therefore, it should be reserved for patients in whom other prophylactic endeavours have failed. Patients must taper the drug and take a 3- to 4-week drug holiday every 6 months.[3]

Other drugs that have been used for migraine prophylaxis but that have not been adequately studied are parthenolide (Tanacet 125 or "feverfew"), pizotyline (Sandomigran), and cyproheptadine (Periactin).[3]

Treat according to char. of migraine
(e. length, acuity of onset (? nasal spray)

❧ REFERENCES ❧

1. Stewart WF, Lipton RB, Celentano DD, et al: Prevalence of migraine headaches in the United States: relation to age, income, race, and other sociodemographic factors, *JAMA* 267:64-69, 1992.
2. Kumar KL, Cooney TG: Headaches, *Med Clin North Am* 79:261-286, 1995.
3. Capobianco DJ, Cheshire WP, Campbell JK: An overview of the diagnosis and pharmacologic treatment of migraine, *Mayo Clin Proc* 71:1055-1066, 1996.
4. Pryse-Phillips WE, Dodick DW, Edmeads JG, et al: Guidelines for the diagnosis and management of migraine in clinical practice, *Can Med Assoc J* 156:1273-1287, 1997.
5. Dahlöf CG, Hargreaves RJ: Pathophysiology and pharmacology of migraine: is there a place for antiemetics in future treatment strategies? *Cephalalgia* 18:593-604, 1998.
6. Lipton RB, Stewart WF, Ryan RE Jr, et al: Efficacy and safety of acetaminophen, Aspirin, and caffeine in alleviating headache pain: three double-blind, randomized, placebo-controlled trials, *Arch Neurol* 55:210-217, 1998.
7. Goldstein J, Hoffman HD, Armellino JJ, et al: Treatment of severe, disabling migraine attacks in an over-the-counter population of migraine sufferers: results from three randomized, placebo-controlled studies of the combination of acetaminophen, Aspirin, and caffeine, *Cephalalgia* 19:684-691, 1999.
8. Hamalainen ML, Hoppu K, Valkeila E, et al: Ibuprofen or acetaminophen for the acute treatment of migraine in children—a double-blind, randomized, placebo-controlled, crossover study, *Neurology* 48:103-107, 1997.
9. New "triptans" and other drugs for migraine, *Med Lett* 40:97-100, 1998.
10. Raja M, Altavista MC, Azzoni A, et al: Severe barbiturate withdrawal syndrome in migrainous patients, *Headache* 36:119-121, 1996.
11. Hoffert MJ, Couch JR, Diamond S, et al: Transnasal butorphanol in the treatment of acute migraine, *Headache* 35:65-69, 1995.
12. Canadian Adverse Drug Reaction Newsletter: Potential abuse of butorphanol nasal spray, *Can Med Assoc J* 156:1054-1056, 1997.
13. Maizels M, Scott B, Cohen W, et al: Intranasal lidocaine for treatment of migraine: a randomized, double-blind, controlled trial, *N Engl J Med* 276:319-321, 1996.
14. Coppola M, Yealy DM, Leibold RA: Randomized, placebo-controlled evaluation of prochlorperazine versus

metoclopramide for emergency department treatment of migraine headache, *Ann Emerg Med* 26:541-546, 1995.

15. Ellis GL, Delaney J, DeHart DA, et al: The efficacy of metoclopramide in the treatment of migraine headache, *Ann Emerg Med* 22:191-195, 1993.

16. Saadah HA: Abortive migraine therapy in the office with dexamethasone and prochlorperazine, *Headache* 34: 366-370, 1994.

17. Shrestha M, Singh R, Moreden J, et al: Ketorolac vs chlorpromazine in the treatment of acute migraine without aura: a prospective, randomized, double-blind trial, *Arch Intern Med* 156:1725-1728, 1996.

18. Drotts DL, Vinson DR: Prochlorperazine induces akathisia in emergency patients, *Ann Emerg Med* 34: 469-475, 1999.

19. Pryse-Phillips WE, Dodick DW, Edmeads JG, et al: Guidelines for the nonpharmacologic management of migraine in clinical practice, *Can Med Assoc J* 59:47-54, 1998.

MULTIPLE SCLEROSIS

Multiple sclerosis (MS) is primarily a disease of young white adults. About 60% of cases occur in women. The disease is more common in northern than in tropical regions, and the incidence seems to be increasing.[1] The lifetime risk for a child whose mother has MS is 3% to 5%; the risk appears to be somewhat lower if the father has the disease.[2] Variations in the gene for myelin basic protein are associated with an increased risk of developing MS.[3]

In 90% of cases MS begins between the ages of 20 and 50. The four most common initial symptoms, which occur with about equal frequency, are optic neuritis, numbness, weakness, and gait imbalance.[2] MS usually has a relapsing or remitting course, but in 10% to 15% of cases the course is progressive from the onset. Primary progressive MS tends to involve only one part of the nervous system, usually the spinal cord, and has a poor prognosis.[2,4] In more than half of patients with relapsing or remitting MS, secondary progressive disease eventually develops. Ten years after the onset of the disease, 50% of patients cannot work, after 15 years 50% cannot walk unassisted, and after 25 years 50% cannot walk at all. In 10% of patients the disease is benign with little evidence of progression.[2]

MRI is the investigation of choice for confirming an MS diagnosis when suspected clinically. However, MRI is negative in up to 10% of cases, and it is not 100% specific. In patients with MS, MRI almost always detects many more lesions than would be expected on the basis of clinical examination.[1] The presence of abnormal evoked potentials alone is not pathognomonic of MS. However, in the context of other clinical and laboratory findings, they may help confirm such a diagnosis. Visual evoked potentials and somatosensory evoked potentials are abnormal in more than three fourths of patients with MS, and brainstem auditory evoked responses are abnormal in more than half of such patients.[1]

Several factors influence the prognosis of relapsing or remitting MS. The prognosis is better in younger patients, females, and those who have only a limited number of neuroanatomical areas affected, have primarily sensory symptoms, experience a complete first remission, and have limited deficits after 5 years. However, even after many years the course may become progressive, and in that case the prognosis for permanent disability is grave.[5]

Acute relapses of MS are usually treated with corticosteroids. This shortens the duration of the relapse, but whether such therapy affects the ultimate course of the disease is unknown.[2,4,6]

Disease-modifying agents for relapsing-remitting MS include interferon and glatiramer. Both interferon beta-1a (Avonex) and interferon beta-1b (Betaseron, Rebif) decrease the number of relapses and plaques found on MRI scanning in patients with relapsing-remitting MS[4,6,7]; however, beta-1b has recently been shown to be somewhat more effective.[6] Interferon 1a, on the other hand, when given after the first dyelinating event, was shown to delay the onset of clinically definite MS.[6,8] The evidence is inconsistent regarding the role of interferon in secondary progressive MS.[6] Glatiramer (Copaxone) reduces the relapse rates over a 2-year period, but does not slow the progression of disability.[6] Newer drugs like Mitoxantrone have been shown to effectively delay the progression of disability in worsening relapsing-remitting or progressive MS; however, significant side effects include leucopenia, arrhythmia, CHF, and sterility.[6,9,10] Other drugs currently under investigation include Natalizumab, an anti-alpha4beta1 integrin antibody, and alemtuzumab, an antileucocyte (CD52) antibody and statins.[9] Drugs such as azathrioprine IV Ig and methotrexate are of little or no benefit to date.[6]

---------- ⌁ **REFERENCES** ⌁ ----------

1. Brod SA, Lindsey JW, Wolinsky JS: Multiple sclerosis: clinical presentation, diagnosis and treatment, *Am Fam Physician* 54: 1301-1311, 1996.

2. Rudick RA: A 29-year-old man with multiple sclerosis, *JAMA* 280:1432-1439, 1998.

3. Guerini FR, Ferrante P, Losciate L et al: Myelin basic protein gene is associated with MS in DR4- and DR5-positive Italians and Russians, *Neurology* 61:520-526, 2003.

4. Rudick RA, Cohen JA, Weinstock-Guttman B, et al: Management of multiple sclerosis, *N Engl J Med* 337: 1604-1611, 1997.

5. Runmarker B, Andersen O: Prognostic factors in a multiple sclerosis incidence cohort with twenty-five years of follow-up, *Brain* 116:117-134, 1993.

6. Boggild M, Ford, H: Multiple sclerosis, *Clin Evid* 10: 1566-1581, 2003.

7. PRISMS (Prevention of Relapses and Disability by Interferon β-1a Subcutaneously in Multiple Sclerosis) Study Group: Randomised double-blind placebo-controlled study of interferon β-1a in relapsing/remitting multiple sclerosis, *Lancet* 352: 1498-1504, 1998.
8. Comi G, Filippi M, Barkof F, et al: Effect of early interferon treatment on conversion to definite multiple sclerosis: randomized study, *Lancet* 357(9268):1576-1582, 2001.
9. Polman CH, Uitdehaag BMJ: New and emerging treatment options for multiple sclerosis, *Lancet* 2:563-566, 2003.
10. Goodin DS, Arnason BG, Coyle PK, et al: The use of mitoxantrone (Novantrone) for the treatment of multiple sclerosis: report of the therapeutics and technology assessment subcommittee of the American Academy of Neurology, *Neuro* 25:1332-1338, 2003.

MYASTHENIA GRAVIS
(See also paraneoplastic syndromes)

Myasthenia gravis (MG) is an acquired autoimmune disorder of the neuromuscular junction resulting from antibodies against the nicotinic acetylcholine receptor (AChR) in 85% of cases (seropositive MG) and other post-synaptic neuromuscular junction antigens in the remaining 15% of cases (seronegative MG). The autoimmune attack leads to a decrease in AChR and damage to the structure of the endplate itself.[1]

The incidence of MG occurs in two peaks. The first is in the second and third decades and involves mostly women; the second is in the sixth and seventh decades and involves mostly men.

The presentation is that of fluctuating muscle weakness (involving eye, facial, oropharyngeal, axial, and limb muscles in varying combinations and severity), which improves with rest and worsens with use.[2]

The traditional diagnostic test for MG is to give the patient an IV dose of 2 mg of edrophonium (Tensilon), a short-acting acetylcholinesterase inhibitor, to see whether muscle strength improves. A positive result is usually seen within 30 to 60 seconds, and the effect lasts about 5 minutes. Another diagnostic test is the repetitive nerve stimulation test in which action potentials are recorded from the innervated muscle. The most specific test is an assay for acetylcholine-receptor antibodies. However, antibodies are found in only 85% of patients and in only 50% of those whose symptoms are limited to ocular muscle weakness.[3]

The goal of MG therapy is induction and maintenance of remission (complete or nearly complete absence of symptoms).[1]

Thymectomy is indicated for any patient found to have a thymoma. Although the benefit of surgery in non-thymomatous autoimmune MG has not been established, thymectomy is an option for patients with moderately severe generalized MG.[2] Thymectomy is most effective when performed in the first 2 years following diagnosis and especially if the patient is under 50 years of age. The effect of thymectomy is not seen until 1 year after the procedure, and the full effect may not be seen until after 5 years.[1] The medical treatment of MG is comprised of symptomatic, immune-directed therapy. Symptomatic therapy consists of anticholinesterase medications, pyridostigmine bromide (Mestinon), and neostigmine chloride (Prostigmin).

Short-term immune-directed therapy, consisting of IV immune globulin and plasma exchange, are used to stabilize the condition of patients in myasthenic crisis or as perioperative therapy for patients undergoing thymectomy.[3] The improvement begins within several days but the effect only lasts 3 to 6 weeks.

A few patients require long-term therapy with immunosuppressive drugs such as corticosteroids, azathioprine, mucophenolate mofetil (Cellcept), cyclosporine, and cyclophosphamide.

◢ REFERENCES ◣

1. Richman DP, Agius MA: Treatment of autoimmune myasthenia gravis, *Neurology* 61(12):1652-1661, 2003.
2. Keesey JC: Clinical evaluation and management of myasthenia gravis, *Muscle Nerve* 29(4):484-505, 2004.
3. Drachman DB: Myasthenia gravis, *N Engl J Med* 330: 1797-1810, 1994.

NEUROPATHY
(See also diabetic neuropathy; herpes zoster)

Bell's Palsy

Bell's palsy is an acute, unilateral, peripheral facial paresis ("incomplete") or paralysis ("complete") of unknown cause; the prognosis is better for patients with the incomplete form and for those under 40 years of age. Most patients recover without treatment; 71% achieve complete recovery, 84% achieve near-normal function.[1] The incidence is about 20/100,000 people per year, or about 1/60 to 1/70 people in a lifetime.[2] Recovery usually commences in 6 weeks, and the median time to complete resolution of paresis is 6 weeks.[3]

A systematic analysis by the Cochrane group found no evidence to support the use of corticosteroids in the management of Bell's palsy.[4] A similar analysis by the Quality Standards Subcommittee of the American Academy of Neurology concluded that corticosteroids (prednisone, 400 to 760 mg per day for 10 to 17 days) were "probably effective" at shortening the duration of paresis.[1]

◢ REFERENCES ◣

1. Grogan PM, Gronseth GS: Practice parameter: steroids, acyclovir, and surgery for Bell's palsy (an evidence-based review), *Neurology* 56:830-836, 2001.
2. Victor M, Martin J: Disorders of the cranial nerves. In: Isselbacher KJ, et al, eds: *Harrison's principles of internal medicine*, ed 13, New York, 1994, McGraw-Hill, 2347-2352.

3. Williamson IG, Whelan TR: The clinical problem of Bell's palsy: is treatment with steroids effective? *Br J Gen Pract* 46:743-747, 1996.
4. Salinas RA, Alvarez G, Alvarez MI, et al: Corticosteroids for Bell's palsy (idiopathic facial paralysis) (Cochrane Review) In: *The Cochrane Library,* issue 1, 2002, Oxford: Updat softaware. Search Date 2000; primary sources Cochrane Neuromuscular Disease Group register, Medline, Embase, Lilacs, hand searches of reference lists, and personal contacts with experts.

Carpal Tunnel Syndrome

The normal pressure within a limb compartment is 7 to 8 mm Hg. In carpal tunnel syndrome the pressure is often 30 mm Hg. With wrist flexion or extension it may be as high as 90 mm Hg.[1]

The prevalence of electrophysiologically confirmed, symptomatic carpal tunnel syndrome is about 3% among women and 2% among men, with peak prevalence in women older than 55 years of age.[2] Work-related carpal tunnel syndrome now accounts for more than 41% of all repetitive motion disorders, and as many as 1/3 of these are associated with concurrent medical conditions, including obesity, pregnancy, hypothyroidism, inflammatory arthritis, amyloidosis, diabetes mellitus, acromegaly, and Colles' fracture;[3] the authors question whether the syndrome is the result of repetitive strain or underlying medical illness.

Diagnosis of carpal tunnel syndrome is often difficult. As many as 15% of an unselected population report pain, numbness, and/or tingling in the median nerve distribution.[2] Many patients with typical symptoms of numbness, tingling, and weakness had normal electrophysiological tests (28/94), and conversely many individuals with electrophysiological evidence of median nerve neuropathy had no symptoms (23/125).[2] To frustrate family physicians even more, trusted physical signs such as the Phalen and Tinel tests have poor sensitivity and specificity. Current thought is that the most precise diagnosis is obtained by combining clinical features with electrodiagnostic confirmation.[4]

About one third of patients will improve with conservative management; this is particularly true in young patients who have mild-to-moderate symptoms of short duration (less than 1 year).[5] NSAIDs, although commonly prescribed, have not been shown to be effective. Splinting of the wrist is the most effective nonsurgical therapy; it does not matter whether the splint is in neutral position or in 20° of extension, or whether the splint is worn full time or only during the night.[6] Local injection of corticosteroid or short courses of oral corticosteroids are effective for the short term, but long-term results are uncertain.[6]

Surgery is the definitive treatment for carpal tunnel syndrome, but it should be a patient-driven decision; however, complaints of constant numbness, symptoms for more than 1 year, sensory loss, or thenar muscle atrophy are clear indications to recommend surgery.[7] Endoscopic carpal tunnel release does not appear to offer any advantage over open carpal tunnel release,[6] and a "mini"-open release (with an incision of 2 to 2.5 cm rather than the traditional 5- to 6-cm incision) is gaining favour.[7] In a randomized clinical trial comparing surgery with splinting, 80% of surgical patients reported good results after 3 months versus 54% of the splinted group; after 18 months, the success rate was reported as 90% in the surgical group versus 75% in the splinted group (but 41% of the splinted patients had undergone surgery by then).[8]

──────────── ❧ **REFERENCES** ❧ ────────────

1. Dawson DM: Entrapment neuropathies of the upper extremities, *N Engl J Med* 329:2013-2018, 1993.
2. Atroshi I, Gummeson C, Johnsson R, et al: Prevalence of carpal tunnel syndrome in a general population, *JAMA* 282:153-158, 1999.
3. Atcheson SG, Ward JR, Lowe W: Concurrent medical disease in work-related carpal tunnel syndrome, *Arch Intern Med* 158:1506-1512, 1998.
4. Rempel D, Evanoff B, Amadio PC, et al: Consensus criteria for the classification of carpal tunnel syndrome in epidemiologic studies, *Am J Public Health* 88:1447-1451, 1998.
5. Gerritsen AAM, Korthals-de-Bos IBC, Laboyrie PM, et al: Splinting for carpal tunnel syndrome: prognostic indicators of success, *J Neurol Neurosurg Psychiatry* 74:1342-1344, 2003.
6. Marshall S: Carpal tunnel syndrome, *Clin Evid* 10:1271-1288, 2003.
7. Katz JN, Simmons BP: Carpal tunnel syndrome, *N Engl J Med* 346:1807-1812, 2002.
8. Cerritsen AAA, de Vet HCW, Scholten RJPM, et al: Splinting vs surgery in the treatment of carpal tunnel syndrome: a randomized controlled trial, *JAMA* 288:1245-1251, 2002.

Guillain-Barré Syndrome

Guillain-Barré syndrome (GBS) is an autoimmune condition of the peripheral nervous system that results in inflammation and demyelination; more recently, the term *acute inflammatory demyelinating polyradiculoneuropathy (AIDP)* has been used to refer to the most common subtype of this condition (85% to 90% of cases).[1] The annual incidence of GBS is approximately 1.3 to 1.9 cases per 100,000 population[2]; its distribution is worldwide and it affects all age groups and both sexes equally. GBS is characterized by rapid and progressive weakness in the extremities and sensory deficit in most patients. Weakness peaks within 4 weeks and recovery is slow; about 25% of patients require assisted ventilation. In an epidemiological study of GBS in southeast England in 1993-1994, the authors confirmed 79 cases; after 1 year, 62% had made a complete functional recovery, 18% were unable to run, 9% were unable to walk unaided, 4% were bed bound and/or ventilated, and 8%

had died. (All deaths occurred in patients older than 60 years.)[3]

In two thirds of cases a respiratory or gastrointestinal infection precedes the disease by 1 to 3 weeks.[1,2] A common precipitant of the syndrome is *Campylobacter jejuni* infection. Cytomegalovirus infections account for the most common viral trigger to GBS. Oral polio vaccine and influenza vaccine have been implicated as possible causes for GBS, but multiple studies have failed to confirm an association or prove causation.[2]

Management of GBS, in addition to supportive and rehabilitative care, involves immunotherapy. In a recent practice parameter, the American Academy of Neurology concluded that plasma exchange and IV immunoglobulins were effective therapies; immunoabsorption, combination treatments, and corticosteroids were of unproven value.[4]

❧ REFERENCES ❧

1. Joseph SA, Tsao CY: Guillain-Barré Syndrome, *Adolesc Med* 13:487-494, 2002.
2. Hahn A: Guillain-Barré syndrome, *Lancet* 352:635-641, 1998.
3. Rees JH, Thompson RD, Smeeton NC, et al: Epidemiological study of Guillain-Barré syndrome in south east England, *J Neurol Neurosurg Psychiatry* 64:74-77, 1998.
4. Hughes RAC, Wijdicks EFM, Barohn R: Practice parameter: immunotherapy for Guillain-Barré syndrome. Report of the Quality Standards Subcommittee of the American Academy of Neurology, *Neurology* 61:736-740, 2003.

Trigeminal Neuralgia

Trigeminal neuralgia (TN) is defined by the International Association for the Study of Pain as "a sudden, usually unilateral, severe, brief, stabbing, recurrent pain in the distribution of one or more branches of the fifth cranial nerve."[1] This disease is relatively rare, with an annual incidence of 3 to 5 per 100,000 population.[2] The incidence increases with age[2] and, in up to 15% of cases, an underlying benign or malignant tumour of the posterior fossa or MS is identified.[3] The maxillary division of the trigeminal nerve is most often affected, and trigger sites are found on the face or in the mouth. TN is marked by attacks separated by variable periods of remission; in one of the few observational studies, the number of episodes varied from 1 to 11, and the length of episodes from 1 day to 4 years.[4] The diagnosis of TN is purely clinical and involves eliminating the other causes of unilateral facial pain.[2] The initial treatment of choice for TN is carbamazepine; it is the only treatment that has been clearly shown to be effective, and provides relief in about two thirds of patients.[5] Unfortunately, the effectiveness of carbamazepine tends to wear off with time; 69% of patients in one study reported initial relief, but only 22% still found it effective 5 to 16 years later.[6] When carba-

mazepine fails, various medications (all the anticonvulsants, baclofen, pimozide, lamotrigine) may be added, but none have proved effective in clinical trials.[5]

The intense pain of TN will convince up to half of patients to seek out a surgical solution.[2] Various procedures to destroy the peripheral nerve (cryotherapy, thermocoagulation, phenol injection, neurectomy, stereotactic gamma knife radiosurgery) or microvascular decompression of the nerve root are available; microvascular decompression carries more risk but leaves nerve function intact, whereas the destructive procedures are safer, but destroy the nerve and carry the risk of anesthesia dolorosa. The surgical therapies are not amenable to randomized controlled trials, and some of the improvement (25% to 80%, depending on the technique) may be a placebo effect, or the result of the natural history of TN.

❧ REFERENCES ❧

1. Merskey H, Bogduk N: *Classification of chronic pain: descriptors of chronic pain syndromes and definitions of pain terms,* Seattle, 1994, IASP Press, 1.
2. Kitt CA, Gruber K, Davis M, et al: Trigeminal neuralgia: opportunities for research and treatment, *Pain* 85:3-7, 2000.
3. Zakrzewska JM: Diagnosis and differential diagnosis of trigeminal neuralgia, *Clin J Pain* 18:14-21, 2002.
4. Katusic S, Beard CM, Bergstralh E, et al: Incidence and clinical features of trigeminal neuralgia, Rochester, Minnesota, 1945-1984, *Ann Neurol* 27:89-95, 1990.
5. Zakrzewska JM, Lopez BC: Trigeminal neuralgia, *Clin Evid* 10:1599-1609, 2003.
6. Taylor JC, Brauer S, Espir MLE: Long-term treatment of trigeminal neuralgia with carbamazepine, *Postgrad Med J* 57:16-18, 1981.
7. Fields HL: Treatment of trigeminal neuralgia (editorial), *N Engl J Med* 334:1125-1126, 1996.

PARKINSON'S DISEASE
(See also neuroleptics; serotonin syndrome; tremors)

Parkinson's disease (PD), a neurodegenerative disorder, affects approximately 100,000 Canadians. Compared with age-matched controls, affected patients have an overall mortality odds ratio of 2.5. No genetic predisposition to the disease has been found for those who acquire it after 50 years of age, but when it develops before 50, those affected have a strong familial history.

The cardinal symptoms include tremor, rigidity, akinesia, and gait disturbance. Although the criteria for diagnosis requires at least two of the above four symptoms, evidence from post-mortem examinations reveals that 25% of patients have an alternate explanation for their parkinsonian symptoms. Unilateral onset of symptoms, tremor plus one of rigidity or akinesia, and a response to L-dopa support a pathological diagnosis of PD.

The differential diagnosis of PD includes essential tremor, progressive supranuclear palsy, multiple system atrophy, neuroleptic drugs, certain antiemetics such as metoclopramide, and Wilson's disease. Wilson's disease should be ruled out in any young individual with parkinsonian-like symptoms. Investigations of such individuals include a slit-lamp examination for Kayser-Fleischer rings, liver function tests, and an assessment of plasma copper and ceruloplasmin levels.

The major pathophysiological defect in PD is a deficit of dopamine in the substantia nigra and other basal ganglia. Although many drugs have been studied, including the monoamine oxidase inhibitor selegiline and dopamine agonists, no therapies to date have been shown to be neuroprotective. Treatment of PD is, therefore, symptomatic. The decision to treat should be based on the patient's functional impairment and preference.

Non-pharmacological treatment includes support for the patient and caregivers, education, and referral to allied health professionals (physiotherapists, occupational therapists, and speech-language pathologists). The patient's ability to drive a motor vehicle is often seriously impaired, even in patients with mild Parkinson's disease. Accurate assessment of this problem is impossible in the usual office setting; formal psychological and psychomotor testing or driving tests are necessary to detect significant driving deficits.

The options for symptomatic treatment of PD include L-dopa, dopamine agonists, anticholinergic agents, and amantadine. Levodopa is combined with a peripheral decarboxylase inhibitor to block its conversion in the periphery (carbidopa in Sinemet and benserazide in Prolopa). This combination remains the most efficacious treatment for PD, and most patients will require it at some point. It is not, however, without problems. As the disease progresses, the duration of symptom relief from each dose of the regular formulation wanes ("wearing-off" effect). Increasing the frequency of L-dopa dosing, using a controlled-release formulation or adding entacapone, amantadine, a dopamine agonist, or selegiline are all options for treating the motor fluctuations that result. In addition, many patients (50% after 5 to 10 years of treatment) develop motor complications induced by L-dopa. These dyskinesias may represent a buildup of L-dopa, and options include stopping entacapone and selegiline or changing to a standard formulation of L-dopa instead of controlled release. Adding a dopamine agonist or amantadine and trying a small decrease in L-dopa dose may also be effective.

Dopamine agonists such as bromocriptine, pramiprexole, pergolide, and ropinirole result in less motor fluctuations and dyskinesias compared with L-dopa. They are also associated with significant side effects and are not as efficacious in the long term. They are recommended as adjunctive treatment to L-dopa or as a first line in younger patients with mild-to-moderate disease who can better tolerate the side effects of nausea, postural hypotension, and drowsiness.

Table 21   Drugs for Parkinson's Disease

Drug	Usual dose
Dopamine precursors	
Levodopa/carbidopa (Sinemet)	100/25 tid-qid; maximum 1000 mg of levodopa per day; controlled-release formulations have about 70% the bioavailability of regular tablets
Levodopa/benserazide (Prolopa)	100/25 tid-qid; maximum 1000 mg levodopa per day
Catechol-o-methyltransferase inhibitors	
Entacapone (Comtan)	200 mg with each dose of levodopa/carbidopa (max 1600 mg/d)
Dopamine agonists	
Bromocriptine (Parlodel)	15-30 mg/d divided tid or qid
Pergolide mesylate (Permax)	1.5-5 mg/day divided tid
Pramipexole (Mirapex)	1.5-5.0 mg/d divided tid
Ropinirole (Requip)	6.0-24 mg/d divided tid
Dopaminergic agents	
Amantadine (Symmetrel)	5-200 mg/d divided bid
Selective monoamine oxidase inhibitor drugs (Type B)	
Selegiline	5-10 mg/d divided bid with breakfast and lunch
Anticholinergic agents	
Trihexyphenidyl (Artane)	1-6 mg divided tid
Benztropine mesylate (Cogentin)	1-6 mg/day divided bid or tid
Antiemetics	
Domperidone (Motilium)	10-20 mg 30-60 min before medications causing nausea

Amantadine, an antiviral medication with mild anti-parkinsonian effects, may also provide symptomatic effect in patients with mild disease severity. It may be used as an adjuvant to L-dopa or to a dopamine agonist.

Anticholinergics such as trihexyphenidyl (Artane) or benztropine mesylate (Cogentin) may decrease tremor but are seldom useful for rigidity or bradykinesia. These drugs may cause confusion and should be avoided or used with caution, especially in the elderly.

Drugs used for the treatment of Parkinson's disease are listed in Table 21. The usual regimen is a low beginning dose followed by a gradual buildup of whatever drug or drugs are chosen. Before treatment begins, the practitioner should ensure that drugs such as metoclopramide or a neuroleptic are not the cause of the clinical syndrome.

Pallidotomy, a stereotactic neurosurgical operation that destroys a portion of the globus pallidus, usually controls dyskinesias on the contralateral side and to a lesser extent on the ipsilateral side, but surgical morbidity is high.[4] In a small number of patients with advanced Parkinson's disease, electrical stimulation of the subthalamic nuclei through electrodes implanted under stereoscopic guidance decreased the "off" periods and dyskinesias and permitted a lower dose of levodopa.[5]

❧ REFERENCES ❧

1. Guttman M, Kish SJ, Furukawa Y: Current concepts in the diagnosis and management of Parkinson's disease, *CMAJ* 168(3):293, 2003.
2. Rascol O, et al: Treatment interventions for Parkinson's disease: an evidence based assessment, *Lancet* 359:1589, 2002.
3. Tarsy D: Treatment of Parkinson's disease, In Rose BD (ed): *UpToDate*, Wellesley, MA, 2004.
4. Scrag A, et al: Unilateral pallidotomy for Parkinson's disease: results after more than 1 year, *J Neurol Neurosurg Psychiatry* 67:511, 1999.
5. Limousin P, et al: Electrical stimulation of the subthalamic nucleus in advanced Parkinson's disease, *NEJM* 339:1105, 1998.

RESTLESS LEG SYNDROME
(See also insomnia, sleep apnea)

Patients with restless leg syndrome (RLS) complain of an aching, cramping, or crawling sensation deep in the legs, usually the calves. These symptoms occur at rest, usually at night, and are relieved by moving or walking. Associated symptoms include periodic limb movements during sleep or involuntary limb movements while awake. Insomnia is a common initial symptom, and in many cases the underlying RLS is not diagnosed. An estimated 2.5% to 15% of the general population is affected.

Patients with primary idiopathic RLS have a positive family history consistent with autosomal dominant inheritance more than 40% of the time. Patients who have an onset of symptoms when they are older than 50 years of age are more likely to have secondary RLS associated with dialysis, iron deficiency, peripheral neuropathy, and rheumatic diseases.

The pathogenesis of RLS is uncertain, but alterations in dopamine functioning appear to be important. For this reason the first line of treatment has often been levodopa/carbidopa or dopamine agonists such as bromocriptine, pergolide, or, more recently, pramipexole[1] and ropinirole.[2,3] Tolerance development is a problem with levodopa, and sometimes a rebound daytime augmentation of symptoms occurs, which may be related to the short half-life of levodopa. Switching to longer-acting drugs such as pergolide, pramipexole, or ropinirole may resolve the problem. When prescribing medications for this condition, practitioners should start with low doses and increase gradually. Gabapentin (Neurontin) has been shown to be effective in a small open-label trial[4] as well as in an RCT.[5] Benzodiazepines such as clonazepam and opioids have been known to suppress symptoms, but run the risk of tolerance and dependence and should be used cautiously as a final or adjunctive option.

The findings regarding the relationship between iron deficiency and RLS are inconclusive. It is reasonable, however, to measure a serum ferritin in patients with RLS, even in the absence of anemia.[6] A low serum ferritin (less than 50 μg/L) has been associated with a greater severity of RLS,[7] and oral iron supplementation in patients with a ferritin less than 18 μgrams/L resulted in improvements in RLS symptoms.[8]

❧ REFERENCES ❧

1. Montplaisir J, et al: Restless leg syndrome improved by pramipexole: a double-blind randomized trial, *Neurology* 52:938, 1999.
2. Ondo W: Ropinirole for restless legs syndrome, *Mov Disord* 13:138. 1999.
3. Adler CH, et al: Ropinirole is beneficial for restless legs syndrome: a placebo-controlled crossover trial, *Neurology,* 60 (Suppl 1): A439, 2003.
4. Happe S, et al: Treatment of idiopathic restless legs syndrome (RLS) with gabapentin, *Neurology,* 57:1717, 2001.
5. Garcia-Borreguero D, et al: Treatment of restless legs syndrome with gabapentin: a double-blind, cross-over study, *Neurology,* 59:1574, 2002.
6. Earley C: Restless leg syndrome, *NEJM* 348:2109, 2003.
7. Sun ER, et al: Iron and the restless legs syndrome, *Sleep,* 21:371-7, 1998.
8. O'Keefe ST, et al: Iron status and the restless legs syndrome in the elderly, *Age Aging* 23:200, 1994.

SEIZURES

(See also alcoholism; anticonvulsants in pregnancy; bipolar disorder; concussion; febrile seizures; motor vehicle accidents; syncope; transient global anemia)

Seizures are classified as follows[1]:

Partial seizures (focal seizures). Partial seizures begin in one part of a cerebral hemisphere and may or may not become generalized. In simple partial seizures, consciousness is preserved and manifestations may include motor, somatosensory or special sensory, autonomic, or psychic symptoms. Complex partial seizures (temporal lobe seizures, psychomotor seizures) may start as a simple partial seizure that is followed by impaired consciousness, or consciousness may be impaired from the onset.

Generalized-onset seizures. Generalized-onset seizures involve both cerebral hemispheres from the beginning. They are subcategorized as tonic-clonic (grand mal), absence (petit mal), atypical absence, myoclonic, tonic, and atonic.

The type of seizure may be determined if a reliable observer provides an accurate description of its course, but in other cases the diagnosis depends on video monitoring combined with electroencephalographic recordings that are often repeated and sometimes recorded while the patient is hyperventilating or subject to visual stimulation.

Recognized precipitating factors for seizures include alcohol and drug abuse, use of certain medications (e.g., neuroleptics, tricyclics), neoplasms, neurocysticercosis, previous head injury, and previous cerebrovascular accident.[1]

The major causes of spontaneous loss of consciousness are seizures, pseudoseizures (conversion reactions), and syncope. Multifocal and generalized myoclonic jerks are commonly seen in syncope.[2] One study found that tongue biting (lacerations observed by a physician) had a sensitivity of 24% and a specificity of 99% for epilepsy. Lateral tongue biting was 100% specific for tonic-clonic seizures.[3]

Brief convulsive episodes immediately following head injury with rapid recovery are usually called posttraumatic seizures. However, the prognosis is excellent and they are probably not true epileptic reactions.

About one third of patients with a single unprovoked seizure have recurrences, whereas three fourths of those with two or three unprovoked seizures have recurrences.[4] Recurrence is more likely if the patient had a previous serious central nervous system injury or has a family history of seizures, if the seizure was of the complex partial type, or if the EEG is abnormal.[5-7] More than 30% of patients continue to have seizures despite pharmacological treatment. Localization-related epilepsies are less likely to be controlled than the idiopathic generalized syndromes. Refractory epilepsy increases the risk of cognitive deterioration, psychosocial dysfunction, and sudden unexpected death. The treatment goal should be prevention of decline in social, vocational, and cognitive performance, and minimization of the risk of injury or death.[8]

Controversy exists regarding required therapy for all patients who have had an unprovoked seizure. The care goal for patients with epilepsy is "no seizures and no side effects equals control." Three steps to achieve this goal include prompt and accurate diagnosis of epilepsy in patients presenting with epileptic seizures; administration of an appropriate first treatment intervention; and adequate monitoring to ensure not only the efficacy and safety of the treatment intervention, but also the accuracy of the initial epilepsy diagnosis. Although evidence supporting the best approach to these steps is limited, physicians should strive to control epilepsy by using sound clinical judgement and applying the best available evidence.[9,10]

The selection of an antiepileptic drug (AED) for initial treatment of epilepsy in infancy, childhood, and adolescence should ideally be made after a clear diagnosis of the patient's seizure disorder.[8] Erroneous diagnosis is a common cause of failure of the first AED. The availability of new-generation AEDs has expanded the choice of available agents with comparable efficacy for most syndromes.[9] Relative toxicity and tolerability of AEDs must also be assessed in making the selection. Appreciation of age-specific organ toxicities is especially important. Moreover, the use of AEDs in childhood requires an understanding of the neurobehavioural effects of the AEDs. Important neuropsychiatric co-morbidities in children with epilepsy include attention deficit/hyperactivity disorder (ADHD), autistic spectrum disorders, depression and anxiety, and thought disorders.

Treatment decreases the frequency of recurrent seizures.[10-12] However, treatment does not alter the long-term prognosis,[13,14] and therefore, if the risk of recurrence is low, the adverse effects of treatment may outweigh the benefits. For low-risk children, withholding treatment may be acceptable in many cases because a single recurrent seizure may not have major adverse social or vocational implications. However, for many adults such an event may be perceived as catastrophic, and such patients may well choose therapy even if they are also at low risk.[15]

The majority of patients with newly diagnosed epilepsy in the developed world are started on prophylactic treatment with an AED. Many patients remain seizure-free on the first or second drug chosen; however, combinations of AEDs are usually prescribed for those patients unresponsive to monotherapy.[8] About 60% of patients are successfully treated with the first or second AED. Response to the first AED is the most powerful predictor of long-term prognosis. Substantial attention should be given to choosing the first AED most suited to the individual patient. The balance of efficacy, tolerability, and safety (i.e., "effectiveness") is critical to making the best choice.

Doses are initially low and are increased gradually as necessary.[5,6] Marks and Garcia suggest some important modifications to such a regimen.[15] They advise increasing the level of the initial drug until complete seizure control is attained or until persistent unacceptable side effects occur, regardless of serum drug levels. They point out that many patients require so-called toxic levels for control and that in general, the term *toxic levels* refers to an increased risk of dose-related adverse effects and not life-threatening situations. If a patient has further seizures once the maximum tolerated dose of a drug is achieved, a second drug should be added. As the dose of the second drug is increased to the maximum tolerated level, the dose of the initial drug is decreased and eventually discontinued so that the patient is once again receiving monotherapy.

Carbamazepine (Tegretol), phenytoin (Dilantin), valproate (Depakene, Depakote, Epival), and lamotrigine (Lamictal) are considered by many to be the first-line drugs for both partial seizures and generalized tonic-clonic seizures.[15-18] Sustained-release variants of carbamazepine

Table 22   Some Aspects of Principal Antiepileptic Drugs

Drug; side effect	Incidence	Avoidance	Management
Carbamazepine (focal and generalized seizures)			
Rash, maculopapular	5%	Introduce drug slowly	Transient dose reduction
Stevens-Johnson syndrome	Very rare (case reports only)	Introduce drug slowly	Admit to hospital; stop drug
Interaction with other antiepileptic drugs	Common, variable	—	Possible dosage adjustments
Transient leukopenia	10%-20%	—	Complete blood count every 3-6 mo in first year
Persistent leukopenia	2%	—	Complete blood count at intervals or change drug
Aplastic anemia	1 in 200,000	—	Stop drug
Lamotrigine (focal and generalized seizures, including absence seizures)			
Rash, mild	3%-5%	Introduce drug very slowly	Dose reduction
Rash, severe	0.1% in adults, 1%-2% in children	Introduce drug very slowly	Admit to hospital; stop drug
Diplopia	Dose dependent	—	Dose reduction
Phenytoin (Dilantin) (focal and generalized seizures)			
Augments metabolism of oral contraceptives, anticoagulants, other antiepileptic drugs, and dexamethasone	Common	—	Dosage adjustment of affected medications
Rash	5%	—	Reduce dose or stop drug
Gingival hypertrophy	25%	Meticulous dental hygiene	Dosage adjustment
Mild hirsutism	75%	—	Stop drug if female patient
Topiramate (focal and generalized seizures)			
Weight loss	10%	—	Reassure patient as levels out; reduce dose
Mental sluggishness	Dose dependent	—	Dose reduction
Fatigue	Dose dependent	—	Dose reduction
Kidney stones	1%-2%	—	Stop drug
Glaucoma	Very rare (case reports only)	—	Stop drug
Valproate (focal and generalized seizures, including absence seizures)			
Weight gain	40%-100%	Exercise	Dose reduction
Hair loss	1%-3%	—	None (side effect usually transient)
Liver failure	0.16% in children < 3 yr; lower in older patients	—	Stop drug
Ethosuximide (absence seizures only)			
Gastrointestinal irritability	20%-33%, usually transient	—	Dose reduction
Depression, psychosis, leukopenia	Very rare (case reports only)	—	Reduce dose or stop drug

Adapted from Brodie MJ, Kwan P, *Neurology* 58(8 Suppl 5):S2-8, 2002.

(Tegretol-XR, Carbatrol) increase seizure control and decrease adverse effects. Valproate is the preferred drug for myoclonic and atonic-type seizures, whereas absence seizures should be treated with ethosuximide (Zarontin) or valproate. Since long-term use of phenytoin is associated with facial coarsening, gingival hyperplasia, and hirsutism, it may not appeal to everyone.

The FDA has approved several new AEDs as add-on treatments for patients with treatment-resistant partial or secondary generalized seizures (Table 22). In clinical trials, many of these drugs have been effective as monotherapy for refractory partial seizures. Felbamate (Felbatol) has been associated with hepatic failure and aplastic anemia, and its use is restricted to patients unresponsive to other therapies. Levetiracetam (Keppra) is a newer AED that is effective for partial-onset seizures, and lacks any of the typical serious side effects involving liver and bone marrow of older AEDs.[17-19]

When AED serum levels are drawn to determine whether therapeutic levels have been achieved, they should be obtained only after steady-state conditions have been reached.[21] For phenytoin this is 6 days after starting or changing the dose, for carbamazepine and valproic acid it is 3 days, and for phenobarbital it is 20 days. Except for phenobarbital, which has an extremely long half-life, trough levels should be obtained. Immediate serum levels are indicated within 6 hours of a seizure or when toxicity or non-compliance is suspected.[21] In some patients, seizures are controlled with subtherapeutic levels, whereas others require "toxic" levels (see earlier discussion).

After a period of good control, patients with epilepsy may be able to stop their medications. A variety of studies suggest that after 2 years of treatment without seizures, a little over two thirds of patients remain seizure free after stopping medications. This does not necessarily mean that 2 years of treatment improves the natural history of the disease; rather, it may be a method of selecting patients who are most likely to remain seizure free with or without medications. Some factors that predict a higher risk of relapse in children who discontinue medications include partial epilepsy, older age at onset, and an epileptiform EEG while receiving medications. Since relapses in children are not harmful, discontinuing medications after 6 to 12 months may be safe for many, especially those at low risk of recurrence. Medications can be restarted if seizures recur.[21,22]

People with temporal-lobe epilepsy should be evaluated for surgery if prolonged anticonvulsant drug therapy proves ineffective.[23]

❧ REFERENCES ❧

1. Veilleux M: The keys to seizure management, *Can J CME* 11:113-123, 1999.
2. Sander JW, O'Donoghue MF: Epilepsy: getting the diagnosis right; all that convulses is not epilepsy (editorial), *BMJ* 314:158-159, 1997.
3. Benbadis SR, Wolgamuth BR, Goren H, et al: Value of tongue biting in the diagnosis of seizures, *Arch Intern Med* 155:2346-2349, 1995.
4. Hauser WA, Rich SS, Lee JR-J, et al: Risk of recurrent seizures after two unprovoked seizures, *N Engl J Med* 338:429-434, 1998.
5. Drugs for epilepsy, *Med Lett* 37:37-40, 1995.
6. Brodie MJ, Dichter MA: Antiepileptic drugs, *N Engl J Med* 334:168-175, 1996.
7. Shinnar S, Berg AT, Moshe SL, et al: The risk of seizure recurrence after a first unprovoked afebrile seizure in childhood—an extended follow-up, *Pediatrics* 98: 216-225, 1996.
8. Sillanpää M, Jalava M, Kaleva O, et al: Long-term prognosis of seizures with onset in childhood, *N Engl J Med* 338:1715-1722, 1998.
9. Sankar R: Initial treatment of epilepsy with antiepileptic drugs: pediatric issues, *Neurology* 63(10 Suppl 4):S30-S39, 2004.
10. Camfield P, Camfield C, Dooley J, et al: A randomized study of carbamazepine versus no medication following a first unprovoked seizure in childhood, *Neurology* 39: 851-852, 1989.
11. First Seizure Trial Group: Randomized clinical trial on the efficacy of antiepileptic drugs in reducing the risk of relapse after a first unprovoked tonic-clonic seizure, *Neurology* 43:478-483, 1993.
12. Gilad R, Lampl Y, Gabbay U, et al: Early treatment of a single generalized tonic-clonic seizure to prevent recurrence, *Arch Neurol* 53:1149-1152, 1996.
13. Musicco M, Beghi E, Solari A (First Seizure Trial Group): Effect of antiepileptic treatment initiated after the first unprovoked seizure on the long-term prognosis of epilepsy, *Neurology* 44(suppl 2):A337-A338, 1994.
14. Shinnar S, Berg AT: Does antiepileptic drug therapy alter the prognosis of childhood seizures and prevent the development of chronic epilepsy? *Semin Pediatr Neurol* 1: 111-117, 1994.
15. Marks WJ, Garcia PA: Management of seizures and epilepsy, *Am Fam Physician* 57:1589-1600, 1998.
16. McCorry D, Chadwick D, Marson A: Current drug treatment of epilepsy in adults, *Lancet Neurol* 3(12):729-735, 2004.
17. Levetiracetam—a new drug for epilepsy, *Drug Ther Bull* -01-APR-2002; 40(4): 30-2 (From NIH/NLM MEDLINE).
18. Blume WT: Diagnosis and management of epilepsy, *CMAJ* 168(4):441-448 2003.
19. Ross S: Management of patients with newly diagnosed epilepsy: a systematic literature review (editorial), *Am Family Physician* 70(5):824, 827-828, 2004.
20. Brodie MJ, Kwan P: Staged approach to epilepsy management, *Neurology* 58(8 Suppl 5):S2-8, 2002.
21. Schoenenberger RA, Tanasijevic MJ, Jha A, et al: Appropriateness of antiepileptic drug level monitoring, *JAMA* 274:1622-1626, 1995.
22. Peters AC, Brouwer OF, Geerts AT, et al: Randomized prospective study of early discontinuation of antiepileptic drugs in children with epilepsy, *Neurology* 50:724-730, 1998.
23. Wiebe S, Blume WT, Girvin JP, et al: A randomized, controlled trial of surgery for temporal-lobe epilepsy, *N Eng J Med* 345(5): 311-318, 2001.

SPASTICITY

Spasticity results from cerebral disorders such as stroke, acquired brain injury, or cerebral palsy; spinal cord injuries, and MS. Treatment is required only when interference with function or risk of injury exists. Certain factors can increase spasticity, including urinary tract infection (UTI), constipation, and ulcers, which must be sought out and treated. PT and OT can play an important role in management. Oral medications include baclofen, dantrolene, tizanidine, and gabapentin. The dosage should be low initially and increased gradually to the usual maintenance dosage, which for baclofen is 40 to 80 mg per day divided three or four times a day, for dantrolene 25 to 100 mg four times a day, for tizanidine 12 to 36 mg per day divided three times a day, and for gabapentin 600 to 800 mg four times a day. Newer therapies requiring referral to a physiatrist include botulinum toxin injection and intrathecal baclofen.

--- ⮚ **REFERENCES** ⮘ ---

1. Rehabilitation medicine: 3. Management of adult spasticity, *CMAJ* 169(11): 1173-1178, Nov 2003.

SUBARACHNOID HEMORRHAGE

(See also cerebrovascular accidents; prevention; screening)

Subarachnoid hemorrhage (SAH) is a neurological condition with a greater prevalence rate than that of primary brain tumours or MS. Incidence ranges from 6 to 16 per 100,000, with approximately 25,000 to 30,000 cases of SAH per year in the United States.[1] SAH is a disease of middle-aged women, with a 3:2 female to male predominance and peak incidence in the sixth decade of life. The only consistently reported risk factors for SAH are hypertension, smoking, and heavy drinking. Other risk factors include a personal history of a previous intracerebral aneurysm; family history of aneurysm; and certain heritable connective tissue disorders such as autosomal-dominant polycystic kidney disease, Ehlers-Danlos syndrome, and Marfan's syndrome.[2]

The characteristic symptom of an SAH is the sudden onset of severe headache, sometimes called the "thunderclap headache."[3] In some patients, severe lower back pain with bilateral radicular pain develops as a result of the irritating properties of blood that has descended into the subarachnoid space surrounding the lower spinal cord. Between one third and one half of patients in whom a significant SAH is found have had an unusual headache, often described as "the worst headache in my life" in the preceding days or weeks, which was caused by a "warning leak;" physicians usually miss the significance of these headaches. Classic physical findings are meningismus, focal neurological signs, and retinal hemorrhages, with the latter found in about a quarter of the patients. CT scans without contrast medium identify 90% to 95% of patients with subarach-noid hemorrhages if obtained within 24 hours, but because blood is rapidly absorbed, the sensitivity of CT detection drops to 80% at 3 days and 70% at 5 days. MRI is not a sensitive way of diagnosing an acute SAH, but is a good technique for detecting intracranial aneurysms.[1] The mortality rate associated with SAH is 50%.[1-3]

Screening

It may be justified to investigate individuals with a strong family history of cerebral aneurysms; that is, patients with two or more affected first-degree relatives, for the presence of intracranial aneurysms. Screening may also be indicated in patients with polycystic kidney disease, particularly those who also have a family history of cerebral aneurysms.

Cerebral angiography is the most sensitive technique for detecting intracranial aneurysms. This procedure is invasive and relatively unpleasant but still carries significant morbidity and occasional mortality, and therefore may not be appropriate for screening of asymptomatic patients. With newly emerging technology, MRI or CT angiography may soon provide good-quality imaging that would detect all intracranial aneurysms.[4-6] At present, very small aneurysms can be missed on MRI and/or CT angiograms. However, these techniques do play a role presently, and may be particularly appropriate when asymptomatic screening appears warranted.

Morbidity and mortality from surgical clipping of aneurysms are considerable, ranging from about 6.5% in those under age 45 to 32% in those age 65 or over.[4] An alternative management protocol is endovascular coil embolization (coiling), in which a neurointerventional radiologist inserts a number of detachable platinum coils into the aneurysm via a femoral artery catheter. Long-term outcomes of this technique have not been determined, but short-term benefits and complication rates are as good as or better than those with surgical clipping.[5]

--- ⮚ **REFERENCES** ⮘ ---

1. Manno EM: Subarachnoid hemorrhage, *Neurol Clin* 22(2) May, 2004.
2. Schievink WI: Intracranial aneurysms, *N Engl J Med* 336:28-40, 1997.
3. American College of Emergency Physicians: Clinical policy: critical issues in the evaluation and management of patients presenting to the emergency department with acute headache, *Ann Emerg Med* 39:108-122, 2002.
4. Wermer MJ, Rinkel GJ, van Gijn J: Repeated screening for intracranial aneurysms in familial subarachnoid hemorrhage, *Stroke* 34(12):2788-2791, Dec 2003.
5. Magnetic Resonance Angiography in Relatives of Patients with Subarachnoid Hemorrhage Study Group: Risks and benefits of screening for intracranial aneurysms in first-degree relatives of patients with sporadic subarachnoid hemorrhage, *N Engl J Med* 341:1344-1350, 1999.

6. Kirkpatrick PJ, McConnell RS: Screening for familial intracranial aneurysms: no justification exists for routine screening (editorial), *BMJ* 319:1512-1513, 1999.
7. Subarachnoid hemorrhage-www.firstconsult.com.
8. International Study of Unruptured Intracranial Aneurysms Investigators: Unruptured intracranial aneurysms—risk of rupture and risks of surgical intervention, *N Engl J Med* 339:1725-1733, 1998.
9. Johnston SC, Dudley A, Gress DR, et al: Surgical and endovascular treatment of unruptured cerebral aneurysms at university hospitals, *Neurology* 52:1799-1805, 1999.

SYNCOPE

(See a brief primary care approach to dizziness)

Syncope is defined as a sudden temporary loss of consciousness with a loss of postural tone and spontaneous recovery. The episodes often have typical precipitants such as pain, hot environment, stress, exercise, coughing, and micturition. Syncope is often associated with nausea, diaphoresis, and pallor and usually lasts less than 5 minutes. Data from Framingham participants demonstrated an incidence of 6.2 events per 1000 person-years, an incidence that increased with age.[1]

The etiology of syncope in descending order of incidence in one study[1] was classified as follows: vasovagal and other (vasovagal, orthostatic hypotension, medication-induced, cough, micturition, situational), unknown cause, cardiac (structural heart disease, arrhythmia), and neurological (migraine, TIA, seizure). History and physical examinations helped to detect the cause in 45% of one series of syncopal patients. The absence of nausea or vomiting before the syncopal episode was a predictor of higher risk for arrhythmic causes of syncope, but no other symptoms were helpful. The likelihood of dying within the year following the syncopal episode was not related to any symptom. No symptoms predicted recurrence of syncope.[2] A more recent study had more success, but used more expert procedures such as tilt test and carotid sinus massage. Patients without palpitations or a cardiac history were less likely to have a cardiogenic cause.[3] In the Framingham cohort, the risk of death was 31% higher in patients with syncope compared with those without syncope.[1] The prognosis is significantly influenced by the etiology, with the most important predictors of poor outcome a year after a syncopal episode being age greater than or equal to 45 years, history of heart failure, history of ventricular arrhythmia, and an abnormal EKG. Therefore, the goal of syncope evaluation is to identify cardiac syncope with structural heart disease or an abnormal EKG.[4] Vasovagal and situational syncope portend a fairly benign prognosis.[1]

Management of syncope is aimed at the underlying cause if identified. Many patients use beta blockers for prevention of vasovagal syncope, but evidence of effectiveness is lacking.[5] There is some data for SSRIs.[6]

REFERENCES

1. Soteriades ES, Evans JC, Larson MG, et al: Incidence and prognosis of syncope, *N Engl J Med* 347:878-885, 2002.
2. OH JH, Hanusa BH, Kapoor WN: Do symptoms predict cardiac arrhythmias and mortality in patients with syncope? *Arch Intern Med* 159:375-380, 1999.
3. Alboni P, Brignole M, Menozzi C, et al: Diagnostic value of history in patients with syncope with or without heart disease, *J Am Coll Cardiol* 37: 1921-1928, 2001.
4. Kapoor WN: Current evaluation and management of syncope, *Circulation* 106 (13):1606-1609, 2002.
5. Flevari P, Livanis E, Theodorakis GN, et al: Vasovagal syncope: a prospective randomized, crossover evaluation of the effect of propranolol, nadolol and placebo on syncope recurrence and patients' well-being, *J Am Coll Cardiol* 40:499-504, 2002.
6. Girolamo ED, Iorio CD, Sabatini P, et al: Effects of paroxetine hydrochloride, a selective serotonin reuptake inhibitor, on refractory vasovagal syncope: a randomized, double-blind, placebo-controlled study, *J Am Coll Cardiol* 33: 1227-1230, 1999.

TOURETTE'S SYNDROME

(See also attention deficit disorder; obsessive-compulsive disorder; sleepwalking)

Tourette's syndrome (TS) is a neurodevelopmental disorder characterized by motor and phonic tics. Simple tics include shoulder jerking, eye blinking, picking movements of hands, sniffing, grunting, and barking. Complex tics include flapping of arms, facial grimaces, kissing self or others, repeating words, and using obscene language.

TS affects 1% to 3% of the general population, although many cases are mild and don't come to medical attention. TS usually begins as simple motor tics in young school-aged children. Boys are affected more often than girls. Symptoms wax and wane, and one type of tic is commonly replaced by another. Patients with TS can often voluntarily suppress tics for hours and are influenced by external events such as stress or excitement. Most patients have a significant decrease in tic severity by age 19 to 20.

The treatment approach of a patient with TS involves a careful history and observation. About half of patients with TS also meet the diagnostic criteria for ADHD. One fourth to one third have obsessive-compulsive disorder or learning disabilities, so symptoms of such comorbidities should be sought out and treated first. It is important to list symptoms in order of their intrusiveness such that treatment of the most distressing symptoms occurs first.

Careful education of parents and teachers about the nature and natural history of TS is essential and often allows the condition to be managed without pharmacological agents. A decision to treat should be based on the impairment of function and the risks and benefits of the proposed treatment. Behavioural treatment that focuses on improving academic and social skills is recommended for all patients. Specifically, habit reversal training has shown significant promise.[1] Drugs that can be used to control symptoms include clonidine (0.025 to 0.05 mg qhs to start) to a daily dose of 0.15 to 0.3 mg twice a day (divided one-third in a.m., two-thirds qhs); guanfacine 0.25 to 1.0 mg twice a day for children over age 12; haloperidol; pimozide; risperidone (olanzapine and quetiapine). Newer therapies with limited evidence include pergolide, locally injected botulinum toxin, nicotinic drugs, and Delta-9-tetrahydrocannabinol. For many patients the agents of first choice are clonidine or guanfacine. These medications have moderate efficacy in controlling tics and are often beneficial for comorbid conditions such as ADHD. The medications should always be started at a low dose and increased gradually. A therapeutic response may not be seen for 2 to 3 weeks or until a therapeutic dose is achieved with clonidine and atypical neuroleptics, respectively. An adequate trial may be as long as 3 months, and the physician must keep in mind the natural history of the disorder (waxing and waning of symptoms) when assessing treatment success.

◣ REFERENCES ◤

1. Wilhelm S, et al: Habit reversal versus supportive psychotherapy for Tourette's disorder: a randomized controlled trial, *Am J Psychiatry* 160(6):1175-1177, 2003.
2. Sandor P: Pharmacological management of tics in patients with TS, *J Psychosom Res* 55:41-48, 2003.
3. Leckman JF: Tourette's syndrome, *Lancet* 360:1577-1586, 2002.

TRANSIENT GLOBAL AMNESIA
(See also seizures; transient ischemic attacks)

Transient global amnesia (TGA) is an unusual neurological syndrome first described in 1958 by Fisher and Adams.[1] TGA is a frightening experience for patients and relatives, marked by a "sudden inability to acquire new information (a deficit of anterograde memory), usually lasting a few hours and not accompanied by any other focal neurologic signs or symptoms."[2] Full recovery usually occurs within a few hours (typically less than 12). The annual incidence has been estimated to range from 5.2/100,000 to 10/100,000 in the general population, but up to 32/100,000 in patients over 50 years; the peak of incidence is in the seventh decade. Patients may appear perplexed and disoriented in terms of time and location but retain immediate memory and the ability to perform complex activities. Upon recovery, the patient is fully functional but has a memory gap regarding the duration of the episode. The etiology of TGA remains elusive; no indications exist that it might be a TIA equivalent, a seizure equivalent, nor that it might be a migraine variant. The annual recurrence rate is approximately

2.5%. There is no increased risk of cerebrovascular accidents.[1]

If patients have no history of head trauma or previous neurological disorders, if a reliable witness is present who can describe the attack, and if a thorough history and physical examination fail to show evidence of other disorders, no investigation is required.[3]

◣ REFERENCES ◤

1. Fischer CM, Adams RD: Transient global amnesia, *Trans Am Neurol Assoc* 83:143-146, 1958.
2. Pantoni L, Lamassa M, Inzitari D: Transient global amnesia: a review emphasizing pathogenic aspects, *Acta Neurol Scand* 102:275-283, 2000.
3. Brown J: Evaluation of transient global amnesia, *Ann Emerg Med* 30:522-526, 1997.

TREMOR

The most common causes of tremor are essential tremor, medication-induced tremor, exaggerated physiological tremor (anxiety, thyrotoxicosis, hypoglycemia, pheochromocytoma, drug withdrawal), and Parkinsonism.

Essential tremor (ET), a genetic, monosymptomatic condition, has an insidious bimodal onset that peaks between 15 to 20 and 50 to 70 years of age, and a kinetic/postural tremor. It most commonly affects the hands (85% to 96% of patients). Less commonly affected in patients are the head (35% to 45%), voice (15% to 20%), leg (10% to 15%), and the chin, jaw, trunk and tongue (less than 5%).

Fifteen percent of patients who seek medical attention for ET do so because of functional impairment or social embarrassment. The tremor itself also progresses over time with an increase in severity and wider distribution throughout the body.

The treatment goal is to minimize functional disability, reduce social handicap, and improve quality of life. Medical therapy improves the condition in 50% of cases. First-line medical therapy consists of beta blockers (propranolol) and primidone or a combination of the two. Second-line treatments include benzodiazapines (episodic, anxiety-related), gabapentin, topiramate, and botulinum toxin (not helpful functionally in hand tremor).

Surgical treatment (thalamotomy or deep brain stimulation) is indicated if medical treatment fails.

◣ REFERENCES ◤

1. Lyons KE, Pahwa R, Comella CL, et al: Benefits and risks of pharmacological treatments for essential tremor, *Drug Safety* 26(7):461-481, 2003.
2. Sethi KD: Tremor, *Curr OpinNeurol* 16(4):481-485, 2003.
3. Chen JJ, Swope DM: Essential tremor: diagnosis and treatment, *Pharmacotherapy* 23(9):1105-1122, 2003.

DENTISTRY

ANTIBIOTIC PROPHYLAXIS

Endocarditis Prophylaxis

(See also prosthetic joint infection prophylaxis; valvular heart disease)

In 1955 the American Heart Association (AHA) first drew up guidelines for the prevention of bacterial endocarditis. The latest revision took place in 1997.[1] The new guidelines state that the only persons requiring prophylaxis are those at high or moderate risk of endocarditis; that is, patients with prosthetic heart valves, a past history of endocarditis, congenital heart disease (except for isolated secundum atrial septal defect), acquired valvular disease, and hypertrophic cardiomyopathy. Patients with mitral valve prolapse (MVP) usually need antibiotics only if they have a regurgitant murmur. (Some patients diagnosed with MVP in the more distant past were falsely labelled and do not have the risk factor when re-examined with new ultrasound technology.) The specific dental procedures for which prophylaxis is recommended include extractions, dental implant placement, periodontal surgery, and scaling or cleaning associated with bleeding. Antibiotic prophylaxis is not recommended for most local anaesthetics, fillings, crowns, or root canals provided the latter do not extend beyond the apex of the tooth. However, if unexpected bleeding is encountered during one of these procedures, antibiotic prophylaxis may be given if the medication is taken no later than 4 hours after the intervention.[1]

Two major antibiotic regimens are recommended by the new guidelines[1]:

Amoxicillin	2 g po 1 hour before the procedure (children 50 mg/kg)
Penicillin Allergic	
Clindamycin	600 mg po 1 hour before the procedure (children 20 mg/kg)
or	
Cephalexin	2 g po 1 hour before procedure (children 50 mg/kg)
or	
Azithromycin *or* Clarithromycin	500 mg taken po 1 hour before the procedure (children 15 mg/kg)

All guidelines for endocarditis prophylaxis are based on expert opinion because no prospective randomized controlled trials have shown that antibacterial prophylaxis for dental procedures is effective.[1-4] Indirect evidence suggests that it is, but even if this is so, only a small proportion of cases (4% to 19%) are related to procedures for which prophylaxis is recommended.[2] A study in the Netherlands estimated that only 6% of cases of endocarditis would be prevented if 100% of patients requiring prophylactic antibiotics received them,[3] while a U.S. case-control study concluded that antibiotic prophylaxis for dental work failed to prevent any infections and that current guidelines should be reconsidered.[4]

❧ REFERENCES ❧

1. Dajani AS, Taubert KA, Wilson W, et al: Prevention of bacterial endocarditis: recommendations by the American Heart Association, *JAMA* 277:1794-1801, 1997.
2. Durack DT: Prevention of infective endocarditis, *N Engl J Med* 332:38-44, 1995.
3. Van der Meer JTM, van Wijk W, Thompson J, et al: Efficacy of antibiotic prophylaxis for prevention of native-valve endocarditis, *Lancet* 339:135-139, 1992.
4. Strom BL, Abrutyn E, Berlin JA, et al: Dental and cardiac risk factors for infective endocarditis: a population-based, case-control study, *Ann Intern Med* 129:761-769, 1998.

Prosthetic Joint Infection Prophylaxis

(See also endocarditis prophylaxis)

Whether patients with prosthetic joints should receive prophylactic antibiotics for dental treatments is controversial. No randomized trials dealing with this issue have been published, so recommendations are based on expert opinion.[1] Rather convincing case reports indicate that prosthetic joint infection may follow invasive dental procedures, particularly in patients at elevated risk of infection because of underlying conditions such as inflammatory arthritis, diabetes, or immunosuppression. However, the numbers involved are small, and how many cases of infection are prevented by antibiotic prophylaxis is unknown. Furthermore, morbidity from reactions to antibiotics might outweigh possible benefits.[2] In 1997 the American Academy of Orthopaedic Surgeons and the American Dental Association recommended against routine antibiotic prophylaxis for patients with joint arthroplasties but advised that prophylaxis might be considered for all patients during the first 2 years after arthroplasty placement and indefinitely for patients at elevated risk of infection. Such prophylaxis should be given only for dental procedures that are associated with an elevated risk of bacteraemia. (See previous discussion of endocarditis prophylaxis.)[3]

_____ ◈ REFERENCES ◈ _____

1. Uyemura MC: Antibiotic prophylaxis for medical and dental procedures: a look at AHA guidelines and controversial issues, _Postgrad Med_ 98:137-140, 147, 151-152, 1995.
2. LaPorte DM, Waldman BJ, Mont MA, et al: Infections associated with dental procedures in total hip arthroplasty, _J Bone Joint Surg [Br]_ 81-B:56-59, 1999.
3. American Dental Association: American Academy of Orthopaedic Surgeons: Advisory statement: antibiotic prophylaxis for dental patients with total joint replacements, _J Am Dent Assoc_ 128:1004-1007, 1997.

ANTICOAGULANTS
(See also anticoagulants in hematology section)

Because of an increased risk of thromboembolism, discontinuing anticoagulants before dental procedures such as extractions or gingival and alveolar surgery may be dangerous. The international normalized ratio (INR) should be maintained in the therapeutic range; any bleeding that occurs can be controlled by local measures.[1,2]

_____ ◈ REFERENCES ◈ _____

1. Wahl MJ: Dental surgery in anticoagulated patients, _Arch Intern Med_ 158:1610-1616, 1998.
2. Dunn AS, Turpie AGG: Perioperative management of patients receiving oral anticoagulants: a systematic review, _Arch Intern Med_ 163:901-908, 2003.

AVULSED TOOTH

An avulsed tooth that is re-implanted within 30 minutes will survive in 90% of cases. After 30 minutes the success rate decreases by about 1% per minute. The patient or physician should hold the avulsed tooth by the crown, rinse it off in water (with a plug in the sink so that it is not lost down the drain), and re-implant it. The patient can hold it in place by biting gently on it through an overlying piece of gauze until he or she is seen by a dentist. If the physician or patient is unable to replace the tooth in the socket, it should be rinsed and transported to the dentist in milk, saliva (either in the vestibule of the mouth or in a container into which the patient spits), physiological saline, or water.[1] Water is the least desirable storage medium because the hypotonic environment causes rapid cell lysis and increased inflammation on replantation.[2] Primary teeth need not be reimplanted.[3]

_____ ◈ REFERENCES ◈ _____

1. Hiltz J, Trope M: Vitality of human lip fibroblasts in milk, Hanks Balanced Salt Solution and Viaspan storage media, _Endod Dent Traumatol_ 7:69, 1991.
2. Blomlof L: Milk and saliva as possible storage media for traumatically exarticulated teeth prior to replantation, _Swed Dent J Suppl_ 8:1, 1981.
3. Clark MM, Album MM, Lloyd RW: Medical care of the dental patient, _Am Fam Physician_ 52:1126-1132, 1995.

DENTAL ABSCESS

A dental abscess can often be diagnosed by percussing the suspected tooth for pain.[1] Physicians should provide appropriate pain medication and refer patients to a dentist as soon as possible, because treatment of a periapical abscess requires incision and drainage plus root canal treatment or extraction of diseased tooth.[2] Antibiotics are adjunctive only and are generally not needed in healthy patients with pulpitis (inflammation of the nerve) alone. For more serious infections, choices of antibiotics include Penicillin VK or Cephalexin 500 mg four times a day for 7 days or Clindamycin 300 mg by mouth every 6 hours for 7 days in patients who are allergic to penicillin.[3]

_____ ◈ REFERENCES ◈ _____

1. Clark MM, Album MM, Lloyd RW: Medical care of the dental patient, _Am Fam Physician_ 52:1126-1132, 1995.
2. Douglass AB. Douglass JM: Common dental emergencies, _Am Fam Physician_ 67(3):511-516, Feb 1 2003.
3. Johns Hopkins Division of Infectious Diseases Antibiotic Guide, accessed April1, 2004 at http://hopkins-abxguide.org/terminals/diagnosis_terminal.cfm?id=943.

INFLUENCES ON ORAL HEALTH
Drugs

Any drug that inhibits salivation is likely to increase the incidence of dental caries, periodontal disease, and oral infections. Antidepressants, particularly tricyclics, are an important cause of this phenomenon. Patients taking such drugs should participate in a regimen of optimal oral hygiene, including use of fluorides. A patient can increase salivary flow between meals by taking vitamin C tablets or chewing sugar-free gum. If the problem is serious, the patient should attempt to change medications.[1]

Bulimia Nervosa

The complications of this disease include enamel erosion of all teeth due to the chronic exposure to acid in vomit; increase in occurrence of cavities due to excessive carbohydrate intake during binge-eating; dry mouth from decreased salivary flow and parotid gland dysfunction, which put the patient at an even higher risk for cavities; small, purplish-red lesions on the palate due to contact with objects used to induce vomiting; and possibility of raised silver fillings due to erosion of the teeth.[2]

Tooth Grinding (Bruxism)

Use of a mouth guard at night is recommended to prevent damage to teeth and jaws during sleep.[3]

Sucking on Citrus Foods, Use of Pacifiers, and Babies Sleeping with Bottles

These activities cause erosion, bacterial growth, and increase in cavities.[4,5]

Severe Infections, Vitamin C Deficiencies

These cause poor oral health, damage to the oral mucosa, and increased periodontal disease.[6,7]

Frequent and Vigorous Tooth Brushing

This causes enamel erosion when done with an improper hard toothbrush or over-abrasive toothpaste.[8]

Discolouration of Teeth by Coffee & Smoking

These are treated by cleaning or whitening, and very occasionally by laminates and caps.[9]

―――――――― ❧ REFERENCES ❧ ――――――――

1. Peeters FP, deVries MW, Vissink A: Risk for oral health with the use of antidepressants, *Gen Hosp Psychiatry* 20:150-154, 1998.
2. Christensen GJ: Oral care for patients with bulimia, *J Am Dent Assoc* 133(12):1689-1691, Dec 2002.
3. Howard HP: Destructive nocturnal bruxing, *Aust Dent J* 48(4):267, Dec 2003.
4. Lussi A, Jaeggi T, Zero D: The role of diet in the aetiology of dental erosion, *Caries Res* 38(Suppl review)1:34-44, 2004.
5. Durward L: Sugar in baby foods, *Dent Update* 18(4):162-165, May 1991.
6. Fontana M: Vitamin C (ascorbic acid): clinical implications for oral health–a literature review, *Compendium* 15(7):916, 918, 920 passim; quiz 930, Jul 1994.
7. Pollack RL, Kravitz E, Litwack D: Nutrition and periodontal health, *Quintessence Int* 15(1):65-69, Jan 1984.
8. Gillette WB, Van House RL: Ill effects of improper oral hygeine procedure, *J Am Dent Assoc* 101(3):476-480, Sep 1980.
9. Reibel J: Tobacco and oral diseases. Update on the evidence, with recommendations, *Med Princ Pract* 12(Suppl review)1:22-32, 2003.

FLUORIDES

The amount of fluoride children should receive and the ages at which it should be administered are controversial issues. Because a significant amount of fluoride is present in toothpaste, mouthwash, and even soft drinks and juices reconstituted with fluoridated water, many young children receive their daily fluoride requirements in this fashion even if their drinking water is not fluoridated. There is fear that excessive supplementation could lead to fluorosis.[1] Degrees of fluorosis vary; most cases in North America are so mild that the alterations in the enamel are visible only to experts.[2,3]

The optimal fluoridation levels of the water supply should be 0.6 or 0.7 to 1.2 ppm.[2-5] The trend has been to initiate fluoride supplementation later in life (at 2 to 3 years of age) and to give lower doses than were previously believed necessary. This is done not only to prevent fluorosis, but also because the traditional view that fluorides had to be incorporated into the tooth enamel before tooth eruption occurred is false; therefore, administration of the agent can be delayed until after tooth eruption.[2,3] The American Academy of Pediatrics advises no supplementation before the age of 6 months regardless of the concentration of fluorides in the water; they recommend that from 6 months to 3 years children receive 0.25 mg/day only if the water supply fluorides are less than 0.3 ppm.[5] The Canadian Dental Association further recommends no supplementation before the age of 3 years regardless of the fluoride concentration of the water.[2,3]

Whether or not fluoride supplements are given, young children should brush their teeth twice daily under adult supervision, using only a pea-sized amount of (fluoridated) toothpaste, and they should be taught to spit it out, not swallow it.[1-3]

The Canadian Task Force on Preventive Health Care updated its evaluation of dental caries in 1995.[6] It gave "A" recommendations for fluoridation of the water supply, the use of fluoride dentifrices, daily fluoride supplementation when the water is not fluoridated, and annual or biannual professional application of topical fluorides. The latter is effective but costly and is therefore not recommended for the general populace. The U.S. Preventive Services Task Force also gives an "A" recommendation to fluoride supplementation if the fluoride concentration in the water supply is inadequate.[7]

―――――――― ❧ REFERENCES ❧ ――――――――

1. Raves J: MDS call for more study before endorsing dentists' new recommendations on fluoride, *Can Med Assoc J* 149:1820-1822, 1993.
2. Clark DC: Appropriate uses of fluorides for children: guidelines from the Canadian Workshop on the Evaluation of Current Recommendations Concerning Fluorides, *Can Med Assoc J* 149: 1787-1793, 1993.
3. Clark DC: Appropriate use of fluorides in the 1990s, *J Can Dent Assoc* 59:272-279, 1993.
4. Jakush J: New fluoride schedule adopted, *ADA News* 25:12, 14, 1994.
5. American Academy of Pediatrics Committee on Nutrition: Fluoride supplementation for children: interim policy recommendations, *Pediatrics* 95:777, 1995.
6. Lewis DW, Ismail AI (Canadian Task Force on the Periodic Health Examination): Periodic health examination, 1995 update. 2. Prevention of dental caries, *Can Med Assoc J* 152:836-846, 1995.
7. U.S. Preventive Services Task Force: *Guide to clinical preventive services,* ed 2, Baltimore, 1996, Williams & Wilkins, 711-721.

PAIN

Non-steroidal anti-inflammatory drugs are, in general, the analgesics of choice for dental pain.[1] A weak opioid may be added in an appropriate quantity to last until the dental appointment.[2]

≥ REFERENCES ≤

1. Seymour RA, Walton JG: Analgesic efficacy in dental pain, *Br Dent J* 153:291-298, 1982.
2. Douglass AB, Douglass JM: Common dental emergencies, *Am Fam Physician* 67(3):511-6, Feb 1 2003.

PERIODONTITIS

Gingivitis is inflammation that is limited to the gums. Periodontitis is inflammation of the gums that has extended into the periodontal area, causing destruction of periodontal ligaments, bone involvement, and eventual loosening (loss of attachment) of affected teeth. As periodontitis advances, the gums recede and retract from around the roots of affected teeth, forming pockets. The process can be localized or generalized. In its most common form, periodontitis is a disease of older individuals. Smoking and diabetes are additional risk factors. Of the hundreds of organisms found in the mouth, attention has recently been focused on gram-negative anaerobic rods and spirochetes. The goal of treatment is good oral hygiene in the form of brushing, flossing, and professional removal of calculus to reduce the bacteria that may populate periodontal pockets. Adjuvant measures are smoking cessation, 2-minute mouthwashes twice a day with agents such as 0.2% chlorhexidine, in some cases antibiotic treatment with one of the tetracyclines, and in more advanced cases surgery.[1]

≥ REFERENCES ≤

1. Watts TL: Periodontitis for medical practitioners, *BMJ* 316: 993-996, 1998.
2. Williams RC, Paquette DW: Understanding the pathogenesis of periodontitis: a century of discovery, *J Int Acad Periodontol* 2(3):59-63, Jul 2000.

DERMATOLOGY

Topics covered in this section

ACNE VULGARIS

(See also oral contraceptives; polycystic ovarian syndrome)

Acne is present in over 80% of adolescents and in 12% of women and 3% of men age 25 to 44. Acne develops earlier in girls than boys but affects boys more frequently and more severely.[1-3]

Pathogenesis

The basic pathogenetic factors in acne are an increased proliferation and abnormal desquamation of epithelial cells, which block the follicular orifices, and an increased production of sebum. Sebum accumulating behind the obstruction favours the growth of *Propionibacterium acnes,* which is a normal commensal within the pilosebaceous units. *P. acnes* secretes lipolytic enzymes, leading to the release of free fatty acids, as well as secreting chemotactic factors that attract neutrophils. The hydrolytic enzymes of the neutrophils damage the follicular wall, and these, as well as the free fatty acids, are released into the tissues, causing inflammation.[2-4]

Clinical Manifestations

A whitehead or closed comedone is caused by accumulation of sebum behind a plugged pilosebaceous follicle. Continued distention leads to a partial protrusion from the follicular opening, which has the clinical appearance of an opened comedone or blackhead. The black colour of a blackhead is due to melanin and oxidized lipids, not dirt. Once the sebaceous contents rupture into the dermis, the pattern becomes one of inflammatory acne with papule, and in more severe cases nodule, or "cyst," formation. Acne usually develops at puberty when androgens stimulate the sebaceous follicles.[2-4] Persistence of acne in adulthood may reflect end-organ hyper-responsiveness as well as absolute levels of androgens.[5] Premenstrual flares of acne are common because the follicular orifices become more obstructed at that time of the cycle.[2,3]

Specific Etiological Factors

Endocrine disorders with excess androgen production such as polycystic ovarian syndrome and Cushing's syndrome can cause acne. Endocrine evaluations may be indicated in women with acne associated with irregular periods, hirsutism, and alopecia. The sulfated form of dehydroepiandrosterone (DHEA-S), total and free testosterone luteinizing hormone/follicle-stimulating hormone (LH/FSH) ratio, prolactin and 17-OH progesterone should be taken in the luteal phase (in the 2 weeks preceding menses).[5] Medications known to be associated with acne include corticosteroids, androgens, certain oral contraceptives containing antiestrogenic progestins, phenytoin, barbiturates, lithium, isoniazid, cyclosporine, iodides, and bromides. Oil-based cosmetics and occupational exposure to oils are other known precipitants.[2]

Treatment

Diet has no influence on acne. Vigorous scrubbing of the affected areas may aggravate rather than ameliorate the situation.[3] Gentle washing is all that is required.[2]

Patients should be instructed that medical treatment will do little for the current "crop" of acne lesions, but will help in prevention of further lesions. This can take a month or more. Antibacterial soaps with the exception of benzoyl peroxide are not indicated. Moisturizers and cosmetics, if used, should be labelled as non-comedogenic, non-acnegenic, or "will not clog pores."[5] Treatment is primarily medical. Acne surgery, such as comedone extraction, cryotherapy, or drainage and intralesional triamcinolone injections for nodules are useful adjuncts. Mild comedonal acne should be treated with a topical retinoid. Treatment of papular/pustular acne should start with topical benzoyl peroxide gel and retinoid and/or topical antibiotic. An oral antibiotic can be included for resistant or more severe cases. Nodular acne can be treated with oral isotretinoin. Oral antiandrogens can be added to conventional therapy for women with resistant acne.[5]

Retinoids

Tretinoin, adapalene, and tazarotene reverse the abnormal desquamation in acne and prevent comedone formation. Applied over the entire affected area, they can significantly reduce lesion counts after 2 to 3 months.

A "flare" in the acne may occur in the first 2 weeks. Treatment should continue after improvement to maintain benefit. Adverse effects include erythema, scaling, burning, and photosensitivity and are dose related. Tretinoin is available (in order of increasing strength) as cream 0.01% to 0.05%, gel 0.01% to 0.05%, and liquid 0.025% to 0.05%. Adapalene is as effective as tretinoin gel 0.025%, but is as well tolerated as tretinoin cream 0.025%.[5,6] The strength of the medication can be titrated upward at 4-week intervals until there is benefit or adverse effects become uncomfortable. Retinoids can be used as first-line treatment of papular/pustular acne in combination with topical antibiotics (antibiotic every morning or twice a day, retinoid at bedtime). Fixed combinations of tretinoin with erythromycin or clindamycin are available in some regions. Retinoids (at bedtime) can also be combined with benzoyl peroxide (every morning) and oral antibiotics for more inflammatory cases.

Benzoyl peroxide

Benzoyl peroxide is antimicrobial but may also have comedolytic and anti-inflammatory effects. Gels are preferred and come in concentrations of 1% to 20%. Adverse effects include erythema, scaling, burning, and bleaching of hair and fabrics. Combination therapy with topical antibiotics is more effective and antibiotic resistance is reduced. Fixed combinations with erythromycin or clindamycin are available.

Topical antibiotics

Clindamycin and erythromycin are effective topically in concentrations of 1% to 3%. Monotherapy should be avoided if possible due to potential for resistance. Pseudomembranous colitis is rare but has been reported with topical clindamycin.[5]

Oral antibiotics

Erythromycin 1 g, tetracycline 1 g, minocycline 100 to 200 mg, doxycycline 100 to 200 mg or TMP/SMX (160/800) daily, given in two divided doses, are commonly used. Topical retinoids or benzoyl peroxide should be added to improve and maintain outcomes. Benzoyl peroxide may also reduce occurrence of resistance. Oral antibiotics should be given for 2 to 4 months, but if improvement cannot be maintained with topical agents, they may be continued indefinitely.[5]

Oral isotretinoin (Accutane)

Accutane is indicated in severe nodular acne and moderate-to-severe acne that scars physically or psychologically and is resistant to other therapies. Accutane decreases the size and secretion of sebaceous glands, normalizes keratinization, and indirectly inhibits *P. acnes* growth and decreases inflammation. The dosage range is 0.1 to 1.0 mg/kg/day for 4 to 6 months for a cumulative

dose of 120 to 150 mg/kg. Accutane is a potent teratogen. Women of child-bearing age must be given verbal and written instructions about this effect. They should start treatment on the third day of a normal menstrual period and preferably use two forms of contraception. Beta-human chorionic gonadotropin (HCG) should be tested before, monthly during, and 1 month after use of Accutane. Patients can be reassured that Accutane will be cleared from the body's system 6 weeks after discontinuation. Adverse effects include dry skin, nosebleeds, mood changes, headaches, and muscle aches. Severe headaches, decreased night vision, or depression call for immediate discontinuation of Accutane. The patient should discuss the possibility of psychiatric side effects with family and friends to aid detection. A negative beta-HCG, serum lipids, and liver function tests should be obtained before treatment and repeated monthly until 1 month after cessation of treatment. Relevant changes may require dosage reduction or discontinuation. Recurrence of some acne within 3 to 5 years occurs in 30% to 60% of cases.[5]

Antiandrogens

Hormonal therapy in women may be used when there are signs of hyperandrogenism, significant perimenstrual exacerbations, if contraception is desired, as a complement to conventional therapy, or as an alternative to repeated courses of Accutane. Hormonal therapy can be beneficial whether or not serum androgens are elevated. Improvement may take 3 to 6 months, and relapses are common after discontinuation.[3-5] Even low-dose estradiol, when paired with a non-androgenic progesterone such as norgestimate or levonorgestrel, can be beneficial.[5] Cyproterone acetate (not available in the United States), usually paired with estradiol (Diane 35), is more effective but may have a higher incidence of deep venous thrombosis (DVT).[7] Concommitant use of oral antibiotics common for acne does not appear to decrease oral contraceptive (OC) efficacy.[8] Spironolactone 25 to 200 mg per day may be used if cyproterone is unavailable or contraindicated.[3] OCs with an antiandrogenic progestin derivative may be slightly more effective than other OCs in improving mild-to-moderate acne. However, nearly half the women in a 2001 trial comparing the antiandrogen OCs to a typical OC had a significant reduction in their acne after 12 cycles of treatment regardless of brand.[9]

─────────────── ❧ **REFERENCES** ❧ ───────────────

1. Goulden V, Stables GI, Cunliffe WJ: Prevalence of facial acne in adults, *J Am Acad Dermatol* 41(4):577-580, 1999.
2. Nguyen QH, Kim YA, Schwartz RA: Management of acne vulgaris, *Am Fam Physician* 50:89-96, 1994.
3. Leyden JJ: Therapy for acne vulgaris, *N Engl J Med* 336:1156-1162, 1997.

4. Brown SK, Shalita AR: Acne vulgaris, *Lancet* 351:1871-1876, 1998.
5. Gollnick H, Cunliffe W, Berson D, et al: Management of Acne, *J Am Acad Dermatol* 49(1)Suppl: S1-S37, 2003.
6. Wolf JE: An update of recent clinical trials examining adapalene and acne, *J Eur Acad Venereol* 15(Suppl 3)23-29, 2001.
7. Wooltorton E: Diane-35 (cyproterone acetate): safety concerns, *CMAJ* 168(4):455-456, 2003.
8. Rasmussen JE: The effect of antibiotics on the efficacy of oral contraceptives, *Arch Dermatol* 125:562-564, 1989.
9. Worret I, Arp W, Zahradnik HP, et al: Acne resolution rates: results of a single-blind, randomized, controlled, parallel phase III trial with EE/CMA (Belara) and EE/LNG (Microgynon), *Dermatology* 203:38-44, 2001.

ACTINIC KERATOSES

Actinic keratosis (AK), also known as *solar keratosis,* is a precancerous skin lesion caused by long-term sun (UV light) exposure. The lesions appear as ill-defined macules, papules, or plaques with a rough, dry, scaly surface. Their colour varies from erythematous to light brown. Risk factors for AK are advancing age, fair skin, and excess sun exposure.[1]

Over a 10-year period, about 10% of actinic keratoses develop into low-grade squamous cell carcinomas.[1,2] Such carcinomas rarely metastasize.[3] Not all actinic keratoses progress; some remain unchanged, and others undergo spontaneous regression.[3] The treatment of choice for isolated lesions is destruction, usually with liquid nitrogen. Multiple lesions may be treated with topical 5-fluorouracil (5-FU, Efudex, Fluoroplex) or topical tretinoin (Retin-A).[2-4]

5-FU is applied twice daily (with gloves or a wooden spatula[2]) in concentrations of 1% to 2% for the face and lips and 5% for the scalp, neck, arms, hands, chest, and back.[3] The usual duration of therapy is 3 weeks for the face and lips and 4 to 8 weeks for other areas of the body.[3] Erythematous and necrotic reactions beginning 5 to 15 days after the onset of therapy are normal. The degree of inflammation is aggravated by sun exposure and can be somewhat ameliorated by applying a moderate-potency topical steroid. One way of decreasing inflammation is to use lower concentrations of 5-FU (0.1% to 0.9%), but if this is done, treatment must continue until the last lesion resolves, which may take 2 to 3 months. Residual lesions may be treated with higher concentrations of 5-FU or by cryosurgery.[2] Another way of decreasing inflammation is to use a "pulsing" schedule in which 5% 5-FU is applied once or twice a week for 6 to 8 weeks.[3]

Newer topical agents available in some countries are diclofenac 3% (Solaraze, U.S.), 5-FU 0.5% (Carac, U.S.), and imiquimod 5% (Aldara, North America). These agents can be used more diffusely on at-risk skin areas with the intention of destroying both existing AK lesions and potential subclinical foci of dyskeratotic cells that may become AK lesions or squamous cell carcinomas.[4]

A once-daily application of 0.1% tretinoin cream may be used to treat actinic keratoses, but applications have to continue for 12 to 15 months or even longer.[3]

❧ REFERENCES ❧

1. Lebwohl M: Actinic keratosis: epidemiology and progression to squamous cell carcinoma, *Br J Dermatol* 149(Suppl 66):31-33, 2003.
2. Schwartz RA: Therapeutic perspectives in actinic and other keratoses, *Int J Dermatol* 35:533-538, 1996.
3. Odom R: Managing actinic keratoses with retinoids, *J Am Acad Dermatol* 39:S74-S78, 1998.
4. Salasche SJ: Update on actinic keratosis and Bowen's disease in clinical trial experience, *Br J Dermatol* 149(Suppl 66):30, 2003.

ALOPECIA

Telogen Effluvium

Telogen effluvium is a common cause of diffuse hair loss. Hair loss results from psychological, physiological, or pathological stress. The disorder usually declares itself 2 to 4 months after the precipitating event, and up to 50% of hair may be lost. Specific causes include childbirth; surgery and anesthesia; crash dieting; infections; hypothyroidism; a variety of drugs, including antidepressants, lithium, beta blockers, angiotensin-converting enzyme (ACE) inhibitors, and anticoagulants; and discontinuation of oral contraceptives. Hair regrowth occurs in 2 to 3 months if the precipitating condition is no longer present.[1]

Trichotillomania and Alopecia Areata

Trichotillomania is a self-inflicted loss of hair, typically from the frontoparietal region progressing backward. Regrowth of up to 1.5 cm may be visible before the hair is long enough to pull again. Patients with alopecia areata have "exclamation point" hairs around the periphery of the bald spots.[1] A variety of treatments may be used for alopecia areata, alone or in combination: intralesional glucocorticoid injections, topical glucocorticoids, 5% topical minoxidil (Rogaine), topical anthralin, and topical immunotherapy (an experimental procedure available in only a few centres).[2] The recurrence rate is 30%, and recurrence usually affects the initial area of involvement.[3]

Male Pattern Androgenic Alopecia

Male pattern alopecia is common; 30% of white men are affected by age 30 and 50% by age 50. Whites are affected four times as often as African Americans.[4] The inheritance pattern is thought to be polygenic.[2]

Topical Vasodilator

The standard topical medication for male pattern baldness is minoxidil (Rogaine) applied to the scalp twice a day. If benefits ensue, they persist only as long as the drug continues to be applied.[2,4] About 15% of treated men have a medium regrowth of hair, 50% notice a delay of further hair loss, and 35% have continuing hair loss. Dense hair growth is rare. In view of the data the main benefit of minoxidil appears to be a delay in further hair loss.[4] Hair counts have shown the 5% solution (Rogaine Extra Strength for Men) to be more effective than the 2% solution,[2] but whether this translates into a clinically important improvement is uncertain.[5] The efficacy of minoxidil can be increased by synergistic use of tretinoin (Retin-A) applied at separate times during the day.[6]

Another pharmacological approach to male pattern baldness is the use of finasteride (Propecia) 1 mg per day orally. This drug decreases the level of circulating dihydrotestosterone by inhibiting the enzyme 5-alpha-reductase, which is necessary for the conversion of testosterone to the more potent dihydrotestosterone. After 2 years of treatment with finasteride, two thirds of men have hair regrowth and almost all of the remaining have no further hair loss.[2,4] Some benefit may be noted within 4 months of initiating treatment, but a full 24-month trial is required to fully assess efficacy. Treatment must be continued indefinitely to maintain benefits, and for some individuals continuing treatment beyond 2 years may lead to even further scalp coverage.[2] Decreased libido, usually reversible, is a rare but significant side effect when the drug is discontinued.[4]

The most frequently used surgical treatment of male pattern baldness is hair transplantation from the occiput to the frontal and vertex areas. The transplanted follicles maintain their resistance to androgenic alopecia. Other surgical techniques involve excision of bald areas and the use of scalp flaps.[4]

Female Androgenetic Alopecia

Female androgenetic alopecia is common and is manifested as diffuse hair loss in the temporoparietal region and a more-than-usually apparent central part. The frontal hairline is usually maintained. Treatment of this condition with 2% minoxidil has resulted in minimal hair growth in about half of patients and moderate hair growth in 13%[7]; 5% minoxidil is no more effective than the 2% solution.[2] Women may also benefit from adjunctive treatment such as estrogen or spironolactone.[6] Because hair loss can be devastating to women, management should include an assessment for psychological effects.[8] Women with androgenic alopecia do not require an endocrinological workup unless there is evidence of virilism. They can be reassured that they will not become bald and that dyes, hair sprays, and permanents will not harm their hair.[2]

≈ REFERENCES ≈

1. Nielsen TA, Reichel M: Alopecia: diagnosis and management, *Am Fam Physician* 51:1513-1522, 1995.
2. Price VH: Treatment of hair loss, *N Engl J Med* 341:964-973, 1999.
3. Goodheart HP: Hair and scalp disorder. Part 2: Alopecia areata, *Women's Health Prim Care* 2:283-287, 1999.
4. Sinclair R: Male pattern androgenetic alopecia, *BMJ* 317:865-869, 1998.
5. Propecia and Rogaine Extra Strength for alopecia, *Med Lett* 40:25-27, 1998.
6. Springer K, Brown M, Stulberg DL: Common hair loss disorders, *Am Fam Physician* 68(1):107-108, 2003.
7. De Villez RL, Jacobs JP, Szpunar CA, et al: Androgenetic alopecia in the female: treatment with 2% topical minoxidil solution, *Arch Dermatol* 130:303-307, 1994.
8. Thiedke CC: Alopecia in women, *Am Fam Physician* 67(5):1007-1014, 2003.

CELLULITIS

Cellulitis typically presents as an acute onset of an inflammatory patch or plaque with erythema, tenderness and pain, warmth, and variable edema. Fever, malaise, and regional lymphadenopathy are common. Erysipelas is a more severe variant with superficial inflammatory process and sharply demarcated borders usually affecting the extremities and, less commonly, the face, scalp, and genitals.[1]

Common diagnostic challenges include abscess, gout, contact dermatitis, eczema, herpes zoster, osteomyelitis, and DVT. Cellulitis is predominantly caused by gram-positive cocci (*Staphylococcus aureus,* group A or B streptococci, viridans streptococci, and *Enterococcus faecalis*).[2] Risk factors, which may predict severity and recurrence, are diabetes, chronic limb edema, peripheral vascular disease, chronic fungal infection, eczema, IV drug abuse, and immunocompromised state. Necrotizing fasciitis must be ruled out, and any underlying abscess should be drained. Initial blood work is not needed except to identify diabetes or renal failure[3] (to decrease antibiotic dose). There is no need for routine blood or tissue cultures because the yield is very poor.[4]

Few studies exist on the optimal treatment of cellulitis because many studies include a variety of more severe skin infections. Additionally, antibiotic resistance varies by geography and is constantly changing.[2] Milder cases can be treated orally with cephalexin (500 mg every 6 hours for 10 to 14 days), clindamycin (300 to 600 mg every 6 to 8 hours for 10 to 14 days) or azithromycin (500 mg loading dose, 250 mg once a day for 4 days).[5,6] Special cases such as bites, IV drug-use–related infections, and diabetic foot require addition of gram-positive coverage, such as fluoroquinolones.[7] Successful treatment must include addressing the underlying disease if present. Determination of failure should not be anticipated for at least 48 hours of antibiotic use, unless a clear progression of infection or worsening systemic signs and symptoms occur. The only validated parameter predicting failure is widening of the diameter of erythema at 72 hours after initial treatment.[8]

The need for IV treatment or switching to IV management is largely a judgement call. Typically, the factors playing a role in making that decision include underlying patient status, severity of systemic signs and symptoms, and reliability of the follow-up. Cefazolin 1 g IM/IV every 8 hours has an excellent success rate of 92% to 100%. (Lower rates were observed only in patients with pre-existing illness.)[9,10] There is good evidence for concurrent use of metabolic inhibitors (Probenecid or Sulbactam 500 mg to 1000 mg orally) in addition to once- or twice-daily dosage.[11] In penicillin-allergic patients, clindamycin 600 mg IV every 8 hours is a suitable alternative. The decision to taper down to the oral therapy is a judgement call as well. IV therapy lasts on average 4 to 5 days. Recurrent cellulitis requires longer treatment.

REFERENCES

1. Martins C: Johns Hopkins Antibiotic Guide. Last update April 7, 2003. (Accessed May 27, 2004, http://hopkins-abxguide.org)
2. Swartz MN: Clinical practice: cellulitis, *N Engl J Med* 350(9):904-912, Feb 26 2004.
3. Simonart T, Simonart JM, Derdelinckx I, et al: Value of standard laboratory tests for the early recognition of group A β-hemolytic streptococcal necrotizing fasciitis, *Clin Infect Dis* 32:E9-12, 2001.
4. Lee PC, Turnidge J, McDonald PJ: Fine-needle aspiration biopsy in diagnosis of soft tissue infections, *J Clin Microbiol* 22:80, 1985.
5. Aly AA, Roberts NM, Seipol KS, et al: Case survey of management of cellulitis in a tertiary teaching hospital, *Med J Aust* 165:553-556, 1996.
6. Robinson JL, Hameed T, Carr S: Practical aspects of choosing an antibiotic for patients with a reported allergy to an antibiotic, *Clin Infect Dis* 35:26-31, 2002.
7. Lipsky BA, Pecoraro RE, Larson SA, et al: Outpatient management of uncomplicated lower-extremity infections in diabetic patients, *Arch Intern Med* 150:790-797, 1990.
8. Murray HE, Steill IG, Wells GA: Defining treatment failure in ED patients with cellulitis, *Acad Emerg Med* 8(5):478, 2001.
9. Nathwani D: The management of skin and soft tissue infections: outpatient parenteral antibiotic therapy in the United Kingdom, *Chemotherapy* 47(Suppl1):17-23, 2001.
10. Campbell SG: The management of cellulitis in adults, *Drugs Ther Maritime Practitioners* 24(6):31-36, 2001.
11. Brown G, Chamberlain R, Goulding J, et al: Ceftriaxone versus cefazolin with probenecid for severe skin and soft tissue infections, *J Emerg Med* 14:547-551, 1996.

CONTACT DERMATITIS

Contact dermatitis can come from a variety of sources, but the common agents are plants, chemicals, metal, and medications. A common cause of contact dermatitis from ear-rings, watches, or eyeglass frames is nickel allergy. One method of preventing the contact is to coat the offending object with clear nail polish and let it dry. Repetition of applications every 2 to 8 weeks is usually required.[1]

REFERENCES

1. Gore BQ: For nickel allergy, *Patient Care Can* 7(3):22, 1996.

ECZEMA

Eczema and *dermatitis* are the general terms that encompass a number of skin conditions including atopic dermatitis, seborrhoeic dermatitis, dyshidrotic eczema, irritant contact dermatitis, and allergic contact dermatitis. In general, eczema is an inflammatory skin disorder that is best characterized by pruritus with exacerbations and remissions. Other cardinal features include a personal or family history of atopic disease as well as typical distribution, which includes the facial and extensor surfaces in infants and young children and flexure lichenification in older children and adults. The presence of extensor distribution in older children and adults indicates a poor prognosis for ultimate cure.[1]

Acute lesions are papules and vesicles on a background of erythema. Subacute lesions may develop scales and lichenification. Chronically involved areas become thick and fibrotic, and nodules often develop within the plaques. Lesions at any stage can develop secondary infections that may resemble impetigo, with crusting and weeping lesions. When the lesions resolve, areas of hyperpigmentation or hypopigmentation may persist. Xerosis (dry skin) is another characteristic skin finding in patients with atopic dermatitis. Reversing xerosis is one of the key elements in the treatment of atopic dermatitis.

Between 50% and 80% of patients with atopic dermatitis have or develop asthma or allergic rhinitis. Nearly 70% of patients have a positive family history of atopy. Even if atopic dermatitis resolves with age, the predisposition for asthma and rhinitis persists.[2]

The pathogenesis of atopic dermatitis is unknown, but the disease seems to be the result of genetic susceptibility, immune dysfunction, and epidermal barrier dysfunction.[3]

Exposure to aeroallergens such as pollens, moulds, mites, and animal dander appears to be important in some patients with atopic dermatitis. Substantial clinical improvement may occur when these patients are removed from environments that contain the allergens to which they react.[4] If food or aeroallergen sensitivity is suspected, patients should be evaluated with in vitro radioallergosorbent test (RAST) or prick skin testing and possibly a withdrawal diet or controlled food challenge test.

Because the skin lesions in atopic dermatitis can take many forms, including papules, vesicles, plaques, nodules, and excoriations, the differential diagnosis of atopic dermatitis is extensive. Conditions that need to be considered in patients with pruritus include seborrhoeic dermatitis, psoriasis, and neurodermatitis. Occasionally, a patient with skin lesions and a history consistent with atopic dermatitis will have contact dermatitis. Systemic illnesses such as malignancy, thyroid disorders, and hepatic or renal failure can also cause pruritus and excoriations. Adults with new-onset pruritus must undergo a thorough history and complete physical examination to exclude systemic disease.[5]

Treatment

The treatment of atopic dermatitis targets underlying skin abnormalities such as xerosis, pruritus, superinfection, and inflammation. Patients should also be educated about the chronic nature of the disease and the need for continued adherence to proper skin care.

A reasonable recommendation for bathing is once daily with warm (not hot) water for approximately 5 to 10 minutes. Soap should not be used unless it is needed for the removal of dirt, and only with a mild cleanser (e.g., Dove, Basis, Kiss My Face, or Cetaphil) should be used. Immediately after bathing (and before the skin is completely dry), patients should apply a moisturizer liberally (e.g., Aquaphor, Eucerin, Moisturel, mineral oil, or baby oil). Ointments are superior to creams and lotions, but they are greasy and therefore poorly tolerated. Creams are effective and better tolerated than ointments. Lotions are least effective because of their alcohol content.

Soaks in sodium bicarbonate or colloidal oatmeal (Aveeno) can treat pruritus. To avoid injury to the skin from scratching, fingernails should be cut short, and cotton gloves can be worn at night.

Large colonization of the atopic dermatitis skin with staphylococci and staphylococcal superantigens is a chronic stimulus for cutaneous inflammation. Oral antibiotics and topical antibacterial treatments can improve atopic dermatitis by reducing the effects of the staphylococcal superantigens.

Corticosteroids

Systemic corticosteroids should be reserved for use in patients with severe treatment-resistant atopic dermatitis. Oral corticosteroids improve the lesions of atopic dermatitis, but a disease flare may occur when these medications are stopped. Topical corticosteroids are effective in patients with atopic dermatitis, but therapy with these agents should not replace the frequent use of moisturizers. The local and systemic side effects of topical steroids are well recognized. Local effects include skin atrophy, striae, telangiectasias, hypopigmentation, rosacea, perioral dermatitis, and acne. Topical corticosteroids are grouped into seven potency categories (Table 23), with group 1 containing the most potent agents and group 7 containing the least potent agents. A general principle in treating atopic dermatitis with topical steroids is to use the least potent agent possible and limit the frequency of application.

Compared with adults, children (especially infants) are at higher risk for the local and systemic side effects of topical corticosteroids. Thus it is reasonable to use a group 6 or 7 steroid initially in infants and for intertriginous areas in patients of any age. If the dermatitis is severe and a more potent steroid is needed, the patient should be followed closely, and the strength of the steroid should be reduced as skin lesions improve.

Use of a midpotency topical corticosteroid (group 4 or 5) is appropriate for non-intertriginous areas in children and adults. Groups 1 and 2 steroids are best reserved for use on thickened plaques and for the palms and soles. Group 1 steroids are generally best avoided in children under 12 years of age or for use with occlusion.

Topical steroids come in many forms, including solutions, lotions, creams, gels, and ointments. The thicker preparations (ointments) penetrate the epidermis better. The same steroid in a different form can differ in potency by one or two classes. Some areas of the body dictate the type of form needed. For example, the scalp is best treated with solutions and lotions. Occlusion should be limited to isolated resistant areas because it significantly increases the absorption of topical steroids.[5]

Tar Preparations

Tar preparations have anti-inflammatory and antipruritic effects on atopic dermatitis lesions. These preparations are effective when used alone or with topical corticosteroids. The disadvantages of tars are their odour and dark staining colour. Using the products at night and covering the treated areas can decrease these problems.

Phototherapy

Phototherapy is effective in treating refractory atopic dermatitis. This treatment may be administered as ultraviolet A (UVA), ultraviolet B (UVB) or combined UVA and UVB. Psoralen plus UVA (PUVA) photochemotherapy may be a treatment option in patients with extensive refractory disease.

Calcineurin Inhibitors

Tacrolimus as 0.1% and 0.03% ointment and Pimecrolimus as 1% cream are new, expensive immunosuppressive medications called *calcineurin inhibitors*. They affect a variety of interleukins and can therefore be effective in the treatment of acute and chronic atopic dermatitis. Several studies have examined the efficacy of topical tacrolimus and Pimecrolimus in adult and pediatric patients with success versus placebo.[6-9] In clinical trials, the most common side effect was a burning sensation of the skin, no laboratory abnormalities were reported, and no skin atrophy was noted. The recommended dosage is twice a day. It is considered safe to use throughout the body surface, including on the face.[10]

Table 23 Selected Topical Steroid Creams

Generic Names	Selected Trade Names
Group I	
Betamethasone dipropionate/ propylene glycol 0.05%	Diprolene
Clobetasol 17-propionate 0.05%	Dermovate, Temovate
Group II	
Desoximetasone 0.25%	Topicort
Fluocinonide 0.05%	Lidex Regular
Halcinonide 0.1%	Halog-E
Group III	
Triamcinolone acetonide 0.5%	Aristocort "C"oncentrate
Group IV	
Amcinonide 0.1%	Cyclocort
Fluocinolone acetonide 0.2%	Synalar HP
Halcinonide 0.025%	Halog
Group V	
Betamethasone-17-valerate 0.1%	Betnovate, Celestoderm-V, Valisone
Fluocinolone acetonide 0.025%	Synalar Regular
Hydrocortisone valerate 0.2%	Westcort
Triamcinolone acetonide 0.1%	Aristocort "R"egular, Kenalog
Group VI	
Desonide 0.05%	Tridesilon
Triamcinolone acetonide 0.025%	Aristocort "D"ilute
Group VII	
Hydrocortisone 1%	Hytone, Synacort, Cortate
Methylprednisolone 0.25%	Medrol

❧ REFERENCES ❧

1. Lookingbill D, Marks JG: Eczematous rashes. In: *Principles of dermatology,* ed 2, Philadelphia, 1993, Saunders, 127-130.
2. Halbert AR, Weston WL, Morelli JG: Atopic dermatitis: is it an allergic disease? *J Am Acad Dermatol* 33:1008-1018, 1995.
3. Cooper KD: Atopic dermatitis: recent trends in pathogenesis and treatment, *J Invest Dermatol* 102:128-137, 1994.
4. Adinoff AD, Tellez P, Clark R: Atopic dermatitis and aeroallergen contact sensitivity, *J Allergy Clin Immunol* 81:736-742, 1988.
5. Correale C, et al: Atopic dermatitis: a review of diagnosis and treatment, *Am Fam Physician* 60:1191-1198, 1209-1210, 1999.
6. Paller A, Eichenfield LF, Leung DY, et al: A 12-week study of tacrolimus ointment for the treatment of atopic dermatitis in pediatric patients, *J Am Acad Dermatol* 44(1 Suppl):S47-57, 2001.
7. Boguniewicz M, Fiedler VC, Raimer S, et al: A randomized, vehicle-controlled trial of tacrolimus ointment for treatment of atopic dermatitis in children, *J Allergy Clin Immunol* 102(4 pt 1):637-644, 1998.
8. Ruzicka T, Bieber T, Schopf E, et al: A short-term trial of tacrolimus ointment for atopic dermatitis. European Tacrolimus Multicenter Atopic Dermatitis Study Group, *N Engl J Med* 337:816-821, 1997.
9. Hanifin JM, Ling MR, Langley R, et al: Tacrolimus ointment for the treatment of atopic dermatitis in adult patients: part I, efficacy, *J Am Acad Dermatol* 44(1 suppl):S28-38, 2001.
10. Russel J: Topical tacrolimus: a new therapy for atopic dermatitis, *Am Fam Physician* 66:1899-1902,1906, 2002.

FOLLICULITIS

Folliculitis is an inflammation of the hair follicles caused by infection (most commonly -coagulase-positive staphylococci) or physical/chemical irritation, which results in obstruction or disruption of individual hair follicles and the associated pilosebaceous units.[1] The primary lesion is a papule or pustule with a central hair. More serious forms of folliculitis involve the deep portion of the hair follicle and may result in a systemic illness with scarring. The most common form of superficial folliculitis is idiopathic.[2] Clinical variants of folliculitis include: *Pseudomonas,* eosinophilic pustular, *Pityrosporum,* gram-negative, tinea barbae, herpetic, and allergic. Differential diagnosis includes keratosis pilaris, which is similar to folliculitis in appearance, but the small papules on the posterolateral aspects of the upper arms and anterior thighs are not associated with hair follicles.[2]

The major predisposing factors are friction, shaving and other skin injuries, perspiration, occlusion, hyperhidrosis, pre-existing dermatitis, and immunocompromised states, especially HIV. The diagnosis is made clinically.[3] Skin biopsy may help if fungus is suspected.

Treatment with topical or oral antibiotics is empiric.[3] Washing with antibacterial soaps prevents or controls mild cases of folliculitis. Erythromycin, clindamycin, mupirocin, or benzoyl peroxide can be used as topical therapy, and a first-generation cephalosporin, penicillinase-resistant penicillin, macrolide, or fluoroquinolone can be used for systemic therapy.[3] If a patient does not improve with a 2- to 4-week course of antibiotics, other variant courses must be investigated. Portions of chronic sufferers are staphylococcal nasal carriers.[4] Nasal culture of family members to look for *S. aureus* colonization may be needed in refractory chronic cases. For recurrent and resistant folliculitis, mupirocin ointment in the nasal vestibule twice a day for 5 days may eliminate the *S. aureus* carrier state.[5] Family members also may need to be treated with mupirocin ointment or rifampin 600 mg per day orally.[5]

❧ REFERENCES ❧

1. Arndt KA, Robinson JK, Wintroub BU, et al: *Dermatology: cutaneous medicine and surgery in primary care,* Philadelphia, 1997, Saunders.
2. Hook EW, et al: Microbiologic evaluation of cutaneous cellulitis in adults, *Arch Intern Med* 146:295, 1986.

3. Stulberg DL, Penrod MA, Blatny RA: Common bacterial skin infections, *Am Fam Physician* 66(1):119-24, Jul 1 2002.
4. Jang KA, Chung ST, Choi JH: Eosinophilic pustular folliculitis (Ofuji's disease) in myelodysplastic syndrome, *J Dermatol* 25(11):742-746, Nov 1998.
5. Piantanida EW, Turiansky GW, Kenner JR: HIV-associated eosinophilic folliculitis: diagnosis by transverse histologic sections, *J Am Acad Dermatol* 38(1):124-126, Jan 1998.

HIRSUTISM
(See also Cushing's syndrome; oral contraceptives; polycystic ovarian syndrome)

Hirsutism affects approximately 8% of adult women. More than 95% of cases of hirsutism are idiopathic, familial, or secondary to polycystic ovarian syndrome.[1] Other causes include late-onset congenital adrenal hyperplasia, Cushing's syndrome, testosterone-secreting tumours, starvation, anorexia nervosa, obesity (sometimes), and drugs, such as progestins in some oral contraceptive pills, danazol, phenytoin, and minoxidil.[1,2]

Source of Androgens
The ovary produces testosterone, androstenedione, and dehydroepiandrosterone (DHEA). The adrenal gland also produces these, as well as the sulfated form of DHEA (DHEA-S). Testosterone is 99% bound to sex hormone-binding globulin, and only the free portion is biologically active. In some obese women, sex hormone-binding globulin is decreased, which allows for more active testosterone to stimulate the receptors.[2]

Investigations
The main purpose of investigating patients with hirsutism is to rule out ominous causes of the condition. In general, investigations are not indicated for patients whose clinical picture is associated with a benign cause of hirsutism. Such patients are usually between the ages of 15 and 25, have had hirsutism for more than a year (not a rapid new onset), and have no evidence of virilization (frontal balding, voice deepening, increased muscle mass, clitoromegaly). Investigations are required for the small group of women who do not have this clinical pattern. In particular, investigations should be carried out if the onset is rapid, if there is hair on the back and shoulders with no family history, if there are signs of virilism, or if Cushing's syndrome is suspected.[1] Idiopathic hirsutism, polycystic ovarian syndrome, and late-onset congenital adrenal hyperplasia all may be associated with mild elevations of testosterone level (usually less than twice the normal value). When indicated, initial investigations should include the following[1,2]:

1. *Total testosterone or free testosterone.* Levels greater than twice the normal value suggest a tumour.[2]
2. *Bioavailable testosterone.* This is used when reduced sex hormone-binding globulin is suspected, such as in obesity or polycystic ovary syndrome (PCOS).
3. *Dehydroepiandrosterone sulfate (DHEA-S).* Levels greater than twice the normal value suggest a tumour.[2]
4. *17α-hydroxyprogesterone.* Blood for this assay should be drawn in the early morning during the first week of the menstrual cycle. The level is usually significantly elevated in patients with the more common and innocuous forms of congenital adrenal hyperplasia.[1]
5. *Dexamethasone suppression test, urine and serum cortisol levels, prolactin* are further tests to consider. If Cushing's syndrome is suspected, appropriate investigations should be conducted. (See discussion of Cushing's disease.) Pelvic ultrasound or adrenal CT should be included if the history suggests a tumour.

Treatment of Benign Forms of Hirsutism
Hirsutism usually requires lifelong treatment. Methods of treating benign forms of hirsutism include weight loss (if obese), electrolysis, birth control pills, and spironolactone (Aldactone). Birth control pills should have a low-androgen progestin, such as desogestrel or norgestimate, which are found in third-generation oral contraceptives. (See discussion of oral contraceptives.) The usual dosage of spironolactone is 50 to 100 mg per day or even 200 mg per day in two divided doses. This drug may cause hyperkalemia. Androgen-suppressing drugs such as flutamide (Euflex) and finasteride (Proscar) have also been used to treat hirsutism. A Cochrane review found spironolactone 100 mg per day is superior to finasteride 5 mg per day and low-dose cyproterone acetate 12.5 mg per day (first 10 days of cycle) up to 12 months after the end of treatment.[2] The patient should be using birth control while on anti-androgen therapy.[3] All treatments will take at least 6 months to become clinically effective. Gonadotropin-releasing hormone analogs such as leuprolide (Lupron) are very expensive and should be reserved for use in women who do not respond to OCs.[1] Eflornithine hydrochloride cream has been indicated for temporarily removing facial hair along with plucking, waxing, and shaving.[4] Ketoconazole cream (Nizoral) has limited evidence of efficacy, many side-effects, and is expensive, but can be used for resistant cases.[1] More permanent treatment includes electrolysis and laser. Electrolysis involves treating hair follicles one at a time, so treatment schedules may go on for weeks or years. A newly developed alternative for dark hairs is laser treatment. The melanin in dark hairs absorbs a spectrum of laser wavelengths, generating heat and selectively destroying the follicles. Fewer sessions are required than with electrolysis. As yet no large, well-designed studies of this procedure have been completed.[3]

♫ REFERENCES ♪
1. Hunter M, Carek P: Evaluation and treatment of women with hirsutism, *Am Fam Physician* 67:2565-2572, 2003.

2. Farquhar C, Lee O, Toomath R, et al: Spironolactone versus placebo or in combination with steroids for hirsutism and/or acne, Cochrane Database Nov 25, 2003.
3. Kalve E, Klein J: Evaluation of women with hirsutism, *Am Fam Physician* 54:117-124, 1996.
4. Hickman JG, Huber F, Palmizsano M: *Curr Med Res Opinion* 16:235-244, 2001.
5. Laser hair removal, *Med Lett* 41:68-69, 1999.

PALMAR HYPERHIDROSIS

Palmar hyperhidrosis (sweaty palms) usually occurs at puberty and often causes personal and professional problems for patients afflicted with the problem. Primary palmar hyperhidrosis is a pathological condition of excessive perspiration caused by overproduction of the eccrine sweat glands, the cause of which is unknown.[1] Following are current treatment options, in order of increasing invasiveness.

1. Topical application of a solution of 20% aluminium chloride hexahidride (Drysol). The usual regimen is to apply the solution to the palms nightly for 3 nights, and wearing polyethylene gloves until morning. Maintenance regimen is to repeat the same program up to twice weekly.[2]
2. Iontophoresis. Hands are placed in a special unit containing tap water while direct current (DC) is administered. Eight sessions can control symptoms in 81.2% of patients with an average remission period of 35 days and minimal adverse effects.[3] Adding anticholinergic substances, such as aluminium chloride salts, to the water produces a more rapid and longer-lasting therapeutic response.[4] Contraindications include pregnancy, cardiac pacemakers, and metallic orthopedic implants. Adverse effects, although uncommon, include pain and burns. Research in using alternating current iontophoresis shows promising results with no reported side effects.[5]
3. Botulinum injection. Botulinum toxin type A (BTX-A), injected intradermally, has been demonstrated as effective and safe in reducing palmar hyperhidrosis for upward of 6 months.[6] One study shows that high-dose (100 U) BTX-A reduces finger pinch strength to a far greater extent than low-dose (50 U), but both doses reduce sweating for at least 2 months in all patients and 6 months in most patients.[7] The injections are uncomfortable, however, and more centres are now performing this procedure under ulnar and median nerve blocks.[8,9]
4. Transthoracic endoscopic sympathectomy. It is the only permanent method of treating palmar hyperhidrosis, but is also the most invasive option. Immediate success rate can be close to 100% for resection and 95.2% for ablation.[10] Ablation is quicker, easier, and results in fewer cases of Horner's syndrome. Other complications include pneumothorax, intercostal neuralgia, chest wall hematoma, and compensatory sweating.[11]

REFERENCES

1. Hashmonai M, Kopelman D, Assalia A: The treatment of primary palmar hyperhidrosis: a review, *Surg Today* 30(3):211-218, 2000.
2. Hurley HF: Questions and answers, *JAMA* 259:3325, 1988.
3. Karakoc Y, Aydemir EH, Kalkan MT, et al: Safe control of palmoplantar hyperhydrosis with direct electric current, *Intern J Dermatol* 41(9):602-605, Sep 2002.
4. Togel B, Greve B, Raulin C: Current therapeutic strategies of hyperhidrosis: a review, *Eur J Dermatol* 12(3):219-223, May-June 2002.
5. Shimizu H, Tamada Y, Shimizu J, et al: Effectiveness of iontophoresis with alternating current in the treatment of patients with palmoplantar hyperhidrosis, *J Dermatol* 30(6):444-449, June 2003.
6. Lowe NJ, Yamauchi PS, Lask GP, et al: Efficacy and safety of botulinum toxin type A in the treatment of palmar hyperhidrosis: a double-blind, randomized, placebo-controlled study, *Dermatol Surg* 28(9):822-827, Sep 2002.
7. Saadia D, Voustianiouk A, Wang AK, et al: Botulinum toxin type A in primary palmar hyperhydrosis: randomized, single-blind, two-dose study, *Neurology* 57(11):2095-2099, Dec 11 2001.
8. Hayton MJ, Stanley JK, Lowe NJ: A review of peripheral nerve blockade as local anaesthesia in the treatment of palmar hyperhidrosis, *Br J Dermatol* 149(3):447-451, Sep 2003.
9. Vadoud-Seyedi J, Heenen M, Simonart T: Treatment of idiopathic palmar hyperhidrosis with botulinum toxin: report of 23 cases and review of the literature, *Dermatology* 203(4):318-321, 2001.
10. Hashmonai M, Assalia A, Kopelman D: Thoracoscopic sympathectomy for palmar hyperhidrosis: ablate or resect? *Surg Endosc* 15(5):435-441, May 2001.
11. Matthews BD, Bui HT, Harold KL, et al: Thoracoscopic sympathectomy for palmaris hyperhidrosis, *South Med J* 96(3):254-258, 2003.

PEDICULOSIS PUBIS AND PEDICULOSIS CAPITIS

Transmission of head lice is usually by direct contact (head to head) and rarely if ever through fomites.[1] Two recent evidence-based reviews found that malathion, permethrin, and pyrethrum insecticides were equally effective in treating head lice infestations.[2,3] A 1% solution of permethrin (Nix Creme Rinse) is the pharmacological treatment of choice for pediculosis pubis and capitis.[4,5] After the area is shampooed, rinsed, and dried, the permethrin solution is applied in sufficient quantities to saturate the area and is left in place for 10 minutes before being rinsed off with water. Although a single treatment is sufficient to kill both the nits and the adult lice, many experts recommend a second treatment 7 to 10 days later as insurance.[1] Unfortunately, in the United States, evidence shows that lice are becoming resistant to permethrin.[5] Although lindane (Kwellada) might be chosen as an alternative to permethrin, one systematic review concluded that there is insufficient evidence of benefit to justify using the drug.[6]

The policy of some schools that children must be free of nits before returning is not based on scientific evidence and should be discouraged. However, if the school insists on this policy, nits can be removed by applying a damp towel to the scalp for 30 to 60 minutes (or by applying a mixture of equal parts water and white vinegar to the scalp, which is then covered with a damp towel soaked in the same material for 15 minutes), followed by combing with a fine-tooth comb.[1]

Pesticides are not always needed to control pediculosis capitis. An alternative is to wash the hair with ordinary shampoo and then add conditioner. Immediately afterward, while the hair is still wet, it is combed thoroughly with a fine-tooth comb. The procedure is repeated every 3 or 4 days for a total of four shampoos and combings over a 2-week period. Wetting the hair slows down the lice, and conditioner makes the hair slippery so they have difficulty gripping the shafts. Thus the initial combing removes all adult and nymphal lice. Subsequent shampooing and combing remove further nymphal lice that have hatched from the nits (incubation period of 7 to 10 days) before they mature, mate, and lay still more eggs.[7]

Ivermectin (an antiparasitic drug) could be effective in cases resistant to standard treatment. Safety trials are ongoing. It is available only as a special release from Health Canada at present.[8]

It is important to wash fomites (bedding, stuffed animals, and recently worn clothing, particularly hats and head bands) in hot water (130°F for 20 minutes) and dry in a hot dryer, and to soak combs and brushes in hot (but not boiling) water, rubbing alcohol, or a phenol solution for at least 1 hour.[9] Recently used clothing, such as shoes that are difficult to wash, can simply be stored for 24 hours, because head lice can only live 15 to 20 hours apart from their host.[10]

◢ REFERENCES ◣

1. Infectious Diseases and Immunization Committee of the Canadian Paediatric Society: Head lice infestations: a persistent itchy "pest," *Paediatr Child Health* 1:237-240, 1996.
2. Dawes M, Hicks NR, Fleminger M, et al: Evidence based case report: treatment for head lice, *BMJ* 318:385-386, 1999.
3. Dodd CS: Interventions for treating head lice, Cochrane Database Syst Rev (3):CD001165, 2001.
4. Drugs for parasitic infections, *Med Lett* 37:99-108, 1995.
5. Pollack RJ, Kiszewski A, Armstrong P, et al: Differential permethrin susceptibility of head lice sampled in the United States and Borneo, *Arch Pediatr Adolesc Med* 153:969-973, 1999.
6. Vander Stichele RH, Dezeure EM, Bogaert MG: Systematic review of clinical efficacy of topical treatments for head lice, *BMJ* 311:604-608, 1995.
7. Ibarra J, Hall DM: Head lice in schoolchildren, *Arch Dis Child* 75:471-473, 1996.
8. Estrada, B: Head Lice: What about Ivermectin? *Infect Med* 15(12):823, 1998.
9. First Consult. (Accessible at http://www.firstconsult.com/home/framework/fs_main.htm)
10. Flinders D, De Schweinitz P: Pediculosis and scabies, *Am Fam Physician* 69:341-348,349-350, 2004.

PSORIASIS
(See also psoriatic arthritis)

The common form of psoriasis is plaque psoriasis. Other variants are guttate, pustular, and arthritic psoriasis. Unless otherwise specified, this section deals with plaque psoriasis. Psoriasis affects between 1% and 3% of all individuals. The two peak ages of onset are the late teens to early twenties and the late fifties to early sixties. The natural history is one of exacerbations and remissions. Factors known to exacerbate psoriasis are trauma to the skin (physical, sunburn, or infection), psychological stress, and use of certain drugs. Drug classes to avoid prescribing for patients with psoriasis include beta blockers, ACE inhibitors, indomethacin, lithium, and antimalarials.[1] Eight percent of patients with psoriasis will develop psoriatic arthropathy.

A variety of treatment options is available for control of psoriasis. Avoidance of precipitating factors is integral to management. If lesions are sparse and do not bother the patient, no treatment is needed. If less than 20% of the body is involved, topical agents are often effective, but if more than 20% is involved, systemic therapy may be required.[1]

Frequently used topical agents are corticosteroids; the vitamin D analogue calcipotriene, which is also called *calcipotriol* (Dovonex); and the retinoid tazarotene (Tazorac). In general, medium-strength corticosteroids are used on the torso and extremities and low-potency drugs on the face, genitals, and flexural areas. High-potency corticosteroids should be used for only short periods on lesions of palms or soles or on individual plaques that do not respond to usual treatment. With continued use the efficacy of corticosteroids diminishes (tachyphylaxis), and sometimes a flare occurs when the drug is discontinued. Tachyphylaxis can be minimized by switching to less potent formulations as soon as possible or by using the corticosteroids intermittently. Lotions or gels should be used for scalp lesions. Calcipotriene is as effective as midpotency corticosteroids, and tachyphylaxis does not occur. It should not be applied to the face or groin. Tazarotene gives excellent results, often with an extended response, and it can be safely used on the face. It may be teratogenic; women of child-bearing age must receive strict precautions to prevent pregnancy. Other topical agents that may be used are coal tar preparations and anthralin; however, both may stain the skin and clothes.[2] Combination therapy can be more effective, such as tazarotene and corticosteroids or calcipotriene and topical corticosteroids.

Systemic therapies and phototherapies are usually administered by or in conjunction with a dermatologist. These therapies include UVB phototherapy combined with topical tars or anthralin, UVA phototherapy combined with the photosensitizing drug methoxsalen, methotrexate, and in some cases cyclosporine.[1] New biological agents that show promise include etanercept, infliximab, alefacept, and efalizumab.[3]

— ❧ **REFERENCES** ❧ —

1. Greaves MW, Weinstein GD: Treatment of psoriasis, *N Engl J Med* 332:581-588, 1995.
2. Federman DG, Froelich CW, Kirsner RS: Topical psoriasis therapy, *Am Fam Physician* 59:957-962, 1999.
3. Weinberg JM: An overview of infliximab, etanercept, efalizumab, and alefacept as biologic therapy for psoriasis, *Clin Ther* 25(10):2487-2505, 2003.

ROSACEA

Acne rosacea is a chronic, progressive inflammatory skin disorder with periods of exacerbation and remission. It occurs in 5% of the population and has a genetic predisposition. It occurs more commonly in women and individuals of Northern and Eastern European descent.[1]

Acne rosacea has four classic phases[1]:

1. Facial flushing
2. Persistent erythema with telangiectasias
3. Inflammatory lesions (papules, pustules, nodules, edema)
4. Rhinophyma (sebaceous gland hypertrophy of the nose)

Ocular involvement such as conjunctivitis, blepharitis, and dry eyes are common. Extrafacial rosacea can occur but is rare.

Rosacea may present similarly to adult acne. However, rosacea differs from acne by the absence of comedones.

Treatment of acne rosacea begins with avoidance of aggravating factors, including exposure to sunlight (encourage sunscreen use), exposure to heat or cold, ingestion of alcohol and hot spicy foods, and emotional stress.

Topical and oral steroids can severely worsen rosacea and must be avoided.

Standard drug therapy is oral antibiotics, which are particularly effective in the papular and pustular phase of rosacea. First-line therapy is tetracycline or tetracycline derivatives such as minocycline (Minocin) and doxycycline (Vibramycin). A suggested initial dosage of tetracycline is 500 mg orally twice a day for 2 to 3 weeks followed by 500 mg orally once a day for another 2 to 3 weeks.

If a good response is not obtained, second-line drugs such as trimethoprim-sulfamethoxazole (Septra, Bactrim) or oral metronidazole (Flagyl) may be used.[2] Adding topical metronidazole to the oral antibiotic regimen is often advisable.[3]

Topical 0.75% or 1% metronidazole cream or gel applied twice a day may be used alone for the treatment of mild or even moderate rosacea. In more severe cases, remission induced by antibiotics and topical metronidazole may be maintained by topical metronidazole alone. With this regimen, both inflammatory lesions and erythema are lessened.[3]

Rosacea unresponsive to oral and topical antibiotic therapy may be effectively treated with oral isotretinoin (Accutane) 0.5 to 1 mg/kg per day for 4 to 5 months.[1,2] Patients must be counselled on teratogenic effects of isotretinoin and the need for reliable contraception in females of child-bearing age. Potential liver side effects must be monitored throughout treatment.

Telangiectasis can be reduced with cosmetics or pulsed-dye laser for more severe cases. Mild or early rhinophyma can be improved with antibiotic treatment. Treatment of severe or late-stage rhinophyma requires surgical intervention, such as dermabrasion, cryosurgery, electrosurgery, or laser.[1,2]

— ❧ **REFERENCES** ❧ —

1. Blount BW: Rosacea: a common, yet commonly overlooked, condition, *Am Fam Physician* 66(3):435-40, 2002.
2. Thiboutot DM: Acne and rosacea: new and emerging therapies, *Dermatol Clin* 18:63-71, 2000.
3. Dahl MV, Katz I, Krueger GG, et al: Topical metronidazole maintains remission of rosacea, *Arch Dermatol* 134:679-683, 1998.

SCABIES

The mite *Sarcoptes scabiei* is an obligate human ectoparasite that causes an intensely pruritic skin eruption. Scabies was one of the first health problems described in humans, and remains one of the most common, with an estimated annual 300 million cases worldwide.[1]

In addition to pruritus, which is usually worse at night, scabies is characterized by specific lesions—the mite's epidermal burrow—and non-specific lesions such as papules, vesicles, and excoriations typically found on the finger webs, wrists, axillary folds, abdomen, buttocks, and genitalia.[2] A hyperkeratotic form of the disease, Norwegian or crusted scabies, occurs in debilitated or immunocompromised individuals.[3] The diagnosis is usually made clinically, but can be confirmed through visualization of mites, eggs, or fecal pellets on light microscopy of skin scrapings from burrows or from under the fingernails of affected individuals.[4]

The infestation is spread through direct contact with affected individuals, either skin-to-skin or through contact with mites or eggs transmitted via clothing or bed linen. The mites can survive 3 to 4 days of separation from a human host, and have been found in the dust fomites generated by affected individuals.[5] Extremes of age and crowded living conditions increase individual susceptibility to scabies.

First-line treatment for scabies is 5% permethrin cream, applied as a single treatment to the whole body, paying particular attention to skin folds, fingernails, toenails, groin, and behind the ears, and is washed off after 8 to 12 hours.[4] Some authorities recommend a repeat treatment 1 week after the first.[5] It is important to remind patients that only the 5% cream formulation of permethrin, not the 1% cream rinse used to treat head lice, is effective against scabies.[4] A second-line treatment is lindane cream or lotion, applied the same way as permethrin, washed off after 12 hours, and reapplied in 24 hours.[4] Significant adverse effects, including neurotoxicity and aplastic anemia, have been reported with lindane in particular.[1]

Neither permethrin nor lindane is recommended for use in infants or pregnant or lactating women. Precipitated sulphur (7%) in petroleum jelly (prepared by a pharmacist) is a safe and effective treatment for these groups. It is applied for 3 consecutive days, left on for 24 hours, and washed off before the next application.[4]

Ivermectin, a veterinary antiparasitic, has been used safely and successfully in human scabies treatment, given as a single oral dose of 200 μg/kg.[2] It is not available for human use in Canada, and not licensed for scabies treatment in the United States. It has been particularly useful in controlling institutional outbreaks, and for the treatment of crusted scabies.[3]

A number of other measures are required to control the spread of scabies and to prevent individual reinfection[4]:

- All household members should be treated at the same time as the index case.
- All bed linen and clothing should be laundered and dried using hot wash and dry cycles.
- If hot water is not available, linen and clothing should be sealed in plastic bags for 5 to 7 days.
- Health care workers in contact with scabies may require prophylactic treatment.
- Children may return to school or daycare the day after treatment is completed.

Itching may last up to 2 weeks after eradication of the scabies mite. During this time oral antihistamines may be used to control pruritus. Occasionally, skin infections requiring antibiotic treatment will occur in excoriated areas. Worsening of itch after scabies treatment may be due to a reaction to the topical preparation. Persistence of symptoms beyond 2 weeks' post treatment generally indicates treatment failure. Retreatment and strict attention to other control measures, especially prophylactic treatment of all household contacts, is necessary.[4]

❧ REFERENCES ❧

1. Walker GJA, Johnstone PW: Interventions for treating scabies, The Cochrane Database of Systematic Reviews, May 2000.
2. Chouela E, Abedano A, et al: Diagnosis and treatment of scabies: a practical guide, *Am J Clin Derm* 3(1):9-18, 2002.
3. Scheinfeld N: Controlling scabies in institutional settings: a review of medications, treatment models, and implementation, *Am J Clin Derm* 5(1): 31-37, 2004.
4. Indian and Inuit Health Committee, Canadian Pediatric Society: Scabies management, *Pediatr Child Health* 6(110): 775-777, 2001.
5. Wendel K, Rompalo A: Scabies and pediculosis pubis: an update of treatment regimens and general review, *Clin Infect Dis* 35: S146-S151, 2002.

SCALP TREATMENTS
Scalp Lotions, Steroid

Some of the available steroid-containing scalp lotions are betamethasone valerate 0.1% (Valisone, Betnovate), betamethasone dipropionate 0.05% plus salicylic acid (Diprosalic), and clobetasol-17-propionate 0.05% (Temovate, Dermovate).

Scalp Shampoos, Medicated

To apply medicated scalp shampoos, shake the bottle thoroughly, rub the shampoo well into the scalp, leave it on for 4 minutes, and then rinse it out. Some of the medicated scalp shampoos available include salicylic acid shampoo (Ionil, Sebcur), salicylic acid/tar shampoo (Ionil T, Sebcur/T), salicylic acid/sulfur shampoo (Sebulex), and salicylic acid, sulfur, and tar shampoo (Sebutone).

SEBORRHEIC DERMATITIS

This chronic inflammatory skin disorder is generally confined to areas of the head and trunk where sebaceous glands are most prominent. *Malassezia yeasts* have been implicated in the development of this condition. It has been suggested that seborrheic dermatitis is an inflammatory response to this organism, but this remains to be proven. Nonetheless, the fact that seborrheic dermatitis often responds to antifungal medications is strongly suggestive of the role of yeast in this disorder. Although seborrheic dermatitis affects only 3% of the general population, the incidence in persons with AIDS may be as high as 85%. Persons with central nervous system disorders, such as Parkinson's disease, cranial nerve palsies, and major truncal paralyses also appear to be prone to the development of seborrheic dermatitis. It has been postulated that seborrheic dermatitis in these patients is a result of increased pooling of sebum caused by immobility. This increased sebum pool permits growth of *Pityrosporum ovale*, which induces seborrheic dermatitis.[1]

The distribution of seborrheic dermatitis is classically symmetrical, and common sites of involvement are the hairy areas of the head, including the scalp, the scalp margin, eyebrows, eyelashes, mustache, and beard. Seborrhea of the trunk may appear in the presternal area and in the body folds, including the axillae, navel, groin, and in the inframammary and anogenital areas.

One of the characteristics of seborrheic dermatitis is dandruff, characterized by a fine, powdery white scale on the scalp. Many patients complain of the scalp itching with dandruff, and because they think that the scale arises from dry skin, they decrease the frequency of shampooing, which allows further scale accumulation. Inflammation then occurs and the symptoms worsen. More severe seborrheic dermatitis is characterized by erythematous plaques frequently associated with powdery or greasy scale in the scalp. If left untreated, the scale may become thick, yellow, and greasy and, occasionally, secondary bacterial infection may occur.

Seborrheic dermatitis is more common in men than in women, probably because sebaceous gland activity is under androgen control. Seborrhea usually first appears in persons in their teens and twenties and generally follows a waxing/waning course throughout adulthood.

Treatment

The primary goals of treatment include controlling itching and scaling, controlling severity and occurrence of future attacks, and educating patients in self-management skills.

Hygiene issues play a key role in controlling seborrheic dermatitis. Frequent cleansing with soap removes oils from affected areas and improves seborrhea. Outdoor recreation, especially during summer, will also improve seborrhea, although caution should be taken to avoid sun damage.

Pharmacological treatment options for seborrhoeic dermatitis include antifungal preparations such as selenium sulfide, pyrithione zinc, azole agents, sodium sulfacetamide, and topical terbinafine, which decrease colonization by lipophilic yeast. These are often started on a daily or every-other-day regimen, either as shampoos or creams for the face and trunk. The regimens are then decreased to twice a week once the initial inflammation is under control. A topical steroid can help with irritation and erythema, but patients should be advised to use potent topical steroids sparingly because excessive use may lead to atrophy of the skin and telangiectasis. For severe disease, keratolytics such as salicylic acid or coal tar preparations may be used to remove dense scale; then topical steroids may be applied. Other options for removing adherent scale involve applying any of a variety of oils (peanut, olive, or mineral) to soften the scale overnight, followed by use of a detergent or coal tar shampoo.[1,2]

An occasional patient with severe seborrhea that is unresponsive to the usual topical therapy may be a candidate for isotretinoin therapy. Isotretinoin can induce up to a 90% reduction in sebaceous gland size, with a corresponding reduction in the production of sebum. Treatment with daily doses of isotretinoin as low as 0.1 to 0.3 mg/kg may result in improvement in severe seborrhea after 4 weeks of therapy. Thereafter, a dose as low as 5 to 10 mg per day may be effective as maintenance therapy over several years. However, isotretinoin has potentially serious side effects, and few patients with seborrhea are appropriate candidates for therapy. This agent must be used cautiously and is only prescribed by physicians who are well versed in all of its adverse effects. Topical tacrolimus may show some benefit for resolution.[3]

A more practical approach to the refractory patient may be to first try different combinations of the usual agents, including a dandruff shampoo, an antifungal agent, and a topical steroid. If these fail, short-term use of a more potent topical steroid in a "pulse fashion" may put some refractory patients into remission and actually decrease the total steroid exposure. Recently, a small trial suggested that topical metronidazole may also be effective.[4] Head-to-head comparisons with topical ketoconazole and low-potency steroids are lacking. Infants frequently have seborrheic dermatitis, commonly known as "cradle cap." Involvement may be extensive, and is very concerning for parents, but this disorder frequently clears spontaneously by 6 to 12 months of age and does not recur until the onset of puberty.

❧ REFERENCES ❧

1. Gupta AK: Sebborheic dermatitis *Dermatol Clin* 21(3): 401-412, Jul 1 2003.
2. Johnson B, Nunley J: Treatment of sebborheic dermatitis, *Am Fam Physician* 61:2703-2710, 2713-2714, 2000.
3. Meshkinpour A: An open pilot study using tacrolimus ointment in the treatment of seborrheic dermatitis, *J Am Acad Dermatol* 49(1):145-147, Jul 1 2003.
4. Parsad D, Pandhi R, Negi KS, et al: Topical metronidazole in seborrheic dermatitis: a double-blind study, *Dermatology* 202:35-37, 2001.

SKIN CANCER

Skin cancer is the most common form of cancer. The three major forms of skin cancer are basal cell carcinoma (76% to 80%), squamous cell carcinoma (16% to 19%), and malignant melanoma (5%).[1] Ninety percent of all skin cancers result from exposure to ultraviolet radiation from the sun, causing DNA damage to tumour suppressor genes.[2,3] The incidence of all three cancers is increasing, likely due to increased recreational sun exposure and diminishing ozone layer. Studies so far have not been able to establish how much and what type of sun exposure (i.e., high intensity/short exposure vs. prolonged consistent exposure) leads to cancer. One severe sunburn before the age of 20 doubles the lifetime skin cancer risk and may be the most preventable risk factor.[1]

Little evidence recommends preventative manoeuvres. The U.S. Preventive Services Task Force in their 2002 update state that there is insufficient evidence to recommend total body screening by physicians for skin cancer detection.[4] A 2003 trial using a theoretical model and existing sources of data estimated that the lifetime risk that a mole will become melanoma in a 50-year-old man is 1 in 2000, and in a 50-year-old woman is 1 in 9000. These findings call into question the cost-effectiveness of surveillance programs and frequent excisions, especially for young or low-risk patients.[5] Daily application of sunscreen in adults seems to be preventive for squamous cell but not for basal cell and melanoma.[6-8] Using sunscreen can lead to a false sense of security. Experts generally recommend avoiding sun exposure between 10 a.m. and 4 p.m.; wearing sun-protective clothing; using sunscreen with a sun-protection factor (SPF) of 15 or higher; and avoiding artificial sources of ultraviolet light.[9,10]

Basal Cell Carcinoma

Basal cell carcinoma (BCC) is the most common malignancy in whites, with a lifetime risk of 30%.[3] It is rarely seen in dark-skinned people. Risk factors include family history (Odds Ratio [OR] 2.2), freckling, severe sunburn, or cumulative sun exposure as a child, fair colouring (OR 1.6), increasing age (Relative Risk [RR] 4-8), male sex (RR 2), geographical location (increasing closer to equator), tanning beds, and immunosuppression (OR 10).[3,11,12] BCC is in itself a risk factor for further BCC, other skin cancers, and possibly other malignancies, such as cancers of the lung, thyroid, mouth, breast, and cervix, and non-Hodgkin's lymphoma.[3]

The characteristic look of BCC is a raised, pearly lesion with rolled borders, telangiectasia, and central indentation (rodent ulcer). Superficial BCC can look like eczema, psoriasis, or Bowens' disease. It can crust, bleed, ulcerate, or present as a sore that does not heal. BCC is most commonly found on the nose, cheek, forehead, and ears but can appear in any sun-exposed area. It rarely metastasizes but can be locally destructive, especially on the face. Treatment options vary depending on size, location, recurrence, and patient factors. A recent Cochrane review was unable to clearly determine the most efficacious treatment approach.[13]

Surgical techniques include curettage and electrodesiccation (scrape tumour and cauterize several times), cryosurgery, excision, and Mohs' micrographic surgery (excision of tumour with serial thin section examinations to determine margins). The latter two allow for a pathological diagnosis, with the Mohs' surgery being superior for recurrent, more aggressive lesions or to preserve appearance. Radiotherapy has been used for large lesions in the frail patient but is inferior to excision.[13] Non-surgical options for superficial BCC include topical 5-fluorouracil cream (Efudex) applied with a spatula or glove twice a day until ulcerating (usually 2 to 4 weeks) (see section on AK), imiquimod 5% cream (Aldara) applied daily for 6 weeks (success rate 87%),[13] or photodynamic therapy (apply photosensitizing solution, then light).[3] In a small study 5-fluorouracil in phosphatidylcholine had a cure rate of 9/10 patients as compared with 4/7 in the commercially available preparation.[14] Regular follow-up and full skin exam are required because the risk of developing additional BCC is greatest in the first year after excision.

Malignant Melanoma

Malignant melanoma (MM) is the least common skin cancer but the most deadly. Risk factors are the same as for the other skin cancers as well as presence of atypical nevi or greater than 50 moles. Early detection increases survival. One out of four MMs arise from a pre-existing mole, so any change in appearance or manifestation of symptoms needs to be investigated.[1,15]

The acronym **ABCDE** helps to detect MM. If a lesion meets one of the following criteria it should be biopsied.

A	is for asymmetry (one half of the lesion is not identical to the other).
B	is for border (outline not smooth).
C	is for colour. MM usually has more than one colour (black, blue, red, brown, white), and pigment can extend beyond the border as opposed to moles that may also be multicoloured, but usually have the same colour combination throughout the body.
D	is for diameter (greater than 6 mm).
E	is for elevation.[11]

One aggressive type of MM, acral lentiginous, occurs under nails or on palms or soles, and is more common in African Americans.[1] MMs are treated with a wide excision down to muscle. Higher-grade tumours and metastases need further treatment with interferon and/or chemotherapy.

Squamous Cell Carcinoma

Squamous cell carcinoma (SCC) is the second most common skin cancer and has the same risk factors as BCC. SCC can develop from actinic keratoses, areas of previous skin injury (burn, radiation treatments), ulcer, or chronic skin disease such as from scars, lichen planus, or epidermolysis bullosa. Human papillomavirus (HPV) has been linked to superficial SCC as well as a number of chemical exposures (arsenic, tar, tobacco).[2,11] Lesions are nodules/plaques on a red base that may ulcerate in the centre. The lesions are firm, raised, opaque, and pink or flesh-coloured. They can be symptomatic (itchy, painful) or resemble warts, eczema patches, or a non-healing sore. The usual sites of occurrence are sun-exposed areas such as the face, neck, exposed scalp, ears, and lips. Most patients with SCC have an excellent prognosis (90% to 95%), yet those that metastasize do poorly; less than 20% have a 10-year survival rate.[2] Metastatic potential (range 5% to 45%) depends on location, size, histology, rate of growth, health status, and previous skin condition. Treatment and follow-up are the same as for BCC.

◣ REFERENCES ◢

1. Schober-Flores C: The sun's damaging effects, *Dermatol Nurs* 13(4):279-286, Aug 2001.
2. Alam M, Ratner D: Primary care: cutaneous squamous-cell carcinoma, *N Engl J Med* 344(13):975-983 Mar 29 2001.
3. Wong CS, Strange RC, Lear JT: Basal cell carcinoma, *BMJ* 327(7418):794-798, Oct 4 2003.
4. Screening for skin cancer: recommendations and rationale, *Am Fam Physician* 65(8):1623-1626, Apr 15 2002.
5. Tsao H, Bevona C, Goggins W, et al: The transformation rate of moles (melanocytic nevi) into cutaneous melanoma, *Arch Dermatol* 139:282-288, 2003.
6. Vainio H, Miller AB, Bianchini F: An international evaluation of the cancer-preventive potential of sunscreens, *Intern J Cancer* 88(5):838-842, Dec 1 2000.
7. Green A, Williams G, Neale R, et al: Daily sunscreen application and betacarotene supplementation in prevention of basal-cell and squamous-cell carcinomas of the skin: a randomised controlled trial, *Lancet* 354(9180):723-729, Aug 28 1999.
8. Huncharek M, Kupelnick B: Use of topical sunscreens and the risk of malignant melanoma: a meta-analysis of 9067 patients from 11 case-control studies, *Am J Public Health* 92(7):1173-1177, Jul 2002.
9. Centers for Disease Control and Prevention, Morbidity and Mortality Weekly Report Recommendations and Reports, vol 52, No. RR-15, October 17, 2003.
10. Skin Cancer Foundation: Sun safety. (Accessed on May 2, 2004 at http://www.skincancer.org/prevention/index.php)
11. Strayer SM, Reynolds PL: Diagnosing skin malignancy: assessment of predictive clinical criteria and risk factors, *J Fam Pract* 52(3):210-218, Mar 2003.
12. Karagas MR, Stannard VA, Mott LA, et al: Use of tanning devices and risk of basal cell and squamous cell skin cancers, *J National Cancer Inst* 94(3):224-226, Feb 6 2002.
13. Bath FJ, Bong J, Perkins W, et al: Interventions for basal cell carcinoma of the skin, *Cochrane Database Syst Rev* (2):CD003412, 2003.
14. Romagosa R, Saap L, Givens M, et al: A pilot study to evaluate the treatment of basal cell carcinoma with 5-fluorouracil using phosphatidyl choline as a transepidermal carrier, *Dermatol Surg* 26(4):338-340, Apr 2000.
15. Goldstein B, Goldstein A: Diagnosis and management of malignant melanoma, *Am Fam Physician* 63:1359-1368, 1374, 2001.

SWIMMER'S ITCH
(See also travel medicine)

Swimmer's itch is caused by the accidental penetration into the skin of the cercarial form of an animal schistosome. (The usual natural cycle of the schistosome is duck–snail–duck.) Since humans are not the definitive host, the cercariae die after penetrating the skin and cause a delayed hypersensitivity reaction. The person often has a brief period of skin stinging when first exposed to the cercariae and perhaps a transient macular or urticarial rash. This is followed by a latent period of 1 to 14 days before the development of the maculopapular-vesicular rash, which is usually seen over body areas not protected by clothing. Resolution begins in a few days and is complete within 2 weeks. Treatment is symptomatic and includes antihistamines, topical antipruritics, and in severe cases corticosteroids.[1,2]

The cercariae are most abundant in warm, shallow, fresh water where children tend to swim and this may account for the more frequent and severe cases in children.[3]

◣ REFERENCES ◢

1. Mulvihill CA, Burnett JW: Swimmer's itch: a cercarial dermatitis, *Cutis* 46:211-213, 1990.
2. Chapman A, Ekelund C, Tominaga J: Rash and pruritus after a camping trip, *Pediatr Infect Dis J* 12:966, 968-969, 1993.
3. Blankespoor HD, Reimink RL: Swimmer's Itch. The Authorized Home Page. (Accessed April 13, 2004 at http://hope.edu/swimmersitch/)

TINEA
Tinea Pedis

Tinea pedis is a common dermatophytic infection of the feet that presents with itching, scaling, and erythema. More severe infections, such as *trichophyton rubrum,* may present in a moccasin distribution or with a secondary bacterial infection (dermatophytosis complex).[1]

Simple tinea pedis is effectively treated with topical fungicidal terbinafine for 1 to 2 weeks with a 70% cure rate. Topical fungistatic medications such as clotriazole or miconazole require 2 to 4 weeks of therapy and while less expensive, they are also less effective (64% cure rate).[1-3] Oral therapy for tinea pedis is only indicated for resistant or severe infections because oral therapy is more expensive and has greater potential for systemic side effects and drug interactions. Terbinafine (250 mg per day) for 2 to 6 weeks, itraconazole (100 mg per day) for 4 weeks, or fluconazole (150 mg per week) for 2 to 6 weeks can be used.[4] All of these medications have proved superior to placebo. A 2001 Cochrane review showed no difference between these medications.[5]

Tinea Versicolour

Tinea versicolour is an infection of the skin by *Malassezia furfur* that results in a macular rash with altered pigmentation, scaling, and possibly mild pruritus.[6] Ketoconazole 2% (Nizoral) shampoo applied to the dampened skin of all affected areas with lathering to both affected and surrounding areas, and left in place for 5 minutes, showed clinical response rates at 1 month of 73%, 69%, and 5% for the 3-day ketoconazole, 1-day ketoconazole, and placebo groups, respectively.[7] Alternatively, topical 2.5% selenium sulfide solution (Selsun) for 10 minutes two times a day for 2 weeks is effective.[8] Oral treatment with fluconazole (single dose of 400 mg) may be effective for severe or recurrent cases.[9] For prophylaxis, itraconazole 200 mg given twice a day for 1 day a month improves mycological outcomes.[10]

Onychomycosis

Onychomycosis is a fungal infection of the nail bed, matrix, or plate. There are a variety of fungal causes (such as non-dermatophyte infections[4]), so it is important to obtain culture results or positive potassium hydroxide smears before initiating oral treatment. The best specimens are obtained from the more proximal portions of the nail.[11] At present, oral agents should be used to treat onychomycosis.[11,12] Part of the reason for the efficacy of the newer oral agents such as terbinafine (Lamisil), itraconazole (Sporanox), and fluconazole (Diflucan) in curing onychomycosis is that these agents bind to nail keratin and persist in the nails for several weeks after oral therapy is discontinued.[11] A 1999 double blind randomized trial of treatment for onychomycosis compared continuous terbinafine (250 mg per day for 16 weeks) with intermittent itraconazole (400 mg per day for 1 week in every 4 weeks for a total of 16 weeks). Fingernails require less treatment, typically 2 to 3 months. After 72 weeks the mycological cure rate was 81% for terbinafine and 49% for itraconazole.[13] These patients were then revisited up to 5 years later, and the advantage continued for oral terbinafine.[14] Several authors suggest that continuous oral terbinafine therapy is the current treatment of choice for onychomycosis.[12,15] It is important to tell patients that the nail will not appear cured at the end of treatment; it can take 4 to 6 months for fingers and even longer for toes to grow a new nail.[4] For patients who cannot tolerate oral medication or as an adjuvant to oral therapy, topical ciclopirox 8% nail lacquer (Penlac) can be used with a cure rate of around 35% to 52% when used alone.[16] The clinical recurrence rate at 2 years (based on one study of 88 patients) was 17% among patients who had disease-free nails at 1 year. Not treating can certainly be an option for some patients.[17] The use of itraconazole has been associated with fetal loss.[18]

Tinea Capitis

Tinea capitis is a fungal infection of the scalp resulting from contact with infected persons or animals. Ninety percent of cases are caused by *Trichophyton tonsurans*, while 10% are caused by *Microsporum species*. Tinea capitis is almost exclusively an infection of prepubertal children.[19] Adenopathy, alopecia, scaling, and characteristic black dots resulting from broken hairs are almost pathognomonic of tinea capitis. Treatment requires oral antifungal therapy with griseofulvin as first choice with ketoconazole, terbinafine, and itraconazole as alternatives.[19,20]

❧ REFERENCES ❧

1. Gupta AK, Chow M, Daniel CR, et al: Treatment of tinea pedis, *Dermatol Clin* 21(3):431-462, Jul 2003.
2. Crawford F, Hart R, Bel-Syer SE, et al: Cochrane Review. In: *The Cochrane Library,* issue 3, Oxford, England, 2001, Update Software.
3. Hart R, Sally E, Bell-Syer SE, et al: Systematic review of topical treatments for fungal infections of the skin and nails of the feet, *BMJ* 319:79-82, 1999.
4. Noble SI, Forbes RC, Stamm PL: Diagnosis and management of common tinea infections, *Am Fam Physician* 58:163-174, 1998.
5. Bell-Syer SE, Hart R, Crawford F, et al: Oral treatments for fungal infections of the skin of the foot, Cochrane Database Syst Rev (2):CD003584, 2002.
6. Gupta AK, Batra R, Faergemann J: Pityriasis versicolor, *Dermatol Clin* 21:413-429, 2002.
7. Lange DS, Richards HM, Guarnieri J, et al: Ketoconazole 2% shampoo in the treatment of tinea versicolor: a multicenter, randomized, double-blind, placebo-controlled trial, *J Am Acad Dermatol* 39:944-950, 1998.
8. First consult. (Accessed April 26, 2004 at http://www.first consult.com)
9. Faergemann J: Treatment of pityriasis versicolor with a single dose of fluconazole, *Acta Derm Venereol* 72:74-75, 1992.
10. Faergemann J, Gupta AK, Mofadi AA, et al: Efficacy of itraconazole in the prophylactic treatment of pityriasis (tinea) versicolor, *Arch Dermatol* 138:69-73, 2002.
11. Gupta AK, Shear NH: Onychomycosis: going for cure, *Can Fam Physician* 43:299-305, 1997.
12. Finlay AY: Skin and nail fungi—almost beaten (editorial), *BMJ* 319:71-71, 1999.
13. Evans EG, Sigurgeirsson B (Lion Study Group): Double blind, randomized study of continuous terbinafine compared with intermittent itraconazole in treatment of toenail onychomycosis, *BMJ* 318:1031-1035, 1999.
14. Sigurgeirsson B, Olafsson JH, Steinsson J, et al: Long-term effectiveness of treatment with terbinafine vs itraconazole in onychomycosis, *Arch Dermatol* 138:353-357, 2002.
15. Crawford F, Young P, Godfrey C, et al: Oral treatments for toenail onychomycosis: a systematic review, *Arch Dermatol* 138(6), 811-816, 2002.
16. Gupta AK, Joseph WS: Ciclopirox 8% nail lacquer in the treatment of onychomycosis of the toenails in the United States, *J Am Podiat Assoc* 90(10):495-501, Nov-Dec 2000.
17. Epstein E: How often does oral treatment of toenail onychomycosis produce a disease-free nail? *Arch Dermatol* 134:1551-1554, 1998.

18. Bar-Oz B, Moretti ME, Bishai R, et al: Pregnancy outcome after in utero exposure to itraconazole: a prospective cohort study, *Am J Obstet Gynecol* 183:617-620, 2000.
19. Temple ME, Nahata MC, Koranyi KI: Pharmacotherapy of tinea capitis, *J Am Board Fam Pract* 12:236-242, 1999.
20. Bergus GR: Tinea capitis. (Accessed April 27, 2004 at http://www.5mcc.com/Assets/SUMMARY/TP0921.html)

ULCERS, DERMAL
(See also venous ulcers)

Management of pressure ulcers involves topical wound care but also a complex interaction of other factors. The Braden scale for predicting risk of ulcer reflects the breadth of the six clinical categories that need to be considered: sensory perception, moisture, activity, mobility, nutrition, and friction and shear.[1] Because excessive pressure for a period of time is causative, a major preventive opportunity consists of removing or redistributing pressure. This can range from repositioning (every 2 hours for bedridden patients and every hour for sitting patients and relieving pressure on bony prominences) and foam, to more expensive interventions such as air-fluidized mattresses. Heels are extremely difficult areas in which to prevent skin breakdown and, if possible, must be floated off the bed at all times. The patient who is incontinent of urine and stool, especially stool, is at greater risk for developing pressure ulcers. Constant exposure of urine to the skin leads to maceration, weakening of the tissue, and breakdown. The enzymes in stool, especially in liquid stool, promote a chemical breakdown of the skin and quickly lead to skin ulceration. If diapers are used to contain urinary or fecal incontinence, the caregiver must apply a moisture barrier to the skin with each diaper change and notify the health care provider at the first sign of skin breakdown. If cost is an issue, petroleum jelly is an inexpensive, effective moisture barrier. Immobility results in many complications for the elderly. If the patient is bedridden, he or she must be repositioned on a regular schedule.[1,2]

Staging of skin ulcers is as follows[3]:

Stage 1: Non-blanchable erythema of the intact skin

Stage 2: Partial thickness loss involving the epidermis or dermis or both; presents clinically as an abrasion, blister, or shallow crater

Stage 3: Full-thickness loss extending into the subcutaneous tissue, but not through the underlying fascia

Stage 4: Full-thickness loss extending to muscle, bone tendons, joint capsule, and supporting structures

Debridement and Cleansing

Removal of devitalized tissue is necessary to allow granulation tissue formation and subsequent re-epithelialization. It is typically done in the family medicine setting in a few ways: with scissors or scalpels, via synthetic dressings (typically hydrocolloids or gels in cases in which the bad tissue is self-digested), by mechanical debridement (wet-to-dry dressing, water irrigation) and, finally, by special enzyme-impregnated dressings.

Irrigation with normal saline may be used to clean most ulcers. Careful use of gauzes and sponges can help reduce the trauma and help adherence of dressing. In general, antiseptic agents can be toxic to wound tissue and should not be used.

Occlusive Dressings

The modern treatment of skin ulcers often involves the use of occlusive dressings, and a confusingly large number of these are on the market. Occlusive dressings not only protect the area, but also maintain a moist wound surface that facilitates autolytic debridement and the formation of granulation tissue and increases the rate of re-epithelialization. Pain is relieved, and the degree of scarring diminished. Although bacterial colonization takes place in this milieu, the rate of clinical infections is actually less than in wounds treated with gauze or other conventional dressings. However, occlusive dressings should not be used if the lesion is clearly infected.[3,4]

Occlusive dressings can be applied only if the surrounding skin is intact and healthy. The dressings should be large enough to give a 2.5-cm or 1-inch margin around the borders. Dressings should be changed when they leak or look as if they are going to leak, or at least once a week. Patients wearing occlusive dressings can bathe or shower with them on. The dressings come in various sizes and shapes, so the physician can keep a list handy to prescribe the specific size required or can tell the pharmacist the size and shape of the ulcer and let him or her dispense the appropriate product.

In general, studies of different types of moist wound dressings have shown no differences. The following are some occlusive dressings and wound fillers that family physicians may use reasonably frequently[3,4]:

- **Transparent polymer films (e.g., Tegaderm Transparent Dressing, Duoderm Extra Thin Dressings and Border Dressings, Opsite Wound Dressing).** In general these are used to cover first- and second-degree ulcers. These dressings are impermeable to water and non-absorbent, so serous fluid may accumulate. This is not in itself harmful, but if enough accumulates, it may break the seal and leak out.
- **Hydrocolloid dressings (e.g., Tegasorb Ulcer Dressing, Duoderm CGF [Controlled Gel Formulation] Dressings, IntraSite Wound Dressing).** These are used for third- and fourth-degree ulcers. They are self-adhering and contain gelling agents. Before application, the wound should be cleaned with normal saline. When the dressing is removed, a viscous gel remains in the ulcer, but it can be easily removed by saline irrigations (not hydrogen peroxide or other antiseptic solutions).
- **Calcium alginate dressings (e.g., Kaltostat Wound Dressing, Algoderm calcium alginate wound packing, Sorbsan).**

Alginates are seaweed-derived polysaccharides that are useful for packing large exuding cavities because they are highly absorbent. Only half of the cavity should be gently packed because these products expand.[3]

- **Hydrocolloid pastes and polyurethane foam (e.g., Cutinova Cavity, Duoderm Hydroactive Paste or Hydroactive Granules, Allevyn Hydrophilic Polymer Foam Dressing, LYOfoam).** These are absorbent agents used for large exuding cavities. About half the wound cavity should be gently packed.

Adjunctive wound therapies are treatment modalities that are used, when available, in conjunction with conventional topical-wound management when the wound response has been marginal. Hyperbaric oxygen is the systemic, intermittent administration of oxygen delivered under pressure. It increases the capacity of blood to carry and deliver oxygen to tissues. Negative-pressure wound therapy (NPWT) is a mechanical wound-care treatment that uses controlled negative pressure to assist and accelerate wound healing. It is also known as vacuum-assisted closure.[2]

REFERENCES

1. Lyder CH: Pressure ulcer prevention and management: contempo update; *JAMA* 289(2): 223-226, 2003.
2. Wooten M: Management of chronic wounds in the elderly, *Clin Fam Pract* 3(3):599-626, 2001.
3. Findlay D: Practical management of pressure ulcers, *Am Fam Physician* 54:1519-1528, 1996.
4. Helfman T, Ovington L, Falanga V: Occlusive dressings and wound healing, *Clin Dermatol* 12:121-127, 1994.

URTICARIA AND ANGIOEDEMA
(See also drug allergy; food allergy)

Urticaria is a cutaneous syndrome characterized by dermal edema (wheal) and erythema (flare) that blanches with pressure. The lesions typically last less than 24 hours and are usually pruritic.[1] Urticaria and angioedema are said to affect 15% to 25% of the population at least once in a lifetime. Among patients with these disorders, 40% have urticaria alone, 10% angioedema alone, and 50% a combination of the two. Urticaria involves swelling of the superficial dermal tissues, whereas angioedema is located in the deep dermal, subcutaneous, or submucosal tissues. The swelling of angioedema is usually found in the extremities, eyelids, and lips, but it may involve the gastrointestinal tract or the respiratory tract. In the latter instance, respiratory obstruction is a real possibility. Patients with angioedema usually complain of burning or tingling rather than itching. Individual lesions of both urticaria and angioedema come on rapidly, usually resolve in 2 to 4 hours, and rarely last more than 24 hours.[2]

Common causes of acute urticaria are *Hymenoptera* insect stings; foods such as nuts, chocolate, shellfish, eggs, and milk; viral infections, including hepatitis B; and drugs, especially antibiotics.[2] In rare cases angioedema may develop months or even years (and may even resolve, then worsen) after a patient starts taking a medication, such as ACE inhibitors.[3]

Chronic urticaria is defined as the presence of widespread wheals daily or almost daily for at least 6 weeks. In about 75% of cases, no etiological factor is found,[2,4] and about half of these patients will be symptom-free after 1 year.[1] Physical urticarias such as cold, solar, pressure, and cholinergic (brought on by exercise or hot shower) should be considered in the differential diagnosis. Urticarial vasculitis is one of the most important conditions to be ruled out. Urticarial vasculitis is associated with connective tissue diseases such as lupus and Sjögren's syndrome. In this condition the individual wheals last more than 24 hours, and often purpura and sometimes skin pigmentation are seen. Fever, arthralgia, nephritis, and abdominal pain may also be present. The diagnosis can be made with a skin biopsy. A rare condition causing recurrent episodes of urticaria or angioedema is deficiency of C1 esterase inhibitor. It is diagnosed by finding a low C4 complement level.[2,4] Routinely ordering elaborate investigations for patients with chronic urticaria or angioedema in an attempt to determine the etiology is not necessary. In one study comparing a careful history plus a few selective investigations with a history plus an exhaustive investigative protocol, the minimal investigations missed only 6% of identifiable causative conditions. For example, all the patients whose urticaria was due to parasites had lived in or been born in tropical countries; these were the only persons who needed to have stools tested for ova and parasites.[5]

The mainstay of therapy for urticaria is avoidance of known triggering agents, judicious use of oral corticosteroids, and treatment with long-acting second-generation antihistamines, H_2-receptor antagonists, tricyclic antidepressants, and anti-inflammatory leukotriene antagonists.[6] In one small U.S. study, patients with acute-onset urticaria, regardless of cause, had better itch control if given a 4-day course of prednisone 20 mg in addition to hydroxyzine (Atarax) 25 mg every 4 to 8 hours as needed compared with those given only hydroxyzine.[5]

Patients with chronic urticaria should avoid taking ACE inhibitors, Aspirin, and other non-steroidal anti-inflammatory drugs.[4] For patients who fail to respond to H_1-receptor antagonists alone, the addition of an H_2 antagonist such as cimetidine or ranitidine may result in control of symptoms.[8] The antidepressant doxepin (Sinequan) has significant H_1 antihistaminic activity and may be used in doses of 25 to 50 mg at bedtime.[4] Patients that have experienced any upper-airway symptoms should be prescribed an Epi-Pen device.

❧ REFERENCES ☙

1. Lee EE, Maibach HI: Treatment of urticaria: an evidence-based evaluation of antihistamines, *Am J Clin Dermatol* 2(1):27-32, 2001.
2. Kulp-Shorten CL, Callen J: Urticaria, angioedema, and rheumatologic disease: rheumatic disease, *Rheum Dis Clin North Am* 22:95-115, 1996.
3. Shionoiri H, Takasaki I, Hirawa N, et al: A case report of angioedema during long-term (66 months) angiotensin converting enzyme inhibition therapy with enalapril, *Jpn Circ J* 60:166-170, 1996.
4. Greaves MW: Chronic urticaria, *N Engl J Med* 332:1767-1772, 1995.
5. Kozel MM, Mekkes JR, Bossuyt PM, et al: The effectiveness of a history-based diagnostic approach in chronic urticaria and angioedema, *Arch Dermatol* 134:1575-1580, 1998.
6. Pollack CV, Romano TJ: Outpatient management of acute urticaria—role of prednisone, *Ann Emerg Med* 26:547-551, 1995.
7. Muller BA: Urticaria and angioedema: a practical approach, *Am Fam Physician* 69(5):1123-1128, Mar 1 2004.
8. Bleehen SS, Thomas SE, Greaves MW, et al: Cimetidine and chlorpheniramine in the treatment of chronic idiopathic urticaria: a multi-centre randomized double-blind study, *Br J Dermatol* 117:81-88, 1987.

WARTS

Between 5% and 10% of children and young adults have warts, which are lesions caused by the human papillomavirus.[1] The peak age is 12 to 16 years.[2] About 70% of warts resolve spontaneously within 2 years (most within 1 year), but because new lesions develop in a number of patients, only about 50% of patients are lesion-free after 2 years if left untreated.[3]

Differential Diagnosis

Common warts are rough, keratotic papules on any skin surface. They may be distinguished from nevi by the presence of black points (thrombosed capillaries) on the warts. Early lesions of molluscum contagiosum may mimic warts, but mature lesions have a characteristic umbilicated centre. Palmar/plantar warts can be distinguished from calluses and corns by the presence of thrombosed capillaries and disturbed dermatoglyphics in warts after paring. Flat or plane warts may be confused with lichen planus except that in the latter, lesions are itchy, violaceous with a white lace-like pattern (Wickham's striae), and often involve the oral mucosa.[4]

Treatment

Evidence supporting efficacy for most wart treatments is weak. A recent Cochrane review concluded that there is a considerable lack of evidence on which to base the rational use of the local treatments for common warts. The reviewed trials are highly variable in method and quality.[5] Since many of the lesions resolve spontaneously, no treatment is often the preferred choice.[2,3] Specific indications for treatment include symptomatic warts, disfiguring or disabling lesions, large numbers of lesions, and an immunocompromised host.[6] The best available evidence of efficacy is for salicylic acid and cryotherapy.[4,7]

If salicylic compounds are used, the lesion should be soaked in water or a shampoo solution for 5 minutes before application. It should be rinsed and dried, and any debris should be mechanically removed from the lesion. The liquid should be applied to the lesion, with care not to include surrounding normal skin. Treatments should be repeated every 24 to 48 hours until the skin lines can be seen over the base of the lesion. Examples of the many available products are salicylic acid 17% (Compound W gel), salicylic acid 20% (Compound W liquid), salicylic acid 30% (Compound W plus), salicylic acid 16.7%/lactic acid 16.7% (Duofilm liquid), and salicylic acid 27% (Duoforte 27). Salicylic acid compounds specifically formulated for plantar warts include 40% salicylic acid disks and plasters (Carnation Callous and Corn Caps, Clear Away Plantar Wart Remover, Scholl Corn Removers), and salicylic acid 25%, lactic acid 10%, and formalin 5% (Duoplant). Disks or plaster should be purchased or cut to fit the lesion exactly so that normal surrounding skin is not affected. The plaster should then be applied and covered with waterproof tape, and treatments should be repeated every 48 hours. Once skin lines can be seen across the base of the lesion, treatment can be stopped. Total duration of treatment varies but may be up to 12 weeks. Liquid salicylic acid products such as Duoplant may be applied to the wart and covered with a waterproof bandage.

Cryotherapy may require repeat treatments every 2 to 3 weeks until the lesions resolve. Liquid nitrogen is preferred because other methods may not reach cold enough temperatures. Hyperkeratotic lesions should be pared prior to freezing. For common and hand warts, a single freeze-thaw cycle lasting 5 to 30 seconds with white margins extending 1 to 3 mm beyond the lesion is usually adequate. Plantar warts may respond better to two cycles.[4] Cryotherapy is painful and may cause blistering but is unlikely to scar.

Cantharidin is supported only by cohort and case-control studies, but weekly use makes it more convenient than salicylic acid and it is less painful than cryotherapy.[7]

Cantharidin is an extract of the blister beetle or "Spanish fly." The method of using cantharidin is as follows: Apply the liquid to the wart, allow it to dry, and cover the wart with non-porous tape for 24 hours. After 24 hours, replace the tape with a loose bandage such as a Band-Aid. After 2 weeks, reassess the wart and remove necrotic tissue. One treatment is usually effective for hand and body warts, but a second application may be given if necessary. Two or more treatments at 2-week intervals are usually required for plantar warts.

Duct tape may be effective and is cheap and painless. In children, occlusion with duct tape (wear continuously for 6 days, remove tape, soak and buff lesion on evening of sixth day, reapply next morning for another 6 days, repeat for 2 months) may be as or more effective than lightly applied cryotherapy.[8] Acceptability may depend on the site of the wart and the patient's fondness for home improvement.

Tretinoin cream 0.05% was more effective for flat warts than placebo in one small RCT.[7] Preliminary results are encouraging for the use of imiquimod 5% cream in plain warts and, in conjunction with cryotherapy, in the treatment of resistant plantar warts.[9,10] Several open trials suggested efficacy for cimetidine, but a controlled trial showed no advantage over placebo.[4,11] Local heat treatment has not been adequately assessed.[4] Cautery, curettage, laser, and bleomycin injections are painful and may scar. Plantar scarring may lead to persistent pain.[4]

✑ REFERENCES ✒

1. Sterling J: Treating the troublesome wart, *Practitioner* 239:44-47, 1995.
2. Siegfried EC: Warts on children: an approach to therapy, *Pediatr Ann* 25:79-90, 1996.
3. Landow K: Nongenital warts: when is treatment warranted? *Postgrad Med* 99:245-249, 1996.
4. Sterling JC, Handfield-Jones S, Hudson PM: Guidelines for the management of cutaneous warts, *Br J Dermatol* 144:4-11, 2001.
5. Gibbs S, Harvey I, Sterling JC, et al: Local treatments for cutaneous warts (Cochrane Review). Cochrane Database Syst Rev (3):CD001781, 2003.
6. Committee on Guidelines of Care: Guidelines of care for warts: human papillomavirus, *J Am Acad Dermatol* 32: 98-103, 1995.
7. Brodell RT, Marchese Johnson S: *Warts, diagnosis and management: an evidence-based approach,* London, 2003, Martin Dunitz.
8. Focht DR, Spicer C, Fairchok MP: The efficacy of duct tape vs cryotherapy in the treatment of verruca vulgaris (the common wart), *Arch Pediatr Adolesc Med* 156:971-974, 2002.
9. Grussendorf-Conen E-I, Jacobs S, Rubben A, et al: Topical 5% imiquimod long-term treatment of cutaneous warts resistant to standard therapy modalities, *Dermatology* 205:139-145, 2002.
10. Sparling JD, Checketts SR, Chapman MS: Imiquimod for plantar and periungual warts, *Cutis* 68:397-399, 2001.
11. Yilmaz E, Alpsoy E, Basaran E: Cimetidine therapy for warts: a placebo-controlled, double-blind study, *J Am Acad Dermatol* 34:1005-1007, 1995.

GASTROENTEROLOGY

ANAL AND ANORECTAL DISORDERS
(See also constipation)

Anal Fissures

Ninety percent of anal fissures (a split in the squamous epithelium) are found at or just inside the anal verge in the posterior midline.[1] Traditionally, trauma to the anus, such as occurs with constipation, was thought to be the cause.[2] The current theory proposes sphincter spasm and accompanying ischemia as the precipitant.[3,4] Fissures outside the midline require evaluation for an underlying diagnosis such as inflammatory bowel disease, sexually transmitted infections, or cancer.[5,6]

Pain is described as sharp, burning, and severe, lasting from minutes to hours and associated with defecation.[5-7] Patients commonly report bright red blood on the toilet paper following a bowel movement as well as rectal itching and discharge.[8]

Acute fissures (present for less than 6 weeks) are best managed conservatively by avoiding hard bulky stools. A high-fibre diet heals over 80% of people presenting with an acute fissure, and relapses can be prevented with continued high fibre (diet or supplements) for 6 to 12 months.[2,4,5] Healing is also promoted by soaking in warm baths for 2 to 5 minutes followed by cold water for 1 minute (reported to relax the anal sphincter),[1,9] or application of 1% hydrocortisone ointment (if no infection is present).[5,6] Five percent lidocaine applied to the anus just before bowel movements provides pain relief for most people.[2,10]

Chronic fissures (present for 6 weeks or longer) can also be treated conservatively but many require further management. A prospective randomized placebo-controlled trial showed that nitroglycerin (glyceryl trinitrate) ointment dramatically increases the healing rate of persistent anal fissures. In this study a 0.2% glyceryl trinitrate ointment was applied to the fissure twice a day for up to 8 weeks.[2] Over half the patients treated with the ointment had headaches that were mostly short lived and mild. The drug is believed to relax the anal sphincter muscle.[7] If prescribing this ointment, the physician should be sure to underline the dosage of 0.2%, since the concentration of nitroglycerin ointment used for angina is generally 2.0%. Kennedy et al showed similar healing rates. Moreover, they reported that the nitroglycerin-treated group had less surgical treatments for the sphincter spasm and at 29-month follow-up, remained fissure free compared with the placebo group.[3] In a randomized control trial the injection of botulinum A toxin into the anal sphincter reduced spasm and promoted healing. Lysy et al reported that the nitroglycerin potentiated the effects of the botulinum toxin in refractory cases.[4] Long-term follow-up studies are needed to assess relapse rates and toxin effect on incontinence.

If conservative treatment fails, surgery is probably indicated. The procedure of choice is a lateral internal sphincterotomy with the goal of breaking the cycle of internal sphincter spasm.[4,7] Digital stretching of the anal sphincter no longer has a role and may in fact cause further tearing and incontinence.[3,4]

In a few children under 6 years of age, anal fissures may be the result of cow's milk intolerance. The parents usually seek treatment for the child's chronic constipation, and in one double-blind crossover study, switching to soy milk caused resolution of the fissures and constipation.[11]

Hemorrhoids

Hemorrhoids may be external or internal. External hemorrhoids lie distal to the dentate line and are covered by skin; internal hemorrhoids are proximal to the dentate line and are covered by mucosa.[8,12]

External hemorrhoids may cause minor discomfort or severe pain if they become thrombosed. Pain peaks in 48 to 72 hours and then gradually resolves over 7 to 10 days. If the patient has intense pain and is seen within 72 hours, incision and evacuation of the thrombus or excision of the lesion with overlying skin may be performed. However, thrombosis generally recurs, and secondary prevention should be stressed.[12] The usual conservative treatment consists of warm baths, increased fibre, and fluids to prevent constipation, weight loss, and good anal hygiene.[8,12] Evidence of the effectiveness of any of the available hemorrhoidal preparations is insufficient, although topical anesthetics and anti-inflammatory products (see Anal Fissures section) might be helpful.

Four categories of internal hemorrhoids have been established. Grade I internal hemorrhoids are small and do not prolapse; grade II hemorrhoids prolapse with bowel movement but return spontaneously; grade III hemorrhoids prolapse but can be replaced manually; grade IV hemorrhoids prolapse and cannot be replaced manually. Internal hemorrhoids usually lie in the right anterior, right posterior, and left lateral positions.[8,12] Anemia from rectal bleeding secondary to internal hemorrhoids is well documented. Among 43 patients with this condition as reported from the Mayo Clinic, the mean hemoglobin concentration was 9.4 g/dl (94 g/L). Eighty-four percent of the patients gave a history of blood squirting from the anus or the passage of clots. Six of the 43 had coagulation defects.[13]

Conservative management of internal hemorrhoids is the initial treatment of choice for grades I to III lesions. This consists of avoiding straining at stool; increasing fibre in the form of fruit, vegetables, and fibre products such as psyllium; and maintaining a high fluid intake (six to eight glasses of caffeine-free fluid per day).[8] Interventional options include rubber band ligation, infrared photocoagulation, and injection sclerotherapy. Hemorrhoidectomy is indicated for grade IV lesions and for other cases that do not respond to less invasive procedures.

Proctalgia Fugax

Proctalgia fugax is characterized by infrequent episodes of severe perianal pain lasting from seconds to a few minutes.[14,15] The etiology remains unclear, although some investigators have suggested it is a variation of irritable bowel syndrome (IBS), pelvic floor myalgia, or internal anal sphincter spasm.[6,14] No serious underlying diseases are associated with this condition, and with a typical history, no investigations are required.[15] Generally, no specific treatment is available, although digital dilatation of the anus by the patient has been reported to give relief, presumably by relaxing the sphincter. Anecdotal reports claim that clonidine (Catapres) 0.15 mg twice a day or diltiazem (Cardizem) 80 mg twice a day is effective for very severe cases.[6,14] In two case reports, Kastinelos et al (2001) reported that botulinum A toxin seemed a promising therapy. They describe two cases of proctalgia fugax associated with exaggerated myoelectrical activity of the anus. Botulinum A toxin injections of the anal sphincter resulted in a decrease in the recorded sphincter hyperkinesis and control of the perineal pain.[16]

Pruritus Ani

Pruritus ani is an intense itching sensation of the rectal area. It has been estimated to occur in about 5% of the population, four times more often in men than women, and occurring in the fourth through sixth decades of life.[6] Itching is more intense after a bowel movement and at bedtime. Most cases of pruritus ani are primary or idiopathic, but can be secondary to benign or malignant anorectal or systemic disorders, including diarrhea, poor hygiene, perspiration, tight fitting underclothes (all resulting in excessive moisture in the area), infections, hemorrhoids, fissures, fistulas, chronic dermatoses, diabetes, rectal carcinomas, Paget's disease, and Bowen's disease.[6] In children the most common cause is pinworms.[9] Anecdotal evidence suggests diet, such as coffee or acidic foods, may contribute to the discomfort.[6] A thorough workup for secondary causes is indicated if suggested by the initial history or physical examination or if the patient fails to respond to treatment within a month or so. Treatment of primary pruritus ani consists of eliminating aggravating nutrients and potentially irritating local agents such as scented soaps. Flushable baby wipes are an excellent alternative to toilet paper and washing after every bowel movement. After a bath, the patient should avoid harsh rubbing and consider the use of a blow drier to ensure complete drying of the anal area. Systemic antihistamines at night may help break the itch-scratch cycle. Cotton underpants and/or a cotton pad placed in the perianal area help absorb excess moisture. Use of zinc protective creams (Zincofax) and in some cases a short course of 1% hydrocortisone cream hastens symptomatic relief. Consider referral to a dermatologist or gastroenterologist if improvement does not occur after 4 weeks of conservative management.[6]

Anal Cancer

Squamous cell cancer of the anus is rare. An important risk factor for both men and women is receptive anal intercourse, which presumably allows transmission of the carcinogenic strains of human papillomavirus.[17]

◢ REFERENCES ◣

1. Nagle D, Rolandelli RH: Primary care office management of perianal and anal disease, *Primary Care* 23(3):609-620, 1996.
2. American Gastroenterological Association medical position statement: Diagnosis and care of patients with anal fissure, *Gastroenterology* 124(1):233-234, 2003.
3. Kennedy ML, Sower S, Nguyen H, et al: Glyceryl trinitrate ointment for the treatment of chronic anal fissure: results of a placebo-controlled trial and long-term follow-up, *Dis Colon Rectum* 42(8):1000-1006,1999.
4. Lysy L, Israelit-Yatzkan Y, Sestiery-Ittah M, et al: Topical nitrates potentiate the effect of botulinum toxin in the treatment of patients with refractory anal fissure, *Gut* 48:221-224, 2001.
5. Lubowski DZ: Anal fissures, *Aust Fam Physician* 29(9):839-844, 2000.
6. Vincent C: Anorectal pain and irritation: anal fissure, anal levator syndrome, proctalgia fugax and pruritus ani, *Prim Care* 26(1):53-68, 1999.
7. Lund JN, Armitage NC, Scholefield JH: Use of glyceryl trinitrate ointment in the treatment of anal fissure, *Br J Surg* 83:776-777, 1996.
8. Hussain JN: Haemorrhoids, *Aust Fam Physician* 30(1):29-35, 2001.

9. Mazier WP: Hemorrhoids, fissures, and pruritus ani, *Surg Clin North Am* 74:1277-1292, 1994.

10. ASCRS, The Standards Task Force: Practice parameters for the management of anal fissure, American Society of Colon and Rectal Surgeons.. 2001. http://www.fascrs.org/displaycommon.cfm?an=1&subarticlenbr=146 Accessed April 20,2005.

11. Iacono G, Cavataio F, Montalto G, et al: Intolerance of cow's milk and chronic constipation in children, *N Engl J Med* 339:1100-1104, 1998.

12. Orkin BA, Schwartz AM, Orkin M: Hemorrhoids: what the dermatologist should know, *J Am Acad Dermatol* 43:449-456, 1999.

13. Kluiber RM, Wolff BG: Evaluation of anemia caused by hemorrhoidal bleeding, *Dis Colon Rectum* 37:1006-1007, 1994.

14. Nidorf DM, Jamison ER: Proctalgia fugax, *Am Fam Physician* 52:2238-2240, 1995.

15. Potter MA, Bartolo DC: Proctalgia fugax, *Eur J Gastrenterol Hepatol* 13(11):1289-1290, 2001.

16. Katsinelos P, Kalomenopoulou M, Christodoulou K, et al: Treatment of proctalgia fugax with botulinum A toxin, *Eur J Gastroenerol Hepatol* 13(11):1371-1373, 2001.

17. Frisch M, Glimelius B, van den Brule AJ, et al: Sexually transmitted infection as a cause of anal cancer, *N Engl J Med* 337:1350-1358, 1997.

CELIAC DISEASE

Celiac disease is a chronic diarrheal condition characterized by malabsorption of nutrients and precipitated by the ingestion of gluten commonly found in foods with wheat, rye, and barley. Celiac disease may be diagnosed at any age but is most common during childhood or in the third to fifth decades.[1-3] A variety of presenting symptoms have been described in the literature, and include diarrhea; weight loss; bone pain from fractures[1,2]; fatigue[2,3]; recurrent aphthous ulcers[2,4] or sore tongue and mouth[2]; unexplained hypocalcemia, anemia,[2] or folate deficiency[1]; and autoimmune thyroiditis.[1] In fact, many if not most patients have few or no gastrointestinal (GI) symptoms, only a small proportion are underweight, and a significant number are overweight.[5]

Pain is not a common symptom associated with celiac disease. Not surprisingly, the diagnosis is often missed or delayed by several years.[6]

Traditional screening tests for celiac disease are serum carotene, fecal fat estimation, D-xylose absorption test, complete blood count, international normalized ratio (INR) and blood chemistry such as; serum iron, calcium, potassium, magnesium, aspartate transaminase (AST), and alanine transaminase (ALT).[7] More sophisticated tests, which are not available in all centres, are antigliadin antibodies (gliadin is a portion of the protein gluten),[8] IgA anti-endomysial antibodies, and antitissue transglutaminase.[2,3,7] Sensitivity and specificity of IgA anti-endomysial antibodies are 85% to 98% and 97% to 100% respectively.[7] Tests for IgA and IgG antigliadin have

moderate sensitivity but are far less specific than tests for IgA anti-endomysial antibodies.[7] Definitive diagnosis is made with a small bowel biopsy.[2,3,8]

Major complications of celiac disease are osteoporosis, fractures, and small bowel lymphoma. A strict gluten-free diet not only relieves symptoms, it diminishes the risks of these complications.[2] Seventy percent of patients see a clinical improvement in symptoms in just 2 weeks after withdrawing food that contains gluten from the diet.

❧ REFERENCES ❧

1. Shaker JL, Brickner RC, Findling JW, et al: Hypocalcemia and skeletal disease as presenting features of celiac disease, *Arch Intern Med* 157:1013-1016, 1997.

2. Feighery C: Coeliac disease, *BMJ* 319:236-239, 1999.

3. Hin H, Bird G, Fisher P, et al: Coeliac disease in primary care: case finding study, *BMJ* 318:164-167, 1999.

4. Srinivasan U, Weir DG, Feighery C, et al: Emergence of classic enteropathy after longstanding gluten sensitive oral ulceration, *BMJ* 316:206-207, 1998.

5. Dickey W, Bodkin S: Prospective study of body mass index in patients with coeliac disease, *BMJ* 317:1290, 1998.

6. Dickey W, McConnell JB: How many visits dose it take before celiac sprue is diagnosed? *J Clin Gastroenterol* 23: 21-23, 1996.

7. Farrell RJ, Kelly CP: Current concepts celiac sprue, *N Engl J Med* 346:181-187, 2002.

8. Chartrand LJ, Agulnik J, Vanounou T, et al: Effectiveness of antigliadin antibodies as a screening test for celiac disease in children, *Can Med Assoc J* 157:527-533, 1997.

COLON

(See also inflammatory bowel disease; irritable bowel disease)

Colon Cancer

(See also anemia; hematochezia)

Epidemiology

Over 150,000 new cases of colorectal cancer are diagnosed yearly in the United States. Colorectal cancer is the third most common cancer in men and women and the second leading cause of death. The incidence increases progressively with age; in North America the lifetime risk of having the disease is estimated between 2.5% and 5.6%, and the lifetime risk of dying of the disease is about 2.6%.[1] The peak incidence is in the seventh decade; only 4% of cases occur in persons under age 50.

The distribution of cancers within the colon has changed over the past few decades; more lesions are now found on the right side and fewer on the left side. Presently at least half of all colonic polyps and cancers are within 60 cm of the anus and so are at least theoretically within reach of the long flexible sigmoidoscope.[2]

A number of risk factors have been recognized or postulated for colon cancer:

1. Patients with familial adenomatous polyposis have an almost 100% risk of developing colorectal cancer by age 40.[1]
2. Autosomal inheritence of the gene for Lynch Syndrome 1 and 2 (hereditary nonpolyposis coli).
3. Personal history of large adenomatous colonic polyps or colon cancer.[1]
4. Personal history of endometrial, ovarian, or breast cancer.[1]
5. Family history of colon cancer. An affected first-degree relative carries a two- to three-fold increased risk. The relative risk is much higher for persons under 45 years of age (Relative risk=5.37) and is negligible for those age 60 and older.[3]
6. Family history of adenomatous polyps. The risk is particularly great if the polyps are diagnosed in patients under age 50.[4]
7. Inflammatory bowel disease. Ulcerative colitis and to a lesser extent Crohn's disease are risk factors. In the case of ulcerative colitis, the risk is greatest if the patient has had extensive colonic involvement for over 7 years. The risk is higher with right-sided colonic involvement but is not increased if the disease is limited to the sigmoid colon and rectum.[5]
8. Cigarette smoking. Carcinogenic agents can cause mutational activation of oncogenes and loss of tumour suppression genes. The induction period appears to be about 35 years.[6,7]
9. Diet. Epidemiological evidence points to an increased risk of colon cancer among those whose diet is high in fat and meat and a decreased risk among those who eat a lot of fruits and vegetables[8] or bread and pasta.[9] High-fibre diets (mainly cereals) have long been thought to protect against colon cancer, and this view is supported by an international prospective cohort study published in 1999.[10] However, a prospective cohort study of nurses, also published in 1999, failed to find such a correlation.[11]
10. Vitamins. A diet high in folate or vitamin E or the long-term use of multivitamins containing folate is associated with a lower risk of colon cancer.[10]
11. Activity and obesity. Both sedentary lifestyle[12] and obesity[12-14] increase the risk of colorectal cancer, whereas leisure-time physical activity decreases the risk.[12]
12. Diabetes. In the Nurses' Health Study, women with type 2 diabetes were found to be at increased risk for colorectal cancer.[15]
13. Constipation. A case-control trial found constipation to be a risk factor.[16]

The overall mortality rate for cancer of the large bowel is 50%. The rate depends on the stage of the cancer. For stage I disease (Dukes' stages A and B-1), in which inva-sion is limited to the muscularis propria without nodal involvement, the cure rate is 90%. For stage II (Dukes' stage B-2), in which cancer has invaded through the muscularis to the serosa but nodes are not involved, the cure rate is 75%. For stage III disease (Dukes' stage C), in which the disease has metastasized to the regional nodes, the cure rate is 35%.[17]

❧ REFERENCES ❧

1. U.S. Preventive Services Task Force: Screening for colorectal cancer: recommendations and rationale, *Ann Intern Med* 137:129-131, 2002.
2. American Gastroenterological Association: Colorectal cancer screening and surveillance: clinical guidelines and rationale—update based on new evidence, *Gastroenterology* 124: 544-560, 2003.
3. Fuchs CS, Giovannucci EL, Colditz GA, et al: A prospective study of family history and the risk of colorectal cancer, *N Engl J Med* 331:1169-1174, 1994.
4. Ahsan H, Neugut AI, Garbowski GC, et al: Family history of colorectal adenomatous polyps and increased risk for colorectal cancer, *Ann Intern Med* 128:900-905, 1998
5. Donald JJ, Burhenne HJ: Colorectal cancer: can we lower the death rate in the 1990s? *Can Fam Physician* 39:107-114, 1993.
6. Giovannucci E, Rimm EB, Stampfer MF, et al: A prospective study of cigarette smoking and risk of colorectal adenoma and colorectal cancer in U.S. men, *J Natl Cancer Inst* 86: 183-191, 1994.
7. Giovannucci I, Colditz GA, Stampfer MJ, et al: A prospective study of cigarette smoking and risk of colorectal adenoma and colorectal cancer in U.S. women, *J Natl Cancer Inst* 86:162-164, 1994.
8. Potter JD: Nutrition and colorectal cancer, *Cancer Causes Control* 7:127-146, 1996.
9. Jansen MC, Bueno-de-Mesquita HB, Buzina R, et al: Dietary fiber and plant foods in relation to colorectal cancer mortality: the Seven Countries Study, *Int J Cancer* 81: 174-179, 1999.
10. Fuchs CS, Giovannucci EL, Colditz GA, et al: Dietary fiber and the risk of colorectal cancer and adenoma in women, *N Engl J Med* 340:169-176, 1999.
11. Giovannucci E, Stampfer MJ, Colditz GA, et al: Multivitamin use, folate, and colon cancer in women in the Nurses' Health Study, *Ann Intern Med* 129:517-524, 1999.
12. Martinez ME, Giovannucci E, Spiegelman D, et al: Leisure-time physical activity, body size, and colon cancer in women: Nurses' Health Study Research Group, *J Natl Cancer Inst* 89:948-955, 1997.
13. Schoen RE, Tangen CM, Kuller LH, et al: Increased blood glucose and insulin, body size, and incident colorectal cancer, *J Natl Cancer Inst* 91:1147-1154, 1999.
14. Ford ES: Body mass index and colon cancer in a national sample of adult U.S. men and women, *Am J Epidemiol* 150:390-398, 1999.
15. Hu FB, Manson JE, Liu S, et al: Prospective study of adult onset diabetes mellitus (type 2) and risk of colorectal cancer in women, *J Natl Cancer Inst* 91:542-547, 1999.

16. Jacobs EJ, White E: Constipation, laxative use, and colon cancer among middle-aged adults, *Epidemiology* 9:385-391, 1998.

17. Dube D, Heyen F, Jenicek M: Adjuvant chemotherapy in colorectal carcinoma: results of a meta-analysis, *Dis Colon Rectum* 4:35-41, 1997. Reviewed in *Clin Evidence* 10:509-517, 2003.

Primary prevention of colon cancer
(See also exercise; healthy user effect)

Diet, exercise, and smoking. In view of the risk factors enumerated in the previous section, a diet that is low in animal fat, containing plenty of vegetables, fruit, bread, and pasta would probably be beneficial, as might taking a multivitamin containing folate. Every effort should be made to be physically active. Smoking should be discouraged. Excessive use of alcohol should be avoided.

One study found that a daily supplement of 3 g of calcium carbonate (1200 mg of elemental calcium) decreased the risk for colonic adenomas. At least in theory this might also decrease the risk of colon cancer.[1]

Hormone replacement therapy. A number of observational studies have shown a decreased risk of colon cancer[2,3] and adenomatous polyps[3] in women on hormone replacement therapy. No randomized controlled trials have been published, so whether these findings represent a "healthy user" effect is not known.

Non-steroidal anti-inflammatory drugs. Several prospective studies involving men and women have shown a significant decrease in the incidence[4-6] and mortality[5] of colon cancer in individuals taking 325 mg of Aspirin at least four to six times a week; this benefit may not become obvious until 10 years have elapsed.[6] However, a 12-year follow-up of the Physicians' Health Study failed to show such a relationship.[7] A retrospective population-based cohort study found that long-term use of non-Aspirin NSAIDs also provided protection against colon cancer. No one class of drugs was better than another, and low doses appeared to be as effective as high ones.[8] NSAIDs reduce the incidence of adenomas in humans, and various NSAIDs inhibit carcinogenesis in the colon in experimental animals.[4,5] One editorial writer has recommended that patients at elevated risk of colon cancer take an Aspirin a day. Elevated risk is defined as having a past history of colonic adenoma or cancer; a family history of colorectal cancer or adenoma; inflammatory bowel disease; or breast, ovarian, or endometrial cancer.[9]

❧ REFERENCES ❧

1. Baron JA, Beach M, Mandel JS, et al: Calcium supplements for the prevention of colorectal adenomas, *N Engl J Med* 340:101-107, 1999.

2. Paganini-Hill A: Estrogen replacement therapy and colorectal cancer risk in elderly women, *Dis Colon Rectum* 42:1300-1305, 1999.

3. Chlebowski RT, Wactawski-Wende J, Ritenbaugh, C, et al: Estrogen plus progestin and colorectal cancer in postmenopausal women, *N Engl J Med* 350:991-1004, 2004.

4. Peleg II, Lubin MF, Cotsonis GA, et al: Long-term use of nonsteroidal antiinflammatory drugs and other chemopreventors and risk of subsequent colorectal neoplasia, *Dig Dis Sci* 41:1319-1326, 1996.

5. Thun MJ, Namboodiri MM, Heath CW Jr: Aspirin use and risk of fatal cancer, *Cancer Res* 53:1322-1327, 1993.

6. Giovannucci E, Egan KM, Hunter DJ, et al: Aspirin and the risk of colorectal cancer in women, *N Engl J Med* 333:609-614, 1995.

7. Stürmer T, Glynn RJ, Lee IM, et al: Aspirin use and colorectal cancer: post-trial follow-up data from the Physicians' Health Study, *Ann Intern Med* 128:713-720, 1998.

8. Smalley W, Ray WA, Daugherty J, et al: Use of nonsteroidal anti-inflammatory drugs and incidence of colorectal cancer: a population-based study, *Arch Intern Med* 159:161-166, 1999.

9. Marcus AJ: Aspirin prophylaxis against colorectal cancer (editorial), *N Engl J Med* 333:656-657, 1995.

Secondary prevention of colon cancer
(See also hematochezia; informed consent; positive predictive value; prevention; relative risk reduction)

Fecal occult blood screening. In a study by Mandel and associates[1] from the University of Minnesota, mortality from colon cancer was decreased by a relative rate of 33% over 13 years by annual Hemoccult testing. (On average each patient submitted samples for 8 years; each test consisted of six specimens obtained from three different stool samples.) The number of individuals who had to be screened over 13 years to prevent one colon cancer death was 360, or put another way, screened individuals decreased their risk of dying of colon cancer by 0.3%.[1,2] Total mortality was not reduced. This relative mortality reduction rate of 33% translates into an absolute mortality reduction rate of 3:1000 or 0.3%. The positive predictive value of the Hemoccult testing for cancer was 2.2%, but for cancer and polyps combined it was 30%.[1] After 18 years of follow-up, the absolute reduction in cancer mortality in this group of patients was 5:1000 or 0.5%, and there was still no reduction in total mortality; analysis of 3200 stool samples for occult blood was required to save one life.[3]

Fecal occult blood testing (FOBT) in the Minnesota trial triggered large numbers of colonoscopies. Among the 15,000 patients in the annual Hemoccult testing group, 4500 had colonoscopies.[4] The reported complications of colonoscopy in this study were four perforations requiring surgery and 11 episodes of serious bleeding, three of which required surgery.[1]

Two large prospective studies of fecal occult blood screening were published in the *Lancet* in 1996, one from

Great Britain[5] and one from Denmark.[6] Both studies screened patients every 2 years, and both showed a small but significant decline in colon cancer-related mortality (but not total cohort mortality) in the screened group. In the British study the 15% relative reduction in colon cancer deaths over 8 years of follow-up meant that 747 patients had to be screened to prevent one colon cancer death,[2] while in the Danish study the 18% relative reduction of colon cancer deaths over 10 years of follow-up meant that 470 patients had to be screened to prevent one colon cancer death.[2] Both these studies are notable in that only about 4% of the screened cohort had full colonoscopies.[5,6] Six major complications of colonoscopy (a rate of 0.5%) were reported in the British study; only one occurred during diagnostic endoscopy, and the other five were associated with therapeutic interventions.[2]

The study by Mandel and associates from the University of Minnesota also analyzed a group of patients screened biennially. At 13 years of follow-up, no decrease in colon cancer mortality was found,[1] but after 18 years, there was a 21% relative reduction in cancer mortality. Screening 1000 patients led to three fewer colon cancer deaths after 18 years.[3]

A systematic review of five major Hemoccult screening studies concluded that Hemoccult screening of 10,000 people every second year for 10 years would result in 8.5 fewer cancer deaths than would occur in a non-screened population of equal numbers (relative reduction of 16%; number needed to screen to prevent one cancer death = 1176).[7]

Fecal occult blood screening for colon cancer or adenomas is neither sensitive (few adenomas bleed and even advanced cancers tend to bleed intermittently) nor specific (most positive occult blood tests are associated with innocuous conditions). In prospective studies of asymptomatic populations comparing fecal occult blood screening with colonoscopy, only 26% of cancers and 12% of large adenomas were associated with positive Hemoccult tests. The low sensitivity explains why two thirds of colon cancers are not detected, and the low specificity explains why many colonoscopies (50 in the Minnesota trial) are required to detect one cancer. The decreased colon cancer mortality seen with fecal occult blood screening is probably due to the detection of early cancers rather than to the detection and removal of adenomas; adenomas rarely bleed, and the incidence of colon cancer is not decreased in screened populations.[8]

Fecal occult blood screening is not innocuous. The high false-negative rate may falsely reassure patients and lead them to ignore symptoms of cancer, and many patients without cancer are subjected to colonoscopy with its attendant complications. (See later discussion.) Possibly, deaths caused by screening cancel out the decreased mortality from colon cancer.[8]

The Canadian Task Force on Preventive Health Care gives FOBT a "C" recommendation,[9] while the U.S.

Preventive Services Task Force gives annual FOBT (with or without sigmoidoscopy, time interval not specified) a "B" recommendation.[10] In 2003, guidelines for screening for colorectal cancer were issued by a multidisciplinary expert panel administered by the American Gastroenterological Association under the auspices of the Agency for Health Care Policy and Research (AHCPR).[11] These guidelines were endorsed by a number of other organizations, including the American Cancer Society. The guidelines recommend that average-risk men and women 50 years and over undergo screening. Although the only screening programs that have been proved to decrease colon cancer mortality in randomized controlled studies are those using FOBT, the new guidelines offer several screening options to be selected by individual patients and their physicians. These are annual FOBT, flexible sigmoidoscopy every 5 years, flexible sigmoidoscopy every 5 years plus FOBT annually, barium enema every 5 to 10 years, and full colonoscopy every 10 years.[12]

In 1999 the Centers for Disease Control and Prevention, the Health Care Financing Administration, and the National Cancer Institute launched a campaign called "Screen for Life" to educate people in the United States about the value of screening for colorectal cancer. The website (http://www.cdc.gov/cancer/screenforlife) does not mention the very small number of individuals who might benefit from or the numerous adverse effects that are intrinsic to such a screening program.

Colonoscopy and sigmoidoscopy screening. No prospective randomized controlled trials have been published to show that screening sigmoidoscopy or colonoscopy decreases colon cancer mortality. However, case-control studies suggest a protective effect from sigmoidoscopy. Selby and co-workers[13] from the Kaiser Permanente Program in Oakland, California, studied a group of patients who died of colon cancer and compared them with a series of matched control subjects who did not have colon cancer. When cancers within reach of the sigmoidoscope were evaluated, 8.8% of the cancer patients had undergone one or more previous rigid sigmoidoscopies, compared with 24.2% of the control group. In contrast, when cancers above the reach of the sigmoidoscope were assessed, the rates of previous sigmoidoscopies were equal in the cancer patients and the control subjects. The protective effect of sigmoidoscopy was apparent even when it had been performed as much as 10 years previously.

In another study suggesting a protective effect of sigmoidoscopy, Atkin and associates[14] in Great Britain found that removal of tubular adenomas at sigmoidoscopy was associated with a low cancer rate at follow-up. Similar results were reported from a case-controlled Veterans Administration study in the United States; the odds ratio of mortality for patients who had a diagnostic procedure of the large bowel was 0.41 compared with control subjects who did not have such procedures. This protective effect was most marked if tissue had been removed.[15]

For flexible sigmoidoscopy or colonoscopy to be used as a screening method for the detection of colon cancer, the frequency of examinations needs to be determined. As noted previously, the AHCPR[11] recommends flexible sigmoidoscopy every 5 years or full colonoscopy every 10 years.[10] Another approach for which suggestive but not definitive evidence has been presented is selective colonoscopy for screening of high-risk patients such as those with a strong family history of colon cancer.[16]

Is the potential value of sigmoidoscopy screening decreased in the elderly? A Norwegian colonoscopy screening study of 193 asymptomatic men and women with a mean age of 67.4 years detected adenomas in 38% of the women and 47% of the men, and in almost half the cases the adenomas were proximal to the sigmoid colon and would not have been detected by sigmoidoscopy. However, since the average time for an adenoma to progress to malignancy is 10 to 15 years, most elderly patients would die of other causes before the development of colon cancer.[17]

The best-known complications of colonoscopy are perforation, major hemorrhage, and death. Both perforation and hemorrhage are more common if a polypectomy is performed during the endoscopy. In 1996 Waye, Kahn, and Auerbach[18] analyzed the combined complication rates of the few prospective studies of colonoscopy complications reported between 1987 and 1994. The perforation rate was 1:2222, the rate of significant hemorrhage was 1:81 if a polypectomy had been performed and 1:1352 if it had not, and the mortality rate was 1:16,745. These rates were lower than those reported in previous decades, a fact that Waye et al attributed to improved physician training and better instruments. They cautioned, however, that reports from centres with extensive experience in endoscopy may not reflect the experience of the broader medical community, since complication rates are known to be higher for inexperienced operators.[18]

Morbidity and mortality after colonoscopy are not limited to the complications of perforation and hemorrhage. The most common cause of death associated with colonoscopy is cardiac, possibly related to stress or to onerous preparatory regimens. The detection of cancers (or adenomas that cannot be resected during endoscopy) leads to surgical interventions—procedures with mortality rates of 1% to 7%. Some patients who die as a result of surgery harboured lesions that would never have manifested clinically had they been left alone.[8]

A rare but serious complication of colonoscopy is found in the report of the transmission of hepatitis C infection to two patients as a result of inadequate cleaning of a colonoscope.[19] That more cases have not been reported may be due to the difficulty in identifying the disease in many cases, because the incubation period is 30 to 90 days, and only 25% of affected persons become jaundiced.[20] Although following the established guidelines for cleaning colonoscopes should prevent such transmission of disease,[21] surveys suggest that inadequate disinfection is common in clinical practice.[22,23] One microbiology study found that 24% of "patient-ready" endoscopes were contaminated.[23]

Waye, Kahn, and Auerbach[18] were unable to find any randomized prospective trials reporting the complications of flexible sigmoidoscopy. Cohen and associates[24] quoted a perforation rate of 1:8795, and a 1996 Swedish report recorded a rate of 1:716.[25] The authors of the latter study attributed their high rate to the initial inexperience of the endoscopists.[25] A survey of British gastroenterologists reported a perforation rate of 1:16,810 for flexible fibre-optic sigmoidoscopy.[26]

A potential barrier to adopting population-based screening by flexible sigmoidoscopy is a lack of adequately trained endoscopists. Non-physician endoscopists might be the answer; two trials comparing endoscopies performed by a nurse[27,28] or physician assistant[28] with those performed by a gastroenterologist found no difference between the groups in the detection of adenomatous polyps or in complications.

Strong evidence suggests that screening by flexible fibre-optic sigmoidoscopy may decrease the incidence and mortality of colon cancer, but whether these probable benefits outweigh the adverse effects remains in question. In considering these issues, both physicians and patients should be aware that the published complication rates of sigmoidoscopy and colonoscopy are mostly from centres with considerable experience in the use of these instruments. Complication rates are almost certain to be higher for practitioners who only occasionally perform these procedures; however, such statistics are not currently available. Physicians should also realize that if such screening is undertaken, any value of repeat screening in negative cases and the time intervals at which it should be performed are unknown.

If screening sigmoidoscopy is undertaken, adequate bowel preparation is necessary. A prospective single-blinded randomized trial found that a light breakfast on the morning of the procedure followed by two Fleet phosphate enemas was as effective as more complex regimens involving oral laxatives, clear liquid dinner the previous evening, and nothing by mouth after midnight.[29]

Barium enema screening. Barium enema is the best radiographic examination, but may have to be followed by colonoscopy. Although no definitive studies have shown a decrease in colorectal mortality associated with double-contrast barium enema screening, the American Gastroenterological Association recommends this procedure every 5 to 10 years as an alternative to fecal occult blood or endoscopy screening. (See previous discussion.)[11] The rationale is that any procedure that can detect polyps and allow their removal should prevent colorectal cancer.

Virtual colonoscopy

A rapidly evolving technology that may play an important role in colon cancer screening is virtual colonoscopy. Bowel preparation is similar to that for conventional colonoscopy. The empty colon is distended with air, and multiple two-dimensional, thin-section images of the colon are rapidly obtained by means of helical computed tomography (CT). The images are then reconstructed off-line to create three-dimensional images simulating what is seen with conventional colonoscopy.[30] A recent study suggested that CT virtual three-dimensional colonoscopy is an accurate screeing method for the detection of colorectal neoplasia in asymptomatic average-risk adults. It compared favourably with optical colonoscopy for the detection of clinically relevant lesions. However, benefits of new diagnostic techniques are often initially overestimated because early reports usually come from centres with expertise that is difficult to replicate in other settings and this study was contradicted in another comparison of CT colonography (CTC) and standard colonoscopy on 615 patients, 50 years or older, from nine major hospital centres in the United States and United Kingdom. After the CTC, patients had conventional colonoscopy within 2 hours. CTC missed two of the eight patients with colon cancer and accuracy varied considerably between different centres and did not improve over time. Interestingly, patients did not report a preference for either technique.[31]

--- ❧ **REFERENCES** ❧ ---

1. Mandel JS, Bond JH, Church TR, et al: Reducing mortality from colorectal cancer by screening for fecal occult blood, *N Engl J Med* 328:1365-1371, 1993.
2. Robinson MH, Hardcastle JD, Moss SM, et al: The risks of screening: data from the Nottingham randomised controlled trial of faecal occult blood screening for colorectal cancer, *Gut* 45:588-592, 1999.
3. Mandel JS, Church TR, Ederer F, et al: Colorectal cancer mortality: effectiveness of biennial screening for fecal occult blood, *J Natl Cancer Inst* 91:434-437, 1999.
4. Mandel JS, Church TR, Ederer F: Screening for colorectal cancer (letter), *N Engl J Med* 329:1353-1354, 1993.
5. Hardcastle JD, Chamberlain JO, Robinson MH, et al: Randomised controlled trial of faecal-occult-blood screening for colorectal cancer, *Lancet* 348:1472-1477, 1996.
6. Kronborg O, Fenger C, Olsen J, et al: Randomised study of screening for colorectal cancer with faecal-occult-blood test, *Lancet* 348:1467-1471, 1996.
7. Towler B, Irwig L, Glasziou P, et al: A systematic review of the effects of screening for colorectal cancer using the faecal occult blood test, Hemoccult, *BMJ* 317:559-565, 1998.
8. Ahlquist DA: Fecal occult blood testing for colorectal cancer: can we afford to do this? *Gastroenterol Clin North Am* 26:41-55, 1997.
9. Canadian Task Force on the Periodic Health Examination: *Clinical preventive health care,* Ottawa, 1994, Canadian Communication Group, 798-809.
10. U.S. Preventive Services Task Force: *Guide to clinical preventive services,* ed 2, Baltimore, 1996, Williams & Wilkins, 89-103.
11. American Gastroenterological Association: Colorectal cancer screening and surveillance: clinical guidelines and rationale—update based on new evidence, *Gastroenterology* 124:544-560, 2003.
12. Winawer SJ, Fletcher RH, Miller L, et al: Colorectal cancer screening and surveillance: clinical guidelines, evidence and rationale, *Gastroenterology* 112:594-642, 1997.
13. Selby JV, Friedman GD, Quesenberry CP Jr, et al: A case-control study of screening sigmoidoscopy and mortality from colorectal cancer, *N Engl J Med* 326:653-657, 1992.
14. Atkin WS, Morson BC, Cuzick J: Long-term risk of colorectal cancer after excision of rectosigmoid adenomas, *N Engl J Med* 326:658-662, 1992.
15. Mueller AD, Sonnenberg A: Protection by endoscopy against death from colorectal cancer: a case-control study among veterans, *Arch Intern Med* 155:1741-1748, 1995.
16. Chen TH-H, Yen M-F, Lai M-S, et al: Evaluation of a selective screening for colorectal carcinoma: the Taiwan Multicenter Cancer Screening (TAMCAS) Project, *Cancer* 86:1116-1128, 1999.
17. Thiis-Evensen E, Hoff GS, Sauar J, et al: Flexible sigmoidoscopy or colonoscopy as a screening modality for colorectal adenomas in older age groups? Findings in a cohort of the normal population aged 63-72 years, *Gut* 45:834-839, 1999.
18. Waye JD, Kahn O, Auerbach ME: Complications of colonoscopy and flexible sigmoidoscopy, *Gastrointest Endosc Clin North Am* 6:343-374, 1996.
19. Bronowicki J-P, Venard V, Botté C, et al: Patient-to-patient transmission of hepatitis C virus during colonoscopy, *N Engl J Med* 337:237-240, 1997.
20. Bronowicki J-P, Bigard M-A: Transmission of hepatitis C virus during colonoscopy (letter), *N Engl J Med* 337:1849, 1997.
21. American Society for Gastrointestinal Endoscopy Ad Hoc Committee on Disinfection: Reprocessing of flexible gastrointestinal endoscopes, *Gastrointest Endosc* 43:540-546, 1996.
22. Spach DH, Silverstein FE, Stamm WE: Transmission of infection by gastrointestinal endoscopy and bronchoscopy, *Ann Intern Med* 118:117-128, 1993.
23. Kaczmarek RG, Moore RM, McCrohan J, et al: Multi-state investigation of the actual disinfection/sterilization of endoscopes in health care facilities, *Am J Med* 92:257-261, 1992.
24. Cohen LB, Basuk PM, Waye JD: *Practical flexible sigmoidoscopy,* New York, 1995, Igaku-Shoin, 117-125.
25. Kewenter J, Brevinge H: Endoscopic and surgical complications of work-up in screening for colorectal cancer, *Dis Colon Rectum* 39:676-680, 1996.
26. Robinson RJ, Stone M, Mayberry JF: Sigmoidoscopy and rectal biopsy—a survey of current UK practice, *Eur J Gastroenterol Hepatol* 8:149-151, 1996.

27. Schoenfeld P, Lipscomb S, Crook J, et al: Accuracy of polyp detection by gastroenterologists and nurse endoscopists during flexible sigmoidoscopy: a randomized trial, *Gastroenterology* 117:312-318, 1999.

28. Wallace MB, Kemp JA, Meyer F, et al: Screening for colorectal cancer with flexible sigmoidoscopy by nonphysician endoscopists, *Am J Med* 107:214-218, 1999.

29. Manoucheri M, Nakamura DY, Lukman RL: Bowel preparation for flexible sigmoidoscopy: which method yields the best results? *J Fam Pract* 48:272-274, 1999.

30. Pickhardt PJ, Choi JR, Hwang I, et al: Computed tomographic virtual colonoscopy to screen for colorectal neoplasia in asymptomatic adults, *N Engl J Med* 349: 2191-2200, 2003.

31. Cotton PB, Durkalski VL, Pineau BC, et al: Computed tomographic colonography (virtual colonoscopy): a multicenter comparison with standard colonoscopy for detection of colorectal neoplasia, *JAMA* 291:1713-1719, 2004.

Colonoscopy versus barium enema for investigation of suspected colon cancer

(See also secondary prevention of colon cancer)

If clinical findings indicate that a patient may have colon cancer, the major investigative techniques of choice are colonoscopy and barium enema. FOBT has little or no value in this context, since further investigation is required regardless of whether the test result is positive.

A complete colonoscopy and a well-performed barium enema are excellent means of detecting cancers and polyps. A double-contrast barium enema likely gives a greater yield for polyps smaller than 1 cm than does a single-contrast study, but for polyps larger than 1 cm, they are equally effective.[1] Both barium enema and colonoscopy detect a few cases that were missed by the other. One review of the radiological literature found that colorectal cancer was detected by barium enema in 90% to 99% of cases.[2] In general, rigid sigmoidoscopy detects about 25% of colonic polyps, and flexible 60-cm fibreoptic sigmoidoscopy detects 50% to 60%.[3]

A clear advantage of colonoscopy is that a biopsy can be performed at once if a cancer is detected and that a polyp, if seen, can be removed during the procedure. Another advantage, according to one survey, is that patients prefer colonoscopy to a double-contrast barium enema, probably because of the sedating and analgesic medications given with the former.[4]

An important factor influencing the choice of any investigative procedure is complication rates. For a barium enema, the perforation rate is 1:10,000 and the mortality rate is 1:50,000.[3] For a full colonoscopy, these numbers are higher. (See discussion of secondary prevention of colon cancer.)

────────   ❧ REFERENCES ❧   ────────

1. Donald JJ, Burhenne HJ: Colorectal cancer: can we lower the death rate in the 1990s? *Can Fam Physician* 39:107-114, 1993.

2. Levine R, Tenner S, Fromm H: Prevention and early detection of colorectal cancer, *Am Fam Physician* 45:663-668, 1992.

3. Gelfand DW, Ott DJ: The economic implications of radiologic screening for colonic cancer, *Am J Roentgenol* 156:939-943, 1991.

4. Van Ness MM, Chobanian SJ, Winters C Jr, et al: A study of patient acceptance of double-contrast barium enema and colonoscopy: which procedure is preferred by patients? *Arch Intern Med* 147:2175-2176, 1987.

Management of colorectal cancer

Adjuvant chemotherapy. A combination of fluorouracil and levamisole has been shown to decrease the rate of recurrence of stage III (Dukes' C) colon cancer by 40% and the death rate by 33%.[1] Chemotherapy also appears to provide a slight benefit in stage II (Dukes' B) disease, but whether it should be prescribed for all patients is not yet clear.[2]

Adjuvant radiation therapy. A randomized prospective study from Sweden compared surgery alone with preoperative radiation plus surgery for resectable rectal carcinoma. After 5 years the local recurrence rate among those who did not receive radiation therapy was 27% compared with 11% among those who were irradiated. The overall 5-year survival was 48% in the surgery-only group and 58% in the surgery plus radiation therapy group.[3]

Resection of hepatic metastases. Resection of hepatic metastases is associated with a 2-year survival rate of 65%. In one study the addition of hepatic arterial chemotherapy infusion combined with systemic chemotherapy led to a 2-year survival rate of 86%.[4]

Alcohol avoidance. A small Japanese study reported a higher rate of liver metastases in patients with colon cancer who consumed alcohol than among those who did not.[5]

Postoperative surveillance. The American Society of Clinical Oncology guidelines for postoperative surveillance advise that the following interventions be undertaken: history and physical examinations every 3 to 6 months for the first 3 years and annually thereafter (expert opinion), colonoscopy every 3 to 5 years, regular flexible sigmoidoscopy for those who had rectal cancer resected but who received no adjuvant radiation therapy, and carcinoembryonic antigen assays every 2 to 3 months for patients with stage II disease provided they would be suitable candidates for resection of hepatic metastases. The Society of Clinical Oncology advises against performing regular complete blood counts, liver function tests, FOBTs, chest X-ray examinations, CT, and pelvic imaging.[6]

────────   ❧ REFERENCES ❧   ────────

1. Moertel CG, Fleming TR, Macdonald JS, et al: Fluorouracil plus levamisole as effective adjuvant therapy

after resection of stage III colon carcinoma: a final report, *Ann Intern Med* 122:321-326, 1995.

2. Harrington DP: The tea leaves of small trials (editorial), *J Clin Oncol* 17:1336-1338, 1999.

3. Swedish Rectal Cancer Trial: Improved survival with preoperative radiotherapy in resectable rectal cancer, *N Engl J Med* 336:980-987, 1997.

4. Kemeny N, Huang Y, Cohen A, et al: Hepatic arterial infusion of chemotherapy after resection of hepatic metastases from colorectal cancer, *N Engl J Med* 341:2039-2048, 1999.

5. Maeda M, Nagawa H, Maeda T, et al: Alcohol consumption enhances liver metastasis in colorectal carcinoma patients, *Cancer* 83:1483-1488, 1998.

6. Desch CE, Benson AB III, Smith TJ, et al: Recommended colorectal cancer surveillance guidelines by the American Society of Clinical Oncology, *J Clin Oncol* 17:1312-1321, 1999.

Diverticulitis

Classic triad: Fever, WBC, resp. abdo Pain [handwritten annotation]

In Western society, diverticula are found in 5% to 10% of individuals over 45 years of age and the vast majority of those over age 80. Diverticulitis develops in only 20% of those with diverticula, and in 85% of cases, the disease involves the descending or sigmoid colon. The most common presenting symptoms and signs are pain and tenderness in the left lower quadrant. If the affected bowel is near the bladder, the patient may have dysuria and frequency, and if it crosses the midline, tenderness may be detected in the right lower quadrant. Diarrhea or constipation may also occur; gross blood in the stool is rare.[1]

The imaging process of choice for diagnosing diverticulitis is CT scanning. Endoscopy may help rule out other conditions but is not useful for making a positive diagnosis of diverticulitis because the inflammatory process in this condition is in the pericolic region and the bowel mucosa is normal.[1]

Treatment of a mild first attack of diverticulitis in patients who can tolerate oral hydration is a 7- to 10-day course of a liquid diet combined with broad-spectrum oral antibiotics (e.g., ciprofloxacin and metronidazole) that cover both aerobic and anaerobic organisms. Sicker patients, or those who do not respond to outpatient management, require admission, nothing by mouth, and IV antibiotics. In many cases abscesses detected by CT scanning can be drained percutaneously with CT guidance. About 20% of patients with diverticulitis require surgery. Once the acute attack has resolved, the patient should be placed on a high-fibre diet.[1]

≈ REFERENCES ≥

1. Ferzoco LB, Raptopoulos V, Silen W: Acute diverticulitis, *N Engl J Med* 338:1521-1526, 1998.

Familial Polyposis

Presymptomatic diagnosis of adenomatous familial polyposis is possible in the majority of cases by a blood test involving molecular genetic diagnosis.[1] Both indomethacin (Indocin, Indocid) and sulindac (Clinoril) have been shown to cause regression of polyps in familial polyposis and are routinely prescribed for patients who have had a total colectomy with ileorectal anastomosis.[2]

≈ REFERENCES ≥

1. Powell SM, Petersen GM, Krush AJ, et al: Molecular diagnosis of familial adenomatous polyposis, *N Engl J Med* 329:1982-1987, 1993.

2. Hirota C, Iida M, Aoyagi K, et al: Effect of indomethacin suppositories on rectal polyposis in patients with familial adenomatous polyposis, *Cancer* 78:1660-1665, 1996.

CONSTIPATION

(See also anal fissures)

According to the "Rome II criteria," constipation is the presence of two or more of the following symptoms for at least 3 months out of the preceding 12 months[1]:

- Three or fewer bowel movements a week
- Hard lumpy stool on more than 25% of occasions
- Straining at defecation on more than 25% of occasions
- Sensation of incomplete evacuation on more than 25% of occasions

An initial approach to a patient with constipation involves a thorough history of diet, exercise, medications (including fibre and previous laxative use) and fluid intake (including caffeine and alcohol consumption). Any relevant medical and surgical history should be obtained to determine such things as neurological disorders, diabetes, hypothyroidism, IBS, hemorrhoids, anal fissure, and previous abdominal surgeries, to mention a few.

Complications of constipation include fecal impaction, obstruction and perforation, urinary incontinence, and psychological disorders.[2] Straining raises intrathoracic pressure, which can lead to reduced coronary and cerebral circulation, development of hernias, worsening gastroesophageal reflux, and transient ischemic attacks (TIAs) and syncope in the elderly.[2]

Management of Constipation in the Community

Once organic disease is ruled out, most patients in the community can be managed with exercise, good hydration, and fibre (25 to 30 g per day). If this does not resolve the problem in approximately 1 month (or less if a rapid response is required), laxatives should be considered. Proof of comparative efficacy between different laxative groups is lacking. Available evidence shows that bulk-forming agents are likely as effective as other groups.[3] Patients can be started on regular supplements of psyllium (Metamucil, Prodiem), beginning with 1 tbsp per day and working up as rapidly as possible to 3 tbsp per day. Each dose should be accompanied or followed by 237 ml (8 oz) of water or other fluid. An osmotic laxative, such as lactulose (Lactulax) 30 to 60 ml at bedtime or magnesium hydroxide (Milk of Magnesia) 15 to 30 ml at bedtime can also be added. Most osmotic laxatives take several days to work. Stimulant laxatives (Senokot 187 mg once a day, Dulcolax 5 to 10 mg every night) work quicker but may cause more nausea and cramping.[4] For many patients, however, laxatives do not provide sustained relief of symptoms. In addition, increasing dietary fibre has been shown to worsen symptoms in many patients by causing increased bloating without an improvement in bowel function.[5]

People with diabetes should avoid lactulose and sorbitol since the metabolites (fructose and lactose) may alter blood glucose levels. People with lactose intolerance may find lactose most effective. Use of other laxatives, including mineral oil, those that cause intestinal secretion (docusate [Colace, Regulex]), and stimulant laxatives (sennosides [Senokot], bisacodyl [Dulcolax], glycerin suppositories), can be used if no improvement occurs. Tegaserod is a colonic prokinetic agent that improves stool consistency in women with IBS characterized by constipation.[6] However, a recent letter to health care professionals from the drug's manufacturer warns of serious adverse events in some cases. Although 1 in 10 patients taking the drug will experience mild diarrhea, about 1 in 250 will have very serious diarrhea complicated by hypovolemia, hypotension, and syncope that sometimes necessitates admission to hospital and IV therapy[7]. Regular reassessment of the patient is critical to avoid laxative abuse syndrome.

Laxatives in Palliative Care

Pharmacological therapy is the mainstay of treatment for the prevention and management of constipation in the palliative care population. Non-pharmacological measures should also be incorporated in parallel. When initiating opioid therapy, the physician should also start the patient on a laxative. Stool softeners and peristaltic stimulants take 6 to 9 hours to work, so they should be given at bedtime. The two should be administered together, because using only a stool softener may cause soft stool to accumulate in the rectum. Suppositories work within the hour, so they should be given half an hour before breakfast or supper.[8] The suppositories should be pushed against rectal mucosa, not into stool. They should be inserted with the "base" and not the pointed end first.

The following sequence of therapeutic interventions for constipation is one physician's guideline for palliative care.[8] Missing here is the osmotic laxative lactulose (Lactulax). Doses of 15 to 60 ml per day are usually very effective.

1. Encourage fluids, fibre, and exercise.
2. Use one of these: standardized sennosides (Senokot) 1 to 2 tablets at bedtime plus docusate sodium (Colace, Regulex) 100 mg twice a day; or bisacodyl (Dulcolax) 5 to 15 mg orally at bedtime plus docusate sodium

(Colace, Regulex) 100 mg twice a day; or magnesium hydroxide (Milk of Magnesia) 15 to 30 ml at bedtime plus docusate sodium (Colace, Regulex) 100 mg twice a day.
3. Increase docusate sodium (Colace, Regulex) to 200 to 300 mg twice a day and double the dose of one of the other three laxatives.
4. Add one glycerin suppository and one bisacodyl (Dulcolax) suppository before breakfast.
5. Prescribe a phosphate enema (Fleet enema).
6. Prescribe an oil enema if the stool is hard or a saline enema if the stool is soft.
7. Disimpact the bowel.

Constipation in Children

One definition of constipation in children is having one bowel movement every 3 to 15 days.[9] Usually the condition is self-limited and responds to increases in dietary fibre and a program encouraging regular bowel habits. If these are unsuccessful, a short trial of Milk of Magnesia in doses of 1 to 2 ml/kg may be tried.[10] In some cases changing from cow's milk to a protein-hydrolysate formula containing 100% whey protein[10] or to soy milk[9] resolves the problem. (See discussion of anal fissures.)

An essential examination in children with chronic constipation or encopresis (because encopresis is often secondary to fecal impaction) is a digital rectal examination (DRE). In a study of 128 children referred to a pediatric gastroenterology centre for chronic constipation, 77% had not had a DRE performed by the referring physicians, and over half had fecal impaction. The treatment of severe fecal impaction is repeated phosphate enemas followed by laxative therapy.[11]

────────────── ❧ **REFERENCES** ❧ ──────────────

1. Thompon WG, Longstretch GF, Drossman DA, et al: Functional bowel disorders and functional abdominal pain, *Gut* 45(Suppl. II):1143-1147, 1999.
2. McCormack J: Gastrointestinal diseases: drug therapy for constipation. In: McCormack J, ed: *Drug therapy: decision making guide,* London, 1996, W.B. Saunders, 60-64.
3. Tramonte SM, Brand MB, Murlow CD, et al: The treatment of chronic constipation in adults: a systematic review, *J Gen Intern Med* 12(1):15-24, 1997.
4. Lembo A, Camilleri M: Chronic constipation, *N Engl J Med* 349:1360-1368, 2003.
5. Kamm MA: Constipation and its management, *BMJ* 327(7413):459-460, Aug 30 2003.)
6. American College of Gastroenterology Functional Gastrointestinal Disorders Task Force: Evidence-based position statement on the management of irritable bowel syndrome in North America, *Am J Gastroenterol* 97:S1-S5, 2002.
7. Health Canada: Important safety update. *Diarrhea and ischemic colitis in patients using Zelnorm (tegaserod hydrogen maleate).* [Letter]. Dorval (QC): Novartis Pharmaceutical Canada Inc, 2004.

8. Van Tilburg EG: Constipation: a frequent iatrogenic complication in cancer patients receiving narcotics, *Can Fam Physician* 36:967-970, 1990.
9. Loening-Baucke V: Constipation in children (editorial), *N Engl J Med* 339:1155-1156, 1998.
10. Iacono G, Cavataio F, Montalto G, et al: Intolerance of cow's milk and chronic constipation in children, *N Engl J Med* 339:1100-1104, 1998.
11. Gold DM, Levine J, Weinstein TA, et al: Frequency of digital rectal examination in children with chronic constipation, *Arch Pediatr Adolesc Med* 153:377-379, 1999.

DIARRHEA

(See also celiac disease; cryptosporidiosis; cyclosporiasis; food borne illnesses; giardiasis; irritable bowel syndrome; lactose intolerance; travellers' diarrhea)

Diarrhea has a variety of causes, including infectious disease, inflammatory bowel disease, malabsorption syndromes, medications, toxins, malignancies, and endocrine abnormalities.

Acute Diarrhea

Most episodes of acute diarrhea are infectious in nature (Table 24).

Laboratory investigation (stool culture and sensitivity, stool for ova and parasites, fecal leukocytes, and occult blood) should be considered for patients presenting with fever, blood (dysentery) or mucus in the stool, dehydration, recent travel or antibiotic use, and diarrhea present for longer than 4 to 5 days.

Most cases of mild-to-moderate diarrhoea (i.e., minimal cramps, no fever, and non-bloody stools) are self-limited. Personal hygiene with hand washing and disinfection of contaminated surfaces should be stressed. Normal feeding should be started as soon as possible in children and adults after a period of oral rehydration therapy with commercially available solutions. There is no evidence that fasting will have any benefit.[3]

Loperamide (Imodium) can be used for the symptomatic control of mild-to-moderate diarrhea in patients over the age of 2 years. In cases of severe diarrhea (dysentery), the use of loperamide has been associated with toxic megacolon and hemoloytic uremic syndrome in children with *Escherichia coli* O157:H7.[3] In adults, the usual dose of loperamide is 4 mg (2 tablets) initially and then 2 mg after each subsequent loose stool. Maximum is 16 mg (8 tablets) per day. Lomitil (diphenoxylate and atropine sulphate) is not recommended because of its habit-forming potential (with a pharmacological similarity between diphenoxylate and meperidine) and its central nervous system effects. Antibiotic therapy is appropriate for patients with positive stool cultures, high-risk patients, or those presenting with dysentery. Randomized controlled trials show that ciprofloxacin reduces the duration of community-acquired diarrhea by 1 to 2 days.[3]

Table 24   Selected Infectious Diseases Causing Diarrhea

Bacterial	Viral	Parasitic
Salmonella	Rotaviruses	*Giardia lamblia*
Shigella	Norwalk viruses	*Entamoeba histolytica*
Campylobacter	Adenoviruses	*Cyclospora cayetanensis*
Yersinia	Astroviruses	Cryptosporidiosis
Enterotoxigenic		
Eschericha coli		
Enteroinvasive *E. coli*		
Verotoxin-producing		
E. coli (hamburger		
disease; hemorrhagic		
colitis)		
Clostridium difficile		
Clostridium perfringens		
Vibrio cholerae		
Vibrio parahaemolyticus		

Chronic Diarrhea

Chronic diarrhea is defined as persistent diarrhea lasting more than 4 weeks. Before being placed into this category, a patient should be on a lactose-free diet for several days, since lactase deficiency may be a result of an infectious agent and cause persistence of symptoms after the organisms themselves have been eradicated.[4]

Excluding irritable bowel disease, lactase deficiency, and diarrhea in HIV-positive patients, the following, in order of frequency, are the most common causes of chronic diarrhea treated by gastroenterologists[4]:

1. Infections (giardiasis, amebiasis, *Clostridium difficile,* cyclosporiasis)
2. Inflammatory bowel disease
3. Steatorrhea (greasy or bulky stools difficult to flush, bad odor, oil in toilet bowel requiring brush for removal, weight loss)
4. Medications (e.g., antibiotics, antihypertensives, magnesium-containing antacids), foods (ethanol, caffeine), sweeteners (sorbitol in gum or mints, fructose in corn syrup)
5. Previous GI surgery
6. Endocrine disease such as hyperthyroidism
7. (Addison's disease, diabetes mellitus, hyperthyroidism, hypothyroidism) Laxative abuse (often concealed by patient or parent)
8. Ischemic bowel disease
9. Radiation enteritis or colitis
10. Colon cancer
11. Idiopathic (functional)

Given the extensive differential diagnosis, referral to a specialist for investigation is warranted. A recent British guideline highlighted the importance of considering celiac disease and laxative abuse.[5]

While waiting for a definitive diagnosis, empirical treatment may include dietary restrictions, increase in dietary or supplemental fibre, or cholestyramine (Questran) 2 to 4 g (a half to a full packet) one to six times a day. Antibiotic use is discussed under "Travellers' Diarrhea."

─────────────── ❧ **REFERENCES** ❧ ───────────────

1. Gorbach SL: Treating diarrhoea (editorial), *BMJ* 314:1776-1777, 1997.
2. Wong CS, Jelacic S, Habeeb RL, et al: The risk of the hemolytic-uremic syndrome after antibiotic treatment of *Escherichia coli* O157:H7 infections, *N Engl J Med* 342:1930-1936, 2000.
3. Farthing M: Treatment and prevention of diarrhea, *Practitioner* 242(1586):388-394, 1998.
4. Donowitz, Kokke FT, Saidi R: Evaluation of patients with chronic diarrhea, *N Engl J Med* 332:725-729, 1995.
5. Thomas PD, et al: Guidelines for the investigation of chronic diarrhoea, *Gut* 52(Suppl V):v1–v15, 2003.

ESOPHAGUS

(See also asthma; chronic cough; esophageal candidiasis; peptic ulcer)

Achalasia

Achalasia is a rare disease caused by inadequate relaxation of the lower esophageal sphincter and aperistalsis of the esophageal smooth muscles. Initial symptoms are dysphagia and heartburn. Aspiration is a complication of the disorder. Patients also have a sixteenfold relative increase in their risk for carcinoma of the esophagus. Surveillance endoscopy for carcinoma is not recommended because the absolute risk is low and because 681 annual endoscopies would be necessary to detect one cancer.[1]

Treatment modalities for achalasia include isosorbide dinitrate or calcium channel blockers, botulinum toxin injections into the sphincter (the effect lasts for less than a year), balloon dilatation, and surgery, which can be performed using a laparoscopic approach.[1]

Dysphagia

Dysphagia may be esophageal or oropharyngeal. If a patient has trouble getting the food bolus out of the mouth or has nasal regurgitation, choking, or coughing upon swallowing, dysphagia is likely to be oropharyngeal, whereas a definite feeling of sticking in the retrosternum indicates esophageal dysphagia. The initial symptom of organic stricture is difficulty swallowing solids, whereas motor disorders such as may be associated with cerebrovascular accidents, amyotrophic lateral sclerosis, myasthenia gravis, or other neurological conditions may be associated with episodic difficulty in swallowing both liquids and solids from the beginning. Idiopathic oropharyngeal neuromuscular dysphagia is common in the elderly, and many such persons never seek medical help for the condition.[2]

Gastroesophageal Reflux Disease

Gastroesophageal reflux occurs mainly from transient relaxation of the lower esophageal sphincter, and less commonly from a low resting sphincter pressure. Other causes include reduced esophageal or gastric acid clearance, reduced resistance of the esophageal mucosa, and increased gastric acid secretion. An associated hiatus hernia enhances reflux.[3] Other causes include pregnancy, diabetes, connective tissue diseases, food, and drugs.

In North America, gastroesophageal reflux disease (GERD) affects 20% of adults at least once a week and 4% to 9% on a daily basis.[4] In Asia GERD is rare, probably because of a high prevalence of chronic gastritis secondary to widespread *H. pylori* infection[5]; chronic gastritis decreases acid secretion and protects against GERD.[5,6]

Coronary artery disease may be difficult to differentiate from GERD. According to one study, coronary artery disease can be ruled out with reasonable certainty if symptoms are controlled by omeprazole (Prilosec, Losec) 40 mg twice a day for 7 days (omeprazole test).[7] Lower doses of omeprazole and ranitidine are ineffective for this purpose.[8] The sensitivity of this test is similar to pH monitoring.

Several reports suggest that reflux sometimes induces "acid laryngitis," which manifests as persistent cough, hoarseness, and a continual need to clear the throat. The existence of this entity is controversial. Believers treat the patients with omeprazole for 2 months,[3] but no randomized controlled studies have been published documenting benefit from this therapy.[9] Other reports suggest that reflux has a role in causing some cases of asthma. (This is discussed under Asthma.)

Guidelines from the American College of Gastroenterology recommend that patients with mild symptomatic GERD be started on empirical therapy without prior endoscopy provided they are less than 50 years old and have no "alarm" features such as weight loss, recurrent vomiting, bleeding or anemia, dysphagia, or odynophagia.[10]

The initial treatment of symptomatic esophageal reflux involves lifestyle changes and over-the-counter medications,[9-11] although few of these measures have been established by well-controlled trials.[11] Most cases with mild symptoms can be successfully controlled by these measures,[9-11] which include the following:

1. Avoid bedtime snacks.
2. Avoid foods that relax the lower esophageal sphincter, such as fats, whole milk, chocolate, orange juice, tomatoes, carminatives (peppermint), and ethanol.
3. Discontinue smoking.
4. Raise the head of the bed by at least 14 cm.
5. Take alginic acids such as Gaviscon Heart Burn Relief Formula (there are Gaviscon products without alginic acid) or Gastrocote. The usual dose is 2 to 4 tablets well chewed three or four times a day.

6. Use antacids such as calcium carbonate (Tums) or aluminum hydroxide/magnesium hydroxide (Maalox).
7. Use over-the-counter H_2-blockers.

For many patients a combination of antacids and alginic acid is more effective than either one alone. Antacids act more quickly than H_2-blockers, but their duration of action is shorter. Patients who can predict activities that are likely to induce reflux should self-medicate prophylactically.[10] However, these medications appear to have no effect on endoscopic healing.

For patients who do not respond to the measures outlined above, the physician can either use "step-up" or "step-down" therapy. The former starts with low-potency drugs such as H_2-blockers and if necessary, the physician replaces them with more potent proton pump inhibitors. Alternatively, therapy can begin with high doses of proton pump inhibitors, which are then titrated down to lower doses and then less potent agents provided the patient remains asymptomatic. Clinicians seem to tend toward step-up therapy when symptoms are mild and tend toward step-down therapy when the symptoms are moderate to severe or there is diagnostic uncertainty as to whether it is an acid problem. In the past, prokinetic agents have been as effective as H_2-blockers, but are currently not recommended for use in family practice.[12] Proton pump inhibitors are preferable in terms of cost, compliance, and safety (see later discussion) when treating erosive esophagitis and probably also non-erosive disease.[13] Over time, patients with mild disease can often discontinue medications or use them only on demand; those with severe disease may require prolonged maintenance therapy.[11] One suggested protocol is to start patients with omeprazole 20 mg per day for 2 weeks or, if symptoms have not completely resolved, for 4 weeks. Thereafter, medications are given only if symptoms recur. Ranitidine 150 to 300 mg twice a day may be used instead of omeprazole, but symptom relief is not as rapid.[14] Tolerance can also occur with H_2-receptor anatagonists; this generally does not occur with proton pump inhibitors.[15]

Frequently used H_2-blockers are cimetidine (Tagamet) 800 mg twice a day or ranitidine (Zantac) 150 mg twice a day. Both omeprazole (Prilosec, Losec) 20 to 40 mg per day and lansoprazole (Prevacid) 30 mg per day are effective proton pump inhibitors for GERD.

Surgical interventions should be considered when medical therapy fails.[10]

Barrett's Esophagus

Barrett's esophagus is the replacement of the squamous epithelium of the lower esophagus with the columnar epithelium of intestinal metaplasia.[4,16,17] It is strongly associated with GERD and is thought to develop as a metaplastic form of healing when acid reflux has eroded the squamous epithelium.[4] Barrett's esophagus is impor-tant because of its association with an increased incidence of adenocarcinoma of the lower esophagus.[4,17-20] Two large prospective endoscopic surveillance studies of patients with Barrett's esophagus in the United States found an adenocarcinoma incidence of 1:208[18] and 1:285[19] patient years. A population-based case-control study in Sweden reported that the risk of esophageal adenocarcinoma was eight times higher for patients who had regurgitation, heartburn, or both at least once a week, and over 20 times higher for those with more frequent or severe symptoms. Although the relative risk is high, the absolute risk is low. The authors of this study calculated that among patients with heartburn and thus a twenty-fold increased risk of cancer, only 1 in 1400 would be found to have malignancy over a 1-year period.[16]

In terms of cancer risk, management of patients with heartburn is controversial. Cohen and Parkman[4] recommend that if heartburn is severe enough to be a primary complaint, the patient be assessed by endoscopy and biopsies. According to these authors, aggressive long-term treatment of erosive lesions with medical therapy should be instituted. They also suggest that ablation of Barrett's tissue by use of laser or thermal techniques may be indicated.[4] Whether endoscopy is feasible or desirable for all patients with heartburn is questionable. Large numbers of patients would be subjected to the anxiety, discomfort, and danger of endoscopy for unproved benefit. As Lagergren and associates[16] point out, there is no proof that intensive medical management of GERD decreases the incidence of either Barrett's esophagus or adenocarcinoma of the esophagus.

Current guidelines recommend that once Barrett's esophagus is diagnosed by endoscopy and biopsy, regular endoscopic and biopsy surveillance to detect dysplasia and early cancer should occur.[17,20] Cancers detected by this means tend to be small and free of nodal metastases, but whether long-term survival is increased is unknown.[20] Identification of mild dysplasia has no clinical value, because 73% of such lesions regress spontaneously.[19] Management of severe dysplasia is controversial; up to 25% of cases regress, but others are associated with undetected carcinomas.[17,20]

Whether long-term intensive acid suppression can lead to regression of Barrett's esophagus is uncertain. One 2-year trial comparing ranitidine 150 mg twice a day with omeprazole 40 mg twice a day found no regression with ranitidine and a slight but statistically significant regression with omeprazole.[21]

Adenocarcinoma of the Esophagus

The incidence of adenocarcinoma of the esophagus has been increasing dramatically in the Western world over the past two decades, especially among white men, in whom its frequency now equals that of squamous cell cancer.[4] This rise has coincided with a marked decrease in the rate of *Helicobacter pylori* infection of the stomach. Preliminary evidence suggests that some strains of *H. pylori* exert a protective effect against gastroesophageal reflux disease, Barrett's esophagus, and adenocarcinoma of the esophagus.[22] The relationship of Barrett's esophagus to adenocarcinoma of the esophagus is discussed in the preceding section.

Most adenocarcinomas of the esophagus have regional lymph node involvement at the time of diagnosis. Stage 1, 2 and 3 disease may undergo curative resection provided there are no comorbidities. The 5-year survival rate after surgical resection is 15% to 20%, and the median survival after resection is 18 months.[23] One study found that preoperative radiation therapy and chemotherapy increased the 3-year survival rate for resectable tumours from 6% to 32%.[24]

Esophageal Varices

The treatment of choice for acute variceal bleeding is endoscopic band ligation of the varices.[25] Both beta blockers and endoscopic variceal ligation have been used to decrease the incidence of recurrent bleeding from esophageal varices; according to one editorial writer, management of first choice is a non-selective beta-adrenergic blocker such as propranolol.[26] One randomized control trial recently found that there was no difference in rebleeding or death in cirrhotic patients treated by beta blockers or endoscopy.[27] In the acute bleed, somatostatin analogues may reduce the number of transfusions required but not necessarily the mortality of this disease.[28] Patients with portal hypertension and esophageal bleeding who do not respond to other therapeutic modalities may be treated with a shunt between the portal and hepatic veins. Interventional radiologists do this by introducing a catheter through the jugular vein and passing it through the liver into the portal vein. This procedure is called a *transjugular intrahepatic portosystemic shunt (TIPS)*.[29]

❧ REFERENCES ❧

1. Spiess AE, Kahrilas PJ: Treating achalasia: from whalebone to laparoscope, *JAMA* 280:638-642, 1998.
2. Paterson WG: Dysphagia in the elderly, *Can Fam Physician* 42:925-932, 1996.
3. Pope CE II: Acid-reflux disorders, *N Engl J Med* 331: 656-660, 1994.
4. Cohen S, Parkman HP: Heartburn–a serious symptom (editorial), *N Engl J Med* 340:878-879, 1999.
5. Wu JC, Sung JJ, Ng EK, et al: Prevalence and distribution of *Helicobacter pylori* in gastroesophageal reflux disease: a study from the East, *Am J Gastroenterol* 94:1790-1794, 1999.
6. El-Serag HB, Sonnenberg A, Jamal MM, et al: Corpus gastritis is protective against reflux oesophagitis, *Gut* 45: 181-185, 1999.
7. Fass R, Ofmann JJ, Sampliner RE, et al: The Omeprazole Test is as sensitive as 24-hour oesophageal monitoring in

diagnosing gastro-oesophageal reflux disease in symptomatic patients with erosive oesophagitis, *Ailment Pharmacol Ther* 14:389-396, 2000.
8. Schindlbeck NE, Klauser AG, Voderholzer WA, et al: Empiric therapy for gastroesophageal reflux disease, *Arch Intern Med* 155:1808-1812, 1995.
9. Kahrilas PJ: Gastroesophageal reflux disease, *JAMA* 276:983-988, 1996.
10. DeVault KR, Castell DO (Practice Parameters Committee of the American College of Gastroenterology): Updated guidelines for the diagnosis and treatment of gastroesophageal reflux disease, *Am J Gastroenterol* 94:1434-1442, 1999.
11. Galmiche JP, Letessier E, Scarpignato C: Treatment of gastro-oesophageal reflux disease in adults, *BMJ* 316: 1720-1723, 1998.
12. Kim C, Harrison V, Heidelbaugh J, et al: *Management of gastro-esophageal reflux disease,* Ann Arbor, MI, 2002, University of Michigan Health System.
13. van Pinxteren B, Numans ME, Bonis PA, et al: Short term treatments with proton pump inhibitors, H_2 antagonists and prokinetics for gastro-esophageal reflux disease-like symptoms and endoscopy negative reflux disease. In: *The Cochrane Library,* issue 3, Oxford, 2003, Update Software.
14. Bardhan KD, Müller-Lissner S, Bigard MA, et al (European Study Group): Symptomatic gastro-oesophageal reflux disease: double blind controlled study of intermittent treatment with omeprazole, *BMJ* 318:502-507, 1999.
15. Caro JJ, Salas M, Ward A: Healing and relapse rates in gastro-oesophageal reflux disease with the newer proton-pump inhibitors compared with omeprazole, ranitidine and placebo: evidence from randomized controlled trials, *Clin Ther* 23:998-1017, 2001.
16. Lagergren J, Bergström R, Lindgren A, et al: Symptomatic gastroesophageal reflux as a risk factor for esophageal adenocarcinoma, *N Engl J Med* 340:825-831, 1999.
17. Sampliner RE and the Practice Parameters Committee of the American College of Gastroenterology: Practice guidelines on the diagnosis, surveillance and therapy of Barrett's esophagus, *Am J Gastroenterol* 93:1028-1032, 1998.
18. Drewitz DJ, Sampliner RE, Garewal HS: The incidence of adenocarcinoma in Barrett's esophagus–a prospective study of 170 patients followed 4.8 years, *Am J Gastroenterol* 92:212-215, 1997.
19. O'Connor JB, Falk GW, Richter JE: The incidence of adenocarcinoma and dysplasia in Barrett's esophagus, *Am J Gastroenterol* 94:2037-2042, 1999.
20. Morales TG, Sampliner RE: Barrett's esophagus: update on screening, surveillance, and treatment, *Arch Intern Med* 159:1411-1416, 1999.
21. Peters FT, Ganesh S, Kuipers EJ, et al: Endoscopic regression of Barrett's oesophagus during omeprazole treatment; a randomised double blind study, *Gut* 45:489-494, 1999.
22. Blaser MJ: *Helicobacter pylori* and gastric diseases, *BMJ* 316:1507-1510, 1998.
23. National Comprehensive Cancer Network: *Clinical practice guidelines in oncology,* vol 1, Jenkintown, PA, 2003, The Network.
24. Walsh TN, Noonan N, Hollywood D, et al: A comparison of multimodal therapy and surgery for esophageal adenocarcinoma, *N Engl J Med* 335:462-467, 1996.

25. Van Dam J, Brugge WR: Endoscopy of the upper gastrointestinal tract, *N Engl J Med* 341:1738-1748, 1999.

26. Burroughs AK, Patch D: Primary prevention of bleeding from esophageal varices (editorial), *N Engl J Med* 340:1033-1035, 1999.

27. Patch D, Sabin CA, Goulis J, et al : A randomized controlled trial of medical therapy vs endoscopic ligation for the prevention of variceal rebleeding in patients with cirrhosis, *Gastroenterology* 123:1013-1019, 2002.

28. Gotzche PC: Somatostatin analogues for acute bleeding oesophageal varices. In: *The Cochrane Library,* issue 4, Chichester, UK, 2003, John Wiley.

29. Miller-Catchpole R: Transjugular intrahepatic portosystemic shunt (TIPS): diagnostic and therapeutic technology assessment (DATTA), *JAMA* 273:1824-1830, 1995.

FLATUS

Alpha-galactosidase (Beano) is available as an over-the-counter tablet or liquid preparation. Its mode of action is to hydrolyze undigestible complex sugars (oligosaccharides) of certain vegetables into their digestible monosaccharides and disaccharides. Most cruciferous vegetables and most legumes have a high content of undigestible sugars. Patients with major flatus would benefit by avoiding beans, cabbage, uncooked broccoli, chickpeas, peas, lentils, brussels sprouts, cabbage, carrots, corn, leeks, squash, onions, parsnips, oats, and wheat.

In a study from San Diego, volunteers took 8 drops of Beano or 8 drops of placebo before a meal of meatless chili consisting of navy, pinto, and kidney beans. Beano decreased the number of times flatulence was passed.[1] No solid evidence has been presented that simethicone relieves the discomfort of "gas,"[2] and activated charcoal is ineffective in reducing the volume or odor of released intestinal gas.[3]

------------------ **⌖ REFERENCES ⌖** ------------------

1. Ganiats TG, Norcross WA, Halverson AL, et al: Does Beano prevent gas–a double-blind crossover study of oral alpha-galactosidase to treat dietary oligosaccharide intolerance, *J Fam Pract* 39:441-445, 1994.

2. Simethicone for gastrointestinal gas, *Med Lett* 38:57-58, 1996.

3. Suarez FL, Furne J, Springfield J, et al: Failure of activated charcoal to reduce the release of gases produced by the colonic flora, *Am J Gastroenterol* 94:208-212, 1999.

GALLSTONE AND GALLBLADDER DISEASE

Cholecystitis is defined as acute or chronic gallbladder inflammation. This can be found with or without gallstones.[1,2] Patients present with steady pain lasting longer than 1 day in the epigastrium and right upper quadrant, fever, chills, nausea and vomiting (70%), Murphy's sign, and a palpable gallbladder (20%). Without gallstones, the pain can be more vague and complications can occur more rapidly.[1-3]

Risk factors for gallstone formation include obesity, a sedentary lifestyle, a diet high in refined sugars and animal fats, rapid weight loss or starvation, pregnancy, and medications such as thiazides, contraceptives, or estrogen.[1,4,5] Gallstones are associated with Crohn's disease, diabetes, increased triglycerides, decreased high-density lipoproteins, alcoholic cirrhosis, chronic hemolysis, duodenal diverticulae, truncal vagotomy, and hyperparathyroidism. It occurs more commonly in women, Pima Indians, and Scandanavians. Positive maternal family history of gallstones is another risk factor.[1]

Gallbladder disease can be complicated by ascending cholangitis as defined by Charcot's triad—pain, jaundice, and chills; refractory sepsis defined by Raynold's pentad —Charcot's triad plus altered mentation and hypotension; and pancreatitis.[1-3]

The pain of gallbladder disease must be differentiated from other causes of abdominal pain. Differential diagnosis includes biliary colic, right lower lobe pneumonia, acute myocardial infarction, abdominal aortic aneurysm, hepatic abscesses, perforated viscus, and gonoccocal perihepatitis. Infection may be the primary cause of acalculous cholecystitis. Polyarteritis nodosa and Kawasaki's disease may also present with acute cholecystitis.[1,2]

Biliary colic tends to be infrequent, episodic, and intense. Short, fleeting pain or continuous pain is usually not due to gallstones.[1] Meperidine (Demerol) has been considered preferable to morphine for controlling the pain of biliary colic on the grounds that morphine causes more constriction of the sphincter of Oddi. This is a myth; morphine is more effective, less toxic, and does not increase the risk of pancreatitis.[5] A non-narcotic alternative available in the United Kingdom is diclofenac (Voltaren) 75 to 150 mg given intravenously, intramuscularly, or rectally.[6]

Routine testing to be done in the assessment of gallbladder disease includes a complete blood count, liver function tests, amylase, and an electrocardiogram.[1,2] Diagnostic imaging should include ultrasonography to confirm or exclude the presence of gallstones. CT or magnetic resonance imaging (MRI) can also be used to detect common bile duct stones as well as rule out abscesses, neoplasms or pancreatitis.[1] Endoscopic retrograde cholangiopancreatography (ERCP) is the best method of diagnosing choledocholelithiasis and provides therapeutic options including sphincterotomy.[7,8] This procedure is complicated by acute pancreatitis or retroperitoneal perforation in 5% to 10% of cases. Biliary scintography (HIDA scan) can also be used to diagnose gallbladder disease; however, it does not demonstrate the presence of gallstones and is best used to exclude acute cholecystitis.[1]

Management of gallbladder disease depends on the specific clinical picture. The presence of asymptomatic gallstones is not an indication for surgery because the incidence of biliary pain in such circumstances is only 1% to 2% per year and decreases over time; serious sequelae are 10 times less frequent in asymptomatic cases. Clear indications for cholecystectomy are acute cholecystitis and gallstone-associated pancreatitis. Even one episode of biliary colic has a high risk of recurrence. In 30% no more episodes of pain occur, but overall risk of recurrent pain is 30% to 50% per year for a few years.[1]

Once the diagnosis of acute cholecystitis is confirmed and the patient is hemodynamically stable, early cholecystectomy is indicated. Advantages of laparoscopic versus open cholecystectomy are less pain, shorter hospital stay, faster return to work (within 10 days), and minimal abdominal scarring. Early laparoscopic cholecystectomy (within 72 hours of hospital admission) is associated with increased safety, fewer conversions to open cholecystectomy, and more socio-economic benefits, such as earlier return to work and decreased hospital stay.[2,9]

If surgical treatment is not possible, the second choice of treatment for gallstones is drug therapy with either ursodiol (ursodeoxycholic acid) or chenodiol (chenodeoxycholic acid).[11] Therapy lasts 6 to 12 months, and stone dissolution rate is under 50%. Unfortunately therapy is often limited by side effects such as nausea, vomiting, diarrhea, and pruritis. Therapy treatments can also interact with other medications and are contraindicated in pregnancy and breastfeeding.

Some patients experience post-cholecystectomy cholecystitis pain syndrome due to the dysfunction of the sphincter of Oddi.[2,7,8] Major symptoms are abdominal pain and the transient elevation of liver enzymes, most frequently diagnosed in women. Treatment is a sphincterotomy by ERCP, but this only relieves symptoms in less than 75% of patients and has a complication rate of 8%.[1]

--- **REFERENCES** ---

1. Ahmed A, Cheung RC, Keefe EB: Management of gallstones and their complications. *Am Fam Physician* 61: 1673-1680, 2000.
2. Moscati RM: Cholelithiasis, cholecystitis, and pancreatitis, *Emerg Med Clin North Amer* 14(4):719-737, 1996.
3. Bateson M: Gallbladder disease, *BMJ* 318:1745-1748, 1999.
4. Misciagna G, Centonze S, Leoci C, et al: Diet, physical activity, and gallstones—a population-based, case-control study in southern Italy, *Am J Clin Nutr* 69:120-126, 1999.
5. Syngal S, Coakley EH, Willett WC, et al: Long-term weight patterns and risk for cholecystectomy in women, *Ann Intern Med* 130:471-477, 1999.
6. Lee F: Meperidine vs morphine in pancreatitis and cholecystitis (letter), *Arch Intern Med* 158:2399, 1998.
7. Brugge WR, Van Dam J: Pancreatic and biliary endoscopy, *N Engl J Med* 341:1808-1816, 1999.
8. Huigregtse K: Complications of endoscopic sphincterotomy and their prevention (editorial), *N Engl J Med* 335:961-963, 1996.
9. Lo C-M, Liu CL, Fan ST, et al: Prospective randomized study of early versus delayed laparoscopic cholecystectomy for acute cholecystitis, *Ann Surg* 227:461-467, 1998.
10. Fletcher DR, Hobbs MS, Tan P, et al: Complications of cholecystectomy: risks of the laparoscopic approach and protective effects of operative cholangiography; a population-based study, *Ann Surg* 229:449-459, 1999.
11. Howard DE, Fromm H: Bile salts: metabolic, pathologic, and therapeutic consideration. Nonsurgical management of gallstone disease, *Gastroenterol Clin* 28:133-144, 1999.

HEMATOCHEZIA, RECTAL BLEEDING
(See also anal and rectal disorders; anemia; colon cancer; sports medicine)

Hematochezia is common, but fortunately the majority of patients with overt rectal bleeding do not have cancer. Differential diagnosis of rectal bleeding commonly includes hemorrhoids, abscesses, fistula, fissures, and cancer. In a British community study, 38% of respondents (4006) to a questionnaire reported at least one episode of rectal bleeding in their lifetimes, and 18% had had such bleeding within the past 12 months. Only 28% of those who had rectal bleeding in the past year sought medical advice. Rectal cancer was diagnosed in only one patient, giving a predictive value of rectal bleeding for colorectal cancer in the community of 1:709.[1] In another study, patients younger than 40 years with non-acute rectal bleeding have a 1% chance of cancer; however, this study was done in a referral centre so the actual risk is likely to be considerably lower.[2]

Such data suggest that rectal bleeding is relatively innocuous. That this might not be the case is indicated by a study of U.S. veterans (almost all male and 80% over age 40). They were specifically asked about a history of rectal bleeding and, if it had occurred in the past 3 months, were given a complete examination of the colon. Colon cancer was detected in 6.5%, polyps in 13%, and inflammatory bowel disease in 4.5%. The character of the bleeding (e.g., frequency of bleeding, on the toilet paper, mixed with stool) did not distinguish innocuous from severe disease. The only two clinical features that correlated with a diagnosis of cancer were age and duration of bleeding of less than 2 months.[3] In primary care, the risk of cancer in patients with rectal bleeding is estimated to be 1:30.[4] In a study of 248 non-anemic patients whose stools were positive for occult blood, the source of GI bleeding was more often the upper than the lower GI tract. In just over half the cases, the source of bleeding could not be identified.[5] In such cases, the prognosis is good.[6] Occult blood in the stool has been found in 20% of marathon runners immediately after the race.[7] Oral iron supplements turn the stool dark green or black but do not cause FOBT to become positive.

The patient complaint of bright red blood per rectum, although suggestive, does not guarantee that a lesion is in the sigmoid colon.[8] Should all patients with hematochezia undergo total colonoscopy? There is some controversy in the literature on this question. Colorectal cancer infrequently presents with rectal bleeding in isolation.[9] A change in bowel habit toward increased looseness or increased stool frequency has a high predictive value for cancer.[10] The probability of colon cancer in those with rectal bleeding also rises with age.[11] In persons with hematochezia at low risk for cancer (less than 40 years of age, negative family history, and no associated symptoms), flexible sigmoidoscopy may be sufficient to rule out colorectal cancer,[12] but may miss other significant disease.[13] In persons older than 40 years of age, colonoscopy appears to be the procedure of choice regardless of associated symptoms, history, or pattern of bleeding.[14]

◈ REFERENCES ◈

1. Thompson JA, Pond CI, Ellis BG, et al: Rectal bleeding in general and hospital practice: 'the tip of the iceberg,' *Colorect Dis* 2:288-293, 2000.
2. Mulcahy HE, Patel RS, Postic G, et al: Yield of colonoscopy in patients with nonacute rectal bleeding: a multicenter database study of 1766 patients, *Am J Gastroenterol* 97:328-333, 2002.
3. Helfand M, Marton KI, Zimmer-Gembeck MJ, et al: History of visible rectal bleeding in a primary care population: initial assessment and 10-year follow-up, *JAMA* 277:44-48, 1997.
4. Thompson MR, Heath I, Ellis BG, et al: Identifying and managing patients at low risk of bowel cancer in general practice, *BMJ* 327:263-265, 2003.
5. Rockey DC, Koch J, Cello JP, et al: Relative frequency of upper gastrointestinal and colonic lesions in patients with positive fecal occult-blood tests, *N Engl J Med* 339: 153-159, 1998.
6. Rockey DC: Occult gastrointestinal bleeding, *N Engl J Med* 341:38-46, 1999.
7. McCabe ME, Peura DA, Kadakia SC, et al: Gastrointestinal blood loss associated with running a marathon, *Dig Dis Sci* 31:1229-1232, 1986.
8. Fine KD, Nelson AC, Ellington T, et al: Comparison of the color of fecal blood with the anatomic location of gastrointestinal bleeding lesions: potential misdiagnosis using only flexible sigmoidoscopy (FS) for bright red blood per rectum, *Am J Gastroenterol* 94:3202-3210, 1999.
9. Douek M, Wickramasinghe M, Clifton MA: Does isolated rectal bleeding suggest colorectal cancer? *Lancet* 354:393, 1999.
10. Hamilton W, Sharp D: Diagnosis of colorectal cancer in primary care: the evidence base for guidelines, *Fam Pract* 21:99-106, 2004.
11. Wauters H, Van Casteren V, Buntinx, F: Rectal bleeding and colorectal cancer in general practice: diagnostic study, *BMJ* 321:998-999, 2000.
12. Eckardt VF, Schmitt T, Kanzler G, et al: Does scant hematochezia necessitate performance of total colonoscopy? *Endoscopy* 34:599-603, 2002.
13. Mehanna D, Platell C: Investigating chronic, bright red, rectal bleeding, *ANZ J Surg*. 71:720-722, 2001.
14. Bond JH: Rectal bleeding: is it always an indication for colonoscopy? *Am J Gastroenterol* 97:223-225, 2002.

INFLAMMATORY BOWEL DISEASE

(See also biliary cirrhosis; colon cancer; diarrhea; psoriatic arthritis)

Crohn's Disease

Crohn's disease can affect any age group but peaks in early and late adulthood. Important exacerbating factors are cigarette smoking and use of NSAIDs.[1] Management protocols vary according to whether the disease is active or in remission and, when active, according to the severity of disease.[1-3] First-line treatment of mild-to-moderate active disease is sulfasalazine (Azulfidine, Salazopyrin) 3 to 6 g per day or mesalamine (Asacol, Mesasal, Pentasa, Salofalk) 3.2 to 4.8 g per day in divided doses, with metronidazole 10 to 20 mg/kg per day as an alternative for those who fail to respond to sulfasalazine.[2] Metronidazole combined with ciprofloxacin is effective, while preliminary studies suggest that ciprofloxacin and a number of other antibiotics such as clarithromycin and rifabutin either alone or in combination are beneficial.[1,3] Moderate to severe disease usually requires corticosteroids such as prednisone 40 to 60 mg per day for 1 to 4 weeks followed by gradual tapering.[1,2] Budesonide controlled release capsules may be used instead of prednisone and have the advantage of causing less adrenocortical suppression.[1] Budesonide is particularly beneficial for ileal or right-sided colon disease.[3] High-dose mesalazine and, for refractory disease, methotrexate and antitumour necrosis factor antibody are emerging therapeutic options. The most effective measure for maintenance of remission is cessation of smoking.[4]

Ulcerative Colitis

Ulcerative colitis is found three to four times as frequently in whites as in other races. Both sexes are equally affected. About 5% of patients have severe disease manifested as fulminating hemorrhagic colitis, toxic megacolon, or severe diffuse colitis. Ulcerative colitis is more common in nonsmokers than in smokers. The onset of the disease often correlates with discontinuing smoking, and smoking may control the symptoms of the disease. These apparently beneficial effects are not seen in Crohn's disease.[5]

One of the long-term complications of ulcerative colitis is colon cancer; risk increases with duration and extent of the disease. After 8 to 10 years the risk of cancer in patients with pancolitis is 0.5% to 1% per year. For those with left-sided colitis the risk reaches 0.5% to 1% per year after 30 to 40 years. Patients with only proctosigmoiditis do not have an increased cancer risk.

Clinical practice guidelines recommend annual surveillance colonoscopy with multiple biopsies starting after 8 to 10 years in patients at risk of cancer. If dysplasia is found on any pathological specimen, colectomy is indicated. These guidelines are based on opinion, since no randomized trials of surveillance have been reported.[6]

Mild and moderate cases of ulcerative colitis can be managed on an outpatient basis. If colitis involves any portions of the colon proximal to the splenic flexure, oral medications are required, whereas for left side lesions, either oral or topical treatments may be used. If topical agents are chosen, enemas are required for disease in the descending colon, foam can be used if involvement is limited to the distal 15 to 20 cm of the large bowel, and suppositories are effective for isolated proctitis that does not extend proximally beyond 10 cm.[6] The mainstays of treatment are rectal and systemic 5-aminosalicylic acid derivatives and corticosteroids, with azathioprine in steroid-dependent or resistant cases.[7] Oral aminosalicylates such as sulfasalazine, mesalamine, or olsalazine (Dipentum) are usually started at relatively low doses and increased to full therapeutic doses at a tolerable rate for the patient. Enemas containing steroids such as hydrocortisone (Cortenema) or 5-acetylsalicylic acid compounds such as mesalamine (Rowasa) are usually given at bedtime, and the patient is instructed to try to retain the enema all night.[8,9] Some of the newer steroid enemas such as tixocortol (Rectovalone) are not readily absorbed and do not suppress the pituitary-adrenal axis.[8] Mesalamine may also be administered as a suppository,[9] and 10% cortisone is available as a foam.[6] Once active disease is controlled, maintenance therapy with oral or topical aminosalicylates should be instituted.[6]

Patients with mild to moderate extensive disease who do not respond to aminosalicylates or patients with severe disease are treated with corticosteroids and sometimes with IV cyclosporine[3] or 6-mercaptopurine or azathioprine.[6]

In a controlled trial, Nicotine patches showed some reduction in symptoms but no other objective benefits were seen.[3]

Extraintestinal Manifestations of Inflammatory Bowel Disease

Peripheral arthritis, involving primarily the hips and ankles, and ankylosing spondylitis are fairly common complications of inflammatory bowel disease. Ocular manifestations are also common and include episcleritis and uveitis.[10] Sclerosing cholangitis is a rare complication of inflammatory bowel disease. Some patients are asymptomatic, but others have fatigue and pruritus. Levels of aspartate aminotransferase (AST or SGOT) and alanine aminotransferase (ALT or SGPT) may be normal or elevated, whereas alkaline phosphatase and gamma-glutamyl transferase (GGT) levels are markedly elevated.[11]

◢ REFERENCES ◣

1. Rampton DS: Management of Crohn's disease, *BMJ* 319: 1480-1485, 1999.
2. Hanauer SB, Meyers S: Practice guidelines: management of Crohn's disease in adults, *Am J Gastroenterol* 92:559-566, 1997.
3. Podolsky DK: Medical progress inflammatory bowel disease, *N Engl J Med* 347:417-429, 2002.
4. Rampton DS: Management of Crohn's disease, *BMJ* 319:1480-1485, 1999.
5. Haunauer SB: Nicotene for colitis—the smoke has not yet cleared (editorial), *N Engl J Med* 330:856-857, 1994.
6. Kornbluth A, Sachar DB: Ulcerative colitis practice guidelines in adults, *Am J Gastroenterol* 92:204-211, 1997.
7. Ghosh S, Shand A, Ferguson A: Ulcerative colitis, *BMJ* 320:1119-1123, 2000.
8. Hanauer SB: Inflammatory bowel disease, *N Engl J Med* 334:841-848, 1996.
9. Botoman VA, Bonner GF, Botoman DA: Management of inflammatory bowel disease, *Am Fam Physician* 57:57-68, 1998.
10. Hastings GE, Wever RJ: Inflammatory bowel disease. I. Clinical features and diagnosis, *Am Fam Physician* 47: 598-608, 1993.
11. Buckley SE, Dipalma JA: Recognizing primary biliary cirrhosis and primary sclerosing cholangitis, *Am Fam Physician* 53:195-200, 1996.

IRRITABLE BOWEL SYNDROME
(See also approach to complementary and alternative medicine; constipation; diarrhea; fibromyalgia; functional somatic syndromes; lactose intolerance)

Irritable bowel syndrome (IBS) has a prevalence of 12%, is twice as common in females, and is typically associated with abdominal pain and discomfort in the absence of mechanical, biochemical, or overt inflammatory conditions.[1] Although the cause of IBS is unknown, a number of cases appear to be precipitated by an episode of acute bacterial gastroenteritis,[2,3] and stress may aggravate symptoms.[3] Lactose intolerance (lactase deficiency) is not a constituent aspect of IBS, but because symptoms of IBS overlap with those of lactase deficiency, the latter should always be considered in the differential diagnosis.[4] Misuse of laxatives and some medications (including selective serotonin reuptake inhibitors [SSRIs], thyroid and antiarrhythmics) may mimic diarrhea-predominant IBS. Up to 40% of patients with IBS have a history of sexual, physical, or emotional abuse.[5]

The diagnosis of irritable bowel is based on positive clinical findings and ruling out alarm symptoms that include hematochezia, weight loss, family history of colon cancer, recurring fever, anemia, and chronic severe diarrhea. (Some physicians would also add being older than 50 years as an alarm symptom.) Also, if the patient has significant diarrhoea, celiac disease can be considered. Patients over age 50 who have new onset of symptoms should undergo a colonoscopy or barium enema, partly because of the rising incidence of insidious causes and partly because new onset of IBS after 50 is rare.[3,6] The Manning and Rome II criteria for diagnosing IBS require at least 12 weeks (not necessarily consecutive) in the preceding year of abdominal pain/discomfort that has at least two of three features[3,7]:

- Relieved by defecation
- Onset associated with change in stool form (usually looser)
- Onset associated with change in frequency (usually more frequent)

Supportive symptoms for a diagnosis of IBS include:

- Abnormal stool frequency (more than 3 per day, or fewer than 3 per week), form, or passage (straining, urgency, feeling of incomplete evacuation)
- Passage of mucus
- Bloating and abdominal distention

Guidelines simplified this and defined IBS as abdominal discomfort with altered bowel habits.[8] The decision to investigate and treat should be based on the severity of symptoms and the degree to which they affect the patient's quality of life. Routine use of flexible sigmoidoscopy, barium enema, colonoscopy, FOBTs, stool for ova and parasites, stool for culture, or thyroid function tests is not recommended for patients without alarm symptoms, since the diseases being considered are no more common in patients with IBS.[9] Management is guided primarily by the symptom profile and by symptom severity, although all patients may benefit from education about IBS and specific reassurance.[3,7] Reinforce the fact that IBS is a chronic and relapsing, but benign, condition that is not caused by dietary factors or emotional stress, although both factors can aggravate symptoms. IBS does not cause intestinal damage and is not a sign of food allergy or intolerance.

A normal diet should be taken, and unless lactase deficiency has been proved, milk need not be limited. A reasonable treatment approach includes avoidance of dietary excesses, caffeine, and dietary triggers that the patient suspects lead to symptoms. Some patients feel better if they cut down on sorbitol, alcohol, or fat,[3] and those who are constipated may improve with gradually increasing fibre supplements,[3,7] such as ½ to 1 cup per day of bran or ½ to 1 tablespoon of psyllium (Metamucil, Prodiem) one to four times a day taken with plenty of fluids.[7] Diarrhea can usually be controlled with loperamide 2 to 4 mg four times a day as needed, and for some patients it can be given prophylactically before trips, social events, and other occasions.[3] Patients with major flatus would do well to avoid eating beans, cabbage, and uncooked broccoli.

Most patients do not need medications. The placebo effect in IBS trials has ranged from 20% to higher than 50% and typically last 3 months.[1] Pain may be treated with antispasmodics such as dicyclomine (Bentyl, Bentylol) 10 to 20 mg three to four times a day, hyoscine butyl bromide (Buscopan) 10 mg three or four times a day, or trimebutine (Modulon) 200 mg three times a day or with smooth muscle relaxants such as the calcium channel blocker pinaverium bromide (Dicetel) 50 mg three times a day with meals.[10] Trial evidence for the antispasmodics is methodologically flawed.[11] For some patients with frequent or continuous pain, tricyclic antidepressants (TCAs) such as amitriptyline (Elavil) 25 to 100 mg at bedtime or low-dose SSRIs appear to be effective for some, but more trials are needed. A 2000 meta-analysis showed 1 in 3 patients may benefit. Finally, Tegaserod (Zelnorm 6 mg twice a day), a 5-HT4 agonist, is helpful in women with constipation-predominant IBS. Alosetron (Lotronex), a 5-HT3 antagonist, is helpful in patients with diarrhea-predominant IBS but was withdrawn from the market after causing ischemic colitis in 1 in 700. It has been re-introduced to the market, partly because of patient lobbying, with specific guidelines by the FDA in late 2002 for patients with severe diarrhea. TCAs seem to have the best response rate over placebo (33%), followed by antispasmodic drugs (22%), followed by the SSRI's such as Tegaserod (9.3% to 13.2%) when IBS drugs are compared.[1]

Complementary therapy enteric-coated peppermint oil has been shown to significantly improve abdominal pain, distention, stool frequency, borborygmi, and flatulence compared with placebo.[12] However, peppermint oil exacerbates GERD by relaxing the lower esophageal sphincter, so it may not produce a net benefit. Cognitive behaviour therapy and hypnotherapy have been effective treatment for IBS.[3,12] No medications have been shown to control bloating.

In the end, consider education reassurance and stress management for all. For diarrhea-predominant IBS, reduce caffeine and lactose, consider Loperamide and TCAs as needed for more severe symptoms, and possibly alosetron with patient insight and very severe cases. For constipation-predominant IBS, start with fibre (although evidence is limited), exercise, and fluid intake. Then consider adding an osmotic laxative such as Milk of Magnesia 2.4 to 4.8 mg once a day, and an antispasmodic agent 30 minutes before meals. TCAs and Tegaserod could be considered for severe cases. Pain-predominant IBS may do best with the antispasmodic agent or TCAs. All patients would do well with coping therapy.

ঌ REFERENCES ঌ

1. Mertz HR: Irritable bowel syndrome, *N Engl J Med* 349: 2136-2146, 2003.
2. García Rodríguez LA, Ruigómez A: Increased risk of irritable bowel syndrome after bacterial gastroenteritis: cohort study, *BMJ* 318:565-566, 1999.
3. Paterson WG, Thompson WG, Vanner SJ, et al: Recommendations for the management of irritable bowel syndrome in family practice, *Can Med Assoc J* 161:154-160, 1999.

4. Tolliver BA, Gerrerea JL, DiPalma JA: Evaluation of patients who meet clinical criteria for irritable bowel syndrome, *Am J Gastroenterol* 89:176-178, 1994.

5. Drossman DA, Leserman J, Nachman G, et al: Sexual and physical abuse in women with functional or organic gastrointestinal disorder, *Ann Intern Med* 113(11):828-833, 1990.

6. American College of Gastroenterology Functional Gastrointestinal Disorders Task Force: Evidence-based position statement on the management of irritable bowel syndrome in North America, *Am J Gastroenterol* 97:S1-S5, 2002.

7. Thompson WG, Longstreth GF, Drossman DA, et al: Functional bowel disorders and functional abdominal pain, *Informed Plus* 45(Suppl II):1143-1147, 1999.

8. IBS Consensus Conference Participants: Recommendations for the management of irritable bowel syndrome in family practice, Queen's University Gastrointestinal Motility Education Centre, Kingston, Ont, *CMAJ* 161(2):154-160, 1999.

9. Cash BD, Schoenfeld P, Chey WD: The utility of diagnostic tests in irritable bowel syndrome patients: a systematic review, *Am J Gastroenterol* 97:2812-2819, 2002.

10. Thompson WG: Irritable bowel syndrome: strategy for the family physician, *Can Fam Physician* 40:307-316, 1994.

11. Akehurst R, Kaltenthaler E: Treatment of irritable bowel syndrome: a review of randomised controlled trials, *Gut* 48: 272-282, 2001.

12. Kennedy TM, Rubin G, Johns R: Irritable bowel syndrome. In *Clinical evidence,* London, 2004, BMJ.

LACTOSE INTOLERANCE

(See also diarrhea; irritable bowel syndrome; celiac disease; Crohn's disease)

The incidence and prevalence of lactose intolerance is 3 out of 10 in non-Caucasians and 1 out of 10 in Caucasians. Frequencies observed between males and females are essentially the same. Racial statistics show that 5% to 12% of American Caucasians; 60% to 75% of African-Americans, Mexican-Americans, and American Jews; 90% of Asian-Americans; and 75% to 100% of Native Americans have lactose intolerance.[1]

Three forms of lactose intolerance are recognized:

1. *Congenital lactose intolerance*, which is a very rare disorder.

2. *Primary lactose intolerance*, which is common in adults, varies among individuals, and appears to be a natural occurrence depending on ethnicity.

3. *Secondary lactose intolerance*, which occurs with intestinal disease that impairs absorption or speeds up transit. This is seen in celiac disease, acute or chronic infections associated with malabsorption, or in reduction in the mucosal surface resulting from surgical resection. GI infections, antibiotic use, colchicines, cancer therapy, and alcohol consumption also cause secondary intolerance.

Many of these diseases will resolve with time.

The most common symptoms of lactase deficiency are abdominal pain, cramps, nausea, diarrhea, bloating, and flatulence 0.5 to 2 hours after intake of dairy products and milk. These symptoms are similar to those in patients with IBS, who have been found in numerous reports to have an increased incidence of lactase deficiency. Lactose intolerance symptoms usually start during teenage years or adulthood. However, lactase production decreases 2 to 5 years after birth in many individuals with primary lactose intolerance. Lactase deficiency is probably responsible for many cases of recurrent abdominal pain in children.[1]

Symptoms vary greatly among individuals with lactose intolerance.

The standard investigation for lactase deficiency is the hydrogen breath test, but considerable false-negatives and false-positives exist with this test.[2] A lactose tolerance test is useful in patients with concurrent disorders such as celiac disease or gastroenteritis. Adult patients are given a 50 g lactose load, and blood glucose and symptoms are monitored.[3] Stool acidity tests assessing the pH of stool samples can indicate lactose intolerance (less than 6.5). According to Thompson and co-workers,[4] a cheaper and equally effective method is to have the patient abstain from all milk products for 1 week and then drink a litre of milk. If significant symptoms result, the test is positive.

A simple treatment for lactase deficiency is avoidance of milk and dairy products containing lactose. A 3-week follow-up appointment is then appropriate to assess for symptom improvement or resolution. Aged cheese and yogurt do not contain lactose because it is destroyed during the fermentation process. However, processed cheeses such as cream cheese, cottage cheese, and ricotta cheese do contain lactose and should be avoided. Whole milk or chocolate milk may be easier to drink than skim milk. The adverse effect of limiting dairy products may be an inadequate calcium intake, so supplementary calcium and vitamin D should be prescribed.

An alternative to avoiding milk products is to have the patients buy milk that has had lactase added, add lactase enzyme (Lactaid) to ordinary milk, or take lactase enzymes before ingesting dairy products. Lactase replacement does not work for all patients with lactose intolerance.[5]

Patients need to learn to read all food and medicine labels. Lactose is used in the production of 20% of all prescription drugs including birth control pills, and 6% of all over-the-counter drugs, including gas-reducing agents, and gastric acid reducing agents. Although 44% of all women with lactose intolerance achieve normal lactose tolerance during pregnancy, it is important to assess dietary needs of mother and fetus carefully to ensure proper nutrient intake. Infants may require a soy-based infant formula to replace breast milk.[6]

Patients must modify dietary habits to prevent future occurrence of symptoms. Dietary modifications may create a potential compliance problem, but many patients have lactose intolerance temporarily and recover their ability to consume lactose-containing products. Evidence exists that lactose-intolerant individuals can adapt to some extent if given gradually increasing amounts of lactose, probably as a result of increased colonic salvage.[7]

---------------- ◢ **REFERENCES** ◣ ----------------

1. Gudmand-Hoyer E: The clinical significance of disaccharide maldigestion, *Am J Clin Nutr* 59(suppl 3):S735-S741, 1994.
2. Romagnuolo J, Schiller D, Bailey RJ: Using breath tests wisely in a gastroenterology practice: an evidence-based review of indications and pitfalls in interpretation, *Am J Gastroenterol* 97:1113-1126, 2002.
3. Olden KW: Diagnosis of irritable bowel syndrome, *Gastroenterology* 122:1701-1714, 2002.
4. Thompson WG, Drossman DA, Whitehead WE: Approaching IBS with confidence, *Patient Care Can* 31: 51-66, 1993.
5. Marteau PR: Probiotics in clinical conditions, *Clin Rev Allergy Immunol* 22:255-273, 2002.
6. National Digestive Diseases Information Clearinghouse. National Institute of Diabetes & Digestive & Kidney Diseases. Lactose Intolerance. Available at :http://digestive.niddk.nih.gov/ddiseases/pubs/lactoseintolerance/Accessed April 20, 2005.
7. Johnson AO, Semenya JG, Buchowski MS, et al: Adaptation of lactose maldigesters to continued milk intakes, *Am J Clin Nutr* 58:879-881, 1993.

LIVER

Alcoholic Hepatitis
(See also alcohol; hepatitis)

The spectrum of illness in patients with alcoholic hepatitis varies from mild non-specific symptoms (fatigue, anorexia, and weight loss) through liver failure with jaundice, ascites, and hepatic encephalopathy. Alcoholic hepatitis is generally limited to persons who drink 80 g or more of ethanol per day. This is more than eight 12-ounce beers, 1 litre (one and a half bottles) of 12% wine, or a half pint of 80-proof whiskey.[1]

Patients may have macrocytic anemia and leukocytosis (white blood cell count usually higher than 15,000/mm^3), elevated prothrombin time, elevated bilirubin level, and mild elevation of liver enzyme levels. The AST:ALT ratio is almost always greater than 2. Long-term treatment is focused on prevention through abstinence. Immediate treatment is directed toward the complications of alcohol abuse, including, but not limited to, dehydration, trauma, GI bleeding, sepsis, spontaneous bacterial peritonitis, and liver failure.[1]

Ascites

Ascites is most commonly the result of liver failure, but other causes include malignancy, renal disease, congestive heart failure (CHF), infection, and portal hypertension. A sodium-restricted diet (88 mmol per day = 2,000 mg per day), together with oral spironolactone and furosemide, effectively controls fluid overload in 90% of patients with cirrhosis and ascites and is also the mainstay of treatment.[2] Treatment is directed toward the cause and often includes paracentesis for diagnostic and therapeutic reasons. The drug of choice for ascites resulting from cirrhosis is spironolactone (Aldactone) because it counters the hyperaldosteronism of this condition. One regimen is to start with 50 mg once daily and increase the dose every 3 or 4 days to a maximum of 400 mg per day. If necessary, a thiazide or loop diuretic may be added (e.g., Lasix at 40 mg to a max of 160 mgevery morning).[1] Amiloride (Midamor) may be used instead of spironolactone, starting with 10 mg every morning and increasing to a maximum of 40 mg per day. Amiloride has a faster action and does not cause painful gynecomastia.[3]

---------------- ◢ **REFERENCES** ◣ ----------------

1. Brater DC: Diuretic therapy, *N Engl J Med* 339:387-395, 1998.
2. Runyon BA: Management of adult patients with ascites caused by cirrhosis, *Hepatology* 27(1):264-272, Jan 1998.
3. Runyon BA: Care of patients with ascites, *N Engl J Med* 330:337-342, 1994.

Cirrhosis
(See also connective tissue diseases; hypothyroidism; inflammatory bowel disease)

Cirrhosis is the final result of hepatic injury from any cause, characterized by fibrosis and varying degrees of inflammatory changes to the liver. Definitive diagnosis and assessment of cause can be confirmed by liver biopsy. A less invasive transjugular approach has significantly decreased the associated morbidity of the procedure. The primary causes of cirrhosis in North America are alcohol abuse and viral hepatitis. Other causes include primary biliary cirrhosis, hemochromatosis, and nonalcoholic steatohepatitis (NASH) (fatty liver). Clinical features of cirrhosis include hepatomegaly (early) or fibrosis (late), spider nevi, palmar erythema, testicular atrophy, and gyenecomastia. Liver function tests (AST, ALT, alkaline phosphatase, GGT, and bilirubin) along with INR and serum protein and albumin levels can help with diagnosis and assess degree of liver failure.

Primary biliary cirrhosis
Ninety-five percent of patients with biliary cirrhosis are women, and most are middle age. The usual clinical presentation is pruritus and fatigue, although many

asymptomatic cases are detected when an unexpectedly elevated alkaline phosphatase level is discovered during biochemical screening procedures. AST and ALT concentrations may be normal or only slightly elevated, whereas alkaline phosphatase and GGT levels are markedly elevated. The diagnosis of primary biliary cirrhosis (PBC) can be made with confidence in a patient with high-titer antimitochondrial antibodies (AMA) (more than 1:40) and a cholestatic pattern of liver biochemistry in the absence of an alternative explanation. A liver biopsy may also be considered.[1,2] Serum lipid levels are often strikingly elevated, with total cholesterol levels as high as 1000 mg/dl (26 mmol/L). However, patients are not at increased risk of cardiovascular disease, probably because HDL cholesterol levels are markedly elevated.[2]

The median survival is between 10 and 16 years for asymptomatic patients and 7 years for symptomatic patients. Although symptoms develop after 2 to 4 years in most asymptomatic patients, approximately a third remain symptom free for many years. Appropriately selected patients with PBC with abnormal liver biochemistry should be advised to take ursodeoxycholic acid (UDCA), 13 to 15 mg/kg daily in either divided doses or as a single daily dose. If cholestyramine is used, 4 hours should elapse between cholestyramine intake and UDCA administration.[3] The most common symptom is pruritus, which can usually be controlled with cholestyramine (Questran) 4 g orally three times a day.[2]

An association has been reported between biliary cirrhosis and immunological disorders such as lupus, rheumatoid arthritis, scleroderma, CREST syndrome (calcinosis, Raynaud's phenomenon, esophageal involvement, sclerodactyly, and telangiectasia), Sjögren's syndrome, and thyroiditis.[1,2] About one fifth of the patients are hypothyroid.[2] Liver transplantation can be offered for uncontrolled pruritus, osteoporosis, and liver failure.

─────────── ◢ REFERENCES ◣ ───────────

1. Buckley SE, Dipalma JA: Recognizing primary biliary cirrhosis and primary sclerosing cholangitis, *Am Fam Physician* 53:195-200, 1996.
2. Kaplan MM: Primary biliary cirrhosis, *N Engl J Med* 335:1570-1580, 1996.
3. Heathcote EJ: Management of primary biliary cirrhosis. The American Association for the Study of Liver Diseases practice guidelines, *Hepatology* 31(4):1005-1013, Apr 2000.

Hepatitis

(See also adoption; alcoholic hepatitis; biliary cirrhosis; colon cancer; hemochromatosis; immunization schedules for children; immunizations)

Viral hepatitis

The common forms of viral hepatitis seen in family medicine, hepatitis A, B, and C, are discussed below. Rare causes include delta, E, G, and other viruses including cytomegalovirus (CMV) and HIV. Other causes of hepatitis that should be ruled out when investigating for the cause of chronic hepatitis are hemochromatosis, alpha$_1$-antitrypsin deficiency, and PBC.[1]

Terminology and clinical correlations of laboratory tests used in investigating hepatitis. A discussion of viral hepatitis requires a knowledge of a number of terms and abbreviations. Some important ones are listed in Table 25.[1]

Hepatitis A. About 20% of patients with hepatitis A have a brief relapse after initial improvement. Fulminant hepatitis occurs in 0.1% of patients with this disease, usually in patients with underlying liver disease. The diagnosis of acute infection may be confirmed by elevated titers of IgM anti-HAV.[2] Treatment of acute disease is supportive.

Travellers from industrialized countries to developing nations are at risk of acquiring hepatitis A even if they stay in luxury hotels. The overall risk if unprotected by passive or active immunization is estimated to be 3 to 6 per 1000 travellers per month, with the risk increasing to 20 per 1000 per month among those eating and drinking under poor hygienic conditions. Less than 20% of persons from industrialized countries born after 1945 have acquired natural immunity.[2]

For travellers, passive immunization with intramuscular immune globulin (human) is effective for 3 to 5 months in 85% to 90% of cases. Active immunization with a two-dose series of inactivated HAV vaccine (Havrix, Vaqta) is available. (In Canada a combination vaccine against hepatitis A and hepatitis B called *Twinrix* is given as a three-dose course at 0, 1, and 6 months.) Hepatitis A vaccination is effective, and immunity is estimated to persist for 7 to 10 years or more.[2] Patients at risk of exposure to hepatitis A within 4 weeks of vaccination may be given immune globulin at the same time as they are vaccinated, but at a different body site.[3] The usual adult dose of immune globulin is 0.02 mL/kg for travel of less than 3 months and 0.06 mL/kg for travel of 3 to 5 months. For post-exposure prophylaxis of household or sexual contacts, the dose of immune globulin is 0.02 mL/kg given as soon as possible and no later than 2 weeks after exposure.[4]

Immunization of the entire population is not generally recommended, but in view of the fact that both widespread and sporadic outbreaks of hepatitis A have been traced to imported foods, a good case could be made for universal vaccination of children.[5]

Hepatitis B. The prevalence of hepatitis B is high in China, Southeast Asia, and Africa. In these regions, up to half the population has been infected and about 8% are chronic carriers. In developed countries, most cases of hepatitis B are a result of sexual exposure or IV drug use; no clear risk factors are found in about one fourth of

Table 25   Hepatitis Terminology

Term or abbreviation	Definition and comments
Liver Enzymes	
Alanine aminotransferase	ALT = SGPT
Aspartate aminotransferase	AST = SGOT
Hepatitis A	
HAV	Hepatitis A virus
IgM anti-HAV	Acute hepatitis A infection
IgG anti-HAV	Previous hepatitis A infection
Hepatitis B	
HBV	Hepatitis B virus
HBsAg	Hepatitis B surface antigen. Elevated in acute infections and in the carrier state.
Anti-HBs	Anti-hepatitis B surface antigen. Develops 1-3 months after recovery from acute infection.
HBcAg	Hepatitis B core antigen.
IgM anti-HBc	Positive in the window phase of acute hepatitis B when HBsAg has declined but anti-HBs has not yet developed.
HBeAg	Hepatitis Be antigen. Present during acute hepatitis B infection and in chronic active hepatitis B infection.
Anti-HBe	Develops after acute infection. Not usually tested.
HBIG	Hepatitis B immune globulin.
Hepatitis C	
HCV	Hepatitis C virus
Anti-HCV	May not develop until 3 months after infection.
Hepatitis D	
HDV	Hepatitis D virus. Occurs only in patients who are carriers of HBsAg.
Anti-HDV	Order only for patients who are HBsAg positive and have clinical symptoms of acute hepatitis.
Hepatitis E	
HEV	Hepatitis E virus. Clinical picture similar to hepatitis A. Uncommon in developed countries.

those affected, but this may be due to reticence in revealing high-risk activities.[6] About half of adults who acquire hepatitis B are asymptomatic, one fourth have jaundice, and one fourth have non-specific symptoms. Complete cure occurs in 90% of cases, and the carrier state develops in about 10%. In a quarter of this 10%, cirrhosis, chronic hepatitis, or liver cancer will develop. Hepatocellular cancer is most likely to develop in patients whose liver biopsies show severe chronic active hepatitis, cirrhosis, or both.[7]

In patients with acute hepatitis B, detectable HBsAg usually develops about 3 weeks before the onset of clinical symptoms. HBsAg declines over the next few weeks as the patient recovers, and shortly thereafter anti-HBs develops. A "window phase" may occur in the recovery stage of hepatitis B when neither HBsAg nor anti-HBs is present; at that time, tests for IgM anti-HBc are usually positive.[1]

A patient with clinical hepatitis who has anti-HBs does not have acute hepatitis B. HBeAg is present during acute hepatitis B infection and in chronic hepatitis B. If a patient from an endemic area has elevated liver enzyme levels and is HBsAg and HBeAg positive, he or she probably has chronic active hepatitis.[1]

A person is defined as a chronic carrier of hepatitis B if two samples of sera taken 6 months apart are both HBsAg positive or if a single serum sample is HBsAg positive and anti-HBc negative. The risk of development of the carrier state depends on the age of the patient at the time of infection. Specific risks are 90% to 95% in infants, 25% to 50% in children under age 5, and 6% to 10% in adults.[8]

Immunization against hepatitis B and post-exposure prophylaxis. (See the section on immunization.)

Treatment of chronic hepatitis B. Practice guidelines from the American Association for the Study of Liver Diseases updated in September 2003 provide for the following level 1 evidence for treatment[9]:

1. Treatment of HbeAg-positive patients with serum HBV DNA greater than 10 copies/mL, elevated ALT greater than 2 times normal or moderate-to-severe hepatitis on biopsy. One option involves interferon alfa-2b (Intron A) given subcutaneously as either 5

million units daily or 10 million units three times a week for 16 weeks.

2. Treatment of HbeAg-negative patients with serum HBV DNA greater than 10 copies/mL, elevated ALT greater than 2 times normal or moderate-to-severe hepatitis on biopsy with interferon for greater than 1 year.

3. Patients who fail prior interferon treatment may be retreated with lamivudine 100 mg orally once daily or adefovir 10 mg orally once daily for at least 1 year. Superinfection with hepatitis A in patients with chronic hepatitis B rarely results in fulminant hepatitis.[10]

Hepatitis C. Before the discovery and implementation of anti-HCV testing in blood banks in 1989, hepatitis C was responsible for 90% of transfusion-related cases of non-A, non-B hepatitis.[11] At present the risk of acquiring hepatitis C from transfusions is estimated to be 1 in 100,000 for each transfused unit.[12] Other recognized risk factors for hepatitis C are IV drug use, transfusions, accidental needle sticks by health care workers, and living in an endemic area. The risk of acquiring infection from an anti-HCV-positive patient via a needle stick is about 3%; there is no effective post-exposure prophylaxis.[11] Between 50% and 80% of IV drug users become hepatitis C positive within a year of beginning usage.[12] In the United States, more than 35% of hepatitis C cases occur without known risk factors and are labelled as sporadic. Transmission of hepatitis C by colonoscopy has been reported. (See discussion of secondary prevention of colon cancer.)

Transmission of infection by close physical contact or through sexual relations may occur but is rare.[12] Both a German[13] and an Austrian[14] follow-up study of long-term monogamous marriages in which only one partner had hepatitis C found that the risk of sexual transmission was non-existent[13] or extremely small.[14] On the other hand, studies from Asia have shown that the risk of a non-infected partner acquiring hepatitis C increases with the duration of marriage[15]; Neumayr and associates[14] suggest that the frequent use of medical injections and acupuncture in Asia could account for this finding.

Vertical transmission of hepatitis C has been reported to occur in 5% to 36% of pregnancies, with the higher figures found in women who were co-infected with HIV. A multicentre Italian study of pregnant women who had antibodies to hepatitis C but who were HIV negative reported a transmission rate to the infant of 5%. Only women with detectable hepatitis C RNA in their blood transmitted the infection to their offspring. Although previous studies had suggested a diminution of transmission if delivery was by Cesarean section, such was not the case in this study. Hepatitis C is not transmitted through breastfeeding.[16]

A systematic review of studies of hepatitis C transmission found that the risk of transmission is extremely low if hepatitis C RNA cannot be detected in the blood when tested by polymerase chain reaction methods. This may be of particular importance in advising patients about sexual practices (whether to use condoms) and risks of transmitting the disease through pregnancy. When the polymerase chain reaction is positive, the risk of transmission from occupational exposure (needle sticks) and pregnancy is about 6%, whereas the risk from blood transfusions is around 80%.[17]

The incubation period of hepatitis C is usually 6 to 7 weeks but varies from 2 weeks to 6 months. Only 20% to 30% of patients are jaundiced, 10% to 20% have non-specific symptoms, and the rest are asymptomatic. Most symptomatic patients have anti-HCV antibody, but in some cases antibodies do not develop until 3 or more months after the onset of infection. More than 85% of infected adult patients have persistent infection, 70% chronic hepatitis, 26% to 50% chronic active hepatitis, and 10% to 20% cirrhosis. Cirrhosis is a risk factor for hepatocellular cancer, a malignancy that affects between 1% and 4% of cirrhotic patients per year. The 20-year mortality rate from liver disease in patients with hepatitis C is 1.6% to 6%.[12] The outcome of children infected with hepatitis C through blood transfusions appears to be considerably better. In one study half the children had no detectable HCV RNA after 20 years, and of those who had detectable HCV RNA, all but one had normal levels of liver enzymes.[18]

Generally, if the liver enzyme levels are consistently normal for 6 months, the patient does not have chronic active hepatitis. Recent studies show this concept to be false. Anti-HCV-positive females who do not drink are particularly likely to have chronic hepatitis without elevated liver enzyme levels. Although the hepatic changes are minimal in most such patients, a few have more advanced changes.[19]

Treatment of chronic hepatitis C. If patients with chronic hepatitis C are superinfected with hepatitis A, fulminant hepatic failure is a common sequelae. All patients with chronic hepatitis C should be immunized against hepatitis A.[9,10]

Hepatitis C patients who consume alcohol dramatically increase their risk of liver damage, cirrhosis, and hepatocellular carcinoma.[20] Abstention from alcohol is mandatory for patients with hepatitis C.[20,21]

Only selected patients with hepatitis C require active drug treatment. The risk of serious liver disease is low in patients with persistently normal ALT levels and liver biopsies showing minimal hepatocellular inflammation and fibrosis. Such patients probably do not require treatment because its efficacy in this form of the disease is uncertain, because progression of the disease is slow, and because treatments that are being developed and will be available in the future may be more effective and less toxic.[21] In line with this reasoning, a National Institutes of Health Consensus Conference recommends treatment for patients who have persistently elevated ALT levels, HCV viremia, and fibrosis and moderate inflammation on biopsy.[22]

Interferon alpha (interferon alfa-2a [Roferon-A] or interferon alfa-2b [Intron A]) has been used for the treatment of chronic active hepatitis C. Pegylated interferons, which allow for fewer injections and more stable levels of drug, have become a more popular choice for treatment. Combination treatment with oral Ribavirin is more effective, and the choice is based on patient factors and HCV genotype. Typical therapy consists of peginterferon alpha-2a 180 μg subcutaneously weekly or peginterferon alpha-2b 1.5 μg/kg subcutaneously weekly combined with Ribavirin 800 mg orally daily.[23] Close patient and biochemical monitoring are required due to potential significant side effects, including depression, autoimmune disease, thrombocytopenia, and neutropenia with interferon and hemolysis with Ribavirin. Combination treatment has led to complete disappearance of HCV RNA and ALT improvement in up to 70% of patients with a sustained response rate of HCV RNA undetectability 6 months post-treatment in 55% of patients versus only 35% of patients treated with monotherapy.[23] Genotypes 2 and 3 have a high response rate (70% to 80%) versus genotype 1 (40% to 50%). Length of combination therapy yields positive results in 24 weeks for genotypes 2 and 3, and 48 weeks for genotype 1. Patients with HIV and HCV should be offered treatment. The role of treatment in the pediatric population is still uncertain. Of note are several small studies that show resolution of infection in patients with acute hepatitis C when treated with interferon.[24]

❧ REFERENCES ❧

1. Friedman G, Sherker AH: The ABCs of hepatitis, *Can J Diagn* 13:85-97, 1996.
2. Steffen R, Kane MA, Shapiro CN, et al: Epidemiology and prevention of hepatitis A in travelers, *JAMA* 272:885-889, 1994.
3. Public health: hepatitis A, *Can Med Assoc J* 156:545, 1997.
4. *Canadian immunization guide*, ed 5, Otawa, 1998, Minister of Supply and Services Canada.
5. Koff RS: The case for routine childhood vaccination against hepatitis A (editorial), *N Engl J Med* 340:644-645, 1999.
6. Lee WM: Hepatitis B virus infection, *N Engl J Med* 337:1733-1745, 1997.
7. Curley SA, Izzo F, Gallipoli A, et al: Identification and screening of 416 patients with chronic hepatitis at high risk to develop hepatocellular cancer, *Ann Surg* 222:375-380, 1995.
8. Mahoney FJ, Burkholder BT, Matson CC: Prevention of hepatitis B virus infection, *Am Fam Physician* 47:865-874, 1993.
9. Lok AS, Mcmahon BJ: Chronic Hepatits B: Update of Reommendations, AASLD Practice Gudelines, *Hepatology* 39(3):857-61, 2004.
10. Vento S, Garofano T, Renzini C, et al: Fulminant hepatitis associated with hepatitis A virus superinfection in patients with chronic hepatitis C, *N Engl J Med* 338:286-290, 1998.
11. Centers for Disease Control and Prevention: Recommendations for follow-up of health-care workers after occupational exposure to hepatitis C virus, *JAMA* 1056-1057, 1997.
12. Moyer LA, Mast EE, Alter MJ: Hepatitis C. I. Routine serologic testing and diagnosis, *Am Fam Physician* 59: 79-88, 1999.
13. Meisel H, Reip A, Faltus B, et al: Transmission of hepatitis C virus to children and husbands by women infected with contaminated anti-D immunoglobulin, *Lancet* 345:1209-1211, 1995.
14. Neumayr G, Propst A, Schwaighofer H, et al: Lack of evidence for the heterosexual transmission of hepatitis C, *Q J Med* 92:505-508, 1999.
15. Kao JH, Hwang YT, Chen PJ, et al: Transmission of hepatitis C virus between spouses–the important role of exposure duration, *Am J Gastroenterol* 91:2087-2090, 1996.
16. Resti M, Azzari C, Mannelli F, et al: Mother to child transmission of hepatitis C virus: prospective study of risk factors and timing of infection in children born to women seronegative for HIV-1, *BMJ* 317:437-441, 1998.
17. Dore GJ, Kaldor JM, McCaughan GW: Systematic review of role of polymerase chain reaction in defining infectiousness among people infected with hepatitis C virus, *BMJ* 315:333-337, 1997.
18. Vogt M, Lang T, Frösner G, et al: Prevalence and clinical outcome of hepatitis C infection in children who underwent cardiac surgery before the implementation of blood-donor screening, *N Engl J Med* 314:866-870, 1999.
19. Gholson CF, Morgan K, Catinis G, et al: Chronic hepatitis C with normal aminotransferase levels: a clinical histologic study, *Am J Gastroenterol* 92:1788-1792, 1997.
20. Bellentani S, Pozzato G, Saccoccio G, et al: Clinical course and risk factors of hepatitis C virus related liver disease in the general population: report from the Dionysos study, *Gut* 44: 874-880, 1999.
21. Levine RA: Treating histologically mild chronic hepatitis C: monotherapy, combination therapy, or tincture of time? *Ann Intern Med* 129:323-326, 1998.
22. National Institutes of Health Consensus Development Conference Panel statement: management of hepatitis C, *Hepatology* 26(suppl 1):2S-10S, 1997.
23. Chronic Hepatitis C: Current Disease Management. National Digestive Diseases Information Clearinghouse. (Accessed May 11, 2004 at http://digestive.niddk.nih.gov/ddiseases/pubs/chroniche pc/indes.htm)
24. Hartman, C., Berowitz, D., et al: The effect of early treatment in children with chronic hepatitis, *J Pediatr Gastroenterol Nutr* 37(3);252-257, September 2003.

Hepatocellular Carcinoma

Although relatively uncommon in developed countries, primary liver cancer is one of the most common malignancies worldwide because of its association with chronic viral hepatitis, particularly B and C. Other causes of hepatic cirrhosis, as well as exposure to aflatoxin, a foodborne mycotoxin, also increase risk.

The most common presenting feature is hepatic mass in the context of cirrhosis. Frequently, the only clue to the presence of malignancy is increasing alpha-fetoprotein (AFP) or alkaline phosphatase (ALP) or rapidly declining liver function. Although often asymptomatic until the disease is well advanced, sometimes symptoms of abdominal pain and bloating, anorexia, fever, edema, and jaundice are manifested.

Surgical resection is potentially curative when the disease is confined to the liver. This treatment option is available to only a very small proportion of affected individuals, however, since the malignancy has usually spread beyond the liver at diagnosis. For this group, prognosis is poor, with fewer than 5% of symptomatic patients surviving 2 years beyond diagnosis. A variety of treatments, such as systemic chemotherapy, arterial cheo-embolization, radio-labelled antibody injection, radio-frequency ablation, and percutaneous ethanol injection have been tried in this group.[1]

REFERENCES

1. National Cancer Institute: Cancer topics: adult primary liver cancer. (Accessed Nov 15, 2004 at http://www.cancer.gov/cancertopics/pdq/treatment/adult-primary-liver/healthprofessional)

PANCREAS
Pancreatic Cancer

Pancreatic ductal carcinoma is one of the most common causes of cancer death in the Western world.[1] Consistent risk factors include advanced age and cigarette smoking.[2] Current smokers have a 2.5-fold increase in relative risk for this malignancy.[3] Family history and several genetic syndromes also have an association.[2] Diabetic patients who have had the disease for at least 5 years have double the risk of pancreatic carcinoma compared with non-diabetic control subjects.[4]

Two-thirds of pancreatic cancers occur in the head of the pancreas.[1] Most will present with obstructive jaundice. Patients with tumours in the tail of the pancreas often present with symptoms consistent with metastatic disease.[2] Patients with suspected pancreatic cancer are usually investigated initially by CT, followed by endoscopic ultrasound-guided biopsy.[2,5] Laparotomy is rarely necessary.[2]

Over 77% of patients with pancreatic cancer die within 1 year of diagnosis. Only 4.4% survive 5 years.[6] Approximately 15% to 20% of patients have resectable pancreatic cancer at diagnosis, with a 5-year survival of 17% to 24%.[7] Operative mortality for the Whipple procedure (pancreaticoduodenectomy) is lower in high-volume referral centres.[8] Adjuvant treatment with 5-fluorouracil or gemcitabine is often recommended; however, the optimum protocol for adjuvant treatment has not yet been established.[2]

REFERENCES

1. Bornman PC, Beckingham IJ: Pancreatic tumours, *BMJ* 322:721-723, 2001.
2. Li D, Xie K, Wolff R, et al: Pancreatic cancer, *Lancet* 363:1049-1057, 2004.
3. Fuchs CS, Colditz GA, Stampfer MJ, et al: A prospective study of cigarette smoking and the risk of pancreatic cancer, *Arch Intern Med* 156:2255-2560, 1996.
4. Everhart J, Wright D: Diabetes mellitus as a risk factor for pancreatic cancer: a meta-analysis, *JAMA* 273:1605-1609, 1995.
5. American Gastroenterological Assocation: Medical position statement: epidemiology, diagnosis, and treatment of pancreatic ductal endocarcinoma, *Gastroenterology* 117:1463-1484, 1999.
6. Ries LAG, Eisner MP, Kosary CL, et al, eds: SEER Cancer Statistics Review, 1975-2000. Bethesda MD, 2003, National Cancer Institute. (Accessed April 12, 2004, at http://seer.cancer.gov/csr/1975_2000.)
7. Raraty MG, Magee CJ, Ghaneh P, et al: New techniques and agents in the adjuvant therapy of pancreatic cancer, *Acta Oncologica* 41:582-595, 2002.
8. Liegerman MD, Kilburn H, Lindsey M, et al: Relation of perioperative deaths to hospital volume among patients undergoing pancreatic resection for malignancy, *Ann Surg* 222:638-645, 1995.

Pancreatitis
Acute pancreatitis

Acute pancreatitis is an acute inflammatory process of the pancreas with variable involvement of surrounding tissues that leads to intrapancreatic activation of enzymes with pain, nausea and vomiting, and associated intestinal ileus. It varies widely in severity, complications, and prognosis. The true incidence of acute pancreatitis remains contentious, and accurate assessments are hampered by geographical, etiological, and diagnostic variations. In the United Kingdom, acute pancreatitis accounts for 3% of all cases of abdominal pain admitted to hospital.[1] Currently about 10% to 33% of patients die in the early phase of an attack from multiple organ failure typically as a result of a major fluid deficit.[2]

Etiology is diverse and includes gallstones in the lower end of the common bile duct (45%), alcohol (35%), idiopathic (10%), and other miscellaneous causes such as hypertriglyceridaemia or drug reaction (10%). Acute pancreatitis typically presents as an acute abdomen with the sudden onset of severe upper abdominal pain, often radiating to the back, and nausea and vomiting. Once a chemical peritonitis is established, pain is felt throughout the abdomen and may be referred to the shoulder tip with involvement of the diaphragmatic peritoneum. Abdominal wall discolouration is pathognomonic and carries a bad prognosis.[3]

Serum amylase is helpful in diagnosis but can be elevated in other abdominal conditions.[4] If available, urinary trypsinogen can be used as a sensitive diagnostic tool to exclude pancreatitis in suspicious patients presenting with abdominal pain.[5] Imaging tests available for the diagnosis of acute pancreatitis include transabdominal ultrasound, endoscopic ultrasound (EUS), CT scan, MRI, and magnetic resonance cholangiopancreatography (MRCP). ERCP is used to diagnose chronic pancreatitis and for non-operative assessment and treatment of choledocholithiasis.[6]

A key step is stratifying risk in pancreatitis. Severity stratification should be made in all patients within 48 hours. A variety of scoring systems include the Glasgow score, C Reactive Protein (CRP), and the APACHE II score.

Patients with mild pancreatitis usually experience resolution of pain within 24 to 48 hours after a regimen of no oral intake, narcotics for pain relief, and IV fluids. Once oral intake is tolerated, patients can be discharged from the hospital. Patients with pancreatitis secondary to gallstones should undergo cholecystectomy during the same hospitalization. Common bile duct obstruction from a stone at the ampulla requires urgent removal of the stone (preferably by endoscopic papillotomy) if there is evidence of cholangitis. Patients with a history of alcoholism should be counselled and encouraged to participate in a detoxification and rehabilitation program, while patients with hyperlipidemia should be placed on appropriate diet and drug therapy. Probably the single most important element in preventing multiple organ failure is vigorous fluid resuscitation with electrolyte solutions to optimize cardiac index and maintain hemodynamic stability.[7]

Chronic pancreatitis

Chronic pancreatitis is characterized by irreversible glandular destruction and permanent loss of endocrine and exocrine function. Calcifications, obstructions, and pseudocysts can result and can affect function. Chronic pancreatitis may follow acute episodes or may occur without an identifiable attack. It can present with abdominal pain, weight loss and anorexia, and secondary effects of lost exocrine (malabsorption of fat, steatorrhea, and hypocalcemia) or endocrine function (impaired glucose tolerance and diabetes). Patients can be jaundiced and exhibit portal hypertension. As with acute pancreatitis, amylase and other markers of exocrine/endocrine function can be helpful, but an ultrasound, CT scan, or ERCP, in ascending order of accuracy, are diagnostic.[8] Alcohol is the dominant etiologic factor and the most widely studied. Although a linear relationship exists between the amount of alcohol ingested and the risk of developing chronic pancreatitis, the fact that fewer than 10% of people with alcoholism actually develop the disease is not understood. Pain relief may be achieved by abstinence from alcohol or enzyme supplementation. Specific measures include narcotics, and referral to a pain clinic may be wise. Morphine is not recommended because it constricts the sphincter of Oddi. However, in severe paroxysms, its potent analgesia may outweigh any risks of

obstruction. Surgical solutions range from a cholecystectomy to Whipple's procedure.

The prognostic factors associated with chronic pancreatitis are age at diagnosis, smoking, continued use of alcohol, and the presence of liver cirrhosis. The overall survival rate is 70% at 10 years and 45% at 20 years.[9]

❧ REFERENCES ❧

1. UK Working Party on Acute Pancreatitis: UK guidelines for the management of acute pancreatitis, *Gut* 42(suppl 2):S1–S13, 1998.
2. Mann D, Hershman M, Hittinger R, et al: Multicentre audit of death from acute pancreatitis, *Br J Surg* 81:890-893, 1994.
3. Steinberg, W: Acute pancreatitis, *N Engl J Med* 330(17):1198-1208, 1994.
4. Chase CW, Barker DE, Russell WL, et al: Serum amylase and lipase in the evaluation of acute abdominal pain, *Am Surg* 62(12):1028-1033, 1996.
5. Kylanpaa-Back M, Kemppainen E, Puolakkainen P, et al: Reliable screening for acute pancreatitis with rapid urine trypsinogen-2 test strip, *Br J Surg* 87(1):49-52, 2000.
6. American College of Radiology (ACR), Expert Panel on Gastrointestinal Imaging: *Acute pancreatitis*, Reston, VA, 2001, American College of Radiology.
7. Society for Surgery of the Alimentary Tract: *Treatment of acute pancreatitis*, Manchester, MA, 2000, The Society.
8. Steer ML, et al: Chronic pancreatitis, *N Engl J Med* 332:1482-1489, 1995.
9. Ammann RW, Akovbiantz A, Largiader F: Course and outcome of chronic pancreatitis. Longitudinal study of a mixed medical-surgical series of 245 patients, *Gastroenterology* 86(5 Pt 1): 820-828, May 1984.

STOMACH AND DUODENUM
Non-steroidal Anti-inflammatory Drug (NSAID) Gastropathy
(See also *Helicobacter pylori*, hypertension; non-steroidal anti-inflammatory drugs; osteoarthritis; peptic ulcer)

NSAIDs are associated with many adverse GI effects, including dyspepsia, peptic ulcers (which may bleed or perforate), esophagitis, small bowel ulceration, small bowel stricture, colonic strictures, and diverticular disease. Dyspepsia affects 10% to 20% of persons taking NSAIDs, but only a small percentage of those with serious GI lesions have antecedent dyspepsia.[1] One study suggests that if a patient is not positive for *Helicobacter pylori* and is not taking NSAIDs, the chance of an ulcer is almost non-existent.[2] Major risk factors for GI complications from NSAIDs are old age, high doses of NSAIDs, concomitant use of corticosteroids, past history of peptic ulcer or GI bleeding, and serious co-existing diseases such as heart, renal, or hepatic failure.[1] The presence of H. pylori does not appear to increase the risk for NSAID-induced gastropathy.[1,3,4] NSAIDs and *H. pylori* are synergistic in increasing the risk of peptic ulcer disease (PUD); it may be advisable to support serological screening of patients for *H. pylori* and eradication treatment for those with positive results before initiating long-term NSAID therapy.[5] If patients taking NSAIDs have proven peptic ulcers, it is probably worth screening for *H. pylori* and treating those who test positive.[4]

The newer NSAIDs include drugs that inhibit cyclooxygenase 2 (COX-2) without inhibiting cyclooxygenase 1 (COX-1). COX-1 facilitates the production of protective prostaglandins in the stomach and kidneys, whereas COX-2 is found in joints and aggravates inflammation.[1,6] Endoscopic studies demonstrate that coxib inhibitors significantly decrease the risk of new ulcer development compared with traditional NSAIDs. The important clinical question is not whether COX-2-selective NSAIDs decrease the incidence of tiny asymptomatic mucosal ulcers but whether they reduce the complications of ulcers; that is, bleeding, perforation, and obstruction.[7] The data remain mixed; in the VIGOR trial, rofecoxib significantly decreased the risk of clinically important and complicated upper GI events as well as GI bleeding events (all endpoints in the VIGOR trial) compared with naproxen, a non-selective NSAID.[7] However, a systematic review evaluating the safety of celecoxib in older patients taking long-term therapy for treatment of osteoarthritis and rheumatoid arthritis showed that, compared with placebo, patients were more likely to stop taking celecoxib, either because of any side effect or due to a GI side effect.[8] Additionally, serious adverse effects, such as perforations, obstructions, and bleeding, were no different between traditional NSAIDs and COX-2s in the CLASS study.[9] Finally, there is some concern that COX-2s may have prothrombotic effects and thus an increased risk of heart disease.[10] The APPROVe trial (Adenomatous Polyp Prevention On Vioxx) was just released in 2004. This study included 2600 patients and was designed to examine the effects of treatment with rofecoxib on the recurrence of neoplastic polyps of the large bowel in patients with a history of colorectal adenoma. This study showed increased cardiovascular events in patients taking rofecoxib (Vioxx) and thus, Vioxx has been withdrawn from the market.[11] Whether other Cox-2 inhibitors share this risk is a key question. COX-2-selective drugs may be the agents of choice for older patients with multiple risk factors for GI complications from NSAIDs, but they seem to offer no advantage for young, healthy individuals requiring short courses of treatment.[6] Prophylactic use of misoprostol (Cytotec) or proton pump inhibitors such as omeprazole (Prilosec, Losec) can reduce the risk of NSAID-induced peptic ulcers.[1] In a comparative study of misoprostol 200 µg twice a day and omeprazole 20 mg per day, omeprazole was more effective.[12] H_2-receptor blockers are minimally effective for preventing peptic ulcers in patients taking NSAIDs.[1]

The optimal treatment of patients who develop GI disorders when taking NSAIDs is to discontinue the NSAIDs. If this cannot be done, the GI disorder should be treated with a proton pump inhibitor, because this class of drugs is the most effective for treating both NSAID-induced dyspepsia[1] and NSAID-related gastroduodenal ulcers.[1,13] An additional strategy would be to switch to a COX-2 selective NSAID.[1]

❧ REFERENCES ❧

1. Wolfe MM, Lichtenstein DR, Singh G: Gastrointestinal toxicity of nonsteroidal antiinflammatory drugs, *N Engl J Med* 340:1888-1899, 1999.
2. Fraser AG, Ali MR, McCullough S, et al: Diagnostic tests for Helicobacter pylori—can they help select patients for endoscopy? *N Zeal Med J* 109:95-98, 1996.
3. Hawkey CJ, Tulassay Z, Szczepanski L, et al: Randomised controlled trial of *Helicobacter pylori* eradication in patients on non-steroidal antiinflammatory drugs: HELP NSAIDs study, *Lancet* 352:1016-1021, 1998.
4. Chiba N, Lahaie R, Fedorak RN, et al: *Helicobacter pylori* and peptic ulcer disease: current evidence for management strategies, *Can Fam Physician* 44:1481-1488, 1998.
5. Huang JQ, Sridhar S, Hunt RH: Role of *Helicobacter pylori* infection and non-steroidal anti-inflammatory drugs in peptic-ulcer disease: a meta-analysis, *Lancet* 359:14-22, 2002.
6. Peterson WL, Cryer B: COX-1-sparing NSAIDs–is the enthusiasm justified? (editorial), *JAMA* 282:1961-1963, 1999.
7. Langman MJ, Jensen DM, Watson KF, et al: Adverse upper gastrointestinal effects of rofecoxib compared with NSAIDs, *JAMA* 282:1929-1933, 1999.
8. Deeks JJ, Smith LA, Bradley MD: Efficacy, tolerability, and upper gastrointestinal safety of celecoxib for treatment of osteoarthritis and rheumatoid arthritis: systematic review of randomised controlled trials, *BMJ* 325:619-623, 2002.
9. Silverstein FE, Faich G, Goldstein JL, et al: Gastrointestinal toxicity with celecoxib vs nonsteroidal anti-inflammatory drugs for osteoarthritis and rheumatoid arthritis: the CLASS study: a randomized controlled trial. Celecoxib Long-term Arthritis Safety Study, *JAMA* 284:1247-1255, 2000.
10. Mukherjee D, Nissen SE, Topol EJ: Risk of cardiovascular events associated with selective COX-2 inhibitors, *JAMA* 286:954-959, 2001.
11. Unpublished data presented from the APPROVe Trial at American College of Rheumatology Annual Scientific Meeting, San Antonio, Texas, Oct. 18, 2004.
12. Hawkey CJ, Karrasch JA, Szczepanski L, et al (Omeprazole Versus Misoprostol for NSAID-Induced Ulcer Management [OMNIUM] Study Group): Omeprazole compared with misoprostol for ulcers associated with nonsteroidal antiinflammatory drugs, *N Engl J Med* 338:727-734, 1998.
13. Yeomans ND, Tulassay Z, Juhász L, et al (NSAID-Associated Ulcer Treatment [ASTRONAUT] Study Group): A comparison of omeprazole with ranitidine for ulcers associated with nonsteroidal antiinflammatory drugs, *N Engl J Med* 338:719-726, 1998.

Dyspepsia *← abdo pain*   *vs heartburn*
(See also peptic ulcer)

Dyspepsia may be defined as persistent or recurrent upper abdominal pain. Associated symptoms include nausea, vomiting, distention, bloating, and early satiety. Forty percent of patients with dyspepsia have underlying organic conditions; the remainder have non-ulcer dyspepsia.[1] The reported prevalence of dyspeptic symptoms in Western countries is 25% to 50%.

In patients with dyspeptic symptoms who have been investigated, four major causes have been identified: peptic ulcer, gastroesophageal reflux disease (with or without espohagitis), cancer, and functional dyspepsia. Up to 60% of patients with dyspepsia have no structural or biochemical explanation for their symptoms. This is non-ulcer, or functional, dyspepsia. The main causes of organic dyspepsia are gastroduodenal ulcers, GERD with esophagitis, and gastric or esophageal cancer. The cause of non-ulcer dyspepsia is unknown. Although claims have been made that *H. pylori* plays a pathogenic role in some cases, recent randomized controlled trials failed to find any benefit from eradicating *H. pylori* in patients with non-ulcer dyspepsia.[2-4]

A major issue in clinical practice is distinguishing peptic ulcer from non-ulcer dyspepsia. Careful history taking and physical exam are a priority for ruling out other causes of dyspepsia. People who are over age 50 and/or have alarm features associated with dyspepsia should undergo further investigation with endoscopy. These alarm features include persistent vomiting, bleeding, anemia, abdominal mass, unexplained weight loss, and dysphagia.[1,5] Arguments favouring endoscopy are that many patients with dyspepsia have organic disease and that a negative result is reassuring and may subsequently decrease the long-term cost of care.

Since dyspepsia is so common, two empiric strategies are acceptable for patients: lifestyle modification and an acid suppression trial, or the *H. Pylori* "test-and-treat strategy." Randomized controlled trials have demonstrated that the test-and-treat strategy is as effective as prompt endoscopy for managing dyspepsia, and is more cost-effective. More than two thirds in the test-and-treat group were not referred for endoscopy during a 1-year follow-up period.[6]

Symptomatic treatment with H_2-blockers, proton pump inhibitors, or prokinetic agents such as metoclopramide (Maxeran) may help some patients who are *H. pylori* negative.[1] Since smoking and the regular use of NSAIDS are associated with an increased risk of non-ulcer dyspepsia, symptomatic patients should avoid these agents.[7]

❧ REFERENCES ❧

1. Fisher RS, Parkman HP: Management of nonulcer dyspepsia, *N Engl J Med* 339:1376-1381, 1998.
2. Talley NJ, Vakil N, Ballard ED II, et al: Absence of benefit of eradicating *Helicobacter pylori* in patients with nonulcer dyspepsia, *N Engl J Med* 341:1106-1111, 1999.
3. Talley NJ, Janssens J, Lauritsen K, et al (Optimal Regimen Cures Helicobacter Induce Dyspepsia [ORCHID] Study Group): Eradication of *Helicobacter pylori* in functional dyspepsia: randomised double blind placebo controlled trial with 12 months' follow up, *BMJ* 318:833-837, 1999.
4. Greenberg PD, Cello JP: Lack of effect of treatment for *Helicobacter pylori* on symptoms of nonulcer dyspepsia, *Arch Intern Med* 159:2283-2288, 1999.
5. Veldhuyzen van Zanten SJ, Flook N, Chiba N, et al: An evidence-based approach to the management of uninvestigated dyspepsia in the era of *Helicobacter pylori*, Canadian Dyspepsia Working Group, *Can Med Assoc J* 162:S3-23, 2000.
6. Heaney A, Collins JS, Watson RG, et al: A prospective randomised trial of a "test and treat" policy versus endoscopy based management in young *Helicobacter pylori* positive patients with ulcer-like dyspepsia, referred to a hospital clinic, *Gut* 45:186-190, 1999.
7. Nandurkar S, Talley NJ, Xia H, et al: Dyspepsia in the community is linked to smoking and aspirin use but not to *Helicobacter pylori* infection, *Arch Intern Med* 158:1427-1433, 1998.

Peptic Ulcer
(See also esophagus; non-steroidal anti-inflammatory agent gastropathy; non-ulcer dyspepsia; stomach cancer)

Bleeding peptic ulcers

Bleeding peptic ulcers account for 50% of upper GI hemorrhages. In 80% of cases the bleeding stops spontaneously and recovery is uneventful. Rebleeding, when it occurs, usually takes place within the first 3 days. NSAIDs appear to be a major risk factor not only for the development of peptic ulcers, but also for bleeding from peptic ulcers.[1]

In patients with uncontrolled bleeding, immediate hemostasis can usually be achieved through endoscopic procedures,[1,2] although rebleeding occurs in 10% to 30% of cases.[2] Intensive therapy with H_2-blockers has not been effective in controlling acute upper intestinal bleeding, but in India a trial of omeprazole (Prilosec, Losec) 40 mg orally twice a day for 5 days for endoscopically documented bleeding peptic ulcers showed a significant decrease in requirements for transfusion or surgery. No endoscopic therapeutic interventions were attempted in this study.[3] Omeprazole has also been shown to be effective in preventing rebleeding after endoscopic control of hemorrhage from peptic ulcers. In one study the drug was begun as a 40-mg IV bolus, was followed by a continuous IV infusion of 160 mg per day for 3 days, and then was given as 20 mg per day orally for 2 months.[2]

Once a patient has stopped bleeding and is in stable condition, medical treatment is aimed at healing the ulcer and preventing recurrences of the ulcer and bleeding. If possible, NSAIDs should be discontinued. If the patient is positive for *H. pylori* (as are about 75% of patients with bleeding peptic ulcers), the organisms should be eradicated. (See later discussion.) Healing is facilitated by omeprazole 20 mg per day for 6 to 8 weeks or by an H_2-receptor antagonist for 2 to 3 months.[1] Many patients remain on high-dose proton pump inhibitors (PPIs) forever, and this is not necessary.

Helicobacter pylori

More than 80% of people with gastric ulcers and more than 90% of those with duodenal ulcers are infected with *H. pylori*. However, ulcers develop in only 15% to 20% of people infected with the organism. Consequently, ulcer recurrence rate is markedly decreased in patients treated for *H. pylori*.[4]

H. pylori infection is recognized as a cause of gastric and duodenal ulcers, as well as gastric carcinoma.[4,5] Interestingly, the incidence of gastric cancer is decreased in patients with a history of duodenal ulcer.[6] The probable explanation is that *H. pylori* acquired in early childhood (as occurs frequently in developing countries) leads to atrophic gastritis, which is both a predisposing factor for malignancy and, because of decreased acid secretion, a defense against duodenal ulcer formation. However, when the infection is acquired later in life, atrophic gastritis is less likely to develop, so acid secretion is not inhibited.[5] Atrophic gastritis also protects against GERD.

Diagnostic procedures for *H. pylori* include gastric biopsies, urea breath tests, and serological tests.[4,7,8] Serological findings remain positive for many months or years after eradication of the organism and cannot be used to measure the efficacy of therapy within the first few months of treatment.[4,8] However, in one small study, serological findings reverted to normal after 18 months in 65% of patients who had documented cure of *H. pylori* infection. The clinical significance is that a negative serological test many months after treatment of *H. pylori* rules out persistent infection, whereas a positive test has no clinical benefit. If earlier documentation of cure is necessary, it can be established with urea breath tests or gastric biopsies.[7,8] An important caveat is that one third of patients who are taking proton pump inhibitors have false-negative results of urea breath tests (temporary suppression of *H. pylori* by the drug). Patients should not take proton pump inhibitors for at least 1 week, and preferably 2 weeks, before the test.[9]

Treatment of *H. pylori* infections leads to faster healing of ulcers and a marked reduction in the relapse rate.[4,5] Since 95% of duodenal ulcers that are not NSAID-related are associated with *H. pylori* infection, a reasonable approach is to treat all such patients with antimicrobial therapy without testing them for the presence of the organism.[4] Recent observations of gastric mucosa-associated lymphoid tissue (MALT) lymphomas have yielded resolution of these tumours by successful eradication of *H. pylori* infection with antibiotics.[10] Because *H. pylori* is difficult to eradicate, two or more antibiotics should be used. The adjunct use of a proton pump inhibitor such as omeprazole (Prilosec, Losec) or lansoprazole (Prevacid) augments the efficacy of the antibiotics. Most studies to date have used omeprazole 20 mg twice a day, but data suggest that other proton pump inhibitors such as lansoprazole 30 mg twice a day or pantoprazole (Pantoloc) 40 mg twice a day are equally effective.[4]

A confusing variety of treatments for *H. pylori* have been used, and some of the more effective ones are listed below.[4,11,12] Cure rates with any of these regimens are approximately 85% to 90%.[4] Most of the studies of bismuth have been with bismuth subcitrate, which is not available in North America; probably bismuth subsalicylate (Pepto-Bismol), which is the standard form in North America, is equally effective when given as combination therapy.[11,12] Although in vitro resistance to metronidazole (Flagyl) is fairly common, this does not appear to affect its efficacy when used as part of combination therapy.[12]

At present, triple therapy appears to be the optimal first option[12,13]:

- Clarithromycin (Biaxin) 500 mg twice a day plus metronidazole (Flagyl) 500 mg twice a day plus omeprazole (Prilosec, Losec) 20 mg twice a day for 7 to 10 days[12]
- Clarithromycin (Biaxin) 500 mg twice a day plus amoxicillin 1 g twice a day plus lansoprazole (Prevacid) 30 mg twice a day for 14 days[13]

If triple therapy fails, the next step should be a bismuth-based quadruple therapy regimen[12]: bismuth subsalicylate 524 mg (Pepto-Bismol, 2 tablets) once a day or bismuth subcitrate 120 mg once a day plus tetracycline 250 or 500 mg once a day plus metronidazole 250 mg once a day plus omeprazole 20 mg twice a day or lansoprazole 30 mg twice a day. Amoxicillin 1 g two or three times a day can be substituted for the tetracycline.

A less expensive regimen uses bismuth, tetracycline, and metronidazole alone[4]: bismuth subsalicylate (Pepto-Bismol) 2 tablets (262 mg each) once a day for 7 to 14 days plus metronidazole (Flagyl) 250 mg four times a day for 7 to 14 days plus tetracycline 500 mg four times a a day for 7 to 14 days.

A recent trial showed that a four-drug, single-day treatment was as effective as 7 days of treatment with three drugs in eradicating *H. pylori* and symptoms in patients with *H. pylori*-positive dyspepsia.[14] The regimen consisted of 2 tablets of 262 mg bismuth subsalicylate (Pepto-Bismol), 500 mg metronidazole (Flagyl), and 2 g amoxicillin (suspension), all taken four times over the course of the day, along with 60 mg lansoprazole (Prevacid) taken once. This has to be confirmed by more

Table 26   Peptic Ulcer Medications

Drug	Usual doses
H$_2$-Blockers	
Cimetidine (Tagamet)	800 mg qhs or 600 mg bid
Famotidine (Pepcid)	40 mg qhs
Nizatidine (Axid)	300 mg qhs
Ranitidine (Zantac)	300 mg qhs or 150 mg bid
Proton Pump Inhibitors	
Lansoprazole (Prevacid)	15 mg qam
Omeprazole (Prilosec, Losec)	20 mg qam
Esomeprazole (Nexium)	20 mg qam
Pantoprazole (Pantoloc)	40 mg qam
Rabeprazole (Aciphex, Pariet)	20 mg once daily
Prostaglandins	
Misoprostol (Cytotec)	200 μg qid or 400 μg bid
Cytoprotectives	
Sucralfate (Sulcrate)	1-2 g qid ac and hs

studies but may be helpful information from a cost perspective for select patients.

Stress

Physiological stress from sepsis, burns, and head injury can cause the stress-related erosive syndrome. Psychological stress is likely to be important in peptic ulcers, whether related to *H. pylori* or NSAIDs. This effect is likely related to an increased acid secretion, which enhances aggravating factors in people predisposed to peptic ulcer or exacerbates pre-existing peptic ulcer by increasing acid load.[15]

Specific ulcer medications

Traditional medications used for the treatment of peptic ulcers are listed in Table 26.

───────────── ❧ **REFERENCES** ❧ ─────────────

1. Laine L, Peterson WL: Bleeding peptic ulcer, *N Engl J Med* 331:717-727, 1994.
2. Lin H-J, Lo W-C, Lee F-Y, et al: A prospective randomized comparative trial showing that omeprazole prevents rebleeding in patients with bleeding peptic ulcer after successful endoscopic therapy, *Arch Intern Med* 158:54-58, 1998.
3. Khuroo MS, Yattoo GN, Javid G, et al: A comparison of omeprazole and placebo for bleeding peptic ulcer, *N Engl J Med* 336:1054-1058, 1997.
4. Veldhuyzen van Zanten SJ, Sherman PM, Hunt RH: *Helicobacter pylori:* new developments and treatments, *Can Med Assoc J* 156:1565-1574, 1997.
5. Parsonnet J: *Helicobacter pylori* in the stomach–a paradox unmasked (editorial), *N Engl J Med* 335:278-280, 1996.
6. Hansson L-E, Nyrén O, Hsing AW, et al: The risk of stomach cancer in patients with gastric or duodenal ulcer disease, *N Engl J Med* 335:242-249, 1996.
7. Blaser MJ: *Helicobacter pylori* and gastric diseases, *BMJ* 316:1507-1510, 1998.
8. Feldman M, Cryer B, Lee E, et al: Role of seroconversion in confirming cure of *Helicobacter pylori* infection, *JAMA* 280:363-365, 1998.
9. Laine L, Estrada R, Trujillo M, et al: Effect of proton pump inhibitor therapy on diagnostic testing for *Helicobacter pylori, Ann Intern Med* 129:547-550, 1998.
10. Du MQ: Gastric MALT lymphoma: from aetiology to treatment, *Lancet Oncol* 3(2):97-104, 2002.
11. Soll AH: Medical treatment of peptic ulcer disease: practice guidelines, *JAMA* 275:622-629, 1996.
12. Salcedo JA, Al-Kawas F: Treatment of *Helicobacter pylori* infection, *Arch Intern Med* 158:842-851, 1998.
13. Schwartz H, Krause R, Sahba B, et al: Triple versus dual therapy for eradicating *Helicobacter pylori* and prevention of ulcer recurrence: a randomized, double-blind, multicenter study of lansoprazole, clarithromycin, and/or amoxicillin in different dosing regimens, *Am J Gastroenterol* 93:584-590, 1998.
14. Lara LF, Cisneros G, Gurney M, et al: One-day quadruple therapy compared with 7-day triple therapy for *Helicobacter pylori* infection, *Arch Intern Med* 163:2079-2084, 2003.
15. Levenstein S, Ackerman S, Kiecolt-Glaser JK, et al: Stress and peptic ulcer disease, *JAMA* 281:10-11, 1999.

Stomach Cancer
(See also peptic ulcer)

The overall incidence of gastric carcinoma has declined rapidly in North America in the past 50 years. However, in developing countries the incidence of gastric carcinoma is much higher and is second only to lung cancer in terms of mortality. In particular, Japan, China, and South America continue to suffer higher incidence of this disease. Many risk factors have been associated with gastric cancer, and the pathogenesis is likely multifactorial. Risks factors include *H. pylori* infection, smoking, and excessive alcohol ingestion. Surgery is the treatment of choice with consideration of adjuvant chemoradiation therapy depending on the stage of the tumour. The 5-year survival of stage I tumour that has not invaded the muscularis, spread to nodes, or metastasized is 50% to 60% in North America, but stage I accounts for less than 10% of North American cases. The 5-year survival for stage II (invasion of muscularis propria but no serosal involvement) is 30%, and stages III and IV have survival rates less than 20%. In Japan, a higher incidence of adenocarcinoma and rigorous screening processes have led to a greater number of cases of gastric cancer being detected at an early stage, and overall the survival rate is better. Recent observations of gastric MALT lymphomas have yielded resolution of these tumours by successful eradication of *H. pylori* infection with antibiotics.[2]

Early gastric cancer can often manifest as an ulcer or dyspepsia. Treatment with proton pump inhibitors may result in the resolution of dyspeptic symptoms and even healing of malignant ulcers, which may mask the true underlying pathology. For this reason some experts recommend endoscopy and biopsy for all patients with new symptoms of dyspepsia over the age of 45, before proton pump inhibitors are prescribed.[3]

❧ REFERENCES ❧

1. Fuchs CS, Mayer RJ: Gastric carcinoma, *N Engl J Med* 333:32-41, 1995.
2. Du MQ: Gastric MALT lymphoma: from aetiology to treatment, *Lancet Oncol* 3(2):97-104, 2002.
3. Griffin SM, Raimes SA: Proton pump inhibitors may mask early gastric cancer: dyspeptic patients over 45 should undergo endoscopy before these drugs are started (editorial), *BMJ* 317: 1606-1607, 1998.

GENERAL GERIATRICS

(See also dementia; exercise; hip fractures; hypertension; non-steroidal anti-inflammatory drugs; osteoarthritis; osteoporosis; prescribing and the elderly; pseudohypertension; urinary tract infections)

Epidemiology

Persons who are 85 years or older are often labelled as the "oldest old." Among this group, half of the men are living with their wives, most of whom are younger than their husbands, whereas only 10% of women in this age group are living with their husbands because most husbands are dead. About half of persons 85 years or older have impaired hearing, and a third have some degree of dementia. In the United States, 25% of women over the age of 84 and 15% of men of similar age live in nursing homes.[1] The average life expectancy of 80-year-old U.S. women is 9.1 years, while for 80-year-old U.S. men it is 7 years.[2] Among 85-year-olds in the United States, the life expectancy is 6.4 years for women and 5.2 years for men.[1] Use of health services by people ages 65 to 74 is little different from that of the general adult population, but for those 75 and older it increases significantly.[3] Middle-age individuals with low health risk factors (non-smokers and non-sedentary and non-obese persons) not only live longer than their counterparts who have these risk factors, but also have less lifetime disability.[4]

Although exercise is well known to decrease mortality rates in the elderly, it appears that social and productive activities also have a protective role. Typical social activities are church attendance; going to movies, sports events, or restaurants; taking short trips; playing cards or other games; and belonging to social groups. Productive activities include preparing meals, shopping, gardening, paid employment, and volunteer community work.[5]

Caregivers

Many persons believe that elderly patients with dementia or terminal illnesses are best looked after at home. Except for the very affluent, this means that family members or close friends must perform most of the care. Considerable literature shows that this process may adversely affect the emotional and even the physical health of the caregivers, but surprisingly little evidence supports the notion that home care is better than institutional care for either the patient or the family caregivers.[6]

Delirium

Five important precipitating factors for delirium in elderly hospitalized patients are malnutrition, physical restraints, bladder catheterization, taking more than three medications, and any iatrogenic event.[7] Optimal treatment is control of precipitating factors. If medications are required, neuroleptics such as haloperidol or droperidol are the drugs of choice. Benzodiazepines as monotherapy are ineffective, although some reports state that they may have value when combined with neuroleptics.[8]

Dry Mouth and Dry Eyes

In a population survey, just over one fourth of elderly patients complained of dry eyes or dry mouth.[9] In another population-based study of participants age 50 or older, 57.5% reported at least one dry eye symptom, and symptoms were more common with female gender and systemic diseases. Systemic factors significantly associated with dry eye syndrome included history of arthritis, asthma, gout, and use of corticosteroids, antidepressants, and hormone replacement therapy.[10] Accurate measurement of symptoms should be included as part of the diagnostic assessment and management of dry eye patients. The Dry Eye Questionnaire has been developed as an effective tool to measure symptoms in patients with dry eye, particularly in the elderly.[11]

Exercise in the Elderly

For middle age and older adults, regular exercise is associated with a decrease in multiple morbidities and mortality. Specific recommendations for any patient are best provided by an exercise prescription consisting of aerobic exercise, strength training, and balance and flexibility exercise.[12] The American College of Sports Medicine recommends exercise stress testing for all sedentary or minimally active older adults who plan to begin exercising at a vigorous intensity. Most elderly patients can safely begin a moderate aerobic and resistance training program without stress testing if they begin slowly and gradually increase their level of activity. A community-based walking program in Massachusetts involving almost 8,000 elderly patients reported no incidence of myocardial infarction or other adverse cardiac events during exercise over an 8-year period.[13] Patients need to be advised to discontinue exercise and seek medical advice if they experience chest pain, palpitations, or light-headedness or other concerning symptoms.

Exercise emphasizing strength and balance decreases the risk of falls in the elderly.[14,15] In one such program for women over age 80, physiotherapists visited the home every 2 weeks for 2 months. The women were taught lower limb–strengthening exercises using 0.5- and 1-kg ankle weights, walking on toes and heels, doing knee squatting, rising from chairs, climbing stairs, walking backward, turning around, walking in tandem, and active range of motion exercises to increase flexibility, such as maximum head turning or hip and knee extension. Patients were asked to follow this routine independently at least three times per week.[15] A small randomized controlled trial showed that participation in a weekly group exercise program with ancillary home exercises can improve balance and reduce the rate of falling for elderly persons who are at risk and living in the community by 40% over a 12-month period.[16]

Falls

Some of the medical risk factors for falls in the elderly are cardiovascular disorders such as postural hypotension, arrhythmias, and pacemaker failure; and visual impairment; muscle weakness; and peripheral neuropathy.[17] Excessive medications in general[18] and the use of benzodiazepines in particular[19] are associated with increased rates of falling and fractures. Reputed environmental factors leading to falls are uneven outdoor surfaces, change in surface level, and inappropriate floor coverings and footwear.[17]

A thorough medical assessment and a home evaluation by an occupational therapist, followed by appropriate therapeutic interventions, reduce the number of falls in elderly patients when compared with control subjects receiving usual care.[17] One of the most effective interventions in preventing falls is an exercise program emphasizing strength, balance, and aerobic fitness.[14,15] Not only is the degree of osteoporosis minimized, but improved balance and gait decrease the frequency of falls. Whether such programs actually decrease the risk of hip fractures has not been established.[14]

Living Alone

The risk of helplessness or death for a person living alone increases with age. The highest risk group is men over age 85 who are living alone. The longer the interval between the onset of helplessness and the time the person is found, the higher the mortality rate.[20] Suggested solutions are frequent checking on such individuals[20,21] and use of electronic-alert devices.[21]

Prescribing and The Elderly

Inappropriate prescription of drugs for the elderly is rampant. A study by Tamblyn and associates[22] determined that over a 1-year period, about one third of elderly Quebec residents received prescriptions for benzodiazepines to be taken for more than 30 consecutive days. A similar type of survey in British Columbia found that over a 1-year period, 17% of non-institutionalized persons over age 65 received at least one prescription for benzodiazepines, and 4% of elderly patients received a prescription for 20 mg of diazepam or its equivalent to be taken daily for more than 2 months.[23] A U.S. report found

that 60% of individuals in the United States who take non-steroidal anti-inflammatory drugs (NSAIDs) are 60 years or older,[24] and in Alberta, 27% of persons over age 65 received at least one NSAID prescription during a 6-month study period.[25] A Canadian study of the prescribing habits of New Brunswick physicians treating elderly patients showed that high prescribers ordered 45% more prescriptions than did low prescribers and that morbidity, hip fracture, and mortality rates were higher among patients of high-prescribing physicians than among those of low prescribers.[18]

Other important adverse consequences of polypharmacy in the elderly are delirium and incontinence.[26] The number of potentially inappropriate drug combinations prescribed for elderly patients increases with the number of prescribing physicians the patient sees.[27] Although polypharmacy is clearly a major problem with drug prescriptions in the elderly, underuse is also important. Examples are failure to prescribe beta blockers for elderly patients who have had a myocardial infarction,[26,28] anticoagulants for those in atrial fibrillation,[26] or adequate medications to control systolic hypertension[28] or fully control cancer pain.[28]

An important aspect of geriatric care is a careful review of medications with the goal of stopping those that are unnecessary. In most cases, discontinuation is accomplished successfully, but in some, the process results in adverse drug withdrawal events. A relatively infrequent type of adverse drug withdrawal event is the physiological withdrawal reaction, which is most frequently seen with beta blockers, benzodiazepines, antipsychotics, antidepressants, and corticosteroids. The solution is to taper the drug reduction slowly. A more common adverse effect is recurrence of the condition for which the drugs were originally prescribed, such as angina, hypertension, or congestive heart failure. Recurrences may not manifest themselves for 3 or 4 months.[29]

≈ REFERENCES ≈

1. Campion EW: The oldest old (editorial), *N Engl J Med* 30:1819-1820, 1994.
2. Manton KG, Vaupel JW: Survival after the age of 80 in the United States, Sweden, France, England, and Japan, *N Engl J Med* 333:1232-1235, 1995.
3. Rosenberg MW, Moore EG: The health of Canada's elderly population: current status and future implications, *Can Med Assoc J* 157:1025-1032, 1997.
4. Vita AJ, Terry RB, Hubert HB, et al: Aging, health risks, and cumulative disability, *N Engl J Med* 338:1035-1041, 1998.
5. Glass TA, de Leon CM, Marottoli RA, et al: Population based study of social and productive activities as predictors of survival among elderly Americans, *BMJ* 319:478-483, 1999.
6. Grunfeld E, Glossop R, McDowell I, et al: Caring for elderly people at home: the consequences to caregivers, *Can Med Assoc J* 157:1101-1105, 1997.

7. Inouye SK, Charpentier PA: Precipitating factors for delirium in hospitalized elderly persons: predictive model and interrelationship with baseline vulnerability, *JAMA* 275:852-857, 1996.

8. Trzepacz P, Breitbart W, Franklin J, et al: American Psychiatric Association Practice Guideline for the treatment of patients with delirium, *Am J Psychiatry* 156:S1-S20, 1999.

9. Schein OD, Hochberg MC, Munoz B, et al: Dry eye and dry mouth in the elderly: a population-based assessment, *Arch Intern Med* 159:1359-1363, 1999.

10. Chia EM, Mitchell P, Rochtchina E, et al: Prevalence and associations of dry eye syndrome in an older population: the Blue Mountains Eye Study, *Clin Exper Ophthalmol* 31(3):229-232, 2003.

11. Begley CG, Caffery B, Chalmers RL, et al: Dry Eye Investigation (DREI) Study Group. Use of the dry eye questionnaire to measure symptoms of ocular irritation in patients with aqueous tear-deficient dry eye, *Cornea* 21(7):664-670, 2002.

12. Nied RJ, Franklin B: Promoting and prescribing exercise for the elderly, *Am Fam Physician* 65(3): 419-426, 2002.

13. Evans WJ: Exercise training guidelines for the elderly, *Med Sci Sports Exerc* 31:12-17, 1999.

14. Kannus P: Preventing osteoporosis, falls, and fractures among elderly people: promotion of lifelong physical activity is essential (editorial), *BMJ* 318:205-206, 1999.

15. Campbell AJ, Robertson MC, Gardner MM, et al: Randomised controlled trial of a general practice programme of home based exercise to prevent falls in elderly women, *BMJ* 315:1065-1069, 1997.

16. Barnett A, Smith B, Lord SR, et al: Community-based group exercise improves balance and reduces falls in at-risk older people: a randomised controlled trial, *Age Ageing* 32(4):407-414, 2003.

17. Close J, Ellis M, Hooper R, et al: Prevention of falls in the elderly trial (PROFET): a randomised controlled trial, *Lancet* 353:93-97, 1999.

18. Davidson W, Molloy DW, Bédard M: Physician characteristics and prescribing for elderly people in New Brunswick: relation to patient outcomes, *Can Med Assoc J* 152: 1227-1234, 1995.

19. Herings RM, Stricker BH, de Boer A, et al: Benzodiazepines and the risk of falling leading to femur fractures, *Arch Intern Med* 155:1801-1807, 1995.

20. Gurley RJ, Lum N, Sande M, et al: Persons found in their homes helpless or dead, *N Engl J Med* 334:1710-1716, 1996.

21. Campion EW: Home alone, and in danger (editorial), *N Engl J Med* 334:1738-1739, 1996.

22. Tamblyn RM, McLeod PJ, Abrahamowicz M, et al: Questionable prescribing for elderly patients in Quebec, *Can Med Assoc J* 150:1801-1809, 1994.

23. Thomson M, Smith WA: Prescribing benzodiazepines for noninstitutionalized elderly, *Can Fam Physician* 41:792-798, 1995.

24. Gurwitz JH, Avorn J: The ambiguous relation between aging and adverse drug reactions, *Ann Intern Med* 114: 956-966, 1991.

25. Hogan DB, Campbell NRC, Crutcher R, et al: Prescription of nonsteroidal anti-inflammatory drugs for elderly people in Alberta, *Can Med Assoc J* 151:315-322, 1994.

26. Hogan DB: Revisiting the O complex: urinary incontinence, delirium and polypharmacy in elderly patients, *Can Med Assoc J* 157:1071-1077, 1997.

27. Tamblyn RM, McLeod PJ, Abrahamowicz M, et al: Do too many cooks spoil the broth? Multiple physician involvement in medical management of elderly patients and potentially inappropriate drug combinations, *Can Med Assoc J* 154:1177-1184, 1996.

28. Rochon PA, Gurwitz JH: Prescribing for seniors: neither too much nor too little, *JAMA* 282:113-115, 1999.

29. Graves T, Hanlon JT, Schmader KE, et al: Adverse events after discontinuing medications in elderly outpatients, *Arch Intern Med* 157:2205-2210, 1997.

DEMENTIA

Dementia is diagnosed when cognitive impairment in multiple faculties has occurred to the extent that it affects daily life functioning.

Eight percent of Canadian elderly (over the age of 65) suffer from dementia, but its prevalence, like many diseases in the elderly, increases with age.[1,2]

As many as 80% of normal elderly have some complaints of memory loss.[3]

Normal aging can be associated with changes in memory (e.g., being unable to recall the name of a distant acquaintance), but some elderly persons show progressive deterioration in cognition beyond what would be accepted as normal but have not yet reached the point of a noticeable decline in function. This cohort has been labelled with many different terms, including benign senescent forgetfulness; late-life forgetfulness; age-associated memory impairment (AAMI); questionable dementia; aging-associated cognitive decline (AACD); cognitive impairment, no dementia (CIND); and most recently, mild cognitive impairment (MCI).

There is no reliable way to predict which patient with MCI will progress to dementia, but in a population study, 78% of patients did not progress over an 8-year follow-up.[4]

Increasing age is the most significant risk factor for Alzheimer's disease (AD). Risk of developing the disease increases with age. First-degree relatives of an affected patient have an increased risk of 2 to 4 times that of people who do not have an affected relative.[5,6]

Early-onset or familial AD shows an autosomal-dominant pattern of transmission in a minority of cases, which usually begin before age 60. The overwhelming majority of AD cases are late-onset (occur after age 65) and occur sporadically.[7]

The presence of genotype 4 of the apolipoprotein E gene (apoE4) on chromosome 19 is associated with increased risk of late-onset AD but with poor sensitivity (50%) and specificity (75%) for the disease, genetic testing is of limited use even in symptomatic cognitive impairment.[8,9] Half the patients with late-onset AD do not even carry the apolipoprotein E4 (apoE4) gene allele, so other unknown risk factors must exist.[10]

Dementia, associated with clear sensorium (usually alert) is distinguished from delirium, which has a fluctuating level of alertness. The two diagnostic criteria accepted for AD include DSM-4 and NINCDS-ADRDA.[11] A cut off of less than 24/30 on the MMSE suggests dementia.[12]

Clinicians must look for symptoms and signs that are inconsistent with the diagnostic criteria of AD and may indicate other types of dementia, especially vascular dementia. These include abrupt-onset, early-onset seizures, history of hypertension or stroke, gait disturbance, or focal neurological signs. Pseudodementia, or depression, needs to be ruled out at this time.

For patients who fit the criteria for AD, relatively few blood tests are indicated, and they include CBC, electrolytes, glucose, calcium, and thyroid-stimulating hormone (TSH). Others that may be indicated in certain circumstances include ammonia, drug levels, erythrocyte sedimentation rate (ESR), folic acid, heavy metals, cortisol, lipids, and tests for B_{12}, VDRL, and HIV.[13,14]

In most cases, computed tomography (CT) scanning is not indicated except when other types of dementia are suspected, such as patients with age less than 60 years, atypical presentation, rapid decline, head trauma, seizures or focal neurological symptoms, possible metastatic cancer, anticoagulants, incontinence and "magnet foot" (normal pressure hydrocepahlus), and gait disturbance.[15]

The first cholinesterase inhibitor, tacrine (Cognex), has significant adverse effects including reversible elevated alanine transaminase (ALT) liver enzyme levels, and there is limited evidence of its effectiveness on cognitive enhancement.[16,17]

The following table lists three cholinesterase inhibitors that have been shown to enhance cognition.[18-20]

It has been difficult to justify prescribing these medications because the research-outcome measures are not easily applied to clinical scenarios in practice. Furthermore, the study subjects are often not primary-care cohorts. Side effects, which can be predicted given the cholinergic function of these medications, include nausea, vomiting, anorexia, diarrhea, bradycardia, gastritis, possible chronic obstructive pulmonary disease (COPD)/asthmatic exacerbation, and seizures.

Table 27 Cholinesterase Inhibitors that Enhance Cognition

Cholinesterase Inhibitor	Dosage	
	Starting dose:	4 week dose escalation:
Aricept (Donepezil)*	5 mg po od	10 mg po od
Exelon (Rivastigmine)†	1.5 mg po bid	3 mg po bid
Reminyl (Galantamine)‡	4 mg po bid	8 mg po bid

*Aricept Product Monograph, PFIZER Canada Inc., May 2000.
†Exelon Product Monograph, NOVARTIS Canada Inc., October 2003.
‡Reminyl Product Monograph, JANSSEN-ORTHO Inc., January 2003.

Deciding on the best cholinesterase inhibitor is difficult. Comparison trials have always favoured the pharmaceutical sponsor's product, and Canadian geriatricians have many concerns about the validity of the trials.[21-24] Cholinesterase inhibitors should be stopped when the clinician feels that the benefits are limited; this could be when the dementia has progressed to a severe stage. Nevertheless, Feldman et al studied donepezil in 290 people ages 48 to 92 years with moderate and severe AD and found that it improved CIBIC-Plus scores at 24 weeks.[25]

In one randomized controlled trial, vitamin E was not found to enhance cognitive function compared with placebo after 2 years of treatment but it did reduce mortality, institutionalization, and loss of functioning.[26]

Other medications, including Ginkgo biloba, selegiline, and propentofylline, have shown little if any benefit and would be considered inappropriate for use as a cognitive enhancer in AD.[27] NSAIDs, estrogen, and HMG-CoA reductase inhibitors (statins) have not been shown to prevent AD.[28-30] A new class of cognitive enhancers available in the United States, N-methyl-D-aspartate (NMDA) blockers such as Memantine have shown to improve cognitive functioning in mild-to-moderate vascular dementia.[31,32] Memantine has also shown to improve global clinical outcome and care dependence in severe AD.[33]

Behavioural problems of dementia can be managed using the PIECES approach, which examines physical, intellectual, emotional, functional (capabilities), environmental, and social causes.[34]

Often times, a non-pharmacological treatment plan is possible. When medication is required, antidepressants should be considered first if agitation is felt to be related to an affective disorder. Atypical neuroleptics such as risperidone have shown to have fewer extrapyramidal side effects compared with older ones like halperidol but seem to be equally effective.[35] In a randomized controlled trial, olanzapine was shown to reduce agitation, hallucinations, and delusions in patients with dementia over a 6-week period compared with placebo.[36] It was postulated that atypical neuroleptics (such as risperidone and olanzapine) may be associated with risk of stroke.[37] However, a recent retrospective population-based cohort study did not find an increased risk of stroke with atypical neuroleptics when compared with typical neuroleptics.[38]

Quetiapine (Seroquel) has been effective in controlling behavioural and psychological symptoms of dementia.[39] Anticonvulsants (e.g., sodium valproate and carbamazepine) may offer some benefit with increasing evidence of effectiveness.[40-43]

In one study, trazodone was shown similar to haloperidol for behaviour management techniques and placebo, but the study may have been too small to find clinically relevant improvements.[44]

❧ REFERENCES ❧

1. Lindsay J, Sykes E, McDowell I, et al: More than the epidemiology of Alzheimer's Disease: contributions of the Canadian Study of Health and Aging, *Can J Psychiatry* 49(2):83-91, Feb 2004.
2. Canadian Study of Health and Aging Working Group: Canadian Study of Health and Aging; study methods and prevalence of dementia, *Can Med Assoc J* 150:899-913, 1994.
3. Sluss TK, Rabins P, Gruenberg EM, et al: Memory complaints in community residing men, *Gerontologist* 20(20):201-218, 1980.
4. Ritchie K, et al: A typology of sub-clinical senescent cognitive disorder, *Br J Psychiatry* 168(4): 470-476, 1996.
5. Blacker D, Tanzi RE: The genetics of Alzheimer's disease, *Arch Neurol* 55:294-296, 1998.
6. Van Duijn CM, Clayton D, Chandra V: Familial aggregation of Alzheimer's disease and related disorders: a collaborative re-analysis of case-control studies, *Int J Epidemiol* 20:S13-20, 1991.
7. Richard F, Amouyel P: Genetic susceptibility factors for Alzheimer's disease, *Eur J Pharmacol* 412(1):1-12, Jan 19 2001.
8. Tilvis RS, Strandberg TE, Juva K: Apolipoprotein E phenotypes, dementia and mortality in a prospective population sample, *J Am Geriatr Soc* 46:712-715, 1998.
9. Kukull WA, Schellenberg GD, Bowen JD: Apolipoprotein E in Alzheimer's disease: risk and case detection: a case-control study, *J Clin Epidemiol* 49:1143-1148, 1996.
10. Myers AJ, Goate AM: The genetics of late-onset Alzheimer's disease, *Curr Opin Neurol* 14(4):433-440, Aug 2001.
11. McKhann G, Drachman D, Folstein M, et al: Clinical diagnosis of Alzheimer's disease: report of the NINCDS-ADRDA Work Group under the auspices of Department of Health and Human Services Task Force on Alzheimer's Disease, *Neurology* 34(7):939-944, 1984.
12. Folstein MF, Folstein SE, Mchugh PR: Mini-mental state: a practical method for grading the cognitive state of patients for the clinician, *J Psychiatr Res* 12:189-198, 1975.
13. Patterson CJS, Gauthier S, Bergman H, et al: The recognition and management of dementing disorders: conclusions from the Canadian Consensus Conference on Dementia, *CMAJ* 160(Suppl 12):S1-S15, 1999.
14. Frank C: Dementia workup: deciding on laboratory testing for the elderly, *Can Fam Physician* 44:1489-1495, 1998.
15. Patterson CJ, Gauthier S, Bergman H, et al: Canadian Consensus, *CMAJ* 160(Suppl 12):S1-S15, 1999.
16. Knapp MJ, Knopman DS, Solomon PR, et al: A 30-week randomized controlled trial of high-dose tacrine in patients with Alzheimer's disease. The Tacrine Study Group, *JAMA* 271:985-991, 1994.
17. Qizilbash N, Birks J, Lopez Arrieta J, et al: Tacrine for Alzheimer's disease. *Cochrane Database Syst Rev* (3): CD000202, 2004.
18. Birks JS, Harvey R: Donepezil for dementia due to Alzheimer's disease, *Cochrane Database Syst Rev* (3): CD001190, 2004.
19. Birks J, Grimley-Evans J, Iakovidou V: Rivastigmine for Alzheimer's disease, *Cochrane Database Syst Rev* (4): CD001191, 2000.
20. Olin J, Schneider L: Galantamine for Alzheimer's disease, *Cochrane Database Syst Rev* (4):CD001747, 2004.
21. Wilkinson DG, Passmore AP, Bullock R, et al: A multinational, randomized 12-week, comparative study of donepezil and rivastigmine in patients with mild to moderate Alzheimer's disease, *Int J Clin Pract* 56:441-446, 2002.
22. Wilcock G, Howe I, Coles H, et al: A long-term comparison of galantamine and donepezil in the treatment of Alzheimer's disease, *Drugs and Aging* 20:777-789, 2003.
23. *Int J Geriatr Psychiatry* 19:58-67, 2004.
24. Hogan DB, Goldlist B, Naglie G, et al: Comparison studies of cholinesterase inhibitors for Alzheimer's disease, *Lancet Neurol* 3(10):622-626, 2004.
25. Feldman H, Gauthier S, Hecker J, et al: A 24-week, randomized, double blind study of donepezil in moderate to severe Alzheimer's disease, *Neurology*, 57:613-620, 2001.
26. Sano M, Ernesto C, Thomas RG, et al: A controlled trial of selegiline, alph-tocopherol, or both as treatment for Alzheimer's disease, *N Engl J Med* 336:1216-1222, 1997.
27. Pryse-Phillips et al: The use of medications for cognitive enhancement, *Can J Neurol Sci* 28(Suppl):1-S108-S114, 2001.
28. In't Veld BA, Ruitenberg A, Hofman A, et al: Nonsteroidal anti-inflammatory drugs and the risk of Alzheimer's disease, *NEJM* 345:1515-1521, 2001.
29. Mulnard RA, Cotman CW, Kawas C, et al: Estrogen replacement therapy for treatment of mild to moderate Alzheimer's disease: a randomized controlled trial. Alzheimer's disease Co-operative Study, *JAMA* 283(8):1007-1015, 2000.
30. Scott HD, Laake K: Statins for the reduction of risk of Alzheimer's disease, Cochrane Database of Systematic Reviews, (3):CD003160, 2001.
31. Wilcock G, Mobius HJ, Stoffler A: A double-blind, placebo-controlled multicentre study of memantine in mild to moderate vascular dementia (MMM500), *Int Clin Psychopharmacol* 17:297-305, 2002.
32. Areosa Sastre A, McShane R, Sherriff F, et al: Memantine for dementia, *Cochrane Database Syst Rev* (4):CD003154, 2004.
33. Reisberg B, Doody R, Stoffler A, et al: Memantine in moderate to severe Alzheimer's disease, *New Engl J Med* 348:1333-1341, 2003.
34. Hamilton P, Harris D, Kessler L, et al: P.I.E.C.E.S. Consultation Team. Revised 03-12-03.
35. Pwee KH, Shukla VK, Hermann N, et al: *Novel antipsychotics for agitation in dementia: a systematic review,* Ottawa, 2003, Canadian Coordinating Office for Health Technology Assessment. Technology report No. 36. Search date 2002; primary sources Medline, Embase, Psychinfo, Ageline, Biosis Previews, Pascal, Toxfile, Health Technology Assessment website and other relevant websites, had searches of bibliographies and conference proceedings, and contact with experts in the field.
36. Street JS, Clark WS, Gannon KS, et al: Olanzapine treatment of psychotic and behavioural symptoms in patients with Alzheimer's disease in nursing care facilities: a double blind, randomized placebo-controlled trial, *J Clin Psychiatry* 64:134-143, 2003.
37. Wooltorton E: Risperidone (Risperdal): increased rate of cerebrovascular events in dementia trials, *CMAJ* 167: 1269-1270, 2002.

38. Herrmann N, Mamdani M, Lanctot KL: Atypical antipsychotics and risk of cerebrovascular accidents, *Am J Psychiatry* 161(6):1113-1115, Jun 2004.

39. Fujikawa T, Takahashi T, Kinoshita A, et al: Quetiapine treatment for behavioral and psychological symptoms in patients with senile dementia of Alzheimer type, *Neuropsychobiology* 49(4):201-204, 2004.

40. Sival RC, Duivenvoorden HJ, Jansen PA, et al: Sodium valproate in aggressive behaviour in dementia: a twelve-week open label follow-up study, *Int J Geriatr Psychiatry* 19(4):305-312, April 2004.

41. Porsteinsson AP, Tariot PN, Jakimovich LJ, et al: Valproate therapy for agitation in dementia: open-label extension of a double-blind trial, *Am J Geriatr Psychiatry* 11(4):434-440, July-Aug 2003.

42. Sival RC, Haffmans PMJ, Jansen PAF, et al: Sodium valproate in the treatment of aggressive behaviour inpatients with dementia-a randomized placebo controlled clinical trial, *Int J Geriatr Psychiatry* 17:579-585, 2002.

43. Tariot PN, Erb R, Podgorski CA, et al: Efficacy and tolerability of carbamazepine for agitation and aggression in dementia, *Am J Psychiatry* 155:54-61, 1998.

44. Teri L, Logsdon RG, Peskind E, et al: Treatment of agitation in AD: a randomized, placebo-controlled clinical trial, *Neurology* 55(9):1271-1278, Nov. 14 2000.

Headaches
- New onset always req. investigation
    - ESR (temporal arteritis)
    - MRI
    - Med. review

Ministry recall at age 80
Private center if liscence revoked
    → DriveAble $400

ANEMIA

(See also aspirin; fecal occult blood screening; hematochezia; hemorrhoids; leukemias; peptic ulcers; restless leg syndrome; sports medicine; vitamin B_{12})

Microcytic Anemias

The differential diagnosis of microcytic anemias includes iron-deficiency anemia, thalassemia, and the anemia of chronic disease (usually normocytic but microcytic in 20% to 30% of cases). Classic findings of these anemias on laboratory examination are as follows[1,2]:

- *Iron deficiency:* Mean corpuscular volume (MCV) usually less than 80, red blood cell distribution width index (RDW) greater than 15, decreased reticulocytes, decreased ferritin level, elevated iron binding capacity, low serum iron level
- *Thalassemia:* MCV often less than 70, normal RDW, normal reticulocyte count, target cells in peripheral smear
- *Anemia of chronic disease:* Hemoglobin level usually greater than 90 g/L (9 g/dl), MCV normal or low but greater than 72, ferritin level normal or elevated

Iron-Deficiency Anemias

Sequence of laboratory changes

Iron deficiency usually develops in the following sequence of changes[1]:
1. Decreased ferritin
2. Decreased MCV
3. Decreased hemoglobin
4. Subjective symptoms (usually when the hemoglobin level reaches 8 g/dl [80 g/L])

The most useful test for diagnosing iron deficiency is the serum ferritin level.[3] Ferritin levels less than 18 μg/L (18 ng/ml) are almost pathognomonic of iron deficiency, while levels above 100 μg/L (100 ng/ml) virtually rule it out.

Ferritin is an acute-phase reactant that tends to rise in cases of inflammatory or neoplastic disease. Patients with iron-deficiency anemias in addition to neoplastic or other chronic disease may have a normal or elevated ferritin level. In such situations, a bone marrow examination may be necessary to assess iron stores, although some studies have questioned the use of bone marrow examination as a gold standard.[4]

Sources of bleeding in iron-deficiency anemia

Gastrointestinal (GI) lesions are a common cause of chronic iron-deficiency anemia, although 38% of adults with this condition have no demonstrable GI lesions. While some experts have recommended performing the initial endoscopic investigation (i.e., upper vs. lower) based on symptoms and forgoing further investigations if a lesion is found, others believe that both the upper and lower intestinal tracts should be investigated regardless of what is found during the initial procedure.[5] A review of this approach performed for iron-deficiency anemia in 89 patients over the age of 60 found that close to half of the 13 with colon cancer also had "acceptable" upper GI causes for their anemia.[6]

The investigation of patients who test positive for fecal occult blood but are not anemic is discussed in the section on hematochezia.

Iron therapy

Numerous formulations of oral iron preparations are available for the treatment of iron-deficiency anemia. The three major ones are ferrous sulfate, ferrous fumarate, and ferrous gluconate. The amount of elemental iron varies among these products. In general elemental iron makes up 20% to 30% of ferrous sulfate, 30% of ferrous fumarate, and 11% of ferrous gluconate. Doses should be calculated on the basis of elemental iron. For the treatment of iron-deficiency anemia, adults usually require elemental iron 100 to 200 mg per day in divided doses, and children 3 mg/kg per day in divided doses.

Upper gastrointestinal tract discomfort, constipation, and sometimes diarrhea are the most frequent adverse effects of iron therapy,[7] and their severity depends on the dose of elemental iron.[8] Methods of minimizing these effects are to take the medication with meals, to increase the dose gradually, and to keep the total daily dose as low as possible.[8] Ferrous gluconate seems to be tolerated better than ferrous sulfate; this may simply be a dose-related phenomenon. A standard dose of ferrous sulfate is 300 mg three times a day, which gives a daily dose of elemental iron of approximately 200 mg, whereas 300 mg of ferrous gluconate three times a day gives approximately 100 mg of elemental iron per day. In general, treatment for iron-deficiency anemia should be continued for 4 to 6 months or until the serum ferritin level reaches 50 μg/L (50 ng/ml).[9]

Treatment with iron should cause reticulocytosis to begin within 3 to 5 days. If no such response is seen, the patient is not being compliant or the diagnosis is wrong.[1] Treatment with ferrous sulfate should raise the hemoglobin level by 2 g/L (0.2 g/dl) per day if there is no continued blood loss.[9]

Macrocytic Anemias

The following are some of the more important causes of macrocytic anemia:

1. Vitamin B_{12} deficiency (pernicious anemia)
2. Folate deficiency (often nutritional in elderly; celiac disease in younger patients)
3. Liver disease (alcoholism)
4. Hypothyroidism
5. Myelodysplasia (refractory anemia, sideroblastic anemia)
6. Acute bleeding or hemolysis with reticulocytosis (reticulocytes are larger than mature red blood cells)

Myelodysplasia is a common cause of macrocytic anemia in the elderly and usually has little clinical import.

Megaloblastic anemias often have oval macrocytosis and an MCV greater than 115 fl (115 μm^3). In chronic liver disease, the macrocytosis is generally between 100 and 110 fl, and oval macrocytes are not seen in the peripheral smear.[1]

Pernicious anemia is an autoimmune disease and may be associated with other autoimmune conditions such as Hashimoto's thyroiditis, Graves' disease, Addison's disease, primary hypoparathyroidism, primary ovarian failure, myasthenia gravis, and vitiligo.[10] The diagnosis of vitamin B_{12} deficiency is complex. Neurological abnormalities may be the only manifestation, as 19% to 28% of patients with B_{12} deficiency are not anemic and 17% to 33% have a normal mean corpuscular volume.[11] Laboratory testing for pernicious anemia is complex because the sensitivity and specificity of many tests are low. Initial clues to the diagnosis often come from the incidental finding of anemia or an elevated MCV in the complete blood count and the presence of oval macrocytes or hypersegmented polymorphonuclear leukocytes on the peripheral smear. When pernicious anemia is suspected, serum cobalamin (vitamin B_{12}) levels should be ascertained. Although the lower limit of normal is usually considered to be 148 pmol/L (200 pg/ml), levels may be decreased in numerous other conditions, including folate deficiency, and many patients with cobalamin deficiency do not have decreased levels. However, if the levels are below 74 pmol/L (100 pg/ml), the odds are high that the patient has cobalamin deficiency. Other useful tests are measurements of serum methylmalonic acid and serum homocysteine levels. Both are usually elevated in patients with cobalamin deficiency, whereas only homocysteine is elevated in folate deficiency. Eighty-five percent of patients with pernicious anemia have antiparietal cell antibodies in the serum, and about 50% have anti-intrinsic factor antibodies. Antiparietal antibodies are not specific, since they are present in 3% to 5% of healthy persons and many individuals with autoimmune endocrinopathies, whereas anti-intrinsic factor antibodies are quite specific. Bone marrow analysis and the Schilling test are rarely indicated.[12] Asymptomatic and milder forms of B_{12} deficiency are increasingly being recognized, and their clinical significance has been debated. Because B_{12} deficiency is common, serious, and easily treated, it should be considered and investigated in patients with unexplained hematological or neuropsychiatric abnormalities.

Treatment of pernicious anemia consists of monthly injections of at least 100 μg of vitamin B_{12}.[12] Since approximately 1% of orally ingested B_{12} is absorbed via simple diffusion (i.e., independently of intrinsic factor), replacement with high doses of oral vitamin B_{12} (1000 to 2000 μg per day) is both effective and safe, regardless of the etiology of B_{12} deficiency, and can be used for patients with newly diagnosed B_{12} deficiency and for those currently receiving injections.[13]

◄ REFERENCES ►

1. Yeo EL: Anemia: a practical approach, *Can J Diagn* 13: 79-92, 1996.
2. Tefferi A: Anemia in adults: a contemporary approach to diagnosis, *Mayo Clinic Proceedings* 78(10):1274-1280, 2003.
3. Guyatt GH, Oxman AD, Ali M, et al: Laboratory diagnosis of iron-deficiency anemia: an overview, *J Gen Intern Med* 7:145-153, 1992.
4. Barron BA, Hoyer JD, Tefferi A: A bone marrow report of absent stainable iron is not diagnostic of iron deficiency, *Ann Hematol* 80(3):166-169, 2001.
5. Goddard AF, McIntyre AS, Scott BB: Guidelines for the management of iron deficiency anaemia. British Society of Gastroenterology, *Gut* 46(Suppl 3-4):IV1-IV5, 2000.
6. Till SH, Grundman MJ: Prevalence of concomitant disease in patients with iron deficiency anaemia, *BMJ* 314:206-208, 1997.
7. Swerdlow PS: A tradition of testing ironclad practices (editorial), *JAMA* 267:560-561, 1992.
8. Wingard RL, Parker RA, Ismail N, et al: Efficacy of oral iron therapy in patients receiving recombinant human erythropoietin, *Am J Kidney Dis* 25:433-439, 1995.
9. Swain RA, Kaplan B, Montgomery E: Iron deficiency anemia: when is parenteral therapy warranted? *Postgrad Med* 100:181-182, 185, 188-193, 1996.
10. Ban-Hock Toh, van Driel IR, Gleeson PA: Pernicious anemia, *N Engl J Med* 337:1441-1448, 1997.
11. Savage DG, Lindenbaum J, Stabler SP, et al: Sensitivity of serum methylmalonic acid and total homocysteine determinations for diagnosing cobalamin and folate deficiencies, *Am J Med* 96(3):239-246, 1994.
12. Snow CF: Laboratory diagnosis of vitamin B_{12} and folate deficiency: a guide for the primary care physician, *Arch Intern Med* 159:1289-1298, 1999.
13. Kuzminski AM, Del Giacco EJ, Allen R, et al: Effective treatment of cobalamin deficiency with oral cobalamin, *Blood* 92(4):1191-1198, 1998.

ANTICOAGULATION

Anticoagulation is recommended for a variety of conditions. (*See atrial fibrillation, cerebrovascular accidents, dentistry, myocardial infarction, prosthetic valves, thrombosis, transient ischemic attacks.)*

For acute indications, use subcutaneous Low Molecular Weight (LMW) heparin; i.e., dalteparin (Fragmin) 200 IU or enoxaparin (Lovenox) 150 IU/kg subcutaneously (both to a maximum of 18,000 IU) daily, and start warfarin (Coumadin) at 5 mg po daily given in the late afternoon. One may wish to titrate by age and give 4 mg per day to patients over 60 and 3 mg per day to those over 70.[1] Because of the increased risk of bleeding and no increase in efficacy, there is no longer a recommendation to "load" with 10 or 15 mg of warfarin.[2] LMW heparin can be discontinued when the international normalized ratio (INR) has been at target for two days (Table 28). Because warfarin is teratogenic, LMW heparin should be used for all pregnancy-related indications. Warfarin is safe in breastfeeding.

Measure a baseline INR if indicated by history (i.e., known liver disease or unknown medications) and measure therapeutic effect every 2 or 3 days starting on day 2 or 3.[3]

While some foods (avocados, broccoli, brussels sprouts) antagonize warfarin,[4] these effects are usually small. Sullivan et al reported an inability of three cans of grapefruit juice concentrate three times a day to budge the INRs in warfarin users.[5]

Medications, however, are of more concern. Common medications that increase INR include acetaminophen, erythromycin, metronidazole (Flagyl), INH, cimetidine (Tagamet), and omeprazole (Losec). Those that commonly lower INR include barbiturates, carbamazepine (Tegretol), chlordiazepoxide (Librium), cholestyramine (Questran) and sucralfate (Sulcrate).[6] All of these medications are safe to take with warfarin as long as the INR is therapeutic. A good rule of thumb is to check the INR on day 3 of any medication change.

Low-dose NSAIDS and alcohol are also safe with warfarin in patients with low GI bleed risk.

Warfarin is an anticoagulant but it does not cause bleeding de novo. Any unexplained bleeding (i.e., GI/GU) requires the appropriate anatomic diagnosis. This is the case even if the INR is excessively elevated.

Table 28 Desirable INR Levels for Anticoagulation with Warfarin

Desirable INR Level	Clinical Condition
0.8-1.2	Normal
2.1-3.0*	All other conditions including mechanical heart valves (some authors recommend that for mechanical heart valves the levels be 2.5 to 3.5)

INR, International normalized ratio.
*As indicated, the therapeutic levels of warfarin for most conditions, including atrial fibrillation, are those that maintain an INR of 2 to 3. This is roughly equivalent to a prothrombin time (PT) of 1.3 to 1.5.

Management of the Excessively Elevated INR[7]

- If the INR is less than 5, omit a dose and resume at a lower dose.
- If the INR is more than 5 and less than 9 with no bleeding or risk of bleeding, omit two doses and resume at a lower dose, monitoring every other day until stable.
- If the INR is more than 5 and less than 9 with minimal bleeding and/or some risk of bleeding, hold warfarin and give vitamin K 1 to 2.5 mg orally (Use the 1 mg or 10 mg vials intended for IM or SC route, draw the fluid up in a syringe, take off the needle, and let the patient drink it). Resume warfarin at a lower dose when the INR is therapeutic.
- If the INR is more than 9 with no bleeding or risk of bleeding, hold warfarin and give vitamin K 3 to 5 mg as above.
- If the INR is more than 20 or there is serious bleeding, hold warfarin and give vitamin K 10 mg IV by slow infusion every 12 hours as necessary.

In all of the above, if the indication for the anticoagulation is severe (recent thrombosis) the patient may require LMW heparin if the vitamin K renders the INR non-therapeutic, which it almost always does.

Reversing Warfarin for Surgery

No reversal is required before dental surgery[7,8] or joint injection[7,9] in low-risk patients.

The ACCP guidelines suggest stopping warfarin 4 days before surgery and giving the following:

- No LMW heparin to low-risk patients (i.e., those with thrombosis more than 3 months into treatment or atrial fibrillation with no history of stroke).
- LMW heparin at prophylactic doses (i.e., dalteparin [Fragmin] 5,000 IU or enoxeparin [Lovenox] 4,000 IU subcutaneously daily to those with intermediate risk).
- LMW heparin at treatment doses (see paragraph 2 above) for patients at high risk (i.e., those with recent thrombosis or mechanical heart valve).[7]

In all of the above, surgery can commence 12 hours after the last dose of LMW heparin. Additionally, in all of the above, warfarin may be restarted postoperatively.

A suggested reading on this topic includes the Seventh ACCP Consensus Conference on Antithrombotic Therapy, in a supplement in *Chest* to be published late 2004 or early 2005.

♬ REFERENCES ♭

1. Ezekowitz MD, Levine JA: Preventing stroke in patients with atrial fibrillation, *JAMA* 281:1830-1835, 1999.
2. Crowther MA, Ginsberg JB, Kearon C, et al: A randomized trial comparing 5 mg and 10 mg warfarin loading doses, *Arch Intern Med* 159:46-48, 1999.
3. Hanna MM, Meuser J: Time to change: rationalizing the daily PT, daily Coumadin order, *Can Fam Physician* 42:513, 1996.

4. Hylek EM, Heiman H, Skates SJ, et al: Acetaminophen and other risk factors for excessive warfarin anticoagulation, *JAMA* 279: 657-662, 1998.

5. Sullivan DM, et al: Grapefruit juice and the response to Warfarin, *Am J Health Syst Pharm* 55:1581-1583, 1998.

6. Wells PS, et al: Interactions of Warfarin with drugs and food, *Ann Intern Med* 121:676-683, 1994.

7. Sixth ACCP Consensus Conference on Antithrombotic Therapy: CHEST, 119/1 January 2001 Supplement.

8. Wahl MJ: Dental surgery in anticoagulated patients, *Arch Intern Med* 158:1610-1616, 1998.

9. Thumboo J, et al: A prospective study of the safety of joint and soft tissue aspirations and injections in patients taking warfarin sodium, *Arthritis Rheum* 41:736-739, 1998.

BLEEDING DISORDERS

Bleeding disorders are suspected on the basis of personal and family history and confirmed by laboratory tests. Standard investigations are a complete blood count and smear, INR, partial thromboplastin time (PTT), thrombin time or fibrinogen level, and bleeding time.[1]

Hemophilia

Two types of hemophilia are recognized. The classic form, or hemophilia type A, is caused by factor VIII deficiency, and the type B form, or "Christmas disease," is caused by factor IX deficiency. Between 80% and 85% of cases are type A. Laboratory tests show a prolonged PTT, but a normal INR. Fifteen to twenty percent of patients with hemophilia A have a prolonged bleeding time. All other patients have a normal bleeding time. Both types of hemophilia can be distinguished by measuring factors VIII and IX. Both variants of the disease are X-linked recessive. For optimal treatment of bleeding episodes, therapy should be initiated at the immediate onset of each incident. Urgent transfusion with factor concentrates and blood may be necessary. This is best done with home therapy in which the parents, other caregivers, or the patients themselves are trained to give replacement-therapy preparations. The effective organization of such a program usually requires a specialized team. Never give hemophiliac patients drugs that contain Aspirin.[2]

Thrombocytopenia

A low platelet count as reported by an automated counter may be an artifact caused by platelet clumping. This is easily determined by ordering a smear. If present, the platelet clumps will be seen.[3]

Immune thrombocytopenic purpura (ITP), which is also called *idiopathic thrombocytopenic purpura,* may occur as an acute (acute ITP) or chronic (chronic ITP) disorder. The chronic form is more common in adults and is often detected incidentally when a low platelet count (less than 100×10^9/L) is reported in a complete blood count.[3,4] It is a diagnosis of exclusion, in which thrombocytopenia exists in the absence of any causative factors, including diseases or drugs. Features include purpura, bleeding from mucous membranes, and prolonged bleeding time. Splenomegaly is rare. About three fourths of adult cases are in women, and most are in persons under age 40.[4] The prognosis for adult cases is excellent.[5]

A harmless, self-limited form of thrombocytopenia is incidental thrombocytopenia of pregnancy. It occurs in the third trimester and does not cause maternal or fetal bleeding.[3] However, pregnant women with a history of ITP who have a platelet count less than 50×10^9/L should be referred to a specialist.

Other causes of thrombocytopenia include drugs, some viral infections (e.g., HIV), hypersplenism, thrombotic thrombocytopenic purpura, autoimmune diseases such as lupus, lymphoproliferative disorders, and myelodysplasia.[4]

Bleeding after trauma or surgery may occur with platelet counts less than 50×10^9/L (50,000/mm^3), and serious spontaneous bleeding develops at levels less than 20×10^9 (20,000/mm^3).[1] Massive GI bleeding and intracerebral bleeding are most often seen with levels less than 5×10^9/L (5000/mm^3). Patients with a platelet count less than 20×10^9/L who have mucous membrane bleeding should be hospitalized.[6]

Treatment of chronic ITP is necessary only if the platelet count decreases to dangerous levels, which are somewhere around 20 to 30×10^9/L (20,000 to 30,000/mm^3). Prednisone at a dose of 1 mg/kg for 2 to 4 weeks is the first line of therapy. Intravenous infusions of immune globulin are very expensive and are reserved for actively bleeding patients.[7] Some patients require a splenectomy.[4] Drugs such as vincristine, azathioprine (Imuran), Danazol, cyclophosphamide, and cyclosporine have been used in severe cases.[8] Non-bleeding patients rarely require platelet transfusions if platelet counts are above 5×10^9/L (5000/mm^3).[6]

A patient with thrombocytopenia must never be given aspirin.[6]

Von Willebrand's Disease

Von Willebrand's disease is the most common inherited coagulopathy, with an incidence of about 1%. It is caused by an abnormality or reduction of von Willebrand's factor, which has the dual function of stabilizing factor VIII levels and promoting normal platelet functioning. The disease has an autosomal dominant inheritance, and most cases are mild. Bruising, nosebleeds, profuse bleeding from cuts, and hemorrhage after dental extractions are common, but hemarthroses are rare. When hemarthroses do occur, the bleeding begins immediately, whereas with coagulation defects such as hemophilia, bleeding is often delayed 12 to 24 hours. Classically the bleeding time is prolonged, and levels of factor VIII and von Willebrand factor are low. Repeated testing may be necessary to detect these abnormalities.[1,2]

≈ REFERENCES ≈

1. Hampton KK, Preston FE: ABC of clinical haematology: bleeding disorders, thrombosis and anticoagulation, *BMJ* 314:1026-1029, 1997.
2. Association of Hemophilia Clinic Directors of Canada: Hemophilia and von Willebrand's disease. 1. Diagnosis, comprehensive care and assessment, *Can Med Assoc J* 153:19-25, 1995.
3. Goldstein KH, Abramson N: Efficient diagnosis of thrombocytopenia, *Am Fam Physician* 53:915-920, 1996.
4. George JN, el-Harake MA, Raskob GE: Chronic idiopathic thrombocytopenic purpura, *N Engl J Med* 331:1207-1211, 1994.
5. Kirchner JT: Acute and chronic immune thrombocytopenic purpura: disorders that differ in more than duration, *Postgrad Med* 92:112-118, 125-126, 1992.
6. Beutler E: Platelet transfusion: the 20,000/microL trigger, *Blood* 81:1411-1413, 1993.
7. Immune Thrombocytopenia Purpura Treatment Guideline. Dr. Jeannie Callum, Toronto Sunnybrook Regional Cancer Center. (Accessed April 27, 2004 at http://www.tsrcc.on.ca/ TreatmentGuidlines/MalignantHaematology/ITP.pdf)
8. Immune Thrombocyotpenic Purpura National Institute of Diabetes and Digestive and Kidney Diseases (NIDDK), Bethesda, MD, USA. (Accessed April 27, 2004, at http:// www.niddk.nih.gov/health/hematol/pubs/itp/itp.htm# treated)

ERYTHROCYTE SEDIMENTATION RATE
(See also connective tissue diseases; polymyalgia rheumatica)

The Erythrocyte Sedimentation Rate (ESR) lacks sensitivity and specificity and therefore is not an appropriate screening test for asymptomatic individuals.[1] Various reference values have been proposed for the upper limits of normal for the ESR (Westergren method). Higher normal ranges are usually between 20 and 30 mm/hr. ESR rises with age and is higher in women than men. Upper limit of normal adjusted for age is: men = age divided by 2, women = age + 10, divided by 2. ESR is also increased by anemia, pregnancy, obesity, and renal failure.

Most cases of elevated ESR are not associated with significant disease,[2] and these elevations may persist for prolonged periods. The exception is an ESR greater than 100 mm/hr, which has a 90% chance of serious disease (infection, collagen vascular disease, metastases).[1] For mild elevations, if the cause is not immediately apparent, first repeat the test in 2 to 3 months before further investigation.[1] Recently an elevated ESR has been identified as most useful in diagnosing polymyalgia rheumatica and temporal arteritis. Only 1% to 2% of patients with temporal arteritis have a normal sedimentation rate[2] compared with one fourth of patients with polymyalgia rheumatica.[4] Sedimentation rates may be useful in following the course of four diseases: polymyalgia rheumatica, temporal arteritis, rheumatoid arthritis, and Hodgkin's disease.[1]

≈ REFERENCES ≈

1. Brigden M: The erythrocyte sedimentation rate. Still a helpful test when used judiciously, *Postgrad Med* 103(5):257-262, 272-274, May 1998.
2. Brigden ML: Clinical utility of the erythrocyte sedimentation rate, *Am Fam Physician* 60:1443-1450, 1999.
3. Andresdottir MB, Sigfusson N, Sigvaldason H, et al: Erythrocyte sedimentation rate, an independent predictor of coronary heart disease in men and women: The Reykjavik Study, *Am J Epidemiol* 158(9):844-851, 2003.
4. Helfgott SM, Kieval RI: Polymyalgia rheumatica in patients with a normal erythrocyte sedimentation rate, *Arthritis Rheum* 39:304-307, 1996.

LEUKEMIAS
Childhood Leukemias

Acute lymphoblastic leukemia (ALL) accounts for 85% of childhood leukemias, and the peak age of incidence is 3 to 4 years.[1] Although claims have been made that long-term exposure to magnetic fields from high-tension power lines is a risk factor, a large case-control study failed to find such a correlation.[2] Over 97% of children with ALL have complete remission after initial therapy, and the cure rate approaches 80%. Colony-stimulating factors given on the completion of induction chemotherapy decrease the duration or neutropenia and reduce the morbidity of therapy.[3] Late sequelae in cured children include acute myeloid leukemia, cardiomyopathy, brain tumours, short stature, and obesity, the latter three particularly prevalent among children who have had cranial irradiation. In most instances, however, intensive systemic chemotherapy and/or intrathecal chemotherapy successfully eradicate leukemic cells from the central nervous system, so cranial radiation is rarely necessary.[4]

Acute Myeloid Leukemia

The overall 4-year survival rate for acute myeloid leukemia in adolescents and adults is 35%. Induction chemotherapy (cytarabine plus daunorbicin or idarubicin) leads to complete remission in 70%. Whether bone-marrow transplant is more effective than chemotherapy alone as post-remission treatment is controversial. A 1998 study found that it was not.[5]

Chronic Lymphocytic Leukemia

The median age of persons with chronic lymphocytic leukemia (CLL) is 65 years, with only 10% to 15% of patients younger than age 50. The prognosis of CLL is variable. The median survival is 9 years. Patients with early stable disease do not require treatment.[6,7] In intermediate and advanced disease, chorambucil is the conventional first-line drug. However, fludarabine can also be used first line and is often used after the failure of chorambucil. Fludarabine has been found to improve progression-free survival, but it has greater toxicity.[8]

Chronic Myeloid Leukemia

Chronic myeloid leukemia (CML) usually affects middle-age adults. Nearly half of all patients are asymptomatic at the time of diagnosis, and the disease is detected only because of an abnormal blood count. An initial stable chronic phase is followed within 3 to 5 years by a rapidly fatal blastic phase. Just preceding the blast phase is an accelerated phase, during which one sees a rapid rise in the white cell count. Optimal treatment of the blastic phase is high-dose chemotherapy and allogeneic bone marrow transplantation from a suitable donor, usually a sibling. With this treatment, up to 70% of patients are alive after 10 years, but unfortunately only 20% to 30% of patients are candidates for bone marrow transplantation.[9]

The chronic phase is usually treated with interferon if bone marrow transplant is not an option.[9] Other chemotherapeutic agents for the chronic phase include busulphan (Myleran) and hydroxyurea (Hydrea), the latter being the preferred choice due do to its more favourable toxicity profile.[9] One of the newer agents, Imatinib mesylate, a tyrosine kinase inhibitor, has been shown to be effective in patients in whom interferon has failed.[10] Imatinib is also better tolerated and has improved progression-free survival when compared with interferon plus low-dose cytarabine in a randomized control trail.[11] In fact, the National Comprehensive Cancer Network now recommends Imatinib as the first-line therapy in the chronic phase of CML.[11] Imatinib is also an option for treating the blast phase of CML.[12] Hydroxyurea is the drug of choice for the accelerated phase.

Myelodysplasia

Myelodysplasia (refractory anemia, sideroblastic anemia) is considered a pre-leukemic condition, although leukemia is by no means an inevitable outcome of the disorder. Bone marrow cellularity is normal or increased, but because of defects in cell maturation, patients may have anemia, neutropenia, or thrombocytopenia. Although some patients have such initial symptoms as dyspnea, infections, bleeding, or bruising, many are clinically well and the disorder is detected as a result of abnormal routine complete blood counts. Most patients with myelodysplasia are elderly. The prognosis is extremely variable and depends in part on the percentage of blast cells in the marrow. Patients with fewer than 5% blasts are likely to remain well for many years and die of other causes, whereas those with more than 5% blasts have a 30% to 75% chance of bone marrow failure or the development of acute myelogenous leukemia.[13]

◆ REFERENCES ◆

1. Liesner RJ, Goldstone AH: The acute leukaemias, *BMJ* 314: 733-736, 1997.
2. Linet MS, Hatch EE, Kleinerman RA, et al: Residential exposure to magnetic fields and acute lymphoblastic leukemia in children, *N Engl J Med* 337:1-7, 1997.
3. Alstair JJ, Wood MD: Acute lymphoblastic leukemia, *N Engl J Med* 339:605-615, 1998.
4. Pui C-H: Childhood leukemias, *N Engl J Med* 332:1618-1630, 1995.
5. Cassileth PA, Harrington DP, Appelbaum FR, et al: Chemotherapy compared with autologous or allogeneic bone marrow transplantation in the management of acute myeloid leukemia at first remission, *N Engl J Med* 339: 1649-1656, 1998.
6. Rozman C, Montserrat E: Chronic lymphocytic leukemia, *N Engl J Med* 333:1052-1057, 1995.
7. Dighiero G, Maloum K, Desablens B, et al: Chlorambucil in indolent chronic lymphocytic leukemia, *N Engl J Med* 338:1506-1514, 1998.
8. Cancer Care Ontario Practice Guidelines Initiative: *Fludarabine in intermediate and high-risk chronic lymphocytic leukemia,* Ontario, 1999, Hamilton Cancer Care.
9. Sawyers CL: Chronic myeloid leukemia, *N Engl J Med* 340: 1330-1340, 1999.
10. Drucker BJ, Talpaz M, Rest DJ, et al: Efficacy and safety of a specific inhibitor of the BCR-ABL tyrosine kinase in chronic myeloid leukemia, *NEJM* 344:1031-1037.
11. National Comprehensive Cancer Network: *Clinical Practice Guideline in Oncology: Chronic Myelogenous Leukemia,* vol 1, 2004 (updated guideline vol 2, 2005). http://www.nccn.org/professionals/physician_gls/PDF/cml.pdf. Accessed April 21, 2005.
12. Drucker BJ, Sawyers CL, Kantarjian H, et al: Activty of a specific inhibitor of the BCR-ABL tyrosine kinase in the blast crisis of chronic myeloid leukemia and acute lymphoblastic leukemia with the Philadelphia chromosome, *N Engl J Med* 344:1038-1042, 2001.
13. Heaney ML, Golde DW: Myelodysplasia, *N Engl J Med* 340:1649-1660, 1999.

LYMPHADENOPATHY

The causes of most cases of lymphadenopathy in primary care are often apparent from the history and resolve without intervention. Unexplained lymphadenopathy is of more concern, but in the primary-care setting only 1% of cases are malignant.[1] Key risk factors for malignancy include older age (over age 40 goes up to 4% on average), firm, fixed nodal character, duration of greater than 2 weeks, and supraclavicular location.[1,2]

If lymphadenopathy is present in two or more non-contiguous areas, it is generalized. If it is limited to one region, it is localized. In general, patients with localized lymphadenopathy of undetermined etiology who are otherwise well may be observed for 1 month. If improvement is noted, no further action is needed. Patients with generalized adenopathy of undetermined etiology usually require further investigation, typically with fine needle aspiration or excisional biopsy.[3]

─────────── ◄ **REFERENCES** ► ───────────

1. Fijten GH, Blijham GH: Unexplained lymphadenopathy in family practice: an evaluation of the probability of malignant causes and the effectiveness of physicians' workup, *J Fam Pract* 27(4): 373-376, Oct 1988.
2. Bazemore AW, Smucker DR: Lymphadenopathy and malignancy, *Am Fam Physician* 66(1): 2103-2110, Dec 1 2002.
3. Ferrer R: Lymphadenopathy: differential diagnosis and evaluation, *Am Fam Physician* 58: 1313-1320, 1998.

LYMPHOMAS

The Ann Arbor staging system for lymphomas is as follows[1]:

Stage I   Single lymphoid or extranodal site
Stage II   Two lymphoid or extranodal sites on the same side of the diaphragm
Stage III   Lymphoid areas (including spleen) on both sides of the diaphragm
Stage IV   Diffuse involvement of extranodal organs (e.g., bone marrow, liver)

Symptoms of lymphomas are categorized as A if the patient has no systemic symptoms or B if the patient has weight loss, fever, or drenching night sweats.[1]

Hodgkin's Disease

Localized Hodgkin's disease is generally treated with radiation therapy, and more widespread disease with chemotherapy. Patients with B symptoms must undergo combined radiation and chemotherapy.[1] The overall cure rate is 70% to 80%.[2]

Second tumours are common among children treated for Hodgkin's disease.[2-4] In one study the cumulative risk was 7% by 15 years.[2] The incidence of leukemia reached a plateau by 14 years, but such a levelling off was not seen with solid tumours. Breast cancer was the most common solid tumour, with a relative risk 75 times that of the normal population. The risk was related to radiation and was greatest in girls treated between the ages of 10 and 16 (when breast tissue was proliferating). Other solid tumours were thyroid cancers, basal cell carcinomas of the skin, brain tumours, bone tumours, and colorectal cancers.[2-4]

Non-Hodgkin's Lymphoma

Low-grade non-Hodgkin's lymphoma is a disease of the elderly. Ninety percent of patients are over age 50. Most of the follicular lymphomas fall into the non-Hodgkin's lymphoma group. These neoplasms have a similar epidemiology and natural course to chronic lymphocytic leukemia. The tumours are often widespread but indolent with slow progression over many years. The median survival is 5 to 8 years, and cure is rarely possible. Patients without symptoms do not necessarily require treatment. As the disease progresses, chemotherapy may be offered, often in the form of chlorambucil (Leukeran),[2,5] cyclophosphamide (Cytoxan), or fludarabine (Fludara). A new therapy, rituximab, an anti-CD20 monoclonal antibody, can be used alone or in combination with other chemotherapeutic agents as first-line therapy or for aggressive lymphoma resistance to other therapies.[6,7] Stem cell transplant is considered in cases in which previous therapies have failed.[6]

Intermediate-grade non-Hodgkin's lymphoma affects all age groups. The most common form is a diffuse large-cell lymphoma that is a B-cell neoplasm. These tumours progress rapidly, are often associated with type B symptoms, and require therapy.[1] The usual therapy regimen involves the initiation CHOP (cyclophophamide, vincristine, prednisolone, and adriamycin), with the addition of rituximab in stages III and IV.[6] Chemotherapy may be combined with radiation therapy.[6] The overall 5-year survival is about 40%,[1] but it exceeds 64% for those with stage I or II disease.[8]

High-grade non-Hodgkin's lymphomas make up only 5% of the non-Hodgkin's lymphomas. The high-grade form is primarily a disease of children and young adults.[1] The cure rate for non-Hodgkin's lymphoma in children is about 70%.[9]

─────────── ◄ **REFERENCES** ► ───────────

1. National Comprehensive Cancer Network: *Practice guidelines for Hodgkins lymphoma: Version 2000,* Hodgkin's Disease vol.1, 2005. http://www.nccn.org/professionals/physician_gls/PDF/hodgkins.pdf. Accessed April 21, 2005.
2. Mead GM: ABC of clinical haematology: malignant lymphomas and chronic lymphocytic leukaemia, *BMJ* 314:1103-1106, 1997.
3. Bhatia S, Robison LL, Oberlin O, et al: Breast cancer and other second neoplasms after childhood Hodgkin's disease, *N Engl J Med* 334:745-751, 1996.
4. Donaldson SS, Hancock SL: Second cancers after Hodgkin's disease in childhood (editorial), *N Engl J Med* 334:792-793, 1996.
5. Rituximab for non-Hodgkin's lymphoma, *Med Lett* 40: 65-66, 1998.
6. National Comprehensive Cancer Network: *Non-Hodkin's Lymphoma Clinical Practice Guidelines in Oncology,* vol 1, 2005. http://www.nccn.org/professionals/physician_gls/PDF/nhl.pdf. Accessed April 21, 2005.
7. Wannesson L, Ghielmini M: Overview of antibody therapy in B-cell non-Hodkin's lymphoma, *Clin Lymphoma* 4s1: s5-12, 2003.

8. Miller TP, Dahlberg S, Cassady R, et al: Chemotherapy alone compared with chemotherapy plus radiotherapy for localized intermediate- and high-grade non-Hodgkin's lymphoma, *N Engl J Med* 339:21-26, 1998.

9. Sandlund JT, Downing JR, Crist WM: Non-Hodgkin's lymphoma in childhood, *N Engl J Med* 334:1238-1248, 1996.

MULTIPLE MYELOMA

Multiple myeloma is a malignancy characterized by the accumulation of malignant plasma cells in the bone marrow producing immunoglobulins, usually IgG or IgA.[1]

The majority of patients with multiple myeloma are over 40 years of age, with a peak around 70 years.[2] Multiple myeloma accounts for approximately 10% to 15% of all hematological malignancies.[3]

The clinical presentation of multiple myeloma can vary. It can include bone pain, which may be present in three-quarters of patients.[4] Osteolytic lesions and compression fractures occur commonly in the axial skeleton.[4] Hypercalcemia may present as lethargy, nausea, and constipation.[4] Renal failure is due to a combination of hypercalcemia, direct damage from paraproteins, or precipitation of light chains in renal tubules.[3] Marrow failure, with resultant anemia, is found in more than 75% of myeloma patients.[4] Compromised cellular and humoral immune system increases the risk of infection. Neurological dysfunction may present as spinal cord compression; hyperviscosity symptoms such as headache, blurry vision, progressive obtundation; or a demyelinating neuropathy as a paraneoplastic manifestation of the myeloma paraproteins.[4]

Monoclonal gammopathy of undetermined significance (MGUS) is a related disorder and is 80 to 100 times more common than multiple myeloma.[4,5] M-protein (paraproteins), as measured by serum electrophoresis, is less than 3g/dl (30g/L), and the bone marrow contains less than 10% plasma cells in MGUS.[5] Other clinical or laboratory findings typical of multiple myeloma are absent. One study found that serious hematological disorders developed in one fourth of patients (multiple myeloma in most). Patients with MGUS require no treatment but should have follow-up examinations at regular intervals.[6]

The three criteria for the diagnosis of multiple myeloma[7] include:

1. Monoclonal plasma cells in the bone marrow greater than or equal to 10% and/or presence of a biopsy-proven plasmacytoma

2. Monoclonal protein present in the serum and/or urine

3. Myeloma related organ dysfunction
   i. Calcium elevation in the blood (serum calcium greater than 10.5mg/L or upper limit of normal)
   ii. Renal insufficiency (serum creatinine greater than 2 mg/dl)
   iii. Anemia (hemoglobin less than 10 g/dl or 2 g less than normal)
   iv. Lytic bone lesions or osteoporosis

The standard evaluation of a patient with suspected myeloma includes[4,7]:
- Complete blood count with differential and peripheral blood smear
- Blood-chemistry profile including calcium, creatinine, LDH, and albumin
- Bone marrow aspirate and biopsy with cytogenetics and plasma cell labelling index
- Complete skeletal survey, including spine, pelvis, skull, humeri, and femurs
- Serum and 24-hour-collection urine electrophoresis with immunofixation to identify the M protein and quantification of the protein
- Serum beta-2 microglobulin and C-Reactive Protein

The treatment of multiple myeloma depends on the symptoms and laboratory findings. Patients who are asymptomatic and who do not have significant anemia, renal failure, or severe bone lesions on the X-ray examination may be followed without treatment.

One systematic review of treatment made the following conclusions[8]:
- Cyclophosphamide is superior to placebo in the management of multiple myeloma
- Progression-free survival is improved with interferon, but survival benefit is minimum
- Autologous bone marrow transplant is better than standard chemotherapy (melphalan)
- If a twin donor is not available for Bone Marrow Transplant (BMT), autologous Stem Cell Transplant is better than allogenic BMT
- If a transplant fails, thalidomide with or without dexamethasone is an effective antitumour therapy
- Biphosphonates have no effect on survival but decrease the probability of vertebral fractures and improve bone pain
- Epoietin alpha improves anemia and reduces transfusion requirements
- PS-341, a novel proteasome inhibitor, is an anticancer agent with evidence of antitumour activity in refractory multiple myeloma

◥ REFERENCES ◤

1. Bataille R, Harousseau JL: Multiple myeloma, *N Engl J Med* 336(23):1657-1664, Jun 5 1997.

2. Durie BG: The epidemiology of multiple myeloma, *Semin Hematol* 38(suppl 3):1-5, Apr 2001.

3. Morgan GJ, Davies FE, Linet M: Myeloma aetiology and epidemiology, *Biomed Pharmacotherapy* 56(5):223-234, Jul 2002.

4. Zaidi AA, Vesole DH: Multiple myeloma: an old disease with new hope for the future, *CA Cancer J Clin* 51(5):273-285, Sep-Oct 2001.

5. Kyle RA: Multiple myeloma: diagnostic challenges and standard therapy, *Semin Hematol* 38(suppl 3):11-14, Apr 2001.

6. Kyle RA: Monoclonal gammopathy of undetermined significance, *Blood Rev* 8:135-141, 1994.

7. Durie BG, Kyle RA, Belch A, et al: Myeloma management guidelines: a consensus report from the Scientific Advisors of the International Myeloma Foundation, *Hematol J* 4(6):379-398, 2003.

8. Kumar A, Loughran T, Alsina M, et al: Management of multiple myeloma: a systematic review and critical appraisal of published studies, *Lancet Oncol* 4(5):293-304, May 2003.

IMMUNOLOGY

Topics covered in this section

Drug Allergy
Food Allergy
HIV and AIDS
Insect Stings and Bites

DRUG ALLERGY

True allergic reactions are IgE-mediated immune reactions (Type I immediate hypersensitivity), and account for only 5% to 10% of drug reactions. The more usual reactions are toxicity, expected side effects, and drug interactions. Although urticaria is often a manifestation of drug allergy, it may also appear in Type II or pseudoallergic reactions. Angioedema, urticaria, or bronchospasm in patients on medications should raise suspicion of an anaphylactic reaction. On the other hand, the predominant aetiology of maculopapular skin reactions to drugs is uncertain.[1]

Skin testing for Type I reactions is a useful diagnostic procedure and can be done safely for a number of drugs. Protocols are standardized for penicillin, and are also well described for local anesthetics, muscle relaxants, high-molecular-weight proteins such as insulin, and vaccines. Skin tests have a good positive predictive value; however, a reliable negative predictive value has only been described for penicillin.[1] Due to cross-reactivity, cephalosporins should be used with caution in patients with a history of penicillin allergy, and skin testing can be done prior to the initiation of cephalosporin therapy.[1]

When a patient gives a history of drug allergy, an alternative drug class can often be prescribed. In most patients, symptoms should resolve within 2 weeks after withdrawal of the drug. Additional therapy for drug hypersensitivity reactions is largely symptomatic and includes corticosteroids and oral antihistamines. Patients with an anaphylactic reaction require prompt treatment.[1]

Desensitization protocols have been described for a few drugs (e.g., penicillin) and should only be attempted under close monitoring.[2] Such protocols have particular value for HIV-positive patients who require prophylaxis against *Pneumocystis carinii* and are allergic to trimethoprim-sulfamethoxazole.[3]

❧ REFERENCES ❧

1. Riedl MA, Casillas AM: Adverse drug reactions: types and treatment options, *Am Fam Physician* 68:1781-1790, 2003.
2. Yates AB, deShazo RD: Allergic and nonallergic drug reactions, *Southern Med J* 96(11):1080-1087, 2003.
3. ieder MJ: In vivo and in vitro testing for adverse drug reactions, *Pediatr Clin North Am* 44:93-111, 1997.

FOOD ALLERGY
(See also insect stings and bites)

General surveys report that 25% to 30% of adults claim to have a food allergy, but when samples of these individuals were investigated, the actual number turned out to be 0.5% to 2.5%.[1] The most common reaction to food is simply "food intolerance," a variety of non-immune reactions, which individuals wrongly attribute to food allergy. Among the many nonallergic reactions to foods are diarrhea from lactose intolerance, flushing from monosodium glutamate, and headaches secondary to tyramine in cheese or red wine.[2,3]

True food allergies are immune-mediated. The majority of these are IgE-mediated, but some are non–IgE-mediated, with an as yet poorly defined contribution from T cells and macrophages.[1,2] Symptoms of IgE-mediated reactions usually come on within minutes of eating the offending agent, whereas non-IgE reactions generally take several hours to appear.[1] Common symptoms of IgE-medicated reactions are itching and swelling of the mouth and pharynx, often associated with symptoms of anaphylaxis, such as urticaria, dyspnea, stridor, wheezing, coughing, nausea, vomiting, diarrhea, and in some cases faintness and syncope.[1]

Foods likely to induce food allergy in children are cow's milk, eggs, peanuts, wheat, tree nuts, and fish; in adults, the common offending foods are peanuts, tree nuts, fish, and shellfish.[2] Food additives such as salicylates, sulfites, tartrazine, and benzoates may also cause allergic reactions. Generally, people with food allergies react to only a few foods. Occasionally a person who is allergic to one food may also cross-react to other related foods. People with a history of eczema or asthma are at higher risk of having a reaction to food and are more likely to have a more severe reaction.[3] Children usually "outgrow" allergies to milk, eggs, soya, and wheat, especially with food avoidance. However, allergies to peanuts, tree nuts, fish, and shellfish are rarely outgrown.[2] An interesting recent trial showed some evidence that children who had their weepy rashes treated with creams that contained peanut oil had significantly higher risk of developing an allergy to peanuts.[4]

The most important tool for making a diagnosis is the history. When the history is suggestive, the next step is skin testing, and if this is positive, the third step is a diagnostic diet in which the suspected allergen is eliminated. The final and definitive test is an oral food challenge, which is often useful because 50% of positive skin tests are false positives. Oral food challenges can be dangerous and should be undertaken only in carefully controlled situations. Diagnosing non–IgE-mediated reactions is more difficult, and elimination diets and supervised oral food challenges are often necessary in these cases.[2]

Immediate treatment of acute food allergy, as for any anaphylactic reaction, is epinephrine. Patients with food allergies not only must be very careful to avoid the offending foods, but also should never be without an epinephrine syringe. (See discussion of insect stings and bites.) Antihistamines, bronchodilators, and corticosteroids can be used as adjunctive treatment.[1,2]

ℳ REFERENCES ℳ

1. James JM: Food allergies, E-medicine. Last updated: 2004. (Accessed on April 10, 2004, http://www.emedicine.com/med/topic806.htm.)

2. Sicherer SH: Manifestations of food allergy: evaluation and management. American Academy of Family Physicians, 1999. (Accessed on April 9, 2004, at http://www.aafp.org/afp/990115ap/415.html.)

3. Singh J, Clark M: Food allergy, E-medicine. Last updated: 2004. (Accessed on April 10, 2004, at http://www.emedicinehealth.com/articles/8567-1.asp.)

4. Lack G, Fox D, Northstone K, et al (Avon Longitudinal Study of Parents and Children Study Team): Factors associated with the development of peanut allergy in childhood, *N Engl J Med* 348:977-985, 2003.

HIV AND AIDS

(See also adoption; cervical cancer; poverty; sexually transmitted diseases)

SECTION 1: INTRODUCTION

Hotlines

Management of human immunodeficiency virus (HIV) disease is constantly evolving and therefore is a significant challenge for most physicians.

Several resources are available on the World Wide Web, including:

- Health Canada's HIV/AIDS web site: http://www.hc-sc.gc.ca/english/diseases/aids.html for general information from a Canadian perspective;
- the Canadian HIV/AIDS Clearinghouse: http://www.aidssida.cpha.ca, for extensive resources on all HIV-related topics
- AIDS Education Global Information System: http://www.aegis.com, probably the best single web site for HIV-related information
- Guidelines for the Use of Antiretroviral Agents in HIV-Infected Adults and Adolescents (http://www.aidsinfo.nih.gov)
- HIV InSite, the University of California at San Francisco: http://hivinsite.ucsf.edu
- the Cochrane Collaborative Review Group on HIV/AIDS: http://www.igh.org/Cochrane
- American Foundation for AIDS Research (AmFAR) HIV/AIDS Treatment Directory: http://www.amfar.org/td

History

The first case of acquired immunodeficiency syndrome (AIDS) was reported in 1981,[2,3] and the virus was isolated in 1984.[3] However, archival serum samples reveal that the disease existed before that time. The disease first became evident when large numbers of gay men in large metropolitan centres in the United States as well as smaller numbers of blood transfusion recipients became ill with and died from unexplained opportunistic infections and malignancies, notably Kaposi's sarcoma.

Stephen Lewis, United Nations Special Envoy for HIV/AIDS in Africa, made the following comment in a keynote speech in San Francisco regarding the pandemic in 2004:

"On the continent of Africa, it is estimated that 4.1 million people need treatment now . . . i.e., their CD4 counts are below 200 . . . and approximately 70,000 to 100,000 are actually in treatment, or roughly two per cent. It's important for everyone here to recognize that you're part of the most significant battle against a disease that has ever been waged in human history . . . and when you're consumed in your laboratories, or wrestling with the esoterica of science, at the end of that long exploratory road there lies the whole fabric of the human family fighting for survival, searching, desperately, for hope. The grieving villages, the funerals, the hospital wards, the orphans, the women at the clinics; it's an hallucinatory nightmare; it should never have come to this."

Distribution of HIV Infection

As of the end of 2001, an estimated 40 million people were living with HIV/AIDS worldwide, including 18.5 million women and 3 million children. Five million were newly infected that year, including 2 million women and 800,000 children. Three million people died of AIDS in 2001 at a rate of over 8000 a day, including 1.1 million women and nearly 600,000 children. Over 14 million children were orphaned by HIV/AIDS in 2001. Over 70% of those living with HIV/AIDS are in sub-Saharan Africa. North America accounts for a little more than 2% of the infected population.[4] The prevalence of HIV infection in Canada in 2003 was estimated at 0.3%.

HIV-1 Virus Strains

Over 99% of cases in the current pandemic of AIDS are caused by the group M strain of the HIV-1 virus.[5] The virus is subclassified into classes, with type B most prevalent in the developing world, types A and D in sub-Saharan Africa, type C in India, and type E in Southeast Asia.

Prognosis

The median elapsed time from the acquisition of HIV infection to the development of AIDS is 10 to 11 years without treatment.[7] The rate of progression seems to be the same for men and women,[8] and pregnancy does not appear to accelerate it.[9] A Swedish study of HIV-positive homosexual men determined that progression was significantly faster in those who had an acute infectious mononucleosis-like illness at the time of seroconversion than in those who had no or only minor symptoms at seroconversion. The authors estimated that a glandular fever-type syndrome occurs in about half of men who become HIV positive.[10]

One important prognostic factor is the plasma viral load in the early months or years of infection, as has been documented in hemophiliacs,[11] African American IV drug users in the United States,[12] and HIV-positive patients living in the community in Switzerland.[13] In the hemophiliac study, for example, progression to AIDS at 10 years correlated with the viral load measured between 12 and 36 months after seroconversion. In patients with fewer than 1000 copies/mL, no progression was found at 10 years.[11]

A surrogate measure of HIV progression is the CD4+ lymphocyte count.[13,14] On average, without treatment, the cell count decreases by 50 to 100/μL per year. The CD4+ count at initiation of therapy is being increasingly recognized as an indicator of long-term survival. In a Vancouver study, survival rates were 97% to 100% for patients who started antiretroviral (ARV) therapy with a CD4+ count of over 350 and 74% for those whose baseline CD4+ count was less than 50.

Opportunistic infections usually start to develop in individuals with CD4+ counts less than 200/μL, although tuberculosis can develop at any stage of HIV infection.[13]

The survival time of patients with AIDS correlates directly with the experience of their physicians in managing this disease. In a study published in 1996, the median survival of patients looked after by inexperienced physicians was 14 months compared with 26 months for those cared for by experienced physicians.[15] Health professionals inexperienced in the care of HIV-positive patients may obtain help from the various hotlines and warmlines or by accessing appropriate sites on the World Wide Web. (See earlier discussion.) While guidelines are helpful, managing HIV infection is increasingly complex, and physicians with little experience in treating patients with HIV infection should comanage them with an experienced physician.

In one series the median survival from the onset of an AIDS-defining illness was 20 months without treatment.[16] However, in developed countries, survival has increased dramatically in the last few years because of the introduction of highly active antiretroviral therapy (HAART), which includes combinations of three, four, or occasionally more drugs. (See Section 5 below.)[3]

The frequency of specific opportunistic infections varies with geographical location. *P. carinii* pneumonia is common in the developed world, whereas tuberculosis is a far more frequent event in developing nations. Furthermore, because patients in the industrialized world are surviving longer, infections associated with more advanced degrees of immunosuppression such as cytomegalovirus retinitis and *Mycobacterium avium* complex infection are becoming more common.[17] For the same reason, HIV-associated malignancies, especially lymphomas, are also being seen more often.

❧ REFERENCES ❧

1. Voelker R: Rural communities struggle with AIDS, *JAMA* 279:5-6, 1998.
2. Klein A: Beyond biases and outdated perceptions: HIV prevention and mentoring (editorial), *Can Fam Physician* 43:133-134, 1997.
3. Fauci AS: The AIDS epidemic: considerations for the 21st century, *N Engl J Med* 341:1046-1050, 1999.
4. Report on the Global HIV/AIDS Epidemic 2002, Geneva, 2002, UNAIDS (Joint United Nations Programme on HIV/AIDS).
5. Centers for Disease Control and Prevention: Identification of HIV-1 group O infection–1996, *JAMA* 276:521-522, 1996.
6. Hooper E: Sailors and star-bursts, and the arrival of HIV, *BMJ* 315:1689-1691, 1997.
7. Gao F, Bailes E, Robertson DL, et al: Origin of HIV-1 in the chimpanzee, *Pan troglodytes troglodytes* (letter), *Nature* 397:436-441, 1999.
8. Pezzotti P, Phillips AN, Dorrucci M, et al: Category of exposure to HIV and age in the progression to AIDS: a longitudinal study of 1199 individuals with known dates of seroconversion, *BMJ* 313:583-586, 1996.
9. Lepri AC, Pezzotti P, Dorrucci M, et al: HIV disease progression in 854 women and men infected through injecting drug use and heterosexual sex and followed for up to nine years from seroconversion, *BMJ* 309:1537-1542, 1994.
10. Alliegro MB, Dorrucci M, Phillips AN, et al: Incidence and consequences of pregnancy in women with known duration of HIV infection, *Arch Intern Med* 157:2585-2590, 1997.
11. Yerly S, Perneger TV, Hirschel B, et al: A critical assessment of the prognostic value of HIV-1 RNA levels and CD4+cell counts in HIV-infected patients, *Arch Intern Med* 158:247-252, 1998.
12. O'Brien TR, Blattner WA, Waters D, et al: Serum HIV-1 levels and time to development of AIDS in the Multicenter Hemophilia Cohort Study, *JAMA* 276:105-110, 1996.
13. Lindback S, Brostrom C, Karlsson A, et al: Does symptomatic primary HIV-1 infection accelerate progression to CDC stage IV disease, CD4 count below 200 × 10 (6)/l, AIDS, and death from AIDS? *BMJ* 309:1535-1537, 1994.
14. Goldschmidt RH, Moy A: Antiretroviral drug treatment for HIV/AIDS, *Am Fam Physician* 54:574-580, 1996.
15. Viahov D, Graham N, Hoover D, et al: Prognostic indicators for AIDS and infectious disease death in HIV-infected injection drug users: plasma viral load and CD4+ cell count, *JAMA* 279:35-40, 1998.
16. Kitahata MM, Koepsell TD, Deyo RA, et al: Physicians' experience with the acquired immunodeficiency syndrome as a factor in patients' survival, *N Engl J Med* 334:701-706, 1996.
17. Mocroft A, Youle M, Morcinek J, et al (Royal Free/Chelsea and Westminster Hospitals Collaborative Group): Survival

after diagnosis of AIDS: a prospective observational study of 2625 patients, *BMJ* 314:409-413, 1997.

18. Beiser C: Recent advances: HIV infection–2, *BMJ* 314: 579-583, 1997.

SECTION 2: CLINICAL HIV INFECTION
Transmission and Epidemiology of HIV Infection

About 95% of HIV-infected people live in the developing world, where HIV is mostly transmitted through heterosexual sex. Canada reflects the situation in the developed world, where the main mode of transmission has been sexual transmission among men who have sex with men. Smaller but increasing numbers of people have been infected through injection drug use and heterosexual sex, with small numbers infected through blood transfusion (prior to implementation of universal testing in 1985) and maternal-child transmission without preventive therapy. The proportion of women among newly infected people has increased from less than 9% prior to 1995 to 24% in 1999.

Acute Retroviral Syndrome

Forty to fifty percent of persons newly infected with HIV will develop an infectious mononucleosis-like syndrome called *acute retroviral syndrome* or *seroconversion reaction*. The incubation period is 4 to 11 days, and the illness usually lasts less than 2 weeks. Progression to AIDS is more rapid among patients who have a prolonged acute retroviral syndrome.[2]

Symptoms and signs of the acute retroviral syndrome may include fever, fatigue, myalgia, headache, a maculopapular rash, lymphadenopathy, and in some cases oral or genital ulcers or neck stiffness (aseptic meningitis). Acute retroviral syndrome is often not diagnosed or misdiagnosed. Laboratory findings may include lymphopenia and thrombocytopenia, a reduction in CD4+ counts, and high levels of viral plasma load (if the possibility of the diagnosis is entertained). The usual HIV antibody serological tests (ELISA) are negative; they become positive in 2 to 3 weeks at the earliest, and up to 12 weeks after the onset of illness. The only investigations that can confirm the diagnosis during the acute phase are p24 antigen testing or HIV-1 RNA testing, although most labs will perform the latter test without a positive p24 antigen or ELISA test.[2]

Diagnosis of the acute retroviral syndrome is important for three reasons:

1. Aggressive treatment of the disease at this stage may be beneficial in preventing seeding of the virus throughout the body, notably in sanctuary sites (e.g., central nervous system [CNS]). However, the benefit of this weighed against the need to take medications for several years when it would not otherwise be necessary raises doubts about the net benefit of early treatment.

2. Identification of the disease during the acute phase, when it is highly contagious, permits education of the patient about the increased risks of transmission at this time.

3. Early contact tracing may also decrease spread of disease.[2]

Occupational Exposure

The risk of HIV infection from a needle-stick injury is estimated at 0.36%. The risk is greater if the exposure is from an object visibly contaminated with blood of the HIV-positive patient, an intravascular device caused the needle stick, or the injury is a deep one. The risk is also higher if the patient is in a terminal phase of AIDS and thus has a higher titer of HIV in the blood. When none of these added risk factors is present, the risk of infection is less than 0.3%.[3] Post-exposure use of zidovudine (ZDV) in doses of approximately 1000 mg per day for 3 to 4 weeks appears to decrease the risk by about 80%.[4]

Recommendations of the Centers for Disease Control and Prevention (CDC) on the management of occupational exposure include the following[5]:

1. Contaminated skin areas should be washed immediately with soap and water, and mucous membranes should be flushed with water.

2. When possible, an expert on retroviral diseases should be consulted. Resources include the CDC risk assessment algorithm found at the resources listed in the Hotlines section above.

3. Post-exposure prophylaxis should be offered to persons exposed to body fluids or tissues known or suspected to be infectious. Blood is the most infectious, but other fluids associated with risk are semen, vaginal secretions, cerebrospinal fluid, and body cavity and joint fluids. Urine, feces, saliva, and sweat are not included in this category unless they are contaminated with blood. Although breast milk is associated with vertical transmission of HIV, it is not a risk factor for health care workers.

4. Post-exposure prophylaxis should be started as soon as possible after exposure, preferably within 1 to 2 hours, and is probably not effective if started after 24 to 36 hours. However, in a case of high-risk exposure, treatment may be worth attempting if started within 2 weeks.

All prophylactic regimens include zidovudine (Retrovir) because this drug has been beneficial in such cases.

Two post-exposure prophylactic regimens are recommended. The basic regimen is suitable for most exposures, and the expanded regimen is recommended for high-risk exposures. Both regimens are administered for 4 weeks.

The basic regimen consists of two nucleoside reverse transcriptase inhibitors–zidovudine (Retrovir) 600 mg per day in divided doses and lamivudine (3TC, Epivir) 150 mg twice daily.

The expanded regimen consists of the basic regimen plus a protease inhibitor, either indinavir (IDV, Crixivan) 800 mg every 8 hours or nelfinavir (Viracept) 750 mg three times daily.

Sexual Transmission

A variety of factors affect the risk of acquiring HIV through sexual contacts. Possibility for infection transmission is greatest in the few weeks after HIV is acquired (before HIV serological tests become positive) and again in the late stages of the disease. In both these situations, viral blood titers are high. Chances of acquiring HIV are greater for persons with genital ulcers or other sexually transmitted diseases such as gonorrhea, *Chlamydia* infection, and trichomoniasis. Intercourse during menstruation increases the risk of infection for both men and women. Systematic reviews provide insufficient evidence as to whether circumcised men are less likely to acquire HIV or transmit it to their partners than are uncircumcised men.[6] Consistent use of condoms can reduce transmission by 80%.[7] A systematic review shows that nonoxynol-9 is actually harmful.[8]

Male-to-female transmission occurs at about twice the rate of female-to-male transmission,[9] but because many more males than females in the North American population are HIV-infected, the overall risk that a North American female will be infected through heterosexual intercourse has been estimated to be 12 times greater than the risk that a male will be infected in this manner.[10] The risk of acquiring HIV from a single act of unprotected vaginal intercourse is estimated as less than 1%.[11] Among 124 couples in which only one partner was HIV positive, no HIV transmission was recorded after 15,000 episodes of intercourse using condoms. In a similar situation in which condoms were used only intermittently, about a 5% conversion rate occurred after 1 year with an estimated cumulative conversion rate of 13% at 2 years.[12]

A study of male homosexual and bisexual men found unprotected receptive anal intercourse to be the highest-risk sexual activity, with an estimated per-contact risk of 0.82% if the partner was known to be HIV positive and 0.27% when partners of unknown serostatus were included in the analysis. The per-contact risk for unprotected insertive anal intercourse with HIV-positive or unknown serostatus partners was 0.06% and for unprotected receptive oral sex was 0.04%.[13]

Should post-exposure treatment be given to individuals exposed to HIV through an isolated sexual or shared needle exposure? No data are available on which to base an answer. Katz and Gerberding[11] argue that treatment should be provided if continued exposure is likely, and that such treatment can be started within 24 hours. Treatment is the same as for occupational exposure. Lurie and associates generally support this approach,[12] with the proviso that if the risk of infection is low, post-exposure prophylaxis may cause more harm than benefit. No data are available on the risk of acquiring HIV infection as a result of sexual assault or on the benefit of postexposure treatment in this case. Current consensus is that treatment (following the protocol for occupational exposure) should be offered to all victims. It should be started within 72 hours and continued for 28 days.[14]

Blood Transfusions

A 1996 U.S. paper calculated the risk of acquiring HIV from a single unit of blood as 1:493,000. (See discussion of transfusions.) This would be possible if someone were infected with HIV just prior to donating blood, before any diagnostic tests became positive.[15]

Household Contacts

HIV transmission through household contacts is rare. As of May 1994, eight such cases in the United States had been reported to the CDC. These were probably the result of contact with blood or body fluids.[16]

Pregnancy

A recent systematic review reported the following effective strategies for reducing fetal maternal transmission of HIV[20]:

- Zidovudine: significantly reduces the risk of transmission compared with placebo (risk reduction (RR) 0.54 95% CI:0.42-0.69)
- Nevarapine: compared with zidovudine, significantly reduces risk (RR 0.58 95% CI: 0.40-0.83)
- Caesarean section: compared with vaginal delivery, significantly reduces risk of transmission (RR 0.17 95% CI: 0.05-0.55)

Breastfeeding

HIV can be transmitted to newborns through breastfeeding. An international (Europe and Africa) pooled analysis estimated that the overall risk of such transmission was 3.2% per each year of breastfeeding. The authors concluded that if breastfeeding had been discontinued by 4 months, none of the 902 infants in the study would have been infected, and if it had been stopped at 6 months, 3 would have been infected.[21] A study from Malawi found the annual transmission rate of HIV through breastfeeding to be a little over 7%, with the highest risk occurring in the first few months. Early weaning would decrease transmission rates, but in much of Africa such a practice would probably result in increased infant mortality from other diseases.[22]

⟋ REFERENCES ⟍

1. Centers for Disease Control and Prevention: AIDS associated with injecting-drug use–United States, 1995, *JAMA* 275: 1628-1629, 1996.

2. Kahn JO, Walker BD: Acute human immunodeficiency virus type 1 infection, *N Engl J Med* 339:33-39, 1998.

3. Cardo DM, Culver DH, Ciesielski CA, et al: A case-control study of HIV seroconversion in health care workers after percutaneous exposure, *N Engl J Med* 337:1485-1490, 1997.

4. Centers for Disease Control and Prevention: Case-control study of HIV seroconversion in health-care workers after percutaneous exposure to HIV-infected blood–France, United Kingdom, and United States, January 1988-August 1994, *JAMA* 275:274-275, 1996.

5. Centers for Disease Control and Prevention: Public Health Service guidelines for the management of health care worker exposures to HIV and recommendations for postexposure prophylaxis, *MMWR* 47(no RR-7):1-33, 1998.

6. Siegfried N, Muller M, Volmink J, et al: Male circumcision for prevention of heterosexual acquisition of HIV in men. [Systematic Review] Cochrane HIV/AIDS Group *Cochrane Database of Systematic Reviews,* 2, 2004.

7. Weller S, Davis K: Condom effectiveness in reducing heterosexual HIV transmission. [Systematic Review] Cochrane HIV/AIDS Group *Cochrane Database of Systematic Reviews,* 2, 2004.

8. Wilkinson D, Ramjee G, Tholandi M, et al: Nonoxynol-9 for preventing vaginal acquisition of sexually transmitted infections by women from men. *Cochrane Database of Systematic Reviews,* 4:CD003939, 2004.

9. Nicolosi A, Leite ML, Musicco M, et al: The efficiency of male-to-female and female-to-male sexual transmission of the human immunodeficiency virus: a study of 730 stable couples, *Epidemiology* 5:570-575, 1994.

10. Padian NS, Shiboski S, Jewell N: The effect of the number of exposures on the risk of heterosexual HIV transmission, *J Infect Dis* 161:883-887, 1990.

11. Katz MH, Gerberding JL: Postexposure treatment of people exposed to the human immunodeficiency virus through sexual contact or injection-drug use, *N Engl J Med* 336:1097-1100, 1997.

12. Lurie P, Miller S, Hecht F, et al: Postexposure prophylaxis after nonoccupational HIV exposure: clinical, ethical, and policy considerations, *JAMA* 280:1769-1773, 1998.

13. Vittinghoff E, Douglas J, Judson F, et al: Per-contact risk of human immunodeficiency virus transmission between male sexual partners, *Am J Epidemiol* 150:306-311, 1999.

14. Bamberger JD, Waldo CR, Gerberding JL, et al: Postexposure prophylaxis for human immunodeficiency virus (HIV) infection following sexual assault, *Am J Med* 106:323-326, 1999.

15. Schreiber GB, Busch MP, Kleinman SH, et al (Retrovirus Epidemiology Donor Study): The risk of transfusion-transmitted viral infections, *N Engl J Med* 334:1685-1690, 1996.

16. Human immunodeficiency virus transmission in household settings–United States, *MMWR* 43:347, 353-356, 1994.

17. Mofenson LM, Lambert JS, Stiehm ER, et al: Risk factors for perinatal transmission of human immunodeficiency virus type 1 in women treated with zidovudine, *N Engl J Med* 341:385-393, 1999.

18. Wade NA, Birkhead GS, Warren BL, et al: Abbreviated regimens of zidovudine prophylaxis and perinatal trans-mission of the human immunodeficiency virus, *N Engl J Med* 339:1409-1414, 1998.

19. Carpenter CC, Fischl MA, Hammer SM, et al: Antiretroviral therapy for HIV infection in 1998: updated recommendations of the International AIDS Society—USA Panel, *JAMA* 280:78-86, 1998.

20. Brocklehurst P: Interventions for reducing the risk of mother-to-child transmission of HIV infection. [Systematic Review] Cochrane HIV/AIDS Group *Cochrane Database of Systematic Reviews,* 2, 2004.

21. Leroy V, Newell M-L, Dabis F, et al: International multi-centre pooled analysis of late postnatal mother-to-child transmission of HIV-1 infection, *Lancet* 352:597-600, 1998.

22. Miotti PG, Taha TE, Kumwenda NI, et al: HIV transmission through breastfeeding: a study in Malawi, *JAMA* 282:744-759, 1999.

SECTION 3: HIV TESTING

The HIV-antibody test was first made widely available in 1985. After infection with HIV, a serological window occurs during which HIV antibodies are undetectable. Among infected persons, 95% become seropositive within 3 months and 99% within 6 months. The traditional screening test is ELISA. If it is positive, the serum is tested twice more with ELISA and, if positive again, is further tested with Western blot, immunoblot, radio-immunoprecipitation, or immunofluorescence. Most results are positive or negative, but a few are indeterminate; in the latter situation the patient should be retested no sooner than 6 weeks after the initial blood was obtained.[1] Antibodies can be detected in saliva, and a commercially available system for doing this is OraSure. It has good sensitivity and specificity. Urine tests are not as sensitive or specific.[2] Rapid HIV test kits can give results in 10 minutes and can be used in the offices of health professionals. In Canada, health care professionals licensed the first such test for use in March 2000. Although positive tests require verification, rapid preliminary results may facilitate counselling. Many commercial kits are available. For most brands, sensitivity and specificity are only slightly less than for standard enzyme immunoassays, but for a few brands results are unacceptable.[3]

False-positive results from HIV testing occur but are rare. In one study of blood transfusion donors, 1 in 250,000 had a false-positive Western blot test. Of all positive Western blot tests, 5% turned out to be false positives when currently acceptable laboratory procedures were used.[4]

A controversial aspect of testing is the use of home sample collection tests. Currently, this is available in the United States but not in Canada. Patients buy a kit, obtain a finger-stick blood sample that they collect on a filter paper, and send the sample to the laboratory. Identification is with an anonymous code number. Patients call for results and receive telephone counselling if the test is positive. If patients do not have a physician, they are offered referrals. Preliminary data suggest that this system attracts a number of individuals who would otherwise not receive testing and that most of those who test positive have sources for medical care or appear willing to accept referrals. Whether they use these resources is unknown. Home sample collection tests for HIV were used by persons who were at risk for HIV and by persons who did not use other testing. Most HIV-positive users either had a source of medical care or received referrals.[5]

⚹ REFERENCES ⚹

1. Expert Working Group on HIV Testing, Canadian Medical Association: *Counselling guidelines for HIV testing,* Ottawa, 1995, Canadian Medical Association.
2. Diagnostic tests for HIV, *Med Lett* 39:81-83, 1997.
3. Giles RE, Perry KR, Parry JV: Simple/rapid test devices for anti-HIV screening: do they come up to the mark? *J Med Virol* 59:104-109, 1999.
4. Kleinman S, Busch MP, Hall L, et al: False-positive HIV-1 test results in a low-risk screening setting of voluntary blood donation, *JAMA* 280:1080-1085, 1998.
5. Branson BM: Home sample collection tests for HIV infection, *JAMA* 280:1699-1701, 1998.

SECTION 4: CLINICAL MANAGEMENT OF PATIENTS WITH HIV INFECTION
Initial Laboratory Investigations for Patients with HIV

Initial laboratory investigations of a patient who is found to be HIV positive should include the following:
- Complete blood count (CBC) and differential, smear, platelets, erythrocyte sedimentation rate (ESR)
- Absolute CD4+ lymphocyte count
- Plasma viral load
- Vitamin B_{12} and folate (AZT may cause macrocytosis)
- Blood urea nitrogen, creatinine, liver function, electrolytes
- Hepatitis A, B, and C screening
- *Toxoplasma* titer
- Cytomegalovirus (CMV) titer
- Tuberculin skin test (repeated annually; may be unreliable in persons with a CD4+ count of less than 300 cells/μL)
- Chest x-ray examination (as a baseline and screening for tuberculosis in persons with a prior history of TB, positive TB skin test, or in whom the TB skin test may be unreliable)
- Papanicolaou smear
- Swabs or serological or urine tests for sexually transmitted diseases (including *Chlamydia*, gonorrhea, and syphilis)

Other baseline lab investigations may be warranted if the patient is initiating ARV therapy or symptoms warrant the need. These may also include:

- Fasting lipid profile (total cholesterol, low-density lipoprotein [LDL], high-density lipoprotein [HDL]), triglycerides
- Random/fasting glucose
- Creatine kinase, amylase, uric acid, L-lactate dehydrogenase (LDH)
- Bioavailable testosterone

Immunizations for HIV-Positive Patients

With the possible exception of measles-mumps-rubella vaccine, patients with AIDS should not receive live vaccines such as oral polio, oral typhoid, or yellow fever. Asymptomatic HIV-positive patients with normal lymphocyte counts may receive such vaccines if they are clinically indicated.[1] Regular immunizations for HIV-positive patients should include the following:
- Inactivated polio vaccine (IPV, Salk) every 10 years
- Diphtheria-tetanus vaccine (Td) every 10 years
- Influenza vaccine annually
- Pneumococcal vaccine every 5 years
- Hepatitis A vaccine for patients at risk
- Hepatitis B vaccine for patients at risk
- Measles-mumps-rubella (MMR) vaccine (if serologically negative for these agents)

Note that patients with a low CD4+ count (over 200/μL) may have a suboptimal response to immunizations. These should be repeated if the patient's immune system is reconstituted through antiviral therapy.

For travel, patients may receive, as indicated:
- Inactivated polio vaccine
- Inactivated typhoid vaccine
- Gamma globulin
- Japanese encephalitis vaccine
- MMR vaccine

⚹ REFERENCES ⚹

1. Canadian communicable disease report: statement on travellers and HIV/AIDS, *Can Med Assoc J* 152:379-380, 1995.

SECTION 5: ANTIRETROVIRAL MANAGEMENT OF HIV INFECTION
Is There a Cure for HIV?

Although HAART treatment of asymptomatic HIV-positive patients may appear to cause complete viral suppression, cure is unlikely.[1-3] A small pool of long-lived memory CD4+ cells continues to harbour replication-competent HIV for at least 2 years,[2] and ultrasensitive techniques reveal the continued presence of low-level replication in both peripheral blood monocytes and so-called sanctuary sites, including the brain, tonsils, testes, and gut.[3]

These latent reservoirs guarantee lifetime persistence of the virus and render HIV incurable with ARV therapy alone.

Initiation of Therapy

The goals of HIV therapy are to maximally suppress viral load, restore and preserve immunological function, improve quality of life, and reduce HIV-related morbidity and mortality. Considerations to include when deciding to initiate ARV therapy are the willingness of the patient to begin and adhere to treatment, the degree of immunodeficiency, plasma HIV RNA, the risk of disease progression, and the overall benefits and risks of treatment.

The 2004 guidelines of the U.S. Panel of the International AIDS Society[1] recommend starting therapy in all patients with symptomatic HIV disease. Clinical benefit has been demonstrated in all patients with CD4+ counts of less than 200 cells/μL. However, most experts would offer therapy at a CD4+ count threshold of less than 350 cells/μL. Treatment is recommended in all asymptomatic patients with a CD4+ of less than 200 cells/μL. In asymptomatic patients with CD4+ count of more than 200 but less than 350, treatment should be offered, although this remains controversial. Treatment may be deferred in asymptomatic patients with CD4+ count of more than 350 cells/μL with a plasma HIV RNA less than 55,000 copies/mL. Decisions about treatment should normally be based on at least two measurements of HIV RNA levels and CD4+ counts unless the CD4+ count is low enough to merit initiation based on that value alone (less than 100 cells/μL).[1]

Classes of Antiretroviral Drugs

There are now 20 approved ARV agents with which to design regimens of three or more agents. These 20 agents belong to four general classes: nucleoside reverse transcriptase inhibitors (NRTIs) and one nucleotide reverse transcriptase inhibitor (NtRTI), protease inhibitors (PIs), non-nucleoside reverse transcriptase inhibitors (NNRTIs), and fusion inhibitors (FIs).

Combination Therapy

Combination therapy with at least three ARV agents has been shown to have a significant effect upon morbidity and mortality in HIV disease.[4] Viral load reduction to below limit of detection usually occurs within the first 8 to 24 weeks of therapy. Monotherapy and certain two or three drug therapies are not currently recommended due to the lack of potency and sustained antiviral activity. Three types of combination regimens may be employed as initial therapy: a combination of two NRTIs and one that avoids or spares PIs, two NRTIs and one or two PIs that spare NNRTIs, and triple NRTI regimens that spare both PIs and NNRTIs; however, these have been shown to be less efficacious in achieving viral suppression. FIs should be reserved for patients who have failed initial regimens.

The goal of a class-sparing regimen is to save one or more classes of drugs for later use and potentially avoid

Table 29   Antiretroviral Drugs and Their Common Abbreviations, Trade Names, and Usual Doses

Nucleoside Reverse Transcriptase Inhibitors (NRTIs)

abacavir (ABC) (Ziagen)	300 mg bid
didanosine, (ddl) (Videx)	200 mg bid or 400 mg od (varies with weight)
lamivudine, 3TC (Epivir)	150 mg bid or 300 mg po od
stavudine (Zerit)	40 mg bid; lower dose for patients < 60 kg
zalcitabine (ddC) (Hivid)	0.375-0.750 mg tid (rarely used now)
zidovudine (ZDV or AZT) (Retrovir)	300 mg bid
Combivir (AZT 300 mg + 3TC 150 mg)	1 tablet bid
Trizivir (AZT 300 mg + 3TC 150 mg + ABC 300 mg)	1 tablet bid

Nucleotide Reverse Transcriptase Inhibitors (NtRTIs)

tenofovir (Viread)	300 mg od

Non-nucleoside Reverse Transcriptase Inhibitors (NNRTIs)

delavirdine (Rescriptor)	400 mg tid (rarely used)
efavirenz (EFV) (Sustiva)	600 mg od
nevirapine (Viramune)	200 mg bid, initiated od for the first 2 weeks

Protease Inhibitors (PIs)

NB: most PIs are combined with small doses of ritonavir (Norvir) to improve their bioavailability, as indicated with a*)

*amprenavir (Agenerase)	1200 mg bid
*indinavir (Crixivan)	800 mg q 8 hours on empty stomach
nelfinavir (Viracept)	750 mg tid or 1250 bid with food
ritonavir (Norvir)	600 mg bid with food
*saquinavir (Invirase)	600 mg tid with food (poor bioavailability without ritonavir)
*saquinavir soft-gel capsules (Fortovase)	1200 mg tid or 1600 mg bid with food (good bioavailability)
lopinavir/ritonavir (Kaletra)	400/100 mg (3 caps) bid
*atazanavir (Reyataz)	400 mg od

Fusion Inhibitors (FIs)

T-20 (enfuvirtide, Fuzeon)	90 mg SC bid

or delay certain class-specific side effects and toxicities. Selection of a specific regimen should be individualized, on the basis of the advantages and disadvantages of each regimen. Factors to consider include patient's preference regarding pill burden, side effect profile, dosing frequency, and food and fluid restrictions. Other factors to consider are comorbid conditions such as hepatitis and tuberculosis, and drug interactions with other medications patients may be taking. Due to the complex nature of HIV care, consultation or referral to experts in the field is advisable in most instances. (See discussion of hotlines and web sites.)

Complications of Antiretroviral Therapy

The effective use of ARV therapy has resulted in significant improvements in morbidity and mortality in HIV-infected patients. However, with the widespread use of these regimens have come increasing reports of metabolic abnormalities, including dyslipidemia, insulin resistance and impaired glucose metabolism, lactic acidosis, and osteopenia. Additionally, morphological changes in body habitus may develop, including lipohypertrophy, which may include accumulation of fat in the abdomen, breast area, and the dorsocervical area (buffalo hump), and lipoatrophy, which is characterized by depletion of subcutaneous fat in the face, buttocks, and extremities. The combination of these morphological changes and ARV-associated metabolic derangements has been referred to as the *lipodystrophy syndrome*. A major concern may be the development of increased cardiovascular morbidity and mortality associated with these metabolic and morphological changes.

The etiology of these changes is not completely understood, but is likely multifactorial including the effect of the HIV virus, the effects of ARV therapy, as well as genetic factors, age (older age), and gender. (Males are more likely to acquire lipoatrophy, whereas females are more likely to have lipohypertrophy). The prevalence of metabolic complications in HIV patients is high and varies according to the treatment regimen. In patients taking PIs, impaired glucose tolerance may occur in 46% of patients and pathological insulin sensitivity in 61%.[2] Between 15% and 30% of HIV-infected patients have dyslipidemia, with close to 60% in patients taking a PI.[3] Body fat abnormalities are common in patients receiving ARV therapy, occurring in 30% to 50% of patients in several large, prospective studies.[5,6] Although early studies focused on the role of PIs in the development of lipodystrophy, it is now evident that lipodystrophy may develop in patients never treated with PIs.[7] The use of NRTIs, in particular stavudine (d4T), has been associated with the development of lipoatrophy.[8] Risk of lipodystrophy increases with the duration of therapy with NRTIs and PIs.

Treatment of the metabolic and morphological complications is still evolving, with no clear standard of care. Lifestyle modification to reduce overall cardiovascular risk and promote a healthy diet, exercise, weight loss, and smoking cessation is crucial. Switching ARV regimens, where PIs or d4T are withdrawn and replaced with different agents, may demonstrate mild improvements in dyslipidemia, insulin resistance, and lipoatrophy. Using pharmacological agents may be required, including metformin and insulin-sensitizing agents such as rosiglitazone to correct insulin resistance and diabetes, and statins and fibrates to treat dyslipidemia. The true incidence, prevalence, and harm associated is not known; toxicities due to ARV therapy have been poorly studied,

analyzed, and reported.[9] This has important implications for the widespread introduction of ARV into the developing world context.

Adherence

The single most significant factor in the success of ARV therapy is adherence. About 80% of patients will achieve complete viral suppression with 95% adherence, whereas only 50% will be successful with 70% adherence. Patient education and commitment, simplification of the regimen (fewer doses, pill and food restrictions), reminders, supports, and provider reinforcement are helpful. Lack of adherence not only leads to failure of the regime but often development of resistance to other drugs in the same class as well, limiting future treatment options.

──────────────────── ✍ REFERENCES ✍ ────────────────────

1. *Guidelines for the use of antiretroviral agents in HIV-1 infected adults and adolescents,* March 23, 2004, Department of Health and Human Services (DHHS).
2. Dube MP, Johnson DL, Currier JS, et al: Protease inhibitor-associated hyperglycemia, *Lancet* 350(9079): 713-714, Sep 6 1997.
3. Shevitz A, Wanke CA, Falutz J, et al: Clinical perspectives on HIV-associated lipodystrophy syndrome: an update, *AIDS* 15(15):1917-1930, Oct 19 2001.
4. Grabar S, Le Moing V, Goujard C, et al: Clinical outcome of patients with HIV-1 infection according to immunologic and virologic response after 6 months of highly active antiretroviral activity, *Ann Intern Med* 133(6):401-410, 2002.
5. Heath KV, Hogg RS, Chan KJ, et al: Antiretroviral treatment patterns and incident HIV-associated morphologic and lipid abnormalities in a population-based cohort, *J Acquir Immune Defic Syndr* 30(4):440-447, Aug 1 2002.
6. Lichtenstein KA, Ward DJ, Moorman AC, et al: Clinical assessment of HIV-associated lipodystrophy in an ambulatory population, *AIDS* 15(11):1389-1398, Jul 27 2001.
7. Saint-Marc T, Partisani M, Poizot-Martin I, et al: A syndrome of peripheral fat wasting in patients receiving long-term nucleoside analogue therapy, *AIDS* 13(13):1659-1667, Sep 10, 1999.
8. Mallal SA, John M, Moore CB, et al: Contribution of nucleoside analogue reverse transcriptase inhibitors to subcutaneous fat wasting in patients with HIV infection, *AIDS* 14(10):1309-1316, Jul 7 2000.
9. Carr A: Toxicity of antiretroviral therapy and implications for drug development, *Nature Rev Drug Disc* 2:624-634, 2003.

SECTION 6: PROPHYLAXIS OF OPPORTUNISTIC INFECTIONS

Perhaps the most widely cited and authoritative guidelines for the prophylaxis of opportunistic infections are those developed by the United States Public Health Service (USPHS) and the Infectious Diseases Society of

America (IDSA).[1] These guidelines are available in multiple formats (free of charge) from the USPHS web site (www.aidsinfo.nih.gov). This section will focus on the USPHS/IDSA recommendations that are the most relevant to the HIV primary care context.

Pneumocystis Carinii Pneumonia

The risk of *Pneumocystis carinii* pneumonia (PCP) is 60% to 70% per year in patients with a prior episode of the disease, and 40% to 50% per year for patients with a CD4+ cell count of less than 0.1×10^9/L (100 cells/μl). PCP prophylaxis reduces both the risk of acquiring PCP and mortality associated with the disease.

No way of preventing exposure to *P. carinii* is known. Evidence is insufficient to support a recommendation that a patient with HIV not share a room with someone who has PCP.

PCP prophylaxis is recommended for all HIV-positive patients with a CD4+ count less than 0.2×10^9/L (200 cells/μL), or a history of oropharyngeal candidiasis. The drug of choice is trimethoprim-sulfamethoxazole. The single strength tablet is better-tolerated; however, the double-strength tablet given once daily confers better cross protection for toxoplasmosis and other bacterial infections. One double-strength tablet can be given three times per week; however, poorer compliance may lead to higher risk of treatment failure.

Unfortunately, Septra is associated with a higher rate of toxicities in HIV-positive patients, and alternative agents may become necessary.

PCP prophylaxis should be discontinued in adult and adolescent patients who have responded to HAART with an increase in CD4+ T-lymphocyte counts to more than 0.2×10^9/L (200 cells/μL) for at least 3 months. Prophylaxis should be reintroduced if the CD4+ T-lymphocyte count decreases to less than 200 cells/μL.

Toxoplasmosis

HIV-infected persons should be tested for immunoglobulin G (IgG) antibody to *Toxoplasma* soon after the diagnosis of HIV infection to detect latent infection with *Toxoplasma gondii*.

Patients who are HIV positive, especially those who do not have antibodies to *Toxoplasma,* should be advised to wash their hands after handling raw meat and to avoid eating rare (pink) or raw meat, especially lamb, pork, or venison. After gardening or other contact with soil, patients should wash hands thoroughly. Cats can transmit the organisms. Strays should be avoided, and pet cats should be kept indoors, never be fed raw or rare meat, and have their kitty litter changed daily, preferably by someone who is HIV negative.

Patients who are seropositive for *Toxoplasma* and have a CD4+ count below 0.10×10^9 (100/μL) should receive

prophylactic trimethoprim-sulfamethoxazole, preferably as one double-strength tablet once a day. Patients who cannot tolerate Septra despite attempts to manage non-life-threatening reactions will require an alternative approach for prophylaxis.

Primary prophylaxis against toxoplasmosis should be discontinued in adult and adolescent patients who have responded to HAART with an increase in CD4+ T-lymphocyte counts to more than 200 cells/μL for at least 3 months. Secondary prophylaxis should be discontinued for patients whose CD4+ T-cell count has increased to more than 200 cells/μL for at least 6 months and the patient is asymptomatic with respect to signs and symptoms of toxoplasmosis. Prophylaxis should be reintroduced if the CD4+ T-lymphocyte count decreases to below those values.

Tuberculosis

When HIV infection is first recognized, the patient should receive a tuberculin skin test (TST). All patients who are HIV positive and have an induration greater than 3 to 4 mm are at high risk for active disease. This constitutes about 10% of patients annually. Patients with a CD4+ count of less than 300 cells/μL should also have a screening chest X-ray because the TB skin test may be unreliable. These patients should receive antituberculosis prophylaxis for 12 months in the form of isoniazid (INH) 300 mg per day plus pyridoxine 50 mg per day (AII), or INH 900 mg twice a week plus pyridoxine 50 mg twice a week. Clinicians should consider repeating the TST for persons whose initial skin test was negative and whose immune function has improved in response to HAART; i.e., those whose CD4+ T-lymphocyte count has increased to greater than 200 cells/μL.

Mycobacterium avium-intracellulare

Mycobacterium avium is omnipresent in soil and water, and there are no known means of preventing exposure. About half of North American patients with AIDS acquire *M. avium* infection. *M. avium* complex prophylaxis should be given to all HIV patients when the CD4+ count drops below 0.05×10^9 (50 cells/μL). The drugs of choice are clarithromycin (Biaxin) 500 mg twice a day or azithromycin (Zithromax) 1200 mg once weekly. Rifabutin 300 mg once per day is an alternative agent for patients who cannot tolerate either clarithromycin or azithromycin. Dosage adjustments of rifabutin are necessary when co-administration with either PIs or NNRTIs occurs. Primary prophylaxis for *M. avium* should be discontinued in adult and adolescent patients who have responded to HAART with an increase in CD4+ T-lymphocyte count to more than 100 cells/μL for at least 3 months. Secondary prophylaxis (maintenance therapy for the treatment of disseminated *M. avium* infection) should be discontinued in adult and adolescent patients who have responded to HAART with an increase in CD4+ T-lymphocyte count to more than 100 cells/μL for at least 6 months, and who have completed a course of at least 12 months of treatment for *M. avium*. Primary and secondary prophylaxis should be reintroduced if the CD4+ T-lymphocyte count decreases to less than 100 cells/μL.

Fungal Infections

Routine primary prophylaxis for fungal infections is not recommended. However, several situations may indicate a need for prophylaxis:

- Patients with frequent or severe (i.e., painful, cannot eat or take other medications) episodes of oropharyngeal or vulvovaginal candidiasis (fluconazole 100 to 200 mg once per day or 200 mg three times per week)
- Patients with a history of recurrent episodes of esophageal candidiasis (fluconazole 100 to 200 mg per day)
- Patients who have completed therapy for acute cryptococcal meningitis (fluconazole 200 mg once per day as suppressive therapy)

Immune reconstitution with HAART is highly effective for the prevention of most infections with *Candida* species, and should be attempted whenever possible as an adjunct to and eventual alternative to chronic antifungal therapy. Suppressive therapy for cryptococcal meningitis can be discontinued with immune reconstitution to a CD4+ count of greater than 100 to 200 cells/mm^3 for at least 6 months with no symptoms of disease.

Cytomegalovirus

Primary prophylaxis for cytomegalovirus (CMV) disease is rarely undertaken. Instead, patients should be made aware of the significance of increased floaters in the eye and should be advised to seek medical attention promptly with any sudden change in vision. Some experts recommend regular funduscopic examinations performed by an ophthalmologist for patients with low CD4+ T-lymphocyte counts.

CMV disease is not cured with courses of the currently available antiviral agents (e.g., ganciclovir, foscarnet, cidofovir, or fomivirsen). Following induction therapy, secondary prophylaxis (chronic maintenance therapy) is recommended for life unless there is immune reconstitution as a consequence of HAART. Discontinuation of prophylaxis can be considered in patients with a sustained (e.g., greater than or equal to 6 months) increase in CD4+ T-lymphocyte count to more than 100 to 150 cells/μL in response to HAART when there is no evidence of active disease. Reinstitution of secondary prophylaxis should occur when the CD4+ T-lymphocyte count has decreased to less than 100 to 150 cells/μL.

Herpes Simplex Virus Disease

Antiviral prophylaxis after exposure to herpes simplex virus (HSV) or to prevent initial episodes of HSV disease in individuals with latent infection is not recommended. Persons who have frequent or severe recurrences can receive daily suppressive therapy with oral acyclovir, oral famciclovir, or oral valacyclovir.

--- ❧ REFERENCES ❧ ---

1. http://www.aidsinfo.nih.gov/

SECTION 7: TREATMENT OF SPECIFIC AIDS-RELATED DISORDERS

The treatment of specific AIDS-related disorders is a vast topic, and only a few entities are covered here.

Aphthous Ulcers

Aphthous ulcers in patients with AIDS can become progressively larger and deeper, causing severe pain and difficulty eating. A randomized prospective trial found that thalidomide 200 mg per day orally ameliorated or healed these lesions. This effect appears to be mediated through the drug's immune-modulating capacity. Thalidomide is available through Health Canada's Emergency Drug Access Program (613-941-2108), which permits the American producer to ship the drug to the physician. The cost of the medication is not covered by any Canadian drug plan and must be paid by the patient. A more practical treatment is the use of so-called "Magic Mouth Wash," a combination of liquid Benadryl, mycostatin, decadurabolin, and erythromycin or tetracycline.[1]

Diarrhea

Diarrhea is the most common gastrointestinal (GI) symptom in patients with HIV.[2] In outpatient studies, the prevalence of diarrhea ranged from 0.9% to 14%.[3] Prevalence is increased in men having sex with men (MSM) and individuals with lower CD4+ counts. A wide variety of protozoal, viral, and bacterial organisms have been implicated as potential causes. The degree of immunodeficiency as expressed by the CD4+ cell count is an important determinant of enteric pathogens. When evaluation of diarrhea reveals an enteric pathogen using stool cultures, specific therapy is indicated. In clinical practice, if the diarrhea is mild or moderate without blood, investigations may be limited to a routine stool culture, and symptomatic treatment may be instituted. Further investigations can be deferred unless the patient's condition deteriorates. Medications are a common cause of diarrhea, especially PIs, including Saquinavir and Nelfinavir. Other causes include small bowel bacterial overgrowth, lactose intolerance, and HIV enteropathy, which is a chronic diarrhea with no identified etiology in patients with advanced HIV disease. HIV patients with chronic diarrhea should be treated symptomatically. Symptomatic treatment consists of short-term bowel rest with clear fluids, bulking agents such as psyllium, and drugs such as diphenoxylate (Lomotil), loperamide (Imodium), or narcotic agents such as codeine phosphate. For patients with uncontrolled profuse diarrhea of unknown etiology, octreotide (Somatostatin) in subcutaneous doses of 50 to 100 mg three times daily may be effective.[3]

Esophageal Candidiasis

The initial treatment of eosphageal candidiasis may be instituted on the basis of clinical suspicion. Endoscopy is reserved for patients who do not respond. The most effective medication at present appears to be fluconazole (Diflucan) 100 to 200 mg per day as a single dose for 3 weeks or for 2 weeks after symptoms have resolved; alternatives are itraconazole (Sporanox) 200 mg per day for 2 to 3 weeks and ketoconazole (Nizoral) 200 to 400 mg per day for 2 to 3 weeks.[4]

Weight Loss

HIV wasting is relatively rare in patients who are receiving highly active combination ARV therapy. Aside from providing optimal ARV drug therapy, interventions that may be helpful for patients with AIDS wasting include nutritional evaluation, drugs, and possibly exercise programs. Appetite-stimulating drugs such as megestrol (Megace) in doses of 800 mg per day may be useful when weight loss is clearly due to reduced food intake; any weight gain achieved is due primarily to increased fat. If androgen deficiency is shown by low levels of serum-free testosterone in HIV-infected men, testosterone therapy may lead to an increase in lean body mass.[5] One study found that a combination of progressive resistance exercise combined with intramuscular administration of testosterone 100 mg per week plus the oral anabolic steroid oxandrolone (Hepandrin, Oxandrin) 20 mg per day increased lean body mass in men with HIV-associated weight loss.[6]

_____ ❧ REFERENCES ❧ _____

1. Jacobson JM, Greenspan JS, Spritzler J, et al: Thalidomide for the treatment of oral aphthous ulcers in patients with human immunodeficiency virus infection, *N Engl J Med* 336:1487-1493, 1997.
2. Wilcox CM, Rabeneck L, Friedman S: AGA technical review: malnutrition and cachexia, chronic diarrhea and hepatobiliary disease in patients with human immunodeficiency virus infection, *Gastroenterlogy* 111(6):1724-1752, Dec 1996.
3. Ulrich R, Riecken EO, Zeitz M, et al: AIDS enteropathy, *Ann Intern Med* 115:328, 1991.
4. Drugs for AIDS and associated infections, *Med Lett* 37: 87-94, 1995.
5. Corcoran C, Grinspoon S: Treatments for wasting in patients with the acquired immunodeficiency syndrome, *N Engl J Med* 340:1740-1750, 1999.
6. Strawford A, Barbieri T, Van Loan M, et al: Resistance exercise and supraphysiologic androgen therapy in eugonadal men with HIV-related weight loss: a randomized controlled trial, *JAMA* 281:1282-1290, 1999.

SECTION 8: OTHER HIV-RELATED TOPICS
Hepatitis C Coinfection

The prevalence of hepatitis C virus infection is increasing worldwide. Chronic infection with this virus is one of the most important causes of chronic liver disease. As part of baseline investigations, one should routinely investigate for hepatitis C (HCV) along with HIV. A substantial number of people are coinfected with HIV and HCV. Approximately 11,194 persons were infected with both HCV and HIV in Canada as of December 1999. Seven thousand nine hundred twenty one injection drug users (IDUs) and 1,648 MSMs who also inject drugs (MSM-IDU) were dually infected, accounting for 71% and 15%, respectively, of dually infected persons in Canada.[1] The vast majority (88%) of dually infected persons in Canada live in Quebec (34%), British Columbia (29%), or Ontario (25%). Genetic analysis of HCV reveals the existence of numerous subtypes or genotypes. Six major genotypes have been identified. Genotype distribution is worldwide. Genotype 1 is the most common in the United States and Canada, accounting for more than 75% of all HCV infections. Hepatitis C genotype does not appear to affect rate of disease progression. Genotype is, however, a predictor of response to therapy. According to the most recent studies in the treatment of chronic HCV in HIV co-infected individuals, sustained virological response (SVR) rates are attainable in up to 40% of individuals.[2] SVR is defined as a negative HCV RNA at 72 weeks. SVR rates for genotype 1 are usually lower. Treatment usually consists of once weekly injections of pegylated interferon along with oral Ribavirin for a total of 48 weeks. Also, the negative predicative value of not achieving an early viral response (defined as either a 2-log drop in HCV-RNA level from baseline or an HCV-RNA level less than 50 IU/L after 12 weeks of therapy) was found to be 100%.

_____ ❧ REFERENCES ❧ _____

1. Health Canada Epidemiology of HIV and HCV co-infection http://www.hc-sc.gc.ca/hppb/hepatitis_c/pdf/hivhcvreport/results2.html.
2. Abstracts from 11th CROI 2004, San Francisco, CA.

HIV and Injection Drug Users

In the early 1980s, the Canadian HIV epidemic was concentrated among MSMs. By the early to mid-1990s, a change toward increasing transmission among IDUs occurred, such that by 1996, approximately 47% of new HIV infections that occurred in Canada were among IDUs.[1] Despite a slight drop in national HIV infections among IDUs, the absolute number of infections in this group remains unacceptably high.[2] A similar trend occurred in the number of positive HIV test reports among adults reported to the Centre for Infectious Disease Prevention and Control (CIDPC).[3] Injection drug use is cited as one of the main modes of transmission for those living with HIV/AIDS in most of the 10 regions of the world, including North America, North Africa, and Middle East, Western Europe, East Asia, and Pacific. In Eastern Europe and Central Asia, where the epidemic began relatively later than in other regions (early 1990s), injection drug use is listed as the single main mode of transmission in that region.[2]

❧ REFERENCES ❦

1. Archibald CP, Remis RS, Farley J, et al: *Estimating HIV prevalence and incidence at the national level: combining direct and indirect methods with Monte-Carlo simulation*, XII International Conference on AIDS, Geneva, June-July 1998 (Abst. 43475).
2. Geduld J, Archibald CP: National trends of AIDS and HIV in Canada, *CCDR* 26:193-201, 2000.
3. Health Canada: *HIV and AIDS in Canada: surveillance report to June 30, 2002*, Division of HIV/AIDS Epidemiology and Surveillance, Centre for Infectious Disease Prevention and Control (CIDPC), 2002, Health Canada.
4. *AIDS epidemic update, December 2002*, Joint United Nations Programme on HIV/AIDS (UNAIDS) and World Health Organization (WHO) 2002.

Reconstitution Syndrome

The advent of highly active ARV therapy has led to evidence of partial immune reconstitution in persons with chronic infection. One of the hallmarks of HIV infection is chronic immune activation, which persists for years. T-cell turnover studies suggested that CD4+ cells were being produced and destroyed at a rate well over threefold.[1] Studies suggest that both an increased destruction of CD4+ cells as well as a block in T-cell production cause lymphopenia in HIV-infected individuals. HAART may alleviate this. A defect in the production of thymic cells may also be involved.[2] In the presence of HAART, dramatic increases in CD4+ cell counts have been documented in some persons, and these increases are associated with a decreased risk of opportunistic infections and death. Patients treated with HAART typically experience an early rise in memory CD4+ cells, followed by a later rise in naive CD4+ cells. The restoration of immune function with HAART can also have adverse consequences, due to augmented immune responses to pathogens that are already present. Such immune reconstitution syndromes are still poorly understood but have

been reported in a variety of settings. Encouragingly, emerging data suggest that most of these cases resolve with continued therapy.[3] Examples include the development of fever and severe lymphadenitis due to previous unsuspected *Mycobacterioum avium* complex infection,[4] immune recovery vitritis associated with CMV retinitis,[5,6] and exacerbation of viral hepatitis associated with the institution of ARV therapy.[7] These and other syndromes of HAART-associated inflammatory disorders indicate that functional immunity is being restored with viremic control and provide the rationale for further attempts to augment pathogen-specific immunity in HIV infection.

❧ REFERENCES ❦

1. Ho DD, Neumann AU, Perelson AS: Rapid turnover of plasma virions and CD4+ lymphocytes in HIV-1 infection, *Nature* 373;123-126, 1995.
2. Teixeira L, Valdez H, McCune JM, et al: Poor CD4 T cell restoration after suppression of HIV-1 replication may reflect lower thymic function, *AIDS* 15:1749-1756, 2001.
3. DeSimone JA, Pomerantz RJ, Babinchak TJ: Inflammatory reactions in HIV-1-infected persons after initiation of highly active antiretroviral therapy, *Ann Intern Med* 133:447-454, 2000.
4. Race EM, Adelson-Mitty J, Kriegel GR, et al: Focal mycobacterial lymphadenitis following initiation of protease-inhibitor therapy in patients with advanced HIV-1 disease, *Lancet* 351:252-255, 1998.
5. Karavellas MP, Plummer DJ, Macdonald JC, et al: Incidence of immune recovery vitritis in cytomegalovirus retinitis patients following institution of successful highly active antiretroviral therapy, *J Infect Dis* 179:697-700, 1999.
6. Nguyen QD, Kempen JH, Bolton SG, et al: Immune recovery uveitis in patients with AIDS and cytomegalovirus retinitis after highly active antiretroviral therapy, *Am J Ophthalmol* 129:634-639, 2000.
7. John M, Flexman J, French MA: Hepatitis C virus-associated hepatitis following treatment of HIV-infected patients with HIV protease inhibitors: an immune restoration disease? *AIDS* 12:2289-2293, 1998.

INSECT STINGS AND BITES

(See also food allergies; tropical medicine; urticaria and angioedema)

Types of Stinging Insects

Most stinging insects are members of the Hymenoptera order of the class Insecta. They include yellow jackets, hornets, wasps, honeybees, bumblebees, and fire ants. In the United States, yellow jackets are responsible for most stings. The stingers of honeybees tend to detach and remain in the skin, while the stingers of other insects do not remain in the skin. The venom of Africanized honeybees or "killer bees" is no more likely to induce anaphylaxis or cause toxicity than is the venom of other members of the Hymenoptera order. However, the Africanized honeybee is more aggressive and more likely to sting than its docile cousin. Anaphylaxis may result from stinging insects but rarely from biting insects.[1]

The longer a bee stinger remains in the skin, the more venom is liberated. Therefore, the stinger should be plucked out with fingers or forceps as rapidly as possible.[2]

Local Reactions to Insect Stings

Reactions to stings vary. In most cases localized pain, swelling, and erythema develop and then subside in a few hours. More extensive localized reactions are common, may reach a maximum size after 48 hours, and may last for up to a week. Extensive erythema is also common and may be mistaken for cellulitis, which in fact is a rare complication of stings.[1]

Treatment of large local reactions is acetylsalicylic acid 650 mg every 4 hours as needed plus an antihistamine. If the reaction is disabling, prednisone 40 mg per day may be given for 2 or 3 days. Persons who have had large local reactions are likely to have similar reactions if stung again; their risk of anaphylaxis with a future sting is 5% per episode. They are not candidates for immunotherapy and therefore are not candidates for venom skin tests. Tetanus prophylaxis is not necessary for insect stings.[1]

Anaphylactic Reactions

Anaphylactic reactions most often occur in persons under age 20 and are twice as common in males, probably because they have greater exposure to stings. The most common symptoms are generalized urticaria, flushing, and angioedema. More serious reactions are upper airway edema, bronchospasm, and circulatory collapse. Most deaths occur in adults. Among unselected patients who have had an anaphylactic reaction and are subsequently stung (without having had venom immunotherapy), only 50% to 60% have a second anaphylactic reaction. The incidence of second anaphylactic reactions is much lower in children, particularly if the initial manifestation was dermal.[1]

Treatment of an acute anaphylactic reaction is 0.2 to 0.5 mL of 1:1000 epinephrine subcutaneously repeated every 30 minutes as needed. If necessary, aerosolized bronchodilators and IV fluids should be added. In most cases, acute symptoms subside in 30 minutes. In the rare cases in which they persist, IV steroids should be given followed by oral prednisone 60 mg per day for 2 days.[1]

Prophylaxis Against Insect Stings

Clothes should be dark-coloured and cover the body fully. For example, gloves are helpful when gardening. Perfumes, cosmetics, and hairsprays should be avoided. Food odours attract yellow jackets.[1]

If patients who have had a large local reaction or a mild generalized reaction are stung again, they should take a rapidly absorbed antihistamine as soon as possible. Backup medication for these patients is epinephrine (adrenaline). Epinephrine is first-line treatment for individuals who have had serious generalized reactions in the past.[3]

Epinephrine is available in kit form either as an EpiPen or as an ANA-Kit. Epinephrine is relatively unstable; it should be stored in the dark and not used after its expiration date.[4] The EpiPen comes as preloaded syringes of epinephrine. At-risk individuals who will be distant from an emergency room should carry more than one. The adult form contains 2 mL of epinephrine 1:1000, and the children's version (EpiPen Jr) contains 2 mL of epinephrine 1:2000. The ANA-Kit contains a preloaded syringe of epinephrine, a tourniquet, alcohol swabs, and two 4-mg chewable chlorpheniramine tablets (Chlor-Trimeton, Chlor-Tripolon). Antihistamines are useful in controlling hives and angioedema.

Venom immunotherapy is indicated for patients who have had severe symptoms of anaphylaxis and have positive venom skin tests. It is not indicated for children (or probably for adults) who have had only dermal reactions, and it is probably not indicated for individuals with relatively mild symptoms such as urticaria plus some shortness of breath.[3,5] The Canadian Society of Allergy and Clinical Immunology currently recommends that immunotherapy be given every 4 to 6 weeks for 5 years.[5] According to a position statement of the American Academy of Allergy, Asthma and Immunology, individuals who have had a mild or moderate reaction may discontinue immunotherapy after 3 to 5 years. Those who have had a severe reaction may be able to safely discontinue treatment after 5 years, although the physician may choose to treat them for longer periods.[6] Recommendations from Britain state that 3 years is long enough for treatment but that this form of therapy should take place only in specialist centres with facilities for resuscitation. Patients must be observed for 1 hour after each dose.[3]

Mosquito Bites
(See West Nile Virus and Tropical Medicine)

Since mosquitoes breed in standing water, such as in old tires, birdbaths, clogged gutters, and empty containers, elimination of these sources may decrease the number of insects in the area. Ultrasonic electronic devices and bug "zappers" are ineffective, and citronella candles are only moderately effective. Symptomatic relief of bites may be obtained with topical corticosteroids or oral antihistamines.[7] DEET repellents are the preferred form of prevention; non-DEET repellents cannot be relied upon for protection for prolonged durations, especially in environments where mosquito-borne diseases are a substantial threat.[8] (See West Nile Virus for a longer discussion of DEET.)

Brown Recluse Spider Bites

Brown recluse spider bites are a common problem in the Southeastern United States. Most bites are asymptomatic or present with pain and erythema. Envenomation can lead to a constellation of systemic symptoms called loxoscelism (fever, chills, arthritic complaints, and blood abnormalities), and/or necrotic arachnidism, which is ulceration or necrosis that occurs as a result of the bite. Mild cases should be treated by a thorough cleansing, elevation of the bitten extremity, analgesics, and administration of tetanus vaccination if indicated. Systemic antibiotics may also be indicated. Immediate hospitalization is required if systemic symptoms develop. If ulcers have formed, skin grafting or amputation of the affected appendage may be necessary, but only after the lesion has stabilized and stopped enlarging. Steroids can be given for severe skin lesions, loxoscelism, and in small children. Topical nitroglycerin may have efficacy in decreasing enlargement of necrotic skin ulcers.[9,10]

◢ REFERENCES ◣

1. Reisman RE: Insect stings, *N Engl J Med* 331:523-527, 1994.
2. Visscher PD, Vetter RS, Camazine S: Removing bee stings, *Lancet* 348:301-302, 1996.
3. Ewan PW: Venom allergy, *BMJ* 316:1365-1368, 1998.
4. Stability of drugs in solution, *Med Lett* 38:90, 1996.
5. Canadian Society of Allergy and Clinical Immunology: Guidelines for the use of allergen immunotherapy, *Can Med Assoc J* 152:1413-1419, 1995.
6. Graft DF, Golden DF, Reisman RE, et al: Position statement: the discontinuation of Hymenoptera venom immunotherapy; report from the Committee on Insects, *J Allergy Clin Immunol* 101:573-575, 1998.
7. Fradin MS: Mosquitoes and mosquito repellents: a clinician's guide, *Ann Intern Med* 128:931-940, 1998.
8. Fradin MS, Day JF: Comparative efficacy of insect repellents against mosquito bites, *N Engl J Med* 347(1):13-8, 2002.
9. Forks TP: Brown recluse spider bites, *J Am Board Fam Pract* 13(6):415-423, 2000.
10. Cacy J, Mold JW: The clinical characteristics of brown recluse spider bites treated by family physicians: an OKPRN Study, *J Fam Pract* 48(7):536-542, 1999.

INFECTIOUS DISEASE

ANTIBACTERIALS, SPECIFIC DRUGS

(See also antibiotic resistance, sexually transmitted infections)

Tables 30 to 35 list the generic names, trade names, and usual doses of selected antibiotics used in the care of ambulatory patients.[1,3] Formulations are for oral use unless otherwise indicated. Optimal doses vary with different clinical conditions, and these are not always indicated in the tables. A reputable drug reference should be consulted before prescribing.

Lincosamides

The most frequently used lincosamide is clindamycin (Cleocin, Dalacin). It is particularly effective against aerobic gram-positive organisms, such as streptococci and staphylococci, and anaerobes. The usual oral dosage is 150 to 300 mg every 6 hours. In pediatrics, the usual dosage is 10 to 30 mg/kg per day orally in 3 to 4 divided doses.

Nitrofurantoin (Macrodantin, MacroBID)

Nitrofurantoin is used for the prevention and treatment of urinary tract infections caused by susceptible *Escherichia coli*, *Klebsiella*, *Enterobacter*, staphylococci, and enterococcus spp. *Pseudomonas*, *Serriata*, and most species of *Proteus* are generally resistant. When used for prophylaxis, the usual adult dosage is 50 to 100 mg once daily and for children is 1 mg/kg per day. When used for treatment, the usual adult dosage is 50 to 100 mg every 6 hours (or if using MacroBid 100 mg twice daily) and for children is 1 mg/kg every 6 hours. Nitrofurantoin should not be used when glomerular filtration rate (GFR) is less than 50 mL/minute.

Trimethoprim (Proloprim)

Trimethoprim is most commonly used in combination with sulfamethoxazole, but is effective on its own for the treatment and prevention of acute, uncomplicated urinary tract infections due to susceptible strains of *E. coli* and *K. pneumoniae*. The normal adult dosage for prevention is 100 mg once daily and for treatment is 100 mg every 12 hours. Its efficacy in pediatrics when used as a single agent has not been established and is therefore not recommended. Dosage adjustment is necessary when GFR is less than 30 mL/minute.

Fosfomycin

Fosfomycin (Monurol) is a broad-spectrum antibiotic that is generally used as a single 3-g dose treatment for uncomplicated urinary tract infections. The product comes in a single dose sachet containing the granules, which are dissolved in one-half cup of water before the medication is taken.

──────────── ◁ REFERENCES ▷ ────────────

1. Rosser WW, Pennie RA, Pilla NJ (and the Ontario Anti-infective Review Panel): *Anti-infective Guidelines for Community-acquired Infections*, Toronto, 2005, MUMS Guideline Clearinghouse.
2. Taketomo CK: *Pediatric Dosage Handbook,* ed 9, Ohio, 2002-2003, Lexi-Comp.
3. Yee CL, Duffy C, Gerbino P, et al: Tendon or joint disorders in children after treatment with fluoroquinolones or azithromycin, *Pediatr Infect Dis J* 21:525-529, 2002.
4. *Compendium of Pharmaceutical Specialities (CPS)*, Ottawa, 2004, Canadian Pharmacists Association.

ANTIMICROBIAL RESISTANCE

Resistance by bacteria to antimicrobial drugs is caused by genetic mutation. This adaptive response is particularly powerful in bacteria because of very large population numbers, short generation times, and the ability of bacteria to transmit genetic information both vertically (mother to daughter) and horizontally (sister to sister). The main factor that selects for these mutations is exposure to antibiotics.[1] Bacteria that are resistant to one antibiotic are more likely to exhibit multidrug resistance.[2] Not surprisingly, decreasing antibiotic use in a community leads to lower levels of resistance.[3]

Agricultural use of antimicrobial drugs accounts for over half of total antibiotic consumption in developed countries, and resistance originating in animals has been demonstrated in human infections.[4] In humans, inappropriate antibiotic prescription for viral upper respiratory tract infections and bronchitis is rampant, on the order

Table 30   Penicillins

Generic name (trade name)	Usual adult dose	Usual pediatric dose
Penicillinase Susceptible		
Benzathine penicillin G (parenteral use only)	1.2 million U IM as a single dose for Group A strep 2.4 million U IM as a single dose for primary or secondary syphilis	25,000-50,000 U/kg IM as a single dose for Group A strep
Penicillin G (benzylpenicillin) (parenteral use only)	2-24 million U/day IM/IV in 4-6 divided doses	50,000 U/kg/day IM/IV in 4 divided doses
Penicillin V potassium, phenoxymethylpenicillin (Pen-Vee)	300 mg (500,000 U) tid-qid	25-50 mg/kg/day (40,000-90,000 U/kg/day) given in 3 or 4 divided doses
Penicillinase Resistant		
Cloxacillin (Orbenin)	250-500 mg qid	25-50 mg/kg/day in 4 divided doses
Aminopenicillins		
Amoxicillin (Amoxil)	250-500 mg q8h	25-50 mg/kg/day in 3 divided doses
Ampicillin	250-500 mg po q6h	50-100 mg/kg/d in 4 divided doses
Pivampicillin (Pondocillin)	500 mg bid	25-35 mg/kg/d in 2 divided doses
Amoxicillin plus clavulanate potassium (Augmentin, Clavulin)	250-500 mg q8h or 875 mg q12h	25-50 mg/kg/day in 3 divided doses

Table 31   Cephalosporins

Generic name (trade name)	Usual adult dose	Usual pediatric dose
First Generation		
Cefadroxil (Duricef)	0.5-1 g po bid	30 mg/kg/day po in 2 divided doses to a max of 2g/d
Cefazolin Sodium (Ancef, Kefzol) *(parenteral use only)*	500 mg-1 g IM/IV bid	50-100 mg/kg/day IM/IV in 3 divided doses
Cephalexin (Keflex)	250-500 po mg qid	20-50 mg/kg/day po in 4 divided doses
Cephalothin sodium (Ceporacin Inj) *(parenteral use only)*	0.5-2 g IM/IV q4-6h	80-150 mg/kg/day IM/IV in 4-6 divided doses
Second Generation		
Cefaclor (Ceclor)	250-500 mg po tid	20-40 mg/kg/day po in 2-3 divided doses
Cefotetan disodium (Cefotan) *(parenteral use only)*	1-2 g IM/IV bid	40-80 mg/kg/day IM/IV in 2 divided doses
Cefoxitin sodium *(parenteral use only)*	1-2 g IM/IV q6-8h	80-100 mg/kg/day IM/IV in 3-4 divided doses
Cefprozil (Cefzil)	250-500 mg po bid	15-30 mg/kg/day po in 2 divided doses
Cefuroxime axetil (Ceftin)	250-500 mg po bid 1 g po single dose for uncomplicated gonorrhea	20-30 mg/kg/day po in 2 divided doses
Cefuroxime sodium (Kefurox) *(parenteral use only)*	750 mg IV tid	30-100 mg/kg/day IV in 2-3 divided doses
Third Generation		
Cefixime (Suprax)	400 mg po once daily 400 mg po single dose for uncomplicated gonorrhea	8 mg/kg/day po as a single dose
Cefotaxime sodium (Claforan) *(parenteral use only)*	1 g IM/IV q12h to 1-2 g IM/IV q8h 1 g IM/IV single dose for uncomplicated gonorrhea	100-200 mg/kg/day IM/IV in 4 divided doses
Ceftazidime pentahydrate (Fortaz) *(parenteral use only)*	1-2 g IM/IV in 2-3 divided doses	100-150 mg/kg/day IM/IV in 3 divided doses
Ceftizoxime sodium (Cefizox) *(parenteral use only)*	0.5-1 g IM/IV q8-12h	150-200 mg/kg/day IM/IV in 3-4 divided doses
Ceftriaxone sodium (Rocephin) *(parenteral use only)*	1-2 g IM/IV q12h 250 mg IM/IV single dose for uncomplicated gonorrhea	50-75 mg/kg/day IM/IV in 1-2 divided doses
Fourth Generation		
Cefepime hydrocholride (Maxipime) *(parenteral use only)*	0.5-2 g IM/IV q12h	50 mg/kg IM/IV q12h

Table 32   Fluoroquinolones

Generic name (trade name)	Usual adult dose	Usual pediatric dose*
Ciprofloxacin (Cipro)	250-500 mg (occasionally 750 mg) bid 100 mg bid for 3 days for uncomplicated urinary tract infections	Not indicated
Levofloxacin (Levaquin)	500 mg once daily	Not indicated
Norfloxacin (Noroxin)	400 mg bid	Not indicated
Ofloxacin (Floxin)	200-400 mg bid	Not indicated

*Based on reports of articular cartilage damage in young beagles, quinolones have not been indicated in young children. However, recent evidence suggests that quinolones appear safe in the human pediatric population. Further evidence is needed to confirm safe prescribing of these drugs for children.[3]

Table 33   Macrolides*

Generic name (trade name)	Usual adult dose	Usual pediatric dose
Azithromycin (Zithromax)	500 mg as single dose on day 1 followed by 250 mg daily on days 2-5 1 g as single dose for *Chlamydia*	10 mg/kg/day on day 1 as single dose followed by 5 mg/kg/day on days 2-5 for otitis media 12 mg/kg/day as single dose for 5 days for pharyngitis or tonsillitis
Clarithromycin (Biaxin)	250-500 mg bid	15 mg/kg/day in 2 divided doses
Erythromycin base	250-500 mg q6-12h or 333 mg (delayed release) tid	30-50 mg/kg/day in 3-4 divided doses
Erythromycin ethylsuccinate	400-800 mg q6-12h	30-50 mg/kg/day in 3-4 divided doses
Erythromycin stearate	250-500 mg q6-12h	30-50 mg/kg/day in 4 divided doses
Erythromycin estolate	250-500 mg q6-12h	30-50 mg/kg/day in 2-4 divided doses
Erythromycin ethylsuccinate-sulfisoxazole (Pediazole)	NA	30-50 mg/kg/day of erythromycin in 3-4 divided doses

*Macrolides are metabolized by the cytochrome P450 system, and as a result, are susceptible to drug interactions with other drugs similarly metabolized (e.g, theophyllines, digoxin, warfarin, some antihistamines and anticonvulsants). It is advised to consult a reputable drug reference before prescribing.

Table 34   Sulfonamides

Generic name (trade name)	Usual adult dose	Usual pediatric dose
Trimethoprim-sulfamethoxazole-TMP-SMX (Septra, Bactrim)	1 DS tablet bid	6 mg/kg/day of trimethoprim and 30 mg/kg/day of sulfamethoxazole in 2 divided doses
Erythromycin ethylsuccinate sulfisoxazole (Pediazole)	NA	30-50 mg/kg/day of erythromycin in 3-4 divided doses

Table 35   Tetracyclines*

Generic name (trade name)	Usual adult dose	Usual pediatric dose
Tetracycline hydrochloride	250-500 mg qid	25-50 mg/kg/day in 4 divided doses for children over 8-12 years of age
Doxycycline (Vibramycin)	100 mg bid on day 1 followed by 100 mg/day	4.4 mg/kg/day on day 1 in 2 divided doses followed by 2.2 mg/kg/day as a single daily dose for children over 8 years of age
Minocycline (Minocin)	200 mg on day 1 followed by 100 mg/day	4 mg/kg/day on day 1 followed by 2 mg/kg/day for children over 8 years of age

*Tetracyclines may cause permanent discoloration of teeth during tooth development and are not recommended in children under 9 years of age (Taketomo, 2003; Rossa, 2005).

of 50% for both adults[5] and children.[6] In the case of children, family physicians are worse offenders than pediatricians.[6]

To the degree that some inappropriate antibiotic prescribing may be due to perceived patient or parental expectations, clinicians can be reassured by a study that demonstrated parental satisfaction is correlated to the quality of physician communication, not with whether antibiotics were prescribed.[7] On a community level, a Canadian study demonstrated that physician and pharmacist education on appropriate antibiotic use, combined with patient and public education programs, resulted in both a decrease in overall antibacterial drug prescribing and a shift to first-line from second- and third-line drugs.[8]

—————————— **≈ REFERENCES ≈** ——————————

1. Arason VA, Kristinsson KG, Sigurdsson JA, et al: Do antimicrobials increase the carriage rate of penicillin resistant pneumococci in children? Cross sectional prevalence study, *BMJ* 313:387-391, 1996.
2. Doern GV, Pfaller MA, Kugler K, et al: Prevalence of antimicrobial resistance among respiratory tract isolates of *Streptococcus pneumoniae* in North America: 1997 results from the SENTRY antimicrobial surveillance program, *Clin Infect Dis* 27:764-770, 1998.
3. Seppälä H, Klaukka T, Vuopio-Varkila J, et al: The effect of changes in the consumption of macrolide antibiotics on erythromycin resistance in group A streptococci in Finland, *N Engl J Med* 337:441-446, 1997.
4. Sirinavin S, Garner P: Antibiotics for treating salmonella gut infections (Cochrane Review). In: *The Cochrane Library,* issue 4, Chichester, UK, 2004, John Wiley & Sons.
5. Gonzales R, Steiner JF, Sande MA: Antibiotic prescribing for adults with colds, upper respiratory tract infections, and bronchitis by ambulatory care physicians, *JAMA* 278:901-904, 1997.
6. Nyquist A-C, Gonsales R, Steiner JF, et al: Antibiotic prescribing for children with colds, upper respiratory tract infections, and bronchitis, *JAMA* 279:875-877, 1998.
7. Mangione-Smith R, McGlynn EA, Elliott MN, et al: The relationship between perceived parental expectations and pediatrician antimicrobial prescribing behavior, *Pediatrics* 103:711-718, 1999.
8. Stewart J, Pilla J, Dunn L: Pilot study for appropriate antiinfective community therapy: Effect of a guideline-based strategy to optimize use of antibiotics, *Can Fam Physician* 46:851-859, 2000.

BITES

Animal Bites

(See also human bites; rabies)

Epidemiology

Bites account for about 1% of emergency room visits. Dog bites are responsible for 80% to 90% of all bites assessed by physicians, cat bites for 5% to 15%, and human bites for 3% to 20%.[1] In the United States each year, approximately 2% of the population is bitten by dogs.[2]

About half of dog bites are trivial; 10% require suturing and follow-up; 6% to 13% that penetrate the skin will get infected;[3] 1% to 2% require hospitalization. Most complications from dog bites occur at the time of initial injury due to the direct trauma, whereas in cat bites most complications arise later as a result of secondary infection of deep tissues.[4] Cat bites are much more likely than dog bites to become infected; the infection rate is 30% to 50%.[1]

In about 50% to 90% of dog-bite cases, the animal belongs to or is known to the victim. Most dog bites involve the extremities except in children under 4, who most commonly have bites to the head and neck. Twenty-five percent of all animal bites occurred in children less than 6 years old; 34% of bites in children 6 to 17 years old.[3] Children under the age of 2 with dog bites to the skull should have imaging to rule out perforation.[4] Risk factors for infection include delay of medical care more than 24 hours, puncture wounds, location: hands (28%) vs facial (less than 4%), and host immune status (e.g., asplenism, diabetes).[3]

Prevention of animal bites begins by selecting only appropriate animals as pets. Ferrets should be banned from homes where infants and small children are present. Non-human primates should be banned from all homes because these animals are prone to vicious attacks on humans. Numerous breeds of dogs are considered dangerous in the presence of small children, but identifying them is difficult because of lack of published data.[5]

Attacks by dogs are considerably decreased by neutering or spaying them and by giving them intensive socialization training between the ages of 7 and 12 weeks. Preventing dogs from roaming free clearly decreases the risk of bites; chaining dogs in the yard or restraining them with buried electric fences is inadequate because such measures do not prevent children from approaching the animal.[5] Infants and toddlers should never be left alone with a dog. Children should be trained to avoid approaching an unknown dog, to stand still and not to scream if approached by a dog, and to avoid eye contact with a dog.[6]

Management principles

Animal bites are managed with meticulous wound cleansing, exploration, irrigation, and if indicated, debridement. Adequate wound cleansing often requires the use of local anesthetics. Wounds should be deeply irrigated with high-pressure flow through a large bore needle (e.g., 19 gauge). Except for the face, devitalized tissue should be debrided. Crushing injury in dog bites creates a large zone of devitalized tissue compared with a laceration.[3] Facial lacerations from cat or dog bites can generally be sutured, if this is possible, within 12 to 24 hours of the injury. Bites to the arms or legs may be sutured if this can be done within 6 to 12 hours.[7] Hand wounds and puncture wounds should not be sutured closed, but rather managed with either loose edge approximation or delayed primary closure with wet dressings. Also, the risk of tetanus and rabies should be assessed.

Microbiology of cat and dog bites

Most infections caused by cat or dog bites are polymicrobial. On average, three to five different organisms are cultured from infected wounds. The most frequently isolated aerobes are *Pasteurella* species (*P. multocida* from cats and *P. canis* from dogs), *Streptococcus* species, *Staphylococcus* species, *Capnocytophaga canimorsus* (in dogs), *Corynebacterium, Moraxella,* and *Neisseria.* The role of anaerobes in infections has been increasingly appreciated. In over two thirds[3] of infected wounds, a variety of anaerobes are found, almost always in conjunction with aerobes. Most of the anaerobes and many of the aerobes are β-lactamase producers.[8]

Antibiotic treatment of infected cat and dog bites

Antibiotics chosen for treatment should be effective against *Pasteurella,* streptococci, staphylococci, and anaerobes and should have activity against β-lactamase-producing organisms.[8] In most cases this can be accomplished by giving a β-lactam antibiotic such as amoxicillin combined with a β-lactamase inhibitor such as clavulanate (Augmentin, Clavulin).[7] Other options are a second-generation cephalosporin, a combination of penicillin and a first-generation cephalosporin, or a combination of clindamycin and a fluoroquinolone. In vitro sensitivities suggest that azithromycin (Zithromax) given alone may be effective. A recent Canadian study looked at the efficacy of treating even moderate-to-severe post-bite infections with once daily parenteral (IV or IM) ceftriaxone as outpatients and reported no treatment failures.[9] Drugs that should not be used as sole treatment are erythromycin, first-generation cephalosporins, anti-staphylococcal penicillins, or clindamycin, because they do not have adequate activity against *Pasteurella.*[8]

A hallmark of *Pasteurella* species infection, in particular in cat bites, is the onset of cellulites within 6 to 24 hours of the bite; cellulites arising more than 24 to 48 hours after the bite are typically other pathogens.[4] *C. canimorsus* is a rare source of overwhelming sepsis after dog bites. It should be suspected if fever, septic shock, and/or disseminated intravascular coagulation (DIC) develop in an immunocompromised patient 2 to 3 days after a dog bite. The organism is sensitive to penicillin.[4,7] If a bite was caused by a healthy dog or cat, the animal can be confined and observed for 10 days to exclude rabies.

Antibiotic prophylaxis of cat and dog bites

Although a 1994 meta-analysis showed that antibiotic prophylaxis after dog bites reduced the relative risk of infection by 44%, this translated into an absolute risk reduction of only 4% (NNT of 25).[10] A more recent meta-analysis concluded that there is no evidence that the use of prophylactic antibiotics is effective for cat or dog bites.[11] Antibiotic prophylaxis is unnecessary for minor wounds, but most experts recommend it for high-risk bites such as deep puncture wounds (a common form of injury in cat bites) and bites involving the hands. Broad coverage for most cases of dog or cat bites may be achieved with amoxicillin-clavulanate (Augmentin, Clavulin).[1,7] An acceptable alternative is cefuroxime (Ceftin)[1] or clindamycin plus a fluoroquinolone.

Snake Bites

Only two families of poisonous snakes live in North America. Pit vipers, which include rattlesnakes, cottonmouths, copperheads, and coral snakes, are found only in the southern United States. In Canada, the only poisonous snakes are rattlesnakes. The term *pit viper* comes from the presence of heat-sensitive pits located between the snake's eyes and the nostrils. Other identifying features of pit vipers are their vertically elliptical pupils (cat's eye pupils), which contrast with the round pupils of non-venomous snakes, and in the case of rattlesnakes, the presence of a rattle on the tail.[11]

Up to 30% of proven snake bites are "dry bites" in which no envenomation occurs. Symptoms and signs of pit viper envenomation are severe pain and burning followed by increasing edema, ecchymosis, and constitutional symptoms.[12]

Dead snakes are not safe snakes. There are several reports of serious envenomation occurring when individuals picked up the heads of decapitated rattlesnakes.[13] Field therapy of poisonous snake bites consists of immobilization and splinting of the bitten appendage, which should be kept below heart level, and removal of the patient to an emergency room as quickly as possible. Constricting bands such as elastic bandages should be applied 5 to 10 cm proximal to the bite and kept sufficiently loose to allow the fifth finger to be slipped between the bands and the skin without causing discomfort. The bands should be periodically loosened and readjusted as edema evolves. The purpose of the bands is to decrease lymph flow without obstructing venous return. Incision and suction of the wound in the field is not recommended.[12]

Hospital treatment consists of supportive care, antibiotics, tetanus booster if necessary, and the IV administration of 4 to 20 vials of antivenin. Antivenin is made from immune horse serum, so skin testing is mandatory before administration. Wyeth's Crotalidae antivenin covers copperheads, cottonmouths, and rattlesnakes, but not coral snakes.

Human Bites
(See also animal bites)

One study found that the infection rate of simple human bites sustained in an institution for developmentally disabled persons was about 18% compared with a rate of 13% for simple lacerations occurring in the same population.[14] Although this infection rate is not very high, the situation is different with bites to the hand where the infection rate is 25% to 50%.[4] Hand bites may be categorized as clenched-fist injuries, sustained by punching someone in the teeth, or as simple bites. Any bite to the hand carries a greater risk of infection than bites elsewhere on the body, but this is particularly so with clenched-fist injuries.[15] The actual skin laceration in hand bites may be small, but in approximately 60% of the cases, the teeth have penetrated closed-hand spaces, tendons, or joints.[16] In clenched-fist injuries, the laceration is often only a 3- to 8-mm puncture wound on the dorsum of the hand or over the third metacarpophalangeal joint.[15] Many times, the extent of the wound depth will be missed when examining the hand in a neutral position, so the hand should be placed in the flexed fist position for proper assessment. Often, the wounds require further opening for adequate cleansing and identification of underlying damaged structures. Primary closure and extensor tendon repair should be delayed.

The affected hand should be splinted in a position of function.[4]

In view of the high incidence of infection and the complexity of the hand, most human bites of the hand require assessment and management by a hand surgeon.[15,16]

In children, approximately 70% of human bites are abrasions, which do not generally become infected. Overall infection rate of human bites in children is 9% to 12%.[4]

Microbiology of human bites

Like cat and dog bites, infections from human bites are almost always polymicrobial. On average, greater than five different organisms are cultured.[15] Compared with animal bites, there is a higher proportion of anerobic isolates.[3] The organisms from human bites are those of the oral flora and include alpha-hemolytic streptococci, beta-hemolytic streptococci, *Staphylococcus aureus, Staphylococcus epidermidis, Eikenella corrodens*, and anaerobes. Predominant aerobes are *S. aureus* and then group A-beta-hemolytic *Streptococcus* and *Eikenella*.

E. corrodens is a gram-negative facultative anaerobe that can be cultured from about 25% of human bite wounds. It causes serious indolent infections. The organism is sensitive to penicillin, amoxicillin-clavulanate (Augmentin, Clavulin), tetracycline, trimethoprim-sulfamethoxazole (Septra, Bactrim), and ciprofloxacin. It is usually resistant to erythromycin, cloxacillin, nafcillin, clindamycin, and first-generation cephalosporins.

Anaerobes can be cultured from nearly 50% of human bite wound infections. Many produce beta-lactamase and are penicillin resistant.

Some consideration should be given to the possibility of transmission of other infections such as Hepatitis B and C, herpes simplex virus (HSV), and theoretical HIV, which may be present in up to 44% of infected patient's saliva, but which the CDC does not consider a source risk unless there is also exposure to source blood.

Antibiotic prophylaxis

Whether all human bites (except the most minimal injuries) require prophylactic antibiotics is controversial. However, if the bite involves the hand, prophylactic antibiotics should certainly be given.[14,17] This approach is supported by a prospective study of uncomplicated human bites of the hand that were treated with mechanical wound care alone or accompanied by prophylactic antibiotics. No infections occurred in those who received antibiotics, whereas the infection rate was 47% in those who did not.[17] Other indications for prophylactic antibiotics are similar to those for cat and dog bites.[14]

Broad coverage for most cases of human bites may be achieved by amoxicillin-clavulanate (Augmentin, Clavulin) 500 mg three times daily or cefuroxime (Ceftin) 500 mg twice daily. Alternatives are penicillin 500 mg four times daily (covers *E. corrodens*) plus dicloxacillin (Dycill, Dynapen, Pathocil) 500 mg four times daily (covers *S. aureus*) or, for those allergic to penicillin, doxycycline 100 mg twice daily or some of the newer quinilones (moxifloxacin and gatifloxacin).[3] Similar to *Pasteurella* in animal bites, *Eikenella* is resistant to many of the typical antibiotics used for cellulitis, including cloxacillin and first-generation cephalasporins. Penicillin needs to be added to these regimens to ensure *Eikenella* coverage.[4] When given prophylactically, these drugs should be used for 3 to 5 days.[14]

─────────────── ❧ REFERENCES ❧ ───────────────

1. Griego RD, Rosen T, Orengo IF, et al: Dog, cat, and human bite: a review, *J Am Acad Dermatol* 33:1019-1029, 1995.
2. Voelker R: Dog bites recognized as public health problem, *JAMA* 277:278-280, 1997.
3. Brook I: Microbiology and management of human and animal bite wound infections, *Prim Care* 1:25-39, 2003.
4. Marx JA: *Rosen's emergency medicine: concepts and clinical practice*, ed 5, St. Louis, 2002, Mosby.
5. Hoff GL, Brawley J, Johnson K: Companion animal issues and the physician, *South Med J* 92:651-659, 1999.

6. Centers for Disease Control and Prevention: Dog-bite-related fatalities—United States, 1995-1996, *JAMA* 278: 278-279, 1997.

7. Fleisher GR: The management of bite wounds (editorial), *N Engl J Med* 340:138-140, 1999.

8. Talan DA, Citron DM, Abrahamian FM, et al: Bacteriologic analysis of infected dog and cat bites, *N Engl J Med* 340: 85-92, 1999.

9. Pennie R, Szakacs T, Smaill F, et al: Short report: ceftriaxone for cat and dog bites, *Can Fam Physician* 50:577-579, 2004.

10. Cummings P: Antibiotics to prevent infection in patients with dog bite wounds: a meta-analysis of randomized trials, *Ann Emerg Med* 23:535-540, 1994.

11. Medeiros I, Saconato H: Antibiotic prophylaxis for mammalian bites, Cochrane review, most recent update: April 11, 2003.

12. Forks TP: Evaluation and treatment of poisonous snakebites, *Am Fam Physician* 50:123-130, 1994.

13. Suchard JR, Lo Vecchio F: Envenomations by rattlesnakes thought to be dead (letter), *N Engl J Med* 340:1930, 1999.

14. Lindsay D, Christopher M, Hollenbach J, et al: Natural course of the human bite wound: incidence of infection and complications in 434 bites and 803 lacerations in the same group of patients, *J Trauma* 27:45-48, 1987.

15. Griego RD, Rosen T, Orengo IF, et al: Dog, cat, and human bite: a review, *J Am Acad Dermatol* 33:1019-1029, 1995.

16. Kelly IP, Cunney RJ, Smyth EG, et al: The management of human bite injuries of the hand, *Injury* 27:481-484, 1996.

17. Zubowicz VN, Gravier M: Management of early human bites of the hand: a prospective randomized study, *Plast Reconstr Surg* 88:111-114, 1991.

CAT SCRATCH DISEASE

Cat scratch disease usually occurs in children. The disease is transmitted by cat (or more often kitten) scratches, licks, or bites. A localized papule is found 2 to 3 days after the contact, often developing into a vesicle or pustule, and within 2 to 3 weeks tender regional lymphadenopathy develops that may persist for weeks or months. Flu-like symptoms are often reported during this period. In about 6% of cases, the site of the inoculum is the conjunctiva, and the initial sign is a polypoid lesion of the palpebral conjunctiva, often associated with preauricular adenopathy. Rarely, patients have central nervous system (CNS) involvement, often manifested as seizures.[1] The organism responsible for most cases is *Bartonella henselae*. Clinical diagnosis can be made on the basis of history, presence of a primary lesion, and persistent tender regional lymphadenopathy. Serological assays can be used to support the clinical diagnosis if necessary.[2] In immunocompetent patients, the disease is usually self-limited, and antibiotic treatment is rarely required.[1,2] Antibiotics are indicated for immunocompromised individuals and for serious complications such as encephalopathy and osteomyelitis. Gentamicin, rifampin, macrolides, and fluoroquinolones have proven efficacious in these cases.[2]

❧ REFERENCES ❧

1. Smith DL: Cat-scratch disease, *Am Fam Physician* 55: 1785-1789, 1997.

2. Conrad DA: Treatment of cat-scratch disease, *Curr Opin Pediatr* 13(1):56-59, 2001.

COMMON COLD
(See also antimicrobial resistance; rhinitis)

The common cold is a ubiquitous upper respiratory infection caused by a variety of viral pathogens, most commonly rhinovirus. Although usually brief (less than 7 days), this infection is responsible for substantial economic costs in lost work time.[1] Another significant social cost is increasing community levels of antibiotic resistance due to needless antibiotic prescriptions for this infection.

Well-conducted reviews show no improvement of common cold symptom resolution or complications with antibiotic treatment compared with placebo, while adverse events were significantly more likely for adults (but not children) in the antibiotic-treated group.[2] Similarly, antihistamines as monotherapy[3] and zinc lozenges[4] are both of unproved benefit for symptom control or hastening resolution. For adults, clinically significant symptom relief is seen with oral decongestants, either as monotherapy[5] or combined with acetaminophen or antihistamines.[6] All patient groups get symptomatic benefit from heated, humidified air.[7] Ipratropium bromide (Atrovent Nasal) has been shown to reduce the amount of nasal secretions during upper respiratory infections, but not nasal congestion.[8] Echinacea has been widely promoted for both prevention and treatment of the common cold. To date, however, it has been impossible to assess actual benefit due to substantial variation in the preparations studied and methodological quality.[9] Prevention with vitamin C has been considerably more thoroughly studied, but no consistent preventive effect has been shown, even with high doses; a modest beneficial effect on symptom duration is evident with vitamin C supplementation during cold episodes.[10] Although a wide range of antiviral drugs is being studied for effectiveness, only intranasal interferon has so far been shown to affect the natural history of the common cold. Its usefulness, however, has been limited by blood-tinged nasal discharge as a side effect.[11]

❧ REFERENCES ❧

1. Heikkinen T, Jarvinen A: The common cold, *Lancet* 361: 51-59, 2003.

2. Arrol B, Kenealy T: Antibiotics for the common cold and acute purulent rhinitis (Cochrane Review). In: *The*

Cochrane Library, issue 2, Chichester, UK, 2004, John Wiley and Sons.

3. De Sutter AIM, Lemeingre M, Campbell H, et al: Antihistamines for the common cold (Cochrane Review). In: *The Cochrane Library*, issue 2, Chichester, UK, 2004, John Wiley and Sons.

4. Jackson JL, Lesho E, Peterson C: Zinc and the common cold: a meta-analysis revisited, *J Nutr* 130: 1512S-1515S, 2000.

5. Taverner D, Bickford L, Draper M: Nasal decongestants for the common cold (Cochrane Review). In: *The Cochrane Library*, issue 2, Chichester, UK, 2004, John Wiley and Sons.

6. Sperber SJ, Turner RB, Sorrentino JV, et al: Effectiveness of pseudoephedrine and acetaminophen for treatment of symptoms attributed to the paranasal sinuses associated with the common cold, *Arch Fam Med* 9(10): 979-985, 2000.

7. Singh M: Heated, humidified air for the common cold (Cochrane Review). In: *The Cochrane Library*, issue 2, Chichester, UK, 2004, John Wiley and Sons.

8. Hayden FG, Diamond L, Wood PB, et al: Effectiveness and safety of intranasal ipratropium bromide in common colds—a randomized, double-blind, placebo-controlled trial, *Ann Intern Med* 125:89-97, 1996.

9. Melchart D, Linde K, Fischer P, et al: Echinacea for preventing and treating the common cold (Cochrane Review). In: *The Cochrane Library*, issue 2, Chichester, UK, 2004, John Wiley and Sons.

10. Douglas RM, Chalker EB, Treacy B: Vitamin C for preventing and treating the common cold (Cochrane Review). In: *The Cochrane Library*, issue 2, Chichester, UK, 2004, John Wiley and Sons.

11. Jefferson TO, Tyrrell D: Antivirals for the common cold (Cochrane Review). In: *The Cochrane Library*, issue 2, Chichester, UK, 2004, John Wiley and Sons.

FEVER

(See also febrile seizures; fever in children)

Normal Temperature Values

In young adults, rectal temperatures exceeded oral readings by 0.4° C (0.7° F), and these in turn exceeded tympanic readings by 0.4° C (0.7° F). Smoking and mastication have been found to increase oral readings, and this effect persists for longer than 20 minutes. Drinking ice water causes a short-term diminution in temperature readings.[1]

What is a normal temperature, and what is the normal range? Mackowiak and associates[2] studied this in a group of healthy young adult men and women between the ages of 18 and 40. The mean oral temperature was 36.8° C (98.2° F), and 37.7° C (99.9° F) was the upper limit of normal. A diurnal variation with an amplitude of variability of about 0.5° C (0.9° F) was normal with the nadir at 6 AM and the zenith at 4 to 6 PM.[2]

Taking Temperatures

Whether axillary temperatures are accurate is controversial. Shann and Mackenzie[3] from Australia studied temperatures taken by various routes in 120 children of different ages. They concluded that axillary temperatures were accurate. In children over 1 month of age, the rectal temperature was very close to 1° C higher than the axillary temperature. During the first 5 weeks of life, rectal temperature exceeded axillary temperature by 0.2° C for every week of life. Forehead temperatures were not as accurate as axillary temperatures.[3] However, most other studies have found the axillary route to have a low sensitivity but a high specificity.[4,5] In other words, if the axillary temperature is elevated, the child is febrile, but if it is not, fever cannot be ruled out.

In the past few years, non-contact tympanic or external auditory canal thermometers that detect infrared radiation from the tympanic membrane have come into widespread use. How accurate are they? In an emergency room study of children under 4 years, the readings of non-contact tympanic thermometers in both the rectal-equivalent mode and the actual-ear mode were compared with rectal temperatures obtained with recently calibrated glass mercury thermometers. With fever defined as at least 38° C (100.4° F) per rectum, the non-contact tympanic thermometer in the rectal-equivalent mode had a sensitivity of 75% and a specificity of 96%. In the actual-ear mode, the sensitivity dropped to just over 50% while the specificity was 100%.[6] These data show that fever in one fourth or more of young children could be missed if only the non-contact tympanic thermometer was used, but if the instrument indicated "fever," it would rarely be wrong. Studies using tympanic thermometers in adult patients have shown significant variations in readings from one ear to the other, as well as among commercial brands.[7,8] At present, tympanic thermometers do not appear to be reliable.

Without measuring their children's temperatures, can parents accurately determine whether young children are febrile? This was assessed in the emergency room study described in the previous paragraph. Parental sensitivity was 82% and parental specificity 77%. The sensitivity of parents' assessment of fever in their children is a bit better than that of the non-contact tympanic thermometer but is considerably less specific; parental opinions should be taken seriously.[6]

Benefits of Fever

Is fever beneficial? Should it be treated? The febrile response to infection is only part of an "acute phase response" involving the activation of numerous cytokines that cause symptoms such as somnolence and anorexia, as well as inducing a wide variety of metabolic and immunological changes that could in theory be beneficial. With few exceptions mammals, reptiles, amphibians, and fish respond to infections with fever, which suggests that such reactions have evolutionary value. One study in humans reported that rhinovirus infections treated with antipyretics were more severe and lasted longer than those not so treated, and another found that treatment of rhinovirus infections with Aspirin increased viral shedding. Circumstantial evidence suggests that fever may be beneficial in some cases, but no useful data are available as to whether treatment with antipyretics causes more harm than good.[9]

Treating Fever

(See discussion of fever in children)

Fever of Unknown Origin

Fever of unknown origin in adults is defined as a temperature higher than 38.3° C lasting at least 3 weeks. A 2003 systematic review shows that infection as a cause was only identified in 28% of the cases. Other identified causes include inflammatory diseases (21%) and malignancies (17%) (and deep vein thrombosis [3%] and temporal arteritis [16%] in the elderly). Still, 19% of patients will never be given a diagnosis; fortunately, 51% to 100% will recover spontaneously. Higher yield investigations ruled out endocarditis, using computed tomography (CT) of the abdomen, a nuclear scan using technetium, and perhaps a liver biopsy.[10]

◾ REFERENCES ◾

1. Rabinowitz RP, Cookson ST, Wasserman SS, et al: Effects of anatomic site, oral stimulation, and body position on estimates of body temperature, *Arch Intern Med* 156: 777-780, 1996.
2. Mackowiak PA, Wasserman SS, Levine MM: A critical appraisal of 98.6 degrees F, the upper limit of the normal body temperature, and other legacies of Carl Reinhold August Wunderlich, *JAMA* 268:1578-1580, 1992.
3. Shann F, Mackenzie A: Comparison of rectal, axillary and forehead temperatures, *Arch Pediatr Adolesc Med* 150: 74-78, 1996.
4. Keeley D: Taking infants' temperatures (editorial), *BMJ* 304:931-932, 1992.
5. Zengeya ST, Blumenthal I: Modern electronic and chemical thermometers used in the axilla are inaccurate, *Eur J Pediatr* 155:1005-1008, 1996.
6. Hooker EA, Smith SW, Miles T, et al: Subjective assessment of fever by parents—comparison with measurement by non-contact tympanic thermometer and calibrated rectal glass mercury thermometer, *Ann Emerg Med* 28:313-317, 1996.
7. Manian FA, Griesenauer S: Lack of agreement between tympanic and oral temperature measurements in adult hospitalized patients, *Am J Infect Control* 26:428-430, 1998.
8. Modell JG, Katholi CR, Kumaramangalam SM, et al: Unreliability of the infrared tympanic thermometer in clinical practice: a comparative study with oral mercury and oral electronic thermometers, *South Med J* 91:649-655, 1998.
9. Mackowiak PA: Concepts of fever, *Arch Intern Med* 158: 1870-1881, 1998.
10. Mourad O, Palda V, Detsky AS: A comprehensive evidence-based approach to fever of unknown origin, *Arch Intern Med* 163:545-551, 2003.

FOOD-BORNE ILLNESS

(See also cryptosporidiosis; cyclosporiasis; giardiasis; infectious diarrhea; travellers' diarrhea)

Food-borne illness (FBI) is caused by ingestion of food contaminated by bacteria, bacterial toxins, viruses, natural poisons, or harmful chemical substances. Global food distribution and production has created new risks. Extremes of age and immunocompromise increase susceptibility and severity. FBI causes approximately 76 million illnesses, 325,000 hospitalizations, and 5000 deaths in the United States each year.[1]

Bacterial Food-borne Illness[1,2]

The common causes are *Staphylococcus, Salmonella* (36% of cases), *Campylobacter* (30%), *Shigella* (23%), *Escherichia coli, Listeria, Yersinia* and *Vibrio* species. The acute symptoms are vomiting, diarrhea, and abdominal pain. Bacterial FBI is generally self-limited, but deaths do occur. Contamination can occur during growing, harvesting, processing, storing, shipping, or final preparation of food.

Botulism

Botulism produces symptoms of diplopia, aphasia, ptosis, and generalized weakness. Common food sources are improperly preserved home-processed foods with low acid content, such as green beans, beets, and corn.

Campylobacter

This infection is acquired from water or undercooked meat and poultry. Besides causing bloody diarrhea, it appears to be a postinfectious cause of Guillain-Barre syndrome.[3]

Escherichia coli O157:H7

Infection with *E. coli* O157:H7 may be asymptomatic, but hemorrhagic colitis and hemolytic-uremic syndrome (HUS) occur due to *Shigella* toxin produced by the organism. The incubation period is 1 to 9 days. Only a few bacteria are needed to cause disease; hence, transmission can occur easily through food, water, and person-to-person spread. Outbreak sources include hamburger, venison, uncooked vegetables, cheese curds, apple cider, and sprouts. An important complication is HUS, which usually affects children who have had bloody diarrhea. The risk of HUS is estimated at 5% to 8%, but may be higher.[4] The role of antibiotics in treating *E. Coli* is unclear. A recent meta-analysis failed to confirm suspicions of increased risk of HUS after antibiotic treatment.[5]

Listerioisis

Associated with unpasteurized dairy products and soft cheeses, listeriosis can cause septic meningitis; maternal–fetal transmission occurs.

Salmonella

Antibiotic treatment of *Salmonella* infection is not recommended because it increases the risk of relapse and adverse reactions.[6] One study reported that alcohol provided protection when consumed with salmonella-contaminated food.[7]

Shigella

As few as 10 bacteria can cause disease. A significant cause of mortality worldwide, *S. dysenteriae* is responsible for 600,000 deaths annually. Hand-washing is highly effective at reducing disease, with a 42% to 47% reduction.

Vibrio (Non-cholera)

This mostly self-limiting infection is acquired from raw or undercooked shellfish.

Fish Poisoning

Ciguatera fish poisoning[8]

Ciguatera toxin is produced by single-celled, free-swimming dinoflagellates, and becomes concentrated in large fish as it passes up the food chain. It occurs primarily in the Caribbean, Australia, and the South Pacific, and in fish that originate in these areas, for example, grouper, king mackerel, red snapper, amberjack, and barracuda. Barracuda are the worst offenders and should never be eaten.[2]

Ciguatera fish poisoning produces a mixture of gastrointestinal (GI) and neurological symptoms. GI symptoms—abdominal cramps, watery diarrhea, vomiting—usually begin within hours. Neurological symptoms include paresthesiae, vertigo, ataxia, myalgia, and weakness. Cold sensation reversal is pathognomonic of ciguatera toxicity. These symptoms usually persist for 2 to 3 weeks, but in some unfortunate persons last for months. Concentration of toxin may vary within a contaminated fish, and therefore not all persons having eaten portions of the same fish may be symptomatic. Although previously considered to be a specific treatment for this condition, IV mannitol has been shown to be ineffective.[9] Patients with ciguatera fish poisoning should avoid nuts and alcohol, which can exacerbate symptoms.

Shellfish food poisoning (SP)[8]

Algal marine dinoflagellates produce ciguatera and other toxins. Toxin levels rise during rapid multiplication of the dinoflagellates ("red tides"). Paralytic SP from saxitoxin causes paresthesiae of the face, tongue, and digits. Death due to respiratory failure can occur within 24 hours. Amnesic SP from the neurotoxin domoic acid can produce permanent memory loss and death due to respiratory failure. Several other forms of SP cause self-limited illness.

Tetrodotoxin poisoning

A neurotoxin produced by bacteria in snails, horseshoe crab eggs, newts, starfish, and puffer fish is responsible for outbreaks in Japan and Southeast Asia. The toxin is heat stable. Symptoms come on rapidly and lead to death from ascending paralysis in about 60% of cases.[10]

Scombrotoxic poisoning

This under-recognized FBI is frequently confused with an allergic reaction. The protein histidine is converted to histamine by a bacterial enzyme in improperly refrigerated tuna, mackerel, or bonito. The peri-intestinal meat is most susceptible. Symptom onset of urticaria, angioedema, vomiting, and headache is rapid and usually lasts 6 to 8 hours. Antihistamines (H1 and 2) are effective in severe cases.[10]

Mushroom Poisoning

Most cases of mushroom poisoning are caused by species of *Amanita*. The toxin, which results in hepatitis, is not destroyed by cooking and is tasteless. Symptoms develop after a latent period of 6 to 12 hours and consist of severe diarrhea and vomiting followed by hepatic and renal failure.[11]

❧ REFERENCES ❧

1. CDC MMWR Weekly: Preliminary FoodNet Data on the Incidence of Foodborne Illnesses—Selected Sites, United States, 2002, 52(15):340-343, 2003.
2. http://digestive.niddk.nih.gov/ddiseases/pubs/bacteria. National Digestive Diseases Information Clearinghouses: *Bacteria and Foodborne Illness*. Accessed April 15th, 2004.
3. Nachamkin I: Chronic effects of *Campylobacter* infection, *Microbes Infect* (4):399-403, 2002.
4. Ochoa TJ, Cleary TG: Epidemiology and spectrum of disease of *Escherichia coli* O157, *Curr Opin in ID* 16(3) 259-263, 2003.
5. Safdar N, Said A, Gangnon RE, et al: Risk of hemolytic uremic syndrome after antibiotic treatment of *Escherichia coli* O157:H7 enteritis: a meta-analysis, *JAMA* 288(8), 996–1001, 2002.
6. Sirinavin S, Garner P: Antibiotics for treating salmonella gut infections, *Cochrane Database of Systematic Reviews,* 2004(1).
7. Bellido-Blasco JB, Arnedo-Pena A, Cordero-Cutillas E, et al: The protective effect of alcoholic beverages on the occurrence of a *Salmonella* food-borne outbreak, *Epidemology* 13(2):228-230, 2002.
8. Brett M: Food poisoning associated with biotoxins in fish and shellfish, *Curr Opin Infect Dis,* 16(5):461-465, 2003.
9. Schnorf H, Taurarii M, Cundy T: Ciguatera fish poisoning: a double-blind randomized trial of mannitol therapy, *Neurology* 58(6):873-880, 2002.
10. Perkins RA, Morgan SS: Poisoning, envenomation, and trauma from marine creatures, *Am Fam Phys* 69(4):885-893, 2004.
11. Hoey J, Todkill AM: Gather ye rosebuds while ye may— but avoid the mushrooms, *Can Med Assoc J* 157:431, 1997.

HERPES SIMPLEX
(See also sexually transmitted diseases)

Herpes simplex infections typically manifest as either orolabial herpes (cold sores, herpes gingivostomatitis) or genital herpes. Either virus can cause eruptions virtually anywhere in the body. Up to 85% of the world's population is seropositive for herpes simplex infection.[1]

Orolabial Herpes

For primary orolabial herpes infections, a randomized double-blind placebo-controlled study of young children found an excellent response to oral acyclovir in doses of 15 mg/kg five times daily for 7 days. Oral lesions resolved in a median of 4 days. Fever and difficulty drinking and eating lasted for a shorter period.[2]

For secondary orolabial herpes infections, a randomized double-blind placebo-controlled trial of patients demonstrated the effectiveness of topical application of 1% penciclovir, improved pain relief, and reduced time to healing and duration of viral shedding.[3]

When eruption of HSV vesicles can be predicted, oral famciclovir can reduce the length of recurrence by 2 days.[4]

Genital Herpes

Genital herpes is increasing in prevalence in the United States.[5] Prevention of transmission is difficult because one third of the episodes of viral shedding are asymptomatic,[6] and condom efficacy is uncertain.

For treatment of primary genital herpes infections, guidelines support acyclovir 400 mg three times daily for 10 days[7] or valacyclovir 1000 mg twice daily for 10 days.[8]

In most patients, recurrence rates decrease with time. The rate decrease in most patients suggests that if prophylactic therapy is prescribed, its continued need should be reassessed periodically.[9] In one study, 239 immunocompetent patients with a history of recurring genital HSV infections (more than 12 episodes per year) received acyclovir (Zovirax) continuously for 6 or more years. During the year after stopping therapy, 86% had at least one infection. After 6 years of therapy the frequency of infection decreased in 72% of the patients.[10]

For the treatment of recurrent genital herpes, acyclovir 800 mg three times daily for 2 days showed a significant improvement in symptoms.[11] Valacyclovir and famciclovir are also effective against recurrent genital herpes infections.[12,13] Topical therapy with acyclovir has not been shown to be effective in genital herpes, but treatment with topical penciclovir has been associated with a modest effect of decreasing time to lesion crusting by 1 day.[14]

Numerous options exist for prophylaxis. Famciclovir 250 mg orally twice daily,[15] valacyclovir at 500 mg daily,[16] and acyclovir at 200 mg five times a day[17] have comparable efficacy.

For prenatal genital herpes eruptions, a systematic review has demonstrated the efficacy of acyclovir pro-phylaxis in the third trimester.[18] Acyclovir is the drug of choice for primary herpetic infection during pregnancy because it has been used longer than other drugs and appears to be safe.[19]

◂ REFERENCES ▸

1. Whitley RJ, Kimberlin DW, Roizman B: Herpes simplex viruses, *Clin Infect Dis* 26: 541-555, 1998.
2. Amir J, Harel L, Smetana Z, et al: Treatment of herpes simplex gingivostomatitis with acyclovir in children: a randomised double blind placebo controlled study, *BMJ* 314:1800-1803, 1997.
3. Spruance SL, Rea TL, Thoming C, et al: Penciclovir cream for the treatment of herpes simplex labialis: a randomized, multicenter, double-blind, placebo-controlled trial, *JAMA* 277: 1374-1379, 1997.
4. Spruance SL, Rowe NH, Raborn W, et al: Perioral famciclovir in the treatment of experimental ultraviolet radiation-induced herpes simplex labialis: a double-blind, dose-ranging, placebo-controlled, multicenter trial, *J Infect Dis* 179:303-310, 1999.
5. Fleming DT, McQuillan GM, Johnson RE, et al: Herpes simplex virus type 2 in the United States, 1976 to 1994, *N Engl J Med* 337:1105-1111, 1997.
6. Wald A, Zeh J, Selke S, et al: Virologic characteristics of subclinical and symptomatic genital herpes infections, *N Engl J Med* 333:770-775, 1995.
7. Centers for Disease Control and Prevention: Sexually transmitted diseases treatment guidelines 2002, *MMWR* 51: RR-6, 2002.
8. Fife KH, Barbarash RA, Rudolph T, et al: Valaciclovir versus acyclovir in the treatment of first-episode genital herpes infection: results of an international, multicenter, double-blind, randomized clinical trial, *Sex Transm Dis* 24: 481-486, 1997.
9. Benedetti JK, Zeh J, Corey L: Clinical reactivation of genital herpes simplex virus infection decreases in frequency over time, *Ann Intern Med* 131:14-20, 1999.
10. Fife KH, Crumpacker CS, Mertz GJ, et al: Recurrence and resistance patterns of herpes simplex virus following cessation of greater-than-or-equal-to-6 years of chronic suppression with acyclovir, *J Infect Dis* 169:1338-1341, 1994.
11. Wald A, Carrell D, Remington M, et al: Two-day regimen of acyclovir for treatment of recurrent genital herpes simplex virus type 2 infection, *Clin Infect Dis*: 34: 944-948, 2002.
12. Bodsworth NJ, Crooks RJ, Borelli S, et al: Valaciclovir versus aciclovir in patient initiated treatment of recurrent genital herpes: a randomised, double blind clinical trial, *Genitourin Med* 73:110-116, 1997.
13. Sacks SL, Aoki FY, Diaz-Mitoma F, et al: Patient-initiated, twice-daily oral famciclovir for early recurrent genital herpes: a randomized, double-blind multicenter trial, *JAMA* 276: 44-49, 1996.
14. Whitley RJ, Roizman B: Herpes simplex virus infections, *Lancet* 357:1513-1518, 2001.
15. Mertz GJ, Loveless MO, Levin MJ, et al: Oral famciclovir for suppression of recurrent genital herpes simplex virus

infection in women: a multicenter, double-blind, placebo-controlled trial, *Arch Intern Med* 157:343-349, 1997.

16. Patel R, Bodsworth NJ, Woolley P, et al: Valaciclovir for the suppression of recurrent genital HSV infection: a placebo controlled study of once daily therapy, *Genitourin Med* 73:105-109, 1997.

17. Douglas JM, Critchlow C, Benedetti J, et al: A double-blind study of oral acyclovir for suppression of recurrences of genital herpes simplex virus infection, *N Engl J Med* 310:1551-1556, 1984.

18. Sheffield JS, Hollier LM, Hill JB, et al: Acyclovir prophylaxis to prevent herpes simplex virus recurrence at delivery: a systematic review, *Obstet Gynecol* 102: 1396-1403, 2003.

19. Balfour HH Jr: Antiviral drugs, *N Engl J Med* 340:1255-1268, 1999.

HERPES ZOSTER

(See also diabetic neuropathy; neuropathy; varicella; viral diseases in pregnancy)

Epidemiology

The incidence of herpes zoster is low in children and adolescents, about 0.5 to 1.6:1000 for persons under age 20, whereas it is 11:1000 in adults over age 80.[1] The incidence is high in HIV-positive patients and those with cancer, including childhood leukemia.[1]

Post-herpetic neuralgia (PHN) is defined in various ways, but a good working definition is persistence of pain for more than a month after the onset of the rash. It is rare in children but occurs in approximately 70% of affected persons over age 70. The pain of PHN may last for months or years.[1]

A study done in Iceland followed all patients with an episode of herpes zoster (n=421) for 7.6 years to determine the natural history of pain following the acute episode. Post-herpetic neuralgia was uncommon in patients younger than 60 years, with only 2% reporting pain 3 months after the outbreak, all of the cases mild. The severity and frequency increased in patients older than 60 years, with 13% reporting pain and 4% reporting moderate-to-severe pain. In patients over age 70, 29% had pain at 3 months. After 12 months, 3.3% of patients reported pain, and most of these reports were of mild pain. Six of these patients had pain that was still present 2 to 7 years following the initial outbreak.[2]

Clinical Presentation

The prodromal pain of herpes zoster may last for a few days or weeks.[1] The distribution of the lesions is as follows[3]:

Location	Percentage of Cases
Thorax	55
Fifth cranial nerve	15
Lumbar roots	14
Neck	12
Sacral roots	3

Crusting occurs in 7 to 10 days, and resolution of the lesions takes 3 to 4 weeks. The area affected is usually hyperesthetic. The pain may be burning or lancinating and is sometimes precipitated by trivial stimuli. Paresthesiae and hypesthesia commonly extend beyond the boundaries of the initial skin lesions.[1]

Treatment of Acute Illness

[handwritten: Pain mild-mod: OTC analgesic Severe: opioids]

Antiviral agents used for the treatment of herpes zoster include acyclovir (Zovirax), famciclovir (Famvir), and valacyclovir (Valtrex). Administration of these drugs within 72 hours of rash onset is associated with a decrease in the herpetic pain of the acute disease. Patients over age 50 with herpes zoster who present within 72 hours of the onset of symptoms may benefit from a course of famciclovir (500 to 750 mg orally three times daily for 7 days) or valacyclovir (1000 mg orally three times daily for 7 to 14 days) to reduce the duration of pain in the event that they develop PHN.[4] The standard dose of acyclovir for this purpose is 800 mg every 4 hours (five times daily) for 7 to 10 days.[5] Keep in mind that patients under age 60 rarely have a problem with PHN. The role of steroids in the management of herpetic pain has been controversial. A systematic review concluded that the combination of steroids and acyclovir decreases pain during the acute phase of illness (first month) but has no effect on PHN.[6]

[handwritten: Calamine or soothing lotion]

[handwritten: +/- Prednisone ✱]

Treatment of Post-herpetic Neuralgia

A 2003 systematic review found the best evidence to support the use of the tricylcic antidepressants amitriptyline, nortriptyline, and desipramine (number needed to treat = 2 to 3). Amitriptyline (Elavil) was the best studied, with a usual dose of 75 mg by mouth at bedtime. Also, evidence from a smaller number of studies supports the use of topical capsaicin (Zostrix), gabapentin (Neurontin titrated upward to doses of 1200 to 3000 mg per day) and controlled-release oxycodone. Lidocaine patch, benzydamine cream, tramadol, and vincristine have not been well studied, while lorazepam, fluphenazine, dextromethorphan, memantine, acyclovir, and acupuncture are unlikely to be beneficial.[7,8]

Two topical treatments that have been assessed are lidocaine gel and capsaicin (Zostrix). In a double-blind trial, 5% lidocaine gel was applied to cranial areas without occlusion for 8 hours and to trunk or limb areas under occlusion for 24 hours. This treatment resulted in significant pain relief.[9] Blinded studies using capsaicin are impossible because of the burning experienced during application of the drug. In a study of 143 patients with PHN treated with either a 0.075% concentration of the drug or a placebo, significant pain relief was reported in the treated cohort.[10] However, an overview of the literature on capsaicin suggests that although the occasional patient receives significant relief, for most it is minor and for many the burning experienced on applying the drug is unacceptable.[1,11]

➤ REFERENCES ✦

1. Kost RG, Straus SE: Postherpetic neuralgia–pathogenesis, treatment, and prevention, *N Engl J Med* 335:32-42, 1996.
2. Helgason S, Petursson G, Gudmundsson S, et al: Prevalence of postherpetic neuralgia after a single episode of herpes zoster: prospective study with long-term follow up. *BMJ* 321:1-4, 2000.
3. Mamdani FS: Pharmacologic management of herpes zoster and postherpetic neuralgia, *Can Fam Physician* 40:321-332, 1994.
4. Alper BS, Lewis PR: Does treatment of acute herpes zoster prevent or shorten postherpetic neuralgia? *J Fam Pract* 49: 255-264, 2000.
5. MacFarlane LL, Simmons MM, Hunter MH, et al: The use of corticosteroids in the management of herpes zoster, *J Am Board Fam Pract* 11:224-228, 1998.
6. Rowbotham MC, Davies PS, Fields HL: Topical lidocaine gel relieves postherpetic neuralgia, *Ann Neurol* 37:246-253, 1995.
7. Alper BS, Lewis PR: Treatment of postherpetic neuralgia: a systematic review of the literature, *J Fam Pract* 51:121-128, 2002.
8. Rowbotham M, Harden N, Stacey B, et al: Gabapentin for the treatment of postherpetic neuralgia: a randomized controlled trial, *JAMA* 280:1837-1842, 1998.
9. Watson CP, Tyler KL, Bickers DR, et al: A randomized vehicle-controlled trial of topical capsaicin in the treatment of postherpetic neuralgia, *Clin Ther* 15:510-526, 1993.
10. Watson CP: Topical capsaicin as an adjuvant analgesic, *J Pain Symptom Manage* 9:425-433, 1994.
11. McQuay HJ, Moore RA: Antidepressants and chronic pain: effective analgesia in neuropathic pain and other syndromes (editorial), *BMJ* 314:763-764, 1997.
12. Tyring S, Barbarash RA, Nahlik JE, et al (Collaborative Famciclovir Herpes Zoster Study Group): Famciclovir for the treatment of acute herpes zoster: effects on acute disease and postherpetic neuralgia; a randomized, double-blind, placebo-controlled trial, *Ann Intern Med* 123:89-96, 1995.
13. Jackson JL, Gibbons R, Meyer G, et al: The effect of treating herpes zoster with oral acyclovir in preventing postherpetic neuralgia: a meta-analysis, *Arch Intern Med* 157: 909-912, 1997.

INFECTIOUS MONONUCLEOSIS

Infectious mononucleosis is primarily a disease of relatively affluent adolescents and young adults. In developing countries and in lower socio-economic groups within developed countries, viral spread is common among young children so that most are infected by the age of 4; in this young group, the disease is mild or asymptomatic. Infectious mononucleosis is rare after age 40.[1-3] The causative organism is most commonly Epstein-Barr virus (EBV), but identical syndromes can be linked to other viral agents, notably cytomegalovirus.[4] Patients who have had infectious mononucleosis acquire lifelong immunity to EBV.

The incubation period of infectious mononucleosis is 1 to 2 months. For most patients the disease is self-limited. The major findings are fever, pharyngitis, and generalized lymphadenopathy. Lymphadenopathy and splenomegaly may persist for weeks,[1,2] and virus can be recovered from throat washings for up to 18 months.[3] Complications of infectious mononucleosis are rare but may be serious, and include splenic rupture, encephalitis, myelitis, Guillain-Barré syndrome, Bell's palsy, cerebellar ataxia, uveitis, thrombocytopenia, hemolytic anemia, and pharyngeal obstruction from enlarged tonsils.[1,2] In over 95% of patients with infectious mononucleosis, a widespread maculopapular rash will develop if they are treated with ampicillin.[3]

Laboratory abnormalities include elevated white blood cell (WBC) count (in the range of 10 to 15 × 10⁹/L [10,000 to 15,000/mm³]) with a relative lymphocytosis. About 10% to 30% of the lymphocytes are atypical; these are not specific for EBV-induced infectious mononucleosis and may be seen in other viral illnesses. The Monospot test has a 10% to 20% false negative rate (higher in young children), and a 5% to 15% rate of false positives.[1,2] Heterophile antibodies begin to develop after a week, peak between weeks 2 and 5, remain detectable for several months after clinical infection subsides, and usually revert to negative within a year.[3,4] Current evidence suggests that it is unlikely that chronic fatigue syndrome results from persistent EBV infection.[4]

Treatment of infectious mononucleosis is generally symptomatic. Strenuous exercises and contact sports should be avoided for 3 to 4 weeks until splenomegaly has resolved. Prednisone 60 to 80 mg per day for 5 to 7 days followed by tapering over 14 days is used for upper airway obstruction, severe hemolytic anemia, and thrombocytopenia.[1-4]

➤ REFERENCES ✦

1. Bailey RE: Diagnosis and treatment of infectious mononucleosis, *Am Fam Physician* 49:879-888, 1994.
2. Strauss SE, Cohen JI, Tosato G, et al: NIH conference: Epstein-Barr virus infections; biology, pathogenesis and management, *Ann Intern Med* 118:45-58, 1993.
3. Auwaerter PG: Infectious mononucleosis in middle age, *JAMA* 281:454-459, 1999.
4. Goodshall SE, Kirchner JT: Infectious mononucleosis: complexities of a common condition, *Postgrad Med* 107(7): 175-179, 183-1844, 186, 2000.

LYME DISEASE

(See also fibromyalgia; functional somatic syndromes)

Etiology and Epidemiology

Lyme disease was initially recognized in 1975.[1,2] The name comes from the initial cluster of cases in children around Lyme, Connecticut. The etiological agent of the disease is the spirochete *Borrelia burgdorferi*. It is transmitted by the *Ixodes ricinus (scapularis)* group of ticks. The larval and nymph forms feed on white-footed mice, and the adult forms on white-tailed deer. The larval form acquires the spirochetes from white-footed mice, and in 90% of the cases the nymph form infects humans. Human infections may occur from May to November, with peak incidence occurring from May to July.

In the United States, Lyme disease has been reported in almost every state but is found predominantly in New England, the Mid-Atlantic region, the Southeast, small endemic areas of Wisconsin and Minnesota, and to a lesser extent on the Pacific coast.[1,2] In 2000, 95% of the 17,730 reported cases were from 12 states, but the disease is infrequent, even in states reporting the highest incidence.[2,3] The only endemic areas of Canada are Long Point, Ontario (a peninsula in Lake Erie), and Vancouver Island and the Gulf Islands in British Columbia.[4] The disease is widespread in Northern and Central Europe and has also been described in Asia.[2]

Early Clinical Manifestations

Erythema migrans is an expanding, annular, erythematous lesion at least 5 cm in diameter with central clearing. It is usually not pruritic or tender. It generally occurs 3 to 30 days after the tick bite (less than one fourth of patients recall this event), although it may develop months later, and usually lasts for 3 to 4 weeks. This rash occurs in 50% to 80% of patients with Lyme disease[2]; in one prospective study of children, 90% had one or more of these lesions.[5] Non-specific viral-like symptoms also occur in about half of patients in the early stage of the illness. Serological tests for Lyme disease are often negative at this stage of the disease and should not be ordered; the diagnosis of erythema migrans is a clinical one.[6] Lesions occurring within 48 hours of exposure are hypersensitivity reactions, not erythema migrans.[1,2]

The standard treatment of erythema migrans is a 2- to 4-week course of oral antibiotics, as highlighted in Table 36.[7] With rare exceptions, appropriate antibiotic treatment of early Lyme disease should prevent the development of late clinical manifestations.[2,5]

Late Clinical Manifestations

The late manifestations of Lyme disease may affect the joints, the CNS, and the heart.[1,2] In 50% of untreated persons with Lyme disease, recurrent (for weeks to months), brief attacks of swelling of one or more joints can develop. The course may also manifest as chronic progressive arthritis preceded by brief attacks. The onset occurs a few weeks to 2 years after the person is infected. Fibromyalgia can be easily mistaken for Lyme disease, particularly in areas where disease incidence is relatively high.[1,2]

Central nervous system involvement occurs in 15% to 20% of persons with untreated Lyme disease. Possible CNS sequelae include lymphocytic meningitis, cranial neuritis, facial palsy, radiculopathy, and, rarely, encephalomyelitis.[1]

The cardiovascular system is affected in 4% to 8% of patients. This usually involves acute onset of atrioventricular conduction defects that resolve in days or weeks.[1]

Laboratory Investigations

For patients presenting with erythema migrans, culture of lesion biopsy specimens offers near 100% specificity, and, at this stage of the disease, is more sensitive than serology.[9] Availability of specialized culture media may be limited. Serology is used to help confirm a diagnosis of Lyme disease. When the clinical picture is typical, the positive predictive value of the serological test is high. It is important to remember that the serological test is not positive until 6 to 8 weeks after a tick bite, and that about 3% to 5% of uninfected persons will also test positive.

Table 36   Recommended Antimicrobial Regimens for Treatment of Patients With Lyme Disease

Recommendation, drug	Dosage for adults	Dosage for children
Preferred Oral		
Amoxicillin	500 mg tid	50 mg/kg/d divided into 3 doses (maximum, 500 mg/dose)
Doxycycline	100 mg bid	Age under 8 y: not recommended; age over or 8 y: 1-2 mg/kg bid (maximum, 100 mg/dose)
Alternative Oral		
Cefuroxime axetil	500 mg bid	30 mg/kg/d divided into 2 doses (maximum, 500 mg/dose)
Preferred Parenteral		
Ceftriaxone	2 g IV once daily	75-100 mg/kg IV per day in a single dose (maximum, 2 g)
Alternative Parenteral		
Cefotaxime	2 g IV tid	150-200 mg/kg/d IV divided into 3 or 4 doses (maximum, 6 g/d)
Penicillin G	18-24 million U IV/d divided into doses given q4h	200,000-400,000 U/kg/d, divided into doses given q4h (maximum, 18-24 million U/d)

From Wormser GP, et al: *Clin Infect Dis* 31(Suppl 1):S7, 2000. © 2000 by the Infectious Disease Society of America. All rights reseved.

Test findings can remain positive long after a patient has been cured. A positive serological test in an asymptomatic person has no clinical significance.[1,2] Serology may provide a helpful baseline in patients seeking treatment because of a recent tick bite if the physician plans simply to observe the patient and obtain a second serology specimen after several weeks.[9] Serological tests should not be ordered for patients with non-specific symptoms of myalgias, arthralgias, and fatigue because a positive result does not increase the probability that the patient has Lyme disease.[6]

Prevention

To avoid infection, patients should be advised to take the following precautions: avoid tick-infested areas; use repellents containing at least 30% DEET; wear protective clothing; and develop the habit of checking for ticks. Long-sleeved shirts and long pants should be worn and kept tight at the wrists and ankles for activities involving possible deer tick exposure.[10]

Prophylaxis After Tick Bites

Prophylactic antibiotic therapy is not indicated after tick bites, even in endemic areas, because of the low transmission rate and the prolonged contact required for infection (see below). In a meta-analysis of three trials of 600 adults and children, Lyme disease never developed in patients given prophylactic antibiotics; whereas the rate of infection in the placebo groups was 1.4%. None of the patients who became infected had serious sequelae.[11]

Vaccinations

Two Lyme disease vaccines, consisting of a recombinant lipidated outer surface protein A (rOspA), have been developed: LYMErix™ and ImuLyme™. Availability of these vaccines will depend on licensing for use in particular jurisdictions.[10]

The Advisory Committee for Immunization Practices in the United States recommends that the vaccine be strongly considered for persons at high *Borrelia* exposure risk, and less strongly for those at moderate risk.[13]

------------------ ❧ REFERENCES ❧ ------------------

1. Verdon ME, Sigal LH: Recognition and management of Lyme disease, *Am Fam Physician* 56:427-436, 1997.
2. Sigal LH: The Lyme disease controversy: social and financial costs of misdiagnosis and mismanagement, *Arch Intern Med* 156:1493-1500, 1996.
3. Centers for Disease Control and Prevention: Lyme disease–United States, *JAMA* 287:1259-1260, 1996.
4. Hamilton J: Zoonotic diseases in Canada: an interdisciplinary challenge, *Can Med Assoc J* 155:413-418, 1996.
5. Gerber MA, Shapiro ED, Burke GS, et al (Pediatric Lyme Disease Study Group): Lyme disease in children in southeastern Connecticut, *N Engl J Med* 1996 335:1270-1274, 1996.
6. Wormser GP, Aguero-Rosenfeld ME, Nadelman RB: Lyme disease serology: problems and opportunities (editorial), *JAMA* 282:79-80, 1999.
7. Wormser GP, Nadelman RB, Dattwyler RJ, et al: Practice guidelines for the treatment of Lyme disease, *Clin Infect Dis* 31(suppl 1): S1-14, 2000.
8. Hengge UR, Tannapfel A, Tyring SK, et al: Lyme borreliosis, *Lancet Infect Dis* 3: 489-500, 2003.
9. Barbour AG: Expert advice and patient expectations: laboratory testing and antibiotics for Lyme disease (editorial), *JAMA* 279:239-240, 1998.
10. National Advisory Committee on Immunization: Statement on immunization for Lyme disease, *Canada Communicable Disease Report* 26: 1-13, 2000.
11. Warshafsky S, Nowakowski J, Nadelman RB, et al: Efficacy of antibiotic prophylaxis for prevention of Lyme disease, *J Gen Intern Med* 11:329-333, 1996.
12. Steere AC, Sikand VK, Meurice F, et al: Vaccination against Lyme disease with recombinant *Borrelia burgdorferi* outer-surface lipoprotein A with adjuvant, *N Engl J Med* 339: 209-215, 1998.
13. Thanassi WT, Schoen RT: The Lyme disease vaccine: conception, development, and implementation, *Ann Intern Med* 132:666, 2000.

MENINGITIS

(See also meningococcal disease, meningococcal immunization, pneumococcal immunization)

Meningitis is broadly divided into aseptic (usually caused by viruses) and septic (caused by bacteria) forms. Septic meningitis is responsible for most of the mortality and morbidity associated with the disease.

The bacteria responsible for meningitis vary with age and immunization practices. Countries that have universal vaccination against *Haemophilus influenzae* type B have experienced a 99% decrease in this type of meningitis.[1] We have yet to see the effects of the new vaccines against *Streptococcus pneumoniae* and *Neisseria meningitidis*. In the neonate, group B *Streptococcus*, gram-negative *enterococci*, and *Listeria monocytogenes* are most common. From 1 to 3 months, these same bacteria, as well as *S. pneumoniae* and *N. meningitides*, are the usual pathogens. In the 3-month-old to 50-year-old population, *S. pneumoniae* and *N. meningitidis* are most common, with *N. meningitidis* more common in persons under age 18. In the geriatric population, there is a rise in the incidence of *L. monocytogenes*.[2-5]

The typical symptoms of fever, headache, and altered mental state occur primarily in older children and adults. In infants, seizures, temperature instability, and listlessness may be present; in the elderly, the onset may be insidious with no fever and variable meningeal signs.[2]

A lumbar puncture is necessary for definitive diagnosis, but if there is to be a significant delay in obtaining a cerebrospinal fluid (CSF) sample, empiric antibiotics should be started, ideally after blood cultures are taken.

Even with prior antibiotic treatment, the CSF will often exhibit signs of meningitis other than a positive culture.[2,3] In a recent study, adverse clinical outcomes were associated with delay in initiation of antibiotic treatment.[3] CT scan prior to the lumbar puncture should be considered if papilledema, focal neurological findings, or altered mentation occur.

A third-generation IV cephalosporin (cefotaxime or ceftriaxone) is the first-line treatment in patients who are between 3 months and 50 years old. Patients under 3 months old or over 50 years should receive IV ampicillin as well. IV vancomycin should be added in cases of suspected or known *S. pneumoniae* resistance.[4] Dexamethasone is now recommended before or with the first dose of antibiotics because it has been shown to decrease long-term sequelae in both adults and children.[5] Chemoprophylaxis for contacts is discussed in the meningococcal disease section.

⊰ REFERENCES ⊱

1. Saez-Llorens X, McCracken Jr., George H: Bacterial meningitis in children, *Lancet,* 361(9375): 2139-2148, 2003.
2. Tunkel Allan R, Scheld W, Michael: Issues in management of bacterial meningitis, *Am Fam Physician* 56(5):1355-1362, 1997.
3. Aronin Steven I, Peduzzi Peter, Quagliarello VJ: Community acquired bacterial meningitis: risk stratification for adverse clinical outcome and effect of antibiotic timing, *Ann Int Med* 129(11):862-869, 1998.
4. Losh D P: Clinics in family practice, 6(1).
5. Van de Beek D, De Gans J, McIntyre P, et al: Corticosteroids in acute bacterial meningitis, *Cochrane Database of Systematic Reviews* (3):CD004305, 2003 (abstract).

NECROTIZING FASCIITIS
(See also streptococcal pharyngitis)

Necrotizing fasciitis, or necrotizing myositis, has existed since the time of Hippocrates. Otherwise healthy individuals may be affected, and the mechanism of entry of the organism is uncertain.[1] An associated toxic shock syndrome is present in about half the cases.[2] The causative organisms are often beta-hemolytic streptococci alone or with staphylococci, but in other instances, mixed aerobic and anaerobic organisms of gut origin are responsible.[3] Case reports suggest that the use of non-steroidal anti-inflammatory drugs (NSAIDs) may mask the symptoms and delay diagnosis, as well as alter the immune response to the detriment of the patient.[4]

Diagnostic findings include pain that is inconsistent with objective findings, hypotension, skin crepitance, bullae, and gas on X-ray examination. A diagnostic model that factored in WBC (greater than 15.4) and serum sodium (less than 135) on admission proved to have high sensitivity and negative predictive value in distinguishing necrotizing fasciitis from other soft tissue infections.[5] Treatment involves antibiotics, surgery, and in a few cases massive doses of IV immune globulins.[5]

Rare cases of secondary infection have been reported in close contacts,[2] but whether contacts should receive antibiotic prophylaxis is uncertain.[6] Based on the results of a prospective study of household contacts of patients with invasive group A *Streptococcus*, prophylaxis (if indicated at all) is probably useful only for those whose contact with the patient exceeded 24 hours during the week before the illness developed.[7]

⊰ REFERENCES ⊱

1. Barza MJ: Case Records of the Massachusetts General Hospital. Case 21-1995, *N Engl J Med* 333:113-119, 1995.
2. Bisno AL, Stevens DL: Streptococcal infections of skin and soft tissues, *N Engl J Med* 334:240-245, 1996.
3. Kingston D, Seal DV: Current hypotheses on synergistic microbial gangrene, *Br J Surg* 77:260-264, 1990.
4. Browne BA, Holder EP, Rupnick L: Nonsteroidal anti-inflammatory drugs and necrotizing fasciitis, *Am J Health Syst Pharm* 53:265-269, 1996.
5. Wall DB, Klein SR, Black S, et al: A simple model to help distinguish necrotizing fasciitis from nonnecrtizing soft tissue infection, *J Am Coll of Surgeons* 191(3): 227-231, 2000.
6. Lamothe F, Damico P, Ghosn P, et al: Clinical usefulness of intravenous human immunoglobulins in invasive group A streptococcal infections—case report and review, *Clin Infect Dis* 21:1469-1470, 1995.
7. Working Group on Prevention of Invasive Group A Streptococcal Infections: Prevention of invasive group A streptococcal disease among household contacts of case-patients: is prophylaxis warranted? *JAMA* 279:1206-1210, 1998.

PARASITOLOGY
(See also diarrhea; food-borne illness; malaria; travellers' diarrhea; tropical medicine)

Amebiasis (Entamoeba histolytica)
Second only to malaria as cause of death from parasitic diseases, amoebiasis causes 50,000 to 100,000 deaths annually worldwide.[1] It has become clear that three species of *Entamoeba* infect humans, and standard microscopy does not distinguish *Entamoeba histolytica* from the nonpathogenic commensals *E. dispar* or *E. moskovski*. To avoid treating aysmptomatic cases of these more common commensals, it is now recommended to confirm *E. histoyltica* by stool antigen or PCR.[1] The luminal treatment agent of choice is paromomycin 30 mg/kg three times daily for 7 days for adults and children. Invasive disease must be treated first with metronidazole 750 mg three times daily (for children 35 to 50 mg/kg three times daily) for 7 days. For amoebic colitis, the sensitivity of microscopy may be as low as 25%, creating a risk of misdiagnosis as ulcerative colitis. Steroid treatment of amoebic colitis can be fatal.[2]

Ascaris lumbricoides

Due to large number of eggs produced by females, a stool smear is sufficient for diagnosis of round worm. This can be confirmed by an upper GI imaging with small bowel follow-through. Round worm infestation caused by *Ascaris lumbricoides* can be treated with mebendazole (Vermox) 100 mg twice daily for 3 days or with a single 500-mg dose in both children and adults. Alternatives are pyrantel pamoate (Combantrin) 11 mg/kg as a single dose or albendazole (Albenza) 400 mg once for adults and children.[3]

Babesiosis

Babesiosis is transmitted by the same tick that transmits Lyme disease, *Ixodes dammini*. *Babesia* species are intraerythrocytic parasites producing a malaria-like illness. In the Americas, babesiosis occurs mostly in the Northeastern United States where seroprevalance is as high as 10%.[4] In Europe, *B. divergens* causes more severe illness. Most infections are asymptomatic; severe illness occurs in immunocompromised, splenectomized, and elderly patients. Treatment guidelines suggest atovaquone 750 mg twice daily for 7 days, plus azithromycin 500 mg once daily, then 250 mg per day for 7 days OR clindamycin 600 mg orally three times daily for 7 days plus quinine 650 mg orally three times daily for 7 days.[5] Transfusion transmission has occurred.[6] For severe illness, IV clindamycin plus oral quinine is recommended.[2,3]

Cercarial Dermatitis

Cercarial dermatitis (swimmer's itch) is a cutaneous inflammatory response caused by penetration of the skin by cercariae of bird schistosomes. Humans are accidental hosts, and the eruption usually occurs under tight-fitting swimwear where the cercariae are trapped. Acquired in brackish or clear water, cases occur worldwide. Previous exposure can intensify the immune response. Corticosteroid cream can be helpful.[7]

Chagas' Disease

Transmitted to humans by blood-sucking triatomine bugs, infection by *Trypanosoma cruzi* is only treatable in the acute phase. The acute phase, however, rarely triggers diagnosis because of the nonspecific presentation. The symptomatic chronic phase occurs years later in 10% to 30% of persons and may involve various organs, with cardiac disease being the most common serious manifestation. Transfusion-related infection has occurred, and screening of all blood donations in the United States is planned. In South America, an estimated 16 million persons are affected.[8-10]

Cryptosporidiosis

Most cryptosporidiosis is caused by *Cryptosporidium parvum* and *Cryptosporidium hominis*, and is a global cause of diarrheal disease. Humans are the host of *C. hominis*, recently distinguished from the bovine *C. parvum*. Life-threatening illness can occur among the malnourished and immunocompromised patients. The diarrhea lasts 1 to 2 weeks. Fecally transmitted oocysts are relatively resistant to water purification programs. Although routinely screened for by some labs, if cryptosporidiosis is suspected in diarrheal illness, testing for it should be specifically requested. Effective treatment is presently limited.[11,12]

Cutaneous Larva Migrans

Cutaneous larva migrans results from erratic migration within human dermis of dog, cat, or cattle hookworm larvae. The larvae hatch from ova in feces and lie in the soil or sand waiting to invade the skin of their definitive hosts. Humans are accidental hosts. In temperate climates, most cases occur in travellers returning from beach holidays in southern climes. The treatment of choice is topical thiabendazole.[1]

Cyclosporiasis

Cyclospora cayetanensis causes watery diarrhea. Outbreaks in the 1990s were linked to imported raspberries, basil, and lettuce. As with cryptosporidiosis, some laboratories require testing for *Cyclospora* to be specifically requested on stool ova and parasite testing.[13] *Cyclospora* infection is sensitive to trimethoprim-sulfamethoxazole.

Cysticercosis

Humans can be infected with *Taenia* (tapeworm) eggs either by ingestion of contaminated food or by autoinfection from reverse peristalsis. The larval forms migrate to muscle, brain, and other organs forming cysticerci. Neurocysticercosis is a significant worldwide problem, and because it has become an increasingly recognized cause of seizures, it has required more widespread use of MRI. The disease is common in Mexico, South America, Africa, India, Asia, and Eastern Europe.[14] A recent randomized controlled trial confirmed improved seizure control after treatment with albendazole. Many endemic areas, however, do not have access to the technology needed to confirm cerebral cysticerci. Prevention by enforcing standards for raising pork, proper cooking, hand-washing, and treatment of taeniasis are more cost-effective.[14,15]

Enterobius vermicularis (Pinworms)

If needed, treatment of pinworms is pyrantel pamoate (Combantrin) 11 mg/kg once, repeated after 2 weeks. Alternatives are mebendazole (Vermox) 100 mg as a single dose or albendazole (Albenza) 400 mg as a single dose repeated after 2 weeks for both children and adults.[1]

Giardiasis

Giardia duodenalis (G. lamblia) has a worldwide distribution and infects wild animals, domestic animals, and humans. Water is a common source of human infection. Cysts are not killed by chlorination but are generally eliminated if the water supply is filtered.[12] A recent Cochrane review found insufficient evidence to support treatment of mild or asymptomatic infection. The review also supported the treatment for more symptomatic giardiasis (abdominal pain, diarrhea, nausea) with a single dose of tinidazole, 2 g for adults and 50 mg/kg (max 2 g) for children.[16] An alternative is metronidazole 250 mg three times daily for adults and 15 mg/kg in three doses for children, both for 5 days.

INTERNET SOURCES

CDC's Division of Parasitic Disease –Laboratory Identification
http://www.dpd.cdc.gov/dpdx/
This is an excellent, 'to-the-point' site that includes disease review, parasitic images, and laboratory issues.

REFERENCES

1. Stanley SL Jr: Amoebiasis, *Lancet* 361:1025-1034, 2003.
2. Kopterides P: Amebiasis, *NEJM* 348:1565–1573, 2003.
3. Anonymous. Drugs for parasitic infections, *Med Lett* 40(1017):1-12, 1998.
4. Krause PJ, McKay K, Gadbaw J, et al: Increasing health burden of human babesiosis in endemic sites, *Am J Trop Med Hyg* 68(4):431-436, Apr 2003.
5. Krause PJ, Lepore T, Sikand VK, et al: Atovaquone and azithromycin for the treatment of babesiosis; *N Engl J Med* 343(20):1454-1458, 2000.
6. http://www.dpd.cdc.gov/dpdx/HTML/Babesiosis.htm Accessed April 15 2004.
7. http://www.dpd.cdc.gov/dpdx/HTML/Cercarial Dermatitis.htm
8. Leiby DA, Herron RM Jr, Read EJ, et al: *Trypanosoma cruzi* in Los Angeles and Miami blood donors: impact of evolving donor demographics on seroprevalence and implications for transfusion transmission, *Transfusion* 42(5):549, May 2002.
9. Conforto: *Top Emerg Med* 25(3): 262-272, July/Aug/Sept 2003.
10. McCarthy M: American Red Cross to screen blood for Chagas' disease: medicine and health policy, *Lancet* 362(9400):1988, Dec 13 2003.
11. http://www.dpd.cdc.gov/dpdx/HTML/Cryptosporidiosis.htm Accessed May 1 2004.
12. Chappell CL, Okhuysen PC: Cryptosporidiosis. *Curr Opin Infect Dis* 15(5): 523-527, Oct 2002.
13. Eberhard ML, Arrowood M: Cyclospora, *J Curr Opin Infect Dis* 15(5):519-522, Oct 2002.
14. Kumar S: A trial of antiparasitic treatment for cerebral cysticercosis, *N Engl J Med* 350:1686-1687, 2004.
15. Maguire JH: Tapeworms and seizures: treatment and prevention *N Engl J Med* 350(3):215-217, 2004.
16. Zaat JOM, Mank TG, Assendelft WJJ: Drugs for treating giardiasis, EBM Reviews: *Cochrane Database of Systematic Reviews,* Cochrane Infectious Diseases Group, 2004.

PERTUSSIS

(See also chronic cough; immunization schedules for children; pertussis immunization)

The classic clinical picture of pertussis is a cough lasting 2 weeks or longer that is often paroxysmal and that may end in vomiting or an apneic episode. There may also be an inspiratory "whoop," especially in infants. The usual clinical course of uncomplicated disease is 6 to 10 weeks. According to the WHO definition, a paroxysmal cough lasting at least 21 days is required as a basis for the diagnosis.[1]

Because immunity acquired from vaccination begins to wane within 3 to 5 years of last immunization, infection with *Bordetella* organisms is common. A significant proportion (7% to 31%) of adolescents and adults with prolonged coughing (6 to 30 days) have an infection with *B. pertussis*.[1] Adults are thus a major reservoir of the disease, infecting both other adults and children.[2] Adults usually have an initial catarrhal phase lasting 1 to 2 weeks, indistinguishable from the common cold. This is followed by paroxysmal coughing lasting 1 to 6 weeks, rarely associated with whooping or cyanosis, but often with vomiting or syncope.[2] In the third or convalescent phase, cough gradually improves over several weeks. The total duration of the disease may be as long as 3 months.[2]

Laboratory diagnosis of *B. pertussis* is traditionally based on culture of nasopharyngeal aspirate or a nasopharyngeal swab. However, *B. pertussis* is fastidious to culture, and the more sensitive polymerase chain reaction and serology tests are quickly becoming the mainstay in diagnosis.[1,2] The diagnosis of pertussis is more likely to be made when it is clustered into epidemics, but in general, *B. pertussis* infection is underreported.[2] Recent publications highlight the increasing incidence of pertussis infection in countries with vaccinated populations.[1-3] Canada, for example, has seen a fourfold increase in pertussis incidence over the last 20 years, with 50% of the cases occurring in adolescents and adults.[2] Pertussis is rarely fatal; however, infants too young to be fully immunized (less than 6 months old) have the highest fatality rate (0.8%).[2]

Standard treatment of affected patients and prophylaxis of contacts (see below) has traditionally been with erythromycin 40 to 50 mg/kg per day for 14 days.[1-3] Clarithromycin for 7 days has recently been shown to be equally efficacious and better tolerated when compared with 14 days of erythromycin.[5] Azithromycin or trimethoprin-sulfamethoxezole (TMP-SMX) are other alternatives.[3] Symptomatic relief and a shorter clinical course with treatment can only be expected if treatment is started during the catarrhal or early paroxysmal stages.[2] Patients with pertussis should be kept home until they have had the disease for 3 weeks, have stopped coughing, or have completed 5 days of antibiotics. Chemoprophylaxis with erythromycin or TMP-SMX is generally reserved for non-immunized contacts and infants less than 1 year of age.[1,2] It should be started within 14 days of initial contact with the primary case.[2,3] Most jurisdictions require pertussis to be reported to public health authorities.[2]

REFERENCES

1. Wirsing von Konig CH, Halperin S, Riffelmann M, et al: Pertussis of adults and infants, *Lancet Infect Dis* 2(12): 744-750, 2002.
2. Hoey J: Pertussis in adults, *CMAJ* 168(4):453-454, 2003.
3. Weir E: Resurgence of *Bordetella pertussis* infection, *CMAJ* 167:1146, 2002.
4. National Advisory Committee on Immunization: Pertussis vaccine. In: *Canadian Immunization Guide,* ed 6, Ottawa, 2002, Canadian Medical Association, 169-176.
5. Lebel MH, Mehra S: Efficacy and safety of clarithromycin versus erythromycin for the treatment of pertussis: a prospective, randomized, single blind trial, *Pediatr Infect Dis J* 20:1149-1154, 2001.

POLIO
(See also immunization schedules for children; polio immunization)

Polio follows infection with one of three related enteroviruses acquired through the fecal-oral route. Following multiplication in the throat and intestines, poliovirus can enter the blood stream and invade the CNS. Within the CNS, the virus destroys motor neurons, often resulting in acute flaccid paralysis. The leg muscles are affected more often than the arm muscles. In the most severe cases (bulbar polio), poliovirus attacks the motor neurons of the brain stem, impairing motor control of breathing, swallowing, and speaking. Without respiratory support, bulbar polio can result in death by asphyxiation.

The incubation period is 4 to 35 days; initial symptoms include fever, fatigue, headaches, vomiting, constipation (or less commonly diarrhea), stiffness in the neck, and pain in the limbs. Over 50% of all cases are children under age 3.[1]

Post-polio Syndrome
WHO estimates that up to 20,000,000 survivors of poliomyelitis are living today.[2] Post-polio syndrome is a neurological disorder characterized by inordinate fatigue, new muscle weakness, or enhanced fatigability with or without loss of muscle bulk, and muscle pain with possible fasciculations, resulting in decreased endurance and diminished function. Other symptoms may include sleeping problems, breathing difficulties, decreased cold tolerance, and joint pains.

The diagnosis is based on the following general criteria, usually accompanied by the health problems listed above:
- Confirmed history of acute paralytic polio. Some clinicians perform an electromyogram (EMG) to document changes compatible with prior polio.
- Recovery followed by 15 years or more of functional stability preceding the gradual or abrupt onset of motor symptoms.
- Exclusion of other medical, orthopedic, and neurological conditions that may cause the same symptoms.

After 40 or more years, over 50% of polio survivors have symptoms (primarily weakness), which often lead to deteriorating gait and occupational and social handicaps.[3]

Specific risk factors for increased muscle weakness are increasing age and the presence of muscle complaints and disabilities during the stable phase. Chronic overuse of muscles has been suggested as a pathogenetic factor in postpolio syndrome.[3]

REFERENCES

1. WHO Global Polio Eradication Initiative (Accessed April 24 2004, at http://www.polioeradication.org/vaccines/polio-eradication/all/background/disease.asp).
2. World Health Organization: Immunization, vaccines and biologicals, WHO Global Polio Eradication Initiative (Accessed April 24 2004, at http://www.who.int/vaccines-polio/all/background/files/PostPolioSyndrom.pdf
3. Ivanyi B, Nollet F, Redekop WK, et al: Late onset polio sequelae: disabilities and handicaps in a population-based cohort of the 1956 poliomyelitis outbreak in the Netherlands, *Arch Phys Med Rehabil* 80:687-690, 1999.

STREPTOCOCCAL PHARYNGITIS
(See also antimicrobial resistance; glomerulonephritis; necrotizing fasciitis; tonsillectomy)

Prospective placebo-controlled double-blind randomized trials in general practice have confirmed that antibiotic treatment of streptococcal pharyngitis hastens symptom improvement by about 1 to 2 days. These studies also indicate that over 90% of both treated and untreated patients are asymptomatic by the end of 1 week, and rates of suppurative complications are extremely low in both groups.[1] Since only a small proportion of primary care patients with sore throats actually have group A streptoccal infections, this modest improvement in symptom resolution must be balanced by awareness of the individual and societal risks of antibiotic over-prescribing, and a natural history of spontaneous, uncomplicated resolution.

Well-validated clinical scorecards and rapid Strep testing have both been shown to aid in improving accuracy of diagnosis and appropriateness of treatment for sore throats.[2,3]

Rapid streptococcal screening tests have a sensitivity of about 86% in children and 77% in adults, and a specificity of 90%.[4] The false-negative rate of a single throat culture

Table 37   Clinical Scorecard for Diagnosing Streptococcal Infection

Criteria	Points
• Fever or history of fever >38°C (101°F)	1
• Tonsillar exudates or tonsillar swelling	1
• Tender enlarged anterior cervical nodes	1
• Absence of cough	1
• Age 3-14 years	0
• Age 15-44 years	0
• Age >44 years	−1

Total points	Sore throat patients in primary care setting (%)[3]	Likelihood of streptococcal infection* (%)[2,3]	Suggested management[3]
0-1	over 50	2-6	No culture No antibiotics
2-3	20-40	10-30	Culture or rapid Strep test Treat with antibiotics if positive
4-5	10-15	38-63	Treat empirically on clinical grounds[†] or Culture /rapid Strep test

*Assuming usual levels of infection in community.
[†]High temperature, clinically unwell, early in course of disease.
Adapted from McIsaac WJ, Kellner JP, Aufricht P, el at: Empirical validation of guidelines for the management of pharyngitis in children and adults, JAMA 291(13):1587-1595, 2004.

sent to a capable microbiology laboratory is about 5%. Between 15% and 20% of children and 5% to 10% of adults are carriers of beta-hemolytic streptococci, as are up to 25% of patients adequately treated with penicillin. Carriers do not appear to be a source of transmission and are not at risk for the complications of streptococcal disease. Further cultures are not needed after treatment.[5]

Treatment of strep throat with antibiotics prevents about 75% of the cases of rheumatic fever that would otherwise follow this infection. However, the actual numbers prevented by such a strategy are low because, in the developed world, rheumatic fever would be expected to develop in only about 3 to 4 persons per 1000 with untreated group A streptococcal pharyngitis.[5] Linkage between group A streptococcal pharyngitis and subsequent development of tic and other neurobehavioural syndromes in children remains unproved.[6] Treating streptococcal disease does not prevent glomerulonephritis.[5]

Antibiotics take about 24 hours to eradicate the organisms. A good working rule is to keep children home from school for 24 hours after beginning antibiotics.[7] Although standard treatment of streptococcal pharyngitis is penicillin V given three times a day, twice daily penicillin V or amoxicillin 750 mg taken once daily has been shown to be equally effective in children.[8]

❧ REFERENCES ❧

1. Del Mar CB, Glasziou PP, Spinks AB: Antibiotics for sore throat (Cochrane Review). In: *The Cochrane Library*, issue 2, Chichester, UK, 2004, John Wiley and Sons.

2. Ebell MH, Smith MA, Henry CB, et al: Does this patient have strep throat? *JAMA* 284:2912-2918, 2000.

3. McIsaac WJ, White D, Tannenbaum D, et al: A clinical scorecard to reduce unnecessary antibiotic use in patients with sore throat, *CMAJ* 158:75-83, 1998.

4. McIsaac WJ, Kellner JP, Aufricht P, et al: Empirical validation of guidelines for the management of pharyngitis in children and adults, *JAMA* 291(13):1587-1595, 2004.

5. Kiselica D: Group A beta-hemolytic streptococcal pharyngitis: current clinical concepts, *Am Fam Physician* 49:1147-1154, 1994.

6. Kurlan R, Kaplan EL: The pediatric autoimmune disorders associated with streptoccal infection (PANDAS) etiology for tics and obsessive-compulsive symptoms: hypothesis or entity? Practical considerations for the clinician, *Pediatrics* 113:883-886, 2004.

7. Snellman LW, Stang HJ, Stang JM, et al: Duration of positive throat cultures for group A streptococci after initiation of antibiotic therapy, *Pediatrics* 91:1166-1170, 1993.

8. Lan AF, Colford JM, Colford JM Jr.: The impact of dosing frequency on the efficacy of 10-day penicillin or amoxicillin therapy for streptoccal tonsillopharyngitis: a meta-analysis, *Pediatrics* 105(2):E19, 2000.

TUBERCULOSIS

Epidemiology

Tuberculosis is the world's leading infectious killer; 8 million people annually develop active disease and 2 million die from the disease. Current estimates indicate that fully one third of the world's population is infected with TB.[1] The most vulnerable populations remain the poor, the homeless, people in and from developing nations and Aboriginal communities, those with HIV infections and other reasons for immunosuppression, substance abusers, and the prison population. Other high-risk groups include health care workers and people with chronic illnesses such as silicosis, chronic renal failure, and diabetes.[2] The interaction of TB and HIV will result in further increases in the rates of TB.

Method of Transmission

Pulmonary TB is transmitted in airborne particles. The number of airborne bacteria produced by an individual with active disease is relatively low, so infection is almost never spread through outdoor contact. Transmission occurs most commonly among persons living in cramped quarters with infected individuals. Tuberculosis that does not involve the lungs or larynx is rarely contagious.[2]

Risk Factors for Spreading Infection

The risk of secondary infection is four to six times greater if the smear of the index case is positive for acid-fast bacilli. Contagiousness is also increased if the index patient is young, has a frequent cough or laryngeal TB, or has extensive cavitation on X-ray examination.[2]

Purified Protein Derivative

The Mantoux test is performed by injecting 0.1 ml of a liquid containing 5 tuberculin units. The reaction is read after 48 to 72 hours, and the degree of induration (not erythema) is measured in millimetres. The definition of a positive purified protein derivative (PPD) reading depends on risk factors and varies from 5 to 15 mm of induration measured in the greatest diameter (Table 38).[2] If the initial PPD test is negative, it should be repeated in 1 week to assess the "booster effect." This second-stage test identifies individuals who are truly tuberculin positive, but whose reactivity has waned. Repeated PPD testing cannot by itself induce sensitization.[3] A negative PPD test does not rule out TB in an individual who has recently been exposed to an active case of TB, because the PPD test takes 3 to 12 weeks to become positive.[3]

Between 20% and 30% of patients with newly diagnosed TB have a negative PPD because of anergy. This is particularly likely in individuals who are immunosuppressed because of HIV infection or chronic corticosteroid use. Anergy can also be induced by recent live virus vaccinations, chronic renal failure, and malnutrition.[2]

Bacille Calmette-Guérin (BCG) vaccinations do not prevent infection but are reasonably effective in preventing clinical disease. Thus they are widely used in many parts of the world. Such vaccinations usually lead to a positive PPD reaction, but this tends to wane with time, although readings of 10 mm or greater may be seen in some individuals even after 25 years. Current guidelines consider a positive PPD test as evidence of present or past tuberculous infection regardless of BCG vaccination status.[2] Non-tuberculous mycobacteria, which are predominantly found in tropical and subtropical

Table 38   Mantoux Test Readings (Induration Maximum Diameter) and Clinical Circumstances Determining the Need for Chemoprophylaxis with Isoniazid in Patients with No Evidence of Active Tuberculosis[2,4]

PPD	Indications for chemoprophylaxis
Negative	Children and adolescents who are close contacts[2,4]: treat for 3 months and repeat PPD. If negative after 3 months of treatment, discontinue treatment.[4]
5-9 mm	Close contacts, HIV positive, upper lobe fibrotic lesion.
10-14 mm	High-incidence groups, IV drug users, high-risk medical groups.
15 mm+	Low-risk group.

regions, may lead to false-positive PPD reactions, but since TB is a far more common cause of positive reactions in individuals from these areas, a positive PPD test is considered evidence of TB infection.[2] The risk of active infection after PPD conversion is greatest in the first 2 years.[3]

Anyone with a positive PPD needs a complete medical assessment and a chest X-ray examination to rule out active disease.[2] Adults over age 35 who are PPD positive but otherwise healthy, who have normal chest X-ray findings, and who are not known to have seroconverted within 2 years do not require INH prophylaxis. Management in adults between 20 and 35 years of age presenting a similar scenario is controversial; some experts recommend treatment and others do not. Anyone under the age of 20 years who is PPD positive requires INH prophylaxis, as does anyone who has recently (within 2 years) seroconverted.[2]

Chemoprophylaxis

The usual method of administering chemoprophylaxis is to give isoniazid at a dose of 300 mg per day for adults and 10 mg/kg to a maximum of 300 mg per day for children. Hepatitis and peripheral neuropathy are important side effects of isoniazid therapy. The risk of liver dysfunction rises with age, so patients over age 35 or any patients who have a history of alcoholism, liver disease, or IV drug use should have liver function studies at the initiation of therapy and monthly for the first 2 to 4 months of treatment. They should also be advised to avoid alcohol and acetaminophen. A doubling of the ALT or AST level is a reason for considering discontinuation of therapy. Peripheral neuropathy is often manifested as paraesthesiae of the hands or feet. Some health care workers recommend giving prophylactic pyridoxine (vitamin B_6) in doses of 6 to 25 mg per day for all patients taking isoniazid.[4]

Treatment of Active Disease

All patients with active TB should be initially treated with a three-drug regimen of isoniazid, rifampin, and pyrazinamide. In addition, patients at high risk of multidrug-resistant disease should receive ethambutol or streptomycin. After 8 weeks of treatment with three or four drugs, the regimen may be cut to isoniazid and rifampin, provided that cultures have not shown resistance to these drugs. These two medications should be continued for another 16 weeks for a total treatment time of 24 weeks or approximately 6 months. Monthly red/green colour discrimination and visual acuity testing is advised for patients taking ethambutol. Regular liver function tests are indicated for the other drugs.[4]

If compliance is uncertain, minor modifications of the preceding regimen may be made so that all medications can be given under direct observation by a health care worker.[5] Directly observed therapy, short course (DOTS) is the standard method of TB control in much of the developing world.

Drug-Resistant TB

Globally, drug-resistant TB is posing challenges for TB control as the proportion of cases increase. Drug-resistant TB is defined as a strain causing illness that is resistant to one of the five major first-line treatments (isoniazid, rifampin, streptomycin, pyrazinamide, and ethambutol). Drug resistance can be primary (when previously uninfected individuals have drug-resistant strains) or acquired (when initially drug-sensitive TB becomes resistant because of inadequate treatment or non-adherence). Drug-resistant TB requires longer treatment duration, resulting in greater difficulties with adherence and more expensive treatment. Primary care providers involved with TB management must take steps to ensure adherence and collaborate with public health and infectious-disease consultants to ensure proper care.

ꙮ INTERNET SOURCES ꙮ

World Health Organization Tuberculosis Program
http://www.who.int/gtb/index.htm
Health Canadian Tuberculosis Standards
http://www.hc-sc.gc.ca/pphb-dgspsp/publicat/cts-ncla00
Centre for Disease Control
http://www.cdc.gov/nchstp/tb/default.htm

ꙮ REFERENCES ꙮ

1. Dye C, Scheele S, Dolin P, et al: Consensus statement: global burden of tuberculosis: estimated incidence, prevalence, and mortality by country. WHO Global Surveillance and Monitoring Project, *JAMA* 282:677-686, 1999.
2. Menzies D, Tannenbaum TN, FitzGerald JM: Tuberculosis. 10. Prevention, *Can Med Assoc J* 161:717-724, 1999.
3. Pennie RA: Mantoux tests: performing, interpreting, and acting upon them, *Can Fam Physician* 41:1025-1029, 1995.
4. McCollister P, Neff NE: Outpatient management of tuberculosis, *Am Fam Physician* 53:1579-1594, 1996.
5. Hershfield E: Tuberculosis. 9. Treatment, *Can Med Assoc J* 161:405-411, 1999.

VARICELLA
(See also herpes zoster; infectious diseases in pregnancy; varicella in children; varicella immunization)

Varicella zoster is a DNA virus that is transmitted mainly through direct contact with open lesions or via the respiratory route. The incidence of varicella is 11 to 12/1000 in the United States. The virus predominantly affects children (90% of cases occur before age 13), with a peak between ages 5 and 9.[1] In the tropics, chickenpox is less common, making immigrants from these areas more susceptible to varicella in adulthood.

The usual incubation period is 10 to 21 days. The disease is infectious for 48 hours before the onset of the rash until the last vesicles crust over (about 1 week). The secondary attack rate among susceptible individuals within a family is 70% to 90%. Varicella infection during the first 20 weeks of pregnancy results in congenital anomalies in about 2% of cases.[2] It is extremely rare for an individual to get chickenpox twice; in most reported cases the original diagnosis was erroneous.[3]

Complications of varicella infection occur in 5% to 10% of all patients. These include impetigo, pneumonia, and viral encephalitis. Hospitalizations for complicated varicella occur in 3/1000 cases, and deaths occur in 1/60,000 cases.[4]

Treatment of uncomplicated varicella in otherwise healthy children is symptomatic only, with antipruritic medications and analgesics. Aspirin should not be used in the treatment of chickenpox due to the association with Reye's syndrome.

Acyclovir, if used within 24 hours of rash onset, reduces time with fever in immunocompetant children by 1 day. The data are inconsistent with respect to number of days to clearance of lesions, maximum number of lesions, and relief of itchiness. In adults, however, acyclovir used within 24 hours of rash onset significantly reduced the maximum number of lesions and time to crusting. There was no difference in time to crusting if given 24 to 72 hours after rash onset. There is no clinically significant difference in rate of complications of varicella or adverse effects of medication between acyclovir-treated and placebo groups.[1]

Theoretical objections to treatment are that it might foster the development of resistance to antiviral drugs, and that either humoral or cellular immunity might be inhibited by treatment. To date, no evidence has been presented that either of these has occurred.[5,6] An important factor to consider in the decision about treatment is the anticipated severity of the disease. Immunocompromised patients, adolescents, and adults tend to manifest more severe symptoms and higher rates of complications; these groups may benefit from treatment, if given within 24 hours. There is no evidence to support the widespread use of acyclovir in healthy children where chickenpox is uncomplicated and self-limiting. Antiviral therapy is not recommended for post-exposure prophylaxis.[1]

The usual dosage of acyclovir is 800 mg orally 5 times a day for 5 to 7 days in adults. Pediatric doses are 20 mg/kg four times daily for 5 days.[5,6]

REFERENCES

1. Klassen TP, Belseck EM, Wiebe N, et al: Acyclovir for treating varicella in otherwise health children and adolescents, *Cochrane Database Review* vol 1, 2004.
2. Pastuszak AL, Levy M, Schick B, et al: Outcome after maternal varicella infection in the first 20 weeks of pregnancy, *N Engl J Med* 330:901-905, 1994.
3. Wallace MR, Chamberlin CJ, Sawyer MH, et al: Reliability of a history of previous varicella infection in adults, *JAMA* 278: 1520-1522, 1997.
4. Centers for Disease Control and Prevention: *The pink book: epidemiology and prevention of vaccine preventable diseases,* ed 8, Atlanta, GA, 2004, CDC.
5. Feldman S: Acyclovir therapy for varicella in otherwise healthy children and adolescents, *J Med Virol* 1(suppl): 85-89, 1993.
6. Levin MJ, Rotbart HA, Hayward AR: Immune response to varicella-zoster virus 5 years after acyclovir therapy of childhood varicella (letter), *J Infect Dis* 171:1383-1384, 1995.

WEST NILE VIRUS

West Nile Virus (WNV) in North America is an emerging, mosquito-borne flavivirus infection that primarily infects birds. Risk of infection to humans increases when local ecological conditions favour virus amplification between birds and mosquitoes and hatching of bridging mosquito vectors that bite both birds and humans. Seroprevalence studies in areas with high levels of WNV activity indicate that between 1% and 4% of residents have antibodies (IgM) to WNV.[1,2] The incubation period for WNV infection ranges between 3 and 14 days. The majority (80%) of infected humans report no symptoms. About 20% develop WNV fever, a self-remitting episode of an abrupt fever accompanied by malaise, anorexia, nausea, vomiting, headache, eye pain, photophobia, arthralgia, myalgia, maculpapular rash, and/or lymphadenopathy.[2,3] After a prodromal fever, about 1 in 80 to 150 infected individuals develop neuroinvasive manifestations (i.e., change in mental status, lower motor neuron dysfunction) and experience a protracted course that may require intensive care in the hospital and home care upon discharge.[2,3] The most significant risk factor for neuroinvasive disease is advanced age (over 55 years).[3]

Enzyme-linked immunosorbent assay (ELISA) detection of IgM antibodies in serum (red tube) within 8 days of symptom onset has a sensitivity of 95% and specificity of 90%.[3] Confirmatory testing, if indicated, should be performed on samples collected in the convalescent phase (10 to 14 days after symptom onset). Treatment is largely supportive; ribavirin and interferon-alpha have been used with mixed results.[4]

Any suspected cases of WNV must be reported immediately to the local medical officer of health. Emphasis is on preventive behaviour and mosquito control. Using a DEET-based insect repellent (no more than 10% for children and 30% for adults and covering babies with netting), a recent trial examined different strengths of DEET versus many products patients swear by, such as citronella, Skin-So-Soft™ oil, wristbands, "botanical agents," and soybean oil, and the DEET was significantly more effective. The 23.8% DEET lasted 5 hours, whereas many of the "natural" therapies lasted 2 to 20 minutes. Other reviews have shown that ingesting vitamin B or garlic or wearing devices that emit sounds are ineffective. The notable exception was 2% soybean oil, which lasted for 1½ hours. The bracelets, whether they had DEET or not, did not work at all. Instead of thinking of the DEET percentage as a reflection of "power," think of it as a function of time. The 25% DEET will work for approximately 5 hours, the 20% for 4 hours, and so on. This is especially important if parents are with children, because the timing for repeat application will be different. DEET has some "solvent" characteristics, which makes it understandably concerning to some. This is also the reason that it has been examined for safety so often over the years. A recent analysis indicated that DEET has been in use for 40 years, that there have been 8 billion applications of DEET, and 50 cases reported of serious adverse effects, of which 75% resolved with no sequelae. A review by the Environmental Protection Agency concluded that "normal use of DEET does not present a health concern to the public."[5] Wearing light-coloured long sleeves and trousers and avoiding outdoors at dusk and dawn reduces the risk of infection.[2]

REFERENCES

1. Mostashari F, Bunning ML, Kitsutani PT, et al: Epidemic West Nile encephalitis, New York, 1999: results of a household-based seroepidemiological survey, *Lancet* 358:261-264, 2001.
2. Loeb M, Elliott S, Gibson B, et al: *Prevalence study for West Nile Virus in Oakville, Ontario: a 2002 hotspot,* 2004. West Nile Virus Seroprevalence Study Report November 7, 2003 at http://www.health.gov.on.ca/english/public/pub/ministry_reports/wnv_rep_2003/wnv_rep03.html
3. Pepperell C, Rau N, Krajden S, et al: West Nile virus infection in 2002: morbidity and mortality among patients admitted to hospital in south central Ontario, *CMAJ,* 168:1399-1405, 2003.
4. Anderson JF, Rahal JJ: Efficacy of interferon alpha-2b and ribavirin against West Nile virus in vitro, *Emerg Infect Dis* 8:107-108, 2002.
5. Fradin M, Day J: Comparative efficacy of insect repellents against mosquito bites, *N Engl J Med* 347:13-18, 2002.

Topics covered in this section

INTRODUCTION TO SUBSTANCE USE DISORDERS

Traditionally, substance dependence has been seen as a social rather than medical problem. More recent evidence is challenging this view. In many ways, substance dependence is similar to other chronic illnesses, such as type 2 diabetes mellitus, hypertension, and asthma.[1] The impact of individual choice, genetics, and environment is comparable in the etiology and treatment of all of these disorders.[2] As with other chronic illnesses, the treatment of substance dependence often requires medication as well as long-term planning and follow-up.

Epidemiology

Approximately 5% to 10% of all North Americans over the age of 12 are ongoing non-medicinal users of prescription psychoactive medications, illicit drugs, and inhalants.[3,4] Roughly, 25% to 30% of North Americans report ever having used illicit drugs.[3,4] The lifetime prevalence of illicit drug abuse and dependence is 6.2%.[5] Patients with substance use disorders are twice as likely to see a primary care physician as those without such problems.[6] In many cases, physicians remain unaware of the substance use disorders in their patients.[7] Less than 70% of primary care physicians reported that they regularly ask new outpatients about drug use.[8]

Substance use can have many serious health consequences. Co-occurring mental health problems are very common in those with substance use disorders. Approximately one third of those with an affective disorder have a comorbid addictive disorder.[9] Of those with co-occurring affective and addictive disorders, in about one third of cases, the affective disorder is directly substance induced.[10] Domestic violence is more common in households where substance-use disorders exist.[11] Some regions of North America, including Vancouver, New Jersey, and New York, have HIV-incidence rates as high as 50% among drug injectors.[3] Drug users have a disproportionate number of medical emergencies, which have become more common over the last decade.[12] Common medical emergencies associated with illicit drug use include overdose,[12] suicide,[3] and acute infection.[13] In addition, more marginalized populations, including aboriginals, street youth, and the inner-city poor not only use drugs disproportionately, they also suffer disproportionate harm from their use of drugs.[3]

Detection and Assessment in Primary Care

Routine screening for substance use disorders in primary care remains somewhat controversial. In their 1996 recommendation, the U.S. Preventive Services Task Force stated that "Clinicians should be alert to the signs and symptoms of drug abuse in patients."[14] However, they conclude that "There is insufficient evidence to recommend for or against routine screening for drug abuse." Since 1996, evidence has been mounting that screening and early intervention is effective, and several more recent guidelines recommend routine screening.[15,16]

The Two-Item Conjoint Screen (TICS) is one of the more well-validated tools used for screening for substance use disorders.[17] Current alcohol or other drug problems can be detected in nearly 80% of young and middle-age patients by asking two questions that are easily integrated into a clinical interview.[17] An affirmative response to *either* of these questions constitutes a positive screening result that should prompt more detailed diagnostics assessments:

- In the last year, have you ever drunk *or used drugs* more than you meant to?
- Have you felt you wanted to cut down on your drinking *or drug use* in the last year?

Laboratory testing may be used to confirm findings from the history and physical. Such testing could include testing of body fluids (e.g., urine, blood, saliva) or tissue (hair) for direct identification of suspected drugs of abuse. It may also include indirect testing for the consequences of use. Accurate interpretation of these tests is essential, given the large personal impact that a misdiagnosis of a substance use disorder could have on patients.[18]

Management of Substance Use Disorders: General Principles

The principles of effective treatment of drug use disorders as defined by the National Institute on Drug Abuse (NIDA) include[19]:

1. Treatment must be readily available, to take advantage of the patient's readiness to change.
2. Counselling and behavioural therapies help patients identify their motivation, build skills to resist urges and solve problems, replace drug-focused activities with constructive activities, and reduce the risk the patients pose to themselves and others.
3. No single treatment is appropriate for all patients, and each patient's situation must be considered.
4. Associated needs, problems, and mental health issues (Info points 3, 4) must be addressed concurrently.

5. The severity of illness guides the level of treatment (e.g., residential programs for patients who need to be removed from their environment).

6. Treatment plans must be reviewed frequently and adapted to changing needs.

7. Patients must stay in treatment long enough (typically more than 3 months) to achieve meaningful improvement.

Brief Interventions

Brief interventions are feasible despite the time limits of primary care practice.[20,21] The FRAMES approach (Table 39) summarizes the key elements included in most primary care brief interventions. (See section on Enhancing Motivation.)

❧ INTERNET SOURCES ❧

Alcoholics/Cocaine/Families/Narcotics/Pills Anonymous
www.AA.org; www.CA.org; www.FamiliesAnonymous.org; www. NA.org;
www.PillsAnonymous.com
  • International, patient-focused information
Centre for Addiction and Mental Health
www.CAMH.net/addiction/index.html
Canadian
  • Health care provider and patient information
Clinical tools and assessment aids available for purchase
Harm Reduction Coalition
www.HarmReduction.org
  • U.S.-based site
  • Patient-focused information
MotheRisk
www.motherisk.org
  • Evidence-based information for health care providers and patients
  • Reliable information on the safety and risks of drugs during pregnancy and lactation
National Institute for Drug Addiction
www.NIDA.NIH.gov
  • Broad range of information for patients and health providers

---

❧ REFERENCES ❧

1. McLellan AT, Lewis DC, O'Brien CP, et al: Drug dependence, a chronic medical illness: implications for treatment, insurance, and outcomes evaluation, *JAMA* 284(13): 1689-1695, 2000.

2. American Psychiatric Association Task Force on DSM-IV, American Psychiatric Association: Diagnostic and statistical manual of mental disorders: DSM-IV-TR, ed 4, Washington, DC, 2000, The Association.

3. Riley D: Drug and Drug Policy in Canada: A brief review and commentary: Canadian Foundation for Drug Policy & International Harm Reduction Association, November 1998. This a report prepared for the Canadian Senate Special Committee on Illegal Drugs. Available online at: http://www.parl.gc.ca/37/1/parlbus/commbus/senate/come/ille-e/library-e/riley-e.htm

4. Substance Abuse and Mental Health Services Administration (SAMSA): 2001 National Household Survey on Drug Abuse (NHSDA), Rockville, 2001, U.S. Depatment of Health and Human Services.

5. Anthony JC, Helzer JE: Syndromes of drug abuse and dependence. In: Robins LN, Reiger DA, eds: *Psychiatric disorders in America,* New York, 1991, Free Press/Macmillan, 116-154.

6. Rush BR: The use of family medical practices by patients with drinking problems, *Can Med Assoc J* 140(1):35-39, 1989.

7. Saitz R, Mulvey KP, Plough A, et al: Physician unawareness of serious substance abuse, *Am J Drug Alcohol Abuse* 23(3):343-354, 1997.

8. Friedmann PD, McCullough D, Saitz R: Screening and intervention for illicit drug abuse: a national survey of primary care physicians and psychiatrists, *Arch Intern Med* 161(2):248-251, 2001.

9. Regier DA, Farmer ME, Rae DS, et al: Comorbidity of mental disorders with alcohol and other drug abuse: results from the Epidemiologic Catchment Area (ECA) Study, *JAMA* 264(19):2511-2518, 1990.

10. Rounsaville BJ, Anton SF, Carroll K, et al: Psychiatric diagnoses of treatment-seeking cocaine abusers, *Arch Gen Psychiatry* 48(1):43-51, 1991.

11. Brookoff D, O'Brien KK, Cook CS, et al: Characteristics of participants in domestic violence: assessment at the scene of domestic assault, *JAMA* 277(17):1369-1373, 1997.

Table 39   Essential Components of Motivational Counselling/Interviewing in Drug Use Disorders

F	Provide **F**eedback about the adverse consequences (current or potential) of the drug use, preferably using any problems already identified (e.g., family issues, financial problems, liver function, respiratory function).
R	Stress personal **R**esponsibility (and desire) for deciding on goals and making changes.
A	Provide **A**dvice—based on realistic goals, and tailored to the patient's situation—to cut down or stop using.
M	Offer a **M**enu of alternative strategies for changing usage patterns. Suggest a general goal, or a range of options, to help find an approach that is appropriate and acceptable to the patient.
E	Use an **E**mpathetic interviewing style. Be friendly, reflective, and understanding. Avoid imposing your own values.
S	**S**elf-efficacy: be encouraging and optimistic, to help the patient feel able to meet the agreed-upon goals.

Adapted from Bien TH, et al: *Addiction* 88(3):315-335, 1993. Reprinted with permission from Blackwell Publishing.

12. Drug Abuse Warning Network (DAWN). Emergency Department Trends From DAWN: Final Estimates 1995-2002: U.S. Department of Health and Human Services; 2003.

13. Sulis CA: HIV, TB and other infectious diseases related to alcohol and other drug use. In: Graham AW, Schultz TK, Mayo-Smith MF, eds: *Principles of addiction medicine,* ed 3, Chevy Chase, Md, 2003, American Society of Addiction Medicine, 1157-1178.

14. U.S. Preventive Services Task Force: Guide to clinical preventive services: report of the U.S. Preventive Services Task Force, ed 2, Baltimore, 1996, Williams & Wilkins.

15. Kahan M, Wilson L: Managing alcohol, tobacco and other drug problems: a pocket guide for physicians and nurses, Toronto, 2002, Centre for Addiction and Mental Health.

16. Management of Substance Use Disorders Working Group: VHA/DoD clinical practice guideline for the management of substance use disordersm, Washington, DC, 2001, Veterans Health Administration, Department of Defense. Available at: National Guideline Clearinghouse. http://www.guideline.gov/summary/summary.aspx?ss=15&doc_id=3169

17. Brown RL, Leonard T, Saunders LA, et al: A two-item conjoint screen for alcohol and other drug problems, *J Am Board Fam Pract* 14(2):95-106, 2001.

18. Wolff K, Farrell M, Marsden J, et al: A review of biological indicators of illicit drug use, practical considerations and clinical usefulness, *Addiction* 94(9):1279-1298, 1999.

19. National Institute on Dug Abuse: Principles of drug addiction treatment: A research-based guide. Bethesda, MD: National Institute on Drug Abuse, National Institutes of Health, 1999. Available at: http://www.nida.nih.gov/PODAT/PODATindex.

20. Bien TH, Miller WR, Tonigan JS: Brief interventions for alcohol problems: a review, *Addiction* 88(3):315-335, 1993.

21. Weaver MF, Jarvis MA, Schnoll SH: Role of the primary care physician in problems of substance abuse, *Arch Intern Med* 159(9):913-924, 1999.

KEY CONCEPTS IN ADDICTIONS
Definition of Addiction

Patients are addicted to a drug when they find its psychoactive effect so pleasurable that they cannot control their urge to use it repeatedly.

Neurobiology of Addiction

The brain reward system maintains important survival behaviours such as eating and sex. It is located in the medial forebrain bundle of the limbic system, and dopamine is its primary neurotransmitter. Alcohol, nicotine, opioids, cocaine, and other stimulants all increase dopamine levels in the reward system, either directly or indirectly.[1]

Abuse Liability of Drugs

Drugs are potentially addicting if they produce a marked contrast between the altered and sober psychic state.

Thus "crack" cocaine enters the central nervous system (CNS) within seconds, has an explosive effect on dopamine concentrations, and wears off within 20 minutes. Benzodiazepines have a much lower abuse potential because they have a slow onset of action and mild anxiolytic properties, and wear off gradually over several hours. Antidepressants lack an immediate pleasurable effect and therefore have virtually no abuse potential.[2] A single cigarette puff has only a slight reinforcing effect, but 200 puffs per day create a powerful cumulative reinforcement. Tolerance and withdrawal enhance the addictive potential of drugs by making it difficult for the addict to stop using.

Tolerance

Tolerance is a neurobehavioural adaptation that enables the CNS to resist a drug's psychoactive effect. For example, alcohol enhances γ-aminobutyric acid (GABA) (a CNS-inhibiting neurotransmitter) and inhibits N-methyl-D-aspartate (NMDA) (an excitatory neurotransmitter). The CNS compensates by decreasing the number and sensitivity of GABA receptors and increasing the NMDA receptors.

Withdrawal

CNS receptors take days or weeks to normalize with abstinence, creating a constellation of symptoms and signs that are opposite of the drug's main effect. Sedative withdrawal creates autonomic hyperactivity with dangerous medical complications. Opioid withdrawal is accompanied by anxiety, powerful cravings, and flu-like symptoms. Stimulant withdrawal consists of depression, insomnia, and cravings.

Clinical Features of Dependence

A simpler description than the DSM-IV is compiled of the 4 Cs: Craving, loss of Control, Compulsion to use, and use despite Consequences. Consider a patient who finds alcohol so pleasurable that he regularly goes to the bar after work (**Craving**). His drinking escalates to overcome tolerance, and he experiences withdrawal when he abstains. He tries and fails repeatedly to cut down (loss of **Control**). He organizes his life to maximize drinking opportunities, neglecting his work and family (**Compulsion**). Eventually his spouse leaves and he loses his job (**Consequences**).

━━━━━━━━━━━━━━ ❧ REFERENCES ❧ ━━━━━━━━━━━━━━

1. Tomkins DM, Sellers EM: *Addiction and the brain: the role of neurotransmitters in the cause and treatment of drug dependence, Can Med Assoc J* 164(6):817-821, 2001.

2. Jaffe JH, Bloor R, Crome I, et al: A postmarketing study of relative abuse liability of hypnotic sedative drugs, *Addiction* 99(2):165-173, 2004.

ALCOHOL DEPENDENCE AND PROBLEM DRINKING
Epidemiology

Alcohol dependence and problem drinking are major causes of morbidity and mortality. In 1999 a study found that 24.2% of Canadian males and 11.7% of females age 20 to 64 exceeded the low-risk drinking guidelines.[1] Alcoholics have a mortality rate 2.5 to 5.5 times higher than age-matched controls.[1a] Prevalence of current alcoholism in medical in-patients is estimated at 6% to 7%;[2,3] alcoholics have more in-patient days per patient than diabetics.[4] Alcohol use accounted for an estimated 6701 deaths, 86,000 hospitalizations, and $7.5 billion in health and social costs in Canada in 1992.[5,6] Risk factors for alcohol problems include male gender, family history, anxiety and mood disorders, antisocial personality disorder, and socio-cultural background.

Role of Primary Care

Research strongly supports the central role of primary care in the management of alcohol problems. Primary care counselling visits may be as effective as cognitive therapy for alcohol dependence.[7] Primary medical care integrated with addiction treatment improves both addiction and health-related outcomes.[8,9]

Low-Risk Drinking Guidelines

Moderate alcohol consumption lowers cardiovascular and total mortality by elevating cardioprotective lipids and inhibiting platelet aggregation. Most of these benefits can be obtained by consumption of less than one drink per day.[10] Above two drinks per day, mortality increases from hypertension, hemorrhagic stroke, and arrhythmias.[11] For younger adults, mortality increases linearly with increasing consumption, due to violence, accidents, and suicide.[12] Moderate alcohol consumption increases the risk of breast cancer.[13]

Low-risk drinking recommendations vary somewhat among countries and agencies. The current Canadian recommendation is no more than 14 drinks per week (men) and 9 per week (women), with no more than two drinks on any 1 day.[14] A lower limit is recommended for women because they have a higher blood alcohol level than men for a given rate of consumption. Abstinence is recommended under the following conditions:

- Pregnancy
- On medications that may interact with alcohol (e.g., sedating medications)
- Medical conditions that may be worsened by alcohol (seizure disorder, cirrhosis, active ulcer)
- Operation of heavy machinery
- Past history of alcohol dependence

Screening
Alcohol consumption history

An alcohol consumption history should be done at baseline, during annual physicals, and with possible alcohol-related presentations. The history should include the following:

- Ask about typical weekly consumption and maximum daily consumption: ("On average, how many days per week do you drink alcohol? On a typical day when you drink, how many drinks do you have? What is the maximum number of drinks you have had on any one day during the past month?"[15]) Patients tend not to count heavy drinking episodes in their estimate of average weekly consumption.
- Convert responses to standard drinks (12 oz bottle of 5% beer, 5 oz table wine, 1½ ounces of liquor).
- Older women, severely addicted patients, patients new to the practice, and patients in the "precontemplation" stage (see Stages of Change Model) are less likely to admit to heavy drinking. If the patient gives vague responses or may be minimizing their consumption:
  - Ask about alcohol consumption in the past week or the past day.
  - Present the patient with a wide range of consumption. "Would you say you drink more like one or two beers per night, or eight or ten beers per night?" This lets the patient know you won't be shocked by heavy consumption.
  - Provide a social or medical excuse for drinking. "Do you ever have a drink to help you sleep at night? Many people have a glass or two to help them sleep. Do you ever have a glass of wine with dinner? How about Christmas, or New Year's?"

Screening questionnaires

The CAGE has a sensitivity of between 45% to 90% in a primary care setting.[16] It is best used in a waiting room questionnaire but can be used in a clinical interview. One "yes" is considered a positive screen for women, two is positive for men.[17] It is retrospective, so a positive CAGE could indicate a past drinking problem.

> Have you ever felt you ought to **CUT DOWN** on your drinking?
> Have people **ANNOYED** you by criticizing your drinking?
> Have you ever felt bad or **GUILTY** about your drinking?
> Have you ever had a drink first thing in the morning to steady your nerves or get rid of a hangover (**EYE OPENER**)?

A number of other screening tests have been developed; perhaps the most useful is the ten-item AUDIT (Alcohol Use Disorders Identification Test).[18] Its advantage over the CAGE is that it incorporates quantity-frequency questions, and it helps determine the severity of drinking. A score of eight or more suggests that the patient is likely alcohol-dependent rather than a problem drinker (see below).

Laboratory markers

Gamma glutamyl transferase (GGT) and mean cell volume (MCV) have a sensitivity of 35% to 60% for detecting heavy alcohol consumption in a primary care setting.[19,20] While not as sensitive as the CAGE, they are useful in confirming a clinical suspicion of heavy drinking and monitoring response to treatment. GGT and MCV have a half-life of about 4 weeks and 3 months respectively. GGT is elevated by diabetes, obesity, enzyme-inducing medication such as phenytoin, and obstructive liver disease. MCV is elevated by hypothyroidism, liver disease, B_{12} and folate deficiency, and medications such as valproic acid.

Common presentations of heavy drinking

Common office presentations include hypertension, trauma, gastritis, insomnia, depression, anxiety, and family dysfunction. These represent important opportunities for identification and intervention.

The At-Risk or Problem Drinker

Most heavy drinkers do not meet criteria for alcohol dependence but are in fact "problem drinkers." They do not experience alcohol withdrawal, they abstain or drink moderately when the occasion warrants, and their consumption has not caused severe social or physical consequences.[21]

Brief advice protocol for problem drinkers

Controlled trials have demonstrated that brief physician advice is effective in reducing alcohol consumption, injuries, emergency room visits, hospital days, and health care costs in problem drinkers.[22-26] A typical brief advice protocol is described below.

- Inform the patient of low-risk guidelines.
- Link the patient's health condition to their alcohol consumption. Point out that almost all alcohol-induced conditions improve substantially within weeks of abstinence or reduced drinking.
- Mention non-specific effects of drinking: fatigue, insomnia, low mood.
- Discuss the effects of alcohol (if any) on family and work. Ask if the spouse/partner has expressed any concerns about drinking.
- Monitor GGT and MCV at baseline and monthly; inform the patient of the results.
- Ask the patient to set a treatment goal: abstinence, or reduced drinking. If a reduced-drinking goal is chosen, ask the patient to specify the number of drinks/day, and the number of days/week.
- Ask patient to keep a daily record of the number of drinks consumed and to bring it in the next office visit.
- Give tips for reducing the patient's alcohol consumption and avoiding intoxication:.

  Drink no more than one standard drink per hour.
  Sip drinks, don't gulp.
  Drink on a full stomach.
  Dilute drinks with mixer.
  Alternate alcoholic with non-alcoholic drinks.
  Put a 20-minute "time-out" between the decision to drink and taking the drink.

- Arrange follow-up visits. If time permits, use the FRAMES counselling approach described in the Introduction to Substance Abuse. If the patient does not respond to brief advice, consider referring for more intensive treatment.

Alcohol Dependence

Clinical features

Alcohol dependence is characterized by:
- Physical dependence (tolerance and withdrawal)
- Loss of control over drinking (continually drinking more than intended, numerous failed attempts at reduced drinking)
- Continued drinking despite knowledge of adverse consequences (physical, psychological, or social)
- Preoccupation with drinking (the patient spends a lot of time drinking, neglecting other activities and responsibilities).

Alcohol withdrawal

Alcohol-dependent patients sometimes attribute withdrawal symptoms to anxiety. Withdrawal should be suspected if the patient reports daily consumption of six or more drinks per day, if drinking begins at a predictable

Table 40   Problem Drinking Versus Alcohol Dependence

	Problem drinking	Alcohol dependence
Withdrawal symptoms*	No	Often
Tolerance	Mild	Marked
Weekly consumption	Above low-risk guidelines	40-60/week or more
Drinks less than 4/day	Often	Rarely
Social consequences†	Nil or mild	Often severe
Physical consequences‡	Nil or mild	Often severe
Socially stable	Usually	Often not
Neglect of major responsibilities	No	Yes

*In almost all cases, the presence of withdrawal symptoms indicates alcohol dependence
†Mild social consequence: Occasional argument with spouse, fatigue at work
Severe: Loss of family or job
‡Mild physical consequence: Hypertension, insomnia, fatty liver
Severe: Cirrhosis, pancreatitis

time in the morning or afternoon, if the patient's anxiety is accompanied by sweating or tremor, or if the patient has a past history of seizures.

Withdrawal can begin as early as 6 to 12 hours after the last drink. Symptoms usually begin to resolve by 3 days, although they can last up to 7 days. The most reliable sign is a postural and intention tremor. Other signs include ataxia, diaphoresis, tachycardia, and hypertension. Subjective symptoms include anxiety, nausea, and headache.

Benzodiazepines are the first-line treatment for withdrawal because they are effective and safe,[27,28] although carbamazepine and other anticonvulsants appear promising.[29,30] Long-acting benzodiazepines such as diazepam may be more effective than short-acting at preventing complications such as seizures.[28] Elderly patients or those with cirrhosis should receive lorazepam rather than diazepam because the latter has a prolonged half-life in these patients.[31]

Withdrawal can be treated as an office procedure using the diazepam loading protocol (Table 41).[32] Advise the patient to have their last drink the night before their appointment. The doctor or nurse should monitor vital signs, and elicit tremor by having the patient reach for an object, hold their arms up, or walk across the room. Treatment is completed when the patient is comfortable with minimal or no tremor. Most patients require only two or three doses of diazepam.

Take-home doses are usually not needed because diazepam continues to act for several days. The common practice of prescribing chlordiazepoxide 25 mg four times a day for home use is not particularly effective, and can be dangerous if patients drink while taking the medication.

Table 41   Diazepam Loading Protocol for Alcohol Withdrawal*:

- Diazepam 20 mg po q 1-2 h until symptoms abate, or CIWA >= 10
- Treatment completed when patient comfortable with minimal tremor, or CIWA < 8 on 2 consecutive readings
- If take-home diazepam is necessary, give no more than 2-3 10 mg tablets
- Thiamine 100 mg IM then 100 mg po for 3 days
- If history of seizures: Diazepam 20 mg q 1 h for a **minimum** of three doses
- If > 65, hepatic dysfunction: Lorazepam SL, PO 1-2 mg q 2-4 h
- To ER if:
  - Still marked withdrawal despite 60-80 mg diazepam
  - Complications (seizures, arrhythmias, DTs)
  - Dehydrated, electrolyte abnormalities, or medically ill

*For CIWA-A score of =>10. Loading protocol will not prevent seizures in patients taking large doses of benzodiazepines or barbiturates in addition to alcohol.
SL, Sublingual.
Adapted from Sellers EM, et al: *Clin Pharmacol Ther* 34(6):822-826, 1983, with permission from the American Society for Clinical Pharmacology and Therapeutics.

Withdrawal scales. The Clinical Institute Withdrawal Assessment (CIWA) scale is a validated instrument for monitoring the severity of withdrawal.[33,34] It can be completed in a few minutes by a nurse or physician. The CIWA consists of ten items measuring the severity of symptoms such as anxiety and hallucinations, and signs such as tremor and sweating. A score of 10 or more indicates the need for benzodiazepines. Treatment is completed when the patient scores less than 8 on two consecutive readings.

Referral to ED. Patients should be referred to the ED for rehydration, monitoring of electrolytes and vital signs, and possible cardiac monitoring if they show marked autonomic signs (diaphoretic, tachycardic, vomiting, severe tremor).

Protracted abstinence syndrome. Some newly abstinent patients experience a prolonged withdrawal syndrome characterized by weeks or months of insomnia, irritability, and cravings for alcohol. Physicians should assess the patient for an underlying mood or anxiety disorder, avoid prolonged use of benzodiazepines, and consider anti-craving medication such as naltrexone. Patients often respond to supportive counselling, AA, and exercise and sleep hygiene.

Complications of withdrawal

Seizures. Alcohol dependence is one of the most common causes of seizures in adults.[35] Typically, seizures occur between 8 and 48 hours after the last drink, and are grand mal, non-focal, and brief.[36] Further investigation is warranted if the seizure has focal features, the neurological examination is abnormal, if the patient is over 40 and has had their first seizure, if the patient has had head trauma, or the seizure occurred outside the expected time frame.

Seizures can be prevented by administering diazepam 20 mg for at least three doses in all patients with a past history of seizures who present for treatment of withdrawal.[37] Lorazepam is also effective in seizure prevention.[35] Treatment should start within 12 hours of the last drink. Phenytoin is ineffective for treating or preventing withdrawal seizures.[38]

Arrhythmias. Patients in withdrawal are at risk for ventricular and supraventricular tacchyarrhythmias. Treatment consists of standard antiarrhythmic therapy, correction of low potassium and magnesium, and identification and management of cardiomyopathy.

Hallucinations. Patients in withdrawal sometimes experience hallucinations, particularly tactile (e.g., bugs crawling under the skin). Hallucinations usually respond to benzodiazepine treatment of withdrawal and low doses of antipsychotics.

Delirium tremens. Delirium tremens (DTs) begins on days 3 to 5 of acute withdrawal. This condition is more common in very heavy drinkers with concurrent medical illnesses such as pneumonia.[39,40] Delirium presents with vivid, frightening hallucinations (visual and auditory), paranoid delusions, extreme disorientation, and fluctuating level of consciousness. It tends to be worse at night (sundowning). Often it is accompanied by severe autonomic symptoms (fever, diaphoresis, vomiting, tremor, tachycardia, hypertension). Death can occur from arrhythmias due to catecholamine excess and hypokalemia.

Management. Delirium may be prevented or shortened by the diazepam loading protocol.[41] Patients experiencing DTs should receive fluid and electrolyte replacement (potassium and magnesium) and cardiac monitoring if necessary. Autonomic hyperactivity should be treated with benzodiazepines; often hundreds of milligrams of diazepam are needed. Delirium responds to antipsychotic medication and reassurance. Restraints should be avoided if possible. If autonomic signs are worsening despite benzodiazepine treatment, ICU admission might be warranted for intubation and infusion of an anesthetic such as propofol.[42]

Medical Complications

Hepatic Complications. *Fatty liver* is reversible with abstinence. It presents with elevated GGT, hepatomegaly on exam, and fatty liver on ultrasound. Alcoholic hepatitis ranges in presentation from asymptomatic to acute liver failure. Transaminases are elevated, with AST higher than ALT. Males have a 10% to 20% risk for cirrhosis if they consume six drinks per day for 10 years, whereas women are at risk with three drinks per day.[43] Diagnosis is made by physical exam (firm liver, stigmata of liver disease) and tests of hepatic function (low albumin, high international normalized ratio (INR) and bilirubin). Ultrasound is not sensitive for detecting cirrhosis, but does detect splenomegaly due to portal hypertension. Biopsy is definitive.

Primary care management of cirrhosis. Abstinence is critical. The 5-year survival in cirrhosis with complications is 60% for abstainers, and 34% for drinkers.[43] Patients should be referred for endoscopy, because beta blockers have been shown to reduce bleeding from esophageal varices in patients with portal hypertension. Ascites is diagnosed on physical exam or ultrasound. It responds to judicious use of diuretics such as spironolactone and a low-sodium diet.

Encephalopathy can be triggered by increased nitrogen in the gastrointestinal (GI) tract due to a protein load, constipation, or GI bleed. It is also triggered by benzodiazepines and other sedation medications,[44] dehydration and electrolyte abnormalities, and infections. Early stages of encephalopathy can be subtle and difficult to diagnose. Patients experience inattention and decreased motor skills, with fatigue, slow responses, poor concentration, day-night reversal, decreased work performance, and increased risk of accidents.[45] A cirrhotic patient who has a change in mental status must be assessed promptly, because untreated encephalopathy can rapidly lead to coma and death.

Encephalopathy is a diagnosis of exclusion, and other causes of altered mental status should be ruled out.[46] Precipitants to encephalopathy should be identified. A rise in blood ammonia level is sometimes helpful in diagnosis. Early encephalopathy responds to osmotic laxatives such as lactulose and a low-protein diet. Benzodiazepines and excessive use of diuretics should be avoided.

Cirrhotic patients with ongoing liver failure are candidates for a liver transplant. Most transplant programs require confirmed abstinence for 6 months to 2 years and participation in an alcohol treatment program. Prognosis is very good, with only 10% to 20% of patients who receive a transplant resuming heavy drinking at a level that could damage the liver.[47-49]

Cardiovascular complications

Risk of hypertension is increased with consumption of three or more drinks per day. Alchol-induced hypertension tends to be refractory to antihypertensive medication, but resolves within weeks of reduced drinking.[50] Heavy alcohol consumption can cause a dilated cardiomyopathy, particularly in women drinkers and in patients with cirrhosis. Patients who abstain from or reduce their consumption have markedly improved outcome, with complete clinical recovery in some cases.[51,52] Heavy drinkers are also at risk for arrhythmias and sudden death, due to intoxication, withdrawal, or cardiomyopathy.

Respiratory complications

Sleep apnea is common. Alcohol-dependent patients are at risk for gram-negative pneumonias and TB, due to aspiration, immunosupression, poor living conditions, and smoking.

Gastrointestinal complications

Gastritis, esophagitis, and pancreatitis respond to standard treatments and abstinence.

Neurological complications

Alcohol-induced dementia is clinically indistinguishable from Alzheimer's disease, but can improve with abstinence. Wernicke's encephalopathy (ataxia, ophthalmoplegia, and encephalopathy) can be prevented with thiamine supplementation (100 mg IM or orally for 3 days). Untreated Wernicke's leads to Korsakoff's syndrome, with permanent, severe loss of short-term memory. Other neurological complications include cerebellar ataxia and *peripheral* neuropathy; both can show partial improvement with abstinence.

Neoplasms. Alcohol is a risk factor for certain types of cancers, including breast, esophageal, hepatic, and colorectal.

Trauma. Brief interventions for alcohol-induced trauma have been shown to reduce alcohol consumption and recurrent trauma.[53] Alcoholics are at risk for subdural hematoma with even minor head trauma, because of cerebral atrophy and stretching of bridging veins. Imaging should be ordered in any alcoholic presenting with a history of head trauma, ataxia, or decreased level of consciousness out of keeping with their level of intoxication.

Reproductive complications (See fetal alcohol syndrome)
Alcohol can cause amenorrhea and irregular cycles. It also causes erectile dysfunction, both acutely and chronically.

Psychiatric complications
Depression is very common in alcohol-dependent patients. A study of 3000 alcohol-dependent patients found that 15% met the criteria for major depression (onset before heavy drinking), while 26% had alcohol-induced depression (depression only with heavy drinking).[54] The lifetime risk of suicide in alcohol dependence is 7%, higher than the risk for affective disorder (6%) or schizophrenia (4%).[55] The high suicide risk is due to depression and to the cognitive impairment associated with acute intoxication.

Treatment. Alcohol-induced depression generally resolves within several weeks of abstinence. Alcohol treatment is effective in reducing both alcohol consumption and suicide attempts.[56] Controlled trials have demonstrated that depressed alcohol-dependent patients will have both improved mood and reduced drinking with SSRIs or TCAs.[57,58]

Other mental health conditions also show a strong association with substance use disorders. An estimated 20% to 30% of schizophrenics have an alcohol use disorder.[59] Alcohol use is also more common with anxiety disorders, bipolar disorder, and antisocial personality disorder, and substantially increases the suicide risk in each of these conditions.[60,61]

Counselling the Alcohol-Dependent Patient
Motivational interviewing strategies have become the standard. An approach to counselling that can be used with both problem drinkers and alcohol-dependent patients is as follows:

- Help the patient to identify high-risk situations (e.g., the bar, drinking buddies, weekends).
- Choose alternate activities (e.g., meet with spouse for dinner right after work).
- Encourage the patient to reconnect with family and rebuild their social network. For many patients, the family is the most powerful motivator for change. Invite supportive family members to office visits. Encourage patients to contact non-drinking friends. AA can be very helpful in helping patients rebuild their social network.

- Develop alternate ways to cope with negative emotions. Anxiety, anger, boredom, loneliness, and depression are common triggers to drinking. Treatment for underlying anxiety and mood disorders may be necessary.
- Have a plan for dealing with strong cravings. The most common plan is to call or meet with an AA sponsor or a close friend. Cravings are usually brief and will often pass with a few words of support.
- Focus on the patient's successes. Ask the patient how they were able to achieve abstinence, even if it was only for a short period.
- Continue to use motivational interviewing strategies. (See An Approach to Enhancing Motivation and Facilitating Change.) Use open-ended questions and reflective listening. Encourage patients to talk about the pros and cons of drinking, and the pros and cons of abstinence. A decisional balance can be helpful.
- Have regular follow-up with alcohol on top of the agenda. Always try to engage the patient in a discussion about their alcohol use, without arguing or lecturing. Don't give up! Some patients take many months before they're ready to change.

Relapse prevention
Primary care physicians have an important role to play in preventing relapse in abstinent drinkers. Encourage continued participation in aftercare groups and AA. Be cautious when prescribing sedatives. Acknowledge anniversaries and dry dates. Be alert to signs of relapse, such as a request for mood-altering drugs, reports of depression, anxiety or insomnia, and missed appointments. If the patient relapses, intervene quickly to treat withdrawal and get the patient into treatment.

Anticraving medications
Several medications have been shown in controlled trials to reduce the frequency and intensity of binges and increase abstinence rates in alcohol-dependent patients. Naltrexone[62-64] blocks the action of endogenous opioids, which may be partly responsible for the reinforcing effects of alcohol. Naltrexone will trigger withdrawal in regular opioid users. Acamprosate[65] antagonizes glutamate, thus relieving protracted withdrawal symptoms and craving. Ondansetron,[66] a selective 5-HT3 receptor antagonist, and topiramate,[67] are presumed to act by attenuating dopamine release in the mesolimbic reward centre.

Although evidence for the effectiveness of disulfiram is equivocal,[68,69] it is sometimes useful in highly motivated, stable patients who take it under the supervision of a spouse. Disulfiram inhibits acetaldehyde dehydrogenase, thus causing the toxic accumulation of acetaldehyde with side effects such as vomiting, flushed face, and headache. Disulfiram can cause death through hypotension and arrhythmias. It should be avoided in patients with severe heart disease, psychosis, severe depression, or severe liver disease.

Other than disulfiram, the above medications are safe and non-addicting, and are probably under-prescribed. Medication should be routinely offered to alcohol-dependent patients, along with psychosocial treatment. Research is underway to determine which combinations of anticraving medications are effective, and which patient subpopulations respond best.

Psychosocial Treatment of Alcohol Dependence
Formal programs
Success rates and cost-effectiveness of formal treatment compare favourably with treatment of other chronic illnesses. For example, a review of controlled trials found a 6-month success rate of 50% (defined as greater than 50% reduction in the Addiction Severity Index).[70] Cognitive therapy, therapist-facilitated AA, and motivational interviewing are all effective,[71] and most programs use a combination of all three approaches.

Outpatient programs are effective for socially stable patients with less severe psychosocial or substance use problems. Inpatient treatment is indicated for patients who have failed at outpatient treatment, require medical management of withdrawal, or live in an unsupportive home environment. Most inpatient programs provide regular follow-up group sessions for up to 2 years.

Physicians can promote entry into treatment by providing information about treatment programs, negotiating a treatment plan acceptable to the patient, assisting with the admission procedure, and addressing practical barriers to attendance.

Alcoholics Anonymous[72]. Alcoholics Anonymous is based on the 12 Steps, a set of principles that emphasize personal responsibility and honesty. Open AA meetings can be attended by the general public; closed meetings are attended only by group members. A group member is encouraged to choose a more senior group member as a sponsor.

Membership in AA has many advantages. AA meetings are free and easily accessible, and membership can be lifelong, making AA important for relapse prevention. Sponsors and experienced members provide practical advice and support, sometimes making themselves available on evenings and weekends. A close bond frequently develops between group members.

Physicians should explain to their patients the importance of attending AA. Encourage patients to try several AA groups until they find one that is right for them. Emphasize that the only requirement for membership is a desire to quit drinking; they do not have to believe in God. If possible, have an AA contact who will accompany patients to their first meeting.

Portions of this article were adapted from: Kahan, M. and L. Wilson, eds: Management of Alcohol, Tobacco and Other Drug problems: A Pocket Guide for Physicians and Nurses. 2002, Centre for Addiction and Mental Health: Toronto[73]

❧ REFERENCES ❧

1. Robson L, Rehm J, et al: Morbidity and mortality attributable to alcohol, tobacco, and illicit drug use in Canada, *Am J Public Health* 89(3):385-390, 1999.
1a. Liskow BI, Powell BJ, Penick EC, et al: Mortality in male alcoholics after ten to fourteen years, *J Stud Alcohol* 61(6):853-861, 2000.
2. Pirmohamed M, Brown C, Owens L, et al: The burden of alcohol misuse on an inner-city general hospital, *QJM* 93(5):291-295, 2000.
3. Schneekloth TD, Morse RM, Herrick LM, et al: Point prevalence of alcoholism in hospitalized patients: continuing challenges of detection, assessment, and diagnosis, *Mayo Clin Proc,* 76(5):460-466, 2001.
4. Fortney JC, Booth BM, Curran GM: Do patients with alcohol dependence use more services? A comparative analysis with other chronic disorders, *Alcohol Clin Exp Res* 23(1):127-133, 1999.
5. Single E, Robson L, Xie X, et al: The economic costs of alcohol, tobacco and illicit drugs in Canada, 1992, *Addiction* 93(7):991-1006, 1998.
6. Single E, Robson L, Rehm J, et al: Morbidity and mortality attributable to alcohol, tobacco, and illicit drug use in Canada, *Am J Public Health* 89(3):385-390, 1999.
7. O'Malley SS, Rounsaville BJ, Farren C, et al: Initial and maintenance naltrexone treatment for alcohol dependence using primary care vs specialty care: a nested sequence of 3 randomized trials, *Arch Intern Med* 163(14):1695-1704, 2003.
8. Friedmann PD, Zhang Z, Hendrickson J, et al: Effect of primary medical care on addiction and medical severity in substance abuse treatment programs, *J Gen Intern Med* 18(1):1-8, 2003.
9. Parthasarathy S, Mertens J, Moore C, et al: Utilization and cost impact of integrating substance abuse treatment and primary care, *Med Care* 41(3):357-367, 2003.
10. Ashley MJ, Ferrence R, Room R, et al: *Moderate drinking and health. Implications of recent evidence, Can Fam Physician* 43:687-694, 1997.
11. Campbell NR, Ashley MJ, Carruthers SG, et al: Lifestyle modifications to prevent and control hypertension. 3. Recommendations on alcohol consumption. Canadian Hypertension Society, Canadian Coalition for High Blood Pressure Prevention and Control, Laboratory Centre for Disease Control at Health Canada, Heart and Stroke Foundation of Canada, *Can Med Assoc J* 160(9 Suppl):S13-20, 1999.
12. Andreasson S, Brandt L: Mortality and morbidity related to alcohol, *Alcohol Alcohol* 32(2):173-178, 1997.
13. Bradley K, Badrinath S, Bush K, et al: Medical risks for women who drink alcohol, *J Gen Intern Med* 13(9):627-639, 1998.
14. Bondy SJ, Rehm J, Ahley MJ, et al: Low-risk drinking guidelines: the scientific evidence, *Can J Public Health* 90(4): 264-270, 1990.
15. Enoch MA, Goldman D: Problem drinking and alcoholism: diagnosis and treatment, *Am Fam Physician* 65(3):441-448, 2002.
16. Fiellin DA, Reid MC, O'Connor PG: Screening for alcohol problems in primary care: a systematic review, *Arch Intern Med* 160(13):1977-1989, 2000.

17. Bradley KA, Boyd-Wickizer J, Powell SH, et al: Alcohol screening questionnaires in women: a critical review, *JAMA* 280(2): 166-171, 1998.

18. Bush K, Kivlahan DR, McDonell MB, et al: The AUDIT alcohol consumption questions (AUDIT-C): an effective brief screening test for problem drinking. Ambulatory Care Quality Improvement Project (ACQUIP). Alcohol Use Disorders Identification Test, *Arch Intern Med* 158(16): 1789-1795, 1998.

19. Girela E, Villanueva E, Hernandez-Cueto C, et al: Comparison of the CAGE questionnaire versus some biochemical markers in the diagnosis of alcoholism, *Alcohol Alcohol* 29(3):337-343, 1994.

20. Wetterling T, Kanitz RD, Rumpf HJ, et al: Comparison of cage and mast with the alcohol markers CDT, gamma-GT, ALAT, ASAT and MCV, *Alcohol Alcohol* 33(4):424-430, 1998.

21. Kahan M, Wilson L, Becker L: Effectiveness of physician-based interventions with problem drinkers: a review, *Can Med Assoc J* 152(6):851-859, 1995.

22. Fleming MF, Barry KL, Manwell LB, et al: Brief physician advice for problem alcohol drinkers. A randomized controlled trial in community-based primary care practices [see comments], *JAMA* 277(13):1039-1045, 1997.

23. Manwell LB, Fleming MF, Mundt MP, et al: Treatment of problem alcohol use in women of childbearing age: results of a brief intervention trial [In Process Citation], *Alcohol Clin Exp Res* 24(10):1517-1524, 2000.

24. Fleming M, Mundt MP, French M, et al: Benefit-cost analysis of brief physician advice with problem drinkers in primary care settings, *Med Care* 38(1):7-18, 2000.

25. Ockene JK, Adams A, Hurley TG, et al: Brief physician- and nurse practitioner-delivered counseling for high-risk drinkers: does it work? *Arch Intern Med* 159(18):2198-2205, 1999.

26. Senft RA, Polen MR, Freeborn DK, et al: Brief intervention in a primary care setting for hazardous drinkers, *Am J Prev Med* 13(6):464-470, 1997.

27. Holbrook AM, Crowther R, Lotter A, et al: Meta-analysis of benzodiazepine use in the treatment of acute alcohol withdrawal, *Can Med Assoc J* 160(5):649-655, 1999.

28. Mayo-Smith MF: Pharmacological management of alcohol withdrawal. A meta-analysis and evidence-based practice guideline: American Society of Addiction Medicine Working Group on Pharmacological Management of Alcohol Withdrawal, *JAMA* 278(2): 144-151, 1997.

29. Malcolm R, Myrick H, Roberts J, et al: The effects of carbamazepine and lorazepam on single versus multiple previous alcohol withdrawals in an outpatient randomized trial, *J Gen Intern Med* 17(5):349-355, 2002.

30. Stuppaeck CH, Pycha R, Miller C, et al: Carbamazepine versus oxazepam in the treatment of alcohol withdrawal: a double-blind study, *Alcohol Alcohol* 27(2):153-158, 1992.

31. Peppers MP: Benzodiazepines for alcohol withdrawal in the elderly and in patients with liver disease, *Pharmacotherapy* 16(1):49-57, 1996.

32. Sellers EM, Naranjo CA, Harrison M, et al: Diazepam loading: simplified treatment of alcohol withdrawal, *Clin Pharmacol Ther* 34(6):822-826, 1983.

33. Sullivan JT, Sykora K, Schneiderman J, et al: Assessment of alcohol withdrawal: the revised clinical institute withdrawal assessment for alcohol scale (CIWA-Ar), *Br J Addict* 84(11):1353-1357, 1989.

34. Reoux JP, Miller K: Routine hospital alcohol detoxification practice compared to symptom triggered management with an Objective Withdrawal Scale (CIWA-Ar), *Am J Addict* 9(2):135-144, 2000.

35. D'Onofrio G, Rathlev NK, Ulrich AS, et al: Lorazepam for the prevention of recurrent seizures related to alcohol, *N Engl J Med* 340(12):915-919, 1999.

36. Ahmed S, Chadwick D, Walker RF: The management of alcohol-related seizures: an overview, *Hosp Med* 61(11): 793-796, 2000.

37. Devenyi P, Harrison ML: Prevention of alcohol withdrawal seizures with oral diazepam loading, *Can Med Assoc J* 132(7):798-800, 1985.

38. Alldredge BK, Lowenstein DH, Simon RP: Placebo-controlled trial of intravenous diphenylhydantoin for short-term treatment of alcohol withdrawal seizures, *Am J Med* 87(6):645-648, 1989.

39. Ferguson JA, Suelzer CJ, Eckert GJ, et al: Risk factors for delirium tremens development, *J Gen Intern Med* 11(7): 410-414, 1996.

40. Schuckit MA, Tipp JE, Reich T, et al: The histories of withdrawal convulsions and delirium tremens in 1648 alcohol dependent subjects, *Addiction* 90(10):1335-1347, 1995.

41. Wasilewski D, Matsumoto H, Kur E, et al: Assessment of diazepam loading dose therapy of delirium tremens, *Alcohol Alcohol* 31(3):273-278, 1996.

42. McCowan C, Marik P: Refractory delirium tremens treated with propofol: a case series, *Crit Care Med* 28(6):1781-1784, 2000.

43. Brands B, Kahan M, Selby P, et al, eds: *Management of alcohol, tobacco and other drug problems: a physician's manual,* Toronto, 2000, Centre for Addiction and Mental Health.

44. Dasarathy S, Mullen KD: Benzodiazepines in hepatic encephalopathy: sleeping with the enemy, *Gut* 42(6):764-765, 1998.

45. Blei AT, Cordoba J: Hepatic encephalopathy, *Am J Gastroenterol* 96(7):1968-1976, 2001.

46. Blei AT: Diagnosis and treatment of hepatic encephalopathy, *Baillieres Best Pract Res Clin Gastroenterol* 14(6):959-974, 2000.

47. Berlakovich GA, Langer F, Freundorfer E, et al: General compliance after liver transplantation for alcoholic cirrhosis *Transpl Int* 13(2):129-135, 2000.

48. Gish RG, Lee A, Brooks L, et al: Long-term follow-up of patients diagnosed with alcohol dependence or alcohol abuse who were evaluated for liver transplantation, *Liver Transpl* 7(7):581-587, 2001.

49. Podevin P, Vidal-Trecan G, Calmus Y: Liver transplantation for alcoholic liver disease, *J Chir* (Paris) 138(3):147-152, 2001.

50. Lang T, Nicaud V, Darne B, et al: Improving hypertension control among excessive alcohol drinkers: a randomised controlled trial in France. The WALPA Group, *J Epidemiol Community Health* 49(6):610-616, 1995.

51. Nicolas JM, Fernandez-Sola J, Estruch R, et al: The effect of controlled drinking in alcoholic cardiomyopathy, *Ann Intern Med* 136(3):192-200, 2002.

52. Spies CD, Sander M, Stangl K, et al: Effects of alcohol on the heart, *Curr Opin Crit Care* 7(5):337-343, 2001.

53. Gentilello LM, Rivara FP, Donovan DM, et al: Alcohol interventions in a trauma center as a means of reducing the risk of injury recurrence, *Ann Surg* 230(4):473-483, 1999.

54. Schuckit MA, Tipp JE, Bergman M, et al: Comparison of induced and independent major depressive disorders in 2,945 alcoholics, *Am J Psychiatry* 154(7):948-957, 1997.

55. Inskip HM, Harris EC, Barraclough B: Lifetime risk of suicide for affective disorder, alcoholism and schizophrenia, *Br J Psychiatry* 172:35-37, 1998.

56. Dinh-Zarr T, Diguiseppi C, Heitman E, et al: Preventing injuries through interventions for problem drinking: a systematic review of randomized controlled trials, *Alcohol Alcohol* 34(4):609-621, 1999.

57. Roy A: Placebo-controlled study of sertraline in depressed recently abstinent alcoholics, *Biol Psychiatry* 44(7):633-637, 1998.

58. Cornelius JR, Salloum IM, Ehler IM, et al: Fluoxetine in depressed alcoholics. A double-blind, placebo-controlled trial, *Arch Gen Psychiatry* 54(8):700-705, 1997.

59. Soyka M, Albus M, Kathmann N, et al: Prevalence of alcohol and drug abuse in schizophrenic inpatients, *Eur Arch Psychiatry Clin Neurosci* 242(6):362-372, 1993.

60. Potash JB, Kane HS, Chiu YF, et al: Attempted suicide and alcoholism in bipolar disorder: clinical and familial relationships, *Am J Psychiatry* 157(12):2048-2050, 2000.

61. Goodwin RD, Hamilton SP: Lifetime comorbidity of antisocial personality disorder and anxiety disorders among adults in the community, *Psychiatry Res* 117(2):159-166, 2003.

62. Anton RF, Moak DH, Waid LR, et al: Naltrexone and cognitive behavioral therapy for the treatment of outpatient alcoholics: results of a placebo-controlled trial, *Am J Psychiatry* 156(11):1758-1764, 1999.

63. Kranzler HR, Van Kirk J: Efficacy of naltrexone and acamprosate for alcoholism treatment: a meta-analysis, *Alcohol Clin Exp Res* 25(9):1335-1341, 2001.

64. Guardia J, Caso C, Arias F, et al: A double-blind, placebo-controlled study of naltrexone in the treatment of alcohol-dependence disorder: results from a multicenter clinical trial, *Alcohol Clin Exp Res* 26(9):1381-1387, 2002.

65. Mason J, Freemantle N, Nazareth I, et al: When is it cost-effective to change the behavior of health professionals? *JAMA* 286(23):2988-2992, 2001.

66. Johnson BA, Roache JD, Javors MA, et al: Ondansetron for reduction of drinking among biologically predisposed alcoholic patients: A randomized controlled trial [In Process Citation], *JAMA* 284(8):963-971, 2000.

67. Johnson BA, Ait-Daoud N, Bowden CL, et al: Oral topiramate for treatment of alcohol dependence: a randomised controlled trial, *Lancet* 361(9370):1677-1685, 2003.

68. Hughes JC, Cook CC: The efficacy of disulfiram: a review of outcome studies, *Addiction* 92(4):381-395, 1997.

69. Garbutt JC, West SL, Carey TS, et al: Pharmacological treatment of alcohol dependence: a review of the evidence, *JAMA* 281(14):1318-1325, 1999.

70. O'Brien CP, McLellan AT: Myths about the treatment of addiction, *Lancet* 347(8996):237-240, 1996.

71. Anonymous: Matching alcoholism treatments to client heterogeneity: Project MATCH three-year drinking outcomes, *Alcohol Clin Exp Res* 22(6):1300-1311, 1998.

72. Chappel JN, DuPont RL: Twelve-step and mutual-help programs for addictive disorders, *Psychiatr Clin North Am* 22(2):425-446, 1999.

73. Kahan M, Wilson L, eds: *Management of alcohol, tobacco and other drug problems: a pocket guide for physicians and nurses,* Toronto, 2002, Centre for Addiction and Mental Health.

BENZODIAZEPINES

Indications

Benzodiazepines are generally not the first-line treatment for any anxiety disorder. They are indicated for severe acute anxiety, severe generalized anxiety disorder, and panic disorder unresponsive to other treatments, and as adjunctive treatment (particularly in the early phases) for depression, bipolar disorder, and schizophrenia. Benzodiazepines are also used in the treatment of alcohol withdrawal, and as anticonvulsants, muscle relaxants, and preprocedure sedation.

Adverse Effects

Benzodiazepine use in the elderly is associated with a higher risk of falls, hip fractures, motor vehicle accidents, confusion, and worsening dementia, although a causal role is difficult to establish.[1-6] Risk is probably somewhat greater with long-acting benzodiazepines such as diazepam, and with initiation of therapy. Benzodiazepines can decrease respiratory drive in patients with severe respiratory disease, particularly early in therapy and in combination with other sedating drugs.

Benzodiazepines can cause or contribute to depression, particularly at higher doses. They can cause disinhibition in patients with psychosis and personality disorders. Rebound insomnia (vivid dreams, fitful sleep) occurs on abrupt cessation of benzodiazepines after 3 weeks of daily therapy.

Benzodiazepine Dependence

Dependence is uncommon. Patients with a current or past history of dependence on other substances are at greatest risk for becoming dependent on benzodiazepines. The treatment approach is similar to other substance dependence. Patients should be tapered under medical supervision. Concurrent treatment for anxiety disorders is often required.

Benzodiazepine Withdrawal

Withdrawal can occur even with therapeutic doses, after daily use for 2 months or more. Withdrawal is more severe with high doses, short-acting agents, long duration of use, and underlying anxiety disorder. Onset of withdrawal is 2 to 4 days for long-acting benzodiazepines, and 1 to 2 days for the short acting. Anxiety-related symptoms include panic attacks, insomnia, and irritability. Neurological symptoms include dysperceptions (harsh sounds, blurry or distorted vision), and tinnitus.[7] Patients who abruptly stop the equivalent of 50 mg of diazepam or more are at risk for seizures, psychosis, delirium, arrhythmias, and hypertension, similar to alcohol withdrawal. Withdrawal can take several weeks or months to resolve.

Tapering is recommended over abrupt cessation unless the patient has only been taking the medication intermittently or for a few weeks.[8] Periodic attempts to taper are warranted even for patients taking therapeutic doses with no apparent adverse effects.[9] Patients sometimes find that they no longer need the drug, feel more alert, energetic, are better able to experience positive emotions such as enthusiasm, and are better able to engage in counselling.

Brief advice and support from a physician and cognitive therapy have both been shown to be effective in benzodiazepine tapering.[10-13] Encourage the patient to become active, rely on their social network, and use stress-reduction techniques. Explore the benefits of tapering (e.g., more energy, increased alertness) as well as withdrawal symptoms. Adjunctive agents such as mood stabilizers and antidepressants may be considered if the taper is difficult,[14,15] although further study is needed on the effectiveness of these agents. Patients with an underlying depression may experience increased anxiety and suicidal ideation during the taper. Taper slowly and halt or reverse taper if necessary.

Approach to tapering
- Slow tapers work better than fast tapers.
- Emphasize need for scheduled rather than as needed doses.
- Halt or reverse taper if severe anxiety or depression occurs.
- Follow-up every 1 to 4 weeks depending on response to taper.

Protocol for tapering patients on therapeutic doses
- Consider tapering with a longer-acting agent such as diazepam or clonazepam, particularly for patients on higher doses.[16] Convert to equivalent dose of diazepam in divided doses.
- Diazepam may cause excessive and prolonged sedation in older patients and those with severe liver or respiratory disease. Taper with an intermediate-acting benzodiazepine (such as lorazepam or clonazepam).
- For patients on alprazolam or triazolam, taper with alprazolam, triazolam, or equivalent dose of clonazepam.[17] (Diazepam may not be effective for alprazolam or triazolam withdrawal.)
- Adjust initial dose according to symptoms. (Equivalence tables are approximate.)

- Taper by no more than 5 mg per week. Adjust rate of taper according to symptoms.
- Slow the pace of the taper once dose below 20 mg of diazepam equivalent (e.g., 2 to 4 mg per week).
- Dispense daily, twice weekly, or weekly depending on dose and patient reliability.

❧ REFERENCES ❧

1. Longo MC, Hunter CE, Lokan RJ, et al: The prevalence of alcohol, cannabinoids, benzodiazepines and stimulants amongst injured drivers and their role in driver culpability: part ii: the relationshipbetween drug prevalence and *drug* concentration, and driver culpability, *Accid Anal Prev* 32(5):623-632, 2000.
2. Lagnaoui R, Begaud B, Moore N, et al: Benzodiazepine use and risk of dementia: a nested case-control study, *J Clin Epidemiol* 55(3):314-318, 2002.
3. Paterniti S, Dufouil C, Alperovitch A: Long-term benzodiazepine use and cognitive decline in the elderly: the Epidemiology of Vascular Aging Study, *J Clin Psychopharmacol* 22(3):285-293, 2002.
4. Ray WA, Thapa PB, Gideon P: Benzodiazepines and the risk of falls in nursing home residents, *J Am Geriatr Soc* 48(6):682-685, 2000.
5. Pierfitte C, Macouillard G, Thicoipe M, et al: Benzodiazepines and hip fractures in elderly people: case-control study, *BMJ* 322(7288):704-708, 2001.
6. Wang PS, Bohn RL, Glynn RF, et al: Hazardous benzodiazepine regimens in the elderly: effects of half-life, dosage, and duration on risk of hip fracture, *Am J Psychiatry* 158(6):892-898, 2001.
7. Marriott S, Tyrer P: Benzodiazepine dependence: avoidance and withdrawal, *Drug Saf* 9(2):93-103, 1993.
8. Rickels K, Case WG, Schweizer E, et al: Benzodiazepine dependence: management of discontinuation, *Psychopharmacol Bull* 26(1):63-68, 1990.
9. Ashton H: The treatment of benzodiazepine dependence, *Addiction* 89(11):1535-1541, 1994.
10. Bashir K, King M, Ashworth M: Controlled evaluation of brief intervention by general practitioners to reduce chronic use of benzodiazepines, *Br J Gen Pract* 44(386):408-412, 1994.
11. Baillargeon L, Landreville P, Verreault R, et al: Discontinuation of benzodiazepines among older insomniac adults treated with cognitive-behavioural therapy combined with gradual tapering: a randomized trial, *Can Med Assoc J* 169(10):1015-1020, 2003.
12. Morgan JD, Wright DJ, Chrystyn H: Pharmacoeconomic evaluation of a patient education letter aimed at reducing long-term prescribing of benzodiazepines, *Pharm World Sci* 24(6):231-235, 2002.
13. Spiegel DA: Psychological strategies for discontinuing benzodiazepine treatment. *J Clin Psychopharmacol* 19(6 Suppl 2):17S-22S, 1999.
14. Ansseau M, De Roeck J: Trazodone in benzodiazepine dependence, *J Clin Psychiatry* 54(5):189-191, 1993.
15. Harris JT, Roache JD, Thornton JE: A role for valproate in the treatment of sedative-hypnotic withdrawal and for relapse prevention, *Alcohol Alcohol* 35(4):319-323, 2000.

16. Harrison M, Busto U, Naranjo CA, et al: Diazepam tapering in detoxification for high-dose benzodiazepine abuse, *Clin Pharmacol Ther* 36(4):527-533, 1984.
17. Albeck JH: Withdrawal and detoxification from benzodiazepine dependence: a potential role for clonazepam, *J Clin Psychiatry* 48 Suppl:43-49, 1987.

OPIOIDS

Opioids and Chronic Pain

Background

In past years, physicians have undertreated chronic pain, even in cancer patients,[1] yet opioid prescribing has risen dramatically in recent years.[2,3] This increase has been accompanied by ambivalence; physicians are concerned about the risk of addiction and uncertain about indications for opioid use.[4,5] Opioids are very safe and have an important role to play in chronic pain. Adherence to a prescribing protocol will minimize the risk of opioid dependence, and lead to a more satisfying and conflict-free clinical practice.

Pharmacology

Opioids attach to endogenous u-receptors in the central nervous system. They are used as analgesics, antitussives, and antidyspneics. Their duration of analgesic action is generally 3 to 6 hours. A number of sustained release preparations are available that extend analgesia to 8 to 12 hours.

Effectiveness

Randomized, placebo-controlled trials have demonstrated the effectiveness of opioids for chronic nociceptive and neuropathic pain.[6-9] Subjective pain ratings have been shown to decrease by 20% to 50% (with a wide variation in individual response). Some trials have also documented improvement in pain-related disability.[9] The quality of life may improve with optimal dosing, less frequent dosing intervals, and aggressive management of constipation and other side effects.[10-11]

Indications

Somatic pain

Opioids are useful for chronic musculoskeletal pain that has not responded adequately to acetaminophen or NSAIDs. Organic pathology should first be documented through physical examination and imaging.

Neuropathic pain

Tricyclic antidepressants and anticonvulsants are first-line treatment for neuropathic pain.[12,13] Opioids are less effective with neuropathic pain than with somatic pain.[14] Higher doses are often needed, and even at high doses some patients don't respond.

Other sources of pain

Opioids are sometimes used for recurrent, severe visceral pain such as pancreatitis. They are not indicated for common GI problems such as irritable bowel syndrome. Opioids should be avoided for isolated tension headaches. In acute migraine treatment, opioids stronger than codeine should be reserved for severe headaches unresponsive to first-line treatments. There is no evidence supporting the use of opioids for fibromyalgia; an exercise program and low doses of amitryptiline are recommended first-line treatments.[15,16]

Adverse Effects and Contraindications

In general, opioids are very safe with virtually no long-term organ toxicity; they are likely considerably safer as a class than NSAIDs.[17]

Gastrointestinal

Opioids very frequently cause constipation. A bowel routine should be suggested at the onset of therapy.

Reproductive

Opioids lower testosterone and increase prolactin. Anovulatory cycles and infertility can occur. Erectile dysfunction is common with high-dose opioid therapy.

Rebound headaches

Regular use of opioid-acetaminophen combinations may cause rebound headaches in migraine patients. Medication discontinuation often results in resolution of the headache.[18,19]

Pain tolerance

Chronic opioid therapy may cause hypersensitivity to pain (hyperalgesia).[20]

Cognitive Effects

Opioids can have subtle cognitive effects such as impaired concentration and calculation. Methadone patients and opioid users have cognitive impairment compared with controls, with recovery of function during abstinence.[21,22] It is difficult to control in such studies for confounders such as alcohol use, previous overdoses, and head injuries. Opioid use is associated with falls and hip fractures in the elderly,[23,24] although the accumulated evidence is weaker than the association with benzodiazepines.

A single oral dose of morphine 15 mg is associated with minimal cognitive impairment in healthy volunteers, significantly less than lorazepam 1 mg.[25] In studies with stable cancer patients on opioids, cognitive impairment was subtle, primarily occurring with initial titration and dose titration.[26] Nonetheless, caution should be exercised with opioids in the elderly and those on sedating drugs. Patients should be advised to limit their driving after a dose increase, or if they are on high doses and on sedating drugs.

Overdose

Symptoms

Opioid overdose is characterized by decreased level of consciousness, decreased respiratory rate, bradycardia, and miosis. Long-acting opioids, particularly methadone, can have a gradual, insidious onset of symptoms.

Risk

The risk of overdose increases with parenteral use, the dose and potency of the opioid, and the patient's underlying tolerance. Other risk factors include age, renal insufficiency, respiratory disease, and use of sedating medications.

Prevention

- Patients who have stopped their opioid for even a few days should be warned to lower their dose if they decide to resume use.
- Try to initiate treatment with the least potent opioid and at the lowest dose. Warn patients not to exceed the prescribed dose.
- Avoid sedating drugs early in therapy.
- Family members should be advised to contact the physician at any sign of sedation and not let the patient "sleep it off." A tolerance check several days after starting therapy (even if by telephone) may be advisable in at-risk patients.

Initiating Treatment

Precautions

Opioids should be used with caution in the following patient populations:
- Acute or chronic respiratory conditions
- Renal insufficiency
- Concurrent use of sedating drugs
- Elderly
- Current or past history of dependence on opioids, alcohol, or other drugs

Screening for substance abuse

Routine screening should be undertaken at the start of therapy, with an alcohol and drug consumption history, the CAGE, GGT and MCV, and urine drug screening. Opioids should be avoided or used with caution if:
- The patient is currently dependent on alcohol or drugs (opioids are usually contraindicated in this circumstance).
- The patient has a past history of dependence (use extreme caution if the patient has a past history of opioid dependence).

- The patient reports having drinks above the low-risk drinking guidelines (14/week for men, 9/week for women), uses over-the-counter (OTC) drugs such as Gravol regularly, or uses cannabis regularly.

Patient expectations

Before starting opioids, explain that the goal of treatment is not the complete elimination of pain but a reduction in pain intensity by 25% to 50%, with improved mood and increased activity. Review the side effects of opioids, including the small risk of dependence and overdose.

Treatment contract

There is evidence that treatment contracts improve compliance and communication between the primary care physician and pain specialist.[27] The contract should include the following:

- I will receive opioids only from my doctor, not from other physicians, friends, or over the counter.
- I will not give my medication to anyone else.
- I will not receive a refill if I run out early.
- I will comply with scheduled visits and consultations.
- I will not use non-authorized drugs such as benzodiazepines, "street drugs" or alcohol in excess.
- I will provide a urine drug screen if requested.
- I understand that if I break these conditions, my physician might choose to modify his or her opioid prescription or cease prescribing opioids.

Opioids as Part of Comprehensive Pain Management

A comprehensive treatment plan often involves other caregivers such as pain specialists and cognitive therapists. Involvement of the family can improve compliance with medications and lifestyle modification.

Comprehensive treatment, which includes education, exercise, and cognitive therapy, improves pain, mood, and activity, and reduces the need for opioids.[28-31] Depression and anxiety can greatly magnify pain perception, so treatment of psychiatric comorbidity is essential. Develop a plan for modifying factors that aggravate pain, particularly physical activity and stress. Encourage the patient to become more active and to rebuild his or her social network.

NSAIDs, anticonvulsants, and tricyclic antidepressants may enhance the analgesic effectiveness of opioids.[32] There is limited evidence for or against the long-term use of modalities such as nerve blocks, acupuncture, chiropractic therapy, and physiotherapy.[33]

Office visits

See the patient frequently (once every 1 to 2 weeks on initiation of treatment and then at least once every 3 weeks until a stable dose is reached). At each visit, document analgesic effectiveness, compliance, adverse effects, and changes in mood and functional status. The amount dispensed depends in part on patient compliance. For example, daily or twice weekly dispensing might be considered in patients who repeatedly run out early.

Dosage titration

Choice of opioid. Codeine is usually the initial treatment choice because it is the least potent opioid. Opioids such as oxycodone, hydrocodone, and hydromorphone have a greater dependence liability and should be avoided if possible in patients at higher risk of opioid dependence. The active metabolites of morphine can accumulate to toxic levels in patients with renal dysfunction.[34] Both the fentanyl patch and hydromorphone are less likely to cause sedation in the elderly and are preferred over morphine.[35,36] Methadone may be indicated for patients with neuropathic pain who have not responded to other opioids. It is the treatment of first choice for patients with both chronic pain and opioid dependence.[37] Demerol has very poor oral bioavailability, and parenteral Demerol is too hazardous for chronic pain management.

Controlled-release (Cr) versus immediate-release (IR). Initial titration should in general be done with IR opioids, with conversion to CR once a stable dose is reached. CR preparations taken twice per day provide equivalent analgesia to IR preparations taken four times daily,[38] and superior analgesia to IR opioids used on an as-needed basis.[39] CR opioids may be less likely to cause psychoactive effects and withdrawal, because of a slower onset and longer duration of action. However, they can be easily converted to short-acting preparations by crushing or biting the tablet. About one-third of patients on long-acting oral preparations require three times a day dosing, and some patients require a slightly higher CR codeine dose than IR dose.[40]

Dose-response; usual dose range. Opioids exhibit a graded analgesic response, with greatest incremental benefit at lower doses and a gradual plateau of response at higher doses. A simple 10-point pain-rating scale can facilitate titration of the opioid dose. With each dosage increase, the patient should report a decline in pain intensity (e.g., from 8 to 7/10) and a longer duration of analgesia per dose. (Note the pain ratings may vary with activity, stress, and other factors). The optimal dose is one in which substantial analgesic benefit has been achieved (e.g., 50% reduction in pain intensity) without major side effects.

This suggests that if partial analgesia is not achieved with several dose increases, the patient should either be switched to another opioid or managed without opioids. In controlled dosing studies of moderate to severe cancer pain, the mean dose for effective analgesia was 100 to 240 mg of morphine per day.[39-42] A consensus statement from a Canadian task force on chronic pain suggested that it was "unusual" for patients to require more than 300 mg of oral morphine per day for chronic non-malignant pain.[33]

Scheduled and breakthrough. Opioids should be taken on a scheduled basis for more consistent pain relief. Use of "breakthrough doses" for musculoskeletal pain can sometimes be minimized through modification of activity, although neuropathic pain is harder to predict and modify. Some suggest that the daily breakthrough dose be no more than one-third of the scheduled dose. If possible, the same opioid should be used for both scheduled and breakthrough use.

Switching opioids

Opioids might be switched because of ineffectiveness, intolerable side effects, or the gradual development of tolerance. Opioid rotatation is often successful at improving analgesia and reducing side effects.[43] Because of unpredictable and incomplete cross-tolerance from one opioid to another, the initial dose of the new opioid should be equivalent to 50% or less of the original opioid. The patient may not receive effective analgesia until the dose of the new opioid is high enough to overcome the analgesic tolerance developed with the previous opioid.

❧ REFERENCES ❧

1. Zenz M, Zenz T, Tryba M, et al: Severe undertreatment of cancer pain: a 3-year survey of the German situation, *J Pain Symptom Manage* 10(3):187-191, 1995.
2. Bell JR: Australian trends in opioid prescribing for chronic non-cancer pain, 1986-1996, *Med J Aust* 167(1):26-29, 1997.
3. Henricson K, Carlsten A, Ranstam J, et al: Utilisation of codeine and propoxyphene: geographic and demographic variations in prescribing, prescriber and recipient categories, *Eur J Clin Pharmacol* 55(8):605-611, 1999.
4. Bendtsen P, Hensing G, Ebeling C, et al: What are the qualities of dilemmas experienced when prescribing opioids in general practice? *Pain* 82(1):89-96, 1999.
5. Deehan A, Taylor C, Strang J: The general practitioner, the drug misuser, and the alcohol misuser: major differences in general practitioner activity, therapeutic commitment, and 'shared care' proposals, *Br J Gen Pract* 47(424):705-709, 1997.
6. Watson CP, Babul N: Efficacy of oxycodone in neuropathic pain: a randomized trial in postherpetic neuralgia, *Neurology* 50(6):1837-1841, 1998.
7. Watson CP, Moulin D, Watt-Watson J, et al: Controlled-release oxycodone relieves neuropathic pain: a randomized controlled trial in painful *diabetic* neuropathy, *Pain* 105 (1-2):71-78, 2003.
8. Moulin DE, Iezzi A, Amireh R, et al: Randomised trial of oral morphine for chronic non-cancer pain, *Lancet* 347(8995):143-147, 1996.
9. Arkinstall W, Sandler A, Goughnour B, et al: Efficacy of controlled-release codeine in chronic non-malignant pain:

a randomized, placebo-controlled clinical trial, *Pain* 62(2):169-178, 1995.

10. Lazarus H, Fitzmartin RD, Goldenheim PD: A multi-investigator clinical evaluation of oral controlled-release morphine (MS Contin tablets) administered to cancer patients, *Hosp J* 6(4):1-15, 1990.

11. McCarberg BH, Barkin RL: Long-acting opioids for chronic pain: pharmacotherapeutic opportunities to enhance compliance, quality of life, and analgesia, *Am J Ther* 8(3):181-186, 2001.

12. Collins SL, Moore RA, McQuay HJ, et al: Antidepressants and anticonvulsants for diabetic neuropathy and postherpetic neuralgia: a quantitative *systematic* review, *J Pain Symptom Manage* 20(6):449-458, 2000.

13. Morello CM, Leckband SG, Stoner CP, et al: Randomized double-blind study comparing the efficacy of gabapentin with amitriptyline on diabetic peripheral neuropathy pain, *Arch Intern Med* 159(16):1931-1937, 1999.

14. Portenoy RK, Foley KM, Inturrisi CE: The nature of opioid responsiveness and its implications for neuropathic pain: new hypotheses derived from studies of opioid infusions: *Pain* 43(3):273-286, 1990.

15. Lautenschlager J, Present state of medication therapy in fibromyalgia syndrome, *Scand J Rheumatol Suppl* 113: 32-36, 2000.

16. Gowans SE, deHueck A, Voss S, et al: Effect of a randomized, controlled trial of exercise on mood and physical function in individuals with fibromyalgia, *Arthritis Rheum* 45(6):519-529, 2001.

17. Langman MJ: Ulcer complications associated with anti-inflammatory drug use. What is the extent of the disease burden? *Pharmacoepidemiol Drug Saf* 10(1):13-19, 2001.

18. Warner JS: The outcome of treating patients with suspected rebound headache, *Headache* 41(7):685-692, 2001.

19. Zed PJ, Loewen PS, Robinson G: Medication-induced headache: overview and systematic review of therapeutic approaches, *Ann Pharmacother* 33(1):61-72, 1999.

20. Compton P, Charuvastra VC, Ling W: Pain intolerance in opioid-maintained former opiate addicts: effect of long-acting maintenance agent, *Drug Alcohol Depend* 63(2): 139-146, 2001.

21. Davis PE, Liddiard H, McMillan TM: Neuropsychological deficits and opiate abuse, *Drug Alcohol Depend* 67(1): 105-108, 2002.

22. Darke S, Sims J, McDonald S, et al: Cognitive impairment among methadone maintenance patients, *Addiction* 95(5):687-695, 2000.

23. Guo Z, Wills P, Viitanen M, et al: Cognitive impairment, drug use, and the risk of hip fracture in persons over 75 years old: a community-based prospective study, *Am J Epidemiol* 148(9):887-892, 1998.

24. Ensrud KE, Blackwell T, Mangione CM, et al: Central nervous system active medications and risk for fractures in older women, *Arch Intern Med* 163(8):949-957, 2003.

25. Hanks GW, O'Neill WM, Simpson P, et al: The cognitive and psychomotor effects of opioid analgesics. II. A randomized controlled trial of single doses of morphine, lorazepam and placebo in healthy subjects, *Eur J Clin Pharmacol* 48(6):455-460, 1995.

26. Lawlor PG: The panorama of opioid-related cognitive dysfunction in patients with cancer: a critical literature appraisal, *Cancer* 94(6):1836-1853, 2002.

27. Fishman SM, Mahajan G, Jung SW, et al: The trilateral opioid contract. Bridging the pain clinic and the primary care physician through the opioid contract. *J Pain Symptom Manage* 24(3):335-344.

28. Covington E, Kotz M: Pain reduction with opioid elimination, *Pain Med* 3(2):183, 2002.

29. Lang E, Liebig K, Kastner S, et al: Multidisciplinary rehabilitation versus usual care for chronic low back pain in the community: effects on quality of life, *Spine J* 3(4):270-276, 2003.

30. Nissen LM, Tett SE, Cramond T, et al: Opioid analgesic prescribing and use—an audit of analgesic prescribing by general practitioners *and* The Multidisciplinary Pain Centre at Royal Brisbane Hospital, *Br J Clin Pharmacol* 52(6):693-698, 2001.

31. Olason M: Outcome of an interdisciplinary pain management program in a rehabilitation clinic, *Work* 22(1):9-15, 2004.

32. Eckhardt K, Ammon S, Hofmann U, et al: Gabapentin enhances the analgesic effect of morphine in healthy volunteers *Anesth Analg* 91(1):185-191, 2000.

33. Tunks E, Mailis A, Moulin DE, et al: *Evidence-based recommendations for the medical management of chronic non-malignant pain,* Toronto, 2000, College of Physicians and Surgeons of Ontario.

34. Osborne R, Joel S, Grebenik K: The pharmacokinetics of morphine and morphine glucuronides in kidney failure, *Clin Pharmacol Ther* 54:158-167, 1993.

35. Payne R: Factors influencing quality of life in cancer patients: the role of transdermal fentanyl in the management of pain, *Semin Oncol* 25(3 Suppl 7):47-53, 1998.

36. Allan L, Hays H, Jensen NH, et al: Randomised crossover trial of transdermal fentanyl and sustained release oral morphine for treating chronic non-cancer pain, *BMJ* 322(7295):1154-1158, 2001.

37. Morley JS, Bridson J, Nash TP, et al: Low-dose methadone has an analgesic effect in neuropathic pain: a double-blind randomized controlled crossover trial, *Palliat Med* 17(7):576-587, 2003.

38. Hale ME, Fleischmann R, Salzman R, et al: Efficacy and safety of controlled-release versus immediate-release oxycodone: randomized, double-blind evaluation in patients with chronic back pain , *Clin J Pain* 15(3):179-183, 1999.

39. Kaiko RF, Grandy RP, Oshlack B, et al: The United States experience with oral controlled-release morphine (MS Contin tablets). Parts I and II. Review of nine dose titration studies and clinical pharmacology of 15-mg, 30-mg, 60-mg, and 100-mg tablet strengths in normal subjects, *Cancer* 63(11 Suppl):2348-2354, 1989.

40. Chary S, Goughnour BR, Moulin DE, et al: The dose-response relationship of controlled-release codeine (Codeine Contin) in chronic cancer pain, *J Pain Symptom Manage* 9(6):363-371, 1994.

41. Brooks I, De Jager R, Blumenreich M, et al: Principles of cancer pain management. Use of long-acting oral morphine, *J Fam Pract* 28(3):275-280, 1989.

42. Parris WC, Johnson BW Jr, Croghan MK, et al: The use of controlled-release oxycodone for the treatment of chronic cancer pain: a randomized, double-blind study, *J Pain Symptom Manage* 16(4):205-211, 1998.

43. Kloke M, Rapp M, Bosse B, et al: Toxicity and/or insufficient analgesia by opioid therapy: risk factors and the impact of changing the opioid. A retrospective analysis of 273 patients observed at a single center, *Support Care Cancer* 8(6):479-486, 2000.

Opioid Misuse and Dependence

Prevalence

Prevalence studies suggest that opioid misuse is common in primary care populations. A retrospective cohort study of two primary care settings in the United States found that 24% and 31% of patients receiving chronic opioid therapy had evidence of opioid misuse (such as double-doctoring) in the past year.[1] A study of 1000 primary care patients with depressive disorders found a 6-month prevalence of 7.2%.[2] Prevalence studies in pain clinics have had wide-ranging results, from 3% to 19%.[3,4] These studies must be interpreted with caution because prevalence may vary among clinics, opiate misuse does not necessarily prove dependence, and results are based on retrospective chart reviews rather than patient assessment.

Clinical features

Tolerance. Tolerance to the analgesic effects of opioids develops over months, whereas tolerance to their psychoactive effects begins within days. Highly tolerant patients can consume opioids in doses that would be fatal in non-tolerant patients.

Withdrawal. Patients taking high doses of opioids for their psychoactive effects often undergo severe and distressing withdrawal symptoms. Opiate withdrawal peaks at 2 to 3 days after the last use, and physical symptoms largely resolve by 5 to 10 days. Opioid-dependent patients may experience insomnia and dysphoria for months afterward.

Psychological symptoms of opiate withdrawal include intense anxiety, craving for opiates, restlessness, insomnia, and fatigue. Physical symptoms consist of myalgias (the most common and reliable symptom), chills, hot and cold feelings, and GI symptoms such as nausea, cramps and diarrhea. Signs resemble a bad case of the flu: lacrimation, rhinorrhea, yawning, mild abdominal and muscle tenderness, vomiting, sweating, and goosebumps. Objective signs are usually not seen except on sudden cessation of high doses of potent opioids.

Unlike alcohol and sedative withdrawal, opiate withdrawal rarely has medical complications. The greatest medical risk is loss of tolerance; patients are at risk for overdose if they resume their opioid use several weeks later. Opioid withdrawal can trigger miscarriage or premature labour in pregnancy.

Screening

A current or past history of substance dependence is a major risk factor for prescription opioid dependence.[1] All patients on chronic opioid therapy should be asked about use of alcohol, cigarettes, cannabis, and street drugs. They should also be asked about current or previous problems with substances, previous substance use treatment, and family history of substance abuse. Valid screening instruments that accurately identify at-risk patients have not yet been developed for clinical use. However, alcohol screening instruments such as the CAGE should be used, as well as a baseline urine drug screen (see below).

Diagnosis of opioid dependence

Diagnosis is made by observing a pattern of behaviour over time. Opioid-dependent patients often take doses well in excess of what is usually required for their pain condition. While all opioids can be addicting, opioid-dependent patients tend to prefer opioids with a stronger psychoactive effect, such as oxycodone, hydrocodone, and hydromorphone. They frequently run out early and are reluctant to try alternatives to their drug of choice. As the opioid wears off, they experience "withdrawal mediated pain" (i.e., dysphoria, diffuse myalgias, and an intensification of the original pain). These patients harass the physician or his/her staff for fit-in appointments, and they acquire opioids from friends or other doctors. They often give dramatic and inconsistent responses to questions about the severity of their pain and the effectiveness of the opioid. They attempt to maximize the opioid's psychoactive effect by binging on it, or (if controlled-release) crushing, biting, or injecting it.

Corroborating information should be obtained from the patient's spouse and previous physician. Spousal reports of intoxication, withdrawal, and neglect of social responsibilities support a diagnosis of dependence. Previous physicians may describe a long history of drug-seeking behaviour. Laboratory tests, such as CBC and liver transaminases, will detect alcohol abuse or hepatitis C.

Urine drug screens are useful for detecting double-doctoring and unauthorized drug use.[5] Immunoassay detects opioids for 3 to 7 days after last use, but cannot distinguish between specific opioids, and semi-synthetic opioids such as oxycodone are easily missed. Poppy seeds and quinolone antibiotics can cause false positives. Chromatography only detects opioids for 1 to 2 days after last use, but will distinguish between different types of opioids and is more reliable for oxycodone.

The physician should inform the patient if a urine drug screen is ordered. The requisition should specify which opioids are to be tested. Codeine is metabolized to morphine, so both will be detected in a patient on prescribed codeine. Prior to the test, the physician must take a careful history of medication use in the past week.

Interpretation. A negative test in a patient could indicate non-compliance or diversion. Presence of a non-prescribed opioid could indicate double-doctoring or street use. Concurrent drug abuse or dependence should be suspected if other drugs such as benzodiazepines, cocaine, and/or cannabis are present.

Approach to the opioid-dependent patient

Opioid-dependent patients experience daily, frightening withdrawal symptoms, opioid-induced depression, anxiety and emotional lability, social isolation, and impaired work and school performance. They may also experience financial and legal difficulties. Yet they often don't ask for help because they are afraid that their pain and withdrawal will be even worse if they are denied opioid therapy. The physician should emphasize that with treatment, the patient's mood and social circumstances will improve, withdrawal symptoms will resolve, and pain will diminish because the patient will no longer experience withdrawal-mediated pain.

Treatment options

Opioid tapering. As a general rule, continued prescribing should only be attempted if the physician knows the patient well, is confident the risk of double-doctoring or street use is minimal, and feels the patient has true organic pain requiring opioids. A treatment contract should be signed specifying the conditions under which opioids will be prescribed. Medications should be dispensed weekly or even daily if necessary. Opioids with a high dependence liability should be avoided, as should the opioid to which the patient has become addicted. Regular urine drug screens must be provided.

The patient's opioid dose should be tapered if it is high (for example, above 300 mg of morphine or equivalent). Tapering can lead to decreased pain levels and improved mood and functioning.[6] The patient should be tapered slowly over several weeks or months, preferably with scheduled doses of a controlled-release preparation.

A consultation should be considered from a pain specialist or addiction medicine specialist, and other pain management modalities should be employed. If problems continue despite this approach, the patient should be referred to an abstinence-based treatment program or agonist therapy (methadone or buprenorphine).

Abstinence-based treatment. Opioid abstinence is a reasonable option for patients who do not have an underlying organic pain condition requiring opioids, who do not wish to participate in methadone or buprenorphine treatment, or who have a relatively short history of opioid dependence and strong social supports.

Opioid withdrawal can be relieved with alpha-adrenergic agents such as clonidine or lofexidine.[7] The clonidine dose is 0.1 mg every 6 hours for up to 5 days. Higher doses can be used for severe withdrawal and in inpatient settings. Clonidine should be discontinued if the patient's blood pressure is less than 90/60 mm Hg after a test dose. Patients should be warned about drowsiness and postural hypotension. Also useful are symptomatic treatments such as trazodone for sleep, NSAIDs for myalgias, and Gravol and loperamide for GI symptoms. Buprenorphine is also effective in the short-term treatment of opioid withdrawal.[8]

Opioid agonist treatment: methadone and buprenorphine. Opioid agonist therapy is indicated for opioid-dependent patients with organic pain requiring opioid treatment, pregnant patients, and patients with a long history of opioid dependence who have failed at abstinence or tapering. Primary care physicians usually must apply for a licence to prescribe methadone, and in many jurisdictions, methadone is only prescribed through formal addiction programs. Because of its more favourable safety profile, buprenorphine is generally available to office-based primary care physicians. Interested physicians should check with their local jurisdiction to determine prescribing requirements.

Methadone. Methadone is an oral opioid agonist with a slow onset and long duration of action. Several large prospective studies and randomized trials have demonstrated that methadone is effective in reducing opioid and illicit drug use, crime rates, rates of HIV and hepatitis C, social costs, and mortality.[9-11] When given to opioid-dependent patients in the appropriate dose, methadone causes minimal euphoria, yet relieves withdrawal symptoms and opioid cravings for up to 24 hours.

The side effects of methadone are similar to other opioids: constipation, diaphoresis, weight gain, and decrease in libido.[12] Methadone overdose can occur with as little as 60 mg in non-tolerant adults, and 10 mg in children.[13] Because of its long half-life, patients suspected of overdose should not be discharged from hospital until they have been observed in the ED for at least 24 hours.

Methadone is dispensed once daily under the observation of a pharmacist, in juice to prevent injection. The initial dose is 5 to 30 mg, and the maintenance dose is usually 50 to 120 mg. Patients in a methadone program are required to provide regular urine drug screens. They are allowed take-home doses when their urine drug tests are negative for illicit drugs. Methadone programs also offer ongoing outpatient counselling and medical care.

Buprenorphine. Buprenorphine is an opioid agonist with partial antagonist properties. Controlled trials have demonstrated that daily doses of up to 16 to 20 mg are as effective as 60 to 80 mg of methadone in reducing illicit opioid use,[14,15] but probably less effective than methadone doses above 80 mg.

Buprenorphine has several advantages over methadone. It has a ceiling effect on μ-receptors and a much lower risk of overdose.[16] Its duration of action is up to 2 or 3 days, allowing alternate-day dispensing. The effective dose can be reached within days rather than weeks, and it has a milder withdrawal than methadone. Because of its side effect profile, buprenorphine can be prescribed safely and effectively by primary care physicians.[17] The National Institute of Drug Abuse in the United States considers buprenorphine a first-line treatment for opioid dependence.[18] As with methadone, buprenorphine is dispensed daily with take-home doses for negative urine tests.

_____ ✦ REFERENCES ✦ _____

1. Reid MC, et al: Use of opioid medications for chronic non-cancer pain syndromes in primary care, *J Gen Intern Med* 17(3):173-179, 2002.
2. Roeloffs CA, et al: Problem substance use among depressed patients in managed primary care, *Psychosomatics* 43(5):405-412, 2002.
3. Chabal C, et al: Prescription opiate abuse in chronic pain patients: clinical criteria, incidence, and predictors, *Clin J Pain* 13(2):150-155, 1997.
4. Nicholson B: Responsible prescribing of opioids for the management of chronic pain, *Drugs* 63(1):17-32, 2003.
5. Gourlay D, Heit HA, Caplan Y: *Urine drug testing in primary care,* San Francisco, CA, 2003, California Academy of Family Physicians.
6. Covington E, Kotz M: Pain reduction with opioid elimination, *Pain Med* 3(2):183, 2002.
7. Kahn A, et al: Double-blind study of lofexidine and clonidine in the detoxification of opiate addicts in hospital, *Drug Alcohol Depend* 44(1):57-61, 1997.
8. Gowing L, Ali R, White J: Buprenorphine for the management of opioid withdrawal (Cochrane Review). In *Cochrane Library*, Oxford, 2001, Update Software.
9. Ball JC, Ross A: *The effectiveness of methadone maintenance treatment: patients, programs, services, and outcome,* New York, 1991 Springer-Verlag.
10. Barnett PG, The cost-effectiveness of substance abuse treatment, *Curr Psychiatry Rep* 1(2):166-171, 1999.
11. Gearing FR, Schweitzer MD, An epidemiologic evaluation of long-term methadone maintenance treatment for heroin addiction, *Am J Epidemiology* 100:101-112, 1974.
12. Kahan M, Sutton N: Opiate-dependent patients receiving methadone. How physicians should manage therapy, *Can Fam Physician* 42:1769-1778, 1996.
13. Brands B, Brands J, eds: *Methadone maintenance: a physician's guide to treatment,* Toronto: 1998, Addiction Research Foundation.
14. Johnson RE, Jaffe JH, Fudala PJ: A controlled trial of buprenorphine treatment for opioid dependence [see comments], *JAMA* 267(20):2750-2755, 1992.
15. West SL, O'Neal KK, Graham CW: A meta-analysis comparing the effectiveness of buprenorphine and methadone, *J Subst Abuse* 12(4):405-414, 2000.
16. Anonymous: Buprenorphine: an alternative to methadone, *Med Lett* 45(1150):13-15, 2003.
17. Vignau J, Brunelle E: Differences between general practitioner- and addiction centre-prescribed buprenorphine substitution therapy in France. Preliminary results, *Eur Addict Res* 4(Suppl 1):24-28, 1998.
18. Bridge TP, et al: Safety and health policy considerations related to the use of buprenorphine/naloxone as an office-based treatment for opiate dependence, *Drug Alcohol Depend* 70(2 Suppl):S79-85, 2003.

OTHER DRUGS OF ABUSE
Classification

Below is a summary of the clinical features of the street or recreational drugs of abuse.

Stimulants

Cocaine. blocks presynaptic uptake of dopamine, epinephrine, and norepinephrine. It is inhaled nasally, injected, or smoked as "crack" (cocaine mixed with sodium bicarbonate). It causes a brief but intense euphoria, characterized by self-confidence and grandiosity. The chronic user experiences a "rush," followed by paranoia and agitation.

Acutely, cocaine causes seizures, delirium and psychosis, as well as vasospasm and hypertension, resulting in stroke, myocardial infarction (MI), ruptured aneurysms, and other cardiovascular events. Withdrawal is primarily psychological. In the "crash" phase, the first 1 to 3 days, the user does little but sleep and eat. In the second phase (1 to 10 weeks), the user experiences depression, irritability, strong cravings, and insomnia with dreams of using. This is followed by months or years of episodic cravings that gradually diminish in intensity and frequency.

Chronic cocaine users are at risk for severe depression, suicide, violence, and drug-induced paranoia and psychosis. Physical signs include weight loss and track marks. Long-term medical complications include respiratory disease and accelerated atherosclerosis, hepatitis C, and HIV.

Amphetamine. such as "ice" (crystal methamphetamine) stimulate the release of dopamine and catecholamines. They can be injected or taken orally. Their acute and chronic effects are similar to cocaine, as are the effects of methylphenidate (Ritalin). MDMA (ecstasy) has stimulant properties, but its main effect is due to serotonin release, generating feelings of empathy and sensuality. Ecstasy causes serotonergic syndrome (high fever, altered mental status) especially when combined with SSRIs. It also causes dehydration, rhabdomyolysis, and renal failure with prolonged physical activity in a hot room. Ecstasy use may cause psychosis and memory impairment due to damage to serotonergic neurons.[1,2]

Cannabis (marijuana and hashish) is the most commonly used illicit drug. It is usually smoked but may be taken orally. Cannabis causes relaxation and a feeling of well-being, accompanied by mild hallucinogenic effects such as perceptual distortions. Withdrawal is not clinically significant, although chronic daily users may experience a rebound anxiety with abstinence. While the risk of dependence is low compared with other illicit drugs such as cocaine, cannabis dependence is a common reason for seeking addiction treatment because its use is so widespread.[3]

Cannabis can induce psychosis and trigger schizophrenia in predisposed patients.[4-6] Adolescents and those with primary psychiatric disorders appear to be particularly vulnerable to the psychiatric and social effects of cannabis.[7,8] Chronic cannabis use may cause COPD, induce premalignant changes in the lungs and other organs, and accelerate coronary artery disease.[9] Currently there is little supportive evidence for the therapeutic use of smoked cannabis in the treatment of pain or other conditions, although controlled trials are underway.[10,11]

Hallucinogens such as LSD, mescaline, and "magic mushrooms" (psilocybin) cause perceptual distortions, hallucinations, and delusions. Long-term consequences include flashbacks and drug-induced psychosis. Dissociative anasthetics (PCP and ketamine, or special K) cause a dream-like state with out-of-body experiences and altered time sense. PCP can cause catatonia and other acute psychotic symptoms, delirium, violence, seizures, hypertension, and arrhythmias. High doses of ketamine cause coma and respiratory depression, especially when mixed with alcohol and other sedatives. Inhalants include glue, gasoline, and varnish remover. Inhalant abuse is more common among disadvantaged youth. Intoxication, withdrawal, and long-term neurological deficits are similar to alcohol, with cerebellar ataxia, memory impairment, and peripheral neuropathy.

Sedatives

Gamma hydroxybutyrate (GHB) is an illicit "club drug," and barbiturates are contained in prescribed medications such as Fiorinal (butalbital and ASA). Both GHB and barbiturates cause disinhibition and euphoria, similar to alcohol. They have a narrow margin of safety, and coma ensues with an excessive dose or when mixed with alcohol. Withdrawal is similar to alcohol but more prolonged (5 to 15 days), characterized by tremor, seizures, hallucinations, paranoia, and delirium.[12] Phenobarbital is the treatment of choice. Antihistamines such as dimenhydrinate cause sedation at therapeutic doses, and hallucinations, delusions, and confusion at high doses. A mild withdrawal (nausea and anxiety) can accompany regular use.

Anabolic steroids

These are used by athletes and by young men to enhance body image. Acute and chronic psychiatric effects include "steroid rage," depression, hypomania, suicidal ideation, and psychosis. Steroid withdrawal consists of fatigue, depression, and craving. Steroids have a variety of hormonal effects, including irregular menses, acne, hirsutism, gynecomastia, testicular atrophy, and premature closure of the epiphysis. Their use has been associated with hepatocellular carcinoma and cardiovascular events. Steroid use can sometimes be detected through decreased serum testosterone levels, and elevated ALT and creatinine phosphokinase (CPK).

Identification and Management
Identification

While screening can be helpful, cases are usually identified by taking a drug history with possible drug-related presentations. Both adolescents and adults should be asked, because many adults are regular users of certain drug classes such as cannabis and cocaine.

Common presentations of drug use
1. Psychiatric (depression, anxiety, insomnia, psychosis): cannabis, cocaine and amphetamines, and hallucinogens are implicated in substance-induced disorders.
2. Infections (due to injection drug use): cellulitis, abscess, hepatitis C, HIV
3. Trauma (accidents, violence, suicide)
4. Social: deterioration in social functioning, family violence
5. Other: weight loss (especially with cocaine use), loss of libido, irregular menstrual cycles

Management

Treatment is the same as that for alcohol: motivational interviewing, self-help groups such as Narcotics Anonymous, and inpatient and outpatient treatment programs. The management of substance-induced depression is similar to that of alcohol-induced depression. Substance-induced psychotic disorders respond to support, follow-up, and antipsychotic medication.

───────────── ❧ REFERENCES ❧ ─────────────

1. Gouzoulis-Mayfrank E, Thimm B, Rezk M, et al: Memory impairment suggests hippocampal dysfunction in abstinent ecstasy users, *Prog Neuropsychopharmacol Biol Psychiatry* 27(5):819-827, 2003.
2. Vecellio M, Schopper C, Modestin J: Neuropsychiatric consequences (atypical psychosis and complex-partial seizures) of ecstasy use: possible evidence for toxicity-vulnerability predictors and implications for preventative and clinical care, *J Psychopharmacol* 17(3):342-345, 2003.
3. Dennis M, Babor TF, Roebuck MC, et al: *Changing the focus: the case for recognizing and treating cannabis use disorders, Addiction* 97 Suppl 1: 4-15, 2002.

4. Basu D, Malhotra A, Bhagat A, et al: Cannabis psychosis and acute schizophrenia: a case-control study from India, *Eur Addict Res* 5(2):71-73, 1999.

5. Caspari D: Cannabis and schizophrenia: results of a follow-up study, *Eur Arch Psychiatry Clin Neurosci* 249(1): 45-49, 1999.

6. Hambrecht M, Hafner H: Cannabis, vulnerability, and the onset of schizophrenia: an epidemiological perspective [In Process Citation], *Aust N Z J Psychiatry* 34(3):468-475, 2000.

7. Fergusson DM, Horwood LJ, Swain-Campbell N: Cannabis use and psychosocial adjustment in adolescence and young adulthood, *Addiction* 97(9):1123-1135, 2002.

8. Fergusson DM, Horwood LJ, Swain-Campbell NR: Cannabis dependence and psychotic symptoms in young people, *Psychol Med* 33(1):15-21, 2003.

9. Henry JA, Oldfield WL, Kon OM: Comparing cannabis with tobacco, *Br Med J* 326(7396):942-943, 2003.

10. Watson SJ, Benson JA Jr., Joy JE: Marijuana and medicine: assessing the science base: a summary of the 1999 Institute of Medicine report, *Arch Gen Psychiatry* 57(6):547-552, 2000.

11. Campbell FA, Tramer MR, Carroll D, et al: Are cannabinoids an effective and safe treatment option in the management of pain? A qualitative systematic review, *Br Med J* 323(7303):13-16, 2001.

12. Dyer JE, Roth B, Hyma BA: Gamma-hydroxybutyrate withdrawal syndrome, *Ann Emerg Med* 37(2):147-153, 2001.

PROCESS ADDICTIONS

Process addictions include gambling, compulsive sexual behaviours, and overeating. Pathological gambling, the most studied of the process addictions, is on the increase throughout the world.[1,2] It shares some of the clinical features of substance dependence, such as continued use despite knowledge of consequences and preoccupation with use. Gamblers have a high prevalence of concurrent substance use, anxiety disorders, and suicide attempts.[3-5] Evidence suggests that gamblers respond to cognitive-based treatment interventions.[6] Preliminary studies suggest that pharmacotherapy may be effective.[7] The role of physicians in identifying and managing gambling requires further study.[2] Physicians should inquire about gambling in patients who present with substance abuse, depression, suicide attempts, or social and family dysfunction.

◢ REFERENCES ◣

1. Miller MM: Medical approaches to gambling issues—I: The medical condition, *Wis Med J* 95(9):623-634, 1996.

2. Potenza MN, Fiellin DA, Heninger GR, et al: Gambling: an addictive behavior with health and primary care implications, *J Gen Intern Med* 17(9):721-732, 2002.

3. Kausch O: Patterns of substance abuse among treatment-seeking pathological gamblers, *J Subst Abuse Treat* 25(4): 263-270 2003.

4. Rodda S, Brown SL, Phillips JG: The relationship between anxiety, smoking, and gambling in electronic gaming machine players, *J Gambl Stud* 20(1):71-81, 2004.

5. Kausch O: Suicide attempts among veterans seeking treatment for pathological gambling, *J Clin Psychiatry* 64(9): 1031-1038, 2003.

6. Toneatto T, Ladoceur R: Treatment of pathological gambling: a critical review of the literature, *Psychol Addict Behav* 17(4):284-292, 2003.

7. Grant JE, Kim SW, Potenza MN, et al: Paroxetine treatment of pathological gambling: a multi-centre randomized controlled trial, *Int Clin Psychopharmacol* 18(4):243-249, 2003.

SMOKING

Detrimental Effects of Smoking

(See also smoking in pregnancy)

Cigarette smoking

Smoking contributes to increased mortality rates from multiple causes. McGinnis and colleagues[1] estimate that smoking accounts for 19% of U.S. deaths, which puts it ahead of all other causes of preventable deaths. Diet and activity patterns are second, accounting for 14% of deaths.[1] In a 40-year study of British physicians, the excess total mortality of continuing smokers between the ages of 45 and 64 was three times that of non-smokers, while for continuing smokers aged 65 to 84 it was twice that of non-smokers. The authors of this study concluded that half of all regular smokers are likely to die from their habit.[2] Extrapolating from a 15-year follow-up of the British Regional Heart Study, Phillips and colleagues[3] concluded that only 42% of 20-year-old smokers who continued to smoke all their lives would still be alive by age 73 compared with 78% of 20-year-old non-smokers who never took up the habit.

Observational studies have shown that mortality rates gradually decrease in smokers who quit and that by 20 years, rates approach those of people who have never smoked. Little if any benefit is observed in the first 5 years after quitting, probably because many smokers who stop do so when they become ill.[4]

In the United States, smoking is responsible for about 30% of all cancer deaths. The overall cancer death rate in smokers is twice that of non-smokers, and the cancer death rate for heavy smokers is four times that of non-smokers. Cancers related to smoking include those of the lung, oral cavity, larynx, esophagus, stomach, pancreas, colon, uterine cervix, bladder, ureter and kidney, and breast. In addition, about 14% of leukemias are thought to be caused by smoking.[5]

Cardiovascular diseases associated with smoking are coronary artery disease, myocardial infarction, sudden death, strokes, subarachnoid hemorrhages, peripheral vascular disease, and aortic aneurysms. Smoking is known to decrease the oxygen-carrying power of the blood because of carbon monoxide production, to activate platelets, and to foster the development of atherosclerosis.[5]

In adults, respiratory diseases caused by smoking include lung cancer, chronic obstructive pulmonary disease (COPD), and pneumonia. Smokers have an increased death rate from influenza.[5] Smoking even as few as five cigarettes a day in adolescence diminishes the normal growth of lung function, particularly in girls.[6]

Smoking during pregnancy is associated with intrauterine growth retardation, low-birth-weight infants, preterm births, placenta previa, abruptio placentae, and a higher incidence of miscarriages of viable infants.[7] Maternal smoking may also be a risk factor for conduct disorder in male offspring and substance abuse in female offspring.[8] Smokers have been reported to have a lower fertility rate than non-smokers,[9] and smokers are more likely to suffer from menopausal hot flashes than are non-smokers.[10]

Smoking has been found to increase the risk of acquiring type 2 diabetes.[11] It also adversely affects thyroid function.[12,13] Smoking is associated with an increased incidence of Graves' disease and even more so with Graves' ophthalmopathy[12] and may also be a contributing factor to the development of subclinical hypothyroidism even if it does not aggravate the clinical manifestations.[13]

Smoking is associated with numerous other maladies. The relapse rate of Crohn's disease is greater in smokers than non-smokers.[14] The risk of age-related macular degeneration is increased in both male[15] and female[16] smokers, and it is likely that smoking is also a risk factor for cataracts.[17] Snoring[18] and hearing loss are more common in smokers than non-smokers.[19] Sun-exposed smokers have a higher incidence of wrinkles and skin cancers than sun-exposed non-smokers.[20] Smokers are at increased risk for periodontal disease.[21] Cigarettes are the leading cause of fire fatalities,[22] smokers are more likely than non-smokers to develop Alzheimer's disease,[23] smokers who are involved in heavy physical work have more low back pain than non-smokers involved in similar activities,[24] and some studies have shown an association between smoking and rheumatoid arthritis.[25]

Passive smoking

Children exposed to passive smoke have a higher incidence of asthma, bronchitis, pneumonia, middle ear effusions, tonsillectomies, adenoidectomies, and deaths (usually from lower respiratory tract infections or fires).[26] They also have an increased rate of respiratory complications after anesthesia.[27] Infants exposed to cigarette smoke have an increased risk of sudden infant death syndrome (SIDS),[28] and exposure of pregnant women to cigarette smoke correlates with an increased risk of fetal growth retardation.[29] Non-smokers exposed to second-hand smoke have an increased incidence of both fatal and non-fatal cardiac events,[30] strokes,[31] lung cancer,[32] breast cancer,[33] and hearing loss.[19]

Pipe and cigar smoking

Regular cigar smokers have a moderately increased risk of coronary artery disease, COPD, and cancers of the oropharynx, nose, larynx, esophagus, and lung.[34] Although elevated, the mortality rates for ischemic heart disease, lung cancer, and COPD are lower among pipe and cigar smokers than among cigarette smokers. In part this is because the former smoke less tobacco and in part because they tend to inhale less. Cigarette smokers who switch to cigars or pipes achieve a decreased mortality rate for these diseases, but to a lesser degree than cigar and pipe smokers who have never smoked cigarettes. This is probably because those who switch inhale more.[35]

--------------------   **REFERENCES**   --------------------

1. McGinnis JM, Foege WH: Actual causes of death in the United States, *JAMA* 270:2207-2211, 1993.
2. Doll R, Peto R, Wheatley K, et al: Mortality in relation to smoking: 40 years' observations on male British doctors, *BMJ* 309:901-911, 1994.
3. Phillips AN, Wannamethee SG, Walker M, et al: Life expectancy in men who have never smoked and those who have smoked continuously: 15 year follow up of large cohort of middle-aged British men, *BMJ* 313:907-908, 1996.
4. Enstrom JE, Heath CW Jr: Smoking cessation and mortality trends among 118,000 Californians, 1960-1997, *Epidemiology* 10:500-512, 1999.
5. Bartecchi CE, MacKenzie TD, Schrier RW: The human costs of tobacco use (first of two parts), *N Engl J Med* 330:907-912, 1994.
6. Gold DR, Wang X, Wypij D, et al: Effects of cigarette smoking on lung function in adolescent boys and girls, *N Engl J Med* 335:931-937, 1996.
7. Brosky G: Why do pregnant women smoke and can we help them quit? (editorial), *Can Med Assoc J* 152:163-166, 1995.
8. Weissman MM, Warner V, Wickramaratne PJ, et al: Maternal smoking during pregnancy and psychopathology in offspring followed to adulthood, *J Am Acad Child Adolesc Psychiatry* 38:892-899, 1999.
9. Bolumar F, Olsen J, Boldsen J (European Study Group on Infertility and Subfecundity): Smoking reduces fecundity: a European multicenter study on infertility and subfecundity, *Am J Epidemiol* 143:578-587, 1996.
10. Staropoli CA, Flaws JA, Bush TL, et al: Predictors of menopausal hot flashes, *J Women's Health* 7:1149-1155, 1998.

11. Rimm EB, Chan J, Stampfer MJ, et al: Prospective study of cigarette smoking, alcohol use, and the risk of diabetes in men, *BMJ* 210:545-546, 1995.

12. Prummel MF, Wiersinga WM: Smoking and risk of Graves' disease, *JAMA* 269:479-482, 1993.

13. Müller B, Zulewski H, Huber P, et al: Impaired action of thyroid hormone associated with smoking in women with hypothyroidism, *N Engl J Med* 333:964-969, 1995.

14. Timmer A, Sutherland LR, Martin F (Canadian Mesalamine for Remission of Crohn's Disease Study Group): Oral contraceptive use and smoking are risk factors for re-lapse in Crohn's disease, *Gastroenterology* 114: 1143-1150, 1998.

15. Christen WG, Glynn RJ, Manson JE, et al: A prospective study of cigarette smoking and risk of age-related macular degeneration in men, *JAMA* 276:1147-1151, 1996.

16. Seddon JM, Willett WC, Speizer FE, et al: A prospective study of cigarette smoking and age-related macular degeneration in women, *JAMA* 276:1141-1146, 1996.

17. West S: Does smoke get in your eyes? (editorial), *JAMA* 268: 1025-1026, 1992.

18. Lindberg E, Taube A, Janson C, et al: A 10-year follow-up of snoring in men, *Chest* 114:1048-1055, 1998.

19. Cruickshanks KJ, Klein R, Klein BE, et al: Cigarette smoking and hearing loss: the Epidemiology of Hearing Loss Study, *JAMA* 279:1715-1719, 1998.

20. Gilchrest BA: A review of skin ageing and its medical therapy, *Br J Dermatol* 135:867-875, 1996.

21. Watts TL: Periodontitis for medical practitioners, *BMJ* 316: 993-996, 1998.

22. McGuire A: Cigarettes and fire deaths, *NY State J Med* 83: 1296-1298, 1983.

23. Ott A, Slooter AJ, Hofman A, et al: Smoking and risk of dementia and Alzheimer's disease in a population-based cohort study: the Rotterdam Study, *Lancet* 351:1840-1843, 1998.

24. Eriksen W, Natvig B, Bruusgaard D: Smoking, heavy physical work and low back pain: a four-year prospective study, *Occup Med* 49:155-160, 1999.

25. Karlson EW, Lee I-M, Cook NR, et al: A retrospective cohort study of cigarette smoking and risk of rheumatoid arthritis in female health professionals, *Arthritis Rheum* 42:910-917, 1999.

26. Difranza JR, Lew RA: Morbidity and mortality in children associated with the use of tobacco products by other people, *Pediatrics* 97:560-668, 1996.

27. Skolnick ET, Vomvolakis MA, Buck KA, et al: Exposure to environmental tobacco smoke and the risk of adverse respiratory events in children receiving general anesthesia, *Anesthesiology* 88:1144-1153, 1998.

28. Klonoff-Cohen HS, Edelstein SL, Lefkowitz ES, et al: The effect of passive smoking and tobacco exposure through breast milk on sudden infant death syndrome, *JAMA* 273:795-798, 1995.

29. California Environmental Protection Agency, Office of Environmental Health Hazard Assessment: *Health effects of exposure to environmental tobacco smoke,* Sacramento, 1997, California Environmental Protection Agency. (http://www.calepa.cahwnet.gov/oehha/docs/finalets. htm).

30. He J, Vupputuri S, Allen K, et al: Passive smoking and the risk of coronary heart disease—a meta-analysis of epidemiologic studies, *N Engl J Med* 340:920-926, 1999.

31. You RX, Thrift AG, McNeil JJ, et al: Ischemic stroke risk and passive exposure to spouses' cigarette smoking, *Am J Public Health* 89:572-575, 1999.

32. Hackshaw AK, Law MR, Wald NJ: The accumulated evidence on lung cancer and environmental tobacco smoke, *BMJ* 315: 980-988, 1997.

33. Lash TL, Aschengrau A: Active and passive cigarette smoking and the occurrence of breast cancer, *Am J Epidemiol* 149:5-12, 1999.

34. Iribarren C, Tekawa I, Sidney S, et al: Effect of cigar smoking on the risk of cardiovascular disease, chronic obstructive pulmonary disease, and cancer in men, *N Engl J Med* 340:1773-1780, 1999.

35. Wald NJ, Watt HC: Prospective study of effect of switching from cigarettes to pipes or cigars on mortality from three smoking related diseases, *BMJ* 314:1860-1863, 1997.

Epidemiology

(See also detrimental effects of alcohol)

The prevalence of smoking in developed countries is declining. However, in the United States, cigarette smoking still kills at least 440,000 annually and costs $157 billion in direct health care costs. Currently, 22.8% of Americans are smokers.[1]

The highest rates of smoking in 1992 to 2001 were in the 18- to 24-year-old group (26.9%) and the 25- to 44-year-old group (31.258%) and among those below the poverty line (35.314%). Slightly more men (29.252%) than women (25.207%) smoked, and smoking incidence declined with years of education.[1] Persons who had not started smoking during adolescence were unlikely ever to become smokers.[2] Rates of adolescent smoking have increased significantly in the 1990s. A study of U.S. college students found that the prevalence of smoking was 22.3% in 1993 and 28.5% in 1997; one fourth of these smokers began to smoke regularly after they entered college.[3]

According to the Canadian Tobacco Use Monitoring Survey,[5] 20% of Canadians are smokers. Smoking is concentrated in lower socio-economic strata of society. The rate for male-dominated, outdoor, blue-collar occupations is 43%, whereas for white-collar workers it is 18%.[4] Among workers who were ill or on disability, the rate was 52%.[4]

Although overall smoking rates have fallen in the already developed world, they have been increasing in the developing world and represent a major public health problem in these regions. For example, in Shanghai, China, 63% of males and 4% of females smoke; most smokers spend a quarter of their income on cigarettes.[5] Physicians in China are heavy smokers as well; in a 1989 survey in Beijing, 68% were found to smoke.[6]

At present, smoking accounts for an estimated 4 million deaths a year split evenly between rich and poor countries. If current patterns of smoking persist, by the year 2030, smoking will be responsible for 10 million deaths annually, 70% of which will be in developing countries.[7] Because alcohol abusers tend to be heavy smokers,[8,9] a history of heavy smoking may alert the clinician to unacknowledged alcohol abuse.[9]

Increases in the price of cigarettes are associated with a decreased prevalence of smoking, particularly among the young, the poor, and members of minority groups.[10]

≈ REFERENCES ≈

1. Centers for Disease Control and Prevention (CDC): Cigarette smoking among adults—United States, 2001, *MMWR* 52:953-956, 2003.
2. Centers for Disease Control and Prevention (CDC): Cigarette smoking among adults—United States, 1992, and changes in the definition of current cigarette smoking, *MMWR* 43:342-346, 1994.
3. Department of Health and Human Services: *Preventing tobacco use among young people: a report of the Surgeon General,* Washington, DC, 1994, U.S. Government Printing Office, 5, 58.
4. Wechsler H, Rigotti NA, Gledhill-Hoyt J, et al: Increased levels of cigarette use among college students: a cause for national concern, *JAMA* 280:1673-1678, 1998.
5. CTUMS 2002: Summary of Results for 2002 (February to December), vol 2003, Health Canada Tobacco Control Programme, 2002.
6. Buske L: Smoking: an occupational hazard, *Can Med Assoc J* 160:630, 1999.
7. Yang G, Fan L, Tan J, et al: Smoking in China: findings of the 1996 National Prevalence Survey, *JAMA* 282:1247-1253, 1999.
8. Skolnick AA: Answer sought for "tobacco giant" China's problem, *JAMA* 275:1220-1221, 1996.
9. Lopez AD: Counting the dead in China: measuring tobacco's impact in the developing world (editorial), *BMJ* 317:1399-1400, 1998.
10. Hurt RD, Offord KP, Croghan IT, et al: Mortality following inpatient addictions treatment: role of tobacco use in a community-based cohort, *JAMA* 275:1097-1103, 1996.
11. Valiant GE, Schnurr PP, Baron JA, et al: A prospective study of the effects of cigarette smoking and alcohol abuse on mortality, *J Gen Intern Med* 6:299-304, 1991.
12. Centers for Disease Control and Prevention: Response to increases in cigarette prices by race/ethnicity, income, and age groups–United States, 1976-1993, *JAMA* 280: 1979-1980, 1998.

Brief Interventions for Smoking Cessation
(See also prevention; ulcerative colitis, enhancing motivation, stages of change)

Quitting smoking is a process, not an event. It is important to remain optimistic with patients and to provide encouragement and support to the smoker who wants to quit. Guidelines based on an extensive literature review have been developed by the U.S. Agency for Health Care Policy and Research (AHCPR).[1] At every visit, the smoking status of every patient should be determined, and all smokers should be assessed in terms of their desire to quit. Patients go through several stages to make lifestyle changes such as quitting smoking, and it is important for the physician to respond to the stage the patient is in (see discussion below on Stages of Change).[2]

The 5 As should be followed:
- *Ask* all smokers about their smoking status and interest in quitting smoking.
- *Advise* all smokers to quit smoking and that you can help.
- *Assess* their readiness to change.
- *Assist* them according to their readiness.
- *Advocate* for decreased rates of smoking in society (i.e., smoke-free bylaws and taxation).

For smokers who do not plan to quit, an attempt should be made to motivate them to do so, and for those who want to quit, a detailed plan should be worked out.

A brief intervention consists of the 5 Rs:
- Explore the *relevance* of smoking and smoking cessation with the patient.
- Then have the patient examine the *risks* and *rewards* of smoking cessation and continued smoking.
- Help them brainstorm for solutions to the *roadblocks* that prevent them from stopping smoking.
- Then use *repetition* to help them stay in the process of quitting smoking.

Education of smokers regarding the health effects of tobacco use is a first step in increasing motivation.

For highly motivated smokers (i.e., those interested in quitting within 30 days), 5 key factors are associated with successful quitting:
- Setting a quit date
- Getting professional help
- Enlisting social support
- Using pharmacotherapy appropriately
- Planning for high-risk situations and developing options to cope with cravings

Several studies have clearly demonstrated that the rate of quitting is increased by psychosocial interventions. Research has demonstrated that a dose-response relationship exists between the dose and intensity of counselling and smoking cessation; pharmacotherapy doubles the chances of a successful quit attempt. This base rate can be doubled by adding pharmacotherapy in the form of either nicotine replacement or antidepressants. Psychosocial therapy may be effectively given face to face or over the telephone. State or provincial "quit lines" are free to all smokers interested in the quitting process, and demonstrate 6-month quit rates of 13%.

Because the chances of stopping smoking are greatly increased by pharmacotherapy (nicotine replacement therapy or antidepressants), some experts in the field recommend that this treatment option be offered to all smokers.[3] However, most randomized controlled trials have been done in those who smoke greater than 10 cigarettes per day.

A systematic review of 188 randomized controlled trials of smoking cessation found that personal advice from a physician during a single consultation resulted in a 2% success rate measured 1 year later. Additional support such as follow-up letters or visits had a positive but variable benefit. Patients at high risk (pregnant patients and those with coronary artery disease) had a cessation rate of about 8%. Behaviour modification techniques in individual or group sessions with a psychologist had a 2% success rate. No data were given for hypnosis, and acupuncture was ineffective. Nicotine replacement therapy led to a 13% success rate.[4]

Two major factors that predict success in quitting are low nicotine dependence and successful abstinence during the first 2 weeks after quitting. One study has even shown that success on the first day of quitting correlates with improved long-term success.[4] Another important variable is patient age; individuals over age 30 are more likely to succeed in quitting than are younger individuals.[5]

Pharmacotherapy

A 4- to 5-year follow-up study of heavy smokers (20 or more cigarettes a day) randomly assigned to 21-, 14-, or 7-mg nicotine patches or placebo patches reported continuous abstinence rates of 20%, 10%, 12%, and 7%, respectively.[6] Regardless of initial treatment, individuals in this trial who were still abstaining at 1 year were unlikely to relapse. Combinations of patches and gum[1] or of patches and nasal spray may also be used. In one trial the abstinence rates among patients who used the patch for 5 months and the spray for 1 year were 27% at 1 year and 16% at 6 years, whereas the rates for the control subjects who used a patch plus placebo spray were 11% and 9%, respectively. Nicotine patches release the drug slowly, and blood levels approximate the trough levels found in smokers. Addition of nicotine nasal spray, gum, or inhalers to patches gives more rapid peaks of nicotine that are similar to those experienced by smokers.[7]

A common consequence of quitting smoking is weight gain. In one study the average excess weight gain at 10 years among persons who had quit smoking compared with control subjects who had never smoked was 4.4 kg (10 lb) for men and 5 kg (11 lb) for women.[5] Among heavy smokers who were evaluated 4 to 5 years after quitting with the help of nicotine patches or placebo, mean weight gain was 10 kg (22 lb) for men and 8 kg (18 lb) for women. Maximum weight gain was 24 kg (53 lb), but 7% of patients actually lost weight.[5] Weight gain may be less in patients taking bupropion (see below).

Increased anxiety is often given as a rationale for not quitting smoking. In fact, after the first week since quitting, anxiety levels tend to decrease.[8]

If all endeavors to give up smoking fail, encouraging the patient to switch to cigars or pipes might be worthwhile. (See discussion of detrimental effects of smoking.)[9] If it appears that the smoker is unable or unwilling to quit, the use of medicinal nicotine (long-term nicotine replacement therapy [NRT]) may be a safer option since the smoker will not be exposed to all the chemicals and carcinogens in smoke. The long-term benefits of this approach have not been studied.

The biggest fraud perpetuated by the tobacco industry under the guise of harm reduction was the introduction of filters and then marketing the concept of light and mild cigarettes. It has been clearly demonstrated that smokers who switch to light and mild cigarettes compensate by smoking more, inhaling more frequently and deeply, and by blocking the vent holes in the filter that are conveniently located where smokers place their lips or fingers while inhaling.[10,11]

One hypothesis to explain why smokers enjoy smoking is that nicotine stimulates the release of dopamine in the brain, and this neurotransmitter then leads to "feeling good" after smoking a cigarette. Other investigations suggest that the brains of smokers have very low levels of monoamine oxidase B (MAO-B), which normally breaks down dopamine, and this too would contribute to the "good feeling" experienced by having a smoke.[12] By extrapolation, it is logical to think that quitting might be facilitated by antidepressants.

A 7-week course of sustained release bupropion (Zyban) in doses of either 150 mg once a day or 300 mg per day (150 mg twice daily) given to smokers with no history of depression resulted in abstinence rates at 1 year of 23% compared with 12% among control subjects. In this study, weight gain among abstainers was greatest for those taking a placebo and least for those taking 300 mg of bupropion daily.[13] Another study compared bupropion 150 mg twice daily, nicotine patch alone, nicotine patch plus bupropion 150 mg twice daily, and placebo over a 9-week period. At the end of 1 year, abstinence rates were 30% in the bupropion-only group, 36% in the bupropion-plus-patch group, and about 16% in the placebo- and patch-only groups.[14] Bupropion has been found effective in smokers not intending to quit[15] as well as those with COPD, cardiovascular disease and those who previously relapsed to smoking after NRT or bupropion.[16]

Nortriptyline (Aventyl, Pamelor) in doses of 50 to 100 mg per day has also been shown to increase abstinence rates among smokers with and without[13]a history of depression.

A relationship between smoking and depression is supported by the observation that smokers with a history of major depression have a high recurrence rate if they quit successfully. In a 3-month follow-up of 126 individuals who had quit smoking successfully, the incidence of major depression was 2% among those with no history of depression, 17% among those with a history of a single episode of depression, and 30% for those with a history of recurrent depressions.[17]

Formulations of nicotine replacement therapy

Nicotine replacement therapy is available in the form of 2- and 4-mg nicotine-containing chewing gum (Nicorette), nicotine-containing transdermal patches with various concentrations of nicotine (Habitrol, Nicoderm, and Nicotrol, and ProStep), and more recently a nicotine-containing nasal spray (Nicotrol nasal spray), Nicotine Lozenge (Commit), and a nicotine inhaler (Nicotrol Inhaler) (Table 42).

Nicotine chewing gum. Nicotine chewing gum is available in 2- and 4-mg formulations. The 2-mg formulation is recommended for those who smoke fewer than 25 cigarettes a day, and the 4-mg formulation is for those who smoke more. Scheduled dosage of one or two pieces of gum per hour gives better results than ad libitum usage. The usual manufacturer's recommendations are to use the gum for 6 weeks and then taper use over another 6 weeks. However, much longer usage has not been associated with an increase in adverse effects, and even use of the drug while the patient continues to smoke has not been associated with an increase in cardiovascular disease.[18] In Canada, the gum has an official indication for temporary abstinence.

Nicotine polacrilex should not be chewed like ordinary gum. The gum should be chewed a few times and then held in the mouth for a minute or so before repeating the cycle. This prevents nicotine rushes. Each piece should be used for about 30 minutes.

Nicotine patches (see Table 42). Nicotine patches are safe for patients with known stable coronary artery disease.[19] Patients smoking more than 10 cigarettes per day should be started on the highest dose patches, while those who smoke less may be started on midrange patches.

Patches should be applied to hairless areas of the skin, and the site changed daily to prevent irritation. Habitrol, Nicoderm, and ProStep are changed every 24 hours, whereas Nicotrol is applied first thing in the morning and removed at bedtime (16 hours of use). Nicotrol is not available in Canada.

Nicotine nasal spray. Nicotine nasal spray results in a more rapid rise in nicotine blood levels than is obtained with patches, gum, or an inhaler. The usual dose of the nicotine nasal spray (Nicotrol NS) is two activations in each nostril (a total of 4 mg) with a maximum of 5 doses an hour or 40 doses a day.

Nicotine inhaler. The nicotine inhaler looks like a cigarette. The patient inserts a 10-mg nicotine cartridge into the mouthpiece and puffs on it to obtain the nicotine. Taking 80 deep puffs over 20 minutes releases 4 mg of nicotine; of this amount, 2 mg is absorbed. The nicotine is deposited on and absorbed from the buccal mucosa (less than 5% reaches the lungs), and therefore the pharmacological effects are similar to those obtained from nicotine gum.

Table 42 Nicotine Replacement Therapy

Drug names	Drug concentrations
Nicotine Polacrilex Chewing Gum	
Nicorette	2 mg
Nicorette DS, Nicorette Plus	4 mg
Nicotine Transdermal Systems	
Habitrol	21, 14, 7 (mg absorbed/24 hr)
Nicoderm	21, 14, 7 (mg absorbed/24 hr)
Nicotrol	15, 10, 5 (mg absorbed/16 hr)
ProStep	22, 11 (mg absorbed/24 hr)
Nicotine Nasal Spray	
Nicotrol NS	0.5 mg per activation
Nicotine Inhaler	
Nicotrol Inhaler	2 mg absorbed from 80 deep inhalations over 20 minutes. *Note: nicotine is absorbed bucally, not in the lungs.*
Commit lozenge 2mg and 4mg	Absorbed buccally over 20 minutes

⊰ INTERNET SOURCES ⊱

http://www.quitnet.com
http://www.quitsmoking.about.com
http://www.gosmokefree.ca/cessation
http://www.surgeongenral.gov/tobacco/default.htm

⊰ REFERENCES ⊱

1. Fiore M, Bailey WC, Cohen SJ, et al: *Treating tobacco use and dependence: clinical practice guideline,* Rockville, Md, 2000, U.S. Department of Health and Human Services.
2. Law M, Tang JL: An analysis of the effectiveness of interventions intended to help people stop smoking, *Arch Intern Med* 155:1933-1941, 1995.
3. Prochaska JO: Why do we behave the way we do? *Can J Cardiol* 11(suppl A):20A-25A, 1995.
4. Westman EC, Behm FM, Simel DL, et al: Smoking behavior on the first 1997 day of a quit attempt predicts long-term abstinence, *Arch Intern Med* 157:335-340, 1997.
5. Flegal KM, Troiano RP, Pamuk ER, et al: The influence of smoking cessation on the prevalence of overweight in the United States, *N Engl J Med* 333:1165-1170, 1995.

6. Daughton DM, Fortmann SP, Glover ED, et al: The smoking cessation efficacy of varying doses of nicotine patch delivery systems 4-5 years post-quit day, *Prev Med* 28: 113-118, 1999.

7. Wald NJ, Watt HC: Prospective study of effect of switching from cigarettes to pipes or cigars on mortality from three smoking-related diseases, *BMJ* 314:1860-1863, 1997.

8. West R, Hajek P: What happens to anxiety levels on giving up smoking? *Am J Psychiatry* 154:1589-1592, 1997.

9. Hurt RD, Sachs DP, Glover ED, et al: A comparison of sustained-release bupropion and placebo for smoking cessation, *N Engl J Med* 337:1195-1202, 1997.

10. Kozlowski LT, O'Connor RJ: Cigarette filter ventilation is a defective design because of misleading taste, bigger puffs, and blocked vents, *Tob Control* 11 Suppl 1:I40-50, 2002.

11. Warner KE: Tobacco harm reduction: promise and perils, *Nicotine Tob Res* 4 Suppl 2:S61-71, 2002.

12. Hall SM, Reus VI, Munoz RF, et al: Nortriptyline and cognitive-behavioral therapy in the treatment of cigarette smoking, *Arch Gen Psychiatry* 55:683-690, 1998.

13. Prochazka AV, Weaver MJ, Keller RT, et al: A randomized trial of nortriptyline for smoking cessation, *Arch Intern Med* 158: 2035-2039, 1998.

14. Henningfield JE: Nicotine medications for smoking cessation, *N Engl J Med* 333:1196-1203, 1995.

15. Hatsukami DK, Rennard S, Patel MK, et al: Effects of sustained release buproprion among persons interested in reducing but not quitting smoking, *Am J Med* 116:151-157, 2004.

16. West R: Bupropion SR for smoking cessation, *Expert Opin Pharmacother* 4:533-540, 2003.

17. Covey LS, Glassmam AH, Stetner F: Major depression following smoking cessation, *Am J Psych* 154:263-265, 1997

18. Hughes JR, Goldstein MG, Hurt RD, et al: Recent advances in the pharmacotherapy of smoking, *JAMA* 281:72-76, 1999.

19. Joseph AM, Norman SM, Ferry FH, et al: The safety of transdermal nicotine as an aid to smoking cessation in patients with cardiac disease, *N Engl J Med* 335: 1792-1798, 1996.

Stages of Change Model
(See also enhancing motivation and changing behaviour)

Prochaska and DiClemente's transtheoretical model of the stages of change (SOC)[1] is familiar to most health care providers. In this model, behavioural change is seen as a process rather than an event—a process that can be broken down into discrete stages through which patients move in making changes in their lives. Originally applied to the process of smoking cessation, it has been incorporated into our way of conceptualizing any change of habitual behaviour.[2] Rather than seeing change as the only goal—quitting smoking, for example—it encourages health care professionals to tailor their interventions to the patient's stage of readiness. The initial goal in the SOC model is simply to move the patient to the next stage. The stages are as follows:

Precontemplation

At this stage patients are not actively considering change. They are not prepared to plan for change, often feel that they are unable to do so, and may rationalize their reluctance by concluding that the cons outweigh the pros. They are often in a state of denial. Interventions appropriate to this stage include:

1. Provide simple advice and information to change, relating the behaviour to current risks or health concerns.
2. Ask whether the patient would be interested in talking about the issue.
3. Offer support and assistance should the patient feel ready to change.

Contemplation

Patients are now considering changing their behaviour, but are not ready to do so. They have conflicting feelings and thoughts about making changes in their lives. This ambivalence is often uncomfortable. They may have low sense of self-confidence regarding accomplishing the task, which prevents them from making a commitment. Interventions could include:

1. Discuss fears, concerns, and potential roadblocks to change.
2. Ask the patient to identify potential risks and rewards associated with change.
3. Observation of patterns in the patient's behaviour (e.g., an eating diary).
4. Offer support and assistance should they feel ready to change.

Preparation

At this stage, patients are seriously considering changing, and are often willing to commit to starting the process. They are generally anxious about their ability to change. Interventions could include:

1. Suggest interrupting or altering current patterns in behaviour.
2. Suggest practicing small elements of the change.
3. Negotiate a change plan.
4. Offer, or refer for, ongoing support and assistance.

Action

This is the point at which observable change begins. While most of the published literature on lifestyle changes deals with this stage, very few patients are at this stage at any given time. This is the point at which nicotine patches are given or serious dieting or regular exercise begins. This stage lasts for several months, the length of time it is thought to take to incorporate a new pattern of behaviour into one's lifestyle. Interventions at this stage include:

1. Positive reinforcement and encouragement for any success achieved.
2. Problem solving regarding barriers or concerns that arise during the process.
3. Relapse prevention strategies for coping with slip-ups or full relapse, and for avoiding triggers to relapse.

Maintenance

This is the stage of continuing the new habit despite the trials and tribulations of life. Ongoing vigilance is continued, often forever. Interventions could include:
1. Encourage maintenance of social supports.
2. Offer assistance and ongoing support as needed.

Relapse

This is the stage of slipping back to one of the earlier stages in the process. Relapse is to some extent an inevitable part of the process in that most attempts at significant behavioural change involve relapse. Interventions could include:
1. Normalize the process, and reframe relapse as an experience from which to learn.
2. Assess where in the change process the patient has relapsed to, and retailor intervention to that stage.
3. Identify the events and thought processes that contributed to the relapse.
4. Offer assistance, referral, and ongoing support.

_____ ⧌ **REFERENCES** ⧍ _____

1. Prochaska JO, DiClemente CC, *The transtheoretical approach: crossing the traditional boundaries of change,* Malabar, Fl, 1984, Krieger.
2. Prochaska JO, et al: Stages of change and decisional balance for twelve problem behaviours, *Health Psychology* 13(1), 39-46, 1994.

Topics covered in this section

Aggression
Anxiety Disorders
Depression
Eating Disorders
Functional Somatic Syndromes
Insomnia (Sleep Disorders)
Mood Disorders
Personality Disorders
Psychotherapy
Schizophrenia

AGGRESSION

(See also abuse; conduct disorder; guns; personality disorders; suicide)

Traditionally high potency antipyschotics and/or short-acting benzodiazepines were used for the short-term management of aggression. However, intramuscular (IM) olanzapine has been shown to result in a greater reduction in acute agitation with fewer adverse events when compared with Haldol.[1] Lithium was one of the first non-sedating therapies used for aggression, making it useful for subacute and chronic treatment.[2] Beta blockers have also been shown to reduce aggressive behaviours in schizophrenic patients and in adults with organic brain injury.[2] More recently, many of the anticonvulsants are thought to help treat aggression by preventing over-stimulation of the brain.[2] Phenytoin was shown to reduce the frequency of impulsive-aggressive behaviours in a randomized controlled trail.[3] Valproate also reduces aggressive behaviours in psychiatric disorders such as conduct disorder[4] and cluster B personality disorders.[5,6] Carbamazepine may also have a role in reducing aggression in patients with head injuries.[2] Selective serotonin reuptake inhibitors (SSRIs)[7] and omega-3 fatty acids[8] can also help with aggression in Axis II disorders, such as borderline personality disorder. Aggression in children and adolescents can be managed with high doses of propranolol or valproate. Finally the atypical antipsychotics, such as risperadol, olanzepine, and clozapine are affective treatment modalities that have fewer extrapyramidal effects when compared with traditional antipsychotics.[2,10]

✒ REFERENCES ✒

1. Wright P, Birkett M, and David SR: Double blind, placebo-controlled comparison of intramuscular olanzapine and intramuscular haloperidol in the treatment of acute agitation in schizophrenia, *Am J Psychiatry* 158(7):1149-1151, 2001.
2. Swann AC: Neuroreceptor mechanisms of aggression and its treatment, *J Clin Psychiatry* 64 Suppl 4:26-35, 2003.
3. Stanford MS, et al: A double blind placebo-controlled crossover study of phenytoin in individuals with impulsive aggression, *Psychiatry Res* 103(2-3) 193-203, 2001.
4. Steiner H, et al: Divalproex sodium for the treatment of conduct disorder: a randomized controlled clinical trial, *J Clin Psychiatry* 64(10)1183-1191, 2003.
5. Hollander E, et al: Divalproex in the treatment of impulsive aggression: efficacy in cluster B personality disorders, N*europsychopharmacology* 28(6) 1186-1197, 2003.
6. Frankenburg FR, Zanarini MC: Divalproex sodium treatment of women with borderline personality disorder and bipolar II disorder: a double-blind placebo-controlled pilot study, *J Clin Psychiatry* 36(5) 442-446, 2002.
7. Kavoussi R, Coccaro E: Psychopharmacologic treatement of hostiliy and aggressive dosoders, *Pyschiatr Clin North Am* 5:53-67, 1998.
8. Zanarini MC, Frankenburg FR: Omega-3 fatty acid treatment of women with borderline personality disorder: a double-blind placebo-controlled pilot study, *Am J Psychiatry* 160(1):167-169, 2003
9. Goodnick PJ, Barrios CA: Use of olanzapine in non-psychotic psychiatric disorders, *Expert Opin Pharmacother* 2(4):667-680, 2001.
10. Brieden T, Ujeyl M, Naber D: Psychopharmacological treatment of aggression in schizophrenic patients, *Pharmacopsychiatry* 35(3):83-89, 2002.

ANXIETY DISORDERS

(See also alcohol; chest pain; depression; fibromyalgia; insomnia; motor vehicle accidents; palpitations; serotonin syndrome, Tourette's syndrome)

Classification

The following conditions are included under the rubric of anxiety disorders:
1. Generalized anxiety disorder (GAD)
2. Panic disorder
3. Phobias (simple, social, agoraphobia)
4. Obsessive-compulsive disorder (OCD)
5. Post-traumatic stress disorder (PTSD)

Non-pharmacological Therapy

Discontinuing or at least decreasing central nervous system stimulants and depressants such as caffeine, alcohol, and hypnotic drugs is an essential initial step in treatment of anxiety disorders.[1] For some, a regular aerobic exercise program is beneficial.[2] Psychotherapy, alone or in combination with pharmacotherapy, is an important therapeutic strategy for all of the anxiety disorders.[3]

Cognitive behavioural therapy (CBT) has been scientifically tested and found to be effective in hundreds of clinical trials. CBT is based on the theory that the way a situation is perceived influences the emotions that we feel, and ultimately our behaviour. CBT helps individuals identify distressing thoughts and recognize distortions in their perceptions.

Medications

The drugs of choice are antidepressants (tricyclics, SSRIs, monoamine oxidase inhibitors (MAOIs), and perhaps buspirone (Table 43). All are at least as effective as benzodiazepines.[1,3-7]

Benzodiazepines may have a limited role in the treatment of anxiety disorders. Dependency and tolerance, with long-term use, are widely recognized potential adverse effects.

Imipramine (Tofranil) and other tricyclic antidepressants, including clomipramine (Anafranil), have been shown to be effective in panic disorders. Because initiation of treatment with this class of drugs is often associated with increased anxiety, the physician should start with low doses such as imipramine 10 mg per day and gradually increase the dose until symptoms are controlled. For some patients, a low dose is sufficient, whereas others may require the full therapeutic dose as used for depression. Clomipramine is the tricyclic of choice for OCD. The dosage should not exceed 250 mg per day because of the risk for seizures.[3]

SSRIs are the pharmacological agents of choice for panic attacks, phobic disorders, OCD, and PTSD. In general, doses are low for phobic disorders and panic attacks and high for OCD.[3] A meta-analysis of the pharmacotherapy of panic disorder found that not only were SSRIs more effective than placebo, they were also more effective than imipramine (Tofranil) or alprazolam (Xanax).[4]

Table 43   Pharmacotherapy of Anxiety Disorders

Drugs	Usual Doses and Comments
Benzodiazepines	Addictive-dependency and tolerance can occur with long-term use; antidepressants preferable
Alprazolam (Xanax)	0.125-0.25 mg tid or qid
Clonazepam (Rivotril)	0.5 mg bid or tid
Diazepam (Valium)	2-10 mg bid-qid
Lorazepam (Ativan)	2-3 mg/day in 3 divided doses
Azapirones	
Buspirone (Buspar)	20-30 mg/day in 2 or 3 divided doses
Tricyclics	
Imipramine (Tofranil)	Panic and phobic disorder (low doses)
Desipramine (Norpramin, Pertofrane)	Panic and phobic disorder (low doses)
Nortriptyline (Aventyl)	Panic and phobic disorder (low doses)
Clomipramine (Anafranil)	OCD (high doses)
Selective Serotonin Reuptake Inhibitors	
Panic and phobic disorder (low doses); OCD (high doses)	
Citalopram (Celexa)	
Fluoxetine (Prozac)	
Fluvoxamine (Luvox)	
Paroxetine (Paxil)	
Sertraline (Zoloft)	
MAO Inhibitors	
Panic and phobic disorders	
Phenelzine (Nardil)	30 mg qam and 15-30 mg at noon
Tranylcypromine (Parnate)	20 mg qam and 10 mg in the afternoon
Azapirones	
Generalized anxiety disorder	
Buspirone (Buspar)	20-30 mg/day in 2 or 3 divided doses
Beta blockers	
Focused social phobias (performance anxiety)	
Atenolol (Tenormin)	Single dose; start low and increase prn
Nadolol (Corgard)	Single dose; start low and increase prn
Oxprenolol (Trasicor)	Single dose; start low and increase prn
Propranolol (Inderal)	Single dose; start low and increase prn

Although rarely used in primary care, the MAOIs phenelzine (Nardil) and tranylcypromine (Parnate) are effective in panic disorders and phobic disorders.[3] Buspirone (Buspar) is a member of a class of antianxiety agents that is not sedative, has little potential for abuse, and is not associated with withdrawal symptoms. Its primary use is for generalized anxiety disorder.[3,6]

Beta blockers are often useful for limited or focused social phobias (performance anxiety) such as may occur before making a speech, performing on a musical instrument, or taking an examination.[3,8,9] Positive results have been reported with single doses of atenolol (Tenormin) 100 mg, nadolol (Corgard) 40 mg, oxprenolol (Trasicor) 40 mg, and propranolol (Inderal) 40 mg.[8] Patients should take a test dose before any important performance to ensure that no unexpected adverse effects occur.[9]

As many as one third of patients on SSRIs develop sexual side effects after several weeks, particularly difficulty achieving orgasm and decreased libido. Buproprion (75 to 150 mg per day) or buspirone (10 to 20 mg twice daily) may reduce these effects.[10]

Generalized Anxiety Disorder (GAD)

The prevalence of GAD is estimated to be 5% of patients in the primary-care setting.[11] It is very often associated with other anxiety disorders, major depression, and substance abuse. One controlled study of patients with newly diagnosed GAD showed that 3 to 6 months of brief supportive counselling by family physicians had similar outcomes to physicians who used benzodiazepines.[12] But several placebo-controlled trials have demonstrated the efficacy of antidepressants for GAD. Effective medications include venlafaxine, imipramine, and trazodone. A review of the literature on GAD suggested that five patients would have to be treated with antidepressants to observe a positive effect.[13]

Obsessive-Compulsive Disorder (OCD)

The lifetime prevalence of OCD is 2% to 3%. It is the fourth most common psychiatric disorder after substance abuse, phobias, and affective disorders. It has a higher prevalence rate than panic disorders or schizophrenia. OCD often begins in childhood, and onset over the age of 40 is rare. Slightly more females than males are affected.[14] The natural history of untreated OCD is improvement in over 80% of cases. Even after several decades, however, only 20% of patients have made a complete recovery, and 28% have "recovered" but continue to have symptoms that do not cause distress or interfere with daily activities.[15]

CBT is almost always an essential component of the treatment of OCD, but medications also play an important role. Patients with OCD are often slow to respond to medications and may require larger doses of antidepres-

sants than are necessary for depression. Once these patients respond, they will probably require long-term or indefinite therapy because of the high relapse rate after discontinuation of medications.[3,16]

The tricyclic antidepressant clomipramine (Anafranil) has long been effective in the treatment of OCD, but SSRIs are equally effective and generally better tolerated. High doses and prolonged treatment are usually required; initial response to the drug may not be evident for up to 3 months. If a patient fails to respond to one SSRI, another should be tried.[3] Clomipramine,[17] fluoxetine,[17] and sertraline[18] have been shown effective in children and adolescents with OCD. The dosage range for fluoxetine in OCD is 20 to 80 mg per day, for fluvoxamine is 100 to 300 mg per day, and for sertraline is 50 to 200 mg per day. It is advisable to start with a low dose and, for non-responders, increase to the maximum dose over 6 to 8 weeks.[3]

Social Phobias

Social phobias are overwhelming irrational fears of being scrutinized or ridiculed by others.[7] Social phobias may be generalized or limited to specific events such as public speaking. Generalized social phobias are incapacitating because affected individuals fear being observed or evaluated by others in a wide range of circumstances. Phobic persons may avoid going to restaurants, have difficulty communicating with others at work or school, withdraw from most social activities, and in more advanced cases drop out of school or the workforce.[7,14]

Social phobia is the third most common psychiatric condition in the United States, exceeded only by major depression and substance abuse.[7,14] The point prevalence of the disorder is 4.5%, but few of those affected are identified by primary-care physicians.[14] Patients with generalized phobias do not voluntarily express their fears. To uncover the disease, the physician must ask specific questions about whether embarrassment or "fear of looking stupid" prevents socializing or other activities.[7] Social phobias almost always begin in adolescence; onset after age 25 is rare. Comorbid psychiatric disorders such as major depression, dysthymia, panic disorder, OCD, and alcohol and other substance abuse disorders are extremely common.[7,14] Some phobic patients use alcohol or other drugs to alleviate their anxieties; 16% are alcoholics.[7]

CBT and medications control social phobias. Effective drugs are MAOIs and SSRIs.[7,14] Paroxetine (Paxil)[14] and fluvoxamine (Luvox)[19] have been beneficial in multicentre randomized placebo-controlled trials. One small study found that when symptoms were controlled with daily fluoxetine (Prozac), remission could be maintained by once weekly doses because of the long half-life of the drug.[17] Tricyclics are not useful,[7] and benzodiazepines should not be used because of the high risk of addiction.[3,7,14]

Panic Disorder

Although benzodiazepines initially relieve symptoms, they are associated with a high incidence of withdrawal symptoms and relapse when discontinued. The drugs of choice for panic disorder are the SSRIs. If benzodiazepines have any role, it is only as very short-term bridge therapy until treatment with antidepressants begins. Alternatives to the SSRIs are tricyclic antidepressants, MAOIs, or in some cases, valproate.[3] Controlled trials have demonstrated that pharmacological treatment and CBT are equally effective in the treatment of panic disorder.[21]

Post-traumatic Stress Disorder (PTSD)

The widespread belief that the intensity and duration of trauma correlate with the frequency of subsequent PTSD may be incorrect. Major stresses are common, and PTSD is rare. More important, a dose-response curve cannot be shown. In many cases the trauma experienced by patients with PTSD is much less severe than that faced by others who did not have psychiatric sequelae. The risk for PTSD is determined predominantly by pre-existing personality traits, especially the tendency to respond to events with negative emotions.[22]

Survivors of the terrorist bombing that destroyed the Alfred P. Murrah Federal Building in Oklahoma City in April 1995 almost all had at least some symptoms characteristic of PTSD, most commonly difficulty concentrating, exaggerated startle response, intrusive memories, and insomnia. These symptoms alone do not fulfill the diagnostic criteria for PTSD and were rarely associated with functional impairment or other psychiatric disorders. Such symptoms are probably best considered a normal reaction to extreme stress and can be managed by education, general support, and reassurance. One third of the victims of the Oklahoma City bombing had PTSD; major risk factors were previous psychiatric disorders, severity of injuries, loss of loved ones, female sex, and pre-existing psychopathological conditions. The symptoms of PTSD came on within hours of the bombing, and in two thirds of those affected, other psychiatric disorders, usually depression, developed.[23] These findings are consistent with previous studies, which have found that most patients with PTSD suffer from other Axis I psychiatric disorders, most often depression, another anxiety disorder, or substance abuse.[24]

Teams of professionals are frequently mobilized to rush to disaster scenes and debrief surviving victims and their families with the hope that this will prevent PTSD. No well-designed controlled studies evaluating the efficacy of such an approach have been published.[22]

The natural history of PTSD is one of spontaneous improvement in most instances, and this makes therapeutic interventions difficult to evaluate unless adequate control subjects are available. Psychotherapy in which patients relive their experiences is not helpful, and in some studies has been found to be harmful. Behavioural and cognitive therapies have been effective in randomized trials.[25]

Few randomized trials of pharmacotherapy have been published. Results of open label trials (in which both patients and physicians are aware of the specific medications that are being taken) suggest that SSRIs, particularly fluvoxamine and sertraline,[26] decrease core symptoms such as numbing, avoidance, and hyperarousal, and some evidence suggests that clonidine (Catapres) ameliorates intrusive recollections, nightmares, hypervigilance, and outbursts of anger. Benzodiazepines decrease anxiety but have no beneficial effect on the core symptoms of PTSD. Because comorbid substance abuse is common, benzodiazepines should rarely be prescribed.[24]

≥ REFERENCES ≤

1. Antony MM, Swinson RP: *Anxiety disorders and their treatment: a critical review of the evidence-based literature,* Ottawa, 1996, Publications Health Canada, 1-101.
2. Petruzello SJ, Landers DM, Hatfield BD, et al: A meta-analysis on the anxiety-reducing effects of acute and chronic exercise, *Sports Med* 11:143-182, 1991.
3. Layton ME, Dager SR: Treatment of anxiety disorders, *Psychiatr Clin North Am* 5:183-209, 1998.
4. Boyer W: Serotonin uptake inhibitors are superior to imipramine and alprazolam in alleviating panic attacks: a meta-analysis, *Int Clin Psychopharmacol* 10:45-49, 1995.
5. Piccinelli M, Pini S, Bellantuono C, et al: Efficacy of drug treatment in obsessive-compulsive disorder: a meta-analytic review, *Br J Psychol* 166:424-443, 1995.
6. Cadieux RJ: Azapirones: an alternative to benzodiazepines for anxiety, *Am Fam Physician* 53:2349-2353, 1996.
7. Bruce TJ, Saeed SA: Social anxiety disorder: a common, under-recognized mental disorder, *Am Fam Physician* 60:2311-2322, 1999.
8. Jefferson JW: Social phobia: everyone's disorder? *J Clin Psychiatry* 57(suppl) 6:28-32, 1996.
9. Jefferson JW: Social phobia: a pharmacologic treatment overview, *J Clin Psychiatry* 56(suppl 5):18-24, 1995.
10. Ashton AK, Rosen RC: Buproprion as an antidote for SSRI induced sexual dysfunction, *J Clin Psych* 59:112, 1998.
11. Roy-Byrne PP, Katon W: Generalized anxiety disorder in primary care: the precursor/modifier pathway to increased health care utilization, *J Clin Psych* 58 (suppl) 3:34, 1998.
12. Catalan J, , *Br J Psych* 144:593, 1984.
13. Kapinski F, Lima MS, Souza JS, et al: Antidepressants for GAD, *Cochrane Database Syst Rev*, CD003592, 2003
14. Stein MB, Liebowitz MR, Lydiard B, et al: Paroxetine treatment of generalized social phobia (social anxiety disorder): a randomized controlled trial, *JAMA* 280:708-713, 1998.
15. Skoog G, Skoog I: A 40-year follow-up of patients with obsessive-compulsive disorder, *Arch Gen Psychiatry* 56:121-127, 1999.
16. Warneke L: Anxiety disorders: focus on obsessive-compulsive disorder, *Can Fam Physician* 39:1612-1621, 1993.

17. Heyman I: Children with obsessive-compulsive disorder should have access to specific psychopharmacological and behavioural treatments (editorial), *BMJ* 315:444, 1997.

18. March JS, Biederman J, Wolkow R: Sertraline in children and adolescents with obsessive-compulsive disorder: a multicenter randomized controlled trial, *JAMA* 280:1752-1756, 1998.

19. Stein MB, Fyer AJ, Davidson JR, et al: Fluvoxamine treatment of social phobia (social anxiety disorder): a double-blind, placebo-controlled study, *Am J Psychiatry* 156: 756-760, 1999.

20. Emmanuel NP, Ware MR, Brawman-Mintzer O, et al: Once-weekly dosing of fluoxetine in the maintenance of remission in panic disorder, *J Clin Psychiatry* 60:299-301, 1999.

21. Barlow DH, Gorman DM, Shear MK, et al: Cognitive behaviour therapy, Imiprimine, or their combination for panic disorder: a randomized trial, *JAMA* 283:2529, 2000.

22. Bowman ML: Individual differences in posttraumatic distress: problems with the DSM-IV model, *Can J Psychiatry* 44:21-33, 1999.

23. North CS, Nixon SJ, Shariat S, et al: Psychiatric disorders among survivors of the Oklahoma City bombing, *JAMA* 282: 755-762, 1999.

24. Friedman MJ: Current and future drug treatment for posttraumatic stress disorder patients, *Psychiatr Ann* 28:461-468, 1998.

25. Ehlers A, Clark DM, Hackman A, et al: A randomized controlled trial of cognitive therapy, a self-help booklet, and repeated assessments as early interventions for posttraumatic stress disorder, *Arch Gen Psych* 60:1024, 2003.

26. Brady K, Pearlstein SM, Tupler LA, et al: Efficacy and safety of sertraline treatment of posttraumatic stress disorder: a randomized controlled trial, *JAMA* 283:1837, 2000.

DEPRESSION

(See also an approach to complementary and alternative medicine; anxiety disorders; bipolar affective disorder; chest pain; cocaine; fibromyalgia; guns; insomnia; pre-menstrual dysphoric disorder; serotonin syndrome; sexual abuse; sexual dysfunction)

Depression is a common psychiatric disorder in children, adolescents, adults, and the elderly. Primary care physicians, not mental health professionals, treat the majority of patients who have symptoms of depression. Identifying patients with depression can be difficult in busy primary care settings where time is limited, but certain depression screening measures may help physicians diagnose the disorder. Patients who score above the pre-determined cut-off levels on the screening measures should be interviewed more specifically for a diagnosis of a depressive disorder and treated within the primary care physician's scope of practice or referred to a mental health subspecialist as clinically indicated. Targeted screening in high-risk patients such as those with chronic diseases, pain, unexplained symptoms, stressful home environments, or social isolation, and those who are post-natal or elderly may provide an alternative approach to identifying patients with depression.[1-5]

The 17-item Hamilton Depression Scale (HAM-D17) has been the criterion standard for objective measurement of depressive symptoms in mood disorders research (level I evidence). The clinical utility of the HAM-D17 is diminished somewhat by the length of time required to administer the interview and by the possible lack of inter-rater reliability. A truncated form of the HAM-D17 with cutoff scores for full remission is useful in family practice settings. On the basis of a sample of 292 patients with major depression who received standard clinical treatment at a university clinic, a 7-item rating scale was derived using the seven items with the greatest frequency and sensitivity to change with treatment (Table 44).

Major depressive disorder (MDD) is a prevalent, progressive, and often chronic disease. It is currently estimated to be the fourth leading cause of disability worldwide and is expected to rise to second behind ischemic heart disease by the year 2020.[1] Researchers estimate that up to 11% of global disability is attributable to depressive symptoms.[2] Frequent users of family physicians' services often manifest syndromal or subsyndromal symptoms of anxiety and depression. The most common ambulatory presentation of MDD is a confluence of anhedonia, non-specific somatic symptoms, and psychic anxiety.

Diagnosis of major depression requires five or more of the following: depressed mood, loss of pleasure and interest in activities, significant weight loss, insomnia or hypersomnia, agitation or retardation, fatigue or loss of energy, feelings of worthlessness or guilt, loss of concentration, recurrent thoughts of death or suicide (Table 45). These symptoms have been consistently present over a 2-week period and have caused significant distress and disturbance in function. For example, depressed individuals may experience interference with work and relationships. Patients who meet these criteria are likely to respond to medical treatment.[1,2] The above are primarily research criteria, and should not be interpreted too rigidly in practice. A patient may still respond to antidepressant treatment if some, but fewer than five, of the criteria are present. If in doubt, and there are no contraindications, it is reasonable to give a trial of antidepressants.[5]

Investigations fall into the following four categories:
- Routine laboratory investigations to exclude other diagnoses. Minimum routine investigations will include hematology, serum biochemistry, urinalysis, liver function tests, thyroid function tests, rhythm strip in patients over age 40. These tests are imperative in view of the high level of association of depression with physical illness (e.g., some 50% in older patients).
- Chest X-ray should be performed on patients who present with depression and unexplained weight loss, particularly in the elderly. Chest X-ray is not routinely performed on all depressed patients.

Table 44   The Ham-D-7 Depression Scale

Depressed mood (sadness, hopeless, helpless, worthless)
Have you been feeling down or depressed this past week? How often have you felt this way and for how long?
0. Absent
1. Indicated only on questioning
2. Spontaneously reported verbally
3. Communicated non-verbally (facial expression, posture, voice, weeping tendency)
4. Patient reports *virtually only* these feeling states in spontaneous verbal and non-verbal communication

Feelings of guilt (self-criticism, self-reproach)
In the past week, have you felt guilty about something you've done, or that you've let others down? Do you feel you're being punished for being sick?
0. Absent
1. Self-reproach (letting people down)
2. Ideas of guilt or ruminating about past errors or sinful deeds
3. Present illness is a punishment. Delusions of guilt
4. Hears accusatory or denunciatory voices or experiences threatening visual hallucinations

Interest, pleasure, level of activities (work and activities)
Are you as productive at work and at home as usual? Have you felt interested in doing the things that usually interest you?
0. No difficulty
1. Fatigue, weakness, or thoughts or feelings of incapacity (related to work, activities, hobbies)
2. Loss of interest (directly reported or indirectly through listlessness, indecision, and vacillation)
3. Decrease in actual time spent in activities or decrease in productivity. (In hospital, rate 3 if patient does not spend at least 3 hours daily in activities exclusive of ward chores.)
4. Stopped working due to current illness. (In hospital, rate 4 if patient only does ward chores or fails to perform ward chores unassisted.)

Tension, nervousness (psychic anxiety)
Have you been feeling more tense or nervous than usual? Have you been worrying a lot?
0. No difficulty
1. Subjective tension and irritability
2. Worrying about minor matters
3. Apprehensive attitude apparent in face or speech
4. Fears expressed without being questioned

Physical symptoms of anxiety (anxiety, somatic)
In this past week, have you had any of these symptoms? Gastrointestinal (dry mouth, wind, indigestion, diarrhea, cramps, belching); cardiovascular (palpitations, headaches); respiratory (hyperventilation, sighing); urinary frequency, sweating
NOTE: DO NOT RATE IF CLEARLY DUE TO MEDICATION
0. Absent
1. Mild
2. Moderate
3. Severe
4. Incapacitating

Energy level (somatic symptoms)
How has your energy been this past week? Have you felt tired? Have you had any aches or pains or felt any heaviness in your limbs, back, or head?
0. None
1. Heaviness in limbs, back, or head (backache, headache, muscle aches; loss of energy and fatigue)
2. Any clear-cut symptoms rate 2 points

Suicide (ideation, thoughts, plans, attempts)
Have you thought life is not worth living or you'd be better off dead? Have you thought of hurting or killing yourself? Have you done anything to hurt yourself?
0. Absent
1. Feels life is not worth living
2. Wishes to be dead (or any thoughts of possible death to self)
3. Suicidal ideas or gestures
4. Attempts at suicide (any serious attempt rates 4 points)

Total score (out of 26)
Depression severity
20+ Severe
12-20 Moderate

Table 44   The Ham-D-7 Depression Scale—cont'd

4-12 Mild
Score ≤3 Indicates full remission
Score ≥4 Indicates no or partial response
Adapted from McIntyre et al.21

A score of 3 or less on the HAM-D7 was found to correlate with the HAM-D17 definition of full remission. Sensitivity (95%), specificity (84%), and positive (94%) and negative (86%) predictive values of this relation were all high. The HAM-D7 takes only a few minutes to complete and could be efficient and practical for enhancing care of people suffering from MDD. There is no prescribed pattern for use of the HAM-D-7, but it is suggested to be used whenever clinical monitoring is required (i.e., 5 to 6 weeks after therapy when dose optimization is being considered) (level III evidence).
From Khullar A, McIntyre RS: *Can Fam Physician* 50:1374-1380, 2004. Reprinted with permission.

Table 45   Diagnostic Criteria for Major Depressive Disorder*

A. The patient has depressed mood (e.g., sad or empty feeling) or loss of interest or pleasure most of the time for 2 or more weeks plus 4 or more of the following symptoms

Sleep	Insomnia or hypersomnia nearly every day
Interest	Markedly diminished interest or pleasure in nearly all activities most of the time
Guilt	Excessive or inappropriate feelings of guilt or worthlessness most of the time
Energy	Loss of energy or fatigue most of the time
Concentration	Diminished ability to think or concentrate; indecisiveness most of the time
Appetite	Increase or decrease in appetite
Psychomotor	Observed psychomotor agitation/retardation
Suicide	Recurrent thoughts of death/suicidal ideation

B. The symptoms do not meet criteria for a mixed episode (major depressive episode and manic episode)
C. The symptoms cause clinically significant distress or impairment in social, occupational, or other important areas of functioning
D. The symptoms are not due to the direct physiological effects of a substance (e.g., a drug of abuse, a medication) or a general medical condition
E. The symptoms are not better accounted for by bereavement

*Adapted from the *Diagnostic and Statistical Manual of Mental Disorders*, 4th edition.[3]
Source: Remick RA, *Can Med Assoc J* 167(11), 2002. Reprinted with permission of the publisher. © 2002 Canadian Medical Association.

- Independent history from relatives/friends.
- Formal psychological testing as necessary.

Epidemiology and Contributing Factors

The incidence of depression is 4/1000 in the United States annually.[5] Reported prevalence of major depression at any given time is approximately 50/1000 of the U.S. population (6.4% of women and 3.2% of men). Prevalence is highest among the elderly, but varies greatly with circumstances, from 2.5% in elderly people with no social or physical problems to 15% if physical illness is present.[4] An additional peak occurs between ages 30 and 40 years. In recent years there has been an increase among subjects age 15 to 19 years. It is believed that this condition is significantly under diagnosed and under reported, and therefore the true incidence and prevalence of depression is significantly higher.[5,6]

Depression is traditionally more common in females, with a female:male ratio of about 2:1. However, depression has become more common among males over the past 20 years. Suicide is three times more common among men. (Women attempt more frequently, but men complete suicide at a higher rate.) Over age 55, the sex difference tends to reverse, with depression becoming more common in men. Prevalence is relatively consistent across races and cultures, although it is greater among recent immigrants and the displaced. The risk of a major depression increases 1.5 to 3.0 times if the illness is present in a first-degree relative as compared with no such illness in a first-degree relative. There is a consistent 10% risk for first-degree relatives of sufferers from major depression, independent of environmental influences, although no major gene locus has been identified. Evidence for inheritance of milder depression is weak, suggesting that environmental influences may be predominant. The incidence of smoking is much higher among individuals who have ever been depressed compared with those who have not, and the success rate in quitting among smokers who have ever been depressed is much lower than among those who have never been depressed.[7]

Depressive illnesses carry significant risks of death and disability. About 15% of patients with a mood disorder die by their own hand, and at least 66% of all suicides are preceded by depression. Rates of suicide in Canada are higher than those in the United States.[8]

Depressive disorders are associated with poor work productivity, as indicated by a threefold increase in the number of sick days in the month preceding the illness for workers with a depressive illness compared with co-workers who did not have such an illness. Depressive illnesses also affect family members and caregivers, and increasing evidence shows that children of women with depression have increased rates of problems in school and with behaviour, and have lower levels of social competence and self-esteem than their classmates with mothers who do not have depression. Depression is the leading cause of disability and premature death among people age 18 to 44 years, and it is expected to be the second leading cause of disability for people of all ages by 2020.[7]

Depressive illnesses have also been shown to be associated with increased rates of death and disability from cardiovascular disease.[7] Among 1551 study subjects without a history of heart disease who were followed for 13 years, the odds ratio for acute myocardial infarction among the subjects who had a major depressive episode was 4.5 times higher than among those who did not have a depressive episode.[9] Among consecutive patients admitted to hospital with an acute myocardial infarction who had their mood measured with a standard depression rating scale, even those with minimal symptoms of depression had evidence of higher subsequent risk of death following their infarction and over the next 4 months. This risk was independent of other major risk factors, including age, ventricular ejection fraction, and the presence of diabetes mellitus.

Depression has a number of contributory or predisposing factors, including older age, but with an additional peak among younger males[10]; physical illness, particularly if debilitating, painful, or life-threatening; multiple sclerosis, HIV/AIDS, and cancer carry especially high risks. Physical illness is the main precipitant of depression in later life.

Other contributing factors include:

- Some medically prescribed drugs (e.g., alpha-methyldopa [an antihypertensive], beta blockers, L-dopa)
- Drug and alcohol misuse   *Steroids*
- Stress, especially recent adverse events, notably divorce or marital adversity
- Vulnerability to adverse events is increased by social isolation and increasing age
- Poverty and unemployment
- Medical illness (e.g., hypothyroidism)

Rule Out Bipolar Disorder

Researchers estimate that up to 25% of people with anxious depression in primary care have bipolar disorder (BPD). Depression is also often the index presentation of bipolar illness, and people with BPD typically present to primary care physicians while experiencing depressive symptoms. Several variables that correlate to higher risk of subsequent bipolarity occur in depressive illness (Table 46). Bipolarity can be assessed easily in family practice settings with rating instruments, such as the MDQ.[11]

Table 46   Factors in Depressed Patients that Increase Suspicion of Past or Future Bipolarity[1]

Onset before age 25
Family history of bipolar illness
History of attention hyperactivity disorder
Pharmacological- or substance-induced mania or hypomania
Seasonal affective disorder
Post-partum depression or psychosis
Episodic comorbid anxiety disorder
Comorbid personality disorder (especially borderline)
Hypersomnia
Substance abuse

From Khullar A, McIntyre RS: *Can Fam Physician* 50:1374-1380, 2004. Reprinted with permission.

Unexplained Medical Symptoms and Frequent Medical Visits

Primary care physicians commonly see depression manifested as physical symptoms, especially when anxiety is also present. One recent trial in a health maintenance organization in the United States screened 7203 patients who heavily used medical care for depression; 20% were found to have a current major depression or major depression in partial remission. In a year, these depressed patients had significantly higher numbers of office visits and days in the hospital than did patients without depression.[12] An international study has also confirmed the relationship between somatic symptoms and depression.[13]

One of the challenges for family physicians is to convert patients to the idea that physical symptoms may have a mental source. One useful practice pearl is to tell patients at the beginning of a medical workup that up to one third of problems seen in family medicine are caused by mental health disorders (a good example is a tension headache or "butterflies") but that the physician will begin by ruling out important physical causes. This gets the possibility of a mental health issue on the table early rather than backing into it. Another approach is to devote one clinical visit to a walk-through diagnostic aid (e.g., the Hamilton Depression Rating Scale). Having an objective score may make the diagnosis more meaningful to patients, as well as further delineate their condition.

Suicide

Some 15% of depression sufferers ultimately commit suicide.[14] Of those who commit suicide, over 60% have consulted their primary care physician within the preceding 6 weeks. Suicidal tendency should be assessed by direct inquiry. Check for serious physical illnesses, which may underlie or mimic depression. In older people, about 50% of depression is associated with physical illness. Check for evidence of severe self-neglect, especially of potential starvation in the elderly. Check for alcohol misuse or drug misuse, both common and hazardous complications of depression. It is important to distinguish bipolar disorder from depression since the therapeutic approach is different.[15]

Although the highest suicide rate is found among men over the age of 69, the incidence of suicide among the young has been increasing in the Western world. This is particularly marked among Aboriginal peoples.[16] The availability of guns appears to increase the risk of suicide. (See discussion of guns.) Over 90% of people who commit suicide have a diagnosable psychiatric illness; depression and alcoholism head the list, but bipolar affective disorder and schizophrenia are also common.[6] Systematic reviews have not found evidence that suicide prevention interventions for ambulatory patients are effective.[12] However, a recent comprehensive program mounted by the U.S. Air Force, involving multiple agencies (mental health, family support centres, child and youth development, health and wellness centres, chaplains, and family advocacy) and a wide spectrum of military personnel, including military leaders, supervisors, attorneys, and health professionals, dramatically decreased the suicide rate of Air Force personnel.[17]

The patient's thoughts of suicide should be taken seriously. The clinician should broach this topic in the first visit and regularly monitor for a change in the patient's intent and lethality. The priority is always the patient's (and others') safety. Detailed lethal plans, social isolation, substance abuse, previous suicide attempts, and a family history of suicide all increase the risk, which may increase the need for careful and close monitoring (i.e., frequent visits, having the patient reside with friends or family, or hospital care).[8]

Treatment

Efficacy of therapies

With all major groups of antidepressant medication, benefit is rarely seen in less than 10 to 14 days. With some antidepressants, however, especially most of the tricyclic antidepressants, there is often an early tranquilizing effect, which may be desirable in agitated depression. Response rate to most groups of antidepressants is 60% to 70%.[5,8] The response to psychotherapy is extremely variable. Most forms of brief psychotherapy, such as counselling, CBT, and interpersonal therapy (IPT), are structured to last for about 10 weeks. However, there may be a wait before these therapies can begin. Studies of CBT, counselling, and interpersonal therapy have quoted 70% to 85% response rates in moderate depression. There is no clear evidence that psychotherapy combined with medication hastens recovery substantially; the combination appears to be more effective in prevention. Response to electroconvulsive therapy (ECT) is usually seen by the fifth treatment; i.e., within about 2 weeks. Some 70% to 80% of patients with severe depres-

sion will respond to ECT. When treatment is successful, recovery is usually complete in 4 to 6 weeks. With light therapy/phototherapy, 75% to 80% of seasonal affective disorder (SAD) sufferers improve within a few days.[2,3]

Review period

Patients who have suffered from major depression should be followed up for at least 6 months following withdrawal of medication.[4] Following the formal review period, the patient or caregiver should always consult the primary care physician if there are any signs of recurrence. Antidepressant therapy can be started right away, without waiting for the results of investigations, provided:

- There is no history of adverse reactions
- There is no serious suicidal risk (a great concern with tricyclic antidepressants; however, SSRIs typically are safe in overdose)
- Physical examination does not reveal any contraindication to antidepressant drugs (e.g., significant cardiac disease in the case of tricyclic antidepressants)
- Patient is receiving no contraindicated medication

A management plan should be negotiated with the patient from the outset.[4] This will involve:

- Regular appointments—ideally weekly initially
- Prescription of only a small quantity of drugs at a time, usually a week's supply; even relatively small overdoses of some antidepressants can be dangerous (especially tricyclic antidepressants)
- The patient having a contact number at all times and a key caregiver

Psychological Treatment

In addition to supportive and psychoeducational techniques, specific psychotherapeutic interventions are as effective as antidepressant therapy in mild-to-moderate major depression and dysthymic disorders.[8]

Cognitive behavioural therapy and interpersonal therapy are the treatment interventions with documented efficacy. Both therapies require specialized training, can be administered individually or in a group setting, and typically require 8 to 16 weekly sessions for efficacy. There is evidence that counselling in the form of CBT and IPT improves short-term outcomes for mental health problems when compared with usual general practitioner care.[8]

The choice of psychotherapy or chemotherapy should be based on patient preference, clinician judgement, and cost as well as the practical issue of availability of psychotherapy. Furthermore, patients who have not responded to their preferred treatment modality should be encouraged to try other interventions.[8]

Psychotherapy, or 'talking treatment'

Some forms of psychotherapy may be as effective as medication in major depression, although there is no evidence that any are more effective. There is also good evidence that psychotherapy enhances the effect of medication in depression.[19-21] Psychotherapy can be a useful alternative for patients who will not take or cannot tolerate medication, or who have a history of overdose.

Cognitive behaviour therapy (CBT)

The main principle of CBT is that patients are harmed by their negative assumptions (e.g., that they are "failures" ["I'm worthless," "I'm fat," "I can't do this"] or that their friends don't like them or want them around). These beliefs are considered to play a part in causing and maintaining depression. CBT is a "here and now" therapy in which past issues are reviewed only to clarify a patient's present observations and attitudes. Treatment aims at challenging and altering these depressive thought patterns. Preliminary studies suggest that CBT may assist the patient in dealing not only with residual symptoms such as anxiety and irritability, but also with maladaptive lifestyles (interpersonal friction, excessive work, inadequate sleep) and a sense of inadequate well-being.[22] Duration of treatment is typically about 10 weeks. Evidence of deteriorating major depression may suggest stopping CBT and/or reviewing antidepressant medication.[8] Cost is relatively high compared with medication. Availability may be low, with a delay before treatment can begin.

Interpersonal therapy (IPT)

Generally, interpersonal therapy (IPT) focuses on the individual's current and past relationships and how these affect mood and self-esteem. Evidence of deteriorating major depression may suggest a review of therapy.[8]
• Cost is relatively high compared with medication
• Availability may be limited, with significant delay before treatment can begin
• Benefit uncertain if used alone in major depression
• Long-term benefit may be limited
IPT can relieve major depression, but is less effective than medication and is best proven in mild-to-moderate depression.

Counselling

Counselling is a broad term, ranging from brief sessions of practical advice to intensive analytical-type sessions. Generally, counselling takes a problem-solving approach, helping the patient to cope better with immediate crises and to make more effective decisions about the future.[23] Evidence of deteriorating major depression may suggest a review of therapy. Counselling may be effective alone in mild-to-moderate depression, but is insufficient treatment for major depression. It may also enhance the effect of medication and improve compliance in major depression.[24] Most patients find counselling helpful, especially in relation to clearly defined problems, such as marital stress.

Self-help groups

A number of organizations help and support depression sufferers. Duration of treatment is variable, and can be indefinite. Anecdotal accounts indicate that many people benefit from attendance at voluntary groups, especially where prevention is concerned. Patients often say that the fellow sufferers they encounter at self-help groups understand depression better than professionals.[8]

Lifestyle therapy

The stresses that have precipitated episodes of depression need to be examined and individually addressed. Exercise and stress relaxation techniques may be helpful.[8]

Antidepressant drug therapy

Therapy with an antidepressant agent is the preferred treatment in cases of moderate-to-severe major depression. The rate of response to an antidepressant trial is about 60% and is close to 80% if therapy with a second drug is tried after an initial antidepressant drug failure.[1,2,8]

Patients should learn that the physiological symptoms of depression (disturbances of sleep, appetite, energy, and motor activity) may resolve before the patient subjectively senses improvement (hence the rationale for "objective" reports from family members). Symptoms typically do not start to resolve until the patient has received an adequate dosage of medication for 2 to 4 weeks. Full remission (i.e., back to baseline and resolution of all SIGECAPS)—the goal of treatment—may take up to 4 months. The risk of recurrence or chronicity, or both, increases if residual symptoms persist.

Reminding the patient that recovery is typically a "sawtooth curve" rather than a linear progression may reassure the patient and family when a few "bad" days occur. Patients need to be aware that side effects are typically transient and that they should not stop therapy, even if they are feeling better, without discussing it with the doctor.

Choosing an Antidepressant Agent

Over 20 antidepressants are commercially available in Canada (Table 47), and this number will certainly increase. Thus, the choice can be daunting in our commercial era, in which television advertisements, gift-laden industry representatives, and distinguished professors at elegant dinners each extol the virtues of a different antidepressant.

The following are basic concepts to consider in choosing an antidepressant[8]:
• If the patient has had a previous positive response to a specific antidepressant, it would be prudent to initiate a trial with this drug. If a family member has had a previous good response with a certain antidepressant, the patient may feel more comfortable starting treatment with that drug. Likewise, if a family member has

Table 47   Daily Dose and Cost of Currently Available Antidepressants

Antidepressant	Usual daily dose, mg	Cost per day, $*
Level I evidence and generally tolerable side effect/safety profile		
Bupropion (Wellbutrin SR)	150-300	0.80-1.60
Citalopram (Celexa)	20-40	1.31-2.32
Fluoxetine (Prozac)	20-40	1.08-2.16
Fluvoxamine (Luvox)	100-200	0.99-1.98
Mirtazapine (Remeron)	15-45	0.69-2.06
Moclobemide (Manerix)	450-600	1.22-2.28
Paroxetine (Paxil)	20-40	1.59-3.18
Sertraline (Zoloft)	50-150	1.60-3.35
Venlafaxine (Effexor)	75-225	1.56-3.21
Level II evidence or level I evidence but less tolerable side effect/safety profile		
Amitriptyline (Elavil)	100-250	0.03-0.08
Clomipramine (Anafranil)	100-250	0.87-2.19
Desipramine (Norpramin)	100-250	0.82-2.06
Doxepin (Sinequan)	100-250	0.63-1.57
Imipramine (Tofranil)	100-250	0.04-0.09
Maprotiline (Ludiomil)	100-250	0.78-1.96
Trazodone (Desyrel)	200-400	0.79-1.58
Trimipramine (Surmontil)	100-250	0.34-1.00
Level III evidence or level I or II evidence and significantly less tolerable side effect/safety profile		
Amoxapine (Asendin)	150-300	0.93-1.86
Nortriptyline (Aventyl)	75-150	0.91-1.82
Phenelzine (Nardil)	30-75	0.60-1.50
Protriptyline (Triptil)	30-60	1.04-2.08
Tranylcypromine (Parnate)	20-60	0.67-2.00

*Derived from the Ontario Drug Benefit Formulary or manufacturers' price lists. Costs do not include professional fees or markups. From Remick RA: *Can Med Assoc J* 167(11): 1253-1260, 2002. Reprinted by permission of the publisher. © 2002 Canadian Medical Association.

had an untoward response to a specific drug (or if the popular press is giving a specific drug a great deal of negative attention), one should consider other drug alternatives.

- Safety considerations should be reviewed. In suicidal patients at risk of overdose, the older-generation antidepressants (i.e., tricyclics and MAOIs) can be lethal, whereas the newer-generation SSRIs and others are relatively safe in overdose.
- Side effect tolerability should be matched to the individual patient. No antidepressant is devoid of side effects, but common class side effects, such as orthostatic hypotension (tricyclics), sedation (trazodone, fluvoxamine, paroxetine), stimulation (bupropion), weight gain (tricyclics, phenelzine, mirtazapine) and sexual dysfunction (SSRIs), may be more or less problematic for a specific patient should that side effect develop.
- Drug interactions are possible due to induction or inhibition of liver enzymes. In patients with coexisting medical disorders who are taking a number of other medications, an antidepressant with few drug–drug interactions (e.g., citalopram, sertraline, venlafaxine, mirtazapine) would be appropriate.
- Unfortunately, physicians seldom consider the cost of drugs for patients; however, cost is often one of the primary factors influencing a patient's decision to continue to take a prescribed medication. Substantial cost differences remain between tricyclic antidepressants, MAOIs, the generic SSRI fluoxetine, and the newer antidepressant agents.

Monotherapy versus augmentation

Sixty percent of patients with major depression or a dysthymic disorder will have a clinical response to an adequate trial (3 to 6 weeks) of an antidepressant. However, if there is no response (i.e., no change in SIGECAPS or HAM_D-7) after 3 weeks, the likelihood of a response is less than 20%, and a switch to an antidepressant of a different chemical class should be contemplated.[8]

If, after 3 to 6 weeks, there is a partial response but not full resolution of symptoms, the physician should consider either raising the antidepressant dose if the patient can tolerate a higher dose with minimal side effects, or augmentation. The addition of a small dose of lithium, liothyronine sodium, or a psychostimulant will quickly (i.e., within 1 to 2 weeks) convert a partial response to a full response in 25% of patients.

Switching antidepressants

If there is no or limited response to an adequate antidepressant trial and increasing the dose or augmentation is either unsuccessful or inappropriate, then switching to a different antidepressant is the appropriate strategy. Current thinking is to switch to a different SSRI or a newer antidepressant, or both. Most clinicians will defer a trial of a tricyclic antidepressant or MAOI until at least two trials of newer medications have failed. In general, there is no need to stop one antidepressant before starting a second drug trial, and typically the dosage of the first drug is tapered as the new antidepressant is started. Classic MAOIs are the exception, requiring a 2-week washout period before therapy with another antidepressant can be initiated. If the patient has not tolerated the first drug well, then a washout period may be prudent to dissipate side effects before a second drug trial.

Special considerations

There are few significant drug–drug interactions with the newer non-tricyclic/non-MAOI antidepressants. All antidepressants are metabolized by one or more of the cytochrome P450 (CYP450) hepatic isoenzymes. For depressive patients taking a number of other medications, antidepressants that have minimal CYP450 inhibitions (e.g., citalopram, venlafaxine, mirtazapine) should be considered.

In elderly people, pregnant women, and breastfeeding women, one should be aware of certain factors. Antidepressants are effective in elderly people. The tenet "start low, go slow" applies, and the use of the newer agents, in particular those with minimal CYP450 inhibition, is appropriate and safer than the use of tricyclic antidepressants or MAOIs. Growing evidence shows that antidepressants are safe during pregnancy, that they do not increase the risk of teratogenesis, and that the risk of depressive relapse may be as high as 75% in pregnant women who stop their antidepressant therapy. These data should be incorporated into discussions with pregnant women as they review the benefits and risks of ongoing antidepressant chemical therapy. Data on the use of antidepressants during breastfeeding are limited, and long-term developmental effects are unknown. Preliminary safety data do not contraindicate the use of several tricyclic antidepressants and SSRIs.[8]

In children and adolescents, caution should be used in light of recent evidence that suggests that children taking SSRIs for depression are more likely to become suicidal than those taking a placebo.[18]

Maintenance therapy. Over 70% of patients experience a recurrence of depression during their lifetime. Most physicians (and their patients) stop antidepressant therapy too early, without discussion as to the risk of relapse and the subsequent risk of disability and death. Current guidelines suggest that, after recovery occurs, antidepressant therapy should be continued at the therapeutic dosage for at least 6 months to significantly lessen the chance of relapse.[8,22] Indefinite antidepressant maintenance therapy should be discussed with patients who have additional risk factors (two or more episodes of depression in 5 years, episodes after the age of 50, and difficult-to-treat episodes). The clinician should review with the patient the benefits (prevention of recurrence) and risks (e.g., cost, side effects, inconvenience of taking medication) of treatment. If antidepressant therapy is stopped, the dosage should be tapered gradually to avoid discontinuation symptoms.

- St John's Wort is an herbal extract that is widely used OTC in the treatment of depression. It has been shown to be effective for the treatment of mild-to-moderate depression, but not for severe depression. There is also considerable purity and quality variation among the several OTC preparations.[25]

Physical treatments. Electroconvulsive therapy (ECT) is used less commonly now, but it still is a valuable treatment, especially in the urgent treatment of a patient who is acutely suicidal, in severely malnourished patients, or for severely depressed patients who do not respond to antidepressants. The usual course of therapy is three times a week for 6 to 12 treatments. ECT is also effective in mania. However, if a patient who responds to ECT is not put on maintenance therapy with antidepressants or lithium, the relapse rate is high. An occasional patient needs maintenance ECT at weekly or monthly intervals.[26] ECT may be administered bilaterally or unilaterally. Amnesia for some events in the weeks following treatment is an important adverse consequence, although in most cases full cognitive function returns within a few weeks. Unilateral ECT causes fewer cognitive disturbances, but 20% of patients do not respond to this form of treatment.[8]

Light box therapy is effective in the management of patients with seasonal affective disorder.[27]

Guidelines and Guidance

- *Guidelines for clinical care: depression,* Ann Arbor, MI, 1998, University of Michigan Health System.
- American Psychiatric Association (APA): Practice guideline for the assessment and treatment of patients with suicidal behaviors, *Am J Psychiatry* 160(11 Suppl): 1-60, 2003.

The following guidelines are available at the National Guideline Clearinghouse:

- American Psychiatric Association (APA): Practice guideline for the treatment of patients with major depressive disorder, *Am J Psychiatry* 157(4 Suppl):1-45, 2000.
- Practice parameters for the assessment and treatment of children and adolescents with depressive disorders, *J Am Acad Child Adolesc Psychiatry* 37(10 Suppl): 63S-83S, 1998. Developed by the American Academy of Child and Adolescent Psychiatry.
- Pharmacologic treatment of acute major depression and dysthymia, *Ann Intern Med* 132:738-42, 2000. Produced by the American College of Physicians.
- *VHA/DOD clinical practice guideline for the management of major depressive disorder in adults,* Washington, DC, 2000, Department of Veterans Affairs (US).
- *Major depression in adults for mental health care providers,* Bloomington, MN, 2002, Institute for Clinical Systems Improvement (ICSI).
- Brigham and Women's Hospital: *Depression: a guide to diagnosis and treatment,* Boston, MA, 2001, Brigham and Women's Hospital.

The American Academy of Family Physicians has produced the following guidance information:

- Cadieux RJ: Practical management of treatment-resistant depression, *Am Fam Physician* 58(9):2059-62, 1998.

Clinical pearl(s)

- It cannot be emphasized enough that the most efficacious treatment for depression is combined treatment, including both psychotherapy and antidepressant medication
- Frequent contacts with the patient initially are highly recommended, especially for that period immediately after prescribing medication when, typically, side effects are most pronounced and efficacy is not well established. Patients require much support and reassurance during this period.
- Terminating antidepressant medication prematurely constitutes a major public and personal health risk.

Never!

- Never prescribe more than a small supply of medication (7 days at most) for a patient with a history of overdose or one who exhibits evidence of tending toward suicide.[24]
- Never prescribe MAOIs without giving clear, printed advice on diet and on which medications to avoid.[23]
- Never forget to ask about other medications, herbal supplements, alcohol, and other drug use.

Bipolar disease and antidepressants

When seeing a depressed patient, the physician should check carefully for a personal or family history of bipolar disorders. Antidepressants should not be prescribed for someone with a bipolar disorder unless the patient is already taking lithium or unless mania may be precipitated. A patient who is depressed but has a family history of bipolar disorder should be watched closely for mania if antidepressants are prescribed. A patient with bipolar disorder may become manic from the rapid withdrawal of antidepressants.[8,11]

Relapses after treatment with antidepressants

Relapses after successful pharmacotherapy for depression are common. In one study of patients with diagnoses of depression alone, dysthymia alone, or dysthymia plus depression (double depression) who had responded to desipramine (Norpramin, Pertofrane), continuation of the drug over a 2-year period resulted in a relapse rate of 11% compared with those assigned at random to receive placebo, whose relapse rate was 52%. Most of the relapses occurred in the 6 months after stopping the active drug. The relapse rate was highest in patients with pure dysthymia or dysthymia plus depression.[28,29]

♪ REFERENCES ♭

1. Khullar A, McIntyre RS. An Approach to managing depression: defining and measuring outcomes, *Can Fam Physician* 50:1374-1380, 2004.
2. Sharp LK, Lipsly MS: Screening for depression across the lifespan: a review of measures for use in primary care settings, *Am Fam Physician* 66:1001-1008,1045-1046,1048, 1051-1052, 2002.
3. Guidelines from: *Diagnostic and statistical manual of mental disorders,* ed 4, Washington, DC, 2000, American Psychiatric Association.
4. Geddes J, Butler R, Hatcher S, et al: Depressive disorders, *Clin Evid* 12:1391-1436, 2004.
5. O'Hanlon K, et al: *Depression,* In: www.firstconsult.com. Elselvier, 2004.
6. Weissman MM, Bland RC, Canino GJ, et al: Cross-national epidemiology of major depression and bipolar disorder, *JAMA* 276:293-299, 1996.
7. Glassman AH: Cigarette smoking: implications for psychiatric illness, *Am J Psychiatry* 150:546-553, 1993.
8. Remick RA: Diagnosis and management of depression in primary care: a clinical update and review, *Can Med Assoc J* 167(11):12531260, 2002.
9. Pratt LA, Ford DE, Crum RM, et al: Depression, psychotropic medication, and risk of myocardial infarction. Prospective data from the Baltimore ECA follow-up, *Circulation* 94:3123-3129, 1996.
10. Weissman MM, Wolk S, Goldstein RB, et al: Depressed adolescents grown up, *JAMA* 281:1707-1713, 1999.
11. Manning JS, Haykal RF, Akiskal HS: The role of bipolarity in depression in the family practice setting, *Psychiatr Clin North Am* 22(3):689-703, 1999.
12. Pearson SD, Katzelnick DJ, Simon GE, et al: Depression among high utilizers of medical care, *J Gen Intern Med* 14: 461-468, 1999.
13. Simon GE, VonKorff M, Piccinelli M, et al: An international study of the relation between somatic symptoms and depression, *N Engl J Med* 341:1329-1335, 1999.

14. APA: Practice guidelines for the assessment and treatment of patients with suicidal behaviors, *Am J Psychiatry* 160(11 Suppl):1-60, 2003.

15. Malchy B, Enns MW, Young TK, et al: Suicide among Manitoba's Aboriginal people, 1988-94, *Can Med Assoc J* 156: 1133-1138, 1997.

16. Geddes J: Suicide and homicide by people with mental illness: We still don't know how to prevent most of these deaths (editorial), *BMJ* 318:1225-1226, 1999.

17. Suicide prevention among active duty air force personnel–United States, 1990-1999, *MMWR* 48:1053-1057, 1999.

18. Meek C: UK psychiatrists question SSRI warnings for under-18s, *Can Med Assoc J* 170(4):455, 17 Feb 2004.

19. Thase ME, Greenhouse JB, Frank E, et al: Treatment of major depression with psychotherapy or psychotherapy-pharmacotherapy combinations, *Arch Gen Psychiatry* 54: 1009-1015, 1997.

20. DeRubeis RJ, Gelfand LA, Tang TZ, et al: Medications versus cognitive behavior therapy for severely depressed outpatients: mega-analysis of four randomized comparisons, *Am J Psychiatry* 156:1007-1013, 1999.

21. Geddes JR, Freemantle N, Mason J, et al. Selective serotonin reuptake inhibitors (SSRIs) versus other antidepressants for depression (Cochrane review). In: *The Cochrane Library*, issue 1, Chichester, UK, 2004, John Wiley & Sons.

22. Fava GA, Rafanelli C, Grandi S, et al: Prevention of recurrent depression with cognitive-behavioral therapy: preliminary findings, *Arch Gen Psychiatry* 55:816-820, 1998.

23. Thase ME, Trivedi MH, Rush AJ: MAOIs in the contemporary treatment of depression, *Neuropsychopharmacology* 12:185-219, 1995. Reviewed in: *Clin Evidence* 10:1121-1144, 2003.

24. Bower P, Rowland N, Mellor Clark J, et al: Effectiveness and cost effectiveness of counselling in primary care (Cochrane Review). In Cochrane Database Syst Rev. (1):CD001025, 2002.

25. Linde K, Mulrow CD: St John's wort for depression (Cochrane Review). In: *The Cochrane Library*, issue 1, Chichester, UK, 2004, John Wiley & Sons.

26. UK ECT Review Group: Efficacy and safety of electroconvulsive therapy in depressive disorders: a systematic review and meta-analysis, *Lancet* 361:799-808, 2003.

27. Lingjaerde O, Foreland AR, Dankertsen J: Dawn simulation vs. lightbox treatment in winter depression: a comparative study, *Acta Psych Scand* 98:73-80, 1998.

28. Barbui C, Hotopf M, Freemantle N, et al: Treatment discontinuation with selective serotonin reuptake inhibitors (SSRIs) versus tricyclic antidepressants (TCAs) (Cochrane review). In: *The Cochrane Library*, issue 1, Chichester, UK, 2004, John Wiley & Sons.

29. Geddes JR, Carney SM, Davies C, et al: Relapse prevention with antidepressant drug treatment in depressive disorders: a systematic review. *Lancet* 361:653-661, 2003.

Treatment-Resistant Depression

In general, 60% to 70% of depressed patients respond to the initial antidepressant used and a further 10% to 15% to a second antidepressant or ECT.[1]

When faced with a depressed patient who fails to respond to treatment, the physician must first reassess the diagnosis and management to date. Is an underlying disease such as hypothyroidism or an interfering co-morbidity such as substance abuse or an anxiety disorder present?[2] According to Joffe[2] and Berber[3] the following are the main options for dealing with truly refractory depression. (These can be remembered with the mnemonic "OSCAR."[3])

- *O*ptimization. The first step is always optimization; that is, to ensure that an adequate dose of the initial antidepressant has been prescribed, that the patient has been compliant in taking it, and that it has been given for a sufficient duration, which is usually 6 weeks. In the case of tricyclic antidepressants, measuring blood levels may be helpful.[2] If a patient is a partial responder, an increase in the dose (if tolerated) may be effective.

- *S*ubstitution. If a patient has no response, a different antidepressant should be considered. The literature suggests that the response rate after switching classes is about 50% to 60% as opposed to 20% to 30% when switching within the same class. However, preliminary evidence based on open trials indicates that this may not be the case with the SSRIs; the response rate from substituting a second SSRI has been reported to be 50% to 60%.[2,4,5]

- *C*ombination. Combination refers to combining two antidepressants from two different classes; for example, an SSRI and a tricyclic.[2] This is a new and promising area of research.

- *A*ugmentation. Augmentation is the addition to an antidepressant of another drug that on its own is not known to have antidepressant effects. Examples are lithium, triiodothyronine or liothyronine (Cytomel), buspirone (Buspar), and psychostimulants such as dextroamphetamine (Dexedrine) or methylphenidate (Ritalin). Most of the studies to date have involved lithium and triiodothyronine.[2]

- *R*eview. This is a general but important concept that reminds physicians to reassess management to date, including mobilization of local resources and psychotherapeutic interventions.[3]

Which strategies should be used? Few controlled trials have been conducted in this area, so the data on which recommendations are based come mostly from open trials. Optimization is obviously the first step for all patients. The traditional second step has been substitution, which can be very effective; the main disadvantage is the time taken to discontinue the first antidepressant and build up the second one to a full therapeutic level. Augmentation has the advantage that time is not lost from stopping one drug and starting another and that if a response is to occur, it sometimes does so within days and usually within 2 to 3 weeks. Combinations of antidepressants can also be effective, and time is not lost; care must be taken that toxicity is not induced through one agent's interference with the metabolism of the other. (See discussion of antidepressants.)[6]

The preceding discussion has been limited to drug therapy for treatment-resistant depression. ECT is an alternative that perhaps should be used at an earlier stage in the therapeutic regimen than is currently the practice.[7]

❧ REFERENCES ❧

1. Warneke L: Management of resistant depression, *Can Fam Physician* 42:1973-1980, 1996.
2. Joffe RT, Levitt AJ, Sokolov ST: Augmentation strategies—focus on anxiolytics, *J Clin Psychiatry* 57(suppl 7):25-33, 1996.
3. Berber MJ: Pharmacological treatment of depression: consulting with Dr. Oscar, *Can Fam Physician* 45:2663-2668, 1999.
4. Joffe RT, Levitt AJ, Sokolov ST, et al: Response to an open trial of a second SSRI in major depression, *J Clin Psychiatry* 57: 114-115, 1996.
5. Thase ME, Blomgern SL, Birkett MA, et al: Fluoxetine treatment of patients with major depressive disorder who failed initial treatment with sertraline, *J Clin Psychiatry* 58:16-21, 1997.
6. Joffe RT, Levitt AJ: Antidepressant failure: augmentation or substitution? (editorial), *J Psychiatry Neurosci* 20:7-9, 1995.
7. Joffe RT, Kellner CH: The role of ECT in refractory depression (editorial), *Convuls Ther* 11:77-79, 1995.

EATING DISORDERS
(See also diabetic retinopathy)

An Australian cohort study found that 8% of 15-year-old girls dieted at a "severe level" and 60% at a "moderate level." The risk for an eating disorder was increased 18-fold in severe-level dieters and 5-fold in moderate-level dieters compared with non-dieters. An additional risk factor for eating disorders was a high level of psychiatric morbidity. The authors recommend exercise rather than dieting as the optimal strategy for weight control in adolescents.[1]

A school survey of thousands of Minnesota adolescents found that those with unhealthy weight loss behaviours as manifested by induced vomiting or the use of diet pills, laxatives, or diuretics had a higher incidence of other maladjusted behaviour patterns such as suicide attempts; alcohol, tobacco, and drug use; unprotected sexual intercourse; and multiple sex partners.[2]

Women with type 1 diabetes have an increased incidence of bulimia and anorexia. Some women skip or reduce insulin doses in an attempt to lose weight.[3] Patients with type 1 diabetes who have eating disorders are at increased risk of retinopathy. (See discussion of diabetic retinopathy.)

❧ REFERENCES ❧

1. Patton GC, Selzer R, Carlin JB, et al: Onset of adolescent eating disorders: population based cohort study over 3 years, *BMJ* 318:765-768, 1999.
2. Neumark-Sztainer D, Story M, French SA: Covariations of unhealthy weight loss behaviors and other high-risk behaviors among adolescents, *Arch Pediatr Adolesc Med* 150:304-308, 1996.
3. Jacobson AM: The psychological care of patients with insulin-dependent diabetes mellitus, *N Engl J Med* 334:1249-1253, 1996.

Anorexia Nervosa
(See also Addison's disease; amenorrhea; bulimia; euthyroid sick syndrome; female athletes)

Four major criteria must be met to make the diagnosis of anorexia nervosa: weight loss, intense fear of gaining weight, disturbance in body image, and amenorrhea.[1,2]

Epidemiology
Anorexia nervosa can be fatal. Crude mortality rates as high as 18% after 30 years have been reported.[1] Suicide accounts for a high proportion of the excess mortality.[2] The ratio of women to men with anorexia nervosa is 10:1 to 20:1. Anorexia is rare in pre-pubertal children, particularly in boys. Tumors affecting the hypothalamus or brainstem may be the cause of an anorexia-like symptom complex, and sometimes, repeated neuroradiological examinations are necessary to detect them.[3]

Negative self-evaluation and perfectionism are character traits predisposing to anorexia nervosa, but unlike patients with bulimia nervosa, those with anorexia are not more likely to have been exposed to dieting by other family members or to have heard negative comments about their eating habits.[4] Patients with eating disorders have an increased incidence of mood, anxiety, and personality disorders.[2]

Physical findings
Physical findings in advanced anorexia are those of starvation: emaciation, bradycardia, hypotension, hypothermia, atrophy of breasts, dry skin, yellow palms and soles from hypercarotenemia, and lanugo hair.[2]

Investigations
Routine laboratory investigations for patients with anorexia nervosa should include a complete blood cell count (increased incidence of anemia, leukopenia, and thrombocytopenia) and measurements of electrolytes (hyponatremia is common, but in the absence of vomiting, laxative, or diuretic abuse, hypokalemia is rare), fasting glucose level (hypoglycemia is common but usually asymptomatic), and bone density (50% of patients have a bone density that is more than 2 standard deviations below normal). Patients with anorexia nervosa may manifest the euthyroid sick syndrome, and a prolonged QT interval is often seen on the electrocardiogram.[2] "Routine" tests performed in an emergency room may produce entirely normal results even though the

patient is in imminent danger of death from a cardiac arrhythmia.

Management

Hospitalization and controlled refeeding are essential for critically ill patients.[1,2] Most individuals whose weight is 75% or less of expected body weight fit in this category.[2] The major therapeutic modality for long-term management is cognitive-behavioural psychotherapy.[1] A randomized trial found that both behavioural family system therapy and ego-oriented individual therapy (plus collateral sessions with the parents) were effective but that more rapid improvement occurred with the behavioural family therapy.[5] Many patients have symptoms of depression, but this is often a direct result of starvation, in which case symptoms usually resolve as weight returns toward normal.[1] Although antidepressants are ineffective for anorexia, they may be useful for associated depression or anxiety disorders or perhaps for preventing relapses, but only when the weight has increased to about 75% of normal.[1,2,3]

The prevention of osteoporosis is another important goal of therapy—amenorrheic women must regain sufficient weight to permit functioning of the hypothalamic-pituitary-ovarian axis. In one study, menses returned within 6 months in most women whose body weight had returned to at least 90% of "standard body weight" charts. The actual weight for return of menses was 2 kg (4.4 lb) more than the weight at which menses ceased. Rise of serum estradiol to levels of 110 pmol/L (30 pg/mL) showed a good correlation with return of menses. Other indicators of improvement are an increase in ovarian size or the presence of a dominant ovarian follicle on ultrasonography.[6] Estrogen replacement therapy has been prescribed to ameliorate bone loss in anorectic women, but its efficacy for this purpose has not been established. Whether bisphosphonates have value is unknown. Expert opinion is that all patients should receive daily calcium supplements of 1000 to 1500 mg plus a multivitamin containing 400 IU of vitamin D.[2]

Prognosis

Predictors of a poor outcome for anorexia nervosa are age at onset over 18 years, vomiting, laxative abuse, alcohol or substance abuse, and numerous hospitalizations. After 10 years, about one fourth of patients have recovered, one fourth are bulimic, one third are functioning reasonably well, and one tenth are still anorectic.[1]

Anorexia nervosa, but not bulimia, often has been cited as a psychiatric illness associated with high mortality.[8] Physicians treating patients with anorexia nervosa on an outpatient basis should carefully assess patterns of alcohol use during the course of care. One of the strongest predictors of fatal outcome has been shown to be alcohol intake during treatment.[9]

♫ REFERENCES ♪

1. Halmi KA: A 24-year-old woman with anorexia nervosa, *JAMA* 279:1992-1998, 1998.
2. Becker AE, Grinspoon SK, Klibanski A, et al: Eating disorders, *N Engl J Med* 340:1092-1098, 1999.
3. Rosenblum J, Forman SF: Management of anorexia nervosa with exercise and selective serotonergic reuptake inhibitors, *Curr Opin Pediatr* 15(3):346-347, Jun 2003.
4. DeVile CJ, Sufraz R, Lask BD, et al: Occult intracranial tumours masquerading as early onset anorexia nervosa, *BMJ* 311: 1359-1360, 1995.
5. Fairburn CG, Cooper Z, Doll HA, et al: Risk factors for anorexia nervosa: three integrated case-control comparisons, *Arch Gen Psychiatry* 56:468-476, 1999.
6. Robin AL, Siegel PT, Moye AW, et al: A controlled comparison of family versus individual therapy for adolescents with anorexia nervosa, *J Am Acad Child Adolesc Psychiatry* 38: 1482-1489, 1999.
7. Golden NH, Jacobson MS, Schebendach J, et al: Resumption of menses in anorexia nervosa, *Arch Pediatr Adolesc Med* 151:16-21, 1997.
8. Sullivan PF: Mortality in anorexia nervosa, *Am J Psychiatry* 152:1073–1074, 1995.
9. Keel PK, et al: Predictors of mortality in eating disorders, *Arch Gen Psychiatry* 60(2):179-183, Feb 2003.

Bulimia

(See also anorexia nervosa)

Bulimia nervosa affects between 1% and 3% of adolescent and young adult females. The course is chronic with remissions and exacerbations. Patients commonly have comorbid psychiatric conditions, particularly affective disorders, personality disorders, and substance abuse.[1] Bulimic individuals are more likely than non-bulimic women and children to have had mothers who were obese during their childhood, to have been exposed to family members who were dieting, and to have been the object of negative remarks about their eating habits, appearance, or weight.[2]

Characteristic physical findings in bulimia include the following[1]:
- Parotid swelling ("chipmunk cheeks") seen in about 25% of patients
- Calluses or red marks on the backs of the hands as a result of trauma from teeth during induced vomiting
- Damaged teeth from acid erosion of enamel; this usually involves the occlusal surfaces of the molars and the lingual surfaces of the other teeth

A number of laboratory tests may be abnormal in patients with bulimia. About 50% have an elevated amylase level. Other common abnormalities reflect a hypokalemic hypochloremic alkalosis induced by vomiting: a urine pH greater than 8 (25% of cases), decreased potassium and chloride levels, and an increased bicarbonate level. The sodium concentration is usually normal. Electrolyte abnormalities may persist for 2 to 7 days after the last binge.

Management

The natural history of bulimia has not been well defined. According to one review of 88 studies in which follow-up took place, about half of bulimic women had fully recovered by 5 to 10 years, 20% still met the criteria for bulimia, and the remainder experienced relapses. Relapses were most common in the first 4 years after diagnosis.[3] Women with substance abuse problems have a lower rate of recovery.[4]

If a bulimic patient also has a substance disorder, the substance disorder has to be treated before bulimia can be effectively managed.

Management is often hampered by high dropout rates.[5] However, proven options for the treatment of bulimia are antidepressants, cognitive-behavioural therapy, or a combination of the two. Antidepressants that have been more effective than placebos include the tricyclics (desipramine [Norpramin, Pertofrane] 150 to 300 mg per day, imipramine [Tofranil] 175 to 300 mg per day), the MAOI phenelzine (Nardil) 60 to 80 mg per day, and fluoxetine (Prozac) 20 to 60 mg per day. In studies of fluoxetine, the best results were reported with 60 mg per day. In the primary care setting, direct comparison between fluoxetine and CBT has shown that there is better retention and an improvement in symptoms when using an SSRI.[5] However, best results are obtained with combination of medications and CBT.[1]

❧ REFERENCES ❧

1. McGilley BM, Pryor TL: Assessment and treatment of bulimia nervosa, *Am Fam Physician* 57:2743-2750, 1998.
2. Fairburn CG, Cooper Z, Doll HA, et al: Risk factors for anorexia nervosa: three integrated case-control comparisons, *Arch Gen Psychiatry* 56:468-476, 1999.
3. Keel PK, Mitchell JE: Outcome in bulimia nervosa, *Am J Psychiatry* 154:313-321, 1997.
4. Keel PK, Mitchell JE, Miller KB, et al: Long-term outcome of bulimia nervosa, *Arch Gen Psychiatry* 56:63-69, 1999.
5. Walsh BT, Fairburn CG, Mickley D, et al: Treatment of bulimia nervosa in a primary care setting, *Am J Psychiatry* 161(3):556-561, Mar 2004.

FUNCTIONAL SOMATIC SYNDROMES

(See also chronic fatigue syndrome; fibromyalgia; hypoglycemia; irritable bowel syndrome; Lyme disease; multiple chemical sensitivities; silicone breast implants; whiplash)

Barsky[1] has lumped together a group of syndromes that are characterized by symptoms of suffering and disability but that do not fit into the categories of specific psychiatric or organic diseases:
- Chronic fatigue syndrome
- Fibromyalgia
- Multiple chemical sensitivities
- Irritable bowel syndrome
- Hypoglycemia
- Candidiasis hypersensitivity
- Gulf War syndrome
- Sick building syndrome
- Systemic reactions to silicone breast implants
- Repetition stress injury
- Chronic whiplash
- Chronic Lyme disease
- Certain food allergies

Symptoms of all these disorders tend to be diffuse and non-specific, and overlap of symptoms among the disorders is common. Identical symptoms are prevalent in healthy populations, but they are often not brought to medical attention, or if they are, they are rapidly resolved with reassurance.[1]

Typical symptoms of functional somatic syndromes are fatigue, insomnia, weakness, headaches, muscle aches, joint pains, nausea and other gastrointestinal complaints, palpitations, shortness of breath, dizziness or lightheadedness, sore throat, dry mouth, decreased concentration, poor memory, irritability, depression, and anxiety. With such a rich choice of complaints many physicians concentrate on those with which they are most familiar; if patients consult a rheumatologist, the diagnosis is likely to be fibromyalgia, whereas if they consult a gastroenterologist, it is likely to be irritable bowel syndrome.[1]

Specific psychiatric diagnoses, particularly depression, anxiety disorders, and somatoform disorder, are more common in patients with functional somatic syndromes than in the general population.[1] A recent meta-analysis reviewed and compared observational studies on the association of medically unexplained physical symptoms, anxiety, and depression with special emphasis on healthy and organically ill control groups and on different types of symptoms, measures, and illness behaviour. The results showed that four functional somatic syndromes (irritable bowel syndrome, non-ulcer dyspepsia, fibromyalgia, and chronic fatigue syndrome) had strong associations with anxiety and depression.[2]

A striking characteristic of functional somatic syndromes is the patient's lack of response to reassurance from negative medical examinations and from explanations of the role of stress in producing body discomfort. Possible explanations are a decreasing trust in science in general and physicians in particular, sensational and alarmist reports in the mass media, litigation and disability issues, and the growing presence of advocacy groups together with clinics and physicians "specializing" in these disorders.[1]

Barsky[1] suggests that functional somatic syndromes originate from the many somatic complaints that are normal experiences of healthy people. A process of amplification perpetuates and aggravates the symptoms in some persons, leading to the development of a "disorder." Prospective patients learn by word of mouth or from the media about a "disease" that would fit their symptoms. They find out about its other manifestations and realize that they are suffering from them as well: "The suspicion of disease heightens bodily awareness, symptom perception, and distress, and these in turn, reinforce the belief that the sufferer is sick."[1]

Management is difficult. The following steps are suggested[1]:

1. Assessment to rule out organic disease (without overinvestigation).
2. Assessment for specific psychiatric disorders.
3. Establishment of a therapeutic alliance with patient.
4. Establishment of restoration of function as the goal of treatment.
5. Limited reassurance.
6. Referral for CBT if the first five steps are unsuccessful.
7. Comorbid psychiatric conditions such as depression may require antidepressants.[1]

─────────────── **❧ REFERENCES ❧** ───────────────

1. Barsky AJ, Borus JF: Functional somatic syndromes, *Ann Intern Med* 130:910-921, 1999.
2. Henningsen P: Medically unexplained physical symptoms, anxiety, and depression: a meta-analytic review, *Psychosom Med* 65(4):528-533, 1 Jul 2003.

INSOMNIA (SLEEP DISORDERS)
(See also anxiety disorders; Creutzfeldt-Jakob disease; hip fractures; hormone replacement therapy; jet lag; prescribing habits; restless leg syndrome; seasonal affective disorder; sleep apnea; alcohol)

Epidemiology
One third of adults indicate some level of insomnia within any given year, and about 10% to 15% indicate that the insomnia is chronic, severe, or both.[1] The prevalence of insomnia increases with age, and is more common in women and in lower socio-economic groups.[2] Periods of sleep difficulty lasting between 1 night and a few weeks are referred to as *acute* or *transient insomnia. Chronic insomnia* refers to sleep difficulty occurring at least 3 nights per week for 1 month or more.[3]

Etiology
Acute insomnia
Acute insomnia is generally related to emotional or physical discomforts such as significant life stresses, acute illnesses, and environmental disturbances involving changes in noise, light, temperature, and place of sleep.

Chronic insomnia
Insomnia is a symptom rather than a disease. Chronic insomnia may be caused by several co-existing factors and often occurs in conjunction with other health problems. In other cases, sleep disturbances are the only complaints and involve abnormal sleep-wake regulation during sleep.[3]

Causes of Insomnia
1. Psychiatric, medical, and neurological disorders
2. Medication/substance use
3. Specific sleep disorders:
    i. Restless leg syndrome
    ii. Periodic limb movement disorder
    iii. Obstructive sleep apnea
    iv. Circadian rhythm sleep disorders
4. Primary or idiopathic insomnia

Depression and anxiety disorders are common psychiatric causes of insomnia. Factors that interrupt sleep, such as pain, urination, difficulty breathing, dementia, and hormone changes associated with pregnancy and menopause, may also result in poor sleep. Other important causes are the use of chemicals such as alcohol, nicotine, and caffeine, and a variety of prescription or non-prescription drugs that have stimulant effects.[4] Even one or two glasses of wine in the evening can cause early awakening as the sedative effect wears off.[2] Sleep in the elderly tends to be more shallow, shorter, and more fragmented. However, older people do not have a decline in the subjective need for sleep. For some, the poor quality of night time sleep leads to daytime somnolence.[4] In the absence of an identified underlying cause, behavioural and conditioned causes of insomnia are referred to as *primary insomnia.*

Screening
Because the majority of people who feel they have insomnia report never discussing it with their physician, attempts should be made to incorporate sleep questions into the routine functional inquiry. In addition to a sleep history, a 1-week sleep diary is often useful in assessing patients with insomnia.[3]

Management
Diagnosis and treatment directed at the underlying cause of insomnia should be the initial goal of management. Many cases of acute insomnia may not require formal treatment. When insomnia begins to affect daily functioning, treatment is often considered. Treatment is generally pharmacological, behavioural, or both. For acute insomnia related to an acute stress, supportive counselling and short-term pharmacological treatment with a hypnotic is a reasonable approach. Education and suggestions regarding sleep hygiene measures are often very helpful.

Chronic insomnia often presents a greater challenge because the causes are often multifactorial, requiring multiple treatment modalities. While treatment of the underlying cause is important, problems are often maintained by poor sleep hygiene even after the initial cause has resolved. Behavioural treatment should be initial management for most cases of chronic insomnia.[3]

Pharmacological interventions

The elimination of many drugs is greatly delayed in the elderly, increasing the risk of side effects.[1] Benzodiazepines are addictive, suppress memory, adversely affect cognition in patients with early dementia, and increase the risk of injury from falls and other accidents.[5] No data from randomized trials have shown that taking hypnotic drugs for more than 35 days provides sustained benefits.[2]

The following are basic principles of the pharmacotherapy of insomnia.[1,6]

1. Use the lowest dose possible.
2. Prescribe for a limited period (no more than 4 weeks on a regular basis).
3. Prescribe intermittent doses (2 to 4 times a week).
4. Discontinue hypnotics gradually.

Available hypnotics are the benzodiazepines (intermediate or short-acting compounds are preferred), zaleplon (Sonata, Starnoc), and chloral hydrate (Noctec). Although zaleplon is not a benzodiazepine, it binds to benzodiazepine receptors.[7] Zopiclone (Imovane) has been touted as being non-addictive in short-term use; case reports of addiction after long-term use are appearing.[8] Amnestic reactions and rebound insomnia with triazolam (Halcion) are common, and like other benzodiazepines, it is addictive.[9]

Antidepressants, especially those that are serotonin specific, have been widely used as hypnotics. No systematic studies of the efficacy of these agents for this purpose have been published. The tricyclic drugs such as amitriptyline (Elavil) or doxepin (Sinequan) have significant anticholinergic side effects. More promising are trazodone (Desyrel), nefazodone (Serzone), and paroxetine (Paxil).[1] Trazodone 50 to 100 mg at bedtime has been used successfully as a hypnotic in depressed patients who had persistent, exacerbated, or new-onset insomnia when being treated with fluoxetine or bupropion.[10]

The value of melatonin for insomnia is unknown because few adequate trials have been published and the purity of some products is questionable.[11] A subgroup of elderly patients with low melatonin levels have benefited from treatment with melatonin.[12] In a 1999 Israeli study, elderly patients who had been taking benzodiazepines daily for at least 6 months were assigned at random to receive a placebo or 2 mg of a sustained release formulation of melatonin taken 2 hours before bedtime. All patients were asked to gradually decrease and then discontinue their benzodiazepines. After 6 weeks, 78% of the melatonin group was no longer taking benzodiazepines compared with 25% of the placebo group.[13]

Table 48 lists a few of the drugs that are approved or used as hypnotics. For all hypnotics, except for the antidepressants, efficacy usually dissipates in a few weeks, and dependency is a major risk.[2]

Behavioural interventions

Behavioural interventions seek to change maladaptive sleep habits, reduce autonomic arousal, and alter dysfunctional beliefs and attitudes, which are presumed to maintain insomnia.[3] Such interventions include:

- *Relaxation Therapy:* To promote the ability to reduce physiological and emotional arousal.
- *Sleep Restriction Therapy:* To limit the amount of time spent in bed to increase sleep quality and efficiency.
- *Stimulus Control Therapy:* To re-associate the bedroom as a place of rapid onset of sleep.
- *Cognitive Therapy:* To identify and shift negative ideas and associations about sleep.

Table 48   Hypnotics

Drugs	Usual doses
Aldehydes and Derivatives	
Chloral hydrate	500-1000 mg qhs
Benzodiazepine Derivatives	
Short acting	
Triazolam (Halcion)	0.125 mg qhs
Intermediate acting	
Oxazepam (Serax)	15-30 mg qhs
Lorazepam (Ativan)	0.5-2 mg qhs
Temazepam (Restoril)	15-30 mg qhs
Long acting	
Diazepam (Valium)	2-10 mg qhs
Flurazepam (Dalmane)	15-30 mg qhs
Cyclopyrrolones	
Zopiclone (Imovane)	3.75-7.5 mg qhs
Pyrazolopyrimidines	
Zaleplon (Sonata, Starnoc)	10 mg qhs
Imidazopyridines	
Zolpidem (Ambien)	5-10 mg qhs
Tricyclics	
Amitriptyline (Elavil)	10-75 mg qhs
Doxepin (Sinequan)	10-75 mg qhs
Modified Cyclic Derivatives	
Trazodone (Desyrel)	50-300 mg qhs
Phenylpiperazine Compounds	
Nefazodone (Serzone)	100-250 mg hs
Selective Serotonin Reuptake Inhibitors	
Paroxetine (Paxil)	20 mg qhs

The following behavioural approach may be helpful:[14]

- Go to bed only when sleepy.
- Do not read, eat, or watch television in bed. Bed is for sleeping and sex.
- If you are in bed and can't sleep, get up, go to another room, and stay up until you are really sleepy and then go back to bed. Do not watch television because the brightness of its light has an arousing effect; instead read with as dim a light as possible. If after returning to bed you still can't sleep, get up again and repeat the cycle.
- Set the alarm for the same time every morning, and get up when it rings regardless of how little sleep you have had.
- Never sleep during the day.

An additional approach is to document the number of hours the patient sleeps and to make bedtime that number of hours (or that number of hours plus 30 minutes) before the fixed morning wakeup time. If, for example, an insomniac sleeps only 5 hours and the morning wake-up time is to be 7 AM, bedtime should be 1:30 or 2 AM. This will probably cause the patient to accumulate a sleep deficit and fall asleep more easily. After a week the bedtime can be made earlier by 15 minutes, and further 15-minute weekly increments of time spent in bed can be added provided that at least 85% of the time in bed is spent sleeping.[2]

In a study from Virginia, elderly patients (mean age 65 years) with primary insomnia were selected at random to participate in one of three therapeutic regimens: an 8-week program of weekly small group sessions for CBT, pharmacotherapy with temazepam (Restoril), and a combination of CBT and either temazepam or place-bo. The behavioural approach was described above, and the cognitive component included rectifying unrealistic expectations about the hours of sleep required (less than 8 hours is OK), clarifying that daytime distress is not entirely the result of insomnia, and correcting fallacious beliefs about how to improve sleep. After 2 years of fol-low-up, excellent results were obtained with CBT, where-as the short-term benefits of temazepam had entirely dissipated. Some of the patients in the combined cogni-tive behavioural and temazepam arm of the study main-tained improved sleep patterns, whereas others did not.[15] This study indicates that although CBT leads to excel-lent results, benzodiazepines have no long-term benefits in treating insomnia in the elderly.

Another study comparing use of similar cognitive-behahioural techniques while tapering benzodiazepines, versus tapering alone, in adults who had used medica-tions for at least 3 months found that patients in the dual modality group were significantly more likely to be off benzodiazepines at the end of the trial and at 1 year of follow-up.[16] A 16-week randomized trial of moderate-intensity aerobic exercises for elderly patients

with sleep disturbances showed a significant improve-ment in self-rated sleep quality. Each subject performed low-impact aerobics, brisk walking, or stationary cycling 4 times a week for 30 to 40 minutes before the evening meal.[7,17]

❧ REFERENCES ❧

1. Mellinger GD, Balter MB, Uhlenhuth EH: Insomnia and its treatment. Prevalence and correlates, *Arch Gen Psychiatry* 42:225-232, 1985.
2. Kupfer DJ, Reynolds CF III: Management of insomnia, *N Engl J Med* 336:341-346, 1997.
3. National Heart, Lung, and Blood Institute Working Group on Insomnia: Insomnia: assessment and manage-ment in primary care, *Am Fam Phys* 59(11):3029-3038, June 1999.
4. Rajput V, Bromley SM: Chronic insomnia: a practical review, *Am Fam Physician* 60:1431-1442, 1999.
5. Bursztajn HJ: Melatonin therapy: from benzodiazepine-dependent insomnia to authenticity and autonomy (edito-rial), *Arch Intern Med* 159:2393-2395, 1999.
6. National Institute for Clinical Excellence: Guidance on the use of zaleplon, zolpidem and zopiclone for the short-term management of insomnia (Technology Appraisal Guidance 77). London, 2004, National Institute for Clinical Excellence. [Online] [access 2005 June]. Available from URL http://www.nice.org.uk/TA077guidance.
7. Zaleplon for insomnia, *Med Lett Drugs Ther* 41:93-94, 1999.
8. Jones IR, Sullivan G: Physical dependence on zopiclone: case reports, *BMJ* 316:117, 1998.
9. Hypnotic drugs, *Med Lett Drugs Ther* 38:59-61, 1996.
10. Nierenberg AA, Adler LA, Peselow E, et al: Trazodone for antidepressant-associated insomnia, *Am J Psychiatry* 151:1069-1072, 1994.
11. Epstein FH: Melatonin in humans, *N Engl J Med* 336:186-195, 1997.
12. Zhdanova IV, Wurtman RJ, Regan MM, et al: Melatonin treatment for age-related insomnia, *J Clin Endocrinol Metab* 86:4727-4730, 2001.
13. Garfinkel D, Zisapel N, Wainstein J, et al: Facilitation of benzodiazepine discontinuation by melatonin: a new clini-cal approach, *Arch Intern Med* 159:2456-2460, 1999.
14. Bootzin RR, Perlis ML: Nonpharmacologic treatments of insomnia, *J Clin Psychiatry* 53(suppl)6:37-41, 1992.
15. Morin CM, Colecchi C, Stone J, et al: Behavioral and phar-macological therapies for late-life insomnia: a randomized controlled trial, *JAMA* 281:991-999, 1999.
16. Baillargeon L, Landreville P, Verrault R, et al: Discontinuation of benzodiazepines among older insom-niac adults treated with CBT combined with gradual tapering: a randomized trial, *Can Med Assoc J* 169:1015, 2003.
17. King AC, Oman RF, Brassington GS, et al: Moderate-intensity exercise and self-rated quality of sleep in older adults: a randomized controlled trial, *JAMA* 277:32-37, 1997.

MOOD DISORDERS

Bipolar Disorder

(See also depression; hypothyroidism; seizures; serotonin syndrome; subclinical hypothyroidism)

The diagnosis of bipolar disorder (BD) is frequently missed in the primary care setting because a prior history of mood elevation is often not clarified in patients presenting with depression.[1] Approximately 1% of people will develop BD at some point in their life,[2] and because a strong familial component exists in the pathogenesis of BD,[3] the risk is significantly increased in patients with a family history of BD. First symptoms of BD usually occur between the ages of 15 and 30, but a 3- to 10-year lag time between the onset of symptoms and treatment is common.[4,5]

Ninety percent of patients with mania will relapse within 5 years,[6] and 90% of individuals with bipolar disorder will require at least one hospitalization.[2] Because substance abuse is very common in individuals with BD, a substance use history is an integral part of the assessment.[5] Twenty five to fifty percent of patients with BD attempt suicide, and 15% of patients are successful,[7] making it a particularly lethal disorder. Inadequately treated patients may have more than 10 episodes of biphasic mood dysregulation during their lifetime, and episodes tend to become more frequent as the patient ages.[8]

BD is divided into two subtypes. A diagnosis of bipolar I disorder requires that the patient has had at least one manic episode with or without a previous depressive episode. The diagnosis of bipolar II disorder implies that the patient has had one or more major depressive episodes, as well as one or more hypomanic episodes, without evidence of prior mania.[4] The term *rapid cycler* is used when there have been four or more periods of mood alteration in the previous 12 months. Seventy to ninety percent of rapid cyclers are women. The term *mixed episode* implies symptoms that meet both the criteria for depression and mania concurrently.

Management

Initial pharmacological therapy for severe acute mania or mixed episodes is lithium or valproate plus an antipsychotic. Atypical antipsychotics are preferable to typicals, and most of the evidence supports the use of olanzapine or risperdal. For milder symptoms, monotherapy with either a mood stabilizer or an antipsychotic is often sufficient.[9] For mania with rapid cycling, either valproate or carbamazepine is the drug of first choice, because these patients are less responsive to lithium.[10]

First-line therapy for patients with bipolar depression is lithium or lamotrigine. In the acute phase of depression, patients may require brief, concomitant use of an antidepressant with lithium, valproate, or carbamazepine.[2] SSRIs and bupropion are the least likely antidepressants to precipitate a manic episode, but all antidepressants carry some risk.[9]

Non-pharmacological therapy. Few studies have examined the efficacy of psychosocial interventions in BD. Only psycho-education, cognitive therapy, and brief inpatient family therapy interventions have been supported by small, randomized control trials. These interventions have been helpful in the depressed or maintenance phases of illness, not the manic phase.[11] Group psycho-education significantly reduced the number of relapses per patient and hospitalizations, and increased the time to depressive, manic, hypomanic, and mixed recurrences compared with non-structured group meetings.[12] An integrated approach involving education, marital and family therapy, substance abuse treatment, and cognitive-behavioural or interpersonal therapy has been used to optimize patient outcomes.[13] A randomized control trial found that bipolar patients who were instructed to identify the specific life situations and prodromal symptoms that preceded their manic or depressive relapses were able to seek earlier treatment than control subjects who received the usual care. Early treatment resulted in fewer manic episodes but had no effect on frequency of depressive episodes.[14]

Lithium. Lithium is effective in controlling acute mania in 70% of patients, but a delay of 1 to 2 weeks is usual before any amelioration of symptoms, and substantial improvement is commonly not evident for 3 to 4 weeks. In practice, antipsychotics or benzodiazepines are usually added to the lithium to control the agitation and excessive activity of acute mania. The starting dose is 300 mg twice a day with increases every 4 to 5 days based on serum levels and side effects. The usual dosage of lithium is 1200 to 1800 mg per day in acute mania and 900 to 1500 mg per day for maintenance therapy. Once an effective level is reached, a single daily dose should be given at bedtime. Aside from convenience, a single dose is thought to decrease the risk of renal damage.

The most common side effect is hand tremor, which can be minimized by lowering the dose or by adding a beta blocker. Other potential side effects are leukocytosis, hypothyroidism, subclinical hypothyroidism, acne, diarrhea, and polyuria because of reduced urinary concentrating ability.[15]

The risk of lithium toxicity increases in clinical situations that involve impairment of lithium excretion: renal insufficiency, volume insufficiency, older age, NSAID use, ACE inhibitor use, and diuretic use. Before commencing lithium therapy, recommended laboratory investigations include a complete blood cell count, urinalysis, an ECG if the patient is over age 40, and measurement of TSH, BUN, creatinine, and electrolytes.

During the initiation of therapy, lithium levels should be assessed every 5 to 7 days, as well as 5 to 7 days after any change in dosage. During maintenance therapy, lithium levels should be checked every 1 to 2 months in the early period and every 6 to 12 months once the patient's condition is stable while receiving the drug. Lithium levels should be measured 10 to 12 hours after the last lithium dose. The therapeutic range for maintenance therapy is 0.6 to 1 mmol/L (0.6 to 1 mEq/L), whereas for acute mania the aim is 0.8 to 1.4 mmol/L (0.8 to 1.4 mEq/L). Toxic levels are 1.2 mmol/L (1.2 mEq/L) or greater. TSH and creatinine levels should be checked annually. Lithium is also useful in cyclothymic disorder and as a potentiating agent for tricyclic or SSRI antidepressants in cases of refractory depression.[9]

Anticonvulsants. Valproic acid (Depakene) or divalproex (Depakote, Epival) is effective for mania.[16] The starting dose is 750 mg per day in divided doses (or 10 to 15mg/kg per day). The dose is increased every few days to achieve trough blood levels of 50 to 125µg/mL or until side effects limit further increases.

Adverse effects include nausea, weight gain, diarrhea, and tremor; the latter can be treated with beta blockers. Patients treated with these drugs should have regular monitoring of serum levels, which should be maintained at the same level as for seizure control. (See discussion of seizures.) Lamotrigine (Lamictal) in doses of 200 mg per day has been shown to be effective monotherapy for the depressive phase of bipolar 1 disorders, and it did not increase the risk of rapid cycling or mania.[17]

Carbamazepine (Tegretol) is usually used as a second-line drug in BD in part due to the increased risk of serious hematological and dermatological side effects. It is initiated at 400 mg per day in divided oral doses, with increases every few days until clinical response or intolerance develops.

The usual dose is 400 to 600 mg per day orally. Topiramate (Topamax) 100 to 400 mg per day in 2 divided doses has also shown promise and has the added advantage of weight loss as a side effect.[14]

Atypical antipsychotics. Evidence shows that atypical antipsychotic agents are effective treatments for bipolar disorder, especially as adjunctive treatments for acute mania. One randomized controlled trial found risperdal to be more effective than lithium in improving symptoms at 4 weeks.[18] A systematic review found that adding olanzapine to lithium or valproate significantly increased the proportion of people who responded at 6 weeks compared with the addition of placebo[1] Level A.[19] Typically, in acute mania, risperdal is started at 1 mg twice daily initially, increasing to 2 mg twice daily on the second day and 3 mg twice daily on the third day, then increased weekly as needed. The usual effective dose is 4 to 8 mg daily. Olanzpine is initiated at 5 to 10 mg once per day orally, which may be increased in 5-mg per day increments at intervals of at least 1 week. The dose generally should not exceed 20 mg per day.

Electroconvulsive therapy. Patients whose disorder is refractory to standard therapy and those who are rapidly cycling often respond to ECT.[20]

The following should always be noted:

- Where there is impaired renal function, never prescribe lithium without consultation.
- In female patients who are, or are likely to become, pregnant, never prescribe lithium, carbamazepine, or valproate unless there is consensus with specialists about the risks/benefits.
- Never prescribe more than a small number of tablets at a time (e.g., enough for 7 days) in acute episodes, especially if there is evidence of leanings toward suicide.
- Never forget the many drug interactions with the mood stabilizers,
- Never prescribe lithium for a patient who is taking diuretics without first discontinuing the diuretic.[21]

✍ REFERENCES ✍ _____

1. Manning JS, Haykal RF, Connor PD, et al: On the nature of depressive and anxious states in a family practice setting: the high prevalence of Bipolar II and related disorders in a cohort followed longitudinally, *Compr Psychiatry* 38:102, 1997.
2. Woods SW: The economic burden of bipolar disease, *J Clin Psychiatry* 61(suppl 13):38, 2000.
3. Craddock N, Jones I: Genetics of bipolar disorder, *J Med Genet* 36:585, 1999.
4. Yatham LN, Kusumakar V, Parikh SV, et al: Bipolar depression: treatment options, *Can J Psychiatry* 42(suppl 2):87S-91S, 1997.
5. Suppes T, Dennehy EB, Gibbons EW : The longitudinal course of bipolar disorder, *J Clin Psychiatry* 61(suppl 9):23, 2000.
6. Hilty DM, Brady KT, Hales RE: A review of bipolar disorder among adults, *Psychiatr Ser* 50:201, 1999.
7. Jamison KR: Suicide and bipolar disorder, *J Clin Psychiatry* 61(Suppl 9):47, 2000.
8. Goldberg JF, Harrow M, Grossman LS: Recurrent affective syndromes in bipolar and unipolar mood disorders at follow-up, *Br J Psychiatry* 166:382-385, 1995.
9. Practice guideline for the treatment of bipolar disorder. Part A: treatment recommendations for patients with bipolar disorder, *Am J Psychiatry* 159 (Suppl):4, 2002.
10. Keck PE Jr, McElroy SL, Arnold LM: Bipolar disorder, *Med Clin North Am* 85:645, 2001.
11. Parikh SV, Kusumakar V, Haslam RS, et al: Psychosocial intervention as an adjunct to pharmacotherapy in bipolar disorder, *Can J Psychiatry* 42(suppl 2):74S-78S, 1997.
12. Colom F, Vieta E, Martinez-Aran A, et al: A randomized trial on the efficacy of group psychoeducation in the prophylaxis of recurrences in bipolar patients whose disease is in remission, *Arch Gen Psychiatry* 60:402, 2003.
13. Rothbaum BO, Astin MC: Integration of pharmacotherapy and psychotherapy for bipolar disorder, *J Clin Psychiatry* 61(suppl 9):68.

14. Perry A, Tarrier N, Morriss R, et al: Randomised controlled trial of efficacy of teaching patients with bipolar disorder to identify early symptoms of relapse and obtain treatment, *BMJ* 318:149-153, 1999.
15. Drugs for psychiatric disorders, *Med Lett Drugs Ther* 39:33-40, 1997.
16. Macritchie K, Geddes JR, Scott J, et al: Valproate for acute mood episodes in bipolar disorder (Cochrane Review). In: *Cochrane Database Syst Rev* (1):CD004052, 2003.
17. Ichim L, Berk M, Brook S: Lamotrigine compared with lithim in mania: a double blind randomized controlled trial, *Ann Clin Psychiatry* 12:5-10, 2000.
18. Poolsup N, Li Wan Po A, de Oliveira IR: Systematic overview of lithium treatment in acute mania, *J Clin Pharm Ther* 25:139-156, 2000. Reviewed in: Geddes J. Bipolar disorder, *Clin Evid* 11:1204-1223, 2004.
19. Rendell JM, Gijsman HJ, Keck P, et al: Olanzapine alone or in combination for acute mania (Cochrane Review). In: *The Cochrane Library*, issue 2, Chichester, UK, 2004, John Wiley & Sons. Reviewed in: *Clin Evidence* 11:1204-1223, 2004. *Level A*
20. Mukerjee S, Sacheim HA, Schnur DB: Electroconvulsive therapy of acute manic episodes: a review of 50 years experience, *Am J Psychiatry* 151:169-176, 1994.
21. First Consult .Bipolar disorder (medical condition file) → Treatment → Never –2004. Available through subscription from: URL: http://www.firstconsult.com/home/framework/fs_main.htm.

Dysthymic Disorder

Dysthymia is a chronic, low-intensity mood disorder generally characterized by anhedonia, low self-esteem, and low energy. Criteria for diagnosis include a depressed mood on most days for 2 years with at least two of the typical symptoms associated with major depression.[1] Despite the prevalence of dysthymia in the primary care setting, there is a paucity of clinical trials on the subject. It has been postulated that this reflects the relative rarity of the condition in psychiatric consultation rooms.

Antidepressants are effective for controlling the symptoms of dysthymic disorder,[2] and for improving psychosocial functioning.[3] Both tricyclics and SSRIs appear to be effective, but SSRIs are generally preferred.[2] Two recent randomized controlled trials conducted in primary care settings support the use of SSRIs and problem-solving therapy in the treatment of dysthymia.

One small study involved paroxetine versus problem-solving therapy versus placebo with six scheduled visits with a family physician. The remission rate for paroxetine (80%) and problem-solving therapy (57%) was significantly higher than for placebo (44%, P=.008).[4] A second 12-week, multicentre, double-blind study involved 310 patients with a DSM-III-R diagnosis of dysthymic disorder without concurrent major depression who were randomly assigned to receive either sertraline (N=158) or placebo. Sertraline-treated patients experienced greater improvement, compared with placebo, in mood and func-

tioning on several structured assessment tools.[5] In a placebo-controlled study, dysthymic patients who responded to desipramine were selected at random to continue the desipramine (Norpramin, Pertofrane) or to take a placebo for a 2-year period. The relapse rate was much higher in the placebo group, and most such events occurred during the first 6 months after stopping the drug.[6]

The long-standing interpersonal and social deficits associated with dysthymic disorder provide a strong rationale for the use of various psychotherapies, including IPT with dysthymic patients, yet no clinical trials have been published to date.

REFERENCES

1. American Psychiatric Association: *Diagnostic and statistical manual of mental disorders,* ed 4, Washington, DC, 2000, American Psychiatric Association.
2. Sansone RA, Sansone LA: Dysthymic disorder: the chronic depression, *Am Fam Physician* 53:2588-2596, 1996.
3. Kocsis JH, Zisook S, Davidson J, et al: Double-blind comparison of sertraline, imipramine, and placebo in the treatment of dysthymia: psychosocial outcomes, *Am J Psychiatry* 154:390-395, 1997.
4. Barrett JE, Williams JW Jr, Oxman TE, et al: Treatment of dysthymia and minor depression in primary care: a randomized trial in patients age 18 to 59 years, *J Fam Pract* 50(5):405-412, May 2001.
5. Ravindran AV, Guelfi JD, Lane RM, et al: Treatment of dysthymia with sertraline: a double-blind, placebo-controlled trial in dysthymic patients without major depression, *J Clin Psychiatry* 61(11):821-827, Nov 2000.
6. Kocsis JH, Friedman RA, Markowitz JC, et al: Maintenance therapy for chronic depression–a controlled clinical trial of desipramine, *Arch Gen Psychiatry* 53:769-774, 1996.

Seasonal Affective Disorder (SAD)

SAD is defined as a pattern of recurring depression with seasonal onset and remission. Though not considered a separate mood disorder, the DSM-IV-TR defines it as a subtype that can occur with both major depressive disorder (80%) or bipolar disorder (20%). While the most common pattern is fall onset, a spring onset pattern has been described. A review of several retrospective and prospective studies suggested a prevalence range in the general population between 0 and 9.7%.[1]

Patients with fall-onset SAD usually have atypical depressive symptoms such as overeating, carbohydrate craving, weight gain, and oversleeping. They show a marked lack of energy, complaining of feelings of physical heaviness, or leadenness, in the limbs. Symptoms usually begin in October or November and are worst in January and February. Spontaneous recovery occurs in April or May. Spring-onset SAD resembles more typical depression, with the vegetative symptoms of weight loss, decreased sleep, and decreased appetite.[2]

While SAD symptoms do respond to antidepressants, "light therapy" is effective for fall-onset SAD. The literature supporting efficacy is limited: one study comparing light therapy of approximately 6000 lux against sham negative ion generator placebos found light therapy to be effective, but benefits were not generally noted until 3 weeks had elapsed.[3] One guideline suggested that light therapy may be considered as first-line therapy when the patient is not suicidal, there are medical reasons to avoid antidepressants, and the patient requests it.[4,5]

The usual protocol involves exposure to a fluorescent light box rated at 10,000 lux for 30 to 45 minutes a day. Light therapy is usually suggested in the morning, but as the evidence is inconclusive, patient convenience should dictate the time of administration.[5,6] Patients should begin with sessions of 10 to 15 minutes and should keep their eyes open without looking directly at the light source. Commercially made units are recommended to ensure safety. Response is usually seen in 1 to 3 weeks but may occur earlier.[7]

Few studies have specifically considered the efficacy of medications for SAD; fluoxetine (Prozac)[8-10] and moclobemide are probably beneficial. One recent study of light therapy combined with exercise demonstrated significant improvement in symptoms, suggesting that the combination of light and behavioural activation may be beneficial.[11]

☙ REFERENCES ❧

1. Magnusson A: An overview of epidemiological studies on seasonal affective disorder, *Acta Psychiatr Scand* 101:176, 2000.
2. American Psychiatric Association: *DSM IV*, Washington, DC, 2000, The Association.
3. Eastman CI, Young MA, Fogg LF, et al: Bright light treatment of winter depression: a placebo-controlled trial, *Arch Gen Psychiatry* 55:883-889, 1998.
4. Saeed SA, Bruce TJ: Seasonal affective disorders, *Am Fam Physician* 57:1340-1346,1351-1352,1998.
5. Terman M, Terman JS, Ross DC: A controlled trial of timed bright light and negative air ionization for treatment of winter depression, *Arch Gen Psychiatry* 55:875-882, 1998.
6. Wirz-Justice A, Graw P, Krauchi K, et al: Light therapy in seasonal affective disorder is independent of time of day or circadian phase, *Arch Gen Psychiatry* 50:929, 1993.
7. Levitt AJ, Wesson VA, Joffe RT, et al: A controlled comparison of light box and head-mounted units in the treatment of seasonal depression, *J Clin Psychiatry* 57:105-110, 1996.
8. Tam EM, Lam RW, Levitt AJ: Treatment of seasonal affective disorder–a review, *Can J Psychiatry* 40:457-466, 1995.
9. Lam RW, Gorman CP, Michalon M, et al: Multicenter, placebo-controlled study of fluoxetine in seasonal affective disorder, *Am J Psychiatry* 152:1765-1770, 1995.
10. Kennedy SH, Bakish D, Evans M, et al: *CANMAT guidelines for the diagnosis and pharmacologic treatment of depression*, Toronto, 1999, Ontario Ministry of Health.
11. Leppamaki SJ, Partonen TT, Hurme J, et al : Randomized trial of light exposure and aerobic exercise on depressive symptoms and serum lipids, *J Clin Psychiatry* 63:316, 2002.

PERSONALITY DISORDERS
Classification

Major personality disorders/Axis II disorders:

Cluster A: Schizotypal, schizoid, paranoid
Cluster B: Borderline, antisocial, narcissistic, histrionic
Cluster C: Dependent, avoidant, obsessive-compulsive [1]

Diagnosis

In general, personality disorders are "an enduring pattern of inner experience and behaviour that deviates markedly from the expectations of the individual's culture." This pattern is seen in at least two areas of an individual's life, be it cognition, affectivity, interpersonal functioning, or impulse control. The personality disorder is long standing, having its origins in adolescence or early adulthood, causes the individual marked distress, and is not better accounted for by another cause (i.e., other psychiatric condition, substance use, or general medical condition).[1]

Prevalence

Estimates of prevalence in community samples range widely from 4.4% to 13.4%.[2-4] Personality disorders seem to be more prevalent in unmarried men, individuals with low socio-economic status, and those without completion of a high-school degree.[3,4]

Risk Factors

Childhood abuse and neglect increase the likelihood of being diagnosed with a personality disorder in early adulthood fourfold.[5] Furthermore, history of personality disorder in adolescence, disruptive disorders, anxiety disorders, and major depression "increase the odds of young adult personality disorder."[6]

Antisocial personality disorder

Criteria for the diagnosis are a consistent disregard for the rights of others and violation of those rights from the age of 15, as well as a history of conduct disorder starting before the age of 15. The individual may commit unlawful behaviour, be deceitful, aggressive, have a disregard for safety, be irresponsible, or show a lack of remorse.[1]

The overall reported prevalence rate of antisocial personality disorder in the Western world is between 2% and 4%, and males outnumber females by a ratio of between 5:1 and 7:1. In most cases, criminal behaviour dies out by middle age, but difficulties in interpersonal relationships persist.[7]

In Europe and North America, important risk factors for the development of antisocial personality disorder are antisocial behaviour in the father, parental alco-holism, childhood physical abuse, and separation from or loss of a parent. The common denominator is lack of parental supervision and discipline. Current evidence suggests that to acquire an antisocial personality disorder, a person must have the genetic potential and then be exposed to an environment conducive to its development.[7] Another significant risk factor for the development of antisocial personality disorder is antecedent attention deficit/hyperactivity disorder.[8]

There is significant debate as to whether antisocial personality disorder is amenable to treatment. In general, the literature does not support treatment as beneficial or cost-effective. However, addressing specific comorbid issues, such as depression or anxiety, may improve prognosis.[9]

Borderline personality disorder

Criteria for diagnosis include unstable relationships, impulsivity, fluctuation in self-image, efforts to avoid abandonment, recurrent self-harm behaviours, anger management difficulty, paranoia, and/or dissociative symptoms.[1]

Prevalence rates in the community range from 0.7% to 2%.[2,4] Axis I comorbid conditions are the norm for patients with borderline personality. In one study, mood disorders were found in 96%, anxiety disorders in 88% (post-traumatic stress disorder in 56%, panic disorder in 48%, and social phobias in 46%), substance use disorders in 64%, and eating disorders in 53%.[10]

Patients with borderline personality disorder are often difficult to manage. Borderline patients obtain a sense of control if they can sabotage the interventions recommended by their physicians.[11]

According to Dawson,[11] an essential aspect of the management of borderline patients is for the physician to refuse to play the role of an ever more powerful paternal figure looking after an increasingly regressing child. The physician should make it clear that the patient is a competent adult who is capable of taking responsibility for his or her own life and health; the physician is a helper but is of secondary importance and cannot take responsibility for the patient's self-destructive behaviour. This process of establishing and maintaining a different type of social contract with the patient is called *relationship management*. Dawson describes a variety of interviewing techniques that may be helpful in establishing and maintaining this contract. A key element is for the physician to refrain from jumping in with empathetic words or gestures when the patient begins to complain about the miseries of life.

Other useful suggestions in the management of borderline patients in primary care are the following[12]:

- Set and observe limits. A verbal contract is often useful in spelling out such items as fixed but limited

appointments, necessity of coming on time and not cancelling, limited number of telephone calls, and contingency plans for overwhelming suicidal ideation.
- Follow a behavioural approach to psychotherapy that focuses on helping the patients understand how to get on with their lives.
- Recognize and treat concomitant Axis I disorders.
- Arrange for judicious psychiatric consultations (not referrals).
- If all the above are unsuccessful, inform the patient that you will not be able to continue being his or her physician.

A recent meta-analysis showed that both psychodynamic therapy and CBT are effective in treating personality disorders; however, further study into specific therapies for specific disorders is required.[13] Pharmacotherapy may also be an option to aid in the treatment of borderline personality disorder. At this time, the data is still preliminary; however, it seems that pharmacotherapy should be aimed at symptom management. For example, atypical antipsychotics seem beneficial to help decrease aggression, impulsivity, self-harm behaviours, and variations in affect. The length of treatment necessary is unclear.[14]

❧ REFERENCES ❧

1. American Psychiatric Association: *Diagnostic and statistical manual of mental disorders*, ed 4, Washington, DC, 1994, The Association, 629-673.
2. Coid J: Epidemiology, public health and the problem of personality disorders, *Br J Psychiatry*, 182, (suppl 44): s3-s10, Jan 2003.
3. Samuels J, Eaton WW, Bienvenu OJ 3rd, et al: Prevalence and correlates of personality disorders in a community sample, *Br J Psychiatry* 180:536-542, Jun 2002.
4. Torgersen S, Kringlen E, Cramer V: The prevalence of personality disorders in a community sample, *Arch Gen Psychiatry* 58(6):590-596, Jun 2001.
5. Johnson JG, Cohen P, Brown J, et al: Childhood maltreatment increases risk for personality disorders during early adulthood, *Arch Gen Psychiatry* 56(7):600-606, July 1999.
6. Kasen S, Cohen P, Skodol AE, et al: Influence of child and adolescent psychiatric disorders on young adult personality disorder, *Am J Psychiatry* 156(10):1529-1535, Oct 1999.
7. Paris J: Antisocial personality disorder: a biopsychosocial model, *Can J Psychiatry* 41:75-80, 1996.
8. Mannuzza S, Klein RG, Bessler A, et al: Adult outcome of hyperactive boys: educational achievement, occupational rank, and psychiatric status, *Arch Gen Psychiatry* 50:565-576, 1993.
9. Ball EM, McCann RA: Antisocial personality disorder. In AM Jacobson AM, Jacobson JL, editors. *Psychiatric Secrets*, ed 2, Philadelphia, 2001, Hanley and Belfus. p. 198-204.
10. Zanarini MC, Frankenburg FR, Dubo ED, et al: Axis I comorbidity of borderline personality disorder, *Am J Psychiatry* 155: 1733-1739, 1998.
11. Dawson DF: Relationship management and the borderline patient, *Can Fam Physician* 39:833-839, 1993.

12. Paré M, Linehan MM, Oldham JM, et al: Dx: personality disorder . . . now what? *Patient Care Can* 7:63-85, 1996.
13. Leichsenring F, Leibing E: The effectiveness of psychodynamic therapy and cognitive behavior therapy in the treatment of personality disorders: a meta-analysis. *Am J Psychiatry*, 160(7): 1223-32. July 2003.
14. Markovitz PJ: Recent trends in the pharmacotherapy of personality disorders, *J Personal Disord* 18(1):90-101, Feb 2004.

PSYCHOTHERAPY

Psychotherapy is defined as "any form of treatment for mental illness, behavioural maladaptions, and/or other problems that are assumed to be of an emotional nature, in which a physician deliberately establishes a professional relationship with a patient for the purposes of removing, modifying, or retarding existing symptoms, or attenuating or reversing disturbed patterns of behaviour, and of promoting positive personality growth and development."

Listening to a person in distress in an empathetic, non-judgemental, supportive, humane way, helps patients cope with calamities and overcome emotional difficulties. Creative listening can empower patients, stimulate growth, and provide encouragement. In addition, psychotherapy can facilitate the removal of existing disabling symptoms, reverse disturbed patterns of behaviour, and promote positive personality maturation and development.

A number of studies show that psychotherapy has positive outcomes in non-psychiatric disorders like asthma,[1] post-myocardial infarction,[2,3] vascular dementia,[4] cancer,[5] mental retardation,[6] and diabetes.[7] In one study, including psychotherapy in a pulmonary rehabilitation program for COPD patients reduced anxiety and depression levels.[8]

There are several forms of psychotherapy. Short-term psychodynamic psychotherapy (STPP), CBT, or behavioural therapy (BT) and generic counselling with antidepressant medication, all have similar outcomes in the treatment of depression.[9,10] Both CBT and psychoeducation delivered via the internet are effective in reducing symptoms of depression.[11] Additionally, reminiscence therapy was shown to reduce depression in older adults.[12] Generic counselling seems to be as effective as antidepressant treatment for mild-to-moderate depressive illness, although patients receiving antidepressants may recover more quickly. General practitioners should allow patients to have their preferred treatment.[13]

Short-term and maintenance empirical data support the effectiveness of using BT and CBT as adjunctive interventions with medications for bipolar I disorder and schizophrenia. Although pharmacotherapy is the foundation of treatment for BD, adjunctive psychosocial Psychoeducation as an adjunct of pharmacotherapy may be beneficial, and family educational interventions have demonstrated encouraging results in relapse prevention. Psychotherapies should be considered early in the course of illness to improve medication compliance and to help patients identify prodromes of relapse in order to take steps for prevention.[14,15]

In major randomized clinical trials, psychotherapy interventions (primarily BT, CBT, and IPT) have been shown to be effective as primary treatments (treatments of choice) for obsessive-compulsive disorder and panic disorder.

Group CBT and Group IPT have been shown helpful in patients with binge-eating disorders.[16] Brief psychodynamic interpersonal therapy helped patients who had deliberately tried to poison themselves.[17] There is accumulated evidence on the efficacy of brief interventions in hazardous drinkers.[11] The sexual offense recidivism rate was lower for those treated with psychological treatment.[18]

Evidence shows that both psychodynamic therapy and CBT are effective treatments of personality disorders.[19]

School-based community-wide screening followed by psychosocial intervention seems to effectively identify and reduce children's disaster-related trauma symptoms and may facilitate psychological recovery.[20] Psychological treatments have been shown to improve psychological symptoms in children who have experienced sexual abuse.[21] Eye movement desensitization and reprogramming (EMDR) therapy has been found useful in post-traumatic stress disorder.[22]

In four behavioural domains, substance abuse, smoking, HIV risk, and diet/exercise, there was substantial evidence that Motivational Interviewing is an effective substance abuse intervention method when used by clinicians who are non-specialists in substance abuse treatment, particularly when enhancing entry to and engagement in more intensive substance abuse treatment-as-usual.[23]

Many other types of psychotherapy have not been tested in randomly assigned, double-blind controlled clinical trials but have been shown to be useful. Hypnotherapy, psychoanalysis, gestalt therapy, family therapy, solution-focused therapy, art therapy, psychodrama, and psychodynamic therapy are just some of the therapies practiced.

❧ REFERENCES ❧

1. Deter HC: Cost-benefit analysis of psychosomatic therapy in asthma, *J Psychosom Res* 30(2):173-182, 1986.
2. Gruen W: Effects of brief psychotherapy during the hospitalization period in the recovery process in heart attacks, *J Consult Clin Psychol* 43:232-233, 1975.
3. Shanfield SB: Return to work after an acute myocardial infarction: a review, *Heart Lung* 19(2):109-117, 1990.
4. Kruglov LS: The early stage of vascular dementia: significance of a complete therapeutic program, *Int J Geriat Psychiatry* 18(5):402-406, May 2003.

5. Newell SA, Sanson-Fisher RW, Savolainen NJ: Systematic review of psychological therapies for cancer patients: overview and recommendations for future research, *J Natl Cancer Inst* 94(8):558-584, 17 Apr 2002.

6. Prout HT, Nowak-Drabik KM: Psychotherapy with persons who have mental retardation: an evaluation of effectiveness; *Am J Ment Retard* 108(2):82-93, Mar 2003.

7. Hampson SE, Skinner TC, Hart J, et al: Effects of educational and psychosocial interventions for adolescents with diabetes mellitus: a systematic review, *Health Technol Assess* 5(10):1-79, 2001.

8. de Godoy DV, de Godoy RF: A randomized controlled trial of the effect of psychotherapy on anxiety and depression in chronic obstructive pulmonary disease, *Arch Physical Med Rehabil* 84(8):1154-1157, Aug 2003.

9. Leichsenring F: Comparative effects of short-term psychodynamic psychotherapy and cognitive-behavioral therapy in depression: a meta-analytic approach, *Clin Psychol Rev* 21(3):401-419, Apr 2001.

10. Craighead WE, Craighead LW: The role of psychotherapy in treating psychiatric disorders, *Med Clin North Am* 85(3):617-629, May 2001.

11. Christensen H, Griffiths KM, Jorm AF: Delivering interventions for depression by using the internet: randomized controlled trial, *BMJ* 328(7434):265, 2004.

12. Hsieh HF, Wang JJ: Effect of reminiscence therapy on depression in older adults: a systematic review; *Int J Nurs Stud* 40(4):335-345, May 2003.

13. Chilvers C, Dewey M, Fielding K, et al: Counselling versus antidepressants in primary care study group, *BMJ* 322(7289):772-775, 31 Mar 2001.

14. Zaretsky A: Targeted psychosocial interventions for bipolar disorder, *Bipolar Disord* 5 (suppl 2):80-87, 2003.

15. Bauer MS: An evidence-based review of psychosocial treatments for bipolar disorder, *Psychopharmacology Bull* 35(3):109-134, 2001.

16. Wilfley DE, Welch RR, Stein RI, et al: A randomized comparison of group cognitive-behavioral therapy and group interpersonal psychotherapy for the treatment of overweight individuals with binge-eating disorder, *Arch Gen Psychiatry* 59(8):713-721, Aug 2002.

17. Arensman E, Townsend E, Hawton K, et al: Psychosocial and pharmacological treatment of patients following deliberate self-harm: the methodological issues involved in evaluating effectiveness, *Suicide Life Threat Behav* 31(2):169-180, Summer 2001.

18. Hanson RK, Gordon A, Harris AJ, et al: First report of the collaborative outcome data project on the effectiveness of psychological treatment for sex offenders, *Sex Abuse J Res Treat* 14(2):169-194, 2002.

19. Leichsenring F, Leibing E: The effectiveness of psychodynamic therapy and cognitive behavior therapy in the treatment of personality disorders: a meta-analysis, *Am J Psychiatry* 160(7):1223-1232, Jul 2003.

20. Chemtob CM, Nakashima JP, Hamada RS: Psychosocial intervention for postdisaster trauma symptoms in elementary school children: a controlled community field study, *Arch Pediatr Adolesc Med* 156(3):211-216, Mar 2002.

21. Ramchandani P, Jones DP: Treating psychological symptoms in sexually abused children: from research findings to service provision, *Br J Psychiatry Suppl* 183:484-490, Dec 2003.

22. Shepherd J, Stein K, Milne R: Eye movement desensitization and reprocessing in the treatment of post-traumatic stress disorder: a review of an emerging therapy, *Psychol Med* 30(4):863-871, Jul 2000.

23. Dunn C, Deroo L, Rivara FP: The use of brief interventions adapted from motivational interviewing across behavioral domains: a systematic review, *Addiction* 96(12):1725-1742, Dec 2001.

SCHIZOPHRENIA

(See also nausea and vomiting; serotonin syndrome; vitamin E)

Schizophrenia is a psychotic disorder that affects approximately 1% of the population. Features include "positive" symptoms such as hallucinations and delusions as well as negative symptoms including poor attention, apathy, social withdrawal, and a loss of will or drive. Most patients also have a history of behavioural dysfunction that may take the form of social or learning difficulties.

The natural course of schizophrenia is deterioration, which is usually greatest in the first few years after diagnosis. Rate of progression varies markedly among individuals. Prognosis is better for women than men, for those who have a later onset of disease, for those who respond well to an initial course of medication, and for those who live in a relatively serene family environment. Prognosis is considerably worse if negative symptoms are prominent, if the patient also has a substance abuse disorder, and if social and cognitive functioning abilities were poor before the onset of illness. The longer the duration of untreated psychosis, the worse the prognosis. The lifetime suicide prevalence is 10%.

There are often comorbid psychiatric conditions, substance abuse or dependence being the most common (10% to 60%). Alcohol use disorder is the most prevalent, and rates of nicotine use range from 58% to 90%.[1]

Early treatment of schizophrenia is recommended in the hope that treatment will improve prognosis. Aside from medications, treatment should include social skills training, family psychoeducational training, and a protected employment environment.

Neuroleptics

The classification and usual dosages of selected neuroleptics are recorded in Table 49.

Typical or "first-generation" antipsychotic drugs have often been divided into two groups: low potency and high potency. The low-potency group, which includes drugs such as chlorpromazine, tends to cause sedation and hypotension but has relatively few extrapyramidal effects. High-potency drugs such as haloperidol are less sedating and cause less hypotension but are associated with greater extrapyramidal effects.[2]

Risperidone, olanzapine, clozapine, and quetiapine are "atypical" or "second-generation" antipsychotics. Atypical

Table 49   Neuroleptics

Drugs	Usual Doses
Typical (First-Generation) Antipsychotics	
Butyrophenone derivatives	
Haloperidol (Haldol)	5-20 mg/day
Phenothiazines, aliphatic	
Chlorpromazine (Thorazine, Largactil)	25-400 mg/day
Methotrimeprazine (Nozinan)	6-75 mg/day
Phenothiazines, piperazine	
Trifluoperazine (Stelazine)	6-20 mg/day
Prochlorperazine (Compazine, Stemetil)	5-10 mg tid or qid; usually used for nausea and vomiting
Fluphenazine enanthate (Prolixin Enanthate, Moditen)	25 mg (12.5-100 mg) IM q 2 weeks
Fluphenazine decanoate (Prolixin Decanoate, Modecate)	25 mg (12.5-50 mg) IM q 3 weeks
Phenothiazines, piperidine	
Thioridazine (Mellaril)	25-400 mg/day
Tricyclic dibenzoxazepine derivatives	
Loxapine (Loxapac)	60-100 mg/day
Atypical (Second-Generation) Antipsychotics	
Clozapine (Clozaril)	100-600 mg/day
Olanzapine (Zyprexa)	5-20 mg/day
Risperidone (Risperdal)	2-10 mg/day
Quetiapine (Seroquel)	100 mg tid-n-200 mg bid

[Handwritten annotations:]
↑ Side effects
- Sedation, anti-cholinergic, EPS
- Acute dystonia
- Parkinsonism
- Akathisia   TD

- first line treatment

↑ Sedation
↑ wt gain
↑ prolactin
Metabolic Syndrome

Aripiprazole Abilify

neuroleptics have been in use for approximately 15 years and are considered first line for treatment of psychoses and schizophrenia. As a group, they improve negative symptoms and may improve cognitive functioning. Their effectiveness equals that of first-generation antipsychotics, and extrapyramidal side effects are less common. Second-generation drugs are chemically diverse, so failure of response to one does not mean that another will not be effective.[3]

Clozapine has been particularly valuable in treating patients who have failed to respond to first-generation neuroleptics. Agranulocytosis has been reported in 1% to 2% of patients, so weekly monitoring of white blood cell counts is necessary. Clozapine also lowers the seizure threshold significantly.[4] *[handwritten: → CBC at any sign of illness]*

The cumulative relapse rate 5 years after a first episode of schizophrenia is 82%; the rate is approximately five times greater in patients who discontinue neuroleptics than in those who continue to take their medications. Robinson and associates[5] advise that after a first psychotic episode, neuroleptics be taken continuously for at least 2 years. Kane[2] recommends neuroleptic treatment for 1 to 2 years after a first episode of schizophrenia and for 5 years or even indefinitely for anyone who has had two or more episodes. The relapse rate while taking medications is 15% to 20% per year.

In outpatient settings, the dosage of neuroleptics should be relatively low initially and should be increased gradually. Maximum control of psychotic thought processes may take weeks or even months, whereas

agitation may be rapidly controlled because of the sedative effects of neuroleptics. Follow-up every 2 weeks is adequate to monitor psychotic thought processes, whereas daily assessments may be necessary to evaluate agitation.

In the past, very large doses of neuroleptics were used for some patients. The current view is that doses greater than 10 to 20 mg of haloperidol or its equivalent add little if any additional therapeutic benefit.[2] Much or all of the neuroleptic dose can be given at bedtime if nocturnal sedation is required. If daytime agitation is a problem, the total daily dose may be divided so that a portion of it is given during the day.

The following are some of the more important adverse effects of neuroleptics:

- Seizures. In general the neuroleptics lower the seizure threshold. The incidence of seizures is particularly high with clozapine (Clozaril).
- Interaction with TCAs. The neuroleptics inhibit the metabolism of tricyclics and so raise their blood levels.
- Hypotension. All of the phenothiazines may cause a marked hypotensive effect through alpha-adrenergic blockade. Phenothiazines should be used with extreme caution in the elderly.
- Anticholinergic effects. The anticholinergic effects of neuroleptics are most marked in the aliphatic phenothiazines (chlorpromazine, methotrimeprazine).
- Sedation. All of the neuroleptics are sedative, but of those commonly used, the most sedative seem to be methotrimeprazine, chlorpromazine, and thioridazine.

- Prolactin elevation. Neuroleptics raise prolactin levels and may cause galactorrhea.
- Tardive dyskinesia (TD). The risk of TD is generally related to dose, treatment duration, and age. TD is three to five times more common in elderly than in young patients treated with conventional antipsychotics, and after 3 years of treatment, the rate of TD surpasses 50%.[6] The most effective treatment is to decrease or withdraw the offending neuroleptic, but TD may be irreversible. TD appears to be less common with second-generation than with first-generation neuroleptics, and if it is caught early during the use of a typical neuroleptic, switching to an atypical neuroleptic may reverse the TD.

[handwritten: 1/3 Permanent]

- Neuroleptic malignant syndrome. The cardinal features of the neuroleptic malignant syndrome are hyperpyrexia, muscle rigidity, altered mental status, and autonomic instability (variations in pulse and blood pressure). Patients may have elevated creatinine kinase levels, myoglobinuria from rhabdomyolysis, and acute renal failure. The mortality rate of untreated persons is 20%. The disorder usually occurs within the first few weeks of starting a neuroleptic or of increasing the dose. Treatment is discontinuation of the neuroleptic, intake of fluids, and administration of dantrolene, bromocriptine, or pergolide.[2] (See also the discussion of serotonin syndrome.)

[handwritten: Cooling, IV fluids]

- Extrapyramidal effects. The extrapyramidal effects of neuroleptics include dystonias, opisthotonos, oculogyric crises, Parkinson-like symptoms, and akathisia. Among first-generation neuroleptics, those commonly causing this type of adverse effect are the butyrophenone derivatives (haloperidol). Extrapyramidal effects are rare with the aliphatic phenothiazine derivatives (chlorpromazine, methotrimeprazine) and are relatively uncommon with the usual oral doses of the piperidine phenothiazine derivatives (thioridazine). The incidence of extrapyramidal side effects with the piperazine phenothiazine derivatives depends on the dosage. These effects are uncommon with the usual outpatient doses of trifluoperazine but very common with the long-acting intramuscular forms (fluphenazine enanthate, and fluphenazine decanoate). Extrapyramidal reactions are relatively rare with the newer atypical antipsychotics. Acute dystonic reactions can be controlled by a single injection of diphenhydramine (Benadryl) 50 mg. Other extrapyramidal effects are controlled by benztropine or procyclidine. At usual outpatient doses, one rarely needs antiparkinsonian drugs with chlorpromazine, methotrimeprazine, trifluoperazine, or thioridazine. Most patients taking haloperidol require them on a regular basis, and patients taking the long-acting intramuscular formulations of fluphenazine enanthate or fluphenazine decanoate require them only during the first week or two after the injections. The usual dosage of benztropine is 1 to 4 mg per day as a single dose or in two divided doses, whereas that of procyclidine is 7.5 to 20 mg per day in three divided doses.

[handwritten: RF - lithium + anti Psychot]

- Akathisia. Akathisia is an extrapyramidal effect that causes the patient to feel extremely restless. The main modality of treatment is to lower the dose of the neuroleptic, but some patients may respond to antiparkinsonian agents, beta blockers (propanolol 20 to 80 mg per day), or benzodiazepines. In view of the high risk of substance abuse in schizophrenic patients, benzodiazepines should be prescribed with caution.
- Weight gain. Weight gain may occur with both first- and second-generation neuroleptics, but is most marked with many of the second-generation agents. Weight gain of up to 20 kg may occur with longer-term treatment, and increased rates of diabetes mellitus have been reported.

[handwritten: Psych: CBT Social: Family therapy, rehab, social skills functioning, Support + accomod.]

✍ REFERENCES ✍

1. Green AI, Canuso CM, Brenner MJ, et al: Detection and management of comorbidity in patients with schizophrenia *Psychiatr Clin North Am* 26(1):115-139, 2003.
2. Kane JM: Schizophrenia, *N Engl J Med* 334:34-41, 1996.
3. Working Group for the Canadian Psychiatric Association and the Canadian Alliance for Research on Schizophrenia: Canadian clinical practice guidelines for the treatment of schizophrenia, *Can J Psychiatry* 43(suppl 2 revised): S25-S40, 1998.
4. Csernansky JG: Psychopharmacologic treatment of schizophrenia, *Psychiatr Clin North Am* 5:161-182, 1998.
5. Robinson D, Woerner MG, Alvir JM, et al: Predictors of relapse following response from a first episode of schizophrenia or schizoaffective disorder, *Arch Gen Psychiatry* 56:241-247, 1999.
6. Kapur S: Receptor imaging studies in the treatment of schizophrenia, *Psychiatry Rounds* 2(1):1-5, 1998.
7. Wood AJJ: Schizophrenia, *N Engl J Med* 349:1738-1749, 2003.

[handwritten notes at bottom of page:
Delusional Disorder.
↓imp. functn Non-bizarre delusions
DDx: Brief Psychotic Episode — Duration of symptoms <1mo, no neg Sx
Schizophreniform — 1 mo, <6mo.
organic — sensory deprivation   Schizophrenia
Dementia   Schizoaffective — schizo + mood dis. in same episode
Delirium   Sub. induced/medical
Hypnogogic/hypnopompic
Bereavement
6 mo — may include prodrome]

ADRENAL DISORDERS
Adrenal Insufficiency

Addison's disease is a rare condition of primary adrenal insufficiency, and causes include autoimmune, infectious, hemorrhagic, and metastatic etiologies. It is more common in females and is mostly diagnosed in young to middle-aged adults. The three cardinal symptoms are weight loss, fatigue, and weakness. Gastrointestinal and psychiatric symptoms are common. Most patients have orthostatic hypotension, and a number are hyperpigmented in creases and pressure areas. Laboratory abnormalities include mild normocytic anemia, mild eosinophilia, hyponatremia, and hyperkalemia.[1] In many cases an 8 A.M. cortisol determination can confirm or rule out the diagnosis. If the level is 83 nmol/L (3 μg/dL) or less, the diagnosis is confirmed, whereas if the concentration is 525 nmol/L (19 μg/dL) or more, it is ruled out (assuming a normal range to be 165 to 662 nmol/L [6 to 24 μg/dL]).[1]

The treatment of choice for chronic adrenal insufficiency is oral hydrocortisone. Although the dosage is variable, most patents receive cortisone 25 to 37.5 mg/day. Usually two thirds of the daily dose is given in the morning and one third at night. In times of stress, such as intercurrent illnesses, injury, or surgery, the maintenance dose is usually doubled. Patients with primary adrenal insufficiency often lose salt and may need to take fludrocortisone (Florinef) 50 to 200 μg as a single daily dose; those with secondary adrenal insufficiency (caused by pituitary disorders) rarely require fludrocortisone.[1] Recent studies suggest that short-term oral dehydroepiandrosterone (DHEA) replacement may improve self esteem, mood, and fatigue symptoms in patients with lower than normal endogenous DHEA/DHEA-S concentrations. A daily dose of 50 mg of DHEA was used.[2]

Prednisone, prednisolone, and dexamethasone are not the drugs of choice for Addison's disease because they have little mineralocorticoid activity. Addison's disease may still develop in patients taking these drugs for other reasons.[3]

Cushing's Syndrome

Cushing's syndrome is a condition of cortisol excess. It is caused by exogenous glucocorticoids, Cushing's disease (adrenocorticotropic hormone [ACTH] hypersecretion by pituitary adenoma), adrenal neoplasms, or ectopic ACTH-secreting tumours. Rapid weight gain is characteristic of Cushing's syndrome. Other characteristics include a rounded "moon" facies, facial plethora, buffalo hump, spraclavicular fat pad, striae, and proximal muscle weakness.[4]

If Cushing's syndrome is suspected, a 24-hour urine study for free cortisol (plus creatinine to assess the adequacy of collection) should be performed and repeated on 1 or 2 consecutive days.[4] Values more than 830 nmol (300 μg) per day are considered diagnostic for Cushing's syndrome (normal < 250 nmol or 90 μg per 24 hours). The reported sensitivity in detecting cortisol excess is 95%, and the specificity is 98%.[5] A dexamethasone suppression test is the standard alternative. This test is performed by giving 1 mg of dexamethasone at 11 P.M. and measuring the serum cortisol by 8 A.M. the next day. If the level is less than 140 nmol/L (5 μg/dL), the diagnosis of Cushing's syndrome is ruled out in 98% of cases. Unfortunately, the dexamethasone suppression test has a high false-positive rate.[5]

Eating disorders, chronic illness, chronic alcoholism and depression can cause false-positive results (pseudo-Cushing's syndrome) on the 1-mg dexamethasone suppression test and the 24-hour urine cortisol collection. If pseudo-Cushing's syndrome is suspected, a midnight serum cortisol level of less than 7.5 μg per dL (207 nmol per L) is strongly suggestive of pseudo-Cushing's syndrome.[5]

Incidentalomas

About 5% of patients who have an abdominal CT scan are found to have an incidental adrenal mass; over 80% of these are benign and hormonally non-functional.[6] All patients should have a hormonal evaluation, including a 1 mg dexamethasone suppression test for hypercortisolism; plasma free metanephrines for pheochromocytoma; and serum potassium, aldosterone, and renin levels in patients with hypertension.[7] Surgery is suggested for patients with pheochromocytoma, functional and clinically apparent adrenal cortex tumours, and any masses > 6 cm.[7] Incidentalomas that are not hormonally active over 4 years, and remain stable on two imaging studies done ≥ 6 months apart do not warrant further follow-up.[7]

⇗ REFERENCES ⇖

1. Oelkers W: Adrenal insufficiency, *N Engl J Med* 335:1206-1212, 1996.

2. Achermann JC, Silverman BL: Dehydroepiandrosterone replacement for patients with adrenal insufficiency. *Lancet* 2001; 357:1381-1382.

3. Cronin CC, Callaghan N, Kearney PJ, et al: Addison disease in patients treated with glucocorticoid therapy, *Arch Intern Med* 157:456-458, 1997.

4. Orth DN: Cushing's syndrome, *N Engl J Med* 332:791-803, 1995.

5. Kirk LF, Hash RB, Katner HP: Cushing's Disease: Clinical Manifestations and Diagnostic Evaluation, *American Family Physician* 62:1119-27,1133-1134, 2000.

6. Ooi TC: Adrenal incidentalomas: incidental in detection, not significance, *Can Med Assoc J* 157:903-904, 1997.

7. Grumbach MM, Biller BM, Braunstein GD, et al: Management of the clinically inapparent adrenal mass ("incidentaloma"), *Ann Intern Med* 138:424-429 2003.

CHRONIC FATIGUE SYNDROME

(See also celiac disease; fibromyalgia; multiple chemical sensitivities)

Myalgic encephalomyelitis/chronic fatigue syndrome (ME/CFS) is a severe systemic, acquired illness that can be debilitating. Symptoms manifest predominantly as neurological, immunological and endocrinological dysfunction. While the pathogenesis is suggested to be multifactorial, the hypothesis of initiation by a viral infection has been prominent.[1] Chronic fatigue syndrome is a diagnosis of exclusion, but many theories[2] concerning etiology are beginning to converge as there is much symptom overlap between it, fibromyalgia, and multiple chemical sensitivities.[3] Given the etiologic and mechanistic uncertainties, it may be useful to view these conditions as multifactorial, with a failure of adaptation, whereby each patient's maximum tolerance for combined stressors, no matter what their source, has been exceeded. An advantage of this framework is that it fits with the patient-centred, bio-psycho-social and spiritual approach of family medicine. There is no specific laboratory test or investigation specifically for ME/CFS yet. One is in the research stage currently.

In general practice, up to 25% of patients present with a symptom of unexplained fatigue.[4] In a large population-based sample of 28,000 adults, the prevalence of CFS was found to be 0.5% of women and 0.3% of men.[5] Most patients in whom the chronic fatigue syndrome is diagnosed are middle-aged women.[6,7]

In 2001, an International Expert Medical Consensus Panel of Health Canada was established. A new detailed clinical working case definition of ME/CFS was developed to encompass the complex symptom complexes of this illness,[1] replacing that of Fukuda et al,[8] created by an international study group and endorsed by the U.S. Centers for Disease Control.

The panel concluded that recognized organic and psychiatric disorders must be ruled out; a process that is quite extensive and may include a sleep study, laboratory work to detect malignancy, nutritional deficiencies, metabolic disorders, endocrine disorders, neurologic disorders such as multiple sclerosis, cardiovascular disorders, connective tissue disease, allergies, pesticide or heavy metal poisoning, drug abuse, or chronic infections.[8] It is important to take a thorough exposure history using the CH2OPD2 mnemonic (community, home/hobby, occupation, personal exposure, diet/drugs).[9]

The new clinical case definition now has seven criteria:

1. New-onset persistent or recurring mental and physical fatigue that substantially reduces the functional level

2. Post-exertional malaise or fatigue with slow recovery lasting over 24 hours

3. Sleep dysfunction

4. Pain in muscles and joints

5. Neurologic/cognitive manifestations

6. At least one symptom from two categories: autonomic, neuroendocrine or immunological

7. Persistence of illness that lasts 6 months or more for adults and three months or more in children[1]

Physical findings co-relate to the clinical history findings, which may include the following: hypotension, tender lymph nodes, subnormal body temperature, crimson (red) crescents in the tonsillar fossae, positive Romberg or tandem test, cognitive symptoms including inability to remember questions, difficulty with serial seven subtraction, positive tender points for fibromyalgia, and symptoms of IBS including increase bowel sounds, mild bloating, and abdominal tenderness.[9]

Patients who have been suffering from fatigue for more than 6 months but have insufficient symptoms to meet the criteria for ME/CFS are said to have "idiopathic chronic fatigue." The term "chronic fatigue" includes both the "chronic fatigue syndrome" and "idiopathic chronic fatigue."[8,10]

A community-based American study reported that 55% of patients with chronic fatigue syndrome had at least one current and 81% at least one lifetime Axis I psychiatric diagnosis secondary to chronic fatigue syndrome and its social consequences.[5]

The natural history of chronic fatigue syndrome has not been fully defined. An 18-month follow-up of 298 self-referred patients meeting the criteria of chronic fatigue syndrome found that 3% reported complete recovery and 17% had improvement.[11] The prognosis is much better in children and adolescents, with 95% improved or completely recovered after 1 to 4 years of follow-up.[12]

As would be expected, optimal treatment for a condition of unknown etiology is uncertain and the illness course can be a repeated "crash and burn" experience if the patient overextends beyond the limitations imposed by the illness. The patient should practice energy conservation and pacing keeping an activity log and filling out a functional capacity scale daily to monitor clinical progress.[9]

The treatment of ME/CFS is symptomatic and supportive.[13] The patient needs to book many appointments to sort out their numerous symptoms. It is helpful to use the Signs and Symptoms Checklist.[9]

Teaching the patient the principles of pacing or energy conservation helps fatigue. Home care assessment is helpful and an occupational therapist visit for an energy conservation assessment is useful. They often need medications to help them sleep. No particular type works for all patients. It is trial and error to find the right type and dosage. Keeping the patient as active as possible within their available energy is the goal. When the pain is severe, medication for the treatment of chronic non-malignant pain may become necessary to enable the patient to have a better quality of life. If narcotic pain medication (including codeine) is necessary, proper records must be kept in your clinical notes as per College requirements. This includes the type of drug, dose and affect the pain medication has on the patient's ability to become more active as better pain control is achieved.[14] The stress of a chronic illness has severe consequences on the spouse and children in the family. The physician can provide long-term emotional support.

A 1996 study from the Netherlands found no benefit from an 8-week treatment regimen of fluoxetine (Prozac) 20 mg.[15] On the other hand, a series of 13[16] or 16[17] weekly or biweekly sessions of cognitive therapy was associated with a satisfactory outcome in about three fourths of treated patients compared with about one fourth of the control subjects who received either relaxation therapy[16] or general medical care from their general practitioners.[17] A randomized controlled trial of graded aerobic exercises versus flexibility exercises and relaxation therapy found a marked improvement with aerobic exercises,[18] while a trial comparing graded aerobic exercises with fluoxetine resulted in improvement in fatigue and work capacity with exercise but not with fluoxetine.[19] A placebo-controlled crossover trial found no benefit from fludrocortisone (Florinef),[20] whereas a randomized crossover trial of patients with no comorbid psychiatric conditions reported subjective benefit from hydrocortisone 5 or 10 mg/day, a benefit that rapidly attenuated when the drug was discontinued.[21]

⚓ REFERENCES ⚓

1. Carruthers BM, Jain AK, De Meirleir KL, et al: Myalgic encephalomyelitis/chronic fatigue syndrome: Clinical working case definition, diagnostic and treatment protocols, *J of Chronic Fatigue Syndrome* 11(1):7-115, 2003.

2. Bested AC, Saunders PR, Logan AC: Chronic fatigue syndrome: Neurologic findings may be related to blood-brain barrier permeability, *Medical Hypothesis*, 57(2):231-7, 2001.

3. Bell IR, Baldwin CM, Schwartz GE: Illness from low levels of environmental chemicals: Relevance to chronic fatigue syndrome and fibromyalgia, *The American Journal of Medicine* 105(3A):74S-82S, 1998.

4. Komaroff AL, Fagioli LR, Doolittle TH, et al: Health status in patients with chronic fatigue syndrome and in general population and disease comparison groups, *Am J of Med* 101(3):281-90, 1996.

5. Jason LA, Richman JA, Rademaker AW, et al: A community-based study of chronic fatigue syndrome, *Arch Intern Med* 159:2129-2137, 1999.

6. Buchwald D, Garrity D: Comparison of patients with chronic fatigue syndrome, fibromyalgia, and multiple chemical sensitivities, *Arch Intern Med* 154:2049-2053, 1994.

7. Wessely S, Chalder T, Hirsch S, et al: The prevalence and morbidity of chronic fatigue and chronic fatigue syndrome: a prospective primary care study, *Am J Public Health* 87:1449-1455, 1997.

8. Fukuda K, Straus SE, Hickie I, et al (International Chronic Fatigue Syndrome Study Group): The chronic fatigue syndrome: a comprehensive approach to its definition and study, *Ann Intern Med* 121:953-959, 1994.

9. Ontario College of Family Physicians: What's New? Communications Publications: Environment and Health. www.ocfp.ca

10. Wessely S, Chalder T, Hirsch S, et al: Psychological symptoms, somatic symptoms and psychiatric disorder in chronic fatigue and chronic fatigue syndrome: a prospective study in primary care, *Am J Psychiatry* 153:1050-1059, 1996.

11. Vercoulen JH, Swanink CM, Fennis JF, et al: Prognosis in chronic fatigue syndrome–a prospective study on the natural course, *J Neurol Neurosurg Psychiatry* 60:489-494, 1996.

12. Krilov LR, Fisher M, Friedman SB, et al: Course and outcome of chronic fatigue in children and adolescents, *Pediatrics* 102:360-366, 1998.

13. Marshall LM, Bested A, Bray RI: Tools to treat chronic fatigue syndrome, fibromyalgia and multiple chemical sensitivity. *The Canadian Journal of CME*, 2003.

14. PAIN Evidence-Based Recommendations for Medical Management of Chronic Non-Malignant Pain Reference Guide for Clinicians, Facilitated by the College of Physicians and Surgeons of Ontario, 2000.

15. Vercoulen JH, Swanink CM, Zitman FG, et al: Randomised, double-blind, placebo-controlled study of fluoxetine in chronic fatigue syndrome, *Lancet* 347:858-861, 1996.

16. Deale A, Chalder T, Marks I, et al: Cognitive behavior therapy for chronic fatigue syndrome: a randomized controlled trial, *Am J Psychiatry* 154:408-414, 1997.

17. Sharpe M, Hawton K, Simkin S, et al: Cognitive behaviour therapy for the chronic fatigue syndrome: a randomized controlled trial, *BMJ* 312:22-26, 1996.

18. Fulcher KY, White PD: Randomised controlled trial of graded exercise in patients with the chronic fatigue syndrome, *BMJ* 314:1647-1652, 1997.

19. Wearden A, Morriss R, Mullis R, et al: A double-blind, placebo-controlled treatment trial of fluoxetine and graded

exercise for chronic fatigue syndrome, *Br J Psychiatry* 172:485-490, 1998.

20. Peterson PK, Pheley A, Schroeppel J, et al: A preliminary placebo-controlled crossover trial of fludrocortisone for chronic fatigue syndrome, *Arch Intern Med* 158:908-914, 1998.

21. Cleare AJ, Heap E, Malhi GS, et al: Low-dose hydrocortisone in chronic fatigue syndrome: a randomised crossover trial, *Lancet* 353:455-458, 1999.

DIABETES MELLITUS

Type 1 Diabetes

Epidemiology

Type 1 diabetes comprises approximately 5% to 10% of all diabetes cases. The mean onset is 8 to 12 years of age, with a rapid decline in incidence after adolescence. The incidence is increased in those who have a first-degree relative with type 1 diabetes (father 6%, mother 2%, sibling 5%, non-identical twin 5%, identical twin 30% to 50%). The highest incidence is in Scandanavians; the lowest incidence is in Asians (especially those from Korea, Japan, and China).[1]

_____ ◖ REFERENCES ◗ _____

1. Atkinson MA, Maclaren NK: The pathogenesis of insulin-dependent diabetes mellitus, *N Engl J Med* 331:1428-1436, 1994.

Diet and type 1 diabetes

The important role of nutrition therapy in improving glycemic control has been well documented.[1] In a recent position statement published by the American Diabetes Association, evidence-based nutrition recommendations were discussed.[2]

The current view of diet in type 1 diabetes is that it should have as few restrictions as possible. Usual food intake should be assessed and used as a basis for adjusting insulin types and doses.[2,3] Sucrose need not be specifically restricted.[3] Patients should monitor glucose levels and use varying doses of short-acting insulins to cover meals (more for a big meal, less for a small meal). Using such an approach, patients have far more flexibility in the timing of meals and may even be able to miss meals safely.[2,3] Individuals receiving fixed doses of insulin should be consistent in day-to-day carbohydrate intake in an effort to maintain optimal control of their diabetes.[2]

_____ ◖ REFERENCES ◗ _____

1. Pastors JG, Warshaw H, Daly A, et al: The evidence for the effectiveness of medical nutritional therapy in diabetes management, *Diabetes Care* 25:608-613, 2002.

2. American Diabetes Association: Nutrition principles and recommendations in Diabetes, *Diabetes Care* 27(suppl S36-S46), 2004.

3. Berger M: To bridge science and patient care in diabetes, *Diabetologia* 39:749-757, 1996.

Exercise and type 1 diabetes

An exercise program is believed to be important for patients with insulin-dependent diabetes because it is thought to improve the quality of their lives and protect against macrovascular disease.[1] However, evidence supporting these hypotheses has not yet been published.[2]

The major risk associated with exercise is hypoglycemia, which may develop during, shortly after, or 6 to 12 hours after exercise. The patient may try to prevent this with a pre-exercise snack or, when exercising is done on a regular basis, by decreasing the appropriate insulin dose. For low-to-moderate-intensity exercise of less than an hour's duration, a pre-exercise snack is usually not required unless the pre-exercise glucose level is less than 5.6 mmol/L (100 mg/dL). For high-intensity exercises, snacks are advised.[3]

Athletes with type 1 diabetes, who exercise regularly should, at least initially, monitor their blood sugar before, during, and for several hours after the exercise. If the exercise is performed in the late afternoon or evening, a 2 A.M. glucose measurement should also be taken. In general, a 30% to 50% reduction in the preprandial insulin dose before exercise is required. To prevent post-exercise nocturnal hypoglycemia, the patient should have only regular insulin before supper and NPH or, even better, Lente at bedtime.[3]

A danger signal for athletes is a pre-exercise glucose level greater than 13.9 mmol/L (250 mg/dL). In this situation, exercise can aggravate hyperglycemia and even cause ketoacidosis. If the glucose level is between 13.9 mmol/L (250 mg/dL) and 16.7 mmol/L (300 mg/dL) and the urine is free of ketones, participation in the athletic event can proceed. If ketones are present or the glucose level is above 16.7 mmol/L (300 mg/dL), the athlete should postpone exercise until better control is achieved.[3]

Exercise of the muscle at the site of an insulin injection increases the rate of absorption and the risk of hypoglycemia, but only if the exercise takes place within 30 minutes of the injection.[4] Absorption from the abdomen is greater than from the thigh, so switching from thigh to abdomen may result in hypoglycemia. The practical significance of these findings is that the athlete should rotate insulin injection sites around one anatomical area and not switch from one body site to another. If there is a choice, the abdomen is probably the preferable site.[3]

_____ ◖ REFERENCES ◗ _____

1. Expert Committee of the Canadian Diabetes Advisory Board: Clinical practice guidelines for diabetes mellitus in Canada, *Can Med Assoc J* 147:697-712, 1992.

2. Berger M, Mühlhauser I: Diabetes care and patient-oriented outcomes, *JAMA* 281:1676-1678, 1999.

3. Fahey PF, Stallcamp ET, Kwatra S: The athlete with type I diabetes: managing insulin, diet and exercise, *Am Fam Physician* 53:1611-1617, 1996.

4. Kemmer FW: Prevention of hypoglycemia during exercise in type I diabetes, *Diabetes Care* 15:1732-1735, 1992.

Intensive treatment in preventing diabetic complications in type 1 diabetes

(Note: For insulin management and review of complications see complications, insulin therapy in diabetes below)

A seminal article dealing with the beneficial effects of tight control in diabetes was the 1993 report of the Diabetes Control and Complications Trial Research Group (DCCT), published in the *New England Journal of Medicine*. It showed that after a mean follow-up of 6.5 years patients with insulin-dependent diabetes mellitus (type 1 diabetes) given intensive therapy had a significant diminution of retinopathy, neuropathy, proteinuria, and microalbuminuria. Specifically, intensive therapy slowed the progression of retinopathy by 54% and reduced the development of proliferative or severe non-proliferative retinopathy by 47%. Clinical neuropathy was reduced by 60%, albuminuria by 54%, and microalbuminuria by 39%. No statistically significant decline occurred in macrovascular disease, but because of the youth of the study population, this was not unexpected.[1]

The improvements in microvascular complications were achieved at a cost. In the DCCT trial, the incidence of severe hypoglycemic reactions increased three-fold and patients had significant weight gain. The mean weight gain over 5 years was 4.6 kg (10 lb) greater than in the conventionally treated control subjects; 33% of the intensively treated group met the criteria for obesity (body mass index >27.8 kg/m^2 for men and >27.3 kg/m^2 for women) compared with 19% of the conventionally treated group.[2,3] Of particular concern was the finding that those in the intensively treated group who became obese met the criteria for the central obesity–insulin resistance syndrome ("syndrome X"). This syndrome, which includes insulin resistance, elevated blood pressure, increased abdominal obesity, and dyslipidemia, is associated with an increased risk of coronary artery disease.[3]

Evidence that establishing complete normoglycemia (a state not achieved by the DCCT trial) may reverse the lesions of diabetic nephropathy comes from a study of eight diabetic patients with this disorder who had pancreas transplants. No improvement was detectable after 5 years, but a reversal of the biochemical abnormalities and histological lesions was achieved by 10 years.[4]

──────────── ❧ **REFERENCES** ❧ ────────────

1. Diabetes Control and Complications Trial Research Group: The effect of intensive treatment of diabetes on the development and progression of long-term complications in insulin-dependent diabetes mellitus, *N Engl J Med* 329:977-986, 1993.

2. Diabetes Control and Complications Trial Research Group: Adverse events and their association with treatment regimens in the Diabetes Control and Complications Trial, *Diabetes Care* 18:1415-1427, 1995.

3. Purnell JQ, Hokanson JE, Marcovina SM, et al: Effect of excessive weight gain with intensive therapy of type 1 diabetes on lipid levels and blood pressure: results from the DCCT, *JAMA* 280:140-146, 1998.

4. Fioretto P, Steffes MW, Sutherland DE, et al: Reversal of lesions of diabetic nephropathy after pancreas transplantation, *N Engl J Med* 339:69-75, 1998.

Type 2 Diabetes

Diagnosis

The American and Canadian Diabetes Association recommend that the diagnosis of diabetes be made if the fasting sugar level is greater than 7 mmol/L (126 mg/dL), a casual plasma glucose is greater than 11.1 in a symptomatic patient or a 2 hour post-prandial plasma glucose exceeds 11.1 after a 75 gram glucose challenge.[1,2] The diagnosis should be validated with a repeat test. Individuals with fasting plasma glucose levels between 6.1 and 7 mmol/L (109 mg/dL and 126 mg/dL) or a 2 hour post-prandial of 8.1-11 have impaired fasting glucose (IFG) or impaired glucose tolerance (IGT). Polyuria, polydypsia, and unexplained weight loss are the key diagnostic symptoms. Although these conditions may not pose an increased risk for microvascular disease, they significantly increase the risk for developing diabetes and are independent risk factors for macrovascular disease.[2]

There are some interesting debates regarding these definitions. Davidson and associates[3] argue that 60% of individuals with fasting plasma glucose levels between 7 mmol/L (126 mg/dL) and 7.7 mmol/L (139 mg/dL) have normal HbA$_1$c and that they are not really diabetic but may be subject to negative psychological, social, employment, and insurance consequences because they are so labelled. An accompanying editorial by Vinicor[4] strongly disagrees. A number of researchers have concluded that using only fasting sugar levels, even lower ones, misses many patients at increased risk of morbidity[5] and death[6] from diabetes-related macrovascular complications but that most of these could be detected by modified glucose tolerance tests. These authors advocate a return to the World Health Organization recommendation that glucose levels above 11.1 mmol/L (200 mg/dL) 2 hours after a 75-g glucose load be considered diagnostic of diabetes.

──────────── ❧ **REFERENCES** ❧ ────────────

1. American Diabetes Association: Standards of medical care for patients with diabetes mellitus, *Diabetes Care* 20(suppl 1):S1-S70, 2004.

2. Canadian Diabetes Association Clinical Practice Guidelines Expert Committee: CDA 2003 Clinical Practice Guidelines

for the Prevention and Management of Diabetes in Canada, *Can J Diabetes* 27(suppl 2):S10-S11, 2003.

3. Davidson MB, Schriger DL, Peters AL, et al: Relationship between fasting plasma glucose and glycosylated hemoglobin: potential for false-positive diagnoses of type 2 diabetes using new diagnostic criteria, *JAMA* 281:1203-1210, 1999.

4. Vinicor F: When is diabetes diabetes? (editorial), *JAMA* 281:1222-1224, 1999.

5. Barzilay JI, Spiekerman CF, Wahl PW, et al: Cardiovascular disease in older adults with glucose disorders: comparison of American Diabetes Association criteria for diabetes mellitus with WHO criteria, *Lancet* 354:622-625, 1999.

6. Tuomilehto J, et al (DECODE_study group on behalf of the European Diabetes Epidemiology Group): Glucose tolerance and mortality: comparison of WHO and American Diabetes Association diagnostic criteria, *Lancet* 354:617-621, 1999.

Epidemiology and prevention

Diabetes affects 4% to 6% of Canadians. About 90% of persons with diabetes are not insulin dependent (type 2) and 5% to 10% are insulin dependent (type 1).

The genetic propensity for type 2 diabetes is greater than for type 1. A person who has one first-degree relative with the disease has twice the risk, and if the person has two first-degree relatives with the condition, the risk is quadrupled. The concordance rate for identical twins is 60% to 80%.[1] Race is also a risk factor; the disease is twice as common in blacks[1] and two-and-one-half to three times as common in Mexican-Americans as in whites.[2] Diabetes among Native Americans was virtually unknown before 1940, but it now has a high prevalence rate.[3] This increase is almost certainly due to a marked increase in the incidence of obesity in this population. In the United States, the incidence of diabetes in Native Americans is five times that of whites.[2] In the northern Canadian community of Sioux Lookout the prevalence of type 2 diabetes in adolescents under 16 was 2.5:1000. Most patients were asymptomatic obese females with a strong family history of type 2 diabetes.[4]

Young women with long or highly irregular menstrual cycles are at an increased risk of developing type 2 DM, independent of their body weight.[5]

A major risk factor, which at least in theory can be controlled, is weight gain. In a prospective cohort study of American nurses, a weight gain after the age of 18 of 5 to 7.9 kg increased the risk of diabetes by 1.9% and a weight gain of 8 to 10.9 kg increased the risk by 2.7%. A weight loss of more than 5 kg decreased the relative risk by 50%.[6] A 2-year study of non-diabetic obese Americans with a mean BMI of 36 compared four management protocols: no specific program (control group), diet, exercise, and diet plus exercise. The mean weight loss in both the diet and diet plus exercise groups was about 10 kg in the first 6 months (compared with 1 to 2 kg in the control and exercise groups), but by 2 years

most of the weight had been regained. In this study, 25% of all patients had a weight loss of 4.5 kg at 2 years and these patients decreased their relative risk of acquiring type 2 diabetes by 30%.[7]

Exercise, such as brisk walking, that leads to improved cardiorespiratory fitness results in a decreased risk of type 2 diabetes[8,9] and impaired fasting glucose.[9] Cigarette smoking[10] and hypertension[11] increase the risk of type 2 diabetes, whereas moderate alcohol intake appears to protect against it.[10]

An estimated 50% of cases of type 2 diabetes in the United States are undiagnosed.[12]

─────────────── ☙ REFERENCES ❧ ───────────────

1. Bennett PH: Epidemiology of diabetes mellitus. In Rifkin H, Porte D Jr, eds: *Ellenberg and Rifkin's diabetes mellitus,* New York, 1990, Elsevier, pp 363-377.

2. Harris MI, Hadden WC, Knowler WC, et al: Prevalence of diabetes and impaired glucose tolerance and plasma glucose levels in the US population, *Diabetes* 36:523-534, 1987.

3. Hall PF: Ironies most bittersweet (editorial), *Can Med Assoc J* 160:1315-1316, 1999.

4. Harris SB, Perkins BA, Whalen-Brough E: Non-insulin-dependent diabetes mellitus among First Nations children: new entity among First Nations people of northwestern Ontario, *Can Fam Physician* 42:869-876, 1996.

5. Solomon CG, Hu FB, Dunaif A, et al: Long or highly irregular menstrual cycles as a marker for risk of type 2 diabetes mellitus, *JAMA* 286:2421-2426, 2001.

6. Colditz GA, Willett WC, Rotnitzky A, et al: Weight gain as a risk factor for clinical diabetes mellitus in women, *Ann Intern Med* 122:481-486, 1995.

7. Wing R, Venditti E, Jakicic J, et al: Lifestyle intervention in overweight individuals with a family history of diabetes, *Diabetes Care* 21:350-359, 1998.

8. Hu FB, Sigal RJ, Rich-Edwards JW, et al: Walking compared with vigorous physical activity and risk of type 2 diabetes in women: a prospective study, *JAMA* 282:1433-1439, 1999.

9. Wei M, Gibbons LW, Mitchell TL, et al: The association between cardiorespiratory fitness and impaired fasting glucose and type 2 diabetes mellitus in men, *Ann Intern Med* 130:89-96, 1999.

10. Rimm EB, Chan J, Stampfer MJ, et al: Prospective study of cigarette smoking, alcohol use, and the risk of diabetes in men, *BMJ* 210:545-546, 1995.

11. Hayashi T, Tsumura K, Suematsu C, et al: High normal blood pressure, hypertension, and the risk of type 2 diabetes in Japanese men: the Osaka Health Survey, *Diabetes Care* 22:1683-1687, 1999.

12. Harris MI: Undiagnosed NIDDM: clinical and public health issues, *Diabetes Care* 16:642-652, 1993.

Insulin resistance, metabolic syndrome, and the pathogenesis of type 2 diabetes

(See also role of intensive treatment in preventing diabetic complications in type 2 diabetes)

Insulin resistance seems to be a necessary, but not sufficient, condition for the development of type 2 diabetes.

The theory is that individuals who develop insulin resistance but have good beta-cell reserves simply produce more insulin (hyperinsulinemia) to maintain normoglycemia. When the reserves of the beta-cells become inadequate, type 2 diabetes supervenes.

Hyperinsulinemia is thought to be responsible for type 2 diabetes, obesity, hypertension, dyslipidemia, and atherosclerotic vascular disease,[1-3] a group of conditions often lumped together as "central obesity–insulin resistance syndrome" or "syndrome X" or "metabolic syndrome". This is one reason that many authorities are reluctant to treat type 2 diabetes with insulin. On the other hand, some workers think that elevated insulin levels are simply markers of insulin resistance and not pathogenetic factors for atherosclerosis.[4]

In a recent editorial on prevention of type 2 diabetes in the BMJ, Meigs wonders whether the concept of metabolic syndrome is a guidepost or detour.[5] The diagnosis of the metabolic syndrome in patients might hold promise for enhanced prevention of diabetes and cardiovascular disease. However, substantial uncertainties remain about the clinical definition of the syndrome and whether risk factor clusters collectively indicate a discrete, unifying disorder. Most importantly, it is unclear whether diagnosing the syndrome will confer benefit beyond risk assessments or treatment strategies associated with diagnosing and treating the syndrome's component traits.[5] At the bedside, the concept of "metabolic" is likely a good one and whether you as a clinician, or your patients, prefer to see this as a "syndrome" or as collective individual risk factors that need to be identified and reduced may matter little. The key is that the big picture of vascular risk reduction is maintained. Modest lifestyle changes, control of raised blood pressure and blood lipids substantially reduces risk of cardiovascular disease events in patients with hypertension or hyperlipidemia.

⊰ REFERENCES ⊱

1. De Fronzo RA, Ferrannini E: Insulin resistance: a multifaceted syndrome responsible for NIDDM, obesity, hypertension, dyslipidemia and atherosclerotic vascular disease, *Diabetes Care* 14:173-194, 1991.
2. Dagogo-Jack S, Santiago JV: Pathophysiology of type 2 diabetes and modes of action of therapeutic interventions, *Arch Intern Med* 157:1802-1817, 1997.
3. Purnell JQ, Hokanson JE, Marcovina SM, et al: Effect of excessive weight gain with intensive therapy of type 1 diabetes on lipid levels and blood pressure, *JAMA* 280:140-146, 1998.
4. Wingard DL, Barrett-Connor EL, Ferrara A: Is insulin really a heart disease risk factor? *Diabetes Care* 18:1299-1304, 1995.
5. Meigs JM: The metabolic syndrome may be a guidepost or detour to preventing type 2 diabetes and cardiovascular disease, *BMJ* 327:12, 61-62, 2003.

Screening and prevention for type 2 diabetes
(See also prevention; screening)

The 2003 AHRQ review on screening did not support mass screening but did support it in patients with hyperlipidemia and hypertension.[1] 2003 Canadian diabetes guidelines reflect that although the relatively low prevalence of diabetes in the general population makes it unlikely that mass screening will be cost-effective, testing for diabetes in people with risk factors for type 2 diabetes or with diabetes-associated conditions is likely to result in more benefit than harm.[2] This can include those with a family history of diabetes, a history of gestational diabetes, or marked obesity, even though early detection has not been shown to affect the ultimate outcome.[3,4] The Canadian Task Force on Preventive Health Care gives screening of the general population for diabetes a "D" recommendation,[3] whereas the U.S. Preventive Services Task Force gives it a "C."[4]

Recent trials involving obese patients with impaired fasting glucose has shown that increasing fibre, reducing saturated fat intake, reduction of weight by 5% to 7%, and activity for 25 minutes 6 days a week reduces progression to frank diabetes by over 50%.[5] This is encouraging as it provides solid evidence for prevention, albeit with a high-risk group. Skepticism remains regarding the general population and of course the limited data in sustainable prevention and treatment of the major risk factor for diabetes: obesity.

⊰ REFERENCES ⊱

1. *Screening for Type 2 Diabetes Mellitus in Adults. What's New from the USPSTF?* AHRQ Publication No. APPIP03-0005, February 2003. Agency for Healthcare Research and Quality, Rockville, MD. http://www.ahrq.gov/clinic/3rduspstf/diabscr/diabscrwh.htm
2. Canadian Diabetes Association Clinical Practice Guidelines Expert Committee: Canadian Diabetes Association 2003 Clinical Practice Guidelines for the Prevention and Management of Diabetes in Canada. *Can J Diabetes* 27(suppl 2), 2003.
3. Canadian Task Force on the Periodic Health Examination: *Clinical preventive health care,* Ottawa, 1994, Canadian Communication Group, pp 602-609.
4. Gerstein HC, Meltzer S: Preventive medicine in people at high risk for chronic disease: the value of identifying and treating diabetes (editorial), *Can Med Assoc J* 160:1593-1595, 1999. (Rebuttal by Marshall KG: *Can Med Assoc J* 160: 1595-1596, 1999.)
5. Tuomilehto J, Lindström J, Eriksson JG, et al: Prevention of type 2 diabetes mellitus by changes in lifestyle among subjects with impaired glucose tolerance. *N Engl J Med.* 344:1343-1350, 2001.

Systematic risk reduction

Historically, management of diabetes has focussed on blood glucose management. This has changed recently as we understand that other risk factors such as blood pressure and cholesterol are at least, and possibly more, important.[1] One review found that hypertension was the most important target.[2,3]

This has changed the paradigm of care from a specific focus to more multi-faceted approach to reduce overall vascular risk (blood pressure, cholesterol, and HbA1c) and microvascular complications (urine albumin, creatine ratio, opthomological assessment, ulcer and foot risk). Systematic risk reduction seems simple but is actually quite challenging to implement, especially in primary care where the incentives for implementation may not be available. Self-management skills in patients, interdisciplinary care, and office system enablers such as flow sheets and reminders, are examples of strategic pathways.[4] Self-management is often best enabled by support from a team and should consider the "big picture" for the individual. For example, those with medium or severe depression are significantly less likely to adhere to diet or medication regimens.[5]

Diet, exercise, and weight-lowering drugs in type 2 diabetes

(See also obesity)

Diet and exercise are essential components of the treatment of type 2 diabetes because of their value in controlling weight, reducing insulin resistance, and preventing coronary artery disease.[6,7] Except in a few symptomatic patients, the initial treatment of patients with type 2 diabetes should be an intensive, individualized diet and exercise program.[7]

As mentioned above, prevention trials involving obese patients with Impaired Fasting Glucose have shown that increasing fibre, reducing saturated fat intake, reduction of weight by 5% to 7%, and activity for 25 minutes six days a week reduces progression to frank diabetes by over 50%.[8]

The role of weight-lowering drugs in type 2 diabetes is uncertain. Anorexiants such as fenfluramine (Pondimin, Ponderal) and dexfenfluramine (Redux) have been associated with lethal adverse effects (see discussion of obesity) and have been taken off the market. Studies of newer antiobesity agents such as orlistat (Xenical) and sibutramine (Meridia) do show some extra weight loss and improved glycemic control, but long-term trials are missing.[9] Studies evaluating the long-term efficacy are lacking and interpretation is limited by high attrition rates.[10] Some clinicians use them as short-term adjunctive therapy to help patients "kick-off" lifestyle change. Many patients are intolerant of these medications. It is important for patients to under-stand that orlistat limits absorption of fat with individual meals. This excess is then transported out of the body (aka loose stools and flatus).

The key message here is that improving the basics (activity, reduced fat intake, preventing or managing depression, and healthy eating) can make a significant impact on diabetes, regardless of stage. When asked, patients often target their "wedding weight" and thus it is important for them to understand that lowering weight by even 5% to 7% can have a significant impact and is likely more sustainable.

✒ REFERENCES ✎

1. Huang ES, Meigs JB, Singer DE: The effects of interventions to prevent cardiovascular disease in patients with type 2 diabetes mellitus *Am J Med* 111:633-642, 2001.

2. Vijan S, Hayward RA: Treatment of hypertension in type 2 diabetes mellitus: blood pressure goals, choice of agents, and setting priorities in diabetes care, *Ann Intern Med* 138:593-602, 2003.

3. Snow V, Weiss KB, Mottur-Pilson C, et al: The evidence base for tight blood pressure control in the management of type 2 diabetes mellitus, *Ann Intern Med* 138:587-592, 2003.

4. Renders CM, Valk GD, Griffin S, et al: Interventions to improve the management of diabetes mellitus in primary care, outpatient and community settings (Cochrane Review), In: The Cochrane Library, Issue 4, Chichester, UK, 2003, John Wiley & Sons, Ltd.

5. Ciechanowski PS, Katon WJ, Russo, JE: Depression and Diabetes: Impact of Depressive Symptoms on Adherence, Function, and Costs, *Arch Intern Med* 160:3278-3285, 2000.

6. Mayer-Davis EJ, D'Agostino R Jr, Karter AJ, et al: Intensity and amount of physical activity in relation to insulin sensitivity: the Insulin Resistance Atherosclerosis Study, *JAMA* 279:669-674, 1998.

7. Expert Committee of the Canadian Diabetes Advisory Board: Clinical practice guidelines for diabetes mellitus in Canada, *Can Med Assoc J*, 147:697-712, 1992.

8. Tuomilehto J, Lindström J, Eriksson JG, et al. Prevention of type 2 diabetes mellitus by changes in lifestyle among subjects with impaired glucose tolerance, *N Engl J Med* 344:1343-1350, 2001.

9. Hollander PA, Elbein SC, Hirsch IB, et al: Role of orlistat in the treatment of obese patients with type 2 diabetes, *Diabetes Care* 21:1288-1294, 1998.

10. Padwal R, Li SK, Lau DCW: Long-term pharmacotherapy for obesity and overweight (Cochrane Review). In: The Cochrane Library, Issue 4, 2003. Chichester, UK, 2000, John Wiley & Sons, Ltd.

Complications of Diabetes Mellitus

Diabetic retinopathy

(See also eating disorders)

Classification. Three types of retinal abnormalities are common in diabetes: non-proliferative or background retinopathy, proliferative retinopathy, and macular edema. Visual loss is caused by either macular edema or proliferative retinopathy. If untreated, half of all patients with proliferative retinopathy will become blind within 5 years, but with argon laser photocoagulation the rate is less than 5%. Photocoagulation is also effective in reducing visual loss in about half of diabetic patients with macular edema.[1] Patients with more severe degrees of retinopathy are at increased risk of death from cardiovascular disease.[2]

Non-Proliferative Retinopathy. The initial and most common manifestation of diabetic retinopathy is microaneurysm formation. As the disease progresses, erythrocytes escape from the lesions, leading to dot and blot hemorrhages. Leakage of serous fluid from the capillaries may lead to the formation of retinal or macular edema and is often associated with the presence of hard exudates and sometimes venous beading. Microaneurysms, dot and blot hemorrhages, and hard exudates are collectively termed background retinopathy or non-proliferative retinopathy. Non-proliferative retinopathy does not lead to loss of vision unless it occurs near the maculae and causes macular edema.[1]

Proliferative Retinopathy. As the diabetic retinal disease progresses, some vessels become occluded, leading to infarcts of the retinae seen as soft or cotton wool exudates. In response to ischemia, new vessels develop and proliferate out of the retina into the vitreous. This is proliferative retinopathy. These attenuated fragile vessels tend to bleed, causing vitreous hemorrhages. Vitreous hemorrhages usually resorb in 1 to 3 months, but subsequent fibrous proliferation can lead to retinal detachment and loss of vision. Aspirin does not increase the frequency or severity of vitreous hemorrhages in patients with non-proliferative or early proliferative retinopathy, and since it is protective against cardiovascular disease, many diabetics should be taking it.[3]

Macular Edema. Direct ophthalmoscopy rarely detects macular edema, but its presence may be suspected if the macula is surrounded by hard exudates. Ophthalmologists detect macular edema by binocular slit-lamp examination or by stereoscopic fundus photography.[1]

Prevalence and Progression. Diabetic retinopathy is the most common cause of new cases of legal blindness in working age North Americans.[1,2] Retinopathy is far more likely to develop in patients with type 1 diabetes than in those with type 2. However, type 2 retinopathy is much more prevelent simply due to the larger burden of disease. If the onset of diabetes occurs before age 30, almost all patients will have some degree of diabetic retinopathy after 20 years and in half the cases, it will be proliferative. In contrast, only 20% of patients with type 2 diabetes who do not

require insulin will have some degree of diabetic retinopathy after 20 years and in only 5% will it be proliferative. Among elderly type 2 patients requiring insulin, 80% will display some degree of retinopathy and 20% will have proliferative retinopathy. After 15 to 20 years about 15% of all diabetics will have macular edema.[1]

In type 1 diabetes, retinopathy rarely develops before puberty and usually only after the patient has had the disease for 3 to 5 years. After 7 years approximately 50% will have some degree of retinopathy.[3]

Although most studies of newly diagnosed type 2 diabetes have reported that about 20% of patients have early-stage retinopathy at the time of diagnosis, a 1998 report found an overall incidence of 39% in men and 35% in women. In 92% of the male cases and 95% of the female cases the disease was early background retinopathy (see above), and in about 20% of cases the retinopathy was so minimal that the diagnosis was based on the finding of three or fewer microaneurysms with no other detectable abnormalities.[4]

Pregnancy[5] and eating disorders[6] are recognized risk factors for the progression of diabetic retinopathy. Between one fourth and one third of adolescent girls with type 1 diabetes also have eating disorders. They tend to vomit, purge, and omit insulin doses, and their metabolic control is poor (some cases of brittle diabetes are probably due to this phenomenon). They have a greatly increased risk for retinopathy.[6]

Diabetic Control and Retinopathy. In both type 1 and type 2 diabetes the degree of retinopathy and the risk of progression correlate with the degree of elevation of the glycosylated hemoglobin level.[7] The Diabetes Control and Complications Trial (DCCT) showed that intensive treatment of type 1 diabetes significantly decreased the incidence of proliferative retinopathy. However, a small proportion of patients displayed early worsening of retinopathy. In about half of these patients, recovery occurred by 18 months, but in the other half it did not. Because of the risk of worsening retinopathy, an ophthalmologist should assess any diabetic patient starting a program of intensive diabetic control before treatment is initiated and the patient should be monitored during the early treatment period.[8]

2003 Canadian guidelines advise that[9]:

1. In people with type 1 diabetes, screening and evaluation for retinopathy by an experienced professional should be performed annually 5 years after the onset of diabetes in individuals over 15 years of age (Grade A, Level 1)

2. In people with type 2 diabetes, screening and evaluation for retinopathy by an experienced professional should be performed at the time of diagnosis (Grade A, Level 1). The interval for follow-up

assessments should be tailored to the severity of the retinopathy. In those with no or minimal retinopathy, the recommended interval is 1 to 2 years (Grade A, Level 1).

3. Screening for retinopathy should be performed by experienced professionals either in person or through their interpretation of photographs (Grade A, Level 1).

✺ REFERENCES ✺

1. Ferris FL III, Davis MD, Aiello LM: Treatment of diabetic retinopathy, *N Engl J Med* 341:667-678, 1999.
2. Klein R, Klein BE, Moss: SE: Epidemiology of proliferative diabetic retinopathy, *Diabetes Care* 15:1875-1891, 1992.
3. Nathan DM: Long-term complications of diabetes mellitus, *N Engl J Med* 328:1676-1685, 1993.
4. United Kingdom Prospective Diabetes Study, 30: diabetic retinopathy at diagnosis of non-insulin-dependent diabetes mellitus and associated risk factors, *Arch Ophthalmol* 116:297-303, 1998.
5. Klein BE, Moss SE, Klein R: Effect of pregnancy on progression of diabetic retinopathy, *Diabetes Care* 13:34-40, 1990.
6. Rydall AC, Rodin GM, Olmsted MP, et al: Disordered eating behavior and microvascular complications in young women with insulin-dependent diabetes mellitus, *N Engl J Med* 336:1849-1854, 1997.
7. Klein R, Klein BE, Moss SE, et al: Relationship of hyperglycemia to the long-term incidence and progression of diabetic retinopathy, Arch Intern Med 154:2169-2178, 1994.
8. Diabetes Control and Complications Trial Research Group: Early worsening of diabetic retinopathy in the Diabetes Control and Complications Trial, *Arch Ophthalmol* 116:874-886, 1998.
9. Canadian Diabetes Association Clinical Practice Guidelines Expert Committee: CDA 2003 Clinical Practice Guidelines for the Prevention and Management of Diabetes in Canada, *Can J Diabetes* 27(suppl 2):S10-S11, 2003.

Diabetic nephropathy

(See also hypertension; microalbuminuria)

Although nephropathy has generally been considered a more common complication of type 1 than type 2 diabetes, this pattern appears to be changing as life expectancy of persons with type 2 diabetes increases. Twenty-five years after the diagnosis of diabetes approximately 50% of both type 1 and type 2 diabetic patients have nephropathy as manifested by proteinuria. Factors known to accelerate the progression of diabetic nephropathy are hypertension, proteinuria, poor glycemic control, and smoking. Whether high-protein diets or elevated lipid levels affect progression is uncertain.[1]

The first evidence of renal damage in diabetes is microalbuminuria, followed by manifest proteinuria. In the case of type 1 diabetes, the mean duration of the disease from the onset of microalbuminuria to the development of proteinuria is 17 years. In half of diabetic patients with proteinuria, end-stage renal failure develops, and the mean time from the onset of proteinuria to azotemia is 5 years.[2] Blacks, Asians, and Native Americans are at greater risk of end-stage renal disease than are whites. The 5-year survival rate for type 2 diabetics with end-stage renal disease is at best 25%.[1]

Microalbuminuria is defined as albuminuria that is too little to be detected by standard urine dipsticks. If the patient has a negative or trace dipstick, then current recommendations prefer sending the patient for a random daytime urine testing for albumin:creatinine ratio (ACR). 2003 Canadian guidelines suggest that two confirmatory tests should be performed between 1 week and 2 months apart. False positives can arise from exercise, fever, heart failure, and urinary tract infections.[3] The test is "positive" if > 2.8 for females and over 2.0 in males. In this instance, capturing a 24-hour urinary albumin excretion is advised, although some feel the ratio is sufficient. Over 300 mg excretion in a day represents overt nephropathy. Rates of 30 to 300 mg in 24 hours, or as 20 to 200 μg/mL or 20 to 200 μg/min represent an opportunity for prevention and needs to be treated.

Type 2 diabetic patients with microalbuminuria are at very high risk for cardiovascular events.[1]

Good control of hypertension may ameliorate diabetic nephropathy or at least slow its progression. Because of this the American and Canadian Diabetes Associations recommend that the target level for blood pressure control in hypertensive diabetic patients be less than 130/80 mm Hg.[4] 2003 Canadian guidelines recommend disruption of the renin-angiotensin system with angiotensin converting enzyme (ACE) inhibitors or angiotensin II receptor antagonists (ARBs) is the preferred method of protecting renal function in people with diabetes, even in the absence of hypertension. Second-line renal-protective agents include the non-dihydropyridine calcium channel blockers (CCBs) (diltiazem, verapamil). Support for controlling hypertension as a way of preventing nephropathy comes from a United Kingdom Prospective Diabetes Study Group (UKPDS) report of patients with type 2 diabetes and hypertension who were treated intensively with either a beta blocker or an ACE inhibitor as first-line therapy (other drug classes were added if necessary). Both drug classes slowed the development of proteinuria compared with that in less intensively treated hypertensive diabetics (see discussion of hypertension).[5] Lifestyle changes such as smoking cessation should be encouraged.

Even in normotensive diabetic patients ACE inhibitors may be valuable.[1,6-9] One study found that lisinopril (Prinivil, Zestril) given to normotensive patients with type 1 diabetes decreased the rate of progression of renal disease as measured by the degree of albuminuria.[6] Similar results in normotensive patients with type 2 diabetes were obtained with enalapril (Vasotec).[7] An expert panel of the U.S. National Kidney Foundation recommends that all diabetics with microalbuminuria be treated with ACE inhibitors.[8] A case can even be made for treating most type 2 diabetics with ACE inhibitors whether or not they have evidence of proteinuria or microalbuminuria.[9]

Tight control of type 1 diabetes has been shown to decrease the incidence of microalbuminuria and proteinuria,[10] but whether this will translate into a decreased incidence of end-stage renal failure is unknown.

Transplantation options for type 1 diabetics with renal failure are renal transplant alone or combined renal and pancreatic transplants. A comparative survey of these two modalities from the Netherlands found mortality rates to be significantly lower in patients who received combined transplants.[11]

The Canadian Task Force on Preventive Health Care recommends screening for microalbuminuria in patients with insulin-dependent diabetes ("A" recommendation),[12] whereas the U.S. Preventive Services Task Force makes no recommendation on the subject.[13] After a thorough literature review, Vijan and associates[14] recommend that patients with type 2 diabetes be screened regularly for microalbuminuria.

≥ REFERENCES ≥

1. Ritz E, Orth SR: Nephropathy in patients with type 2 diabetes mellitus, *N Engl J Med* 341:1127-1133, 1999.
2. Nathan, DM: Long-term complications of diabetes mellitus, *N Engl J Med* 328:1676-1685, 1993.
3. Canadian Diabetes Association Clinical Practice Guidelines Expert Committee: Canadian Diabetes Association 2003 Clinical Practice Guidelines for the Prevention and Management of Diabetes in Canada. *Can J Diabetes* 27(suppl 2), 2003.
4. American Diabetes Association: Clinical practice recommendations 1996: diagnosis and management of nephropathy in patients with diabetes mellitus, *Diabetes Care* 19(suppl 1):S103-S106, 1996.
5. UK Prospective Diabetes Study Group: Tight blood pressure control and risk of macrovascular and microvascular complications in type 2 diabetes: UKPDS 38, *BMJ* 317:703-713, 1998.
6. EUCLID study group: Randomised placebo-controlled trial of lisinopril in normotensive patients with insulin-dependent diabetes and normoalbuminuria or microalbuminuria, *Lancet* 349:1787-1792, 1997.
7. Ravid M, Lang R, Rachmani R, et al: Long-term renoprotective effect of angiotensin-converting enzyme inhibition in non-insulin-dependent diabetes mellitus, *Arch Intern Med* 156:286-289, 1996.
8. Bennett PH, Haffner S, Kasiske BL, et al: Screening and management of microalbuminuria in patients with diabetes mellitus: recommendations to the Scientific Advisory Board of the National Kidney Foundation from an ad hoc committee of the Council on Diabetes Mellitus of the National Kidney Foundation, *Am J Kidney Dis* 25:107-112, 1995.
9. Golan L, Birkmeyer JD, Welch HG: The cost-effectiveness of treating all patients with type 2 diabetes with angiotensin-converting enzyme inhibitors, *Ann Intern Med* 131:660-667, 1999.
10. Diabetes Control and Complications Trial Research Group: The effect of intensive treatment of diabetes on the development and progression of long-term complications in insulin-dependent diabetes mellitus, *N Engl J Med* 329:977-986, 1993.
11. Smets YF, Westendorp RG, van der Pijl JW, et al: Effect of simultaneous pancreas-kidney transplantation on mortality of patients with type-1 diabetes mellitus and end-stage renal failure, *Lancet* 353:1915-1919, 1999.
12. Canadian Task Force on the Periodic Health Examination: *Clinical preventive health care,* Ottawa, 1994, Canadian Communication Group, pp 436-445.
13. US Preventive Services Task Force: *Guide to clinical preventive services,* ed 2, Baltimore, 1996, Williams & Wilkins.
14. Vijan S, Stevens DL, Herman WH, et al: Screening, prevention, counseling, and treatment for the complications of type II diabetes mellitus: putting evidence into practice, *J Gen Intern Med* 12:567-580, 1997.

Diabetic neuropathy
(See also herpes zoster; neuropathy)

Diabetic peripheral neuropathy eventually develops in almost half of all diabetics.[1] Diagnostic strategies for sensation include Pressure with 10 g monofilament (not detected=impaired), Vibration of 128 Hz tuning fork over medial malleolus (perception of <5 s = impaired), and assessment of ankle jerk with tendon hammer (less reliable in the elderly).[2]

Treatment for neuropathic pain includes tricyclic antidepressants, such as amitriptyline (Elavil) (dose range 25 to 200 mg daily), carbamazepine (Tegretol), neurontin (Gabapentin), opiods, mexiletine and isosorbide dinitrate spray.[3] Capsaicin 0.075% cream (Zostrix H.P.) has also been reported to give pain relief.[1,3-5]

Focal motor neuropathies also occur in diabetic patients. These may be cranial or peripheral and usually resolve spontaneously in 2 to 12 months.

Autonomic neuropathies are common. The most frequent manifestation is impotence, which affects up to 45% of men with diabetes.[6] Erectile dysfunction may now be treated with type 5 phosphodiesterase inhibitors (Viagra, Cialis), with the usual nitroglycerin precautions.

Other features of autonomic neuropathy are diabetic gastroparesis, orthostatic hypotension, and diarrhea.[4]

Treatment options for gastroparesis include metoclopramide (Maxeran) 10 mg tid ac meals, or domperidone (Motilium). Cisapride and erythromycin are no longer utilized because of toxicity and poor efficacy respectively.[7]

One treatment method for the diarrhea of autonomic neuropathy is one or two doses of tetracycline (200 or 500 mg) at the onset of symptoms. The mechanism of action is unknown. A more traditional treatment is diphenoxylate with atropine (Lomotil).[4]

Postural hypotension caused by autonomic neuropathy is difficult to treat; increasing salt intake, wearing elastic tights, and sleeping with the head of the bed elevated might be tried. In some cases fludrocortisone (Florinef) is indicated.[4]

The Diabetes Control and Complications Trial has shown that intensive insulin treatment of patients with type 1 diabetes decreases the incidence of peripheral neuropathy measured after 5 years (13% versus 5%).[8] Intensive treatment of patients with type 2 diabetes in the United Kingdom Prospective Diabetic Study (UKPDS) did not result in a lower rate of impotence than in the conventionally treated control subjects.[9]

─────────── ❧ REFERENCES ❧ ───────────

1. Backonja M, Beydoun A, Edwards KR, et al: Gabapentin for the symptomatic treatment of painful neuropathy in patients with diabetes mellitus: a randomized controlled trial, *JAMA* 280:1831-1836, 1998.
2. Perkins BA, Olaleye D, Zinman B, et al: Simple screening tests for peripheral neuropathy in the diabetes clinic, *Diabetes Care* 24:250-256, 2001.
3. Yuen KCJ, Baker NR, Rayman G: Treatment of chronic painful diabetic neuropathy with isosorbide dinitrate spray. A double-blind placebo-controlled crossover study, *Diabetes Care* 25:1699-1703, 2002.
4. Clark CM Jr, Lee DA: Prevention and treatment of the complications of diabetes mellitus, *N Engl J Med* 332:1210-1217, 1995.
5. McQuay HJ, Moore RA: Antidepressants and chronic pain: effective analgesia in neuropathic pain and other syndromes (editorial), *BMJ* 314:763-764, 1997.
6. McCulloch DK, Campell IW, Wu FC et al. The prevalence of diabetic impotence. *Diabetologia* 18:279-283, 1980.
7. Prescrire: Evidence-based drug reviews: erythromycin and gastroparesis? *Can Fam Physician* 45:1887-1891, 1999.
8. Diabetes Control and Complications Trial Research Group: The effect of intensive diabetes therapy on the development and progression of neuropathy, *Ann Intern Med* 122:561-568, 1995.
9. UK Prospective Diabetes Study (UKPDS) Group: Intensive blood-glucose control with sulphonylureas or insulin compared with conventional treatment and risk of complications in patients with type 2 diabetes (UKPDS 33), *Lancet* 352:837-853, 1998.

Diabetic foot

Foot ulcers develop in at least 15% of diabetics, and the underlying cause is almost always a sensory neuropathy.[1] Many diabetologists argue that if clinicians could detect sensory neuropathy in diabetic patients and institute appropriate preventive foot care, the incidence of foot ulcers would decrease.[2]

Current screening guidelines for peripheral neuropathy suggest using a 10-g monofilament at the great toe or checking for loss of sensitivity to vibration at the great toe annually, starting at diagnosis for type 1 and after 5 years for type 2. A simple approach is to ask the patient: 1) if they have had any prior problems with foot or lower leg infections and 2) to "Take off your shoes, roll up your pants" and inspect for ulcer, thickened, horny toenails, corns, or calluses (biomechanical problems, fissures, clawed toes). Advise regarding proper fitting footwear, early assessment of any lesions, moisturizers, and consideration of foot care specialist assessment.

Diabetic foot ulcers heal slowly. A systematic review of standard treatment of uninfected ulcers (avoidance of weight bearing, debridement if indicated, and saline-moistened gauze dressings) found that 24% had healed by 12 weeks and 31% by 20 weeks.[1]

Infected foot ulcers may be categorized into limb-threatening and non–limb-threatening infections. Non–limb-threatening infections are superficial, and the erythema extends less than 2 cm from the edge of the ulcer. Organisms causing non–limb-threatening infections are usually gram-positive cocci, such as streptococci or staphylococci, and these infections may be treated on an outpatient basis if the home situation is adequate and follow-up every 24 to 48 hours can be arranged. Weight bearing must be avoided, and in most cases oral antibiotics such as clindamycin (Cleocin, Dalacin), cephalexin (Keflex), dicloxacillin (Dycill, Dynapen, Pathocil), or cloxacillin (Tegopen, Orbenin) are effective as single agents. Limb-threatening infections are generally polymicrobial, involving gram-positive aerobes, gram-negative aerobes, and anaerobes, and patients with such a condition require hospitalization and IV antibiotics.[2]

With deep ulcers, the presence of an underlying osteomyelitis is often difficult to determine. If bone can be detected in the base of the ulcer by probing with a metal probe, the odds are high that osteomyelitis is present. If the infection is not limb threatening, bone cannot be detected on probing, and initial X-ray findings are negative, the duration of treatment can be that for soft tissue infection (10 to 14 days), with reassessment after it is completed.[3]

─────────── ❧ REFERENCES ❧ ───────────

1. Margolis DJ, Kantor J, Berlin JA: Healing of diabetic neuropathic foot ulcers receiving standard treatment, *Diabetes Care* 22:692-695, 1999.

2. Canadian Diabetes Association Clinical Practice Guidelines Expert Committee. CDA 2003 Clinical Practice Guidelines for the Prevention and Management of Diabetes in Canada, *Can J Diabetes* 27(suppl 2):S72-73, 2003.

3. Caputo GM, Joshi N, Weitekamp MR: Foot infections in patients with diabetes, *Am Fam Physician* 56:195-202, 1997.

Erectile dysfunction and diabetes

(See erectile dysfunction)

Erectile dysfunction (ED) affects approximately 34% to 45% of men with diabetes.[1] Risk factors include increasing age, duration of diabetes, poor glycemic control, cigarette smoking, hypertension, dyslipidemia, and cardiovascular disease; therapy (penile prosthesis) may be considered for these men.[2]

Type 5 phosphodiesterase (PDE5) inhibitors have proven to be effective for ED in the patient with diabetes albeit less so than in the general population. In one trial using Sildenafil (Viagra), at 12 weeks 56% of men in the sildenafil group reported improved erections compared with 10% of men in the placebo group. Because of the potential for silent ischemia in this population, an accompanying editorial recommends an exercise stress test before prescribing sildenafil.[3]

──────────── ⚓ **REFERENCES** ⚓ ────────────

1. Bacon CG, Hu FB, Giovannucci E, et al: Association of type and duration of diabetes with erectile dysfunction in a large *Diabetes Care* 25:1458-1463, 2002.

2. Canadian Diabetes Association Clinical Practice Guidelines Expert Committee: CDA 2003. Clinical Practice Guidelines for the Prevention and Management of Diabetes in Canada, *Can J Diabetes* 27(suppl 2):S10-S11, 2003.

3. Rendell MS, Rajfer J, Wicker PA, Smith MD: Sildenafil for treatment of erectile dysfunction in men with diabetes. A randomized controlled trial, *JAMA* 281:421-426, 1999.

Macrovascular complications of diabetes mellitus

(See also hypertension; secondary prevention of coronary artery disease, vascular risk reduction)

Cardiovascular disease is the major cause of the increased morbidity and mortality associated with diabetes,[1] and the risk for both strokes and myocardial infarcts is greater in diabetic women than in diabetic men.[2,3] In type 2 diabetes the risk of cardiovascular disease is two to three times that of the non-diabetic population[1,3] and is equivalent to the risk of non-diabetics who have had a previous myocardial infarction.[4]

Specific risk markers for coronary artery disease in patients with type 2 diabetes include elevated levels of low-density lipoprotein (LDL) cholesterol, low levels of high-density lipoprotein (HDL) cholesterol, hypertension, and hyperglycemia.[1] Because approximately 80% of diabetics will die from a vascular cause (myocardial infarctions and strokes), aggressive treatment of hypertension and lipid abnormalities is essential (see

discussion of hypertension).[5] Vijan and associates[6] advise daily Aspirin in doses of 81 to 325 mg for all patients with type 2 diabetes over the age of 50, as well as for those under 50 who show evidence of cardiovascular disease. Fagan and Sowers[3] support the American Diabetes Association's view that any evidence of cardiovascular disease in a diabetic is an indication for Aspirin therapy unless strictly contraindicated.[7] It should be noted that recent analysis of the Women's Health Study pointed to possible gender differences in effect of Aspirin. The analysis showed that Aspirin might not affect the incidence of myocardial infarctions or all cause mortality. There was some effect on stroke and more benefit for women over 65. It should be noted that the women in this trial were generally at low risk for cardiac disease, whereas diabetes invokes high risk.[8] A large multicentre international study found that the ACE inhibitor ramipril (Altace) 10 mg once daily led to a decrease in both macrovascular and microvascular complications in diabetics that was greater than could be expected from the small decrease in blood pressure resulting from this treatment.[9] Haffner and associates,[4] underlining the importance of assiduously treating risk factors in diabetes, recommend that all patients with type 2 diabetes be managed in the same way as patients who have had myocardial infarctions.

The United Kingdom Prospective Diabetes Study (UKPDS) found no evidence that tight control of patients with type 2 diabetes treated with sulfonylureas or insulin decreased the incidence of macrovascular events,[10] (Level A) although such a decrease was reported in a subgroup of obese patients treated with metformin.[11] Tight control does decrease microvascular disease (see earlier discussion).

──────────── ⚓ **REFERENCES** ⚓ ────────────

1. Turner RC, Millns H, Neil HA, et al: Risk factors for coronary artery disease in non-insulin dependent diabetes mellitus: United Kingdom Prospective Diabetes Study (UKPDS 23), *BMJ* 316:823-828, 1998.

2. Howard BV, Cowan LD, Go O, et al: Adverse effects of diabetes on multiple cardiovascular disease risk factors in women, *Diabetes Care* 21:1258-1263, 1998.

3. Fagan TC, Sowers J: Type 2 diabetes mellitus: greater cardiovascular risks and greater benefits of therapy (editorial), *Arch Intern Med*, 1033-1034, 1999.

4. Haffner SM, Lehto S, Rönnemaa T, et al: Mortality from coronary heart disease in subjects with type 2 diabetes and in nondiabetic subjects with and without prior myocardial infarction, *N Engl J Med* 339:229-234, 1998.

5. Barret-Connor E, Pyorala K: Long-term complications: diabetes, coronary heart disease, stroke and lower extremity arterial disease. In: Ikoe J-M Zimmet P, Williams R, eds. The Epidemiology of Diabetes Mellitus: An international Perspective. Chichester, UK: John Wiley & Sons, Ltd.; 2001:301-319

6. Vijan S, Stevens DL, Herman WH, et al: Screening, prevention, counseling, and treatment for the complications of type II diabetes mellitus: putting evidence into practice, *J Gen Intern Med* 12:567-580, 1997.

7. American Diabetes Association: Aspirin therapy in diabetes, *Diabetes Care* 21(suppl 1):S45-S49, 1998.

8. Ridker PM, Cook NR, Lee IM, et al: A randomized trial of low dose asprin in the primary prevention of cardiovascular disease in women, *N Engl J Med* 352:1293-1304, 2005.

9. Heart Outcomes Prevention Evaluation (HOPE) Study Investigators: Effects of ramipril on cardiovascular and microvascular outcomes in people with diabetes mellitus: results of the HOPE study and MICRO-HOPE substudy, *Lancet* 355:253-259, 2000.

10. United Kingdom Prospective Diabetes Study (UKPDS) Group: Intensive blood-glucose control with sulphonylureas or insulin compared with conventional treatment and risk of complications in patients with type 2 diabetes (UKPDS 33), *Lancet* 352:837-853, 1998.

11. United Kingdom Prospective Diabetes Study (UKPDS) Group: Effect of intensive blood-glucose control with metformin on complications in overweight patients with type 2 diabetes (UKPDS 34), *Lancet* 352:854-865, 1998.

Target Levels for Glucose in the Control of Diabetes Mellitus

Target levels for glucose control as set by various expert committees have become more stringent since the publication of the Diabetes Control and Complications Trial in 1993 (see below). According to the current position statement of the American Diabetes Association, the optimal preprandial glucose level is 5.2 to 7 mmol/L (89 to 130 mg/dL) and remedial action should be taken if values are above 7.8 mmol/L (140 mg/dL) or below 4.4 mmol/L (80 mg/dL). Bedtime glucose should be between 5.6 and 7.8 mmol/L (100 to 140 mg/dL), and remedial action is indicated if the levels are below 5.6 mmol/L (100 mg/dL) or above 10 mmol/L (160 mg/dL). The ideal HbA$_1$c level is below 7%.[1] Canadian guidelines are almost identical.[2] If felt to be safe, a more aggressive target range may be implemented.

Although the United Kingdom Prospective Diabetes Study (UKPDS) has shown that intensive treatment of type 2 diabetes lowers the rate of microvascular disease, the mean levels of HbA$_1$c did not fall below 7%. It also showed us that despite interventions the HbA1c climbed over time. In the opinion of the authors of the UKPDS study, levels lower than 7% have been obtained only in small groups of obese patients receiving large doses of insulin in the context of intensive short-term trials and may be unrealistic for the majority in the community setting.[3] Current guidelines challenge this somewhat and push for more aggressive treating to target to optimize outcomes.

◈ REFERENCES ◈

1. American diabetes association: standards of medical care for patients with diabetes mellitus, *Diabetes Care* 20(suppl 27):s5-10, 2004

2. Canadian diabetes association clinical practice guidelines expert committee: Canadian diabetes assocciation 2003 clinical practice guidelines for the prevention and management of diabetes in Canada. *Can J Diabetes* 27(suppl2):S19, 2003.

3. United Kingdom Prospective Diabetes Study (UKPDS) Group: Intensive blood-glucose control with sulphonylureas or insulin compared with conventional treatment and risk of complications in patients with type 2 diabetes (UKPDS 33), *Lancet* 352:837-853, 1998.

Pharmacological Treatment of Type 2 Diabetes

(See also intensive treatment in preventing diabetic complications in type 1 diabetes; type 1 diabetes)

Oral hypoglycemic agents

As with most chronic diseases, multiple low-dose medications seem to be the best strategy to manage diabetes and the target levels for glucose control set by the American[1] and Canadian[2] diabetes associations are stringent. Therefore a good working knowledge of hypoglycemic agents is important. The usual protocol for trying to reach these goals in patients with type 2 diabetes is to start with life-style changes, followed by oral hypoglycemic agents, then a combination of oral agents and insulin, and then insulin alone.

When oral therapy is indicated, the physician has the choice of starting with one of the sulfonylureas, a biguanide, an alpha-glucosidase inhibitor,[3] or even a thiazolidinedione (Table 50).[4] Since the United Kingdom Prospective Diabetes Study (UKPDS) has demonstrated that tight control with sulfonylureas or insulin does not decrease macrovascular complications of diabetes[5] whereas treating obese persons with type 2 diabetes with metformin alone does,[6] metformin is the drug of first choice for obese patients. The typical maintenance dose is 1000 mg bid and patients are titrated there by starting at 500 mg od, then bid. The biguanides, of which the only one currently available in Canada and the United States is metformin (Glucophage), act primarily by decreasing glucose output from the liver but also by increasing the insulin sensitivity of muscle. Metformin leads to weight loss and decreases levels of triglycerides, total cholesterol, and LDL cholesterol.[7] Metformin is as effective as the sulfonylureas and rarely induces hypoglycemia.[3] Disadvantages of the drug are that it has to be given two or three times a day and that 5% to 20% of patients have transient gastrointestinal effects, usually diarrhea. Metformin should not be given to persons with impaired liver, renal function or active cardiac failure because of the risk of lactic acidosis. Specifically, physicians should

Table 50   Oral Hypoglycemic Agents

Drugs	Usual doses
Sulfonylureas, Second Generation	
Glyburide (Diabeta, Glynase, Micronase)	5-10 mg qam or 10 mg bid
Gliclazide (Diamicron)	40-160 mg bid
Glimepiride (Amaryl)	1-8 mg qam
Glipizide (Glucotrol)	5-40 mg qam or 10-20 mg bid
Glipizide extended release	5-10 mg qam
Biguanides	
Metformin (Glucophage)	500 mg tid-qid or 850 mg bid-tid
Alpha-Glucosidase Inhibitors	
Acarbose (Precose, Prandase)	25-100 mg tid
Miglitol (Glyset)	50 mg tid at beginning of each meal
Thiazolidinediones	
Pioglitazone (Actos)	15-45 mg once daily
Rosiglitazone (Avandia)	4-8 mg once daily
Troglitazone (Rezulin)	Withdrawn from market
(Avandamet) Combined formulation of rosiglitazone and metformin	
Meglitinides	
Repaglinide (GlucoNorm, Prandin)	0.5-4 mg tid-qid ac

be wary of prescribing the drug to someone with a creatinine level above 150 mmol/L (1.7 mg/dl).

The primary action of sulfonylureas is to increase insulin output from the pancreatic beta-cells. These agents may cause hypoglycemic reactions, weight gain, and hyperinsulinemia[3] and should not be given to patients who are allergic to sulfonamides. The insulin secretagogues include gliclazide (Diamicron) glimepiride (Amaryl), glyburide (Diabeta, Euglucon), and the non-sulfonylureas nateglinide (Starlix) and repaglinide (GlucoNorm). (NOTE: Chlorpropamide and tolbutamide are still available in Canada, but rarely used.) Hypoglycemia and weight gain are especially common with glyburide, whereas the postprandial glycemia is reduced by nateglinide and repaglinide. Consider using other class(es) of antihyperglycemic agents first in patients at high risk of hypoglycemia (e.g., the elderly).

Acarbose (Prandase, Precose) is an alpha-glucosidase inhibitor that is taken three times daily immediately before meals. It acts by inhibiting the hydrolysis of dietary disaccharides and thus inhibits the absorption of monosaccharides. It has been used for both type 1 and type 2 diabetes. Acarbose is usually not recommended as initial therapy in people with severe hyperglycemia (A1C ≥9.0%) and is mostly used in combination with other oral antihyperglycemic agents. The main adverse effects are flatulence, distention, cramps, and diarrhea, and these are of sufficient importance to cause many patients to discontinue the drug.[8] Acarbose may be used as the only pharmacological agent for type 2 diabetes or may be given in conjunction with one or more oral agents or insulin. The UKPDS found that acarbose alone or added to other medications improved glycemic control in patients with type 2 diabetes.[8]

A new class of agents is the thiazolidinediones, which include troglitazone (Rezulin), rosiglitazone (Avandia), and pioglitazone (Actos). These agents act by increasing insulin sensitivity so that liver and muscle cells increase their consumption of glucose. The first of these agents, troglitazone, has been associated with a number of cases of hepatotoxicity, and because of this, the drug was withdrawn from the market in Great Britain in 1997 and the manufacturer voluntarily withdrew the drug from the U.S. market in early 2000. Rosiglitazone and pioglitazone do not appear to lead to serious adverse hepatic effects, but long-term safety and benefits have not been determined.[9]

The thiazolidinediones can be added to metformin and sulfonylureas. Six to twelve months is often required to see full blood glucose lowering effect. When combined with insulin there may increase risk of edema and CHF. The combination of a TZD plus insulin is currently not an approved indication in Canada. Thiazolidinediones are contraindicated in patients with hepatic dysfunction (ALT >2.5 times ULN) or significant cardiac failure.

One of the newest non-sulfonylurea oral agents is repaglinide (Gluconorm, Prandin), which belongs to the meglitinide class.[10] It stimulates the release of insulin from the pancreas and can be used as monotherapy or in combination with metformin.

If adequate control of glucose cannot be obtained with one class of oral hypoglycemic medication, a member of another class can be added, or insulin can be added to or replace the oral agents (see below).[3] Most patients with type 2 diabetes require polytherapy if they are to achieve an HbA_{1c} below 7%. In the UKPDS study, 50% of patients required two or more pharmacological agents 3 years after diagnosis and 75% required multiple therapies after 9 years. This is undoubtedly a reflection of a progressive decline in beta-cell function over time.[11]

Temporary insulin therapy
Patients with type 2 diabetes often require temporary insulin therapy if they become pregnant, undergo surgery, or have intercurrent illnesses such as acute myocardial infarction or pneumonia. A widespread hospital practice in such cases is to use sliding insulin scales so that the patient is given regular insulin q6h with the doses changed frequently on the basis of regularly measured capillary blood glucose levels. The origin of this practice is unclear, and its net effect is poor control of glycemia.[12,13]

There is some evidence that for patients undergoing major surgery (that requires post-operative ICU) that continuous IV infusion may improve outcomes. However, there is no evidence of better outcomes in minor or moderate surgery.[2] Patients are far better off continuing with oral hypoglycemic agents or standard combinations of long- and short-acting insulins.[12-14]

Insulin plus oral hypoglycemic agents

A 1-year randomized controlled trial of obese patients whose type 2 diabetes was inadequately controlled with oral hypoglycemic agents alone compared bedtime isophane insulin (NPH) for all patients plus either glyburide and placebo, metformin and placebo, glyburide and metformin, or a second dose of isophane insulin given in the morning. In patients taking insulin plus metformin, glycosylated hemoglobin dropped from 9.7% to 7.2%, there was no weight gain, and hypoglycemic reactions were rare. All other groups gained weight and had poorer glycemic control and more hypoglycemic reactions. In this study patients adjusted their own insulin doses, starting with a dose equivalent to the fasting blood glucose level measured in millimoles per litre and increasing by 4 IU per day if the fasting levels exceeded eight mmol/L on three consecutive measurements and by 2 IU per day if they exceeded 6 mmol/L. The dose of metformin was 1000 mg before breakfast and 1000 mg before supper and that of glyburide 3.5 mg before breakfast and 7 mg before supper. Bedtime insulin was given at 9 P.M.[16] It is likely that both clinicians and patients overestimate the negative consequences of adding early insulin therapy and instead reserve it as a "final measure."

Home glucose monitoring

Home glucose monitoring of patients with type 2 diabetes has rarely been shown to improve glycemic control. Although some patients feel empowered when they use this technique, anxiety, helplessness, and guilt are much more common reactions.[18] A comparison of blood and urine glucose monitoring in patients with newly diagnosed type 2 diabetes found no difference between the two in glycosylated hemoglobin levels at 6 and 12 months, although urine testing was six times less expensive.[19]

HbA1c is a better way to assess glucose management. The notable exception is patients on insulin who, depending on their dosing strategy, would seem to benefit to provide feedback for therapy.

White coat hyperglycemia

In a British study of patients with non–insulin-dependent diabetes, glucose levels monitored at home were often lower than those measured in the clinic even when technical errors in home readings were ruled out. The authors labelled this phenomenon "white coat hyperglycemia."[20]

❧ REFERENCES ❧

1. American Diabetes Association: Standards of medical care for patients with diabetes mellitus, *Diabetes Care* 20(suppl 1):S1-S70, 1997.
2. Canadian Diabetes Association Clinical Practice Guidelines Expert Committee: CDA 2003 Clinical Practice Guidelines for the Prevention and Management of Diabetes in Canada, *Can J Diabetes* 27(suppl 2):S10-11, 2003.
3. Dagogo-Jack S, Santiago JV: Pathophysiology of type 2 diabetes and modes of action of therapeutic interventions, *Arch Intern Med* 157:1802-1817, 1997.
4. Troglitazone for non-insulin-dependent diabetes mellitus, *Med Lett* 39:49-51, 1997.
5. United Kingdom Prospective Diabetes Study (UKPDS) Group: Intensive blood-glucose control with sulphonylureas or insulin compared with conventional treatment and risk of complications in patients with type 2 diabetes (UKPDS 33), *Lancet* 352:837-853, 1998.
6. United Kingdom Prospective Diabetes Study (UKPDS) Group: Effect of intensive blood-glucose control with metformin on complications in overweight patients with type 2 diabetes (UKPDS 34), *Lancet* 352:854-865, 1998.
7. Robinson AC, Burke J, Robinson S, et al: The effects of metformin on glycemic control and serum lipids in insulin-treated NIDDM patients with suboptimal metabolic control, *Diabetes Care* 21:701-705, 1998.
8. Holman RR, Cull CA, Turner RC, et al: A randomized double-blind trial of acarbose in type 2 diabetes shows improved glycemic control over 3 years (U.K. Prospective Diabetes Study 44), *Diabetes Care* 22:960-964, 1999.
9. Rosiglitazone for type 2 diabetes mellitus, *Med Lett* 41:71-73, 1999.
10. Repaglinide for type 2 diabetes mellitus, *Med Lett* 40:55-56, 1998.
11. Turner RC, Cull CA, Frighi V, et al: Glycemic control with diet, sulfonylurea, metformin, or insulin in patients with type 2 diabetes mellitus: progressive requirement for multiple therapies (UKPDS 49), *JAMA* 281:2005-2012, 1999.
12. Queale WS, Seidler AJ, Brancati FL: Glycemic control and sliding scale insulin use in medical inpatients with diabetes mellitus, Arch Intern Med 157:545-552, 1997.
13. Sawin CT: Action without benefit: the sliding scale of insulin use (editorial), *Arch Intern Med* 157:489, 1997.
14. Jacober SJ, Sowers JR: An update on perioperative management of diabetes, *Arch Intern Med* 159:2405-2411, 1999.
15. Reference deleted in pages.
16. Hannele Y-J, Ryysy L, Nikkilä K, et al: Comparison of bedtime insulin regimens in patients with type 2 diabetes mellitus: a randomized controlled trial, *Ann Intern Med* 130:389-396, 1999.
17. Reference deleted in pages.
18. Gallichan M: Self monitoring of glucose by people with diabetes: evidence based practice, *BMJ* 324:964-966, 1997.
19. Miles P, Everett J, Murphy J, et al: Comparison of blood or urine testing by patients with newly diagnosed non-insulin dependent diabetes: patient survey after randomised crossover trial, *BMJ* 315:348-349, 1997.

20. Campbell LV, Ashwell SM, Borkman M, et al: White coat hyperglycaemia: disparity between diabetes clinic and home blood glucose concentrations, *BMJ* 305:1194-1196, 1992.

Insulin Therapy in Diabetes
(See also glucose monitoring; hypoglycemia)

Classification of insulins

Through the use of recombinant DNA technology, insulin is prepared either as chemically identical to human insulin or as a modified version of human insulin (insulin analogues) intended to improve pharmacokinetics. Animal insulins are infrequently used and are becoming less commercially available. A variety of insulins are available in North America, including ultra-short-acting, short-acting, and long-acting insulins. Insulin is also available as pre-mixed preparations, which are combinations of long- and short-acting insulins, as well as human insulins, pork insulins, insulins in vials and insulins in pens.[1]

Trade names of human insulins

Trade names of human insulins available in Canada or the United States are Humulin, Novolin, Humalog and Lantus. Humalog is the trade name for lispro, which is an analogue of human insulin. It is ultra-short acting. At present, pork insulin has been virtually replaced by human insulin.

Duration of action of insulins

Insulins are subclassified according to their duration of action (Table 51),[1,2] and the figures given vary from one source to another. The table gives a rough approximation of the time of onset, peak effect, and duration of action of various human insulins. It is important to note that rates of absorption of insulin–and therefore their durations of action–vary widely from one patient to another.[2]

Lispro (Humalog) is a synthetic analog of human insulin that is very rapidly absorbed. One of its main advantages is that it can be injected up to 15 minutes before a meal, which increases the flexibility of mealtimes.[3] (If regular insulin is used preprandially, the "lag time" between injection and eating is usually 20 to 30 minutes.[2]) Preprandial lispro does not lead to better control than preprandial regular insulin, but among patients with type 1 diabetes who are aiming for very tight control it decreases the frequency of nocturnal hypoglycemic reactions.[3]

Another insulin analogue is glargine (Lantus), which is a basal (long-acting) insulin that lasts for 24 hours in a steady state. Comparative trials with NPH, which does have an insulin peak, show some reduction in the rate of nocturnal hypoglycemia in patients taking glargine insulin. However, effect on HbA1c and micro-vascular/macro-vascular outcomes has yet to be shown.[3a]

Insulin vials, pens, cartridges, and syringes

All insulins, regardless of the format in which they are supplied and whether they are premixed, contain 100 units/mL. Insulin can be administered by a syringe, pen, or a continuous subcutaneous insulin infusion (CSII) pump.

In Canada the figures given for mixtures have regular insulin first followed by NPH insulin. Thus 30/70 means 30% regular insulin and 70% NPH. In the United States the order may be reversed so that the above mixture might be written 70/30. The practitioner can avoid confusion by remembering that except for a 50/50 mixture (in which the order does not matter), the smaller figure is always regular insulin and the larger one is NPH. In this text the convention of putting regular insulin first is used. In Canada a full range of mixtures of regular and NPH insulins from 10/90 to 50/50 is available, whereas in the United States

Table 51   Classification of Human Insulins by Time of Action

Type of Insulin	Time of Action			Trade Names
	Onset	Peak	Duration	
Rapid acting analogue	10-15min	60-90min	4-5hr	Humalog (lispro) NovoRapid (aspart)
Fast-acting	0.5-1hr	2-4hr	5-8hr	Humulin-R Novolin ge Toronto
Intermediate-acting	1-3hr	5-8hr	up to 18hr	Humulin-L Humulin-N Novolin ge NPH
Long-acting	3-4hr	8-15hr	22-26hr	Humulin-U
Extended long-acting anlg	90min	24hr		Lantus (glargine)
Pre-mixed		variable		Humalog Mix 25 Humulin (20/80, 30/70) Novolin ge (10/90, 20/80, 30/70, 40/60, 50/50)

Used with permission from *Can J Diabetes* 27(suppl 2):S32, 2003.

the 30/70 and 50/50 mixtures are marketed as well as availability of 75% lispro protamine + 25% lispro (Humalog 75/25 mix), 70% NPH + 30% aspart.

A variety of cartridges for dial-a-dose insulin pens that contain regular or NPH insulin or mixtures of regular and NPH insulin (as 30/70 in the United States and in various proportions from 10/90 to 50/50 in Canada) may be purchased. Pens take 1.5-mL cartridges (containing 150 units of insulin) or 3-mL cartridges (containing 300 units of insulin), and the correct dose can be dialed. Disposable pens are also available. Before using an insulin pen, patients should suspend the NPH insulin by tipping the pen 20 times.[4]

Human regular insulin, and human NPH insulin (lispro and aspart) are available in premixed formats, whether as vials, insulin pen cartridges, or disposable dispensing devices. Patients who are receiving pork insulins or Lente or Ultralente insulins (human or animal) and require mixtures of regular and longer acting insulins have to mix their own. Glargine is clear, as opposed to cloudy like other insulins, and cannot be mixed with other insulins.

Insulin syringes have a 1-mL capacity and are graduated in 0.01-mL portions. Since all commercial insulins are supplied as 100 units/mL, 0.01 mL = 1 unit.

Insulin injection sites. Intramuscular injections are more rapidly absorbed than subcutaneous ones. Injections into an extremity that has been exercising, massage of the injection site, or application of heat to the injection site increases the rate of insulin absorption and may lead to hypoglycemia.[2] It is safe to exercise the muscles at the injection site after an elapsed period of half an hour.[5] Absorption of insulin varies with the anatomical site of injection; it is most rapid in the abdomen, intermediate in the arm, and slowest in the thigh or hip. Sites should be rotated in the same general anatomical area, such as the abdominal wall, rather than using the thigh one day, the arm the next, and so on.[2] Injecting insulin through clothes is both safe and convenient.[6]

Glucose monitoring

Self-monitoring of blood glucose has many potential benefits for patients on insulin, including an improved HbA1c, avoiding hypoglycemia, and enhancing lifestyle flexibility. In type 1 diabetes, monitoring blood glucose levels three or more times per day has been associated with a 1% reduction in HbA1c levels.[7] Blood glucose measurements taken after lunch, after dinner and at bedtime have the highest correlation to HbA1c.[8]

Numerous glucometers are available. Modern ones are compact reflectance meters that are operated in one step by drawing fingertip capillary blood onto the strips by osmosis.

The new guidelines of the American[9] and Canadian[10] diabetes associations recommend preprandial glucose levels of 4 to 7 mmol/L and 4 to 6 for patients in whom it can be achieved safely.[10] These goals can be achieved only by monitoring glucose levels three to four times a day, usually before meals and at bedtime.[2] The bedtime measurement is particularly important as a check for hypoglycemia; nocturnal hypoglycemia may be unrecognized and lead to convulsions or coma.[11]

Devices that facilitate continuous monitoring of interstitial glucose concentrations are now available. Analytical standards for this method of glucose analysis are not currently available and insufficient evidence exists to support its widespread use.[12,13]

Glycosylated or glycated hemoglobin is monitored to assess the efficacy of diabetic control over a 2- to 3-month period, whereas fructosamine is used for a 2- to 3-week period. Glycated hemoglobin is measured either as HBA_{1C} or as total glycated hemoglobin.[14] Ideal levels are below 0.07 (7%).[9,10] Measurements should be taken every 3 months. An elevation of 0.01 (1%) corresponds to a rise of about 1.7 mmol/L (30 mg/dl) in the average glucose level.[14]

Initial insulin dose

The usual total daily dose of insulin for a patient with type 1 diabetes is 0.5 to 1 unit/kg. Patients are started on 0.2 to 0.6 unit/kg/day, and on the basis of frequent glucose readings the dose is increased gradually as necessary.[2] In type 2 diabetes there are three general choices for starting insulin:

1. Bedtime insulin regimen
   - Continue oral hypoglycemics
   - Start insulin NPH at 0.1 to 0.2 units/kg each evening
2. Twice daily insulin regimen
   - Discontinue oral hypoglycemic therapy and NPH insulin
   - Start insulin 30/70 at 0.5 units/kg
   - Give ~ ⅔ 30 min before breakfast
   - Give ~ ⅓ 30 min before dinner
3. Intensive insulin therapy
   - Discontinue oral hypoglycemic therapy and/or NPH insulin
   - Start insulin at 0.5 units/kg
   - Give 40% of total dose as basal insulin NPH at bedtime
   - Give 20% of total dose 3 times/day as mealtime insulin (fast or rapid acting), 15 to 30 min before meals (60% of total dose at mealtime)

The usual protocol for tight glycemic control involves a morning and bedtime injection of NPH or Lente insulin to cover the basal insulin needs plus regular insulin or insulin lispro before each meal.[2,11] The evening dose of NPH is given at bedtime rather than suppertime to help prevent nocturnal hypoglycemia and to better control pre-breakfast hyperglycemia.[2] Doses of preprandial insulin are determined by preprandial sugar levels and an estimation of the number of calories to be ingested. Approximately 10 units of insulin is required for every 500 calories.[11] Variations of this basic insulin regimen are possible; a common one for patients who use regular insulin before meals is to omit the morning intermediate-acting insulin. If insulin lispro is used before meals, both morning and evening doses of intermediate insulin are required.[2]

An alternative to multiple insulin injections is continuous subcutaneous insulin infusion (CSII). Regular or lispro insulin is used, and infusion rates can be varied from hour to hour. A meta-analysis of 12 small randomized controlled trials comparing CSII to optimized insulin injection therapy found that the mean blood glucose was 1.0 mmol/L lower and the HbA1c was 0.51% lower in the CSII group.[15]

Adjusting insulin doses. The insulin dose may be increased or decreased at any time by 1 to 2 units (or for higher doses by 10%). The particular insulin to be modified is determined by the blood sugar levels at different times during the day.[16] Assuming a twice a day insulin regimen with a mixture of regular and NPH insulin at each dose, the theoretical relationship would be as shown in Table 52.

Before insulin doses are adjusted, it is important to ensure that exogenous factors such as illness, unusual exercise, irregularity of meal and snack schedules, or non-compliance with the insulin doses is not responsible for the inadequate control.

Hypoglycemic reactions. In individuals with type 1 diabetes, the primary barrier to attaining optimal glycemic control is the risk of severe hypoglycemic reactions.[17] Severe, asymptomatic, spontaneously resolving nocturnal hypoglycemia appears to be common in young diabetic children, but as far as can be determined, cognitive functioning is unaffected by these events.[18] Missed meals, exercise without a snack, and erroneous insulin doses are some of the causes of clinically evident hypoglycemic reactions.

Evidence suggests that 15 g of glucose (e.g., 3 teaspoons of table sugar dissolved in water, 175 mL of juice or regular soft drink, 1 tablespoon of honey) can result in an increase in blood glucose of approximately 2.1

mmol/L within 20 minutes, with an alleviation of symptoms in most individuals.[19]

First-line treatment of hypoglycemia is glucose by mouth if the patient is conscious or applied to the buccal mucosa if the patient is not. Alternatives are a glucagon injection (1 mg for adults and older children and 0.5 mg for children under 5) or IV glucose. Glucagon 1 mg subcutaneously or intramuscularly has been shown to increase blood glucose from 3.0 to 12.0 mmol/L within 60 minutes.[18]

❧ REFERENCES ❧

1. Burge MR, Schade DS: Insulins, *Endocrinol Metabol Clin North Am* 26:575-598, 1997.
2. Hirsch IB: Type 1 diabetes mellitus and the use of flexible insulin regimens, *Am Fam Physician* 60:2343-2356, 1999.
3. Heller SR, Amiel SA, Mansell P (U.K. Lispro Study Group): Effect of the fast-acting insulin analog lispro on the risk of nocturnal hypoglycemia during intensified insulin therapy, *Diabetes Care* 22:1607-1611, 1999.
3a. Hirsch IB: Drug therapy: insulin analogues, *N Engl J Med* 352:174-183, 2005.
4. Jehle PM, Micheler C, Jehle DR, et al: Inadequate suspension of neutral protamine Hagedorn (NPH) insulin in pens, *Lancet* 354:1604-1607, 1999.
5. Fahey PF, Stallcamp ET, Kwatra S: The athlete with type I diabetes: managing insulin, diet and exercise, *Am Fam Physician* 53:1611-1617, 1996.
6. Fleming DR, Jacober SJ, Vandenberg MA, et al: The safety of injecting insulin through clothing, *Diabetes Care* 20: 244-247, 1997.
7. Karter AJ, Ackerson LM, Darbinian JA, et al: Self-monitoring of blood glucose levels and glycemic control: the northern California Kaiser Permanente Diabetes Registry, *Am J Med* 111:1-9, 2001.
8. Rohlfing CL, Wiedmeyer HM, Little RR, et al: Defining the relationship between plasma glucose and HbA1c: analysis of glucose profiles and HbA1c in the Diabetes Control and Complications Trial, *Diabetes Care* 25:275-278, 2002.
9. American Diabetes Association: Standards of medical care for patients with diabetes mellitus, *Diabetes Care* 20(suppl 1):S1-S70, 1997.
10. Canadian Diabetes Association Clinical Practice Guidelines Expert Committee: 2003 Clinical practice guidelines for the prevention and management of diabetes, *Can J Diabetes* 27 (suppl 2), 2003.
11. Havas S: Educational guidelines for achieving tight control and minimizing complications of type 1 diabetes, *Am Fam Physician* 60:1985-1998, 1999.
12. Sacks DB, Bruns DE, Goldstein DE et al: Guidelines and recommendations for laboratory analysis in the diagnosis and management of diabetes mellitus, *Clin Chem* 48: 436-472, 2002.
13. Monsod TP, Flanagan DE, Fire F, et al: Do sensor glucose levels accurately predict plasma glucose concentrations during hypoglyceemia and hyperinsulinemia? *Diabetes Care* 25:889-893, 2002.

Table 52 Relationship Between Glucose Levels and Insulin Dose Adjustments in Patients Taking Mixture of Regular and NPH Insulins

Suboptimal Glucose Reading	Recommended Insulin Adjustment
Before lunch	Before breakfast: regular
Before supper	Before breakfast: NPH
Bedtime	Before supper: regular
Before breakfast	Before supper: NPH

14. Koch B: Glucose monitoring as a guide to diabetes management: critical subject review, *Can Fam Physician* 42:1142-1152, 1996.

15. Pickup J, Mattock M, Kerry S: Glycaemic control with continuous subcutaneous insulin infusion compared with intensive insulin injections in patients with type I diabetes: meta-analysis of randomised controlled trials, *BMJ* 324:1-6, 2002.

16. Hirsch I: Intensive insulin therapy. II. Multicomponent insulin regimens, *Am Fam Physician* 45:2141-2147, 1992.

17. Cryer PE: Banting lecture. Hypoglycemia: the limiting factor in the management of IDDM, *Diabetes* 43:1378-1389, 1994.

18. Matyka KA, Wigg L, Pramming S, et al: Cognitive function and mood after profound nocturnal hypoglycaemia in prepubertal children with conventional insulin treatment for diabetes, *Arch Dis Child* 81:138-142, 1999.

19. Slama G, Traynard PY, Desplanque N, et al: The search for optimized treatment of hypoglycemia. Carbohydrates in tablets, solutions, or gel for the correction of insulin reactions, *Arch Int Med* 150:589-593, 1990.

20. Reference deleted in pages.

HEAT-RELATED ILLNESSES

(See also travel medicine)

Heat stroke is a medical emergency defined as a core body temperature of at least 40° C (104° F) with acute neurological changes.[1] Tachycardia and tachypnea are also present. Progressive multi-organ failure can result in significant morbidity, and mortality is at least 10%.[1,2] In contrast, heat exhaustion is due to volume and/or sodium depletion brought about by heat. Symptoms include sweating, dizziness, confusion, headache, nausea, vomiting, and muscle weakness. The body temperature does not have to be elevated. Many patients with heat exhaustion can be adequately treated with oral fluids and cool sponging.[2] The elderly and young children are particularly vulnerable to both conditions, while athletes and recreational sports enthusiasts are at increased risk.[2,3] There is a growing concern for some poorly acclimated athletes who "hyper-hydrate" by means of maintaining volume status with water but failing to replace sodium lost in sweat.[2]

Drugs may interfere with thermoregulation in a variety of ways. Some act by increasing muscle activity and heat production (amphetamines and cocaine), and some by blocking the parasympathetic system and thus inhibiting sweating (tricyclic antidepressants and phenothiazines). Others decrease blood flow to the skin by decreasing cardiac output (e.g., beta-blockers), by causing vasoconstriction (vasoconstrictors in decongestants), or by inducing volume depletion (diuretics, alcohol).[2]

Heat-related mortality can be decreased by increasing fluid intake (8 oz per hour regardless of thirst), decreasing physical exertion, exercising only during cool times of the day, spending more time in air-conditioned environments, and taking cool water baths.[4,5] Fans are not protective at temperatures above 32.3° C (90° F) with a relative humidity greater than 35%.[4]

In a study of excess deaths in Midwestern U.S. heat waves in 1995 and 1999, increased risk was observed for persons who were confined to bed for known medical problems, who had mental illness, who did not have air conditioners, or who were socially isolated.[4,5]

❧ REFERENCES ❧

1. Bouchama A, Knochel JP: Heat stroke, *N Engl J Med* 346:1978-1988, 2002.

2. Wexler RK: Evaluation and treatment of heat-related illness, *Am Fam Physician* 66:2307-2314, 2002.

3. Committee on Sports Medicine and Fitness, American Academy of Pediatrics: Climactic heat stress and the exercising child and adolescent, *Pediatrics*, 106:158-159, 2000.

4. Blum LN, Bresolin LB, Williams MA (Council on Scientific Affairs of the AMA): Heat-related illness during extreme weather emergencies, *JAMA* 279:1514, 1998.

5. Heat-related illnesses, deaths and risk factors – Cincinnati and Dayton, Ohio, 1999, and United States, 1979-1997, *MMWR* 49:470-473, 2000.

HEMOCHROMATOSIS

Hemochromatosis is a genetic disorder of iron metabolism, characterized by abnormally increased dietary iron absorption and deposition in multiple organs. It is transmitted as an autosomal recessive, single gene mutation designated C282Y, with variable penetrance. It has an incidence of 1 in 250 to 300 among Caucasians with a carrier state of 1 in 10.[1,2]

There is increased incidence of hemochromatosis in people of Northern European descent, particularly those of Nordic and Celtic ancestry.[3–5]

The disease is frequently asymptomatic before age 40. The classic presentation triad of cutaneous hyperpigmentation, diabetes mellitus and liver cirrhosis is a late finding. Currently, emphasis is on clinical suspicion and early diagnosis in patients presenting with non-specific features which may include fatigue, joint pains and increased serum ferritin. Due to multiple organ involvement presentation may include cardiac arrhythmias, cardiomyopathy, unexplained liver disease, hepatomegaly with elevated liver enzymes, hypothyroidism, primary hypogonadism and sepsis.[6]

Diagnosis is by clinical and laboratory parameters including fasting.

$$\text{Transferrin saturation} = [\text{Serum Ferritin/Total Iron binding Capacity}] \times 100.$$

Transferin saturation greater than 45% is highly suspicious. Genotype is required to confirm the diagnosis and should be performed on all first-degree relatives of patients. Liver biopsy should be done in patients above 40 years with evidence of liver disease.[7]

Management requires a multidisciplinary approach due to multiple organ involvement. There is overwhelming evidence that institution of phlebotomy therapy before cirrhosis and/or diabetes develops will significantly reduce disease morbidity and mortality.[8] Cirrhosis is irreversible and decompensated liver disease is an indication for orthotoptic liver transplantation.

The commonest cause of death is sudden cardiac death from arrhythmias and congestive heart failure. Hepatocellular carcinoma is the cause of death in 30% of patients with hemochromatosis. Earlier studies suggest that this risk is not improved with phlebotomy. Regular screening for hepatocellular carcinoma with liver ultrasound and serum alfa fetoprotein is recommended in these patients (Rating: II A, B, C, D, and E).[7] Differential diagnosis includes other causes of iron overload: sideroblastic anemia, thalasemias, chronic hemolytic anemias, and multiple blood transfusions.

_____ ⅍ **REFERENCES** ⅊ _____

1. McDonnell SM, Hover A, Gloe D, et al: Population based screening for hemochromatosis using phenotypic and DNA testing among employees of health maintenance organizations in Springfield, Missouri, *Am J Med* 107: 30-37, 1999.
2. Beutler E, Felitti V, Gelbart T, Ho N: The effect of HFE genotypes on measurement of Fe overload in patients attending a health appraisal clinic. *Ann Intern med* 133:329-337, 2000.
3. Merry-Weather-Clarke AT, Pointon JJ, Shearman JD, Robson KJ: Global prevalence of putative hemochromatosis mutations, *J Med Genet* 34: 275-278, 1997.
4. Lucotte G: Cellic origin of the c282y mutation of haemochromatosis, *Blood Cells Mol Dis* 24:433-438, 1998.
5. Olynyk J K, Cullen D J, Aquila S, et al: A population based study of the clinical expression of the haemochromatosis gene, *N Engl J Med* 341:718-724, 1999.
6. Brandhagen DJ, Fairbanks VF, Baldus W, Mayo Medical School Rochester, Minesota: Recognition and management of hereditary hemochromatosis, *Am Fam Physician* 65:853-860, 865-866, 2002.
7. Tavill AS: Diagnosis and management of hemochromarosis, *Hepatology* 33: 1321-1328, 2001.
8. Niederau C, Fischer R, Purschel A, et al: Long term survival in patients with hemochromatosis, *Gastroenterology*; 110:1107-1119, 1996.

HYPOGLYCEMIA

(See also diabetes mellitus; functional somatic syndromes)

The diagnosis of hypoglycemia is made when a patient has a serum blood glucose of < 2.8 mmol/L while experiencing classical autonomic and neuroglycopenic symptoms, which resolve with the intake of glucose.[1] The two classifications widely used are fasting (post-absorptive) and post-prandial hypoglycemia. A number of conditions may cause fasting hypoglycemia. Insulin and oral hypoglycemic reactions in diabetic patients are the most common. Insulinomas, severe illness, and drugs are other well-recognized causes of hypoglycemia. Hormonal deficiencies such as adrenal insufficiency and hypopituitarism may also result in the syndrome.[1,2]

Post-prandial hypoglycemia usually occurs within 4 hours of food intake. Well-documented causes include fructose intolerance and galactosemia in children, and gastric resection leading to alimentary hypoglycemia in adults.[1]

Idiopathic reactive hypoglycemia has been documented in only a few patients after a 5 hour oral glucose tolerence test (OGTT) and by measuring glucose levels following mixed meals.[1,2] The existence of such an entity is debatable because the diagnosis of post-prandial hypoglycemia should not be based on an OGTT, since values as low as 2.4 mmol/L can be seen in healthy people.[1,2] Several interventions have been suggested for these patients, including frequent low-carbohydrate, high-protein meals; anticholinergic drugs, propranolol, acarbose, and miglitol.[1]

_____ ⅍ **REFERENCES** ⅊ _____

1. Hanna A: Hypoglycemic disorders: endocrinology rounds, 3(10), 2003 (Accessed at www.endocrinology rounds.ca)
2. Service FJ: Hypoglycemic disorders, *N Engl J Med* 332: 1144-1152, 1995.

LIPID DISORDERS

CONVERSION FROM SYSTÉME-INTERNATIONAL UNITS TO TRADITIONAL UNITS

To convert cholesterol readings from Systéme International (SI) units (mmol/L) to traditional units (mg/dl), divide by 0.0259. To convert cholesterol readings from traditional units (mg/dl) to SI units (mmol/L), multiply by 0.0259.

Epidemiology of Lipid Disorders

(See also risk factors for coronary artery disease)

Wide variation is seen in the rates of coronary heart disease (CHD) in different geographical areas, and this is not fully explained by differences in cholesterol levels. For example, men with cholesterol levels in the range of 5.45 mmol/L (210 mg/dL) had CHD mortality rates varying from between 4% and 5% in Japan and Southern Europe to 12% in the United States and 15% in Northern Europe. Within any one culture, CHD risk correlates well with cholesterol levels.[1] Elevated triglyceride levels have been shown to be an independent risk factor for ischemic heart disease,[2-4] and have shown to have an association with increased risk especially when associated with low HDL-C, hypertension, increased fasting glucose, and abdominal obesity (metabolic syndrome).

The PROSPER study evaluated 5804 men and women age 70 to 82 years randomized between pravastatin 40 mg daily and placebo over a 3.2-year follow-up. Results showed 408 events in the treatment group against 473 events in the placebo group. The reduction appeared limited to coronary events as stroke events were not affected. Mortality from coronary disease fell by 24%. The suggestion is that, at least for coronary heart disease, pravastatin proved a benefit in the elderly population.[5]

⊿ REFERENCES ⊾

1. Verschuren WMM, Jacobs DR, Bloemberg M, et al: Serum total cholesterol and long-term coronary heart disease mortality in different cultures: twenty-five-year follow-up of the seven countries study, *JAMA* 274:131-136, 1995.
2. Sattar N, Packard CJ, Petrie JR: The end of triglycerides in cardiovascular risk assessment? Rumours of death are greatly exaggerated (editorial), *BMJ* 317:553-554, 1998.
3. Jeppesen J, Hein HO, Suadicani P, et al: Triglyceride concentration and ischemic heart disease: an eight-year follow-up in the Copenhagen Male Study, *Circulation* 97:1029-1036, 1998.
4. Coresh J, Kwiterovich PO Jr: Small, dense low-density lipoprotein particles and coronary heart disease risk: a clear association with uncertain implications (editorial), *JAMA* 276:914-915, 1996.
5. Shepherd J, Blauw GJ, Murphy MB, et al, for the PROSPER study group: Pravastatin in elderly individuals at risk of vascular disease (PROSPER): a randomized controlled trial, *Lancet* 360:1623-1630, 2002.

Variability of Cholesterol Levels

(See also prevention; screening)

A person's cholesterol levels vary substantially from one day to another independent of diet and laboratory testing procedures. In an Ontario study of cholesterol levels any patient whose initial total cholesterol level was greater than 6.2 mmol/L (240 mg/dL) was asked to give a second sample. On the basis of the initial results patients were divided into three risk categories[1]:

Normal risk	<6.2 mmol/L (240 mg/dl)
Moderate risk	6.2-6.9 mmol/L (240-266 mg/dl)
High risk	>6.9 mmol/L (266 mg/dl)

When a second sample was obtained, the two results were averaged and the patient's risk category was reassigned. The results were striking. Fifty percent

of patients initially classified as at high risk were reclassified to moderate risk, 10.5% of those initially classified as at moderate risk were reclassified to the normal category, and 4.8% of those initially classified as at moderate risk were moved up to a high-risk category.[1] From the findings of this and other studies, no one should be treated for an elevated cholesterol reading on the basis of one sample. When making treatment decisions, borderline lipid levels should lead to a careful risk assessment before drug intervention is initiated.

⊿ REFERENCES ⊾

1. Speechley M, McNair S, Leffley A, Bass M: Identifying patients with hypercholesterolemia: more than one blood sample is needed, *Can Fam Physician* 41:240-245, 1995.

Primary Prevention

(See also exercise; relative risk reduction)

Diet and exercise

The common belief that low-fat and low-cholesterol diets will lower LDL-C is based on observational studies, cross-sectional population-based studies, and metabolic ward–based studies.[1,2] No randomized controlled trial has shown that diet in ambulatory patients lowers coronary artery disease risk, and most studies have shown only small effects on cholesterol levels.[2] For example, a randomized prospective trial of ambulatory patients with elevated LDL-C and low HDL-C who were put on the National Cholesterol Education Program (NCEP) Step 2 diet found that diet alone did not alter lipid profiles. However, when this diet was combined with a regular aerobic exercise program, LDL-C levels fell and HDL-C levels rose. Exercise alone did not bring about these changes.[1]

Patients with elevated cholesterol levels are often advised to decrease their consumption of red meats and increase their consumption of white meats (poultry and fish). A 36-week trial in which hypercholesterolemic subjects were selected at random to eat 80% of their meat as lean pork, beef, or veal or to eat 80% as lean poultry or fish found no differences in LDL-C or HDL-C between the two groups.[3]

Drugs

Table 53 lists six major cholesterol-lowering studies of the effects of lipid-lowering drugs in individuals with elevated cholesterol levels but without known coronary artery disease (CAD).[4-9] With the exception of the AFCAPS/TexCAPS, these studies enrolled primarily middle-aged men with high cholesterol levels but without clinical evidence of CAD. The AFCAPS/TexCAPS enrolled men (82%) and post-menopausal women (18%) with normal or only slightly elevated lipid levels. All of these studies showed a statistically significant decline in coronary events, but only the WOSCOPS demonstrated a statistically significant decrease in cardiovascular mortality. In the World Health Organization (WHO) clofibrate study, total mortality of the treated group was increased by a relative rate of 47%.

The two most relevant studies for current practice are those that used HMG-CoA reductase inhibitors (statins). In WOSCOPS approximately 3300 middle-aged men with very high cholesterol levels but without known CAD received pravastatin 40 mg per day for an average of 4.9 years, while an equal number in the control group received a placebo. Prominently presented figures in the abstract of this *New England Journal of Medicine* report were a relative reduction of 31% in definite non-fatal and fatal myocardial infarctions and a 22% relative reduction in death from all causes in the treated cohort. By careful reading of the text it is possible to calculate that the absolute reduction in definite non-fatal and fatal myocardial infarctions was 2.4% and that more than 200 men had to be treated for 1 year to prevent one such adverse event. The absolute reduction in total cohort mortality was 0.9%, and this required the treatment of 555 men for 1 year to prevent one death.[8] Although WOSCOPS is usually thought of as a primary prevention study, 5% of the men in both the placebo and treatment groups had stable angina.[8] Because of this, purists question whether a reduction in mortality through pharmacotherapy of hypercholesterolemic men without CAD can truly be claimed.

In the AFCAPS/TexCAPS study approximately 3300 middle-aged men and women without known CAD and with normal or slightly elevated lipid levels received lovastatin 20 to 40 mg/day for an average of 5.2 years while an equal number received placebos. Lipid entry requirements were a total cholesterol of 4.65 to 6.82 mmol/L (180 to 264 mg/dL), LDL-C of 3.36 to 4.91 mmol/L (130 to 190 mg/dL), and HDL-C of 1.16 mmol/L (45 mg/dL) or less for men and 1.22 mmol/L (47 mg/dL) or less for women. The reported relative reduction in total cardiac events in the treated group (fatal and non-fatal myocardial infarction, unstable angina, or sudden cardiac death) was 37%. The absolute reduction was 4.1:1000 or 0.4%, and 250 individuals had to be treated for 1 year to prevent one event.[9]

No long-term lipid-lowering studies of young adults have been published,[10] and therefore the value of screening young asymptomatic individuals for cholesterol and treating them if it is elevated is unknown. Hulley and associates[11] point out that the mortality rate from cardiovascular disease is so low in persons under 40 that treatment would be unlikely to have beneficial results, whereas the adverse effects of treatment would continue unabated. They argue that delaying treatment until after age 40 would be unlikely to do any harm.

Data on the effects of cholesterol-lowering programs on women are inconclusive; too few women have been studied to generate enough statistical power to give meaningful results.[12]

WOSCOPS and AFCAPS/TexCAPS clearly show that statins can reduce the incidence of cardiovascular events in asymptomatic middle-aged and elderly individuals. The WOSCOPS results prove that cardiovascular mortality can be reduced, while those of the AFCAPS/TexCAPS indicate that statins may be beneficial even in individuals whose LDL-C levels are below those recommended by the National Cholesterol Education Program for the initiation of treatment (treat anyone over 35 who has no additional risk factors and has an LDL-C ≥4.9 mmol/L [190 mg/dl] and anyone with two or more additional risk factors if the LDL-C is 4.1 to 4.9 mmol/L (160 to 190 mg/dl]). At present, little or no evidence has shown that statins are beneficial for asymptomatic young individuals (except those with inborn errors of lipid metabolism) or for women of any age.

Given the building evidence NCEP ATP III states "Primary prevention of CHD offers the greatest opportunity for reducing the burden of CHD." The report emphasizes therapeutic lifestyle changes and risk assessment for all. For those with two or more risk factors, a 10-year Framingham risk assessment is done to establish a more accurate risk level. Additional drug therapy is dependant on the risk assessment and the LDL level. In the CHD or CHD risk equivalent, drug treatment is initiated with an LDL ≥3.37 mmol/L

Table 53   Cholesterol-Lowering Drug Studies in Patients Without Coronary Artery Disease

Drug studies	Drug
Lipid Research Clinics Program trial (LRC)[4]	Cholestyramine (Questran)
Helsinki Heart Study (HHS)[5]	Gemfibrozil (Lopid)
World Health Organization (WHO)[6]	Clofibrate (Atromid-S)
Upjohn's Colestipol Study (UCS)[7]	Colestipol (Colestid)
West of Scotland Coronary Prevention Study Group (WOSCOPS)[8]	Pravastatin (Pravachol)
Air Force/Texas Coronary Atherosclerosis Prevention Study (AFCAPS/TexCAPS)[9]	Lovastatin (Mevacor)

(130 mg/dL) with drug treatment considered optional with LDL between 2.59 and 3.34 mmol/L (100 and 129 mg/dL), in persons with 2+ risk factors (10-year risk ≤20%) drug therapy is initiated at 3.37 mmol/L (130 mg/dL) if Framingham risk is 10% to 20%, or 4.14 mmol/L (160 mg/dL) if Framingham risk is <10%. In the 01 risk factor group, drug therapy is initiated if the LDL ≥4.92 mmol/L (190 mg/dL) although it is considered optional if the LDL is between 4.14 and 4.90 mmol/L (160 and 189 mg/dL).

───────────────── ❧ **REFERENCES** ❧ ─────────────────

1. Stefanick ML, Mackey S, Sheehan M, et al: Effects of diet and exercise in men and postmenopausal women with low levels of HDL cholesterol and high levels of LDL cholesterol, *N Engl J Med* 339:12-20, 1998.
2. Steinberg D, Gotto AM Jr: Preventing coronary artery disease by lowering cholesterol levels, *JAMA* 282:2043-2050, 1999.
3. Davidson MH, Hunninghake D, Maki KC, et al: Comparison of the effects of lean red meat vs lean white meat on serum lipid levels among free-living persons with hypercholesterolemia, *Arch Intern Med* 1331-1338, 1999.
4. Lipid Research Clinics Coronary Prevention Trial. 1. Reduction in incidence of coronary heart disease, *JAMA* 251:351-374, 1984.
5. Frick MH, Elo O, Haapa K, et al: Helsinki Heart Study: primary prevention trial with gemfibrozil in middle-aged men with dyslipidaemia; safety of treatment, changes in risk factors, and incidence of coronary heart disease, *N Engl J Med* 317:1237-1245, 1987.
6. Heady JA, Morris JN, Oliver MF: WHO Clofibrate/Cholesterol Trial: clarifications, *Lancet* 340:1405-1406, 1992.
7. Dorr AE, Gundersen K, Schneider JC Jr, et al: Colestipol hydrochloride in hypercholesterolemic patients–effect on serum cholesterol and mortality, *J Chron Dis* 31:5-14, 1978.
8. Shepherd J, Cobbe SM, Ford I, et al: Prevention of coronary heart disease with pravastatin in men with hypercholesterolemia, *N Engl J Med* 333:1301-1307, 1995.
9. Downs JR, Clearfield M, Weis S, et al: Primary prevention of acute coronary events with lovastatin in men and women with average cholesterol levels: results of AFCAPS/TexCAPS, *JAMA* 279:1615-1622, 1998.
10. Sox HC Jr: Preventive health services in adults, *N Engl J Med* 330:1589-1595, 1994.
11. Hulley SB, Newman TB, Grady D, et al: Should we be measuring blood cholesterol levels in young adults? *JAMA* 269:1416-1419, 1993.
12. Rich-Edwards JW, Manson JE, Hennekens C, et al: The primary prevention of coronary heart disease in women, *N Engl J Med* 332:1758-1766, 1995.

Secondary Prevention

(See also cholesterol-lowering studies in children without known coronary artery disease; diets and exercise; coronary artery disease; exercise; myocardial infarction; prevention; smoking; treatment of elevated lipid levels)

Lipid-lowering strategies in patients with known CAD are effective, and far fewer patients need to be treated in order that one individual benefits than is the case with patients who have elevated lipid levels but no known CAD.

A Scandinavian randomized placebo-controlled trial of patients with a history of angina or myocardial infarction (Scandinavian Simvastatin Survival Study [4S]) treated patients with either simvastatin (Zocor) 20 to 40 mg or a placebo. There was a 30% relative and 3.3% absolute reduction in all-cause mortality (8.2% in the treated group versus 11.5% in the placebo group), which was due almost entirely to a 42% decrease in coronary events. Another way of looking at these figures is that 150 patients had to be treated for 1 year to prevent one death. The rates of non-cardiovascular deaths were the same in the treatment and placebo groups (no increase in violent deaths occurred in the treated group).[1] A 1995 Dutch study of 885 men with angiographically proven coronary artery disease compared treatment with pravastatin (Pravachol) to a placebo. At the end of 2 years 19% of patients in the placebo group had had vascular events compared with 11% in the treated group. More than twice as many in the placebo group as in the control group required angioplasty.[2]

In patients with known coronary artery disease, "normal" cholesterol levels may be too high. The Cholesterol and Recurrent Events (CARE) trial showed that cholesterol-lowering drugs were beneficial in post–myocardial infarction patients with "average" cholesterol and LDL-C levels. In a 5-year study of more than 4000 patients (mostly men), half were given pravastatin (Pravachol) 40 mg/day and half placebo. At the onset of the study all patients had a cholesterol level less than 6.2 mmol/L (240 mg/dL) with a mean of 5.4 mmol/L (209 mg/dL). At the end of the study the fatal coronary and non-fatal myocardial infarct rates were 10.2% in the pravastatin group and 13.2% in the placebo group for an absolute reduction of risk of 3% (relative risk reduction of 24%). The absolute reduction in the mortality rate of the treated group was 0.8%, which meant that 640 men had to be treated for 1 year to prevent one death. Fewer treated patients required angioplasty or coronary artery bypass surgery, and fewer had strokes.[3] Diabetic patients in the CARE study who received pravastatin experienced a greater absolute reduction in cardiovascular events than did non-diabetics.[4] The Long-Term Intervention with Pravastatin in Ischemic Disease (LIPID) study, which enrolled patients who had had a myocardial infarction or who had unstable angina, also observed benefits in patients with a broad range of initial cholesterol levels.[5]

Data on the benefits of cholesterol-lowering programs in women with proven CAD are limited. On the basis of the information available, this treatment seems to be beneficial.[6]

The prime goal of lipid-lowering agents in patients with proven CAD is to reduce the LDL-C level, and the best drugs for this purpose are HMG CoA reductase inhibitors.[7] The goal of therapy is to lower the LDL-C to 2.6 mmol/L (100 mg/dL) if possible.[8] In some patients with CAD the LDL-C concentration is not elevated but the HDL-C level is low (1 mmol/L [40 mg/dL]). One double-blind placebo-controlled trial found that in these circumstances treatment with slow release gemfibrozil (Lopid SR) 1200 mg once daily increased HDL-C level, decreased triglyceride levels, and decreased the risk of myocardial infarctions, coronary artery deaths, and strokes.[9]

The efficacy of dietary interventions in patients with CAD is controversial. In a 4-year study a very small number of patients with proven CAD were treated with intensive life-style changes, including a vegetarian diet limited to a 10% fat intake. The treated group had a decrease in coronary events and a small degree of regression of coronary artery lesions (determined by angiography) compared with the control group.[10] That more palatable selective diets may be effective is suggested by a French study of 302 post–myocardial infarction patients placed on a Mediterranean diet (see discussion of treatment of elevated lipid levels) and 303 control patients following the usual post–myocardial infarction "prudent" diet. At the end of 2 years 59 control patients had died of cardiovascular causes, had had another myocardial infarction, or had been found to have unstable angina, stroke, heart failure, or thromboembolism. In the Mediterranean diet group only 14 patients experienced similar events. This represents a 76% relative reduction rate and a 15% absolute reduction rate. Between six and seven patients had to be treated for 2 years to prevent one event.[11] A 4-year follow-up of these patients found that the benefits of the Mediterranean diet were maintained.[12] These results are better than those reported in the 1994 Scandinavian simvastatin study of patients with known CAD. The nature of the Mediterranean diet is discussed below in the section on treatment of elevated cholesterol levels. An examination of adherence to the Mediterranean diet and outcomes was assessed in 22,000 Greek adults aged 20 to 86 years. A two-point increment in the Mediterranean diet score reduced the risk of death by about 25%. Effects were important for older people, those taking less exercise, and any level of BMI, as well as cause of death or coronary heart disease or cancer.[13]

The Heart Protection Study[14] looked at 3280 adults with cerebrovascular disease and another 17,256 with other occlusive arterial disease or diabetes. Participants were randomized between simvastatin 40 mg daily or placebo. There was a significant 25% proportional reduction in the first-event rate for stroke. This included subcategories including those with coronary disease or diabetes, aged under or over 70, differing levels of blood pressure or lipids (even for pre-treatment LDL < 3.0 mmol/L).

The Myocardial Ischemia Reduction with Aggressive Cholesterol Lowering Study[15] (MIRACL) studied patients treated using high dose atorvastatin within 24 to 96 hours of admission for unstable angina or non-ST segment elevation MI. Recurrent ischemic events were reduced by 16% over a 16-week period independentntly of baseline lipid levels.

The ASCOT trial[16] showed that cholesterol lowering with atorvastatin 10 mg daily reduced the risk of cardiovascular events in hypertensive patients with normal cholesterol levels (TC <6.5 mmol/L) and three risk factors for CVD. The treatment group was followed for 3.3 years and had a 36% reduction in fatal/non-fatal MI, a 29% reduction in total coronary events and a 27% reduction in stroke.

Given these results, there would appear to be a trend towards treating high risk patients more aggressively.

REFERENCES

1. Scandinavian Simvastatin Survival Study Group: Randomised trial of cholesterol lowering in 4444 patients with coronary heart disease: the Scandinavian Simvastatin Survival Study (4S), *Lancet* 344:1383-1389, 1994.
2. Jukema JW, Bruschke AVG, Vanboven AJ, et al: Effects of lipid lowering by pravastatin on progression and regression of coronary artery disease in symptomatic men with normal to moderately elevated serum cholesterol levels: the Regression Growth Evaluation Statin Study (REGRESS), *Circulation* 91:2528-2540, 1995.
3. Sacks FM, Pfeffer MA, Moye LA, et al: The effect of pravastatin on coronary events after myocardial infarction in patients with average cholesterol levels, *N Engl J Med* 335:1001-1009, 1996.
4. Goldberg RB, Mellies MJ, Sacks FM, et al: Cardiovascular events and their reduction with pravastatin in diabetic and glucose-intolerant myocardial infarction survivors with average cholesterol levels: subgroup analyses in the Cholesterol and Recurrent Events (CARE) Trial, *Circulation* 98:2513-2519, 1998.
5. Long-Term Intervention with Pravastatin in Ischaemic Disease (LIPID) Study Group: Prevention of cardiovascular events and death with pravastatin in patients with coronary heart disease and a broad range of initial cholesterol levels, *N Engl J Med* 339:1349-1357, 1998.
6. Walsh JM, Grady D: Treatment of hyperlipidemia in women, *JAMA* 274:1152-1158, 1995.
7. Kantner T: HMG CoA reductase inhibitors for treatment of hyperlipidemia, *Am Fam Physician* 47:1623-1627, 1993.
8. National Cholesterol Education Program: *The second report of the Expert Panel on Detection, Evaluation, and Treatment of High Blood Cholesterol in Adults (Adult Treatment Panel II)*, Bethesda, Md, 1993, National Heart, Lung, and Blood Institute, National Institutes of Health, NIH Pub No 93-3095.

9. Rubins HB, Robins SJ, Collins D, et al: Gemfibrozil for the secondary prevention of coronary heart disease in men with low levels of high-density lipoprotein cholesterol, *N Engl J Med* 341:410-418, 1999.

10. Ornish D, Scherwitz LW, Billings JH, et al: Intensive lifestyle changes for reversal of coronary heart disease, *JAMA* 280:2001-2007, 1998.

11. De Lorgeril M, Salen P, Martin J-L, et al: Effect of a Mediterranean type diet on the rate of cardiovascular complications in patients with coronary artery disease–insights into the cardioprotective effect of certain nutriments, *J Am Coll Cardiol* 28:1103-1108, 1996.

12. De Lorgeril M, Salen P, Martin J-L, et al: Mediterranean diet, traditional risk factors, and the rate of cardiovascular complications after myocardial infarction: final report of the Lyon Diet Heart Study, *Circulation* 99:779-785, 1999.

13. Trichopoulou A, et al: Adherence to a Mediterranean diet and survival in a Greek population, N Engl J Med 348:2599-2608, 2003.

14. Heart Protection Study Collaborative Group: MRC/BHF Heart Protection Study of cholesterol lowering with simvastatin in 20,536 high risk individuals: a randomized placebo-controlled trial. *Lancet* 360:7-22, 2002.

15. Kinlay S, Schwartz GG, Olsson AG, et al: Myocardial ischemia reduction with aggressive cholesterol lowering, *Circulation* 108(13):1560-1566, 2003.

16. Server PS, Dahlof B, Poulter NR, et al: Prevention of coronary and stroke events with atorvastatin in hypertensive patients who have average or lower than average cholesterol concentrations, in the Anglo-Scndinavial Cardiac Outcomes Trial—Lipid Lowering Arm (ASCOT-LLA): a multicentre randomized controlled trial. *Lancet* 361:1149-1158, 2003.

Cholesterol-Lowering Studies in Children without Known Coronary Artery Disease

In 1992 an expert panel on blood cholesterol levels in children and adolescents convened by the National Heart, Lung, and Blood Institute recommended that all Americans over the age of 2 years reduce their dietary fat intake.[1] This same organization sponsored the Dietary Intervention Study in Children (DISC) with the goal of assessing the efficacy and safety of lowering LDL-C levels in pubescent children. The results of the study were reported in 1995.[2]

Dietary intervention study in children

The children enrolled in the DISC study were between the ages of approximately 8 and 11.[2] They were initially assessed by capillary blood cholesterol measurement, and if it was above the 75th percentile, a fasting venous sample for LDL-C was obtained. If the LDL-C level was between the 70th and 99th age- and sex-specific percentiles, a second fasting venous sample was obtained. If the average of the LDL-C levels from the two venous samples was between the 70th and 99th percentiles, the children were randomly assigned to ordinary care or dietary intervention with a 3-year follow-up. The parents of children in both groups were told that their children's cholesterol levels were high, and in both groups body mass index was calculated and the hip, waist, and skinfold thickness at various sites were measured. In the dietary intervention group 28% of energy was obtained from fat, of which 9% was polyunsaturated (Step 2–type diet). Over the 3-year study period, children and families of the intervention group attended approximately 27 group and individual meetings and received monthly phone calls between meetings. Capillary blood cholesterol measurements were obtained periodically during individual meetings, and at the termination of the study venous samples were obtained for the measurement of a variety of parameters. The report does not mention the children's physical activities.[2]

The primary outcome of the DISC study was a decrease in LDL-C in both the intervention group and the ordinary care group. The reduction was 0.09 mmol/L (3.3 mg/dL) greater in the intervention group, which is a statistically significant difference. The intervention group showed no evidence of decreased growth or decreased ferritin levels, and in fact there was no difference in any of the anthropomorphic measurements, including sexual maturation, between the groups. Psychological measurements showed a lower adjusted mean depression score for the intervention children at 3 years.[2]

The clinical significance of the DISC trial is hard to comprehend. Normal children were labelled as having high cholesterol, and a vast amount of time and energy was devoted to altering the diets of the intervention group. One fact is obvious; even if the physician believes that measuring cholesterol levels in children and instituting a dietary program if they are high is desirable, this clinical trial has no applicability to ordinary clinical practice. What family physician or pediatrician could possibly offer 27 group and individual meetings plus interval phone calls over a 3-year period as a part of his or her regular practice?

Epidemiological data suggest that children of parents with early CAD are more likely to be obese than control subjects and that other indices of CAD risk such as elevated LDL levels appear as they grow older.[3] The benefits and drawbacks of life-style preventive interventions directed toward such children are unknown; one study reports success in controlling obesity in children with an intensive behavioural therapy program.[4]

Guidelines for cholesterol screening

The Expert Panel on Blood Cholesterol Levels in Children and Adolescents of the National Heart,

Lung, and Blood Institute's National Cholesterol Education Program, the American Academy of Family Physicians, the American Academy of Pediatrics, and the American Medical Association do not recommend universal screening of cholesterol levels in children. However, if the child is over 2 and has a parent with a cholesterol level greater than 6.25 mmol/L (240 mg/dL) or if the parents or grandparents have a history of premature (under age 55) cardiovascular disease, screening is recommended.[5] Both the U.S. Preventive Services Task Force[6] and the Canadian Task Force on Preventive Health Care[7] give a "C" recommendation to general cholesterol screening of children and adolescents. The U.S. Preventive Services Task Force qualifies this by stating that a family history of very high cholesterol levels, premature coronary heart disease in a first-degree relative (before age 50 in males and before age 60 in females), or other major risk factors for coronary heart disease may be reasons for measuring cholesterol levels in adolescents or young adults.[6]

────────────── ◙ **REFERENCES** ◙ ──────────────

1. Expert Panel on Blood Cholesterol Levels in Children and Adolescents: National Cholesterol Education Program report, *Pediatrics* 89(suppl):525-584, 1992.
2. Dietary Intervention Study in Children (DISC): Efficacy and safety of lowering dietary intake of fat and cholesterol in children with elevated low-density lipoprotein cholesterol, *JAMA* 273:1429-1435, 1995.
3. Bao W, Srinivasan SR, Valdez R, et al: Longitudinal changes in cardiovascular risk from childhood to young adulthood in offspring of parents with coronary artery disease: the Bogalusa Heart Study, *JAMA* 278:1749-1754, 1997.
4. Epstein LH, Valoski, Wing RR, et al: Ten-year follow-up of behavioral, family-based treatment for obese children, *JAMA* 264:2519-2523, 1990.
5. US Public Health Service: Cholesterol screening in children, *Am Fam Physician* 51:1923-1927, 1995.
6. US Preventive Services Task Force: *Guide to clinical preventive services,* ed 2, Baltimore, 1996, Williams & Wilkins, pp 15-38.
7. Canadian Task Force on the Periodic Health Examination: *Canadian guide to clinical preventive health care,* Ottawa, 1994, Canada Communication Group—Publishing, pp 650-669.

Adverse Effects Associated with Low Cholesterol Levels

Low cholesterol as a marker of increased mortality risk

A number of malignancies such as those of the lung, pancreas, rectum, bladder, liver, and kidney, as well as some non-malignant diseases such as chronic lung disease and strokes, are associated with low cholesterol levels.[1-3] Total mortality in middle-aged and elderly patients is increased among those with the lowest cholesterol levels,[3,4] and this appears to be particularly so in those who have both a low albumin and a low cholesterol level.[5] The accepted explanation for these findings is that the disease processes themselves cause the cholesterol levels to drop even if the diseases have not yet manifested themselves clinically.[5]

Carcinogenic potential of cholesterol-lowering drugs

A well-established but rarely discussed aspect of cholesterol-lowering agents is that many of them, including the fibrates such as gemfibrozil and clofibrate and the HMG-CoA reductase inhibitors such as lovastatin and pravastatin, are carcinogenic in rodents. However, recent analysis[6] reveals that meta-analysis of the first five large statin trials shows no difference in cancer rates between statin-treated and placebo patients.[7] As well, the Heart Protection Study reported the incidence of primary new cancers to be equal between simvastatin and placebo over a 5-year follow-up.[8] A meta-analysis of pravastatin trials including PROSPER and CARE did not suggest any increase of cancer.[9]

────────────── ◙ **REFERENCES** ◙ ──────────────

1. Wannamethee G, Shaper AG, Whincup PH, et al: Low serum total cholesterol concentrations and mortality in middle aged British men, *BMJ* 311:409-413, 1995.
2. Davey Smith G, Shipley MJ, Marmot MG, et al: Plasma cholesterol concentration and mortality: the Whitehall study, *JAMA* 267:70-76, 1992.
3. Manolio TA, Ettinger WH, Tracy RP, et al: Epidemiology of low cholesterol levels in older adults, *Circulation* 87:728-737, 1993.
4. Staessen J, Amery A, Birkenhager W, et al: Is a high serum cholesterol level associated with longer survival in elderly hypertensives? *J Hypertens* 8:755-761, 1990.
5. Reuben DB, Ix JH, Greendale GA, et al: The predictive value of combined hypoalbuminemia and hypocholesterolemia in high functioning community-dwelling older persons: MacArthur Studies of Successful Aging, *J Am Geriatr Soc* 47:402-406, 1999.
6. Waters D: Statins and safety: applying the results of randomized trials to clinical practice, *Am J Cardiology.* 92:692-695.
7. Bjerre LM, LeLorier J: Do statins cause cancer? A meta-analysis of large randomized clinical trials, *Am J Med* 110:716-723, 2001.
8. Heart Protection Study Collaborative Group. MRC/BHF Heart Protection Study of cholesterol lowering with simvastatin in 20,536 high risk individuals: a randomized placebo-controlled trial, *Lancet* 360: 7-22, 2002.
9. Shepherd J, Blauw GJ, Murphy MB, et al, for the PROSPER study group: Pravastatin in elderly individuals at risk of vascular disease (PROSPER): a randomized controlled trial, *Lancet* 360:1623-1630, 2002.

Guidelines for Cholesterol Screening
(See also coronary artery disease)

Canadian Guidelines[1] recommend screening men over age 40, women who are menopausal or over 50, and those with the following risk factors:

- Diabetes
- Presence of hypertension, smoking, or abdominal obesity
- Strong family history of premature CAD
- Manifestations of hyperlipidemia (such as xanthelasma, xanthoma, arcus)
- Evidence of symptomatic or asymptomatic atherosclerosis
- Patients of any age where lifestyle changes are indicated

Three risk levels are identified: low (≤ 10% 10-year risk of CVD event), moderate (10% to 20% 10-year risk of CVD event), and high (≥ 20% 10-year risk of CVD event). Targets are identified for LDL-C (2.5 mmol/L, 3.5 mmol/L, and 4.5 mmol/L for high, moderate, and low risk) and TC:HDL-C ratio (4.0, 5.0, and 6.0 for high, moderate, and low risk). The triglyceride target is 1.7 mmol/L for all risk levels.

The National Cholesterol Education Program (NCEP) Adult Treatment Panel III (ATP III)[2] recommends screening for all adults 20 years of age every 5 years. They list three risk categories: CHD or CHD equivalent (10 year risk of event > 20%), ≥ 2 risk factors (10 year event risk ≤ 20%), and 0 to 1 risk factor. Criterion for CHD and CHD risk equivalent are: patients with established CHD, patients with non-coronary atherosclerosis (symptomatic CAD, abdominal aortic aneurism, PAD), patients with diabetes, and patients with 10-year risk > 20%. NCEP ATP III uses LDL-C as the primary target: CHD or equivalent risk— LDL-C < 100 mg/dL, ≥ 2 risk factors < 130 mg/dL, and 0 to 1 risk factor < 160 mg/dL. They list the major risk factors as cigarette smoking, hypertension (BP ≥ 140/90 or on antihypertensive medication), family history of premature CHD (CHD in male first-degree relative < 55 years or CHD in female first-degree relative < 65 years), or age (men≥ 45 years or women ≥ 55 years).

Both guidelines[1,2] recommend identification and treatment of metabolic syndrome and the identifying criterion are very similar: 3 of 5 risk factors: abdominal obesity (waist circumference > 102 cm or 40 inches in men and 88 cm or 35 inches in women), triglycerides ≥ 150 mg/dL (1.7 mmol/L), HDL-C < 40 mg/dL (1.0 mmol/L) in men or < 50 mg/dL (1.3 mmol/L) in women, blood pressure ≥ 130/≥85, and fasting glucose ≥ 110 mg/dL (6.2 to 7.0 mmol/L).

──────────────── ◢ **REFERENCES** ◣ ────────────────

1. Genest, et al: Recommendations for the management of dyslipidemia and the prevention of cardiovascular disease: summary of the 2003 update, *CMAJ* 169(9):921, 2003.

2. Grundy SM, Cleeman JI, Merz CN, et al: Implications of recent clinical trials for the National Cholesterol Education Program Adult Treatment Panel III guidelines, *Circulation* 110(2):227-239, 2004.

Treatment of Elevated Lipid Levels
(See also cardiac arrest; cholesterol-lowering studies in children without coronary artery disease; prevention)

Guidelines for who should be treated

Canadian Lipid Guidelines recommend drug therapy for those at high risk for coronary artery disease (>20% Framingham Risk Assessment or history of diabetes mellitus or any atherosclerotic disease) in addition to lifestyle measures. The goal is to reduce the LDL-C to 2.5 mmol/L or below a TC/HDL-C ratio < 4.0. With reference to the HPS study, they suggest the equivalent of 1.04 mmol/L (40 mg/dL) of simvastatin. For those with moderate risk (10% to 19%) a target LDL is 3.5 mmol/L or TC/HDL-C ratio < 5.0, and for those at low risk (<10%) a target is 4.5 mmol/L or a TC/HDL-C ratio < 6.0.[1] NCEP ATP III sets similar targets but uses only LDL as a primary target. For patients with 0-1 risk factor the goal is an LDL of 4.14 mmol/L (160 mg/dL). For the patient with 2+ risk factors (≤20%) the LDL goal is 3.37 mmol/L (130 mg/dL) and for the high-risk patient (CHD or CHD risk equivalent) (>20% risk) the LDL goal is <2.59 mmol/L (100 mg/dL).

European guidelines for management of lipid levels are relatively simple. If patients' 10-year risk of CHD is >20% and LDL-C is >3.0 mmol/L (116 mg/dL), they should maintain lifestyle changes and be started on lipid-lowering therapy. Patients with 10-year risk of CHD >20% or LDL-C <3.0 mmol/L (116 mg/dL) are directed to change lifestyle.[2]

U.S. guidelines for management of lipid levels are more complex. Cutoffs for treatment again depend on the patient's 10-year risk of CHD and LDL-C levels. Based on U.S. guidelines, a wider portion of the patient population is eligible for pharmacological treatment than based on European guidelines.

NCEP ATP III emphasizes therapeutic lifestyle changes and risk assessment for all. For those with two or more risk factors, a 10-year Framingham risk assessment is done to establish a more accurate risk level. Additional drug therapy is dependant on the risk assessment and the LDL level. In the CHD or CHD risk equivalent, drug treatment is initiated with an LDL ≥3.37 mmol/L (130 mg/dL) with drug treatment considered optional with LDL between 2.59 and 3.34 mmol/L (100 and 129 mg/dL), in persons with 2+ risk factors (10-year risk ≤20%) drug therapy is initiated at 3.37 mmol/L (130 mg/dL) if Framingham risk is 10% to 20%, or 4.14 mmol/L (160 mg/dL) if Framingham risk is <10%. In the 0-1 risk factor group, drug therapy is initiated if the LDL ≥4.92 mmol/L (190 mg/dL) although it is considered optional if the LDL is between 4.14 and 4.90 mmol/L (160 and 189 mg/dL).[3]

Diet

The usual protocol for lowering blood cholesterol is to begin with a 3- to 6-month trial of diet and to add drugs only if dietary changes are unsuccessful. While studies from metabolic wards have shown that diet can lower cholesterol by 10% to 15%, dietary advice in outpatient settings usually results in only about a 5% decrease.[4]

The Mediterranean diet that was so effective in decreasing cardiovascular events and deaths in post–myocardial infarction patients did not change the serum concentration of total, low-density, or high-density cholesterol.[5,6] The diet was high in linolenic and oleic acid, relatively low in saturated fatty acids and linoleic acid, and high in some antioxidant vitamins.[6,7] The reason for its efficacy is unknown, but constituents such as omega-3 fatty acids, oleic acid, and antioxidant vitamins may be cardioprotective (see discussion of antioxidants).[7,8]

A Mediterranean diet has a high content of oil, particularly olive oil or canola (rapeseed) oil, complex carbohydrates such as bread and pasta, fruits, vegetables, fish, and poultry. It has a low content of beef, pork, and other meats, and the amount of cheese and wine consumed is moderate. More specifically, patients on this diet are instructed to eat the following[5]:

- More bread
- More vegetables
- More fish
- Less beef, lamb, and pork (to be replaced with poultry)
- Fruit daily
- No butter or cream (in the study a special margarine based on canola oil was provided)
- Olive oil or canola oil (rapeseed without erucic acid) to be used exclusively for preparing foods and salad dressings

A number of studies have shown that fish consumption (which does not lower LDL levels) is associated with a decreased rate of sudden cardiac death. This is discussed under the section Cardiac Arrest.

Pharmacotherapy

The treatment of elevated lipids with any class of drugs is a lifelong undertaking. When medications are stopped, cholesterol levels almost always rise to pretreatment levels.[9] The bulk of evidence strongly supports the use of cholesterol-lowering drugs in patients with known CHD or CHD equivalent risk.

A wide variety of lipid-lowering drugs are available (Table 54), and the choice depends on numerous variables. All the lipid-lowering drugs lower LDL-C, and niacin (nicotinic acid) and the fibrates such as gemfibrozil are particularly effective in lowering triglycerides. The HMG-CoA reductase inhibitors are potent and can be taken once daily. Nicotinic acid is inexpensive, available over the counter, and often effective. It not only lowers total cholesterol, LDL-C, and triglycerides, but also is more effective in raising HDL than any other drug.[9] However, for many patients its side effects are unacceptable for long-term treatment. In one study 43% of patients discontinued the drug for this reason.[10] The efficacy of nicotinic acid is related to the dose, but even doses as low as 1.5 g/day may be effective in raising HDL.[11] Flushing caused by nicotinic acid can be diminished by pretreatment with Aspirin or ibuprofen (Advil, Motrin), and adverse effects may be diminished by using an extended-release formulation (Niaspan).[9,11] Adaptation to side effects may be improved by initiating treatment with small doses and increasing them gradually. A new addition to the armamentarium is ezetimibe. Addition of ezetimibe to simvastatin, atorvastatin, and pravastatin therapy decreased LDL 15% to 20% at all doses of statin used. Simvastatin 10 mg plus ezetimibe 10 mg produced a 44% reduction in LDL-C, similar to that of simvastatin 80 mg alone.[12,13]

Soluble fiber such as psyllium (Metamucil) in doses of 5 to 15 g/day (1 to 3 rounded teaspoons) may reduce cholesterol by a small amount.[14,15] The drug appears to be most effective if given with rather than between meals.[16]

Table 54   Lipid-Lowering Drugs

Drugs	Usual doses
Bile Acid Sequestrants	
Cholestyramine (Questran)	4 g 1-6 times per day
Fibrates	
Fenofibrate (Lipidil)	100 mg tid with meals
Micronized fenofibrate (Tricor)	67-201 mg once daily with a meal
Gemfibrozil (Lopid)	600 mg bid
HMG-CoA Reductase Inhibitors	
Atorvastatin (Lipitor)	20-80 mg/day, with evening meal
Cerivastatin (Baycol)	0.2-0.3 mg/day in the evening
Fluvastatin (Lescol)	20-40 mg/day in the evening
Lovastatin (Mevacor)	20-80 mg/day with the evening meal
Pravastatin (Pravachol)	10-40 mg/day in the evening
Simvastatin (Zocor)	20-40 mg/day in the evening
Rosuvastatin (Crestor)	10-40 mg/day any time of day with or without meals.
Niacin Derivatives	
Niacin, nicotinic acid	1-6 g/day in 2-4 divided doses
Niacin extended release (Niaspan)	1-3 g hs
Other Lipid-Lowering Drugs	
Ezetimibe (Zetia, Ezetrol)	10 mg daily with a statin.
Psyllium (Metamucil)	5-15 g/day (1-3 rounded teaspoons)

❧ REFERENCES ❧

1. Genest J, Frohlich J, Fodor G, McPherson R (the Working Group on Hypercholesterolemia and Other Dyslipidemias): Recommendations for the management of dyslipidemia and the prevention of cardiovascular disease: summary of the 2003 update. *CMAJ* 169(9):921-924, 2003.

2. Wood D, De Backer G, Faergeman O, et al: Prevention of coronary heart disease in clinical practice: recommendations of the Second Joint Task Force of European and other Societies on Coronary Prevention, *Atherosclerosis* 140:199-270, 1998.

3. Expert Panel on Detection Evaluation and Treatment of High Blood Cholesterol in Adults: Executive summary of the third report of the National Cholesterol Education Program (NCEP) Expert Panel on Detection, Evaluation, and Treatment of High Blood Cholesterol In Adults (Adult Treatment Panel III), *JAMA* 285:2486-2497, 2001.

4. Tang JL, Armitage JM, Lancaster T, et al: Systematic review of dietary intervention trials to lower blood total cholesterol in free-living subjects, *BMJ* 316:1213-1220, 1998.

5. Renaud S, de Lorgeril M, Delaye J, et al: Cretan Mediterranean diet for prevention of coronary heart disease, *Am J Clin Nutr* 61(suppl):1360S-1367S, 1995.

6. De Lorgeril, Renaud S, Mamelle N, et al: Mediterranean alpha-linolenic acid-rich diet in secondary prevention of coronary heart disease, *Lancet* 343:1454-1459, 1994.

7. De Lorgeril M, Salen P, Martin J-L, et al: Effect of a Mediterranean type of diet on the rate of cardiovascular complications in patients with coronary artery disease: insights into the cardioprotective effect of certain nutriments, *J Am Coll Cardiol* 28:1103-1108, 1996.

8. National Cholesterol Education Program: *The second report of the Expert Panel on Detection, Evaluation, and Treat-ment of High Blood Cholesterol in Adults* (Adult Treatment Panel II), Bethesda, Md, 1993, National Heart, Lung, and Blood Institute, National Institutes of Health, NIH Pub No 93-3095.

9. Choice of lipid-lowering drugs, *Med Lett* 38:67-70, 1996.

10. Gibbons LW, Gonzalez V, Gordon N, et al: The prevalence of side effects with regular and sustained-release nicotinic acid, *Am J Med* 99:378-385, 1995.

11. Guyton JR, Goldberg AC, Kreisberg RA, et al: Effectiveness of once-nightly dosing of extended-release niacin alone and in combination for hypercholesterolemia, *Am J Cardiol* 82:737-743, 1998.

12. Davidson MH et al: Ezetimibe coadministered with simvastatin in patients with primary hypercholesterolaemia. *J Am Coll Cardiol* 40:2125-2134, 2002.

13. Gagne C, et al. Efficacy and safety of ezetimibe added to ongoing statin therapy for treatment of patients with primary hypercholesterolaemia, *Am J Cardiol* 90:1084-1090, 2002.

14. Glore SR, Van Treeck D, Knehans AW, et al: Soluble fiber and serum lipids: a literature review, *J Am Dietetic Assoc* 94:425-436, 1994.

15. Wolever TM, Jenkins DJ, Mueller S, et al: Psyllium reduces blood lipids in men and women with hyperlipidemia, *Am J Med Sci* 307:269-273, 1994.

16. Wolever TM, Jenkins DJ, Mueller S, et al: Method of administration influences the serum cholesterol-lowering effect of psyllium, *Am J Clin Nutr* 59:1055-1059, 1994.

MULTIPLE CHEMICAL SENSITIVITIES

(See also approach to complementary and alternative medicine; breast implants; chronic fatigue syndrome; fibromyalgia)

In the 1970s, an apparently mild form of multiple chemical sensitivity, dubbed "sick building syndrome" (SBS), came into prominence as buildings became tighter and ventilation rates lowered to save energy. As well, new "off-gassing" synthetic products were increasingly being used indoors. The World Health Organization described SBS as a set of multi-system symptoms occurring with increased frequency in buildings with indoor climate problems that improved or resolved on leaving the buildings.[1]

Such sensitivities have been reported worldwide in a variety of patient populations.[2] Synonyms for multiple chemical sensitivities (MCS) include environmental illness, 20th-century disease, total allergy syndrome, sick building syndrome, and immune dysregulation. MCS does not appear to be an uncommon problem.[3] Population-based studies in New Mexico and California revealed 2% to 6% of participants, respectively, had been diagnosed with MCS. In the California study, 16% reported they were "unusually sensitive to everyday chemicals." Between 85% and 90% of patients are women, usually between the ages of 30 and 50.[4]

According to the 1999 Consensus, case criteria defined MCS as follows: symptoms are reproducible with exposure; they are chronic; lower levels of exposure than previously or commonly tolerated result in symptom manifestations; symptoms improve or resolve when incitants are removed; responses occur to multiple, chemically-unrelated substances; and symptoms involve multiple organ systems.[6]

Symptoms commonly include having a stronger sense of smell (hyperosmia) than others; difficulty concentrating, feeling dull or groggy, and "spacey."[7] In MCS there will usually be some physical signs, but there are no consistently abnormal physical findings nor laboratory results. In an attempt to avoid the putative offending environmental agents many patients stop working or seeing friends and isolate themselves in their homes. The link between exposures to each patient's triggers and his or her symptoms may be obscured if the patient has frequent, relatively low-dose exposures. An addiction phenomenon may develop as the person's physiology struggles to adapt. The true trigger-symptom relationship will become apparent with accidental or deliberate environmental changes.[2]

Common symptoms that appear to overlap with multiple chemical sensitivities, chronic fatigue syndrome, and fibromyalgia include cacosmia, hyperosmia, headache, fatigue, trouble concentrating, depression, sleep disturbances, poor concentration, memory loss, dizziness, weakness, joint pains, headaches, and heat intolerance. Other associated conditions include irritable bowel syndrome, atypical connective tissue disease after silicone breast implants, hypoglycemia, and Gulf War illness.[8]

It is important to take a thorough exposure history using the CH2OPD2 mnemonic (community, home/hobby, occupation, personal exposures, diet/drugs).[9] Avoidance of identified triggers has been observed to be helpful.[10] It is helpful to have a scent-free policy in your office and to offer patients with MCS the first appointment of the day (before other patients arrive wearing scented products). Teach relaxation techniques and educate about sleep hygiene, exercise, and good nutrition. If you suspect workplace contamination, ask the patient to obtain Material Safety Data Sheets (MSDS) and ask them to inform their supervisor, health and safety committee, and union representative. As necessary avoidance of triggers may lead to isolation, ensuring an adequate support system for MCS patients is crucial.

───────────── ◄ **REFERENCES** ► ─────────────

1. WHO: *Indoor Air Quality Research.* Euro-Reports and Studies No. 103. Copenhagen: WHO Regional Office for Europe. 1984.
2. Ashford NA, Miller CS: *Chemical exposures, low levels and high stakes,* ed 2, New York, 1998, John Wiley.
3. Kreutzer R, Neutra RR, Lashuay N: Prevalence of people reporting sensitivities to chemicals in a population-based survey, *Am J Epidemiol* 150:1-12, 1999.
4. Magill MK, Suruda A: Multiple chemical sensitivity syndrome, *Am Fam Physician* 58:721-728, 1998.
5. Reference deleted in pages.
6. 1999 Consensus on Multiple Chemical Sensitivity, *Arch Env Health* 54(3):147-149, 1999.
7. McKeown-Eyssen GE, Baines CJ, Marshall LM, et al: Multiple chemical sensitivity: Discriminant validity of case definitions, *Arch Env Health* 56(5):406-412, 2001.
8. Kipen HM, Fiedler N: Invited commentary: sensitivities to chemicals—context and implications (editorial), *Am J Epidemiol* 150:13-16, 1999.
9. Marshall L, Weir E, Abelsohn A, et al: Identifying and managing health effects: Taking an exposure history, *CMAJ* 166(8):1049-1055,2002. www.ocfp.ca
10. Lax MB, Henneberger PK: Patients with multiple chemical sensitivities in an occupational health clinic: Presentationa and follow-up, *Arch Env Health* 50(6):425-431, 1995.

OBESITY
Definition
The World Health Organization (WHO) has defined "overweight" as a body mass index (BMI) of 25 to 29.9 and "obese" as a BMI greater than 30 (Table 55).[1]

Similar guidelines have been adopted by the United States,[2] Canada,[3] and many other nations.[4] For seniors (age 65 and over) there is evidence to suggest that their relative risk of mortality begins to increase only in the upper levels of the overweight range.[5]

There is good evidence that the BMI is a valid and reliable measure for identifying adults at increased risk for mortality and morbidity due to overweight and obesity.[6]

Waist circumference is correlated with abdominal fat and is also a practical indicator of health risk associated with abdominal obesity. [3,7-9] The WHO considers a waist circumference of 102 cm (40 inches) in men and 88 cm (35 inches) in women to indicate a high risk for diabetes, hypertension, and coronary heart disease.[1,5] The Nurses' Health Study reported that women with waist circumferences of 76.2 cm (30 inches) or greater had over twice the risk for coronary artery disease compared with thinner women.[8]

The waist/hip ratio (WHR) is another clinical measure of obesity; however, it is not included in most guidelines. According to Lean and associates,[7] health risks are significant if the values are above 0.95 for men and 0.80 for women. The Nurses' Health Study found that women with a waist/hip ratio greater than 0.75 had over twice the risk for coronary artery disease as those with a lower ratio.[8] A recent study comparing waist circumference, waist-hip ratio, and BMI in an Australian population concluded that WHR was most strongly correlated with CVD risk factors in the general population.[10]

Table 55   Classification of Adults According to BMI

Classification	BMI (kg/m²)	Risk of Comorbidities
Underweight	<18.50	Low (but risk of other clinical problems increased)
Normal Range	18.50-24.99	Average
Overweight	>25.00	
Preobese	25.00-29.99	Increased
Obese Class I	30.00-34.99	Moderate
Obese Class II	35.00-39.99	Severe
Obese Class III	>40.00	Very severe

From *Obesity: preventing and managing a global epidemic.* Report of a WHO Consultation. Geneva, 2000, World Health Organization (WHO Technical Report Series No.894). Reprinted with permission.

❧ REFERENCES ❧

1. *Obesity: preventing and managing a global epidemic.* Report of a WHO Consultation. Geneva, World Health Organization, 2000 (WHO Technical Report Series, No. 894)
2. Expert Panel on the Identification, Evaluation, and Treatment of Overweight and Obesity in Adults: Executive summary of the clinical guidelines on the identification, evaluation, and treatment of overweight and obesity in adults, *Arch Intern Med* 158:1855-1867, 1998.
3. Health Canada. Canadian guidelines for body weight classification in adults. Avaliable at: http://www.hc-sc.gc.ca/hpfb-dgpsa/onpp-bppn/weight_book_e.pdf, Accessed March 30, 2004.
4. Health Canada. Review of weight guidelines. Available at: http://www.hc-sc.gc.ca/hpfb-dgpsa/onpp-bppn/review_weight_guide_e.pdf, Accessed March 30, 2004.
5. Taylor DH, Ostbye T: The effect of middle and old age body mass index on short term mortality in older people, *J Am Geriatr* Soc 49(10):1319-1326, 2001
6. US Preventative services task force. Screening for obesity in adults: recommendations and results, *Ann Int Med* 139(11):930-932, 2003.
7. Lean MEJ, Han TS, Morrison CE: Waist circumference as a measure for indicating need for weight management, *BMJ* 311:158-161, 1995.
8. Rexrode KM, Carey VJ, Hennekens CH, et al: Abdominal adiposity and coronary heart disease in women, *JAMA* 280:1843-1848, 1998.
9. Lean ME, Han TS, Seidell JC: Impairment of health and quality of life in people with large waist circumference, *Lancet* 351:853-856, 1998.
10. Dalton M, Cameron AJ, Zimmet PZ et al: Waist circumference, waist-hip ratio and body mass index and their correlation with cardiovascular disease risk factors in Australian adults. *J Int Med* 254:555-563, 2003.

Epidemiology of Obesity

The prevalence of obesity (BMI 30 or greater) has increased dramatically in the United States during the 1990s, with nearly one third (30.5%) of adults classified as obese in the 1999-2000 National Health and Nutrition Examination Survey. Since 1960, the prevalence of obesity in American adults has increased by 17.5%.[1] Increases have occurred in both sexes, all age groups, all races, and all educational levels, but the greatest degree of increase has been among Hispanics, persons with some college education, men and women in their twenties, and residents of the Atlantic Coast states in the South.[2] When rates of "overweight" and "obesity" are combined, the estimated prevalence among U.S. adults is 64.5%.[1] The trend of increasing obesity has been noted worldwide.[3] A Canadian population survey of individuals over the age of 12 (Aboriginal people excluded) found that one fourth of all women and one third of all men were obese (BMI 27 or greater).[4]

One explanation for the trend toward obesity is an increasingly sedentary life-style[3,5,6] coupled with a high intake of energy-dense foods.[3] The WHO has also identified heavy marketing of energy-dense foods, high intake of sugar-sweetened soft drinks, and adverse socio-economic conditions as probable contributors to the worldwide obesity epidemic.[3]

Childhood obesity is also increasing. The prevalence of overweight among children and teens in the United States aged 6 to 19 has tripled between 1990 and 2000.[1] Rates of childhood obesity have increased similarly in Canada[7] and the United Kingdom.[8] As with adults, obesity in childhood may lead to diabetes, hypertension, dyslipidemia, endothelial dysfunction, and hyperinsulinemia.[8]

❧ REFERENCES ❧

1. Ogden CL, Carroll MD, Flegal KM: Epidemiologic trends in overweight and obesity, *Endocrinol Metab Clin North Am* 32(4):741-60, 2003.
2. Mokdad AH, Serdula MK, Dietz WH, et al: The spread of the obesity epidemic in the United States, 1991-1998, *JAMA* 282:1519-1522, 1999.
3. Diet, nutrition and the prevention of chronic disease. Report of a WHO Consultation. Geneva, World Health Organization, 2003 (WHO Technical Report Series, No. 916).
4. Trakas K, Lawrence K, Shear NH: Utilization of health care resources by obese Canadians, *Can Med Assoc J* 160:1457-1462, 1999.
5. Samaras K, Kelly PJ, Chiano MN, et al: Genetic and environmental influences on total-body and central abdominal fat: the effect of physical activity in female twins, *Ann Intern Med* 130:873-882, 1999.
6. Jeffery RW, French SA: Epidemic obesity in the United States: are fast foods and television viewing contributing? *Am J Public Health* 88:277-280, 1998.
7. Tremblay MS, Katzmarzyk PT, Willms JD: Temporal trends in overweight and obesity in Canada 1981-1996, *Int J Obesity* 26:538-543, 2002.
8. Ebbeling CB, Pawlak DB, Ludwig DS: Childhood obesity: public-health crisis, common sense cure, *Lancet* 360:473-482, 2002.

Pathophysiology of Obesity

(See also exercise)

Obesity results from an imbalance between energy input and energy expenditure.[1] Energy is expended in a variety of ways: basal metabolic rate, post-prandial thermogenesis (the excess energy required to digest and absorb food), and physical activity thermogenesis. Physical activity thermogenesis may in turn be subdivided into volitional exercise and non-exercise activity thermogenesis (NEAT). NEAT includes all physical activity except planned exercise programs, including activities of daily living and maintenance of posture, spontaneous muscle contraction, and fidgeting.[2]

Although overeating is commonly believed to be the major cause of obesity, evidence supporting this hypothesis is not definitive. Decreased physical activity is also an important factor.[1,3] Surveys show that although Americans have become fatter, they have been eating fewer calories and less fat.[4] Approximately 70% of U.S. adults either do not undertake physical activity or are underactive and nearly half of U.S. youth (aged 12 to 21) are not active on a regular basis.[3] Although some individuals may be participating in more leisure-time exercise programs, declining household and occupational physical activity results in decreased total energy expenditure.[4] Levine, Eberhardt, and Jensen[2] studied 16 non-obese volunteers who were fed 1000 excess kcal per day for 8 weeks and whose volitional exercise was strictly controlled. Weight gain ranged from 1.4 to 7.2 kg, and there was a 10-fold variation between individuals in fat storage. Basal metabolic rate and post-prandial thermogenesis increased by a small amount in all subjects, but there was little interindividual variation. However, wide variations in NEAT accounted for the striking differences in fat accumulation.

Obese persons tend to have a higher fat content in their diets than do normal weight individuals.[5] While energy from fat is no more fattening then the same amount of energy from carbohydrate or protein, "passive over-consumption" occurs when the diet is high in energy-dense foods, which tend to be highly processed, micronutrient poor, and high in fats, sugars, or starch.[6] A meta-analysis of 16 trials of ad libitum high-fat versus low-fat diet suggested that a reduction in fat content by 10% corresponds to a reduction in 3 kg of body weight.[7]

The optimal foraging theory offers an evolutionary explanation for our current epidemic of obesity. Animals are programmed to expend a minimum amount of energy to take in a maximum amount of high-energy food. This is beneficial when food is scarce but is harmful when no activity is required to obtain meals.[8] In many individuals the body adjusts its energy output as weight changes. Those who have purposely lost weight have a decreased resting energy output, whereas those who have purposely gained weight have an increased resting energy output[9] The mechanism by which the "set point" for body fat is modulated has not been clearly established, however, the molecular mechanisms involved in the regulation of energy balance are being extensively studied. In general, it is found that the body is better protected against weight loss than weight gain.[10] Even leptin, discovered in 1994 by Friedman, and originally thought to be a satiety hormone, is now regarded to primarily protect against weight loss in times of deprivation rather than weight gain in times of plenty.[11]

Susceptibility to obesity is considered to be a polygenic trait. There is a subset of the population in whom, under conditions of high fat intake or reduced energy expenditure, bodyweight will increase more than in the rest of the population.[12]

❧ REFERENCES ❧

1. Bennett WI: Beyond overeating (editorial), *N Engl J Med* 332:673-674, 1995.
2. Levine JA, Eberhardt NL, Jensen MD: Role of nonexercise activity thermogenesis in resistance to fat gain in humans, *Science* 283:212-214, 1999.
3. Chakravarthy MV, Joyner MJ, Booth FW: An obligation for primary care physicians to prescribe physical activity to sedentary patient to reduce the risk of chronic health conditions, *Mayo Clin Proc* 77(2):165-173, 2002
4. Heini AF, Weinsier RL: Divergent trends in obesity and fat intake patterns: the American paradox, *Am J Med* 102: 259-264, 1997.
5. Toubro S, Astrup A: Randomized comparison of diets for maintaining obese subjects' weight after major weight loss: ad lib, low fat, high carbohydrate diet v fixed energy intake, *BMJ* 314:29-34, 1997.
6. Diet, nutrition and the prevention of chronic disease. Report of a WHO Consultation. Geneva, World Health Organization, 2003 (WHO Technical Report Series, No. 916).
7. Astrup A, Grunwald GK, Melanson EL, et al: The role of low fat diets in body weight control: A meta-analysis of ad-libitum dietary intervention studies, *Int J Obes Relat Metab Disord* 24(12):1545-1552, 2000.
8. Foreyt J, Goodrick K: The ultimate triumph of obesity (editorial), *Lancet* 346:134-135, 1995.
9. Leibel RL, Rosenbaum M, Hirsch J: Changes in energy expenditure resulting from altered body weight, *N Engl J Med* 332:621-628, 1995.
10. Hofbauer KG: Molecular pathways to obesity, *Int J Obesity* 26;S18-S27, 2002.
11. Marx J: Cellular warriors at the battle of the bulge, *Science* 299:846-849, 2003.
12. Barsh GS, Farooqi IS, O'Rahilly S: Genetics and body weight regulation, *Nature* 404:391-404, 2000.

Adverse Medical Consequences of Obesity

(See also exercise; poverty)

A number of medical conditions are associated with obesity. These include the following:

- Hypertension[1,2]
- Coronary heart disease[1-5]
- Type 2 diabetes mellitus[1-5]
- Gallbladder disease[1]
- Sleep apnea[1]
- Respiratory problems such as cough and wheezing[1,6]

- Cancers of the endometrium,[1] breast,[1] prostate,[1] colon,[1,7] and pancreas[8]
- Osteoarthritis[1]
- Congestive heart failure[2]
- Ischemic stroke[2]
- Non-alcoholic steatohepatitis[2]
- Low back pain[6]
- Increased total mortality[1,5,9-11]
- Complications of pregnancy[12,13]
- Emotional distress, discrimination, and social stigmatization[14]

A progressive relationship was found between increasing BMI and coronary artery disease (CAD) in the Nurses' Health Study. The relative risk was lowest for women with a BMI less than 21 and was 3.5 for women whose BMI was greater than 29. Weight gain after the age of 18 was also a risk factor, even if the weight remained well within the "normal" limits.[4] A progressive increase in CAD risk with a BMI over 20 has also been demonstrated in British men.[5] Obesity is now thought to pose as great a risk for coronary heart disease as smoking, a sedentary life-style, and elevated blood cholesterol.[3] Furthermore, it is estimated that 60% to 90% of all patients with type 2 diabetes are or have been obese.[15] Women with BMI of 24-25 have a fivefold increase of developing diabetes than women with a BMI <22. Those with BMI >35 have a 93-fold increase risk.[16] Weight loss has been shown to reduce the incidence of type 2 diabetes, while deliberate weight loss in obese diabetics has been associated with 30% to 40% reduction in diabetes related mortality.[17] Obese individuals who lose 5% to 10% of their body weight may decrease their blood pressure and cholesterol levels[2] but whether this will translate into a reduced risk of cardiovascular disease remains unknown. Analysis of the Framingham Heart Study data showed a 3 to 7 year decrease in life expectancy among obese individuals compared to persons of normal weight. Obese individuals were found to be 81% to 115% more likely to die prematurely.[11] The Nurses' Health Study found sharp increases in total cohort mortality for BMI >27 and weight gain over 10 kg after age 18. Although cardiovascular disease accounted for most of the excess mortality, cancers were also contributing factors.[9] Among British men, total cohort mortality was increased when the BMI was 30 or more.[5]

Maternal obesity is a risk factor for the development of gestational diabetes. Increased body weight is associated with menstrual irregularities and is found to be a risk factor for primary ovulatory infertility.[2] Perinatal mortality[13] and the incidence of neural tube defects[12] are both elevated among the offspring of obese women.

➷ REFERENCES ➴

1. Expert Panel on the Identification, Evaluation, and Treatment of Overweight and Obesity in Adults: Executive summary of the clinical guidelines on the identification, evaluation, and treatment of overweight and obesity in adults, *Arch Intern Med* 158:1855-1867, 1998.
2. National task force on the prevention of overweight and obesity. Overweight, obesity and health risk, *Arch Int Med* 160:898-904, 2000.
3. Eckel RH, Krauss RM (AHA Nutrition Committee): American Heart Association call to action: obesity as a major risk factor for coronary heart disease, *Circulation* 97:2099-2100, 1998.
4. Willett WC, Manson JE, Stampfer MJ, et al: Weight, weight change, and coronary heart disease in women: risk within the "normal" weight range, *JAMA* 273:461-465, 1995.
5. Shaper AG, Wannamethee G, Walker M: Body weight: implications for the prevention of coronary heart disease, stroke, and diabetes mellitus in a cohort study of middle aged men, *BMJ* 314:1311-1317, 1997.
6. Lean ME, Han TS, Seidell JC: Impairment of health and quality of life in people with large waist circumference, *Lancet* 351:853-856, 1998.
7. Ford ES: Body mass index and colon cancer in a national sample of adult US men and women, *Am J Epidemiol* 150:390-398, 1999.
8. Silverman DT, Swanson CA, Gridley G, et al: Dietary and nutritional factors and pancreatic cancer: a case-control study based on direct interviews, *J Natl Cancer Inst* 90:1710-1719, 1998.
9. Manson JE, Willett WC, Stampfer MJ, et al: Body weight and mortality among women, *N Engl J Med* 333:677-685, 1995.
10. Calle EE, Thun MJ, Petrelli JM, et al: Body-mass index and mortality in a prospective cohort of U.S. adults, *N Engl J Med* 341:1097-1105, 1999.
11. Peeters A, Barendregt JJ, Willekens F et al: Obesity in adulthood and its consequesnces for life expectancy: a life-table analysis, *Ann Int Med* 138:24-32, 2003.
12. Goldenberg RL, Tamura T: Prepregnancy weight and pregnancy outcome (editorial), *JAMA* 275:1127-1128, 1996.
13. Cnattingius S, Bergström R, Lipworth L, et al: Prepregnancy weight and the risk of adverse pregnancy outcomes, *N Engl J Med* 338:147-152, 1998.
14. Lyznicki JM, Young DC, Riggs JA, Davis RM: Obesity: Assessment and management in primary care, *Am Fam Phys* 63:2185-2196, 2001.
15. Felber JP, Golay A: Pathways from obesity to diabetes. *Int J Obesity* 26:S39-S45, 2002
16. Colditz GA, Willett WC, Rotnitzky A, Manson JAE: Weight gain as a risk factor for clinical diabetes mellitus in women, *Ann In Med* 122:481-486, 1995.
17. Astrup A. Healthy lifestyles in Europe: prevention of obesity and type II diabetes by diet and physical activity, *Public Health Nutr* 4(2):499-515, 2001.

Obesity Screening
(See also screening)

Recommendations and guidelines regarding obesity screening vary widely. The U.S. Preventative Services Task Force (USPSTF) published updated clinical guidelines in December 2003, giving a "B" recommendation to screening all adult patients for obesity using the BMI measurement.[1] The Canadian Task Force on Preventive Health Care gives a "C" recommendation to calculating the BMI as part of the periodic health examination.[2] The American College of Preventative Medicine recommends periodic measurement of BMI for all adults.[3] A National Institutes of Health expert panel recommends calculating the BMI and measuring waist circumference in individuals with two or more obesity-related diseases or risk factors (see below).[4]

──────────── ☙ REFERENCES ❧ ────────────

1. US Preventative Services Task Force: Screening for obesity in adults: recommendations and results, *Ann Int Med* 139(11):930-932, 2003.
2. Douketis JD, Feightner JW, Attia J, et al: Periodic health examination, 1999 update. 1. Detection, prevention and treatment of obesity, *Can Med Assoc J* 160:513-525, 1999.
3. Nawaz H, Katz DL: American College of Preventative Medicine Practice Policy Statement: Weight management counseling of overweight adults, *Am J Prev Med* 21(1):73-78, 2001.
4. Clinical guidelines on the identification, evaluation, and treatment of overweight and obesity in adults—the evidence report, *Obesity Res* 6(suppl 2):51S-209S, 1998.

Risk Assessment and Decision to Treat

Weight classification using BMI and/or waist circumference (see above) can be used as an initial tool to identify individuals at increased relative risk or morbidity and mortality from obesity. BMI is determined using a nomogram. Waist circumference (WC) is measured at the end of normal expiration, while the person is standing with feet hip width apart, midway between the lower costal margin and the iliac crest.[1]

Health Canada recommends that the BMI and WC be used as a component of a more comprehensive health assessment including the presence of other chronic disease risk factors such as hypertension, dyslipidemia, diabetes, and individual behaviours such as eating habits and physical activity.[1] The NIH Guidelines recommend assessment of underlying diseases associated with obesity as well as risk factors for cardiovascular disease and diabetes, including cigarette smoking, hypertension, high LDL, low HDL, impaired fasting glucose, positive family history, physical inactivity, and elevated triglycerides.[2,3]

The decision to treat overweight and obese individuals is based on the BMI and WC in the presence or absence of risk factors (see above). The NIH guidelines suggest treatment of all individuals with BMI >30 and of individuals with BMI 25.0 to 29.9 or those with increased WC who have two or more risk factors.[2,3] The Canadian Task Force on Preventative Health Care gives a "B" recommendation for weight reduction therapy of obese adults with obesity related diseases.[4] For patients without obesity related disease or with BMI <30 and no other comorbidities or risk factors, the Canadian Task Force gives a "C" recommendation to treatment,[4] and the NIH recommends continuation of periodic weight checks and assessment of risk factors as well as advice to maintain weight.[2,3]

──────────── ☙ REFERENCES ❧ ────────────

1. Health Canada: Canadian guidelines for body weight classification in adults. Available at: http://www.hc-sc.gc.ca/hpfb-dgpsa/onpp-bppn/weight_book_e.pdf. Accessed March 30, 2004.
2. Lyznicki JM, Young DC, Riggs JA, et al: Obesity: Assessment and Management in Primary Care. *Am Fam Phys* 63:2185-96, 2001.
3. Expert Panel on the Identification, Evaluation, and Treatment of Overweight and Obesity in Adults: Executive summary of the clinical guidelines on the identification, evaluation, and treatment of overweight and obesity in adults, *Arch Intern Med* 158:1855-1867, 1998.
4. Douketis JD, Feightner JW, Attia J, et al: Periodic health examination, 1999 update. 1. Detection, prevention and treatment of obesity, *Can Med Assoc J* 160:513-525, 1999.

Treatment of the Obese Patient

Treatment options for obesity include diet, exercise, behaviour therapy, medication, and surgery. The goal of therapy is to initially reduce body weight by approximately 10% from baseline. Weight loss should occur at a rate of 0.5 to 1 kg/week (1 to 2 lbs/week) over a 6-month period.[1]

Lifestyle modification: diet, exercise and behaviour therapy
(See also pathophysiology of obesity)

As obesity and overweight results from an imbalance between energy input and energy expenditure, restriction of calories and increased physical activity are central to most strategies for weight loss reduction.[2] However, without long-term behavioural change, dieting rarely leads to long-term weight loss. A combination of controlled energy intake, increased physical activity, and behaviour therapy provide the most successful treatment for weight loss and the maintenance of that weight loss.

Dietary Therapy. The recent proliferation of popular diets (see below) has led to much confusion for patients regarding healthy eating and weight control. Traditionally, a healthy diet contains about 20% to 35% fat, 10% to 35% protein and 45% to 65% carbohydrates,[3] and it is recommended that a diet low in fat is needed to lose weight.[4] However, regardless of the final nutritional composition of a diet, patients need to decrease their caloric intake to lose weight. Reductions of 500-1000 kcal/d are needed to produce weight loss at the recommended level of 0.5 to 1 kg/week (1 to 2 lbs/week).[1]

Patients should be made aware of the size of average servings and the caloric content of various food classes:

Proteins	4 kcal/g
Carbohydrates	4 kcal/g
Fats	9 kcal/g
Alcohol	7 kcal/g

Once they understand the principles of caloric content and serving size, patients can recognize and try to avoid foods with a high caloric content. Fat intake can be lowered by removing visible fat from meat, avoiding fast foods and fried foods, minimizing margarine, butter, nuts, mayonnaise, sauces, and rich desserts. However, patients should be made aware that many "low fat" products are high in refined sugar and flour,[2] and therefore may still be calorie-rich. A food diary, in which patients record everything they eat or drink for 3 days, can assist their practitioners to identify hidden or unexpected sources of excess calories.

Low-Fat Diets versus Low-Carb Diets and the Mediterranean Diet. Low-fat diets have been found to be effective in producing weight loss when compared to control groups. The principal factors that predicted weight loss were the degree of the reduction in dietary fat and the pre-treatment body weight.[5] When low-energy and low-fat diet are combined, weight loss is greater than with low-fat diet alone; however, those on ad libitum low-fat diets are more likely to maintain their weight loss after 2 years.[6]

Low-carbohydrate diets have been popularized by the success of the Atkins diet,[7] which has been on the New York Times best seller list consistently since its publication. Advocates claim that diets higher in protein and lower in carbohydrates promote the metabolism of adipose tissue in the absence of avaliable dietary carbohydrate. However, there are concerns that low-carbohydrate diets may lead to abnormal metabolic functioning.[8,9] Bravata et al[10] systematically reviewed studies describing adult outpatient recipients of low carbohydrate diets. They found that weight loss was principally associated with decreased caloric intake and increased diet duration rather then with reduced carbohydrate content. They did not find that lower carbohydrate diets were associated with adverse effects on serum lipids levels, fasting glucose or blood pressure. However, due to limitations of the studies they found, it was concluded that there was insufficient evidence to recommend for or against the use of lower carbohydrate diets.

The Mediterranean diet, although not low fat, may contribute to the prevention and treatment of obesity,

provided it is controlled in calories.[11] The Mediterranean diet is high in fruits, vegetables, legumes and whole grains. It includes fish, nuts and low-fat dairy products. It is not restricted in total fat, but emphasizes vegetable oils, principally olive oil, and is low in saturated fats and partially hydrogenated oils. The Mediterranean diet has been shown to reduce total mortality, as well as mortality from heart disease and cancer.[12]

Olestra. Olestra (Olean), a non-absorbable fat substitute, was approved for use in certain snack foods by the U.S FDA in 1996.[13] Olestra has been reported to cause abdominal cramps and diarrhea, particularly if large quantities are taken, and it absorbs fat-soluble vitamins. To prevent vitamin deficiencies, the manufacturer has added vitamins A, D, E, and K to snack foods containing olestra. According to one author no long-term clinical trials of the product have been conducted, so the full spectrum of possible adverse effects is unknown. A 6-week randomized double-blind placebo-controlled trial (funded by the manufacturer)[14] of ad libitum eating of ordinary potato chips or olestra-containing potato chips did not reveal any differences in gastrointestinal complaints. Those who ate the most olestra chips had slightly more frequent and looser bowel movements, but this did not interfere with their activities of daily living. No oil or fecal leakage occurred. Olestra is not currently approved for use in Canada.

Efficacy and Harm of Dieting. Dieting is a significant preoccupation in the developed world. U.S. studies have shown that at any one time 40% of women and 20% of men are dieting.[15,16] However, in most studies one third to two thirds of any initial weight loss is regained within a year and almost all of it within 5 years.[17] This lack of efficacy has led to questions about the harm of dieting.

Negative effects of dieting include fatigue, dizziness, hair loss, menstrual irregularities, cholelithiasis and cardiac arrhythmias (associated with very low calorie (<800 kcal/d) diets). Weight reduction interventions have also been associated with major depression, bulimia and other eating disorders.[17] However, systematic reviews of the literature have found no evidence that weight cycling has adverse effects or that dieting induces eating disorders.[2] As a result, the NIH has concluded that the concerns about possible harms do not outweigh the potential benefits of weight reduction.[18] The Canadian Task Force on Preventive Health Care[14] concluded that in obese patients with obesity related disease, there is sufficient evidence to recommend weight loss, as even <5kg of weight loss may improve quality of life and reduce drug therapy requirements for obesity-related diseases.[17]

For those who initially lose weight the best predictor of the maintenance of weight loss is the frequency of exercise after the completion of dieting, and a good predictor for regaining weight is the amount of television watched.[19] Patients who have lost weight, whether through dieting, exercise, drugs, or a combination of these modalities, must realize that because of a change in their set point their caloric requirements for maintaining this "normal" weight will be about 15% less than the calories required by someone of the same weight who was never obese (see discussion of pathophysiology of obesity).[20]

Physical Activity. Physical activity contributes to weight loss and maintenance, may decrease abdominal fat and increases cardio-respiratory fitness.[1-3] The magnitude of weight loss with regular exercise alone is less than that achieved with caloric restriction; however, exercise in combination with caloric restriction leads to relatively greater fat loss and preserves lean body mass. The increased muscle mass that results may partially counteract the decline in basal metabolic rate that typically accompanies weight loss and confer some protection against weight regain.[21]

Current recommendations suggest that physical activity should be an integral part of weight loss therapy and weight maintenance. Initially 30 to 40 minutes of moderate activity, 3 to 5 times per week, should be encouraged. A long-term goal of 30 minutes of moderate physical activity 7 days per week should be set. A life-style program emphasizing increased physical activity such as walking to the corner store rather than driving or taking stairs rather than the escalator is as effective as traditional exercise programs, at least over a 1-year period.[22] One study of women with a mean BMI of 32.8 found that daily brisk walking (or other equivalent aerobic exercises) increased weight loss and helped maintain the loss. Women who exercised for 30 minutes a day or more (either as a single long bout or as several short bouts) achieved greater weight loss than those who exercised for 20 minutes a day. The presence of a home treadmill increased compliance with repeated short bouts of exercise.[23]

Perhaps the most important reason to make exercise part of a weight control program is that active obese individuals have lower morbidity rates than do the sedentary obese.[24] Even in the absence of significant weight loss, regular exercise has considerable health benefits including improvement in the lipid profile, improved cardiovascular fitness, and enhanced psychological well being.[20,25]

Behaviour Therapy. Cognitive behavioural therapy is effective in producing negative energy balance through maintenance of healthy behaviours during active therapy periods. Generally, however, weight is regained after the program of behavioural intervention is terminated.[20] Interventions include patient motivation,[1] patient self-monotoring,[2] regular eating schedules, focusing on the meal and eating slowly, avoiding second helpings, using small plates, and avoiding distractions while eating.[3]

❧ REFERENCES ❧

1. Lyznicki JM, Young DC, Riggs JA, Davis RM: Obesity: Assessment and Management in Primary Care, *Am Fam Phys* 63:2185-96, 2001.
2. Noel PH, Pugh JA: Management of overweight and obese adults, *BMJ* 325:757-761, 2002.
3. Institute of Medicine. Dietary reference intakes for energy, carbohydrate, fiber, fat, fatty acids, cholesterol, protein and amino acids: Executive Summary. 2002. Avaliable at: http://books.nap.edu/html/dri_macronutrients/reportbrief.pdf. Accessed: April 16th, 2004.
4. Wolf C, Tanner M: Obesity, *West J Med* 176:23-28, 2002.
5. Jequier E, Bray GA: Low fat diets are preferred, *Am J Med* 113(9B):41S-46S, 2002.
6. Toubro S, Astrup A: Randomized comparison of diets for maintaining obese subjects' weight after major weight loss: ad lib, low fat, high carbohydrate diet vs. fixed energy intake, *BMJ* 314:29-34, 1997.
7. Atkins RC: *Dr. Atkins New Diet Revolution*: New York, NY, 1998, Avon Books.
8. Stein K: High-protein, low carbohydrate diets: do they work? *J Am Diet Assoc* 100:760-761, 2000.
9. American Heart Association. High Protein Diets: AHA recommendation. Avaliable at: http://www.americanheart.org/presenter.jhtml?identifier=11234 Accessed April 02, 2004
10. Bravata DM, Sanders L, Huang J, et al: Efficacy and safety of low-carbohydrate diets: A systematic review. *JAMA* 289:1837-1850, 2003.
11. Dietary Fat Consensus Statements, *Am J Med* 113(9B):5S-8S, 2002.
12. Hu F: The Mediterranean diet and mortality—olive oil and beyond, *N Engl J Med* 348(26):2595-2596, 2003.
13. Blackburn H: Olestra and the FDA, *N Engl J Med* 334:984-986, 1996.
14. Sandler RS, Zorich NL, Filloon TG, et al: Gastrointestinal symptoms in 3181 volunteers ingesting snack foods containing olestra or triglycerides: a 6-week randomized, placebo-controlled trial, *Ann Intern Med* 130:253-261, 1999.
15. Serdula M, Collins ME, Williamson DF, et al: Weight control practices of US adolescents and adults: Youth Risk Behavior Survey and Behavioral Risk Factor Surveillance System, *Ann Intern Med* 119:667-671, 1993.
16. Horm J, Anderson K: Who in America is trying to lose weight? *Ann Intern Med* 119:672-676, 1993.
17. Douketis JD, Feightner JW, Attia J, et al: Periodic health examination, 1999 update. 1. Detection, prevention and treatment of obesity, *Can Med Assoc J* 160:513-525, 1999.
18. Executive summary of the clinical guidelines on the identification, evaluation and treatment of overweight and obesity in adults, *Arch Int Med* 158:1855-67, 1998.
19. Grodstein F, Levine R, Troy L, et al: Three-year follow-up of participants in a commercial weight loss program, *Arch Intern Med* 156:1302-1306, 1996.
20. Rosenbaum M, Leibel RL, Hirsch J: Obesity, *N Engl J Med* 337:396-407, 1997.
21. Nawaz H, Katz DL: American College of Preventative Medicine Practice Policy Statement: Weight Management Counselling of Overweight Adults, *Am J Prev Med* 21(1):73-78, 2001.

22. Andersen RE, Wadden TA, Bartlett SJ, et al: Effects of lifestyle activity vs structured aerobic exercise in obese women: a randomized trial, *JAMA* 281:335-340, 1999.

23. Jakicic JM, Winters C, Lang W, et al: Effects of intermittent exercise and use of home exercise equipment on adherence, weight loss, and fitness in overweight women: a randomized trial, *JAMA* 282:1554-1560, 1999.

24. Blair SN: Evidence for success of exercise in weight loss and control, *Ann Intern Med* 119(7 pt 2):702-706, 1993.

25. Chakravarthy MV, Joyner MJ, Booth FW: An obligation for primary care physicians to prescribe physical activity to sedentary patients to reduce the risk of chronic health conditions, *Mayo Clin Proc* 77(2):165-173, 2002.

Pharmacotherapy

(See also exercise; prevention; type 2 diabetes)

The drugs used to promote weight loss are anorexiants or appetite suppressants and lipase inhibitors. The NIH Guidelines recommend that pharmacologic therapy should be considered only when a 6-month regimen of diet, exercise and behaviour therapy fails. Then it should only be offered to individuals with a BMI >30 or those with BMI >27 who have obesity related disease such as coronary artery disease, diabetes, hypertension, hyperlipidemia or sleep apnea.[1] In those patients with a lower level of obesity risk, non-pharmacological therapy is the treatment of choice.[2]

There are few long-term studies evaluating the safety or effectiveness of many currently approved weight loss medications.[2] A review of weight loss trails >1 year in duration found both orlistat and sibutramine modestly effective in promoting weight loss.[3] In most studies, weight gain occurs with the cessation of pharmacotherapy.[2]

Clinicians should also know that high quality behavioural therapy alone has been shown to lead to weight loss in the order of 8.5 kg (19 lb.) at 21 weeks and 5.6 kg (12 lb.) at 1 year. Benefits claimed for pharmacotherapy, therefore, need to be compared against this standard, not baseline weights. Not every patient responds to drug therapy. Initial responders tend to continue to respond, while non-responders are less likely to respond even with an increase in dosage. If a patient does not lose 2 kg in the first 4 weeks after initiating therapy, the likelihood of long-term response is very low.[2]

Sibutramine (Meridia). Sibutramine inhibits norepinephrine and serotonin uptake.[4] It is an anorexiant that was originally developed as an antidepressant, but has been approved for the long-term treatment of obesity since 1997. The usual dosage is 5 to 10 mg/day. Adverse effects include increases in blood pressure tachycardia, dry mouth, insomnia, headache and constipation. It should not be used in patients with uncontrolled hypertension, CHD, congestive heart failure, arrhythmias, or history of stroke.[4] All patients taking the medication should have their blood pressure monitored on a regular

basis.[2] Sibutramine inhibits serotonin uptake, therefore it should not be used with other SSRIs or MAOIs.

The efficacy of sibutramine has been recently reviewed. Patients have been shown to lose 3 to 4 kg (5% to 8% of their body weight) more then patients on placebo medication.[4] Pooling of three long-term studies found that patients taking sibutramine had 4.6% more weight loss than those on placebo. No mortality of cardiovascular morbidity data were available; there was no significant effect on total cholesterol, LDL or glyemic control.[3] Sibutramine has also been found to be useful in maintaining diet-induced weight loss. 75% of patients treated for 1 year after diet therapy sustained 100% of the weight they lost, compared to 42% of patients on placebo.[4]

Phenteramine (Ionamin). Phenteramine is a noradrenergic agent that can lead to appetite suppression for 12-14 hours. No long-term large scale studies of weight loss on phenteramine have been performed.[4] Side effects include insomnia, dry mouth, restlessness, constipation, tachycardia and hypertension. Phenteramine is contraindicated in patients with cardiovascular disease, hypertension, hyperthyroidism, and those on MAOIs.

"Fen/Phen". The combination of fenfluramine and phentermine known as "Fen/Phen," was a particularly popular product, although studies supporting its efficacy were limited and involved small numbers of patients.[5] In September 1997 fenfluramine and dexfenfluramine were voluntarily withdrawn from the market after the U.S. Food and Drug Administration (FDA) had received 33 reports of significant valvular insufficiency (usually involving multiple valves).[6] Two articles subsequently appeared in the *New England Journal of Medicine,* reporting valvular insufficiencies in 24 women after taking fenfluramine-phentermine therapy[7] and a case of fatal pulmonary hypertension in a woman who had taken fenfluramine-phentermine for only 23 days.[8] Patients who have taken fenfluramine or dexfenfluramine in the past should have a careful clinical examination and those with a murmur and all who took the drugs for more than 3 months should have echocardiograms. Those with murmurs or significant regurgitation should receive standard prophylaxis for endocarditis.[9]

Lipase Inhibitors

Orlistat (Xenical). Orlistat inhibits gastrointestinal lipases, including pancreatic lipase, preventing up to 30% of dietary fat absorption at maximun dosing.[4] Orlistat is taken by mouth in doses of 100 to 400 mg tid. Two 2-year placebo-controlled trials[10,11] reported greater weight loss in those treated with orlistat in the first-year (weight loss phase) and less weight gain in the treated group in the second-year (maintenance phase). In the U.S. study the group taking orlistat 120 mg three times per day lost an extra 3.5 kg during the first year and regained 2.25 kg less during the second year. Half the patients in both the placebo and orlistat arms of the study dropped out, and no attempt was made to assess the weight of either dropout group.[12] The longest published trial of orlistat has been 2 years. Gastrointestinal side effects of the drug are common, and an increase in breast cancer has been reported.[13] Although failure to absorb fat may account for some of the weight loss in patients taking orlistat, avoidance of dietary fat because of symptoms of induced steatorrhea probably accounts for most of it.[14]

Over-the-Counter and Herbal Products. Over-the-counter and herbal products marketed as weight control agents include herbal caffeine and ephedrine, bitter orange, green tea, capsaicin, conjugated linoleic acid, hydroxy-citric acid, fiber and chitosan. Serious adverse effects, including stroke and seizures, have been reported with the use of supplements containing ephedra.[15]

──────────── ≈ **REFERENCES** ≥ ────────────

1. Executive summary of the clinical guidelines on the identification, evaluation and treatment of overweight and obesity in adults, *Arch Int Med* 158:1855-1867, 1998.
2. Guidelines on Overweight and Obesity: Electronic textbook.http://www.nhlbi.nih. gov/guidelines/obesity/e_txtbk/txgd/4325.htm. Accessed April 04/2004
3. Padwal R, LI SK, Lau DCW: Long term pharmacotherapy for overweight and obesity: a systematic review and meta-analysis of randomized controlled trials, *Int J Obesity* 27:1437-1446, 2003.
4. Thearle M, Aronne LJ: Obesity and pharmacologic therapy, *Endocrinol Metab Clin North Am* 32(4), 2003.
5. National Task Force on the Prevention and Treatment of Obesity: Long-term pharmacotherapy in the management of obesity, *JAMA* 276:1907-1915, 1996.
6. Food and Drug Administration: Health advisory on concomitant fenfluramine and phentermine use, *JAMA* 278:379, 1997.
7. Connolly HM, Crary JL, McGoon MD, et al: Valvular heart disease associated with fenfluramine-phentermine, *N Engl J Med* 337:581-588, 1997.
8. Mark EJ, Chang HT, Evans RJ, et al: Fatal pulmonary hypertension associated with short-term use of fenfluramine and phentermine, *N Engl J Med* 337:602-606, 1997.
9. Devereux RB: Appetite suppressants and valvular heart disease (editorial), *N Engl J Med* 339:765-766, 1998.
10. Sjöström L, Rissanen A, Andersen T, et al: Randomised placebo-controlled trial of orlistat for weight loss and prevention of weight regain in obese patients, *Lancet* 352: 167-173, 1998.
11. Davidson MH, Hauptman J, DiGirolamo M, et al: Weight control and risk factor reduction in obese subjects treated for 2 years with orlistat: a randomized controlled trial, *JAMA* 281:235-242, 1999.
12. Williamson DF: Pharmacotherapy for obesity (editorial), *JAMA* 281:278-280, 1999.
13. Prescrire: Orlistat; no hurry . . . , *Can Fam Physician* 45: 2330-2338, 1999.
14. Garrow J: Flushing away the fat: weight loss during trials of orlistat was significant, but over half was due to diet (editorial), *BMJ* 317:830-831, 1998.
15. Heber D: Herbal preparations for obesity: Are they useful? *Prim Care* 30(2):441-463, 2003.

Surgical treatment of obesity

Standard surgical techniques for treating intractable morbid obesity (BMI of 40 or more or BMI of 35 or more if comorbid conditions are present) are vertical banded gastroplasty, in which a synthetic band is stapled on the stomach to decrease the gastric outlet, or a Roux-en-Y gastric bypass, in which the distal stomach is resected and the proximal pouch is anastomosed to the jejunum.[1]

Surgical procedures can induce substantial weight loss, and serve to reduce weight-associated risk factors and comorbidities. Compared to other interventions available, surgery has produced the longest period of sustained weight loss.[2] Since surgical procedures result in some loss of absorptive function, the long-term consequences of potential nutrient deficiencies must be recognized and adequate monitoring must be performed, particularly with regard to vitamin B_{12}, folate, and iron. Some patients may develop other gastrointestinal symptoms such as "dumping syndrome" or gallstones.[2]

──────────── ≈ **REFERENCES** ≥ ────────────

1. Semchenko A, Seim HC, Pi-Sunyer FX: *Management of obesity.* Kansas, 1999, American Academy of Family Physicians..
2. Guidelines on Overweight and Obesity: Electronic textbook.http://www.nhlbi.nih.gov/guidelines/obesity/e_txtbk/txgd/4325.htm. Accessed April 04, 2004

OSTEOPOROSIS   *Look at 2010 Guidelines [OP Canada]*

(See also celiac disease; geriatrics; hip fractures; hormone replacement therapy; tamoxifen)

Epidemiology

(See also hip fractures)

Osteoporosis is a skeletal disorder characterized by compromised bone strength predisposing a person to an increased risk of fractures.[1]

Peak bone mass is reached at about age 25 and is about 20% less in women than in men. After age 35, bone mass declines by about 0.5% to 1% per year in both men and women. Between ages 50 and 80 a woman's bone density decreases 30%. In the first 10 years after menopause the decline is about 3% to 5% per year. Men lose about two thirds as much bone mass as women; their rate of bone loss increases after age 65.[2]

Osteoporotic fracture occurs in an estimated 25% of white women over the age of 60. The common sites are the distal radius, hip, ribs, and vertebral bodies. Vertebral fractures in women 50 to 60 years of age are 10 times as common as they are in men of similar age, and hip fractures occur twice as often in women as in men. Patients with osteoporotic hip fractures are usually over 75, and the median age for such fractures in post-menopausal women is 80.[3] Mortality from hip fractures is between 10% and 25% in the first year, many patients lose mobility, and up to 25% require nursing care.[4]

❧ REFERENCES ❧

1. Osteoporosis prevention, diagnosis and therapy. NIH consensus statements 2000;17(10:1-45)
2. Scientific Advisory Board, Osteoporosis Society of Canada: Clinical practice guidelines for the diagnosis and management of osteoporosis, *Can Med Assoc J* 155:1113-1133, 1996.
3. Lees B, Molleson T, Asnett T: Differences in proximal femur bone density over two centuries, *Lancet* 341:673-675, 1993.
4. Kelly PJ, Eisman JA, Sambrook PN: Interaction of genetic and environmental influences on peak bone density, *Osteoporosis Int* 1:56-60, 1990.

Identifying People at Risk for Osteoporosis

Screen if ≥ 65 M/W or if RF

(See also anorexia nervosa; vitamin A)

Recognized risk factors for osteoporosis are listed in Table 56.

There is poor correlation between many of these risk factors and the bone density of individual patients. A recent review of the literature identified four key factors as predictors of fracture related to osteoporosis: low

Table 56   Risk Factors for Osteoporosis

Major Risk Factors
- Age>65 years
- Vertebral compression fracture
- Fragility fracture after age 40
- Family history of osteoporotic fracture (especially maternal hip fracture)
- Systemic glucocorticoid therapy of >3 months duration
- Malabsorption syndrome
- Primary hyperparathyroidism
- Propensity to fall
- Osteopenia apparent on X-ray film
- Hypogonadism
- Early menopause (before age 45)

Minor Risk Factors
- Rheumatoid arthritis
- Past history of clinical hyperthyroidism
- Chronic anticonvulsant therapy
- Low dietary calcium intake
- Smoker
- Excessive alcohol intake
- Excessive caffeine intake
- Weight <57 kg
- Weight loss > 19% of weight at age 25
- Chronic Heparin Therapy[1]

BMD, prior fragility fracture, age, and family history of osteoporosis.[1]

The 2002 clinical practice guidelines for the diagnosis and management of osteoporosis in Canada recommend that people with one major risk factor or two minor risk factors should be screened for osteoporosis with central dual-energy X-ray absorptometry (DXA) measurement (BMD).[1] In addition, it is recommended that people receiving >7.5 mg of prednisone daily for more than three months should be assessed for initiation of bone saving therapy.[1,2]

❧ REFERENCES ❧

1. Scientific Advisory Council of the Osteoporosis Society of Canada: Clinical Practice guidelines for the diagnosis and management of osteoporosis in Canada, *Can Med Assoc J* 167(10 suppl)S1-S34, 2002.
2. Adache JD, Olszynski WP, Hanley, et al:. Management of corticosteroid –induced osteoporosi, *Semin Arthritis Rheum* 200:29.
3. Reference deleted in pages.

Diagnosis of Osteoporosis

The World Health Organization defines osteoporosis as a bone mineral density (BMD) measurement with a T-score lower than –2.5.[1] Due to this definition, diagnosis depends on the measurement of BMD.

-1 to -2.5 = osteope

The evidence that bone densitometry can identify individuals who will sustain fractures is not well established.[2,3] The arguments against using bone density measurements as a screening tool are that a great overlap exists between the bone densities of those who have fractures and those who do not, compliance with such a screening program is unknown, and the effectiveness of preventive interventions for fractures is not well established.[3] The U.S. Preventive Services Task Force gives a "C" recommendation to bone density screening of all post-menopausal women,[4] while the Canadian Task Force on Preventive Health Care gives it a "D" recommendation.[5] Still, the 2002 Canadian practice guidelines cited above clearly recommend using dual-energy X-ray absorptiometry (DXA) for bone densitometry measurement, citing Level 1 evidence that it is the most effective way to estimate fracture risk in post-menopausal Caucasian women.[6-9]

Screening is thus recommended for all persons over the age of 65 as this is a major risk factor in Table 56.[6,8-10]

According to the 2002 Canadian bone densitometry recommendations, the dose of radiation from DXA is very small and studies have not shown any ill effects from such small doses.[7]

--- ❧ **REFERENCES** ❧ ---

1. *Guidelines for preclinical evaluation and clinical trials in osteoporosis.* Geneva, 1998, WHO, p 59.
2. Wilkin TJ: Changing perceptions in osteoporosis, *BMJ* 318:862-865, 1999.
3. Marshall D, Johnell O, Wedel H: Meta-analysis of how well measures of bone mineral density predict occurrence of osteoporotic fractures, *BMJ* 312:1254-1259, 1996.
4. US Preventive Services Task Force: *Guide to clinical preventive services,* ed 2, Baltimore, 1996, Williams & Wilkins, pp 509-516.
5. Canadian Task Force on the Periodic Health Examination: *Canadian guide to clinical preventive health care,* Ottawa, 1994, Canada Communication Group, pp 620-631.
6. Scientific Advisory Council of the Osteoporosis Society of Canada: Clinical Practice guidelines for the diagnosis and management of osteoporosis in Canada, *Can Med Assoc J* 167(10 suppl):S1-S34, 2002.
7. Khan A, et al: The 2002 Canadian bone densitometry recommendations: take-home messages, *CMAJ* 167(10): 1141-1145, 2002.
8. Marshall D, Johnell O, Wedel H: Meta-analysis of how well measures of bone mineral density predict occurrence of osteoporotic fractures, *BMJ* 312:1254-1259, 1996.
9. Torgerson DJ, Campbell MK, Thomas RE, et al:. Prediction of perimenopausal fractures by bone mineral density and other risk factors, *J Bone Miner Res* 11:293-297, 1996.
10. National Osteoporosis Foundation: Osteoporosis: review of the evidence for prevention, diagnosis, and treatment and cost-effectiveness analysis, *Osteoporosis Int* 8(suppl4): S7-S80, 1998.

Prevention of Osteoporosis

(See also exercise; hip fractures; hormone replacement therapy; prevention of corticosteroid-induced osteoporosis)

Any reversible medical or life-style risk factors for osteoporosis should be eliminated if possible; smoking and excessive alcohol use are high on the list. Other specific interventions that may be used are discussed in the ensuing paragraphs.

Calcium and vitamin D supplementation

Whether calcium supplementation inhibits the development of osteoporosis is controversial, but the bulk of the evidence suggests that it does. For example, Reid and associates[1] in New Zealand studied 122 healthy women who were at least 3 years post-menopausal and whose mean dietary calcium intake was 750 mg/day. They treated one cohort with calcium supplements of 1000 mg/day. At the end of 4 years the rate of appendicular and axial bone loss was significantly lower in the calcium-treated group.[1] There is also evidence that supplementation with both vitamin D and calcium may decrease the risk of osteoporosis.[2,3]

The 2002 Canadian Guidelines cite level 1 evidence that adequate calcium and vitamin D through diet or supplementation are essential adjuncts for the prevention of osteoporosis.[4,5]

The National Institutes of Health has recommended the following daily allowances of calcium[6]:

Children 1-10 years	800-1200 mg/day
Adolescents and young adults 1-24	1200-1500 mg/day
Pregnant and lactating women	1200-1500 mg/day
Adult men ages 25-65	1000 mg/day
Adult women ages 25-50	1000 mg/day
Post-menopausal women 51-65 on estrogens	1000 mg/day
Post-menopausal women 51-65 not taking estrogens	1500 mg/day
Everyone over the age of 65	1500 mg/day

[handwritten note: 1200mg OP - Calcium + diet   Vit D 800-2000iu   Wt bearing]

The basic North American diet without dairy products provides a daily intake of 300 to 400 mg of calcium. One 250 mL (8 oz) glass of 1% or 2% milk contains 300 mg of calcium. Other good sources of calcium, supplying about 300 mg per serving, are firm cheeses (45 g or 1½ ounces), canned salmon (125 ml or ½ cup), and canned sardines (seven medium sized) if the bones are eaten. In addition, 125 mL (or ½ cup) of tofu has about 150 mg, 250 mL (or 1 cup) of cooked soy beans about 200 mg, and 125 mL (or ½ cup) of dry-roasted almonds about 200 mg.[7]

It would seem reasonable to recommend that all post-menopausal women, as well as all men over the age of 65, take daily supplements of 1000 to 1500 of "elemental" calcium and 400 to 800 IU of vitamin D (most multivitamins contain 400 IU of vitamin D). A large number of calcium products are available without prescription. Most of them are in the form of calcium carbonate. In choosing a product or prescribing a dose, it is important that the dose be based on the milligrams of "elemental calcium" in each tablet, not the milligrams of calcium carbonate. Absorption of calcium supplements is most effective if no more than 500 mg is taken at one time and if the tablets are taken with meals.[8] Calcium supplements are available in liquid form, as tablets to be dissolved in water, as chewable tablets, or as tablets or capsules to be swallowed. Some of the tablets are large, so many patients prefer chewable forms such as Tums, Os-Cal, and Caltrate.

Exercise

Femoral neck bone densities of the skeletons of pre-menopausal and post-menopausal women buried in the crypt of Christ Church, Spitalfields, London, between 1729 and 1852 were significantly greater than those of present-day women. The probable explanation was a greater degree of physical activity in these 18th- and 19th-century women.[9] Studies of living 20th-century women confirm that exercise correlates with a decrease in hip fractures.[10,11] High-intensity strength training has been shown to increase bone density, muscle mass, overall strength, overall physical activity levels, and dynamic balance.[10] Probably the observed decrease in hip fractures among physically active women is due not only to greater bone density, but also to improved balance, muscle strength, reaction time, and coordination.[11]

Hormone replacement therapy

Hormone replacement therapy with oral estrogens and progestins not only decreases the rate of bone loss but also increases bone density.[3,12,13]

Until recently, there was only one double-blind placebo-controlled RCT of estrogen replacement that demonstrated vertebral fracture prevention.[14]

The Women's Health Initiative (a large prospective randomized placebo-controlled trial finally demonstrated that a continuous estrogen-progesterone regimen significantly reduces the risk of fractures at all sites, including the hip.[15] Unfortunately, this study was terminated early because of an unfavourable risk-benefit ratio with the estrogen-progesterone combination therapy. There was a significant increase in the relative risk for coronary artery disease, invasive breast cancer, stroke, and venous thromboeombolism[14] This has resulted in the 2002 Canadian guidelines recommending HRT as a first-line preventative therapy in post-menopausal women with low bone density with the proviso that the risks may outweigh the benefits.[4,15] Hormone replacement therapy is still recommended as a first-line preventive therapy for women who experience menopause before the age of 45, though this is a grade "D" recommendation.

Even if prolonged estrogen replacement therapy is desirable, it may be difficult to achieve. In one British study 39% of the women for whom hormone replacement therapy was recommended because of low bone density either stopped the therapy prematurely or never started it.[16]

Bisphosphonates

Bisphosphonates are considered first-line preventive therapy in women with a low bone density.[4,17-21] There is level 1 evidence that alendronate and risedronate prevent both vertebral and non-vertebral fractures.[4,17,19-21] There is level 2 evidence that etidronate is efficacious in preventing vertebral fractures.[18] In elderly women who have already sustained one or more osteoporotic fractures, alendronate has been shown to increase bone density and markedly reduce the number of subsequent fractures.[22]

Selective estrogen receptor modulators

Raloxifine is the only selective estrogen receptor modulator that has been approved for the prevention and treatment of osteoporosis. It was proven to be efficacious in preventing vertebral fractures in post-menopausal women with osteoporosis in a large RCT.[22] The Canadian 2002 recommendations consider Raloxifine first-line therapy for prevention of further bone loss in post-menopausal women with low bone density.[4,22]

❧ REFERENCES ❧

1. Reid IR, Ames RW, Evans MC, et al: Long-term effects of calcium supplementation on bone loss and fractures in postmenopausal women: a randomized controlled trial, *Am J Med* 98:331-335, 1995.
2. Dawson-Hughes B, Harris SS, Krall EA, et al: Effect of calcium and vitamin D supplementation on bone density in men and women 65 years of age or older, *N Engl J Med* 337:670-676, 1997.
3. Recker RR, Davies M, Dowd RM, et al: The effect of low-dose continuous estrogen and progesterone therapy with calcium and vitamin D on bone in elderly women: a randomized, controlled trial, *Ann Intern Med* 130:897-904, 1999.
4. Scientific Advisory Council of the Osteoporosis Society of Canada: Clinical Practice guidelines for the diagnosis and management of osteoporosis in Canada, *Can Med Assoc J* 167(10 suppl):S1-S34, 2002
5. Baeksgaard L, Anderson KP, Hyldstrup L: Calcium and vitamin D Supplementation increases spinal BMD in healthy, postmenopausal women, *Osteoporos Int* 8:255-260, 1998.
6. NIH releases consensus statement on optimal calcium intake, *Am Fam Physician* 50:1385-1387, 1994.
7. Miller A: 10 practical answers in dietary counselling, *Patient Care Can* 6:22-49, 1995.
8. Calcium supplements, *Med Lett* 38:108-109, 1996.
9. Lees B, Molleson T, Asnett T: Differences in proximal femur bone density over two centuries, *Lancet* 341:673-675, 1993.
10. Nelson ME, Fiatarone MA, Morganti CM, et al: Effects of high-intensity strength training on multiple risk factors for osteoporotic fractures: a randomized controlled trial, *JAMA* 272:1909-1914, 1994.
11. Gregg EW, Cauley JA, Seeley DG, et al: Physical activity and osteoporotic fracture risk in older women, *Ann Intern Med* 129:81-88, 1998.
12. Writing Group for the PEPI Trial: Effects of hormone therapy on bone mineral density: results from the Postmenopausal Estrogen/Progestin Interventions (PEPI) Trial, *JAMA* 276:1389-1396, 1996.
13. Speroff L, Rowan J, Symons J, et al (CHART Study Group): The comparative effect on bone density, endometrium, and lipids of continuous hormones as replacement therapy (CHART Study), *JAMA* 276:1397-1403, 1996.
14. Lufkin EG, Wahner HW, O'Fallon WM, et al: Treatment of postmenopausal osteoporosis with transdermal estrogen, *Ann Intern Med* 117:1-9, 1992.
15. Writing Group for the Women's Health Initiative Investigators: Risks and benefits of estrogen plus progestin in healthy postmenopausal women: principal results from the Women's Health Initiative Randomized Controlled Trial, *JAMA* 288:321-333, 2002.

16. Ryan PJ, Harrison R, Blake GM, et al: Compliance with hormone replacement therapy (HRT) after screening for post menopausal osteoporosis, *Br J Obstet Gynaecol* 99:325-328, 1992.

17. McClung MR, Geusens P, Miller PD, et al. Effects of risedronate on the risk of hip fracture in elderly women, *N Engl J Med* 334:333-340, 2001.

18. Storm T, Thamsborg G, Steiniche T, et al: Effect of intermittent cyclical etidronate therapy on bone mass and fracture rate in women postmenopausal osteoporosis, *N Engl J Med* 322:1265-1271, 1990.

19. Black DM, Cummings SR, Karpf DB, et al: Randomised trial of effect of alendronate on risk of fracture in women with existing vertebral fractures. Fracture Intervention Trial Research Group, *Lancet* 348:1535-1541, 1996.

20. Cummings SR, Black DM, Thompson DE, et al: Effect of alendronate on risk of fracture in women with low bone density but without vertebral fractures: results from the Fracture Intervention Trial, *JAMA* 280:2077-2082, 1998.

21. Harris ST, Watts NB, Genant HK, et al: Effects of risedronate treatment on vertebral and nonvertebral fractures in women with postmenopausal osteoporosis: a randomized controlled trial, Vertebral Efficacy With Risedronate Therapy (VERT) Study Group. *JAMA* 282:1344-1352, 1999;

22. Ettinger B, Black DM, Mitlak BH, et al: Reduction of vertebral fracture risk in postmenopausal women with osteoporosis treated with raloxifene: Results from a 3-year randomized clinical trial, *JAMA* 282:637-645, 1999;

Prevention of Corticosteroid-Induced Osteoporosis

According to one study, treatment with calcium carbonate 1000 mg/day plus 500 IU of vitamin D_3 to patients receiving long-term corticosteroids prevented bone loss.[1] A similar study showed equivocal benefits.[2] The 2002 Canadian Guidelines for the diagnosis and management of osteoporosis recommend that people receiving 7.5 mg or more of daily prednisone for more than 3 months should be assessed for initiation of bone sparing therapy.[3-6]

The guidelines also cite grade "A" evidence that the bisphosphonates alendronate,[5] risedronate[6], and etidronate[4] are first-line therapy for the prevention of glucocorticoid induced osteoporosis.

The 1996 American College of Rheumatology Task Force on Osteoporosis Guidelines recommended preventive therapy for all patients likely to be taking long-term corticosteroids in doses of 7.5 mg or more of prednisone daily. Bone density measurements are indicated for most patients. Everyone should take calcium and vitamin D supplements and maintain a program of weight-bearing exercises, and women should receive hormone replacement therapy, especially if their bone density is low. Thiazide diuretics increase the absorption of calcium from the gastrointestinal tract and decrease its urinary excretion. Therefore the addition of hydrochlorothiazide in doses of 25 mg or less may be helpful, especially in patients excreting more than 300 mg of calcium in their urine over a 24-hour period. The guidelines also suggested that if post-menopausal women were unable to take replacement hormones, consideration be given to a bisphosphonate such as etidronate or alendronate or to use of calcitonin (Calcimar).[7]

Recent guidelines from Great Britain also target individuals taking 7.5 mg of prednisone or the equivalent per day. Treatment is recommended for all patients over 65 years of age and anyone taking 15 mg or more of prednisone or the equivalent per day. Other patients require treatment if bone densities are decreased. The treatment of choice is bisphosphonates. The role of hormone replacement therapy is less clear; according to one editorial writer it should only be considered for women who do not respond to bisphosphonates.[8]

──────── ❧ **REFERENCES** ❧ ────────

1. Buckley LM, Leib ES, Cartularo KS, et al: Calcium and vitamin D-3 supplementation prevents bone loss in the spine secondary to low-dose corticosteroids in patients with rheumatoid arthritis—a randomized, double-blind, placebo-controlled trial, *Ann Intern Med* 125:961-968, 1996.

2. Adachi JD, Bensen WG, Bianchi F, et al: Vitamin D and calcium in the prevention of corticosteroid induced osteoporosis—a 3 year follow-up, *J Rheumatol* 23:995-1000, 1996.

3. Scientific Advisory Council of the Osteoporosis Society of Canada: Clinical Practice guidelines for the diagnosis and management of osteoporosis in Canada, *Can Med Assoc J* 167(10 suppl):S1-S34, 2002.

4. Adachi, JD, Bensen WG, Brown J, et al: Intermittent etidronate therapy to prevent corticosteroid-induced osteoporosis, *N Engl J Med* 337:382-387, 1997.

5. Saag KG, Emkey R, Schnitzer TJ, et al: Alendronate for the prevention and treatment of glucocorticoid-induced osteoporosis. Glucocorticoid-Induced Osteoporosis Intervention Study Group, *N Engl J Med* 339:292-299, 1998.

6. Cohen S, Levy RM, Keller M, et al: Risedronate therapy prevents corticosteroid-induced bone loss: a twelve month, multicenter, randomized, double-blind, placebo-controlled, parallel-group study. *Arthritis Rheum* 42:2309-2318, 1999.

7. Hochberg MC, Prashker MJ, Rogers EN, et al: Recommendations for the prevention and treatment of glucocorticoid-induced osteoporosis: American College of Rheumatology Task Force on Osteoporosis guidelines, *Arthritis Rheum* 39:1791-1801, 1996.

8. Lips P: Prevention of corticosteroid induced osteoporosis (editorial), *BMJ* 318:1366-1367, 1999.

Treatment of Established Osteoporosis

(See also amenorrhea; metastatic breast cancer; multiple myeloma; prevention of osteoporosis)

Bisphosphonates

Bisphosphonates are the pharmacological agents of choice for the treatment of established osteoporosis.

They bind to bone and inhibit osteoclast activity, thus decreasing bone removal. Post-menopausal women treated with alendronate (Fosamax)[1-3] or risedronate (Actonel)[4] have an increase in bone density and a decrease in vertebral and non-vertebral fracture rates. The 2002 Canadian osteoporosis guidelines state that bisphosphonates are first-line therapy for the treatment of osteoporoses citing grade "A" evidence for alendronate and risedronate and grade "B" evidence for etidronate.[5]

Both alendronate and risidronate can be taken via either daily or weekly doses.[6,7]

Calcitonin

Calcitonin has an analgesic effect and may give rapid pain relief from compression fractures.[1,8] The usual dose of the parenteral formulation (Calcimar) for the pain relief of osteoporotic vertebral fractures is 50 IU subcutaneously or intramuscularly daily, increasing to 100 IU daily if 50 IU is ineffective. Pain relief may be noted within a few days and almost always within 2 weeks. The dose can be tapered after 4 to 6 weeks, and in some cases pain relief persists for months after discontinuing the medication.[8] The nasal spray formulation (Miacalcin) is administered as one spray of 200 IU in one nostril daily (alternate nostrils each day). The PROOF study demonstrated a reduction in fracture rates in persons treated with a daily dose of 200 IU of calcitonin.[9] The guidelines classify this as level 2 evidence only because of concerns about the absence of a dose response with a daily dose of 400 IU.[5,9]

Hormone replacement therapy

Estrogen treatment of post-menopausal women with established osteoporosis has been reported to increase bone density[10] and to decrease the incidence of vertebral fractures (see discussions of amenorrhea and prevention of osteoporosis).[11] Given the results of the Women's Health Initiative (see section on prevention of osteoporosis), HRT is only a second-line treatment for osteoporosis. The significant risks of cardiovascular disease, stroke and invasive breast cancer may lead to an unfavourable risk-benefit ratio with this treatment option.[12]

Selective estrogen receptor modulators

A randomized controlled trial of raloxifene (Evista) 60 mg/day for post-menopausal women with osteoporosis found that after 3 years the women had fewer radiologically evident vertebral fractures than in the control group. No difference in extremity fractures was observed, and most vertebral fractures were asymptomatic. Both the treated and control groups took supplemental calcium and vitamin D.[7,13] Raloxifene is considered a first-line treatment for post-menopausal women with osteoporosis.[5]

Other treatment modalities

Important life-style changes in the treatment of established osteoporosis are stopping smoking, avoiding excessive alcohol intake, and walking for exercise. Calcium supplements of 1500 mg/day should be given, and for those who are housebound 800 mg vitamin D daily is essential.[1]

──────────── ◢ REFERENCES ◣ ────────────

1. Eastell R: Treatment of postmenopausal osteoporosis, *N Engl J Med* 338:736-746, 1998.
2. Black DM, Cummings SR, Karpf DB, et al: Randomised trial of effect of alendronate on risk of fracture in women with existing vertebral fractures, *Lancet* 348:1535-1541, 1996.
3. Karpf DB, Shapiro DR, Seeman I, et al: Prevention of nonvertebral fractures by alendronate: a meta-analysis, *JAMA* 277:1159-1164, 1997.
4. Harris ST, Watts NB, Genant HK, et al: Effects of risedronate treatment on vertebral and nonvertebral fractures in women with postmenopausal osteoporosis: a randomized controlled trial, *JAMA* 282:1344-1352, 1999.
5. Scientific Advisory Council of the Osteoporosis Society of Canada: Clinical Practice guidelines for the diagnosis and management of osteoporosis in Canada, *Can Med Assoc J* 167(10 suppl):S1-S34, 2002.
6. Schnitzer, T, Bone HG, Crepaldi G, et al: Therapeutic equivalence of alendronate 70 mg once-weekly and alendronate 10 mg daily in the treatment of osteoporosis. *Aging (Milano)* 12:1-12, 2000.
7. Hodsman AB, Hanley DA, Josse R: Do bisphosphonates reduce the risk of osteoporotic fractures? An evaluation of the evidence to date, *CMAJ* 166:1426-1430, 2002.
8. Maksymowych WP: Managing acute osteoporotic vertebral fractures with calcitonin, *Can Fam Physician* 44: 2160-2166, 1998.
9. Recurrence of Osteoporotic Fractures Study, *Am J Med* 109:267-276, 2000.
10. Lindsay R, Tohme JF: Estrogen treatment of patients with established postmenopausal osteoporosis, *Obstet Gynecol* 76: 290-295, 1990.
11. Lufkin EG, Wahner HW, O'Fallon WM, et al: Treatment of postmenopausal osteoporosis with transdermal estrogen, *Ann Intern Med* 117:1-9, 1992.
12. Writing Group for the Women's Health Initiative Investigators: Risks and benefits of estrogen plus progestin in healthy postmenopausal women: principal results from the Women's Health Initiative Randomized Controlled Trial, *JAMA* 288:321-333, 2002.
13. Ettinger B, Black DM, Mitlak BH, et al (Multiple Outcomes of Raloxifene Evaluation [MORE] Investigators): Reduction of vertebral fracture risk in postmenopausal women with osteoporosis treated with raloxifene, *JAMA* 282:637-645, 1999.

PARATHYROID DISORDERS
(See also osteoporosis; renal colic)

Ninety percent of patients with hyperparathyroidism have a parathyroid adenoma. The diagnosis is usually suspected because an elevated serum calcium level is detected in a "routine" biochemical screen, and is confirmed by finding an elevated serum parathyroid hormone level. The major complications of hyperparathyroidism—hypercalcuria, nephrolithiasis, renal insufficiency, and osteopenia—are rare.[1] The definitive treatment is parathyroidectomy in the case of symptomatic hyperparathyroidism and asymptomatic individuals under the age of 50.[2] The decision to pursue surgery should be based on the following factors: elevated serum calcium, elevated urine calcium, creatinine clearance, and poor bone mineral density.[2] If surgery is not an option, then close medical surveillance should be maintained. It is recommended that all individuals undergoing surgery should have nuclear imaging with sestambi scanning, as it will allow for localization of the hyperfunctioning parathyroid tissue permitting unilateral neck dissection, in turn reducing operative time and patient morbidity.[3]

_____ ◾ **REFERENCES** ◾ _____

1. Utiger RD: Treatment of primary hyperparathyroidism (editorial), *N Engl J Med* 341:1301-1302, 1999.
2. Bilezikian JP, et al: Summary statement from a workshop on asymptomatic primary hyperparathyroidism: A perspective for the 21st century, *J Clin Endo Metab* 87(12):5353-5361, 2001
3. Gupta VK, et al: 99m-technetium sestamibi localized solitary parathyroid adenoma as an indication for limited unilateral surgical exploration, *Am J Surg* 176:409-412, 1998.

PITUITARY DISORDERS

(See also practice patterns; screening)

Acromegaly

The initial treatment of choice for acromegaly is surgical removal of the pituitary tumour. Results are vastly better if the operation is performed by a surgeon experienced in this subspecialty.[1]

Hypopituitarism

Pituitary adenomas, which may be secreting or nonsecreting, are the most common cause of hypopituitarism. Postpartum hemorrhage with hypovolemia may lead to hypopituitarism (Sheehan's syndrome) either immediately or after a delay of several years.[2]

Clinical manifestations

The clinical manifestations of hypopituitarism are often subtle and variable. The variability depends in large part on which target endocrine glands are deficient and whether the deficiency is mild or severe.[2]

Symptoms of corticotropin deficiency include weakness, headache, orthostatic hypotension, fatigue, anorexia, nausea, vomiting, abdominal pain, and weight loss. In long-standing cases patients may have thinning or loss of axillary and pubic hair. On examination the patient often appears pale because of decreased pigmentation, and this contrasts with the hyperpigmentation of Addison's disease. Deficiency of gonadotropins results in decreased libido and erectile function in men and menstrual irregularities or amenorrhea in women. In addition, women may have decreased libido and even hot flashes. Deficiency of TSH results in the symptoms of hypothyroidism. Adults with growth hormone deficiency have nonspecific symptoms such as decreased energy and decreased exercise tolerance. If the cause of the hypopituitarism is a prolactin-secreting adenoma, the patient may have galactorrhea.[2] Finally one should look for signs of an expanding pituitary adenoma including: bitemporal hemianopsia, reduced visual acuity, visual field defects, and third nerve palsy with ptosis.

Laboratory investigations

If hypopituitarism is suspected, a family physician may order some initial blood tests as discussed below. Imaging of the pituitary gland and sella is the next level of investigation and is probably best done in conjunction with a consultant.[2]

The most important point about basal serum hormone measurements is that they may be entirely normal even in patients with symptomatic hypopituitarism. Test results are helpful only if they are abnormal, particularly with hormones secreted in pulsed fashion, such as luteinizing hormone, follicle-stimulating hormone, and growth hormone. Initial blood tests should include complete and differential blood cell counts, electrolytes, prolactin, morning serum cortisol, T_4 and TSH, and follicle-stimulating and luteinizing hormones. Some patients have normocytic normochromic anemia and eosinophilia because of corticotropin deficiencies. Hyponatremia may also be found, but not hyperkalemia as occurs in Addison's disease because the adrenocortical production of aldosterone is not dependent on corticotropin.[2]

Pituitary Incidentalomas

A pituitary incidentaloma is a lesion of the pituitary gland that is neurologically and endocrinologically inapparent and is discovered incidentally during magnetic resonance imaging or computed tomography of the brain. Almost all such lesions are adenomas, and if they are under 10 mm in diameter (microadenomas), only about 1 in 200 will eventually lead to neurological or endocrinological dysfunction. There is no consensus on the optimal investigation and management of asymptomatic patients with incidentally discovered pituitary microadenomas. Conclusions based on an analytical decision model indicate that the only endocrinological parameter that might be worth assessing is prolactin and that other endocrine panels or regular magnetic resonance imaging examinations would probably lead to more harm than good.[3]

The most common form of functioning pituitary adenoma is a prolactinoma; treatment of these lesions with bromocriptine leads to decrease in tumour size and control of endocrinologically mediated symptoms.[3]

——————— ≈ REFERENCES ≈ ———————

1. Clayton RN, Stewart PM, Shalet SM, et al: Pituitary surgery for acromegaly: should be done by specialists (editorial), *BMJ* 319:588-589, 1999.
2. Vance ML: Hypopituitarism, *N Engl J Med* 330:1651-1662, 1994.
3. King JT Jr, Justice AC, Aron DC: Management of incidental pituitary microadenomas: a cost-effectiveness analysis, *J Clin Endocrinol Metab* 82:3625-3632, 1997.

THYROID DISORDERS
Thyroid Tests

In outpatient practice a sensitive thyroid-stimulating hormone (sTSH) measurement is sufficient to screen for a hyperthyroid or hypothyroid state. Free thyroxine (FT_4) determinations are required only if the sTSH result is abnormal.[1]

——————— ≈ REFERENCES ≈ ———————

1. Bauer DC, Brown AN: Sensitive thyrotropin and free thyroxine testing in outpatients: are both necessary? *Arch Intern Med* 156:2333-2337, 1996.

Euthyroid Sick Syndrome

The euthyroid sick syndrome occurs in three forms. In all of them triiodothyronine (T_3) or thyroxine (T_4) concentrations are abnormal but the TSH level is normal or near normal. The normal TSH is the clue to the diagnosis. These syndromes can be seen in chronic illness or with use of corticosteroids and dopamine.[1]

Low T_3 Syndrome

Normally T_4 is converted in almost equal amounts to T_3 and reverse (inactive) T_3. In severe catabolic states, or with carbohydrate restriction, the enzyme catalyzing T_3 formation is inhibited, resulting in increased production of the metabolically inactive reverse T_3. This causes a state of functional hypothyroidism that helps to prevent nitrogen loss during stress. Hypothyroidism is rapidly reversible once the stress (illness, surgery) is removed. In the low T_3 syndrome, the T_4 level is normal and the T_3 level is low. The diagnosis is made by measuring TSH concentration, which is normal or near normal (except in the rare cases of pituitary or hypothalamic failure as the cause of low T_3).

Low T_3, Low T_4 syndrome

The low T_3, low T_4 syndrome is seen in severely ill patients and indicates a poor prognosis. Both T_3 and T_4 levels are low, but the TSH level is normal.

High T_4 syndrome

In the high T_4 syndrome the T_4 level is elevated because of excessive iodine intake, as occurs with recent gallbladder studies and occasionally from drugs such as amiodarone. The high iodine inhibits the conversion of T_4 to T_3, leading to a buildup of T_4. TSH concentrations are normal or near normal.

Hyperthyroidism

Smokers have an increased incidence of Graves' disease and particularly Graves' ophthalmopathy.[2] Lithium therapy, which is known to be a risk factor for hypothyroidism, may also be associated with an increased risk of hyperthyroidism.[2]

Subclinical hyperthyroidism

Subclinical hyperthyroidism may be defined as undetectable or extremely low sTSH level in association with normal levels of free thyroxine. It affects 1% of men and 1.5% of women over the age of 60. Patients with this condition are at increased risk for progression to overt hyperthyroidism, atrial fibrillation, and possibly osteoporosis.[1] Treatment of subclinical hyperthyroidism is not generally recommended. There is limited evidence that treatment may improve bone mineral density if TSH levels are less than 0.1 mIU/L.[1]

Overview of the treatment of thyrotoxicosis

Therapy for hyperthyroidism is targeted at either immediate control of symptoms (adjunct treatment), usually with beta blockers, or modification of the disease through the use of drugs or radioactive iodine.

Beta Blockers and Calcium Channel Blockers. A number of beta blockers can be used to control the symptoms of tachycardia and palpitations. Examples are propranolol (Inderal) 20 to 40 mg qid, nadolol (Corgard) 80 to 240 mg/day as a single dose, atenolol (Tenormin) 50 to 100 mg/day as a single dose, and metoprolol (Lopressor) 50 to 100 mg bid. Treatment usually starts with low doses that are increased as necessary. Symptomatic beta blocker treatment should be continued for 4 to 6 weeks, overlapping with the definitive treatment. For patients who cannot take beta blockers, the calcium channel blocker diltiazem (Cardizem) 30 to 120 mg tid is often effective.[4]

Radioactive Iodine. Radioactive iodine (^{131}I) is the treatment of choice for Graves' Disease in the United States.[5] ^{131}I is used when antithyroid drugs fail to achieve remission at 6 months to 2 years.[5] It is particularly indicated in patients with risk factors for relapse such as those with severe symptoms or a large goiter.[4] It is contraindicated in pregnancy and breastfeeding and is of no use in the treatment of amiodarone-induced hyperthyroidism.[5]

Antithyroid Drug Therapy. The two major antithyroid drugs in use are propylthiouracil (Propyl-Thyracil) and methimazole (Tapazole). Methimazole is the active metabolite of a third antithyroid drug, carbimazole.[4,6]

The goals of antithyroid drug treatment in Graves' disease are the control of symptoms and the attainment of long-term remission.[4,6] Factors weakly associated with good remissions are small size of goiter and recent onset of hyperthyroidism.[2] More important is the duration of treatment. Long-term remissions have been reported to be much more common after 2 years of treatment than after 6 months of treatment.[7]

Antithyroid drugs are the treatment of choice in pregnancy and are preferred when treating hyperthyroidism in children. It can also be used in the elderly prior to ^{131}I-therapy.[5] Even when use of radioactive iodine is selected, patients may initially be given antithyroid drugs for a short period to control symptoms.[6]

Standard protocol in North America is to treat patients with antithyroid drugs for 1 to 2 years, since attempts at longer treatment are associated with prolonged monitoring and poor compliance. Relapses are most likely to occur in the 6 months after discontinuing therapy but may take place after many years.[6]

The choice of antithyroid drug seems to be arbitrary. In North America propylthiouracil (Propyl-Thyracil) is used more often than methimazole (Tapazole) for unclear reasons. According to Franklyn,[6] methimazole has several advantages and should be the drug of choice. A randomized control trial demonstrated that methimazole was better than propylthiouracil at achieving euthyroidism at 12 wks of therapy.[8] It also requires only once a day dosage and in moderate doses is associated with a lesser risk of agranulocytosis.[6]

The major side effect of both propylthiouracil and methimazole is agranulocytosis. It is an idiosyncratic reaction that is slightly more common in patients over the age of 40. Since it comes on rapidly, routine blood counts are not helpful; instead patients should be warned to report fever or sore throat immediately.[6] A baseline complete blood count before the initiation of therapy may be helpful.[4]

Propylthiouracil is usually started with doses of 75 to 100 mg tid. After 4 to 6 weeks the dose should be decreased by about one third if the TSH has risen to a normal or above normal level or if the T_4 or T_3 level has returned to normal. After another 4 to 6 weeks the dose may have to be reduced again. The usual maintenance dose is about 50 mg tid. The patient should then be examined clinically and have TSH and T_4 determinations every 2 months for 6 months, then every 3 months for 6 months, then twice a year for 1 year, and then annually. Treatment is generally continued for 1 to 2 years.[4,6]

Treatment with methimazole is usually begun with 10 to 20 mg once a day. After 4 to 6 weeks the dose should be decreased by about one third if the T_4 or T_3 has returned to normal or if the TSH has risen to a normal or above normal level. Since the TSH level may take weeks or even months to return to normal, doses are usually adjusted according to the T_4 and T_3 levels. After another 4 to 6 weeks the dose may have to be reduced once again. The usual maintenance dose is about 5 to 10 mg of methimazole a day. TSH and T_4 levels should be determined every 2 months for 6 months, then every 3 months for 6 months, then twice a year for 1 year, and then annually. Treatment is generally continued for 1 to 2 years.[4,6]

Ophthalmopathy. In patients with Graves' disease ophthalmopathy develops before thyroid disease in about 20% of patients, at the same time in 40%, and afterward in 40%. In most cases the disorder improves spontaneously. Ophthalmopathy is more likely to develop in smokers. Treatment of Graves' disease with radioiodine is associated with an increased incidence or a greater rate of progression of ophthalmopathy than is treatment with antithyroid drugs. However, only a few patients are so affected and for them the condition can be controlled with prednisone.[9,10] Prudence dictates avoiding the use of radioactive iodine for most patients with clinically apparent ophthalmopathy.[11]

⚜ **REFERENCES** ⚜

1. Surks MI, et al: Subclinical thyroid disease: Scientific review and guidelines for diagnosis and management, JAMA 29(2):228-238, 2004.
2. Prummel MF, Wiersinga WM: Smoking and risk of Graves' disease, *JAMA* 269:479-482, 1993.
3. Reference deleted in pages.
4. Singer PA, Cooper DS, Levy EG, et al: Treatment guidelines for patients with hyperthyroidism and hypothyroidism, *JAMA* 273:808-812, 1995.
5. Baskin HJ, et al: American association of clinical endocrinologists medical guidelines for clinical practice for the evaluation and treatment of hyperthyroidism and hypothyroidism Endocrine Practice, 8(5) 457-469, 2002.
6. Franklyn JA: The management of hyperthyroidism, *N Engl J Med* 330:1731-1738, 1994.
7. Tamai H, Nakagawa T, Fukino O, et al: Thionamide therapy in Graves' disease: relation of relapse rate to duration of therapy, *Ann Intern Med* 92:448-490, 1980.

8. Homsanit M, Sriussadaporn S, Vannasaeng S, et al: Efficacy of single daily dosage of methimazole vs. propylthiouracil in the induction of euthyroidism, *Clin Endocrinol* 54:385-390, 2001.

9. Bartalena L, Marcocci C, Bogazzi F, et al: Relation between therapy for hyperthyroidism and the course of Graves' ophthalmopathy, *N Engl J Med* 338:73-78, 1998.

10. Wiersinga WM: Preventing Graves' ophthalmopathy (editorial), *N Engl J Med* 338:121-122, 1998.

11. Walsh JP, Dayan CM, Potts MJ: Radioiodine and thyroid eye disease (editorial), *BMJ* 319:68-69, 1999.

Hypothyroidism

(See also biliary cirrhosis; celiac disease; smoking; thyroiditis)

Epidemiology

Lithium therapy is an important risk factor for hypothyroidism; 5% of patients receiving lithium have overt hypothyroidism, and 25% have subclinical hypothyroidism.[1] Smoking probably aggravates both the clinical and the biochemical effects of overt hypothyroidism.[2]

Hypercholesterolemia

Hypercholesterolemia may be a clue to hypothyroidism. In a retrospective analysis of hypercholesterolemic patients referred to a lipid clinic, 4.2% were hypothyroid; correction of the hypothyroidism lowered the lipid levels only if the TSH was at least 10 mU/L (10 μU/mL). Although there is a link between hypothyroidism and lipids, there is no evidence treating patients with slightly lower levels of thyroid hormone may influence the development of coronary artery disease.[3]

Guidelines for screening

The Canadian Task Force on Preventive Health Care recognizes the high prevalence of hypothyroidism among perimenopausal and post-menopausal women but gives screening for this disorder with thyroid function tests a "C" recommendation,[4] and the U.S. Preventive Services Task Force gives screening of asymptomatic adults and children a "D" recommendation.[5] For high-risk groups, including the elderly, the U.S. Preventive Services Task Force gives screening a "C" recommendation.[5]

The 1998 guidelines of the American College of Physicians recommend screening of women over the age of 50 for thyroid disease using a sensitive TSH test. If the TSH is either undetectable or greater than 10 mU/L, a free thyroxine test should be ordered. If the TSH is above 10 mU/L and the free thyroxine level is low, the patient has overt hypothyroidism and should be treated; if the free thyroxine level is in the normal range, the patient has subclinical hypothyroidism (see below).[6]

Treatment

The initial thyroxine dosage ranges from 12.5 ug daily to full replacement dosing, 16 ug/kg/day. Dosing should be adjusted downwards based on age (i.e., >50yrs) and cardiac status. Every 6 weeks one should Reassess and titrate therapy, based on TSH levels. Once TSH is within the normal range follow-up should occur at 6 months and then yearly.[7]

Thyroxine replacement therapy that does not suppress the TSH to below normal limits does not cause osteopenia. If the TSH is suppressed below the normal levels, there is an increased risk of osteopenia, but whether this will translate into an increased fracture rate is unknown.[8] The practical point for family physicians is that when hormone replacement therapy is prescribed for hypothyroidism, the TSH level should be kept in the normal rather than the subnormal range.

REFERENCES

1. Prummel MF, Wiersinga WM: Smoking and risk of Graves' disease, *JAMA* 269:479-482, 1993.

2. Müller B, Zulewski H, Huber P, et al: Impaired action of thyroid hormone associated with smoking in women with hypothyroidism, *N Engl J Med* 333:964-969, 1995.

3. Thyroid function is associated with presence and severity of coronary atherosclerosis, *Clin Cardiol* 26(12):569-573, 2003.

4. Canadian Task Force on the Periodic Health Examination: *Canadian guide to clinical preventive health care,* Ottawa, Canada Communication Group, pp 612-618, 1994.

5. US Preventive Services Task Force: *Guide to clinical preventive services,* ed 2, Baltimore, 1996, Williams & Wilkins, pp 209-218.

6. American College of Physicians: Clinical guideline. 1. Screening for thyroid disease, *Ann Intern Med* 129:141-143, 1998.

7. Baskin HJ et al: American association of clinical endocrinologists medical guidelines for clinical practice for the evaluation and treatment of hyperthyroidism and hypothyroidism, *Endocrine Practice* 8(5): 457-469, 2002.

8. Gharib H, Mazzaferri EL: Thyroxine suppressive therapy in patients with nodular thyroid disease, *Ann Intern Med* 128:386-394, 1998.

Subclinical hypothyroidism

(See also smoking; thyroiditis)

Subclinical hypothyroidism is diagnosed when the TSH is 4.5 mU/L or higher and the free thyroxine is in the normal range.[1] Subclinical hypothyroidism is much more common than overt hypothyroidism and may affect up to 8% of women over the age of 35. In only a small percentage of detected cases is the TSH level 10 mU/L or higher, which is clinically important because the risks of complications are greatest in patients with higher levels of TSH.[2] Risk factors for progression to overt hypothyroidism are older age, TSH levels of 10 mU/L or higher, and the presence of positive microsomal antibody tests.[2,3] In some susceptible subjects, subclinical hypothyroidism may be precipitated by smoking.[4]

The treatment of subclinical hypothyroidism is controversial.[2,3] Subclinical hypothyroidism was thought to contribute to cardiac dysfunction, atherosclerotic disease, increase cardiovascular mortality, elevation in total and LDL cholesterol and neuropsychiatric symptoms.[1] However, a review of the most current evidence failed to adequately demonstrate any relationship.[1] There is also no evidence that treatment prevents progression to overt disease.[1] However, according to some authorities, treatment may be indicated in the following circumstances[2,3]:

- The TSH level is unequivocally elevated (greater than twice the upper limit of normal)
- There are high levels of microsomal antibodies
- The cholesterol level is elevated

───────────── **⊸ REFERENCES ⊱** ─────────────

1. Surks MI, et al: Subclinical thyroid disease: Scientific review and guidelines for diagnosis and management, *JAMA* 29(2): 228-238, 2004.
2. Helfand M, Redfern CC: Clinical guideline. 2. Screening for thyroid disease: an update, *Ann Intern Med* 129:144-158, 1998.
3. Weetman AP: Hypothyroidism: screening and subclinical disease, *BMJ* 314:1175-1178, 1997.
4. Müller B, Zulewski H, Huber P, et al: Impaired action of thyroid hormone associated with smoking in women with hypothyroidism, *N Engl J Med* 333:964-969, 1995.

Thyroid Nodules
(See also screening)

In most clinical series in which patients were examined for the presence of thyroid nodules, only 5% to 8% of patients were found to have clinically palpable nodules and less than 10% of these nodules were cancerous.[1] However, in one California study in which a special effort was made to look for thyroid nodules by palpation in asymptomatic patients, 9% were found to have solitary nodules and 12% had multiple nodules for a total of 21%. When assessed by ultrasound, 67% of these patients were found to have nodules; none was malignant.[2] A Mayo Clinic evaluation comparing palpation and ultrasonography found that nodules less than 1 cm in diameter were rarely palpable and that about 50% of glands thought to have a solitary nodule on palpation were actually multinodular on ultrasonography.[3]

If a low-functioning ("cold") nodule is found in a woman living in an iodine-deficient area, the chance that it is malignant is about 1.5%.[4] On the other hand, a solitary nodule in an elderly man has a greater than 50% chance of being malignant.[5] Thyroid nodules are four times as common in females as in males, and their incidence increases in direct proportion to age.[6]

The vast majority of thyroid cancers are relatively non-aggressive papillary or follicular carcinomas; papillary carcinomas are the more common. Although regional lymph node metastases are reasonably common with these forms of cancer, cure is usually possible with surgery, often in conjunction with therapeutic doses of radioactive iodine. Distant metastases occur in only 10% to 15% of patients with well-differentiated follicular or papillary carcinomas, and if these tumour deposits take up radioactive iodine, complete long-lasting remissions may be expected in close to 50% of cases.[7]

Fine needle aspiration is the investigative procedure of choice for clinically solitary thyroid nodules. When this technique is used, about 70% of nodules will be cytologically benign (with a false-negative rate of 1% to 2%), 4% are malignant, and the remainder either have insufficient cellular material for a diagnosis or are inconclusive.[8] The aspiration is done with a 10- or 25-ml syringe and a 22- to 27-gauge needle. Three to six passes with the needle are generally made to ensure adequate sampling.[1]

About 15% to 25% of aspirated nodules are found to be cysts. Most cysts are benign, but 15% have been reported to be necrotic papillary carcinomas.[6] If the nodule disappears permanently after aspiration, no further testing is required even if no cytological diagnosis has been made.[8]

If a thyroid nodule is smaller than 1 cm, the chances of its being malignant are very low. In this situation a reasonable management plan is simply follow-up observation.[9]

Hyperfunctioning (hot) nodules (detected by thyroid scan) are almost never malignant.[1]

Treatment of benign thyroid nodules with levothyroxine (Synthroid) to suppress thyroid nodule growth is controversial. Some studies have shown no benefit and others only slight benefit. Since this treatment is associated with decreased bone density and possibly an increased risk of atrial fibrillation, there seems little indication for using it.[8]

───────────── **⊸ REFERENCES ⊱** ─────────────

1. Ridgway EC: Clinical review 30: clinician's evaluation of a solitary thyroid nodule, *J Clin Endocrinol Metab* 74:231-235, 1992.
2. Ezzat S, Sarti DA, Cain DR, et al: Thyroid incidentalomas: prevalence by palpation and ultrasonography, *Arch Intern Med* 154:1838-1840, 1994.
3. Tan GH, Gharib H, Reading CC: Solitary thyroid nodule: comparison between palpation and ultrasonography, *Arch Intern Med* 155:2418-2423, 1995.
4. Belfiore A, La Rosa GL, La Porta GA, et al: Cancer risk in patients with cold thyroid nodules: relevance of iodine intake, sex, age and multinodularity, *Am J Med* 93:363-369, 1992.

5. Mazzaferri EL: Thyroid cancer in thyroid nodules: finding a needle in the haystack (editorial), *Am J Med* 93:359-362, 1992.

6. Mazzaferri EL: Current concepts: management of asolitary thyroid nodule, *N Engl J Med* 328:553-559, 1993.

7. Schlumberger MJ: Papillary and follicular thyroid carcinoma, *N Engl J Med* 338:297-306, 1998.

8. Hermus AR, Huysmans DA: Treatment of benign nodular thyroid disease, *N Engl J Med* 338:1438-1447, 1998.

9. Gharib H, James EM, Charboneau JW, et al: Suppressive therapy with levothyroxine for solitary thyroid nodules, *N Engl J Med* 317:70-75, 1987.

Thyroiditis

(See also hypothyroidism; subclinical hypothyroidism)

Classification

Thyroiditis can be classified as follows[1,2]:
- Acute thyroiditis (bacterial, fungal, or parasitic)
- Subacute thyroiditis (subacute granulomatous thyroiditis [de Quervain's or painful thyroiditis], painless thyroiditis, postpartum thyroiditis)
- Chronic lymphocytic thyroiditis (Hashimoto's disease)
- Riedel's thyroiditis (invasive fibrous thyroiditis or chronic sclerosing thyroiditis)

Acute thyroiditis and Riedel's thyroiditis are very rare. Symptoms of acute infectious thyroiditis are anterior neck pain, swelling, fever, dysphagia, and dysphonia. Riedel's thyroiditis is found in middle-aged or elderly women and consists of a fibrous replacement of the gland that turns the gland into a stony hard mass.

Subacute granulomatous thyroiditis. Subacute granulomatous thyroiditis was described by de Quervain in 1904. It is thought to be secondary to a viral infection. It affects women four times as often as men, most patients are middle aged, and cases are most likely to occur in the summer and fall.[1,2]

The usual symptoms are either those of thyrotoxicosis (about 50% of patients), resulting from the excessive release of thyroid hormone by the damaged gland, or anterior neck pain. Granulomatous thyroiditis is the most common cause of anterior neck pain in the region of the thyroid gland. Patients may have low-grade fever and general malaise. The thyroid gland tends to be firm and tender.[1,2]

The symptoms of granulomatous thyroiditis often develop rapidly, and this is a distinguishing point from Graves' disease. If the distinction between these two conditions is not obvious clinically, it can be resolved by measuring ^{131}I uptake. This is significantly increased in Graves' disease but very low (less than 5%) in granulomatous thyroiditis.[1,2]

The initial phase of inflammation and pain usually lasts 3 to 6 weeks. About one third of patients subsequently enter a hypothyroid stage that persists for several weeks before the euthyroid state is restored.

Approximately 5% of patients become permanently hypothyroid.[1,2] A number of patients have elevated antithyroid antibody levels, which suggests the development of an autoimmune process during the disease.[1,2]

Treatment of granulomatous thyroiditis is symptomatic. Non-steroidal anti-inflammatory drugs are usually effective in relieving the neck pain, but sometimes prednisone 20 to 40 mg/day in divided doses and tapered over 2 to 4 weeks is required. Thyrotoxic symptoms can be controlled by beta blockers (see discussion of hyperthyroidism), and the subsequent hypothyroid state may need temporary thyroid replacement therapy.[1,2] Antithyroid drugs such as propylthiouracil or methimazole have no role in treating any of the forms of subacute thyroiditis (granulomatous, painless, or postpartum), since the pathogenesis is leakage of preformed hormone, not its excessive production.[1,2]

Painless thyroiditis. Painless thyroiditis may be sporadic or postpartum. Both forms are believed to be autoimmune disorders, since thyroid antibodies are present in 50% of patients with painless thyroiditis and 80% of those with postpartum thyroiditis.[1,2]

The sporadic form of painless thyroiditis is concentrated in the Great Lakes region of North America and accounts for about one third of cases of thyrotoxicosis in this area. Outside of the Great Lakes region it constitutes only about 5% of thyrotoxicosis cases.[1,2]

Like granulomatous thyroiditis, painless thyroiditis affects women four times as often as men and most patients are 40 to 50 years of age. Symptoms are those of thyrotoxicosis and tend to come on abruptly. Patients do not have neck pain. The thyroid gland is slightly enlarged but non-tender.[1,2]

Also like granulomatous thyroiditis, painless thyroiditis usually begins with a thyrotoxic phase, passes through a hypothyroid phase, and ends with a recovery phase. In a few patients only the hypothyroid phase is seen. About 6% of patients become permanently hypothyroid, but this may take years to develop. Thus annual TSH testing is indicated for all patients with painless thyroiditis.[1,2]

Painless thyroiditis can be differentiated from Graves' disease by radioactive iodine uptake (RAIU). It is high in Graves' disease and usually less than 3% in painless thyroiditis.[1,2]

Treatment of painless thyroiditis is directed at the symptoms. Some patients require no treatment, whereas others benefit from beta-blockers in the thyrotoxic phase and a temporary course of levothyroxine if symptomatic hypothyroidism ensues.[1,2]

Postpartum thyroiditis. As indicated previously, postpartum thyroiditis is a variant of painless thyroiditis. It occurs in 4% to 5% of women and is usually self-limited. The disorder begins with symptoms of hyperthyroidism, which are classically followed by a period of hypothyroidism and finally a return to the euthyroid state. The entire sine wave cycle may last 6 to 9 months. The syndrome is likely to recur with subsequent pregnancies,[1,2] and about 25% of those who have recovered from the disorder are found to be overtly hypothyroid 4 years later.[3,4]

RAIU scanning shows no or little uptake in patients with postpartum thyroiditis. The test should not be performed if the mother is nursing.[1,2]

Treatment of postpartum thyroiditis is symptomatic. Beta blockers may be needed in the hyperthyroid stage and short-term levothyroxine in the hypothyroid stage.[1,2]

Chronic lymphocytic thyroiditis. Chronic lymphocytic thyroiditis was described by the Japanese physician Hashimoto in 1912. It is the most common cause of hypothyroidism. Up to 95% of patients are women,[1] and most are over the age of 45 when the diagnosis is made.[5] A small to medium-sized goiter is usually found. Antithyroid antibodies (antimicrosomal or antithyroglobulin) are present in 90% of patients, and the titers of these, particularly the antimicrosomal antibodies, are usually high. The usual replacement dose of levothyroxine (Synthroid, Eltroxin) is 75 to 150 μg/day. Initial doses are low (12.5, 25, and 50 μg), especially in the elderly or those with coronary artery disease. Increments, based on TSH levels, are made every 4 to 6 weeks (see discussion of hypothyroidism above).[1] If a patient with chronic lymphocytic thyroiditis becomes pregnant, she will probably require a dose increase of 25% to 50%.[5]

In one study 11% of patients with Hashimoto's thyroiditis had a spontaneous remission. Levothyroxine was withdrawn after 1 year of treatment, and thyroid function remained normal for up to a year.[6]

──────────── ◢ **REFERENCES** ◣ ────────────

1. Sakiyama R: Thyroiditis: a clinical review, *Am Fam Physician* 48:615-621, 1993.
2. Morrison A: Guidelines for the diagnosis of common thyroid disorders, *Can J CME,* pp 79-85, 1992.
3. Othman S, Phillips DI, Parkes AB, et al: A long-term follow-up of postpartum thyroiditis, *Clin Endocrinol* 32:559-564, 1990.
4. Tachi J, Amino N, Tamaki H: Long-term follow-up and HLA association in patients with postpartum hypothyroidism, *J Clin Endocrinol Metab* 66:480-484, 1988.
5. Dyan CM, Daniels GH: Chronic autoimmune thyroiditis, *N Engl J Med* 335:99-107, 1996.
6. Comtois R, Faucher L, Lafleche L: Outcome of hypothyroidism caused by Hashimoto's thyroiditis, *Arch Intern Med* 155:1404-1408, 1995.

TOXICOLOGY
(See also lead poisoning; screening)

The approach to the overdose patient requires attention to specific uniqueness of resuscitation, stabilization, decontamination, specific antidote therapy and supportive care. Attention should also be paid to see if the patient presents with evidence of a specific toxidrome. Physicians should be familiar with the clinical manifestations of opioid, anticholinergic, cholinergic, sympathomimietic, serotonin syndrome and sedative-hypnotic withdrawl toxidromes. The initial lab tests should include routine hematology and electrolytes (with anion gap), serum osmolality (with osmole gap), glucose, liver and renal profile, coagulation, ASA and Acetaminophen levels, urinalysis, pregnancy test in all women of child bearing age, and EKG. Specific drug levels should be ordered based on ingestion. Other "routine" drug screens have limited utility.[1]

Pharmacological agents that are particularly dangerous for children (where 1 tablet or 1 teaspoon could be fatal in a 2-year-old) are camphor, chloroquin, tricyclics, phenothiazine, quinine, methyl salicylate, theophylline, sulfonoureas, essential oils (from aspiration), calcium channel blocker, and methadone.[2]

Options for decontamination include oral activated charcoal (AC), whole bowel irrigation and gastric lavage.[2] Syrup of ipecac has very little to no role in the management of the overdosed patient and is effectively obsolete.[3] If the patient cannot protect the airway, decontamination should be given after the airway is secured regardless of the option chosen.

A single dose of AC without cathartic (50 g for adults and 1 g/kg for children up to 12 years of age) is the treatment of choice for most poisonings that are likely to cause moderate or severe toxicity. Ideally, activated charcoal should be administered within 1 hour of toxin ingestion and perhaps withheld if greater than 2 hours have passed since ingestion.[3] AC should be withheld in non-toxic ingestions, or if there is evidence of an ileus. AC does not bind the following and should not be given: corrosive products, heavy metals, hydrocarbons, and alcohols.

Whole-bowel irrigation with polyethylene glycol solutions (GoLYTELY, Colyte PEG-ES) is very useful in the management of the ingestion of Enteric coated or extended release preparation, toxins that are not bound by AC, and in body stuffers.[4,5]

Gastric lavage still continues to have a role in massive ingestions of a potentially lethal nature.[4]

Specific antibodies for overdose are available for digoxin, and colchicine (Europe only). Special mention is made for the following therapies in overdose settings: sodium bicarbonate for tricyclics, ASA, cocaine, and for rhabdomyolysis, which can complicate certain overdoses; fomepizole for ethylene glycol; insulin for calcium channel blockers; glucagon for beta blockers; deferoximine for iron overdoses; hyperbaric oxygen for carbon monoxide; and octreotide for sulfonylureas.[3] Reversal agents such as naloxone for Narcotic ingestion or flumazenil for benzodiazepines should be used cautiously if at all because of the risk of precipitation withdrawal and seizures.[6] The specific antidote for acetaminophen overdose is *N*-acetyl-cysteine (NAC), which is administered on the basis of levels of plasma acetaminophen drawn greater than 4 hours post-ingestion on the Rumack-Matthew nomogram. Ideally this should be administered within 8 hours of ingestion. Evidence of hepatotoxicity is also an indication for NAC administration. Intravenous administration is as effective as oral administration.[7] Given the shorter duration (20 vs 72 hours) and safety,[8] it is the preferred route of administration.

―――――――――― ∂ **REFERENCES** ∠ ――――――――――

1. Montague RE et al: Urine drug screens in overdose patients do not contribute to immediate clinical management, *Therapeutic Drug Monitoring* 23:47-50, 2001.

2. Koren G: Medications which can kill a toddler with one tablet or teaspoonful, *J Toxicol Clin Toxicol* 331:407-413, 1993.
3. Bateman DN: Gastric decontamination: a view for the millennium, *J Accid Emerg Med* 16:84-86, 1999.
4. Canadian Association of Emergency Physicians: *The Toxicology Roadshow,* Course Manual, ed 2, 2003 Series.
5. Farmer JW, et al: Whole bowel irrigation for contraband bodypackers, *J Clin Gastroenterol* 37(2):147-150, 2003.
6. Gueye PN, et al: Emperic use of flumazenil in comatose patients: Limited applicability of criteria to define low risk, *Ann Emerg Med* 27(6):730, 1996.
7. Perry HE, et al: Efficacy of oral vs intravenous *N-J Pediatr* 132(1):149-152, 1998.
8. Yip L, et al: Intravenous administration of oral N-acetylcysteine, *Crit Care Med* 23(1) 40-43, 1998.

VITAMINS AND MINERALS (Table 57)

Table 57 Vitamins and Minerals[1-4]

Vitamin/Mineral	Dietary Sources	Signs of Deficiency	Signs of Toxicity
Thiamine (Vitamin B₁)	Dried yeast, whole grain and enriched grains, wheat germ, pork, liver, dried peas and beans, soy foods	Parethesias, nystamugus, impaired memory, congestive heart failure, lactic acidosis, Wernicke's encephalopathy	Rare irritability, headache, insomnia, interferes with B2 and B6, rapid pulse, weakness, anaphylaxis
Riboflavin (Vitamin B₂)	Milk, liver, enriched grains, meat, eggs, nuts, legumes, green leafy vegetables	Mucositis, dermatitis, cheilosis, angular stomatitis, glossitis, corneal vascularization, photophobia, lacrimation, visual impairment, impaired wound healing, normocytic anemia, amblyopia	None known, yellow discolouration of urine
Pantothenic Acid (Vitamin B₃)	Yeast, organ meats, egg, milk, peanuts, legumes, whole grains, liver, salmon, mushrooms	Fatigue, malaise, headache, insomnia, vomiting, abdominal cramps, growth failure, hypoglycemia, decreased immune function	Diarrhea
Niacin (Vitamin B₅)	Dried yeast, liver, meat, fish, poultry, legumes, enriched whole grains	Dermatitis, dementia, diarrhea, death, loss of memory, headache, glossitis, tremor, insomnia, anorexia, peripheral neuropathy, encephalopathy	Liver damage, vasodilation, flushing, irritation, itching, GI irritation, glucose intolerance
Pyridoxine (Vitamin B₆)	Organ meats, pork, fish, seeds, legumes, nuts, dried yeast, whole grains	Dermatitis, neuritis, convulsions, microcytic anemia, renal calculi	None known from foods; sensory neuropathy, unsteady gait, decreased phenytoin levels
Folate (Vitamin B₉)	Green leafy vegetables, organ meats, dried yeast, dried beans, legumes, citrus, fortified grains	Macrocytic anemia, diarrhea, glossitis, lethargy, stomatitis	None known from foods; seizures
Cyanocbalamin (Vitamin B₁₂)	Meats, organ meats, beef, pork, eggs, milk, cheese, fish	Megoblastic anemia, glossitis, leukopenia, weakness, short of breath, spinal cord degeneration, peripheral neuropathy	None known from foods

Continued

Table 57   Vitamins and Minerals—cont'd

Vitamin/Mineral	Dietary Sources	Signs of Deficiency	Signs of Toxicity
Biotin	Organ meats, egg yolk, yeast, nuts, legumes	Rare dermatitis, depression, alopecia, lassitude, anorexia, glossitis, somnolence, paresthsias, pallor, lethargy	None known
Ascorbic Acid (Vitamin C)	Citrus fruits, tomatoes, potatoes, red berries, peppers	Scurvy, enlargement and keratosis of hair follicles, impaired wound healing, anemia, depression, lethargy, bleeding, ecchymosis, gingivitis	Osmotic diarrhea, nausea, vomiting, oxalate kidney stones, interference with anticoagulation therapy
Vitamin A	Fish liver oils, egg yolk, dairy products, green leafy or orange, yellow vegetables and fruit	Dermatitis, night blindness, keratomalacia, xeroptbalmia	Nausea, vomiting, headache, dizziness, deep bone pain, peeling skin, gingivitis, alopecia, hepatotoxiciy
Vitamin D	Fish, fish liver oils, fortified milk and margarine, liver, egg yolk, UV radiation	Osteomalacia, muscle weakness, bone pain, hypophosphatemia, hypocalcemia	Excess bone and soft tissue calcification, kidney stones, hypercalcemia, anorexia, renal failure
Vitamin E	Polyunsaturated vegetable oils, nuts, eggs, wheat germ, whole grains	Rare hemolysis, anemia, neuronal axonopathy, myopathy	Prolonged clotting time, impaired neutrophil function
Vitamin K	Green leafy vegetables, liver, vegetable oils, intestinal flora (after newborn period)	Bleeding, purpura, bruising, prolonged clotting time	Jaundice
Zinc	Red meats, oysters, poultry, sesame seeds, sunflower seeds, nuts, dried beans, soy foods	Dermatitis, altered taste and smell, alopecia, diarrhea, apathy, depression, impaired wound healing and immune function, immunosuppression, growth retardation, anorexia	Nausea, vomiting, metallic taste, chills, headache, pancreatic damage
Copper	Shellfish, nuts, organ meats, whole grain cereals, dried legumes	Neutropenia, microcytic anemia, osteoporosis, decreased hair and skin pigmentation, dermatitis, hypotonia, leukopenia	Nausea, vomiting, epigastric pain, diarrhea, jaundice, renal tubular swelling, liver cirrhosis
Chromium	Brewer's yeast, meat, cheese	Glucose intolerance, peripheral neuropathy, hyperlipidimia-increased serum cholesterol and triglycerides, insulin resistance	None known from diet or supplement
Manganese	Grains fruit	Rare poor reproductive performance, nausea, vomiting, dermatitis, colour changes in hair, slow hair growth, hypocholesterolemia, growth retardation, skeletal abnormalities, prolonged clotting time	Extrapyramidial symptoms, encephalitis-like symptoms, hyper-irritability
Selenium	Fish, meats, nuts, legumes	Muscle weakness and pain, cardiomyopathy, RBC fragility	Hair loss, nausea, vommittingder-matitis, garlic odour, brittle nails, fatigue
Molybdenum	Meats, grains, legumes	Tachycardia, tachypnea, altered mental status, vision changes, night blindness, headache, nausea, vomiting	Increased copper excretion, gout, hyperuremia

Table 57   Vitamins and Minerals—cont'd

Vitamin/Mineral	Dietary Sources	Signs of Deficiency	Signs of Toxicity
Calcium	Dairy products, dark, green and leafy vegetables, fortified soy foods, fortified orange juice	Tetany, arrythmias, congestive heart failure, altered nerve conduction, osteomalacia	Metastatic calcification, weakness, renal failure, psychosis
Magnesium	Soybeans, clams, wheat germ, almonds, dairy products, green leaves, nuts, cereal grains, seafood	Weakness, convulsions, neuromuscular irritability and dysfunction, failure to thrive	Hypotension, cardiac disturbances, respiratory failure
Phosphorus	Milk products, meat, fish, poultry, nuts, legumes	Osteomalacia, muscle weakness, cardiac failure, red blood cell dysfunction, metabolic acidosis, gastrointestinal tract and renal dysfunction	Arrhythmia, leg weakness, skeletal demineralization
Potassium	Meat, milk, bananas, prunes, raisins, orange, grapefruit, potatoes, legumes	Polyuria, impaired muscle contraction, ECG changes, peritoneal distention, dyspnea, paralysis, cardiac disturbances	Mental confusion, hypotension, weakness, ECG changes, paralysis, cardiac disturbances
Iron	Meat, fish, poultry, organ meats, eggs, prunes, peas, beans, lentils, soy foods, raisins, fortified grain products	Glossitis, fatigue, tachycardia, microcytic hypochromic anemia, koilonychias, enteropathy, impaired behaviour	Nutritional hemosiderosis, organ damage

⚶ REFERENCES ⚶

1. American Dietetic Association & Dietitians of Canada: *Manual of Clinical Dietetics,* 6th ed. Chicago, Il: American Dietetic Association, 2000.
2. Gottschlich MM, Fuhrman MP, Hammond KA, et al, editors: *The science and practice of nutrition support: a case-based core curriculum.* Dubuque, IA, 2001, Kendall/Hunt.
3. Merritt, R.J. (Coordinating ed.) *Nutrition Support Practice Manual.* Silver Spring, MD, 1998, American Society for Parenteral and Enteral Nutrition.
4. Ontario Dietetic Association: *Nutrition Care Manual.* Don Mills, ON, 1989, Ontario Hospital Association.

CHRONIC RENAL FAILURE

(See also diabetic nephropathy; hypertension; microalbuminuria; non-steroidal anti-inflammatory drugs; restless leg syndrome)

Chronic renal failure (CRF) is characterized by persistently abnormal glomerular filtration rate. While the rate of progression varies, the common end result is persistent and progressive damage to the kidneys. Treatments to delay progression are aimed at treatment of primary disease (for example, strict glycemic control in diabetics), aggressive treatment of hypertension and proteinuria and early referral to a nephrologist.[1] Additionally, anemia correction with erythropoietin, acid-base balance maintenance, dyslipidemia treatment and bone-loss prevention with low-phosphate diets and calcium-based phosphate binders, also play a role.[1,2]

CRF is caused by diabetes in 37% of cases, hypertension in 30%, and by chronic glomerulonephritis in 12%. Other important causes include poly-cystic kidney disease, obstructive nephropathy (ureteric or bladder outlet), drug-induced nephropathy (such as non-steroidal anti-inflammatory drugs), and ischemic renal disease.[3] End-stage renal failure is more common in black than in white men, and this correlates with an increased incidence of hypertension and lower socio-economic status.[4]

When presented with an elevated creatinine level, physicians must try to determine the etiology of the renal disease and in particular rule out reversible conditions such as urinary obstruction and volume depletion. In addition to creatinine measurements, the basic work-up of renal failure includes ultrasonography of the urinary tract; urinalysis; 24-hour urine collection for protein and creatinine clearance; a complete blood count with ESR; measurement of electrolytes, urea, calcium, phosphorus, glucose, total protein, and albumin; and serum protein electrophoresis. Rapidly progressive renal failure (a condition that requires emergency consultation) should be ruled out by measurement of creatinine levels at reasonably short intervals.[5]

Elective nephrology consultation is probably indicated for any patient with creatinine levels of 120 to 150 µmol/L (1.4 to 1.7 mg/dl) or higher, levels that represent greater than 50% loss of glomerular filtration function.

Early nephrology consultation is a priority since it may lead to better management of underlying diseases and allows more time for the lengthy period of preparation that usually must precede long-term dialysis or renal transplantation.[5] Additionally, early referral has also been shown to be associated with lower mortality, better pre-dialysis care and is cost effective[1]

One of the most important therapeutic interventions for decreasing the progression of CRF is adequate blood-pressure control. Target levels should be 130/80 to 130/85 mm Hg or, for those with proteinuria of greater than 1 g/day, 125/75 mm Hg.[3] Some authors recommend a mean arterial pressure of 98 mm Hg or lower when proteinuria is between 0.25 and 1.0 g/day and low 90's when higher.[1] Angiotensin-converting enzyme (ACE) inhibitors are the agents of first choice in type 1 diabetic patients (hypertensive and normotensive) since it can prevent the occurrence and progression of diabetic nephropathy.[6] They are also first line agents in non-diabetic patients with CRF since they decrease the rate of progression of CRF.[7] The benefit is independent of blood-pressure lowering and antiproteinuric effects.[6] In the presence of CRF, ACE inhibitors can be used with careful monitoring of renal function and serum potassium levels.[1] Angiotensin receptor blockers (ARBs) diminish proteinuria and protect against renal function decline in patients with type 2 diabetes and also my be beneficial in patients with advanced CRF.[1,6]

Low-protein diets have a small effect on the rate of decline of GFR, but malnutrition is a concern. The issue is still under debate, but a low-protein diet should be considered when the GFR is less than 30 mL/min/1.73m^2 in consultation with a dietician.[8]

End-stage renal disease has a very high mortality and the leading cause of death is CVD. The risk in dialysis patients is age-dependant with a mean of fifteenfold compared to baseline.[6] With the high risk of cardiovascular disease in CRF, many authors recommend aggressive lipid lowering therapy.[6] Statins are often used since they have additional actions that may help slow the progression of disease additional to their lipid-lowering effects.[1]

The decision of when to initiate dialysis is controversial. It is not clear that early dialysis improves outcome, increases survival time or improves quality of life.[9,10]

Renal Transplantation

The 3-year survival rate for transplanted cadaveric kidneys in the United States is 70%. The survival rate is higher among living unrelated donors: for wife-to-husband grafts it is 87%, and for husband-to-wife grafts it is the same provided the wife has never been pregnant. If she has been pregnant, the survival rate is 76%. Good survival in spite of relatively poor histocompatibility is attributed to healthier kidneys.[11] In the United States

27% of transplanted kidneys come from living related donors, whereas in France the figure is only 4%.[12]

The long-term survival rate of recipients of renal transplants is greater than that of patients on long-term dialysis who are suitable candidates for transplants but have not received them.[13]

_____ ◢ **REFERENCES** ◣ _____

1. Yu HT: Progression of renal failure, *Arch Intern Med* 163:1417-1429, 2003

2. Kopes-Kerr CP: A simplified approach to the management of early chronic renal failure, *Family Practice* 19:563-565, 2002.

3. Rahman M, Smith MC: Chronic renal insufficiency: a diagnostic and therapeutic approach, *Arch Intern Med* 158:1743-1752, 1998.

4. Klag MJ, Whelton PK, Randall BL, et al: End-stage renal disease in African-American and white men, *JAMA* 277:1293-1298, 1997.

5. Meddlesome DC, Barrett JB, Brownscombe LM, et al: Elevated levels of serum creatinine: recommendations for management and referral, *Can Med Assoc J* 161:413-417, 1999.

6. Henckes M: Management of the patient with chronic renal failure in the evidence based era, *Acta Clinica Velgica*, 57-5, 257-265, 2002.

7. Ruggenenti P, Perna A, Gherardi G, et al: Renoprotective properties of ACE-inhibition in non-diabetic nephropathies with non-nephrotic proteinuria, *Lancet* 354:359-364, 1999.

8. K/DOQI Clinical practice guidelines for chronic kidney disease: evaluation, classification and stratification. *Am J Kidney Dis* : 39:S1-S266 (suppl 1), 2002.

9. Korevaar et al: Evaluation of DOQI guidelines: early start of dialysis treatment is not associated with better health-related quality of life. National Kidney Foundation-Dialysis Outcomes Quality Initiative *Am J Kidney Dis* 39(1):108-115, 2002.

10. Korevaar JC et al: When to initiate dialysis: effect of proposed US guidelines on survival, The *Lancet* 358(9287) 1046-1050, 2001.

11. Terasaki PI, Cecka JM, Gjertson DW, et al: High survival rates of kidney transplants from spousal and living unrelated donors, *N Engl J Med* 333:333-336, 1995.

12. Soulillou J-P: Kidney transplantation from spousal donors (editorial), *N Engl J Med* 333:379-380, 1995.

13. Wolfe RA, Ashby VB, Milford EL, et al: Comparison of mortality in all patients on dialysis, patients on dialysis awaiting transplantation, and recipients of a first cadaveric transplant, *N Engl J Med* 341:1725-1730, 1999.

GLOMERULONEPHRITIS

(See also hematuria; streptococcal pharyngitis; urinalysis)

Glomerulonephritis (GN) is a group of diseases characterized by inflammatory changes in glomerular capillaries. There are accompanying signs and symptoms of an acute nephritic syndrome; such as hematuria, protein-uria, diminished renal-function hypertension, and edema.[1] Worldwide, it is the most common cause of end-stage renal disease (ESRD). For every patient with clinically apparent disease, there are 5 to 10 with undiagnosed sub-clinical disease. The hallmark of GN is red cell casts in the urine. This differentiates glomerular from extra-glomerular sources of hematuria. GN secondary to systemic disease (e.g., hepatitis B/C, collagen vascular disease) is not discussed in this section.

IgA Nephropathy

IgA nephropathy is the most common cause of GN worldwide. In 50% of patients, the presentation is one of abrupt onset of gross hematuria, and occasionally flank pain, 24 to 48 hours after a viral infection (upper-respiratory or gastrointestinal). Edema and hypertension are less commonly seen. The prognosis is variable with some patients having one isolated event, some with repeated exacerbations and up to 50% with ESRD, which occurs over a chronic period. Treatment is symptomatic. No therapy is recommended for isolated hematuria without proteinuria. These patients should be monitored regularly (every 3 to 12 months) for the development of proteinuria. ACE inhibitors are effective in blood-pressure control and slowing progression. Fish oil capsules and corticosteroids have both been used with some positive results.[2,3]

Post-Streptococcal Glomerulonephritis (PSGN)

PSGN is preceded by an infection with nephritogenic strain of group A hemolytic streptococci by 2 to 3 weeks. Symptoms are those of an acute nephritic syndrome with hematuria, proteinuria, active urine sediment, fluid retention, hypertension and reduced renal function. In the vast majority of patients the condition resolves with spontaneous recovery. In the absence of acute renal failure, only supportive therapy with antihypertensives and diuretics are required. Over 95% of patients recover spontaneously with return to normal renal function within 3-4 weeks with no long-term sequelae, even when renal failure is severe enough to require dialysis.[1] It has been suggested that misdiagnosis, racial differences in the risk of progression of renal disease, and differences in the natural history of sporadic and epidemic glomerulonephritis may be a factor in rate of spontaneous recovery.[4]

Rapidly Progressive Glomerulonephritis (RPGN)

Patients who have signs and symptoms of GN accompanied by rapid loss of renal function associated with >50% glomerular crescents are said to have RPGN. ESRD results in days to weeks. This can follow any form of GN or can occur as a primary disorder (Goodpastures syndrome). It can also be secondary to a systemic disease (antinuclear cytoplasmic antibody-positive vasculitis). Unless associated with systemic disease, the disorder may have an insidious onset with non-specific symptoms such as malaise and lethargy. The condition should be treated aggressively and early, in an attempt to decrease the risk of ESRD and increase the likelihood of recovery. Corticosteroids and cyclophosphamide and occasionally plasmapheresis are the mainstays of therapy.[4]

Membranoproliferative Glomerulonephritis (MPGN)

MPGN can present with the nephrotic syndrome, nephritic syndrome, or, most often, a mixture of the two. Nephrotic syndrome is characterized by heavy proteinuria (greater than 3 g/day), hypoalbuminemia and edema. There are three distinct types based on histology. MPGN is associated with a number of systemic diseases; however, a causal relationship may exist between hepatitis C infection and MPGN. Hepatitis C may be responsible for up to 60% of so called idiopathic cases.[4] Spontaneous remission is rare and a chronic progressive course is common. However, ESRD may take 10 years or longer to occur. Therapy is generally supportive.

─────────── ◢ REFERENCES ◣ ───────────

1. Couser W: Glomerulonephritis, Lancet 353:1509-1515, 1999.
2. Pozzi C: Corticosteroids in IgA nephropathy: a randomised controlled trial, *Lancet* 353:883-887, 1999.
3. Donadio JV Jr, Grande JP, Bergstralh EJ, et al: The long-term outcome of patients with IgA nephropathy treated with fish oil in a controlled trial, *J Am Soc Nephrol* 10:1772-1777, 1999.
4. Hricik DE, Chung-Park M, Sedor JR: Glomerulonephritis, *N Engl J Med* 339:888-899, 1998.

HEMATURIA

(See also bladder cancer; IgA nephropathy; urinalysis)

In a study from the Mayo Clinic, microscopic hematuria (defined as the presence of any red blood cells in a high-power field) occurred in 13% of asymptomatic men and post-menopausal women. Younger women were excluded from the study because of the high rate of contamination of the urine with menstrual flow. After a 5½-year follow-up, only 0.5% of the patients were found to have renal-cell cancer or bladder cancer.[1]

In a study from a British "hematuria clinic," no diagnosis was reached in 20% of the cases. In the same clinic, infections accounted for the most cases (25%), followed by benign prostatic hyperplasia (22%).[2]

One study examined 115 patients presenting to a urology clinic with asymptomatic microhematuria. Each patient underwent both CT and IVP before cystoscopy. Overall, abnormalities were identified in 38 patients (33%). In 77 patients no cause for hematuria was found on either study. False-positive results were reported by the CT and IVP in 2 and 7 of these cases, respectively. The sensitivity and specificity of the CT scan was 100% and 97.4%, respectively. The sensitivity

and specificity for the IVP was less accurate, 60.5% and 90.9%, respectively. Forty non-urological diagnoses were made by CT including abdominal-aortic and iliac-artery aneurysms.[6] Not all red urine is caused by blood. Aside from myoglobinuria and hemoglobinuria, a variety of ingested substances can give a reddish urine. These include beets, berries, food colouring, cascara-containing laxatives, ibuprofen (Motrin, Advil), phenazopyridine (Pyridium), phenytoin (Dilantin), quinine, sulfamethoxazole (Septra, Bactrim), chloroquine (Aralen), and rifampin.[3]

Exercise-Induced Hematuria

Exercise-induced hematuria is a common condition that is usually microscopic but may be macroscopic.[3,4] It affects both sexes and is associated both with contact sports such as boxing and football and with non-contact sports such as swimming, track, and rowing. There are a variety of pathophysiological explanations—ischemic damage to the nephrons from renal vessel constriction, more marked constriction of the efferent than the afferent glomerular arterioles, and repeated trauma to the bladder mucosa caused by the posterior wall slapping against the base.[4]

The differential diagnosis includes exercise-induced rhabdomyolysis and march hemoglobinuria. In neither of these cases are red blood cells found in the urine. In exercise-induced hematuria a urine-dipstick test is positive for blood and the urinalysis reveals red blood cells. The diagnosis can be safely made in asymptomatic individuals under the age of 40 with microscopic hematuria if there are red blood cells, no red blood cell casts, and clearance of hematuria within 72 hours of the precipitating physical activity.[3,5] The presence of gross hematuria raises the question of urothelial neoplasm, and the presence of red blood cell casts suggests a glomerular disease. Patients with exercise-induced hematuria will not damage their kidneys if they continue participating in the activities that elicit the phenomenon.[3]

─────────── ◢ REFERENCES ◣ ───────────

1. Mohr DN, Offord KP, Owen RA, et al: Asymptomatic microhematuria and urologic disease: a population-based study, *JAMA* 256:224-229, 1986.
2. Paul AB, Collie DA, Wild SR, et al: An integrated haematuria clinic, *Br J Clin Pract* 47:128-130, 1993.
3. Gambrell RC, Blount BW: Exercise-induced hematuria, *Am Fam Physician* 53:905-911, 1996.
4. Abarbanel J, Benet AE, Lask D, et al: Sports hematuria, *J Urol* 143:887-890, 1990.
5. Cianflocco AJ: Renal complications of exercise, *Clin Sports Med* 11:437-451, 1992.
6. Sears CLG, Ward JF, Sears ST, et al: Prospective comparison of computerized tomography and excretory urography in the initial evaluation of asymptomatic microhematuria. *J Urology* 168:2457-60, 2002.

MICROALBUMINURIA
(See also diabetes mellitus and hypertension; diabetic nephropathy)

Microalbuminuria is a urinary albumin excretion of 30 to 300 mg/24 hours. The gold standard is a 24-hour urine measurement, but because this may be difficult to achieve, and some debate the utility over a urine sample for random albumin:creatinine ratio.[1] A dipstick specific for microalbuminuria may be used instead. If the dipstick is used on a first morning specimen and the patient does not have a febrile illness, it is reasonably accurate. Other causes of false-positive results include exercise within 24 hours and congestive heart failure. A second dipstick reading should be performed within a few months to verify the results. Microalbuminuria is an important abnormality in a number of renal conditions, but particularly diabetic nephropathy. There has not been a systematic assembly of the literature to assess the risk relation between tests assessing the presence of microalbuminuria with cardiovascular, peripheral-vascular, renal, and neurological outcomes (all of which represent end-organ effects of long-term diabetes, however the detection of microalbuminuria and the subsequent treatment of the patient with ACE inhibitors slow the progression of diabetic nephropathy (see discussion of diabetic nephropathy).[2] Dietary reduction of animal protein has also been found to reduce the progression to overt nephropathy.[3] If ACE inhibitors are not well-tolerated, angiotensin-receptor antagonists are good second-line agents. Combination therapy of ACE-ARB is currently being looked at and shows promise.[5]

REFERENCES
1. *Use of Glycated Hemoglobin and Microalbuminuria in the Monitoring of Diabetes Mellitus.* Summary, Evidence Report/Technology Assessment: Number 84. AHRQ Publication No. 03-E048, July 2003. Agency for Healthcare Research and Quality, Rockville, MD.
2. Cattran DC: Microalbuminuria urine dip tests: recognize limits, *Patient Care Can* 7:8-9, 1996.
3. Pedrini MT, et al: The effect of dietary protein restriction on the progression of diabetic and non-diabetic renal diseases: a meta-analysis. *Annals of Internal Medicine,* 124: 627-632, 1996.
4. Lewis EJ, et al.: Renoprotective effect of the angiotensin receptor antagonist irbesartan in patients with nephropathy due to Type 2 diabetes. *New England Journal of Medicine,* 345: 851-860, 2001.
5. Nakao N, Yoshimura A, Morita H et al: Combination treatment of angiotensin-II receptor blocker and angiotensin-converting enzyme inhibitor in non-diabetic renal disease (COOPERATE): a randomised controlled trial. *Lancet* 361: 117-124, 2003.

POSTURAL PROTEINURIA
Patients with postural proteinuria have proteinuria only in the erect position. The diagnosis can be easily made by collecting urine samples immediately on arising in the morning and after being erect for a few hours. In some patients with postural proteinuria, protein excretion is present whenever the patient is erect, and in others it is intermittent.[1,2]

REFERENCES
1. Trempe D: L'analyse d'urine: bandelettes réactives ou sédiment urinaire? *Med Quebec* 29:25-31, 1994.
2. Rapoport A, Richardson RMA: How to tell it's proteinuria, *Patient Care Can* 5:13-18, 1994.

URINALYSIS
(See also bacteriuria and pyuria in the elderly; bladder cancer; diabetic nephropathy; exercise-induced hematuria; exertional rhabdomyolysis; fever without source; hematuria; IgA nephropathy)

Little is gained by a microscopic examination of urine that is dipstick-negative provided the dipstick is capable of detecting leukocytes.[1] Some important features of the urinalysis are described in the following paragraphs.

Specific Gravity
The usual specific gravity of an early morning urine sample is 1014 to 1028. Heavy proteinuria or glucosuria can elevate the specific gravity.

Glucose
False-negative glucose readings may occur if the patient has taken large quantities of Aspirin or vitamin C.

Blood
Dipsticks can detect as few as two or three red blood cells (RBCs) per high-power field.[1] If the dipstick is positive for blood but RBCs are not seen on microscopic examination, the explanation might be myoglobinuria or hemolysis of RBCs. False-negative readings may result if the patient has ingested large quantities of vitamin C or sometimes as a result of captopril (Capoten) therapy. Healthy people have up to three RBCs per high-power field in a centrifuged specimen.[2]

If the dipstick reading is positive for blood, microscopy to look for RBC casts is important. If such casts are found, the origin of the hematuria is the kidney and in the majority of cases there is underlying glomerular disease. RBC casts lyse quickly, so the urine should be examined by an experienced observer within 2 hours. The casts are better preserved in acid urine.[2]

Intermittent microscopic or even gross hematuria may be a result of vigorous exercise. In asymptomatic persons under the age of 40 with microscopic hematuria, the diagnosis can be safely made if microscopy shows RBCs but no RBC casts and if the hematuria clears within 72 hours of the precipitating physical activity.[3] If after vigorous exercise the urine is positive for blood, no RBCs are found with microscopy, and the patient is complaining of muscle pain or swelling, acute exercise-induced rhabdomyolysis should be considered. If the patient has this condition, the creatine kinase level is very high.[4]

Whether the incidental finding of microscopic hematuria in asymptomatic individuals merits a complete urological and nephrological workup is controversial. A fairly high incidence of significant disease has been reported from referral clinics where most of the patients were over 40 years of age,[2] but in a population survey the incidence of serious disease was only 2.3%.[5]

Both the Canadian Task Force on Preventive Health Care[6] and the U.S. Preventive Services Task Force[7] give a "D" recommendation for dipstick assessment of urine as a screening tool for bladder cancer in the general population.

Leukocytes

The dipstick detects neutrophils by reacting to some of the esterases these cells possess. This reaction takes place even if the white cells have lysed and are therefore not visible on microscopy.[1,2] The test is sensitive and can detect as few as three to five white blood cells (WBCs) per high-power field.[1]

Pyuria is usually defined as five or more WBCs per high-power field in a centrifuged specimen.[2] The presence of WBC casts suggests pyelonephritis or an autoimmune disease such as lupus.[1]

Asymptomatic pyuria and asymptomatic bacteriuria are common in elderly women and usually resolve spontaneously.[8]

Nitrites

The presence of nitrites in the urine occurs when certain bacteria convert nitrates to nitrites. This requires time, so a first-voided morning specimen is the ideal specimen for testing. Ascorbic acid may cause false-negative readings.[2]

Protein

The comments that follow should not be construed as advocating routine urinalysis of asymptomatic persons. The Canadian Task Force on Preventive Health Care recommends against routine protein dipstick analysis of the adult population as a screen for chronic renal disease ("D" recommendation).[6] The reason behind this is that no effective treatment is known for the majority of serious conditions that may cause proteinuria. An exception is diabetic nephropathy in persons with insulin-dependent diabetes. For this group of patients the Canadian Task Force Preventive Health Care recommends screening for microalbuminuria ("A" recommendation).[6]

The Ames dipstick is sensitive primarily for albumin and can detect as little as 15 to 20 mg/dl of protein. Results are classified as negative, trace (10 to 20 mg/dl), 1+ (30 mg/dl), 2+ (100 mg/dl), 3+ (300 mg/dl), and 4+ (1000 mg/dl).[9] Healthy persons may excrete a trace of protein,

particularly if the urine is concentrated. False-positive tests may be seen with highly alkaline urine (pH 7.5 to 8.0), with very concentrated urine, and in patients with gross hematuria.[2,9] False-negative findings occur with dilute urine.[2,9,10] Further investigations are probably unnecessary in a clinically healthy person whose only abnormality on more than one urinalysis is proteinuria of 30 mg/dl or less. Anyone with 100 mg/dl or more has significant proteinuria and needs further tests.[2,10] The dipstick will not detect Bence Jones protein or microalbuminuria.[10] Detection of the latter is important in follow-up of diabetic patients and is discussed under "Diabetic Nephropathy."

Aside from tests for blood urea nitrogen and creatinine and a complete blood count, an important investigation for a patient with proteinuria is a 24-hour urine protein excretion. Creatinine excretion should be measured at the same time to ensure adequacy of the sample. Normal values of 24-hour urine creatinine excretion are 1.3 to 2.2 mmol/kg (15 to 25 mg/kg) for men and 0.9 to 1.9 mmol/kg (10 to 22 mg/kg) for women. The average excretion of protein in the urine is 40 to 80 mg/day, and the upper limit of normal is 150 mg/day or 8 to 10 mg/dl (0.08 to 0.10 g/L). Proteinuria of 3 g/day or more is always the result of glomerular disease, and patients with this test result often have the nephrotic syndrome. (Patients with the nephrotic syndrome usually excrete more than 3.5 g of protein in the urine per day.) Patients with lesser degrees of proteinuria may have glomerular or tubular disease. If urinary protein is less than 1 g/day in an otherwise healthy person and urinalysis shows no other abnormalities, serious disease is unlikely and the patient simply requires follow-up at intervals of 3 to 6 months.[2,10]

Whether the proteinuria is persistent or intermittent is an important determination. Intermittent or transient proteinuria is generally benign and may be induced by fever, exercise, emotional stress, or posture. Postural proteinuria may be diagnosed if a voiding first thing in the morning is negative for protein whereas voidings in the erect position later in the day are positive.[10]

Screening Urinalysis

Screening urinalysis of healthy adults and children is of little value. The positive predictive value of abnormal dipstick results on screening urinalysis is approximately 12% to 16%. Considerable psychological and physical harm ensues to the many individuals who require further investigations to prove that they are normal.[11] Both the Canadian Task Force on Preventive Health Care[6] and the U.S. Preventive Services Task Force[7] give "D" or "E" recommendations for routine urinalysis during the pediatric years, as well as for such screening of the general adult population and the elderly. For pregnant women a urine culture between 12 and 16 weeks of pregnancy is recommended, and dipstick urinalysis is not an adequate substitute.[6,7]

❧ REFERENCES ❧

1. Kiel DP, Moskowitz MA: The urinalysis: a critical appraisal, *Med Clin North Am* 71:607-624, 1987.

2. Misdraji J, Nguyen PL: Urinalysis: when–and when not–to order, *Postgrad Med* 100:173-192, 1996.

3. Gambrell RC, Blount BW: Exercise-induced hematuria, *Am Fam Physician* 53:905-911, 1996.

4. Line RL, Rust GS: Acute exertional rhabdomyolysis, *Am Fam Physician* 52:502-506, 1995.

5. Mohr DN, Offord KP, Owen RA, et al: Asymptomatic microhematuria and urologic disease: a population-based study, *JAMA* 256:224-229, 1986.

6. Canadian Task Force on the Periodic Health Examination: *Canadian guide to clinical preventive health care,* Ottawa, Canada Communication Group, pp 826-836, 1994.

7. US Preventive Services Task Force: *Guide to clinical preventive services,* ed 2, Baltimore, Williams & Wilkins, pp 181-186, 1996.

8. Monane M, Gurwitz JH, Lipsitz LA, et al: Epidemiologic and diagnostic aspects of bacteriuria: a longitudinal study in older women, *J Am Geriatr Soc* 43:618-622, 1995.

9. Larson TS: Evaluation of proteinuria, *Mayo Clin Proc* 69:1154-1158, 1994.

10. Rapaport A, Richardson RM: How to tell it's proteinuria, *Patient Care Can* 5:13-18, 1994.

11. Kaplan RE, Springate JE, Feld LG: Screening dipstick urinalysis: a time to change, *Pediatrics* 100:919-921, 1997.

Topics covered in this section

CATARACTS

(See also macular degeneration)

Epidemiology

Cataracts account for the single largest cause of blindness worldwide. The distribution between the sexes is approximately equal. Cataracts are more common in black than white populations.[2] Diabetes[2,3] and oral and inhaled corticosteroids are risk factors in adults. Hypertension,[2] central obesity,[2] and smoking are probable[4] risk factors for cataracts.[3] An association has been reported between excessive exposure to ultraviolet B (UV-B) light and cataracts.[4] Effective protection against UV-B may be obtained by wearing sunglasses. A wide-brimmed hat cuts the exposure by 30% to 50%.[5] The majority of cataracts are senile- or age-related. Other etiologies include traumatic, metabolic, toxic, and secondary associations with other disease processes.

Symptoms and Signs

Several symptoms suggest cataracts as the cause of visual changes. Visual acuity progressively diminishes over time, manifested by cloudy or blurry vision, glare, halos, decreased night vision, faded colours, double vision, need for brighter light when reading and frequent changes in eyeglasses.[6] One sign that can occur early is "second sight" in far-sighted individuals because the cataract may change the refractive index of the lens so that the patient can begin to read without glasses.

Lens opacity may be evident by direct observation. Most cataracts can be detected with direct ophthalmoscopy. The examiner should set the lens wheel to 4+ diopters and examine the red reflex with the ophthalmoscope 15 to 20 cm from the patient's eye. Cataracts are usually seen as dark specks or a haze against the red reflex.[4]

Treatment

Before cataract surgery it is important to try to predict the degree of visual recovery that can be expected. Such surgery is pointless if macular degeneration will prevent visual acuity from being improved by the procedure. Ophthalmologists use two techniques for assessment: potential acuity measurement (PAM) and laser interferometry. Both procedures are painless and test macular function through small "windows" in the cataracts.[7]

Generally, cataract removal is indicated if there is interference with daily activities.[6] Cataracts can be removed at any stage of their development; it is a myth that surgery must wait until the cataract is "ripe."[7]

Cataract removal in developed countries use an extracapsular approach that removes the lens content but leaves the posterior lens capsule intact. The contents can be removed by direct extraction or phacoemulsification, which involves fragmenting the cataract with ultrasound. An intra-ocular lens is implanted in the capsular bag. If no lens is implanted then contact lenses or aphakic glasses are needed. One common complication is posterior capsule opacification (PCO) which can occur in the first few weeks or months after surgery. Clear vision is instantly re-established by use of a laser beam (yttrium aluminum garnet [YAG]) to cut a hole in the capsule.[7] Recent evidence suggests that the shape of the lens implanted influences the rate of PCO.[8,9] There is very little evidence to determine which is the best surgical approach for cataracts.[1]

Multifocal intra-ocular lenses which correct near vision as well as distance are now available. In a recent Cochrane review, multifocal lenses were equal to unifocal lenses for distance vision and visual acuity but improved near vision and a larger incidence of freedom from glasses was obtained. Adverse effects included reduced contrast sensitivity and the subjective experience of haloes around lights.[10] After surgery patients are usually given a combination of eyedrops to insert: antibiotics (fluoroquinolones) to prevent infection, steroids (prenisolone acetate 1%) to control inflammation and non-steroidal anti-inflammatory drops (ketorolac tromethamine 0.5%) to prevent macula edema. New eyeglasses are usually prescribed about 2 weeks after an uncomplicated extraction.[6]

≈ REFERENCES ≈

1. Snellingen T, Evans JR, Ravilla T, et al: Surgical interventions for age-related cataract. Cochrane Eyes and Vision Group, *Cochrane Database of Systematic Reviews* (2):CD001323, 2002.
2. Leske MC, Wu S-Y, Hennis A, et al: Diabetes, hypertension, and central obesity as cataract risk factors in a black population: the Barbados Eye Study, *Ophthalmology* 106:35-41, 1999.
3. West S: Does smoke get in your eyes? (editorial), *JAMA* 268:1025-1026, 1992.
4. Chylack LT Jr: Cataracts and inhaled corticosteroids (editorial), *N Engl J Med* 337:46-48, 1997.

5. West SK, Duncan DD, Munoz B, et al: Sunlight exposure and risk of lens opacities in a population-based study: the Salisbury Eye Evaluation Project, *JAMA* 280:714-718, 1998

6. Solomon R. Donnenfeld ED: Recent advances and future frontiers in treating age-related cataracts, *JAMA* 290(2): 248-51, July 9, 2003.

7. Fowler JH: Investigating cataracts–unveiling vision loss, *Can J Diagn* 11:64-77, 1994.

8. Prosdocimo G, Tassinari G, Sala M, et al: Posterior capsule opacification after phacoemulsification: silicone CeeOn Edge versus acrylate AcrySof intraocular lens. *J Cataract Refract Surg* 29(8):1551-1555, 2003.

9. Ernest PH: Posterior capsule opacification and neodymium: YAG capsulotomy rates with AcrySof acrylic and PhacoFlex II silicone intraocular lenses, *J Cataract Refract Surg* 29(8):1546-1550, 2003.

10. Leyland M, Zinicola E: Multifocal versus monofocal intraocular lenses after cataract extraction. Cochrane Eyes and Vision Group *Cochrane Database of Systematic Review* 2, 2004.

CONGENITAL LACRIMAL OBSTRUCTION

This is perhaps better termed *delayed canalization of the nasolacrimal duct*. Congenital lacrimal duct obstruction is common, with 6% to 20% of neonates manifesting symptoms of this condition.[1] In 80% of cases, the obstruction is unilateral. Symptoms are watering of the eye, and crusting of the lids so they are stuck together in the morning. The globe remains white, except in the case of a secondary infection. In 90% of cases, the obstruction spontaneously resolves within a year, and in the remaining cases, obstruction usually resolves spontaneously in the second year of life.[1] Treatment is to reassure the parents, clean the lids regularly, and apply topical antibiotics if obvious secondary conjunctivitis occurs (red eye and increased exudate). Probing of the lacrimal system during the first year is usually unnecessary[2] and may cause strictures. One study has shown that massaging the lacrimal sac while occluding the canaliculi opens the canal in some cases.[1]

❧ REFERENCES ❧

1. Young JD, MacEwen CJ: Managing congenital lacrimal obstruction in general practice, *BMJ* 315:293-296, 1997.
2. Robb RM: Congenital nasolacrimal duct obstruction, *Ophthalmol Clin North Am* 14(3):443-446, 2001.

CONJUNCTIVITIS: RED EYE

Red eye is the most common ocular problem presenting to the family doctor.[1] While most are benign conditions not every red eye is conjunctivitis. The differential diagnosis of a red eye is broad and can include pathology of lids, orbit, lacrimal system, conjunctiva, sclera, cornea, or the anterior chamber. It can be divided into two categories: traumatic and non-traumatic. Causes of traumatic red eye include corneal abrasion, foreign body (on cornea, intraocular, or under the lid), hyphema, ultraviolet keratitis, chemical injury, blow-out fracture and corneal laceration. Non-traumatic causes include conjunctivitis (viral, bacterial or allergic), subconjunctival hemorrhage, iritis, orbital or periorbital cellulites, herpes simplex keratitis, acute glaucoma, episcleritis and scleritis.[2] Always begin with a visual acuity.[3] A few key questions will help distinguish the cause of a red eye (Table 58).

Non-pharmacological treatment of the red eye include application of cold wet compresses for allergic or viral conjunctivitis[4] and hot wet compresses for blepharitis or styes.[3] For blepharitis practice lid hygiene daily at bedtime. This involves warm water compresses applied to closed eyelids for 5 to 10 minutes followed by gentle scrubbing of lid margins with a commercial eyelid scrub or a few drops of baby shampoo in a small amount of warm water.[5] Patients with contact lenses should not wear them until the problem has resolved (depending on the cause the lenses may need to be replaced). Makeup should be avoided.

Many eyedrops used in therapy, themselves are capable of causing irritation and can have serious side effects.[6] Corticosteroids may worsen herpetic/fungal keratitis. Long-term use of topical corticosteroids may cause glaucoma and/or cataracts. Topical decongestants/vasoconstrictors may provoke angle-closure glaucoma in those predisposed.

❧ REFERENCES ❧

1. Leibowtiz HM: The red eye, *N Engl J Med* 343(5):345-351, 2000.
2. Canadian Ophthalmological Society: Self-directed learning modules. Assessment of the red eye. Available from: http://www.eyesite.ca/7modules/Module2/html/Mod2_TOC.html. Accessed May 17, 2004.
3. Garcia GE: Management of ocular emergencies and urgent eye problems, *American Family Physician* 53(2):565-574, Feb 1, 1996.
4. Bielory L: Update on ocular allergy treatment, *Expert Opinion on Pharmacotherapy* 3(5):541-553, 2002.
5. Key JE: A comparative study of eyelid cleaning regimens in chronic blepharitis, *CLAO J* 22(3):209-212, 1996.
6. Ventura MT, Di Corato R, Di Leo E: Eyedrop-induced allergy: clinical evaluation and diagnostic protocol, *Immunopharmacol Immunotoxicol.* 25(4):529-538, 2003.

CORNEA

(See also refractive errors; topical ophthalmic medications)

Corneal Lesions

The two most common corneal lesions are abrasions and foreign bodies. Foreign bodies may result in corneal abrasions, infection or scarring if not removed promptly.

Table 58 Differential Diagnosis of the Red Eye

	Conjunctivitis	Acute Iritis	Acute angle closure glaucoma	Keratitis
Discharge	Bacteria: purulent Virus: serous Allergy: mucous	No	No	Profuse tearing
Pain	No	++ (tender globe)	+++ (nauseating)	++ (on blinking)
Photophobia	No	+++	+	++
Blurred Vision	No	++	+++	Varies
Pupil	Normal	Smaller	Fixed in mid-dilation	Same or smaller
Injection	Conjunctiva with limbal pallor	Ciliary flush	Diffuse	Diffuse
Cornea	Normal or opacified	Keratitis precipitates	Cornea steamy	Infiltrate edema, epithelial defects
Intraocular Pressure	Normal	Varies	Increased markedly	Normal or increased
Anterior chamber	Normal	Cells plus flare	Shallow coloured halos	Cells plus flare or normal
Other	Large tender pre-auricular node if viral	Posterior synechiae	Nausea and vomiting	
Treatment	Bacterial: topical broad spectrum AB Viral: usually self limiting, supportive Rx Allergic: antihistamine, mast cell stabilizer	Mydriatics to dilate pupil, refer to ophthalmologist for confirmation of diagnosis and steroid treatment	Refer to ophthalmologist for immediate treatment to preserve vision. Treatment may include miotic drops, steroids, laser treatment	Refer to ophthalmologist. Treatment may include topical or systemic antivirals. May require steroids.

Corneal abrasions are epithelial defects usually due to trauma (i.e., fingernails, paper, twigs) or contact lenses. Symptoms include pain, redness, tearing, photophobia and foreign body sensation. Clinical signs may include foreign body, conjunctival injection, corneal edema or anterior chamber cell/flare. The de-epithelialized area will stain with fluoroscein dye. Pain is relieved with topical anesthetic, which should only be used to facilitate examination and never as the treatment for this condition.

Antibiotic ointment is not necessary in the routine treatment of corneal abrasions, and there is no published evidence supporting its use. Simple corneal abrasions do not require eye patching.[1] Abrasions 1 cm in diameter or smaller heal faster and with less pain when no patch is used.[2] Cold compresses and oral non-steroidal anti-inflammatory drugs (NSAIDs) may give adequate pain relief.[3] A good alternative is topical ophthalmic NSAID drops such as ketorolac tromethamine (Acular) 0.5%, four times per day.[4] A topical mydriatic such as homatropine or cyclopentolate (Cyclogyl) may also be used for pain relief.

The wearing of contact lenses may be associated with corneal lesions that appear to be simple abrasions (see discussion of contact lenses), but are actually infectious keratitis caused by *Pseudomonas aeruginosa*, or a protozoan of the *Acanthamoeba* species. This type of keratitis is more common in persons wearing overnight contact lenses or extended-wear contact lenses. Patching is contraindicated in patients with infectious keratitis. Immediate ophthalmological consultation is highly desirable.[5] *Pseudomonas*

infection is treated by the frequent instillation of antibiotics such as an aminoglycoside (gentamicin [Garamycin Ophthalmic] or tobramycin [Tobrex]) or a quinolone (ciprofloxacin [Ciloxan], norfloxacin [Chibroxin], or ofloxacin [Ocuflox]) and follow-up within 24 hours. Steroid drops should never be used.[6]

Care should be taken not to misdiagnose a corneal herpetic infection as a corneal abrasion. Herpetic lesions have a dendritical appearance, and because of decreased corneal sensitivity in the region of the lesion, the corneal reflex is diminished. Treatment may include topical or systemic antivirals like acyclovir and dendritical debridement. Referral to an ophthalmologist is advisable. Steroids should only be prescribed by an ophthalmologist.

Corneal Transplants

Corneal transplant is the single most common type of human transplant surgery. As such, it is important for family physicians to make their patients aware of the possibility of cornea donation. In a study done of corneal transplants in British Columbia, Canada, 12 months after the procedure visual acuity improved in 69.9% of patients, remained the same in 20.8%, and worsened in 5.9%.[7]

────────── ◢ REFERENCES ◣ ──────────

1. NHS Centre for Reviews and Dissemination: Should we patch corneal abrasions, *Database of Abstracts of Reviews of Effectiveness* (2), 2004.

2. Kaiser PK (Corneal Abrasion Patching Study Group): A comparison of pressure patching versus no patching for corneal abrasions due to trauma or foreign body removal, *Ophthalmology* 102:1936-1942, 1995.
3. Mindlin AM: Treatment of corneal abrasions (letter), *JAMA* (275):837, 1996.
4. Brown MD, Cordell WH, Gee AS: Do ophthalmic nonsteroidal anti-inflammatory drugs reduce the pain associated with simple corneal abrasion without delaying healing?, *Ann Emerg Med* 34:526-534, 1999.
5. Sharma S: Ophthaproblem: contact lens *(Acanthamoeba)* keratitis, *Can Fam Physician* 44:1605, 1615, 1998.
6. Jampel HD: Patching for corneal abrasions, *JAMA* 274:1504, 1995.
7. Saunders PP, Sibley LM, Richards JS, et al: Outcome of corneal transplantation: can a prioritization system predict outcome? *British Journal of Ophthalmology* 86(1):57-61, Jan. 2002.

GLAUCOMA
Acute Angle-Closure

(See also glaucoma, open-angle)

Epidemiology

Acute angle-closure glaucoma occurs when the peripheral iris blocks the outflow of aqueous humor at the trabecular meshwork in the anterior chamber. Acute angle-closure glaucoma has an incidence ranging from 4.1 to 10.4 per 100,000[1,2] peaking at ages 50 to 69.[3] Hypermetropic eyes (long-sighted eyes) are at increased risk because the globe is smaller and has a shallower anterior chamber. Other risk factors include family history, female sex, and being of Inuit, South Asian or Chinese descent.[3]

Prodromal symptoms

Patients with acute angle-closure glaucoma usually have had prodromal symptoms resulting from temporary increases in intraocular pressure. Such preliminary symptoms include slight blurring of vision, mild headaches, and occasionally seeing haloes around objects. Precipitating factors are those causing pupillary dilation such as the dim light of a movie theater, the adrenergic response to anger or anxiety, mydriatics and anticholinergic medications such as tricyclic antidepressants.[4]

Symptoms and signs

Acute angle-closure glaucoma is characterized by sudden and extreme increase in intraocular pressure. The patient complains of agonizing eye pain, blurred vision, and often headache. Nausea and vomiting are common, and sometimes the patient has abdominal and chest pain. The eye is red with a ciliary flush, the cornea is steamy/cloudy, and the pupil is dilated, fixed, and usually vertically oval. Ballottement of the globe often reveals a stony hard consistency, although failure to detect this sign does not rule out acute glaucoma. Visual acuity is markedly diminished.[4] Untreated, optic nerve damage occurs. The diagnosis is best made with a slit lamp, but in the office one can perform the oblique flashlight test. In this test, a penlight or flashlight is held on non-nasal side and parallel to the iris of the eye. When the beam is shone across the anterior chamber, if the whole iris is illuminated, the angle can be considered open. If a shadow is cast on the iris near the nose, then the angle can be assumed to be narrow or closed. The sensitivity of this test was 80% and specificity 69% in one study.[3]

Management

Acute angle-closure glaucoma is considered a medical emergency. Immediate management of acute angle-closure glaucoma is directed toward lowering the intraocular pressure with medication. One three-stage protocol is as follows[4]:
1. Instill 2 drops of a topical beta blocker such as timolol (Timoptic 0.5%) plus 2 drops of pilocarpine 2%.
2. If the attack has not stopped in 15 minutes, give acetazolamide (Diamox) 200 to 500 mg plus an osmotic diuretic, such as glycerol solution in orange juice, 1.5 to 2 g/kg, or mannitol 1 g/kg IV over a 20 minute period. This step may be repeated twice at 2-hour intervals.
3. Perform surgery, usually in the form of laser iridotomy for definitive treatment. A recent review of 33 trials of treatment for angle-closure glaucoma found the only evidence-based treatment to be laser peripheral iridotomy of both the affected and unaffected eye.[5]

REFERENCES
1. Ivanisevic M, Erceg M, Smoljanovic A, Trosic Z: The incidence and seasonal variations of acute primary angle-closure glaucoma, *Collegium Antropologicum* 26(1):41-45, 2002.
2. Lai JS, Liu DT, Tham CC, et al: Epidemiology of acute primary angle-closure glaucoma in the Hong Kong Chinese population: prospective study *Hong Kong Medical Journal* 7(2):118-123, 2001.
3. Coleman AL: Glaucoma. *Lancet* 354(9192):1803-1810, 1999 20.
4. Balazsi AG: Looking into the signs of glaucoma, *Can J Diagn* 10:65-85, 1993.
5. Saw SM, Gazzard G, Friedman DS: Interventions for angle-closure glaucoma: an evidence-based update, *Ophthalmology* 110(10):1869-78; quiz 1878-1879, 1930, 2003.

Open-Angle

(See also asthma; glaucoma, acute angle-closure; screening)

Terminology

Glaucoma is the second most common cause of blindness in the United States and the leading cause among blacks. In open-angle glaucoma there is progressive damage to the optic nerve seen by increasing optic disc cupping and visual field loss. The outflow of aqueous humor is decreased relative to its production and intraocular pressure (IOP) rises.[1] Vision loss is irreversible. Ocular hypertension and glaucoma are not synonymous. Although most patients with glaucoma have elevated intraocular pressures (greater than 21 mm Hg), at least 15% of patients have normal pressures (normal-tension glaucoma). However more than two thirds of individuals who have elevated intraocular pressures have no evidence of glaucoma (ocular hypertension).[1]

Risk factors

Recognized risk factors for open-angle glaucoma include the following:

1. Elevated intraocular pressure
2. Age over 65
3. Family history of glaucoma, especially siblings
4. Black race
5. Severe myopia
6. Diabetes
7. Previous eye trauma
8. Previous eye surgery
9. Corticosteroid use (topical, inhaled, systemic)
10. Vasospasm (migraines, Raynaud's)

Screening

Standard screening techniques are tonometry and funduscopy, but they are neither sensitive nor specific. Perimetry (formal visual-field testing) is too complex to be a practical screening tool.[1] Both the Canadian Task Force on Preventive Health Care[2] and the U.S. Preventive Services Task Force[3] give a "C" recommendation to screening manoeuvres for glaucoma. An alternative strategy is to limit screening to those at high risk, blacks over 40, whites over 65, patients with a family history, diabetes or severe myopia.[1]

Clinical signs

Patients are usually asymptomatic until more than 40 percent of the optic nerve is lost and then they can experience "tunnel vision" (peripheral field loss) and decreased visual acuity.[1] Signs include the following[4]:

1. Visual field defects, especially in the nasal quadrants
2. Elevated intraocular pressure measured with Schiötz or applanation tonometry
3. Cup/disc ratio greater than 0.7
4. Difference of more than 0.2 in the cup/disc ratio between the two eyes
5. Oval cup with the vertical diameter greater than the horizontal diameter
6. Notching of the cup
7. Occasionally splinter hemorrhages at the disc margins
8. Afferent pupillary defect (Marcus Gunn pupil)

Treatment

The principle underlying treatment of glaucoma is that lowering IOP will arrest the progression of the disease. Two ongoing randomized control trials confirm that early treatment (medical and/or surgical) can delay progression of the disease by half.[5,6] Even patients with normal tension glaucoma will benefit from lowering IOP.[7] A wide variety of topical drugs are available for lowering IOP by either decreasing aqueous production (beta blockers, carbonic anhydrase inhibitors), increasing aqueous outflow (prostaglandin analogues, cholinergic agonist) or both (alpha agonists) (Table 59).[1] Non-selective beta blockers or prostaglandin analog drops are used first line. Beta blockers, which decrease IOP by 20% to 25%, were the traditional drugs of first choice, but respiratory and cardiovascular adverse effects are common. One drop of 0.5% timolol solution in each eye is equivalent to a 10 mg oral dose. Specific adverse effects include diminished pulmonary function in about one fourth of patients, bradycardia and a significantly increased incidence of falls.[8] They are contraindicated in patients with reactive airways, congestive heart failure or conduction defects. A simple technique for decreasing systemic absorption while at the same time increasing ophthalmic absorption is to occlude the nasolacrimal duct with pressure from a finger or simply by closing the eyes firmly for 5 minutes after applying the drops.[9]

Latanoprost (Xalatan), a topical prostaglandin analog, is now the number one prescribed glaucoma medication in the world. It is only needed once a day and is more effective than beta blockers in lowering IOP with less serious side effects.[10] Side effects include increased eyelash growth, and iris/eyelash pigmentation.[1] Alpha$_2$-adrenergic agonists are useful as adjunctive therapy but are limited by the incidence of allergic reactions.[1] The cholinergic agonist pilocarpine is rarely used now as it must be taken four times a day, has local side effects, and can cause confusion.[8] If one drug does not work, one from another class or a combination of topical drugs can be used.[9]

While oral carbonic anhydrase inhibitors are usually prescribed for acute angle-closure glaucoma, they are occasionally used for patients with chronic open-angle glaucoma. Caution is needed because they can cause metabolic acidosis, paresthesias, altered taste, and, rarely, aplastic anemia and other blood dyscrasias.[9] The two most frequently used drugs in this class are acetazolamide (Diamox) 250 mg to 1 g daily in divided doses and methazolamide (Neptazane) 50 to 100 mg bid or tid.

If medical therapy fails or the adverse effects are unacceptable, the next option is either laser trabeculoplasty, which has about a 50% 5-year success rate in the elderly, or surgical incisional trabeculectomy.[11] In laser trabeculoplasty a low-power argon laser beam is focused on the trabecular meshwork. This usually increases the

Table 59   Topical Medications for Chronic Open-Angle Glaucoma

Drugs	Usual dose
Topical Non-Selective Beta Blockers	
Carteolol (Ocupress) 1%	1 drop bid
Levobunolol (AK Beta, Betagan) 0.25% and 0.5%	1 drop bid
Metipranolol (Optipranolol) 0.3%	1 drop bid
Timolol (Betimol, Timoptic) 0.25% and 0.5%	1 drop bid except for Timoptic-XE, which is 1 drop daily
Topical Cardioselective Beta Blockers	
Betaxolol (Betoptic) 0.25% and 0.5%	1 drop bid
Topical Alpha$_2$-Adrenergic Receptor Agonists	
Apraclonidine (Iopidine) 0.5% and 1%	1 drop tid
Brimonidine tartrate (Alphagan) 0.2% and 0.15%	1 drop tid
Brimonidine tartrate (Alphagan) 0.2% and 0.15%	1 drop tid
Topical Cholinergic Myopics	
Pilocarpine 1%, 2%, 4% and 6%	1-2 drops qid
Topical Carbonic Anhydrase Inhibitors	
Brinzolamide (Azopt) 1%	1 drop tid
Dorzolamide (Trusopt) 2%	1 drop tid
Topical Prostaglandin Analogues	
Latanoprost (Xalatan) 0.005% (50 μg/ml)	1 drop qhs
Bimatoprost (Lumigan) 0.03%	1 drop od
Travoprost (Travatan) 0.004%	1 drop od
Unoprostone (Rescula) 0.15%	1 drop bid

outflow of aqueous humor with a resultant decrease in the intraocular pressure of about 30%.[12] The advanced glaucoma intervention study compared different sequences of trabeculoplasty (laser:incision:incision versus incision:laser:incision) for medically uncontrolled glaucoma. Long-term visual function was better in blacks with the first sequence and for whites with the second.[13]

❧ REFERENCES ❧

1. Distelhorst JS, Hughes GM: Open-angle glaucoma. *American Family Physician* 67(9):1937-1944, 2003.
2. Canadian Task Force on the Periodic Health Examination: Periodic health examination, 1995 update. 3. Screening for visual problems among elderly patients, *Can Med Assoc J* 152:1211-1222, 1995.
3. US Preventive Services Task Force: *Guide to clinical preventive services,* ed 2, Baltimore, 1996, Williams & Wilkins, pp 383-391.
4. Balazsi AG: Looking into the signs of glaucoma, *Can J Diagn* 10:65-85, 1993.
5. Kass MA, Heuer DK, Higginbotham EJ, et al: The Ocular Hypertension Treatment Study: a randomized trial determines that topical ocular hypotensive medication delays or prevents the onset of primary open-angle glaucoma, *Arch Ophthalmol* 120 (6)701-713, 2002.
6. Leske MC, Heijl A, Hussein M, Bengtsson B, Hyman L, Komaroff E: Factors for glaucoma progression and the effect of treatment: the Early Manifest Glaucoma Trial, *Arch Ophthalmol* 121(1):48-56, 2003.
7. Anderson DR: Collaborative normal tension glaucoma study, *Curr Opin Ophthalmol* 14(2):86-90, 2003.
8. Brimonidine—an alpha-2-agonist for glaucoma, *Med Lett* 39:54-55, 1997.
9. Alward WL: Medical management of glaucoma, *N Engl J Med* 339:1298-1307, 1998.
10. Diestelhorst M, Schaefer CP, Beusterien KM, et al: Persistency and clinical outcomes associated with latanoprost and beta-blocker monotherapy: evidence from a European retrospective cohort study. *European Journal of Ophthalmology 13 Suppl 4*:S21-29, 2003.
11. Diggory P, Franks W: Medical treatment of glaucoma—reappraisal of the risks, *Br J Ophthalmol* 80:85-89, 1996.
12. Tucker JB: Screening for open-angle glaucoma, *Am Fam Physician* 148:75-80, 1993.
13. Ederer F, Gaasterland DA, Dally LG, et al: AGIS Investigators. The Advanced Glaucoma Intervention Study (AGIS): 13. Comparison of treatment outcomes within race: 10-year results. *Ophthalmology* 111(4):651-664, 2004.

MACULAR DEGENERATION
(See also cataracts; vitamin A)

Age-related macular degeneration (AMD) is the leading cause of blindness in the Western world.[1] In AMD, the retinal pigment epithelium and neurosensory receptors degenerate especially affecting the macula.[2] As certain types of macular degeneration are treated effectively with laser, it is important to recognize its occurrence and to refer appropriately. Clues that the cause is macular degeneration rather than cataracts are loss of colour discrimination and spontaneous use of a magnifying glass by the patient.[3]

Age-related macular degeneration is the most common cause of irreversible blindness among persons over the age of 52. Its incidence is about 1% in 55-year-olds and rises to 15% by age 80.[4] Smoking, hypertension and a positive family history are risk factors.[1] Macular degeneration is often divided into two groups; the more common (85%) *dry* form and the more sight-threatening *wet* (exudative). The wet form accounts for 90% of severe visual loss in the elderly.

In the dry form, drusen (yellow amorphous deposits), pigment cell abnormalities and geographic atrophy are seen. In the wet form (also called exudative), Bruch's membrane is broken and new blood vessels from the choroid grow into the deeper layers of the retina (choroidal neovascularisation). The new blood vessels are leaky and cause edema from extravasation of blood and lipid materials. The end result is a dense fibrovascular scar that may involve the entire macular area.

Symptoms include blurring of central vision, meta-morphopsia (distortion of central vision), reduced vision and recent onset of a scotoma, or blind spot. The main symptom in dry macular degeneration is a gradual difficulty in performing fine discriminate tasks and in the wet form is central blurring and sudden onset of visual distortion.

AMD is detected with an ophthalmoscope. The macula is examined for drusen, subretinal exudates, hemorrhages, neovascularization, or pigment stippling. Visual acuity and Amsler grid testing should be conducted. A simple office test is used to show the patient a piece of graph paper. With AMD, the squares may look distorted and the lines wavy.[1] In the wet form, retinal angiography is performed using fluorescein and/or indocyanine green dyes to detect and follow choroidal neovascularization.

Wet macular degeneration was originally treated with thermal laser photocoagulation but this method was found to be useful in only a select group (10%) of patients.[2] Photodynamic therapy using a non-thermal laser and the photosensitizing drug verteporfin is more widely applicable. In one study, 31% of eyes with classic neovascularisation (well defined and leaks dye) treated with photodynamic therapy, at 2 years had moderate or worsening of visual loss compared with 59% of the placebo-treated eyes.[5] Laser treatment cannot restore vision that is already lost. Future therapies being investigated involve antivascular endothelial growth factor medications administered systemically or intravitreally to try and prevent new vessel formation.[2]

Some studies have suggested that certain carotenoids, especially lutein and zeaxanthin, which are found in dark green leafy vegetables such as spinach and collard greens, have a protective effect against age-related macular degeneration.[1] In a randomized placebo-controlled trial of 1193 healthy volunteers, Vitamin E (500 IU) for four years was not found to prevent formation of AMD.[6] In a National Institutes of Health study in patients with AMD four groups were compared: Zinc oxide (80 mg) versus beta-carotene (15 mg), vitamin C (500 mg) and vitamin E (400 IU) versus both versus placebo. Those at highest risk for advancing AMD in the combination group as compared to placebo, lowered their risk of disease progression by about 25%. These results cannot be extrapolated to the general public and smokers.[7] Studies are being conducted to determine if prophylactic laser treatment of drusen will prevent progression to wet AMD.[2]

The U.S. Preventive Services Task Force[8] and the Canadian Task Force on Preventive Health Care[4] give a "C" recommendation to fundoscopy for the detection of age-related macular degeneration. Both these organizations give a "B" recommendation to visual acuity testing in the elderly.[4,8]

◢ REFERENCES ◣

1. Chopdar A, Chakravarthy U, Verma D: Age-related macular degeneration *BMJ* 326(7387):485-488, 2003.
2. Gottlieb JL: Age-related macular degeneration, *JAMA* 288(18):2233-2236, 2002.
3. Fowler JH: Investigating cataracts–unveiling vision loss, *Can J Diagn* 11:64-77, 1994.
4. Canadian Task Force on the Periodic Health Examination: Periodic health examination, 1995 update. III. Screening for visual problems among elderly patients, *Can Med Assoc J* 152:1211-1222, 1995.
5. Bressler NM: Treatment of Age-Related Macular Degeneration with Photodynamic Therapy (TAP) Study Group. Photodynamic therapy of subfoveal choroidal neovascularization in age-related macular degeneration with verteporfin: two-year results of two randomized clinical trials-tap report 2. *Archives of Ophthalmology* 119(2):198-207, 2001.
6. Taylor HR, Tikellis G, Robman LD, et al: Vitamin E supplementation and macular degeneration: randomized controlled trial, *BMJ* 325:11-14, 2002.
7. Age-Related Eye Disease Study Research Group: A randomized, placebo-controlled clinical trial of high dose supplementation with vitamins C and E, beta-carotene and zinc for age-related macular degeneration and vision loss: AREDS report no. 8, *Arch Ophthalmol* 119:1417-1436, 2001.
8. US Preventive Services Task Force: *Guide to clinical preventive services,* ed 2, Baltimore, 1996, Williams & Wilkins, pp 373-391.

REFRACTIVE ERRORS
Contact Lenses

Approximately 1 out of every 20 contact lens wearers develops a contact lens–related complication each year. Complications range from mild to sight-threatening and can involve the lids (ptosis, fibrosis, abcess) conjunctiva (contact dermatitis, giant papillary conjunctivitis) or cornea (abrasion, hypoxia, keratitis).[1] A rare but serious complication of contact lens use that may lead to blindness is microbial keratitis or corneal ulceration, which is usually caused by *Pseudomonas* or *Staphylococcus* species. A study from the Netherlands found the annual incidence among daily-wear soft contact lens wearers was 3.5 per 10,000 users.[2] Microbial keratitis can occur with daily-wear lenses or disposable lenses even when they are used correctly and taken out at night,[2,3] but the risk is much greater if the lenses are worn overnight.[2] Symptoms usually present acutely with pain, photophobia, tearing, purulent discharge, and reduced vision.[1] Traditional treatment consists of frequent (every 15 to 30 minutes) instillation of a combination of topical antibiotics such as cefazolin 50 mg/mL and tobramycin 14 mg/mL). Ciprofloxacin 0.3% and ofloxacin 0.3% alone may be as effective.[1] Patients travelling to remote areas may be advised to include topical ophthalmic antibiotics in an emergency medical kit.[3]

❧ REFERENCES ❧

1. Contact Lens Complications from eMedicine Dr.John Stamler (Accessed on April 27, 2004 at http://www.emedicine.com/oph/topic651.htm#section~corneal_endothelium_and_summary)
2. Cheng KH, Leung SL, Hoekman HW, et al: Incidence of contact-lens-associated microbial keratitis and its related morbidity, *Lancet* 354:181-185, 1999.
3. Donzis PB: Corneal ulcers from contact lenses during travel to remote areas (letter), *N Engl J Med* 338:1629-1630, 1998.

Refractive Laser Surgery

The two classes of surgical techniques for refractive error correction are: laser shaping of the cornea—LASIK (Laser In Situ Keratomileusis) or PRK (Photorefractive Keratectomy) and intraocular lens implants such as phakic IOLs. LASIK and PRK can correct hyperopia and myopia of +5.00 D to −10.00 with astigmatism between −0.25 D and −6.00 D. Low myopia up to −5.00 D is amenable to PRK, and high myopia of over −7.00 D is best treated by LASIK, with both procedures being acceptable between −5.00 and −7.00 D. They are performed with an excimer laser that emits ultraviolet light, which photoablates the superficial tissue layers without causing significant thermal damage to surrounding tissues.

PRK and LASIK are outpatient procedures that take only a few minutes to perform. They are generally contraindicated in persons under the age of 18.[1]

In PRK, the surface corneal epithelium and part of the stroma is albated. The more advanced from of PRK called ASA (Advanced Surface Ablation) reduces the risk of corneal haze by administration of mitomyocin, an antiproliferative chemotherapeutic agent at the time of the procedure and using more precisely controlled lasers. The patient is left with a large iatrogenic corneal abrasion that takes several days to heal. A disposable bandage contact lens is applied. Immediate complications include significant tearing, photophobia, blurred vision and pain.[1]

Topical antibiotics and NSAIDs are used until the abrasion is healed and steroid eyedrops are given for 1 to 3 months. Eyesight fluctuates until around three months post-operatively. Glare, halos and dry-eye symptoms are common during the first month but usually are gone by 6 months post-operatively.[1]

LASIK involves cutting a corneal flap with a microtome. The flap is flipped over and the excimer laser ablates a thin layer of corneal stroma. The flap is then replaced. Healing is faster than PRK because the epithelium is intact. An antibiotic and steroid eyedrop is given for 5 days post-operatively. LASIK does not produce stromal haze but flap complications can occur. In both procedures complications include under/over correction, astigmatism, regression, glare, halos, dryness and reduced contrast sensitivity. Conditions such as large pupils and high degrees of myopia and hyperopia put some patients at greater risk for night vision problems (complication rate 1%).

For higher degrees of myopia or hyperopia (more than −10.00 D or 5.00 D), a different surgical technique is used: Phakic IOL, Intraocular contact LENs (ICL), or Refractive Lens Exchange. In phakic IOL a lens is inserted in the anterior chamber attached to the iris. For ICL a soft lens is placed behind the iris and in front of the crystalline lens. Accommodation is preserved and the procedure is highly reversible. However, patients with large pupils and/or shallow anterior chambers are contradicted.[2] A refractive lens exchange is a lens extraction with insertion of a foldable posterior chamber lens implant, similar to a cataract lens extraction (but without a cataract). It can correct from +20.00 D to −30.00 D. This results in a lost accommodation, so it is better for older patients who would require reading glasses. If both eyes are done, monovision is an option with one eye for distance viewing and the other for reading.[2] The main risk is endophthalmitis but rare at 1 in 10,000 eyes.

A suitable patient should be 18 years of age, with a stable refractive error (no more than 0.5D in spherical or cylinder) and in good health. Contraindications are cataract, herpes simplex, retinal disease, diabetic retinopathy, glaucoma, and pregnancy. Correction of refractive errors following other ocular surgery, including cataract surgery, can be performed. LASIK appears to be preferable since a significant risk of corneal haze formation exists if PRK is performed on an eye with any previous corneal surgery. It is preferable to wait at least 6 months after the procedure for the correction to stabilize before performing an "enhancement" surgery in the event of over or under correction.

❧ REFERENCES ❧

1. Bower KS, Weichel ED, Thomas JK: Overview of refractive Surgery. *Am Fam Physician* 2001;64:1183-90,1193-1194.
2. Stein R: The optometrist's role in co-managing refractive surgery: patient selection, counseling, preop exam and postop care, *Clinical & Refractive Optometry* 14(9) 265-275, 2003.

TOPICAL OPHTHALMIC MEDICATIONS
(See also allergic rhinitis; glaucoma)

While the majority of a topically applied medication to the eye is wasted, some medications can penetrate as far back as the retina.[1] Research is ongoing into new drug delivery methods.[2] Topical application can result in allergy to the drug itself or the preservative.[3] A study comparing instillation of room temperature saline solution with warmed solution showed decreased pain with the warmed solution.[4]

Eyedrop Instillation in Children

Instilling eyedrops in recalcitrant children is difficult. Confrontation may be avoided by having the child lie supine with eyes closed while the drops are applied to the lids near the medial canthus. When the eyes are opened, most of the drops flow onto the conjunctiva. A British ophthalmologist evaluated this technique using pilocarpine. When the degree of pupillary dilatation was measured, it was calculated that 66% of the drug entered the eye.[5]

Anesthetics

A frequently used topical anesthetic is proparacaine (Alcaine, Ophthaine, Ophthetic). The usual dose for removing corneal foreign bodies and other procedures is 1 or 2 drops of a 0.5% solution.

Antibacterials

A variety of topical antibiotics are available, and a number of them are listed in Table 60. These are all available in the form of ophthalmic drops and ointments. Dosages vary slightly among products, but as a general rule for severe conjunctivitis, 1 or 2 drops is instilled every 1 to 2 hours while the patient is awake for the first 1 to 2 days and the dose is then reduced to q4-6h for the next few days. If the infection is mild, drops are applied q4-6h. Ointments may be applied at bedtime. Sulfacetamide sodium (Sodium Sulamyd) comes as a 10% and a 30% solution; most family physicians use the 10% solution. Tobramycin ophthalmic products are safe for children of all ages. The safety of fluoroquinolone ophthalmic preparations for children under 1 year of age has not been established. Although the odds are slim that chloramphenicol eyedrops would cause aplastic anemia, 23 cases of serious hematological toxicity have been reported in a U.S. national register.[3] Since other antibiotic drops are available, prudence dictates reservation in the use of chloramphenicol.[6] Some clinicians prefer ointments when there is significant eyelid involvement.

Antihistamines, Vasoconstrictors, and Mast Cell Stabilizers

Topical antihistamines or antihistamines combined with vasoconstrictors may give relief to some patients with allergic conjunctivitis. Emedastine difumarate (Emadine) 1 to 2 drops qid, Levocabastine (Livostin) 1 drop daily, olopatadine (Patanol) 1 to 2 drops bid, epinastine (Elestat)1 drop bid, azelastine (Optivar) 1 drop bid and ketotifen (Zaditor) 1 drop q8h to q12h are examples of ophthalmic antihistamines.

Many antihistamine-vasoconstrictor combinations are available over the counter. The use of these agents has

Table 60   Topical Ophthalmic Antibacterials

Generic names	Trade names
Aminoglycosides	
Gentamicin	Garamycin
Tobramycin	Tobrex, AKTob
Fluoroquinolones	
Ciprofloxacin	Ciloxan
Gatifloxacin	Zymar
Lecofloxacin	Quixin
Norfloxacin	Chibroxin
Ofloxacin	Ocuflox
Moxifloxacin	Vigamox
Sulfonamides	
Sulfacetamide sodium	Sodium Sulamyd
Other	
Bacitracin	
Chloramphenicol	Chloroptic
Fusidic Acid	Fucithalmic
Combinations	
Gramicidin/neomycin/polymixin B	Neosporin
Polymixin B/trimethoprim	Polytrim

been associated with induction of both acute and chronic conjunctivitis.[7] Examples of these combination drugs are naphazoline plus pheniramine (Naphcon-A) and naphazoline plus antazoline (Vasocon-A). The usual dose is 1 or 2 drops in each eye every 3 to 4 hours.

Topical vasoconstrictors alone decrease redness of the eyes in patients with allergic conjunctivitis, and many of these are available over the counter. Examples are phenylephrine (Neo-Synephrine), tetrahydrozoline (Visine), and naphazoline (Clear Eyes, Naphcon).

Mast cell stabilizers that may relieve symptoms of allergic conjunctivitis are cromolyn sodium (Crolom, Opticrom)1 to 2 drops qid, lodoxamide (Alomide) 1 to 2 drops qid and nedocromil (Alocril) 1 to 2 drops bid. Ketorolac (Acular), a topical ophthalmic NSAID, has been used for treatment of allergic conjunctivitis.

Cycloplegic Mydriatics

Drugs that paralyze the ciliary muscle and thus inhibit accommodation are cycloplegics, and those that dilate the pupils are mydriatics. Many agents do both. Short-acting cycloplegic mydriatics such as tropicamide (Mydriacyl) 0.5% or 1% are generally used by family physicians for dilating the pupil to facilitate fundoscopy. Longer-acting drugs such as cyclopentolate (Cyclogyl) 1% or 2%, atropine (IsoptoAtropine) 1% or homatropine 2% or 5% may be used to relieve ciliary spasm (and pain) from corneal abrasions or for the treatment of iritis or uveitis.

Glaucoma Medications

Glaucoma medications are discussed in the earlier section on glaucoma.

Non-Steroidal Anti-Inflammatory Drugs

Ophthalmic NSAIDs relieve the pain of corneal abrasion. Some of the available agents are flurbiprofen (Ocufen), diclofenac (Voltaren), and ketorolac (Acular).

Tears and Lubricants

A large number of artificial-tear preparations are available without prescription for symptomatic treatment of dry eyes. The usual dose is 1 to 2 drops q1-4h. Examples are hydroxypropyl methylcellulose (Isopto Tears, Lacril, Tears Naturale), polyvinyl alcohol (Hypotears, Liquifilm, Tears Plus), and polysorbate (Teardrops). Lubricating ointments containing white petrolatum and mineral oil may be applied to dry eyes at bedtime. They are often used in cases of Bell's palsy to prevent the cornea from drying. Examples are DuraTears and Lacri-Lube.

✑ REFERENCES ✍

1. Koevary SB: Pharmacokinetics of topical ocular drug delivery: potential uses for the treatment of diseases of the posterior segment and beyond. *Current Drug Metabolism* 4(3):213-22, 2003.
2. Kaur IP, Garg A, Singla AK, et al: Vesicular systems in ocular drug delivery: an overview. *Int J Pharmaceutics,* 269(1):1-14, 2004.
3. Robert PY, Adenis JP: Comparative review of topical ophthalmic antibacterial preparations, *Drugs* 61(2):175-85, 2001.
4. Ernst AA, Thomson T, Haynes M, et al: Warmed versus room temperature saline solution for ocular irrigation: a randomized clinical trial. *Ann Emerg Med* 32:676-679, 1998.
5. Smith SE: Eyedrop instillation for reluctant children, *Br J Ophthalmol* 75:480-481, 1991.
6. Doona M, Walsh JB: Topical chloramphenicol is an outmoded treatment (letter), *BMJ* 316:1903, 1998.
7. Soparkar CN, Wilhelmus KR, Koch DD, et al: Acute and chronic conjunctivitis due to over-the-counter ophthalmic decongestants, *Arch Ophthalmol* 115:34-48, 1997.

EAR
External Ear
Foreign bodies

Many foreign bodies may be removed from the external auditory canal by syringing. This method should not be used for organic materials (e.g., peas, beans) because they may absorb the water and swell. It should not be used for disk batteries such as those in watches and hearing aids because when exposed to water they may leak and cause severe tissue damage. Small children often require a general anesthetic before removal of foreign bodies.[1]

Instilling mineral oil or 2% lidocaine into the canal will kill live insects. The remains may then be gently syringed out.[1]

Otitis externa

Seborrheic dermatitis and other skin conditions can affect the ear canal and cause otitis externa. A common treatment for these conditions is steroid drops alone such as betamethasone (Betnesol Otic) or steroid drops combined with other ingredients such as hydrocortisone plus acetic acid and propylene glycol (VoSol HC Otic).

A variety of bacterial organisms, especially *Staphylococcus aureus* and *Pseudomonas aeruginosa,* have been associated with otitis externa, but in many cases an infectious etiology cannot be ascertained. The most consistently observed predisposing factor is frequent water exposure,[2,3] and one reported method of preventing the condition is to instill 2 to 4 drops of an equal mixture of vinegar (5% acetic acid) and rubbing alcohol (70% isopropyl alcohol) into the ear canals immediately after coming out of the water.[3] Swimming in freshwater lakes has led to outbreaks of *P. aeruginosa* otitis externa.[4] Fungal infections, whether caused by *Candida* or *Aspergillus niger,* are rare in North America.

Medications for bacterial otitis externa often include aminoglycosides (gentamicin, neomycin, or framycetin). Ototoxicity from the use of gentamicin (Garasone Otic) drops has been reported in patients with perforated drums. In patients with perforations, topical drugs containing aminoglycosides should not be used or should be used for as short a time as possible, applied to an ear wick (gauze strip) rather than directly into the canal, and

discontinued immediately if tinnitus, hearing loss, vertigo, or imbalance develops.[5]

Most of the topical antibiotics used for otitis externa are combinations of antibiotics and steroids; the corticosteroids are used to diminish inflammation and prevent obstruction of the canal. Combinations of hydrocortisone, neomycin, and polymyxin B (e.g., Cortisporin Otic) and hydrocortisone and ciprofloxacin (Cipro HC Otic) are available in both the United States and Canada. In Canada combinations of betamethasone and gentamicin (Garasone Otic) or of dexamethasone, framycetin, and gramicidin (Sofracort) are also on the market, and chloramphenicol drops without steroids (Chloromycetin Otic) and ofloxacin (Floxin Otic) drops without steroids may be obtained in the United States. In a 2003 trial with adult patients suffering from OE for less than 3 weeks and done in the primary care setting, steroid and acetic acid combinations work as well as steroid and antibiotic combination drops in uncomplicated otitis externa. Acetic acid eardrops, however, result in longer recovery time and more treatment failures than treatments that include a steroid with an antibiotic or acetic acid. With drops containing steroid with antibiotic or acetic acid, half of otitis externa patients will recover within a week. Most of the other half will recover within 2 weeks.[6]

Indications for systemic antibiotics in the treatment of external otitis are few. According to one U.S. survey, however, 40% of patients with external otitis received both topical and systemic medications, and in most cases the systemic antibiotics were not active against *S. aureus* or *P. aeruginosa.*[7]

Wax

An effective ceruminolytic is a liquid formulation of docusate (Colace, Regulex). Between 8 and 10 drops should be instilled into the canal and left for 10 minutes, followed by instrumental or lavage removal of the cerumen.[8] A 2000 trial randomized docusate (Colace) versus 1 ml triethanolamine oleate (Cerumenex) placed in the ear. After 15 minutes there was no difference but post-irrigation with water, 82% of the docusate-treated subjects had completely visualized ears as compared with 35% of the triethanolamine oleate-treated ears.[9]

_____ ❧ **REFERENCES** ❧ _____

1. Ansley JF, Cunningham MJ: Treatment of aural foreign bodies in children, *Pediatrics* 101:638-641, 1998.
2. Russell JD, Donnelly M, McShane DP, et al: What causes acute otitis externa? *J Laryngol Otol* 107:898-901, 1993.
3. Larimore WL, Hartman JR, Shupe TB, et al: Diary from a week in practice, *Am Fam Physician* 55:2651, 1997.
4. van Asperen IA, de Rover CM, Schijven JF, et al: Risk of otitis externa after swimming in recreational fresh water

lakes containing *Pseudomonas aeruginosa*, *BMJ* 311:1407-1410, 1995.

5. Canadian Adverse Drug Reaction Newsletter: Aminoglycoside ear drops and ototoxicity, *Can Med Assoc J* 156:1056, 1997.
6. Van Balen RAM, Smit WM, Zuithoff NPA, et al: Clinical efficacy of three common treatments in acute otitis externa in primary care: randomised controlled trial, *BMJ* 327:1-5, 2003.
7. Halpern MT, Palmer CS, Seidlin M: Treatment patterns for otitis externa, *J Am Board Fam Pract* 12:1-7, 1999.
8. Chen DA, Caparosa RJ: A nonprescription cerumenolytic, *Am J Otol* 12:475-476, 1991.
9. Singer AJ, Sauris E, Viccellio AW: Ceruminolytic effects of docusate sodium: a randomized, controlled trial, *Ann Emerg Med* 36:228-32, 2000.

Middle Ear

(See also aviation medicine; scuba diving)

Otitis media

(See also middle ear effusion; tonsillectomy)

Acute Otitis Media. Based on tympanocentesis as the gold standard, at least 40% of patients in whom acute otitis media is diagnosed on the basis of clinical findings do not have the disease. Pneumatic otoscopy may increase the specificity of diagnosis but is not commonly used in practice.[1]

Symptoms of upper respiratory tract infection such as cough or rhinorrhea are seen in 94% of children with acute otitis media. In the absence of such symptoms the diagnosis of otitis media is unlikely.[2] In one study the positive predictive value of ear pain as a symptom of acute otitis media in children with upper respiratory tract symptoms was 83%; however, 40% of children with otitis media did not have pain.[3]

Viruses alone or in combination with bacteria are the major causes of otitis media.[4,5] The most common viruses are respiratory syncytial viruses, rhinoviruses and influenza viruses.[4] The most common bacterial pathogens are *Streptococcus pneumoniae*, *Haemophilus influenzae*, and *Branhamella (Moraxella) catarrhalis*.[4,5]

About 30% to 40% of *Haemophilus* and 50% to 90% of *Branhamella* organisms produce β-lactamase and are resistant to amoxicillin in vitro. In some areas 15 to 50% of pneumococci are resistant to penicillin due to alterations of the penicillin-binding protein.[5] However, this in vitro resistance does not usually translate into clinical ineffectiveness.

Reputed advantages of routinely using antibiotics for acute otitis media are that these drugs decrease the duration of symptoms and the rate of complications. Careful review of the literature does not substantiate this. Some studies found no improvement in outcomes with antibiotics,[6] and others reported only a slight advantage.[7] Three separate meta-analyses have found that 80% of

children with acute otitis media had spontaneous relief of symptoms within 2 to 14 days. In children less than 2 years, spontaneous resolution of symptoms was suggested to be 30%.[7] A 2001 trial randomized 315 children to either an immediate prescription versus "wait and see" for 3 days before parents could fill the prescription. Most (75%) did not get the wait-and-see prescription filled. On average, symptoms resolved in both groups within 3 days of the visit. Some outcomes resolved more quickly with therapy: fewer days of illness (1.1 days less per child), less acetaminophen use (½ dose, on average, per child), fewer days of crying, and less night disturbance. Other outcomes did not differ: mean pain scores, episodes of distress, or absence from school. Ten percent more of the children in the immediate treatment group had diarrhea. As well, the parents that waited may employ more self-care the next time around.[8]

The option of observing the patient without the use of antibiotics is now recommended by the American Academy of Pediatrics. This option is available for healthy children, 2 years and older without severe symptoms or when the diagnosis is uncertain. It is also available to children 6 months to 2 years with non-severe illness at presentation *and* an uncertain diagnosis. Caregiver reliability and follow up at 48 to 72 hours (either by phone or appointment) must be assured and antibiotics prescribed if symptoms do not improve or worsen.[5] If the decision is made to use an antibiotic then the American Academy of Pediatrics recommends, as first line therapy, amoxicillin at the higher dose of 80 to 90 mg/kg per day.[5] If severe illness is present (defined as moderate to severe otalgia or fever = 39° C) or β-lactamase coverage is required (for *H. influenzae* or *M. catarrhalis*) high-dose amoxicillin-clavulanate should be initiated. Suggested indications for using β-lactamase-stable drugs, such as amoxicillin-clavulanic acid (Augmentin, Clavulin), erythromycin-sulfisoxazole (Pediazole), or a second- or third-generation cephalosporin, are persistent symptoms for more than 48 to 72 hours while the patient is taking the initial antibiotic, development of otitis media while the patient is taking amoxicillin, or an episode of otitis media within the previous 2 months that did not respond to amoxicillin.[5,9] If amoxicillin allergy is present, other treatment options include trimethoprim-sulfamethoxazole, clarithromycin, azithromycin or erythromycin-sulfisoxazole. In patients unable to tolerate oral medication, a single dose of intramuscular ceftriaxone (50 mg/kg) has been shown to be an effective treatment.[5]

No solid guidelines for optimal duration of treatment with antibiotics have been established. Good results have been reported with 2, 3, 5, and 10 days.[10] One meta-analysis concluded that for uncomplicated acute otitis media in children a 5-day course was as effective as a 10-day course. The power of the study was insufficient to determine whether this was true for children under

2 years of age or those with perforated drums,[10] and therefore 10 days should probably be used in these circumstances.[1]

Persistent ear pain in children with otitis media is not necessarily due to persistent bacterial infection. One study of children treated with antibiotics found that 62% had persistent symptoms even when bacteriological cure was shown by tympanostomy cultures.[11] Viral infection is probably a major cause of this phenomenon.[12] All children should receive adequate analgesia (Acetaminophen or Ibuprofen).[7] A recent Cochrane review of antihistamines and/or decongestants for acute otitis media found no benefit for either medication alone and only a small decrease in persistent otitis media at 2 weeks for the combination. Due to increased side effects they recommend against either medication alone or in combination.[13]

Recurrent Otitis Media. The first-line management of recurrent otitis media is to make sure that environmental risk factors are eliminated. Important ones are eliminating exposure to tobacco smoke, using small rather than large daycare facilities,[15] and if feasible, taking pacifiers away from the children. (A Finnish prospective study of children under 3 years attending daycare found that those who used pacifiers had 25% more episodes of acute otitis media than those who did not.[16])

According to some experts three episodes of otitis media occurring within a 6-month period are an indication for prophylactic antibiotics.[15] These are usually given daily for several months, especially during the winter. Some physicians give antibiotics only at the onset of an upper respiratory tract infection, but this does not seem to be as effective. Prophylactic regimens include amoxicillin 20 mg/kg/day as a single dose or in two divided doses or sulfisoxazole 75 mg/kg/day as a single dose or in two divided doses. Prophylactic antibiotics are at least as effective as ventilation tubes in preventing further infections.[17]

How strong is the evidence supporting the prophylactic administration of antibiotics for otitis media? A 1993 meta-analysis of a number of trials found a small benefit,[18] whereas a more recent randomized placebo-controlled trial found none.[19]

Results of clinical trials have documented that myringotomy and tympanostomy tube insertion are effective for prevention of recurrent AOM.[20] Adenoidectomy or adenotonsillectomy leads to a slight short-term decrease in recurrence rates, but in view of the surgical morbidity, few indications exist for such interventions.[21]

A pneumococcal 7-valent conjugate vaccine was made available in the United States in 2000 and in Canada in 2001. This new vaccine is effective for children less than two years of age as opposed to the pneumococcal polysaccharide vaccine, which was effective only in older children.[22] There was hope that this new vaccine when administered in infancy would decrease the incidence

of otitis media. Thus far, trials show it does reduce pneumococcal invasion but other bugs take over likely resulting in no net benefit. A systematic review of four trials involving the pneumococcal conjugate vaccine in infants vaccinated as early as two months of age and toddlers attending daycare as well as toddlers with recurrent AOM showed only a small effect on prevention of AOM.[23]

❧ REFERENCES ❧

1. Pichichero ME: Changing the treatment paradigm for acute otitis media in children (editorial), *JAMA* 279: 1748-1750, 1998.
2. Ruuskanen O, Heikkinen T: Otitis media: etiology and diagnosis, *Postgrad Med* 13(suppl 1):S23-S26, 1994.
3. Heikkinen T, Ruuskanen O: Signs and symptoms predicting acute otitis media, *Arch Pediatr Adolesc Med* 149:26-29, 1995.
4. Heikkinen T, Thint M, Chonmaitree T: Prevalence of various respiratory viruses in the middle ear during acute otitis media, *N Engl J Med* 340:260-264, 1999.
5. American Academy of Pediatrics: Clinical practice guideline: diagnosis and management of acute qtitis media, *Pediatrics* 113:1451-1465, 2004.
6. Froom J, Culpepper L, Jacobs M, et al: Antimicrobials for acute otitis media? A review from the International Primary Care Network, *BMJ* 315:98-102, 1997.
7. Maroeska M, Schilder A, Zielhuis G, et al: Otitis Media, *The Lancet* 363: 465-473, 2004.
8. Little P, Gould C, Williamson I, et al: Pragmatic randomised controlled trial of two prescribing strategies for childhood acute otitis media, *BMJ* 322:336-342, 2001.
9. Paradise JL: Treatment guidelines for otitis media: the need for breadth and flexibility, *Postgrad Med* 14:429-435, 1995.
10. Kozyrsky J AL, Hildes-Ripstein E, Longstaffe A, et al: Treatment of acute otitis media with a shortened course of antibiotics: a meta-analysis, *JAMA* 279:1736-1742, 1998.
11. Marchant CD, Carlin SA, Johnson CE, et al: Measuring the comparative efficacy of antibacterial agents for acute otitis media: the "Polyanna phenomenon," *J Pediatr* 120:72-77, 1992.
12. Arola M, Ziegler T, Ruuskanen O: Respiratory virus infection as a cause of prolonged symptoms in acute otitis media, *J Pediatr* 116:697-701, 1990.
13. Flynn, CA, Griffin, G, Tudiver, F: Decongestants and antihistamines for acute otitis media in children. Cochrane Acute Respiratory Infections Group *Cochrane Database of Systematic Reviews. 1,* 2004.
14. Aronoff SC: Antimicrobials in children and the problem of drug resistance (editorial), *Am Fam Physician* 54:44-56, 1996.
15. Giebink GS: Preventing otitis media, *Ann Otol Rhinol Laryngol* 163(suppl):20-23, 1994.
16. Niemela M, Uhari M, Mottonen M: A pacifier increases the risk of recurrent acute otitis media in children in day care centers, *Pediatrics* 96:884-888, 1995.
17. Berman S: Otitis media in children, *N Engl J Med* 332:1560-1565, 1995.

18. Williams R, Chalmers T, Stange KC, et al: Use of antibiotics in preventing recurrent acute otitis media and in treating otitis media with effusion, *JAMA* 270:1344-1351, 1993.

19. Roark R, Berman S: Continuous twice daily or once daily amoxicillin prophylaxis compared with placebo for children with recurrent acute otitis media, *Pediatr Infect Dis J* 16:376-381, 1997.

20. Klein J: Nonimmune strategies for prevention of otitis media, *Pediatr Infect Dis J* 19:S89-92, 2000.

21. Paradise JL, Bluestone CD, Colborn DK: Adenoidectomy and adenotonsillectomy for recurrent acute otitis media, *JAMA* 282:945-953, 1999.

22. Infectious Diseases and Immunization Committee, Canadian Pediatric Society: Pneumococcal vaccine for children, *Paediatrics and Child Health* 6:214-217, 2002.

23. Straetemans M, Sanders EAM, Veenhoven RH, et al: Pneumococcal vaccines for preventing otitis media, *Cochrane Database of Systematic Reviews*, 1, 2004

Middle ear effusion
(See also otitis media)

The management of otitis media with effusion has traditionally involved the insertion of ventilation tubes. This is the second most common surgical procedure in U.S. children, superseded only by circumcision.[1]

Risk factors for otitis media with effusions include bottle-feeding, exposure to passive smoke, and attendance at daycare or other group infant facilities.[2]

Longitudinal studies of young children with middle ear effusions have shown that by 3 months 50% of effusions have resolved spontaneously and that resolution continues thereafter at a constant rate so that by 1 year few children still have an effusion.[2]

Suggested initial treatment is observation and probably antibiotics. Antibiotics have been shown to increase the resolution rate by 14%.[2] Spontaneous resolution rates of 20% to 56% coupled with a very slight benefit of antibiotic therapy favours the watchful waiting of otherwise healthy children for three months before considering intervention.[3,4] A cogent reason for avoiding antibiotics whenever possible in the treatment of serous otitis media is to slow the development of antibiotic-resistant organisms.[5]

The rationale for myringotomy with tube insertion is primarily to improve hearing and prevent difficulties in language development. However, no conclusive evidence has been presented to support or reject this hypothesis. The American Academy of Pediatrics (AAP) Clinical Practice Guideline identifies the following as candidates for surgery: children with OME lasting 4 months or longer with persistent hearing loss or other signs and symptoms; recurrent or persistent OME in children at risk regardless of hearing status; and OME and structural damage to the tympanic membrane or middle ear.[4]

Tympanostomy tubes are recommended as initial surgery as randomized trials have shown a relative decrease of 62% in effusion prevalence.[3,4] In a study in the United Kingdom, children who met these criteria were selected at random either to receive immediate placement of ventilation tubes or to be observed for a further 9 months with placement of tubes at that time if hearing deficits persisted. Eighty-five percent of children in the watchful waiting arm of the study required tubes (15% were spared surgery). Expressive language scores were slightly lower in the watchful waiting group at 9 months, but by 18 months no differences between the groups were detectable.[6]

Treatments that are not recommended include antihistamines, decongestants, corticosteroids, and tonsillectomy.[2,4]

Adenoidectomy is a controversial issue. Some experts, as represented by the Otitis Media Panel,[2] believe there is almost no indication for adenoidectomy in the treatment of serous otitis media, others that it has a role in primary treatment with or without ventilation tubes,[7,8] and still others that it is indicated if treatment with ventilation tubes is unsuccessful.[4,5,9]

❧ REFERENCES ❧
---

1. Berman S: Otitis media in children, *N Engl J Med* 332:1560-1565, 1995.

2. Otitis Media Guideline Panel: Managing otitis media with effusion in young children, *Am Fam Physician* 50:1003-1010, 1994.

3. Rovers M, Schilder A, Rosenfeld R: Otitis Media, *Lancet*, 363:465-473, 2004

4. American Academy of Pediatrics subcommittee on Otitis Media with Effusion: Otitis media with effusion, *Pediatrics*, 113:1412-1429, 2004.

5. Paradise JL: Managing otitis media: a time for change (editorial), *Pediatrics* 96:712-715, 1995.

6. Maw R, Wilks J, Harvey I, et al: Early surgery compared with watchful waiting for glue ear and effect on language development in preschool children: a randomised trial, *Lancet* 353:960-963, 1999.

7. Bicknell PG: Role of adenotonsillectomy in the management of pediatric ear, nose and throat infections, *Postgrad Med* 13:S75-S78, 1994.

8. Maw AR: Tonsils and adenoids: their relation to secretory otitis media, *Acta Otorhinolaryngol* 40:81-88, 1988.

9. Paradise JL, Bluestone CD, Rogers KD, et al: Efficacy of adenoidectomy for recurrent otitis media in children previously treated with tympanostomy-tube placement: results of parallel randomized and nonrandomized trials, *JAMA* 263:2066-2073, 1990.

Inner Ear

Hearing impairment
Audiological Assessment of Children. It is estimated that 1 in every 1000 children is born with profound bilateral

deafness (> 90 dB) and 5 in every 1000 with other forms of deafness (> 40 dB). Reduced hearing during the first years of life can interfere not only with the acquisition of language but also with a child's psychological and intellectual development, with subsequent repercussions on his or her overall development.[1]

Conventional audiometry can rarely be performed on children under 4 years of age, but a variety of other techniques can assess hearing capabilities even in infants. Two important tests are otoacoustic emissions (OAE) and auditory brainstem responses (ABR). In response to environmental sounds the cochlea generates very soft sounds of its own which can be detected by a small probe placed in the ear canal (with young infants this is best done when they are asleep). The threshold of hearing loss is then determined by the auditory brainstem response.[2]

Evidence suggesting that intervening (e.g., amplification via hearing aids or cochlear implant, sign language, total communication programs) at 3 or 6 months of age improves the development of language and speech have led some bodies to recommend universal early detection programs.[1] The U.S. Preventive Services Task Force (USPSTF) concludes the evidence is insufficient to recommend for or against routine screening of newborns for hearing loss during the postpartum hospitalization.[3] A cost-effective analysis of universal screening showed equal benefit with selective screening although further analysis needs to be done.[4]

Cochlear implants

Modern cochlear implants use multielectrode arrays that provide several channels of stimulation. The electrodes are implanted into the cochlea near the auditory nerve. At present, 2 years is the lower age limit for implants. Most cochlear implants may be damaged by magnetic resonance imaging.[5] The value of cochlear implants is controversial.[6] It is claimed that both adults and children with profound sensorineural hearing loss receive significant benefit, including improved speech and reading ability because of supplemental information from the implant.[5] On the other hand, many deaf people function well in society and do not consider themselves to have a disability requiring medical therapy (see discussion of cultural aspects of deafness below).[6,7]

Hearing aids

Digital hearing aids not only amplify specific frequencies, but also distinguish speech from background noise.[8] Traditional hearing aids are behind-the-ear models, but improved technology has allowed the development of in-the-ear, in-the-canal, and completely-in-the-canal models. Behind-the-ear aids are generally used for children because changes in the canal with growth would require up to four changes a year for in-the-canal types.[2]

Screening for hearing loss in the elderly

A Dutch study found that the sensitivity and specificity of the whispered voice test were excellent compared with formal audiograms for detecting hearing losses greater than 30 dB (a level of loss causing social disability). Screening audiograms and auriscopes with built-in audiometric devices had high sensitivities for losses greater than 40 dB, but specificities were low. The whispered voice test is much less expensive.[9]

The Canadian Task Force on Preventive Health Care[10] gives a "B" recommendation to screening elderly patients by enquiring, whispered voice test, or audioscope. The USPSTF[11] also gives a "B" recommendation to screening elderly people for hearing impairment by periodically questioning them about their hearing while routine screening with audiometry is not recommended ("C" recommendation).

Smoking

Both active smoking and passive smoking are associated with an increased risk of hearing loss.[12]

Cultural aspects of deafness

Many deaf people, particularly those who were born deaf, identify with the "Deaf" community. This community uses American Sign Language and tends not to use vocal speech or to lip read. Members have some concern that cochlear implants, if proven effective and popular, would marginalize this culture of communication.[7]

❧ REFERENCES ❧

1. Puig T, Municio A, Medà C: Universal neonatal hearing screening versus selective screening as part of the management of childhood deafness (Protocol for a Cochrane Review). In *The Cochrane Library,* Issue 2, Chichester, UK, 2004, John Wiley & Sons.

2. Papaioannou V: Audiological assessment and (re)habilitation in children, *Patient Care Can* 10(1):32-41, 1999.

3. US Preventive Services Task Force *Guide to Clinical Preventive Services*, 3rd Edition, Periodic Updates.

4. Keren R, Helfand M, Homer C, et al: Projected cost-effectiveness of statewide universal newborn hearing screening *Pediatrics* 110(5):855-864, 2002.

5. NIH Consensus Conference: Cochlear implants in adults and children: NIH Consensus Development Panel on Cochlear Implants in Adults and Children, *JAMA* 274:1955-1961, 1995.

6. Swanson L: Cochlear implants: the head-on collision between medical technology and the right to be deaf, *Can Med Assoc J* 157:929-932, 1997.

7. Lane H, Bahan B: Ethics of cochlear implantation in young children: a review and reply from a deaf-world perspective, *Otol Head Neck Surg* 119:297-313, 1998.

8. Werner J, Gottschlich S: Recent advances: otorhinolaryngology, *BMJ* 315:354-357, 1997.

9. Eekhof JA, de Bock GH, de Laat JA, et al: The whispered voice: the best test for screening for hearing impairment in general practice? *Br J Gen Pract* 46:473-474, 1996.
10. Canadian Task Force on the Periodic Health Examination: *Canadian guide to clinical preventive health care,* Ottawa, 1994, Canada Communication Group—Publishing, pp 954-963.
11. US Preventive Services Task Force: *Guide to clinical preventive services,* ed 2, Baltimore, 1996, Williams & Wilkins, pp 393-405.
12. Cruickshanks KJ, Klein R, Klein BE, et al: Cigarette smoking and hearing loss: the Epidemiology of Hearing Loss Study, *JAMA* 279:1715-1719, 1998.
13. Barnett S: Clinical and cultural issues in caring for deaf people, *Fam Med* 31:17-22, 1999.

Motion Sickness

The traditional medications for motion sickness are H_1 receptor antagonists such as dimenhydrate (Dramamine, Gravol) 50 to 100 mg qid, preferably given 1 to 2 hours before onset of motion, and scopolamine patches (Transderm-Scop, Transderm-V) applied to the post-auricular area 12 hours before onset of motion and changed every 72 hours.[1] There have some small studies on the use of acupressure at the wrist to control motion sickness but the results have been mixed.[2,3]

Anecdotal advice includes eating light meals low in dairy and high protein, avoid alcohol, increase ventilation, avoid visual stimuli (e.g., reading, watching videos), focus on a stable horizon or object, limit head movements, stay in a central location on boat or plane or front seat of a car, or lie down.[4]

REFERENCES

1. Nicholson AN, Pascoe PA, Spencer MB, et al: Jet lag and motion sickness, *Br Med Bull* 49:285-304, 1993.
2. Miller KE, Muth ER. Efficacy of acupressure and acustimulation bands for the prevention of motion sickness, *Aviat Space Environ Med.* 75(3):227-234, 2004.
3. Stern RM, Jokerst MD, Muth ER, Hollis C: Acupressure relieves the symptoms of motion sickness and reduces abnormal gastric activity, *Altern Ther Health Med* (4):91-94, 2001.
4. Gahlinger PM: Motion sickness: How to help your patients avoid travel travail, *Postgrad Med* 106:4, 1999.

Tinnitus

Healthy individuals frequently experience intermittent tinnitus lasting a few minutes. Although tinnitus lasting weeks, months, or years may occur in individuals with normal hearing, it is usually associated with hearing loss. The most frequent causes of such hearing loss are sensorineural loss as occurs in presbycusis, noise-induced hearing loss, and Ménière's disease. Tinnitus may also be induced by middle ear disease such as otitis media, serous otitis media, and otosclerosis, external ear disease such as an occluding wax plug, and certain drugs such as Aspirin as well as intracranial disease like acoustic neuroma. With time, most people become less bothered by their tinnitus. The most important therapeutic intervention is reassurance and supportive therapy for symptoms. Consider a consult or further investigations in patients with unilateral subjective tinnitus, in the presence of an audible bruit by auscultation of the skull or carotid, in patients with vibratory tinnitus with clicking or popping sounds, which may be indicative of neoplasms and which should be diagnosed using angiography, CT, or radiography and in patients who do not respond to treatment, particularly those with severely bothersome symptoms.[1] For some patients with hearing impairment as well as tinnitus, hearing aids ameliorate both symptoms. A few patients benefit from tinnitus-masking devices that can be worn in or behind the ear.[2]

REFERENCES

1. Crummer RW, Hassan GA: Diagnostic approach to tinnitus, *Am Fam Physician* 69:120-126,127-128, 2004;.
2. Vesterager V: Tinnitus—investigation and management, *BMJ* 314:728-732, 1997.

MOUTH
Aphthous Ulcers
(See also treatment of specific AIDS-related disorders; dentistry)

There are multiple causes for aphthous ulcers of the mouth including:

- Infections (e.g., Coxsackie, HSV, syphilis)
- Trauma
- Chemicals (including medications)
- Malignancies
- Nutritional deficiencies
- Associations with systemic illnesses (e.g., HIV, SLE, Crohn's and ulcerative colitis).

About 4% of patients with recurrent oral ulcers have a gluten enteropathy. The ulcers respond to a gluten-free diet.[1]

History is very helpful in determining the cause and will direct appropriate investigations. Recurrent ulcers suggest a systemic illness or recurring trauma. The following blood tests may be helpful: CBC, ferritin, vitamin B_{12}, folate, zinc, ESR, routine liver and chemistry tests. Further tests for systemic diseases, swabs or a biopsy may be needed.

Most ulcers resolve without therapy. First-line treatment is supportive and usually topical. Topical anesthetics are available such as a lidocaine solution; half a teaspoon xylocaine to two teaspoons water swished around the mouth for a few minutes, or benzocaine gel. The cheapest, most available, and most effective treatment for symptom relief is diphenhydramine, 5 mL in 10 mL of water, which the patient swishes in the mouth and then expectorates or swallows. This provides a local anesthetic action and some relief of local inflammation.

The application of a solution of sucralfate (Sulcrate) to aphthous ulcers four times a day using an applicator stick not only decreased the duration of pain and the time until healing, but also increased the duration of remissions.[2]

Amlexanox (Aphthasol), an inhibitor of inflammatory mediators, is marketed as a 5% oral paste to be applied to the ulcers four times a day. Controlled trials have shown it to be effective.[3] For more severe lesions, corticosteroids (e.g., Kenalog in Orabase) will help but are contraindicated if the ulcer is caused by an infection. A number of studies have suggested that thalidomide (Synovir) in doses of 50 to 200 mg/day is effective in treating and preventing severe aphthous ulcers in both HIV-negative and HIV-positive patients.[4]

≥ REFERENCES ⮜

1. Srinivasan U, Weir DG, Feighery C, et al: Emergence of classic enteropathy after longstanding gluten sensitive oral ulceration, *BMJ* 316:206-207, 1998.
2. Rattan J, Schneider M, Arber N, et al: Sucralfate suspension as a treatment of recurrent aphthous stomatitis, *J Intern Med* 236:341-343, 1994.
3. Khandwala A, Vaninwegen RG, Alfano MC: 5-Percent amlexanox oral paste, a new treatment for recurrent minor aphthous ulcers. 1. Clinical demonstration of acceleration of healing and resolution of pain, *Oral Surg Oral Med Oral Pathol* 83:222-230, 1997.
4. New uses of thalidomide, *Med Lett* 38:15-16, 1996.

NOSE
Allergic Rhinitis
(See also topical ophthalmic medications; vasomotor rhinitis)

Allergic rhinitis is characterized by paroxysmal sneezing, clear nasal secretions often with a decreased sense of smell. It is usually either seasonal, with pollens or perennial often with dust or animal dander. Differential diagnosis includes vasomotor rhinitis (may be caused by irritant and primarily obstruction and rhinorrhea), upper respiratory tract infections, and nasal polyps. Symptoms include nasal obstruction, itch and rhinorrhea, often with associated conjunctival symptoms, and paroxysmal sneezing. History typically includes a seasonal pattern (warm weather) or perennial pattern (dust mites or animal danders) and is diagnostic.

Environmental control
Environmental control is the most frequently forgotten therapeutic manoeuvre.

House Dust Mites. Fecal residue from the house dust mite is the major source of allergen in house dust.[1] Mites can be killed by washing bedding in hot water. Other appropriate steps to reduce levels of mite antigen include removing rugs; encasing mattresses and pillows in allergen-proof plastic; keeping household humidity below 50%; not using humidifiers; and dusting frequently with a damp cloth. High-efficiency particulate air (HEPA) filters are often recommended to further reduce dust in the bedroom, but rigorous evidence of their benefit is lacking.[2,3]

Moulds. Moulds are another important allergen. In general, homes with reduced ventilation and higher degrees of ambient humidity favour the proliferation of mould. Surfaces such as basement walls, shower stalls and sinks can be wiped down regularly with products that contain chlorine bleach and other fungicides (e.g., Clorox or Lysol). Air conditioning units can harbour significant amounts of mould and should be inspected and cleaned regularly.[1]

Animals. Pets, primarily cats and dogs but also birds and other warm-blooded animals, are a significant source of allergens. Removing the pet from the home is the most effective way to reduce symptoms, although doing so will not confer an immediate cure. In the case of cats, it may take as long as 20 weeks for the allergen levels to reach those of a home that has never had a cat.[1] Bathing cats weekly may reduce the amount of airborne allergen; whether doing the same for dogs has the same effect is unknown.

Pollen. Exposure to pollen can be reduced somewhat by staying indoors as much as possible during the relevant allergy season, by keeping home and vehicle windows and doors closed (use air conditioning), and by showering at bedtime to remove accumulated pollen from skin and hair. In general, sunny, windy days when the humidity is low are considered the worst.

Pharmacotherapy
The two major drug classes used for treating allergic rhinitis are topical nasal corticosteroids (Table 61) and oral antihistamines (Table 62). Maximum efficacy for both is seen if they are started before contact with the offending allergen and are given continuously throughout the period of exposure; they are less effective as "rescue" medications.[4]

Nasal steroids (see Table 61) maximum efficacy is seen only after 1 to 2 weeks of treatment. A meta-analysis found that intranasal steroids are more effective for the treatment of nasal blockage and discharge, sneezing, post-nasal drip, and nasal itch than antihistamines.[5] Other trials show that combining intranasal steroids and antihistamines is more effective than either alone.[6]

For patients with rhinorrhea who do not respond adequately to inhaled corticosteroids, the addition of ipratropium bromide (Atrovent Nasal), two sprays per nostril three times per day (tid), can also result in significant improvement, although nasal hypersecretion appears to be the only symptom of allergic rhinitis that is improved by ipratropium bromide; sneezing or congestion are not affected.[7]

Intranasal cromolyn (sodium cromoglycate, Rynacrom) controls nasal itching, sneezing, or rhinorrhea in some patients but is not as potent as the antihistamines or nasal steroids.[8] This drug is also available as ophthalmic drops (Crolom, Opticrom).

As a group, first-generation antihistamines tend to be dismissed as unsuitable because they are more sedating than second-generation agents and may be hazardous for persons involved in occupational or recreational activities requiring optimal cognitive or psychomotor functioning.[4] However, sedation is not always a problem, especially with children and young adults, and drugs such as chlorpheniramine (Chlor-Trimeton, Chlor-Tripolon) are usually well tolerated, effective, and inexpensive.[9] The usually recommended dose for chlorpheniramine is 4 mg q4-6h, but 4 to 8 mg once daily qhs is equally effective in most cases and causes less sedation.[11] There are several classes of first-generation antihistamines (see Table 62); if a drug from one class is ineffective, it is worth trying one from another class.

Second-generation antihistamines are also listed in Table 62. Terfenadine was withdrawn from the U.S. market in 1997 because of reports of arrhythmias and deaths attributed to the drug. Its active metabolite, fexofenadine (Allegra), does not induce arrhythmias. Cetirizine has been found to be beneficial in numerous studies.[14]

Two RCT's have shown a benefit over placebo for the antileukotriene drugs such as zafirlukast (Accolate) in doses of 20 mg bid or montelukast (Singulair) in doses of 10 mg once daily.[15] In terms of combination therapy, there are two conflicting trials, one showing a benefit to combining the antileukotriene with loratidine and another showing no improvement compared with loratadine alone.[16,17]

At present they should probably be used for patients who do not respond adequately to antihistamines or nasal steroid sprays although there are recent reports of rare cases of fulminant hepatitis.[18]

A number of antihistamine-vasoconstrictor ophthalmic drops can be used as adjuncts to nasal steroids or antihistamines in the treatment of allergic rhinitis. These include antazoline-naphazoline (Vasocon-A), pheniramine-naphazoline (Naphcon-A), and pheniramine-phenylephrine (Ak Vernacon). Use of such topical ophthalmic agents has caused acute and chronic conjunctivitis.[19]

The long-term use of topical nasal vasoconstrictors has no role in the treatment of vasomotor or allergic rhinitis. However, they may be useful for a few days

Table 61   Topical Nasal Steroids

Drug	Usual adult dose
Beclomethasone dipropionate (Beconase, Vancenase)	Two sprays each nostril bid
Budesonide (Rhinocort)	Two doses each nostril bid or four sprays each nostril once daily
Flunisolide (Nasarel, Nasalide, Rhinalar)	Two sprays each nostril bid
Fluticasone propionate (Flonase)	Two sprays each nostril once daily or one spray each nostril bid
Mometasone furoate (Nasonex)	Two sprays each nostril once daily
Triamcinolone acetonide (Nasacort)	Two sprays each nostril once daily

during the initiation of topical steroid therapy if the nose is completely blocked. The vasoconstrictor may be given a few minutes before the steroid to open up the nasal passages. Prolonged use may lead to rhinitis medicamentosa.[8] A short-acting topical decongestant is pheniramine-phenylephrine (Dristan Nasal Mist/Spray), and longer acting products include oxymetazoline HCl (Dristan Long Lasting Nasal Mist/Spray) and xylometazoline HCl (Otrivin).

Immunotherapy

Guidelines of the Canadian Society of Allergy and Clinical Immunology state that immunotherapy for seasonal allergic rhinitis caused by the pollens of trees, grasses, or ragweed is a third-line treatment to be undertaken only if an intensive program of allergen avoidance and symptomatic control with medications has been unsuccessful over a 2-year period.[20] Adverse reactions to

Table 62   Oral Antihistamines

Class and Drug	Usual Adult Dose
First-Generation Antihistamines	
Alkylamines	
Chlorpheniramine (Chlor-Trimeton, Chlor-Tripolon)	4-8 mg qhs as single daily dose[7]
Dexchlorpheniramine (Polaramine)	2 mg qid
Ethanolamines	25-50 mg tid-qid
Diphenhydramine (Benadryl)	
Ethylenediamines	
Tripelennamine (Pyribenzamine, PBZ)	25-50 mg qid
Piperazine derivatives	
Hydroxyzine (Atarax)	10-50 mg tid-qid
Piperidine derivatives	
Azatadine (Optimine)	1-2 mg bid
Second-Generation Antihistamines	
Cetirizine (Zyrtec, Reactine)	10 mg/day
Loratadine (Claritin)	10 mg/day
Fexofenadine (Allegra)	60 mg bid
Desloratadine (Aerius Clarinex)	5mg/day

immunotherapy vary from minimal local reactions to death. Risk factors for serious adverse reactions include patients with asthma, immunotherapy during the season when pollens to which the patient is allergic are present, and first doses from a new vial.[21]

Short preseasonal courses of immunotherapy using absorbed serum have been developed for allergies to trees, grasses, and ragweed. Only six to 11 shots are required.[9]

❧ REFERENCES ❧

1. Dykewics MS, Fineman S, Skoner DP, et al: Diagnosis and management of rhinitis: complete guidelines of the Joint Task Force on Practice Paramaters in Allergy and Immunology, *Ann Allergy Asthma Immunol* 81:478-518, 1998.
2. Wood RA, Johnson EF, Van Natta ML, et al: A placebo-controlled trial of a HEPA air cleaner in the treatment of cat allergy, *Am J Respir Crit Care Med* 158:115-120, 1998.
3. Sheikh A, Hurwitz B: House dust mite avoidance measures for perennial allergic rhinitis (Cochrane Review). In *The Cochrane Library*, 1, Chichester, UK, 2004, John Wiley
4. Kay GG, Berman B, Mockoviak SH, et al: Initial and steady-state effects of diphenhydramine and loratadine on sedation, cognition, mood, and psychomotor performance, *Arch Intern Med* 157:2350-2356, 1997.
5. Weiner JM, Abramson MJ, Puy RM: Intranasal corticosteroids versus oral H1 receptor antagonists in allergic rhinitis: systematic review of randomized controlled trials, *BMJ*;317:1624-1629, 1998.
6. Juniper EF, Guyatt GH, Ferrie PJ: First-line treatment of seasonal (ragweed) rhinoconjunctivitis: a randomized management trial comparing a nasal steroid spray and a nonsedating antihistamine, *CMAJ* 156(8):1123-1131, 1997.
7. Lee NP, Arriola ER. How to treat allergic rhinitis, *West J Med* 171:31-34, 1999.
8. Freedman SO: First-line treatment of hay fever: what is the best option? (editorial), *Can Med Assoc J* 156:1141-1143, 1997.
9. Tkachyk SJ: New treatments for allergic rhinitis, *Can Fam Physician* 45:1255-1260, 1999
10. Dockhorn R, Aaronson D, Bronsky E, et al: Ipratropium bromide nasal spray 0.03% and beclomethasone nasal spray alone and in combination for the treatment of rhinorrhea in perennial rhinitis, *Ann Allergy Asthma Immunol* 82:349-359, 1999.
11. Simons FE, Simons KJ: The pharmacology and use of H₁-receptor-antagonist drugs, *N Engl J Med* 330:1663-1670, 1994.
12. Fexofenadine, *Med Lett* 38:95-96, 1996.
13. Azelastine nasal spray for allergic rhinitis, *Med Lett* 39:45-47, 1997.
14. Sheikh A, Panesar S, Dhami S: Seasonal allergic rhinitis, *Clinical Evidence* 10:621-633, 2003.
15. Philip G, Malmstrom K, Hampel FC Jr, et al for the Montelukast Spring Rhinitis Investigator Group: Montelukast for treating seasonal allergic rhinitis: a randomized, double-blind, placebo-controlled trial performed

in the spring, *Clin Exp Allergy* 32:1020-1028, 2002. Reviewed in *Clinical Evidence* 10:621-633, 2003:
16. Nayak A, Philip G, Lu S, et al, and the Montelukast Fall Rhinitis Investigator Group: Efficacy and tolerability of montelukast alone or in combination with loratadine in seasonal allergic rhinitis: a multicenter, randomized, double-blind, placebo-controlled trial performed in the fall. *Ann Allergy Asthma Immunol* 88:592-600, 2002.
17. Philip G, Malmstrom K, Hampel FC Jr, et al, for the Montelukast Spring Rhinitis Investigator Group: Montelukast for treating seasonal allergic rhinitis: a randomized, double-blind, placebo-controlled trial performed in the spring, *Clin Exp Allergy* 32:1020-1028, 2002.
18. Health Canada Public Advisory, Subject: Important safety information concerning liver problems for patients taking ACCOLATE® (zafirlukast), 2004.
19. Soparkar CN, Wilhelmus KR, Koch DD, et al: Acute and chronic conjunctivitis due to over-the-counter ophthalmic decongestants, *Arch Ophthalmol* 115:34-48, 1997.
20. Canadian Society of Allergy and Clinical Immunology: Guidelines for the use of allergen immunotherapy, *Can Med Assoc J* 152:1413-1419, 1995.
21. Craig T, Sawyer AM, Fornadley JA: Use of immunotherapy in a primary care office, *Am Family Physician* 57:1888-1894, 1998.

Vasomotor Rhinitis

Vasomotor rhinitis is a heterogeneous disease, which is characterized by nasal hyperreactivity that results in symptoms of nasal blockage, rhinorrhea, and sneezing, which are often indistinguishable from nasal symptoms of allergic rhinitis. Diagnosis of the disease is established on the basis of persistent symptoms throughout the year after exclusion of infection, any anatomical or medical disorder of the nose, and negative skin prick testing for IgE-mediated sensitivity to relevant aeroallergens.[1] Pharmacotherapy involves use of either decongestants in patients whose main symptom is nasal congestion, or intranasal anticholinergics (ipratropium bromide nasal spray 2 sprays each nostril bid) in patients whose predominant symptom is rhinorrhea.[2,3] For some patients a combination of topical nasal steroids and nasal ipratropium bromide gives results.[4] Recent studies have shown benefit with the antihistamine, Aseltizine, in treating vasomotor rhinitis.[5] Despite being commonly prescribed, there is no evidence for oral antihistamines in vasomotor rhinitis.[6]

❧ REFERENCES ❧

1. Garay R: Mechanisms of vasomotor rhinitis, *Allergy*. 59(suppl 76):4-9; discussion 9-10, 2004.
2. Ciprandi G: Treatment of nonallergic perennial rhinitis, *Allergy* 59(suppl76):16-22; discussion 22-23, 2004.
3. Proceedings of the Canadian Rhinitis Symposium: assessing and treating rhinitis; a practical guide for Canadian physicians, *Can Med Assoc J* 151(suppl):S1-S27, 1994.

4. Dockhorn R, Aaronson D, Bronsky E, et al: Ipratropium bromide nasal spray 0.03% and beclomethasone nasal spray alone and in combination for the treatment of rhinorrhea in perennial rhinitis, *Ann Allergy Asthma Immunol* 82:349-359, 1999.
5. Lieberman PL, Settipane RA. Azelastine nasal spray: a review of pharmacology and clinical efficacy in allergic and nonallergic rhinitis. *Allergy Asthma Proc* 24(2):95-105, 2003.
6. Long A, McFadden C, DeVine D, et al. Management of allergic and nonallergic rhinitis. (Evidence Report/Technology Assessment No. 54. By New England Medical Center Evidence-based Practice Center, contract No. 290-97-0019). AHRQ Pub. No. 02-E024. Rockville, Md: Agency for Healthcare Research and Quality. May 2002. Available at http://www. ahrq.gov/clinic/rhininv.htm.

PHARYNX
Pharyngitis
(See also streptococcal pharyngitis, otitis media)

Most pharyngitis is viral in etiology. A score has been developed to rule out streptococcal infection (see streptococcal infections. Symptomatic relief of the symptoms of pharyngitis may be obtained by gargling with 15 ml (1 tbsp) of benzydamine (Tantum) every 1½ to 3 hours and especially before meals as well as sips of hot water, flavoured non-caffeinated teas, and oral acetaminophen or non-steroidal anti-inflammatory drugs (NSAIDs).

Tonsillectomy
(See also otitis media; streptococcal infections)

The evidence supporting tonsillectomy for recurrent sore throat is controversial and there is no evidence to establish clear indications for surgery.[1] The Scottish Intercollegiate Guidelines Network recommends that tonsillectomy be preformed when patients meet all of the following criteria: sore throat due to tonsillitis, symptoms lasting > 1 year, 5 or more episodes/year and episodes are disabling and prevent normal functioning.[2] Other indications as recommended by the American Academy of Otolaryngology-Head and Neck Surgery are: 3 or more episodes/year despite adequate therapy, hypertrophy causing upper air way obstruction (sleep apnea), cor pulmonale, severe dysphagia or dental malocclusion, recurrent peritonsillar abscess, foul breath/taste, recurrent tonsillitis in a streptococcal carrier and unilateral hypertrophy suspicious for malignancy.[3] Recurrent otitis media and glue ear are not recognized indications for tonsillectomy

◢ REFERENCES ◣

1. Burton MJ, Towler B, Glasziou P: *Cochrane Database of Systematic Reviews*, Issue 2, Oxford, England, 2001.
2. Scottish Intercollegiate Guidelines Network (SIGN), Scottish Cancer Therapy Network: Management of sore throat and indications for tonsillectomy, (SIGN publication no. 34). Edinburgh: SIGN, 1999.
3. American Academy of Otolaryngology-Head and Neck Surgery: Clinical indications for tonsillectomy and adenoidectomy, American Academy of Otolaryngology-Head and Neck Surgery, *Bulletin* 19 (6), 2000 [Accessed: June 25, 2005]. Available from: URL: http://www.entusa.com/tonsillectomy_surgery.htm

SINUSES
Sinusitis

Acute sinusitis lasts 3 to 4 weeks. In chronic sinusitis, symptoms last for 3 to 8 weeks or longer, and are accompanied by CT or MRI findings. Recurrent sinusitis is defined as three or more episodes of acute sinusitis per year.[1]

Making a clinical diagnosis of acute bacterial sinusitis is difficult. The vast majority of sinusitis that we see are likely secondary to a viral cold or allergies. Symptoms and signs of particular value for bacterial sinusitis are "double sickening," in which a patient with a cold begins to improve and then finds that symptoms worsen; facial pain, particularly if unilateral; maxillary toothache; purulent nasal secretions; and poor response to decongestants.[2] Transillumination is variably performed and does not always correlate with disease, but use of a "Mini-Mag Lite™" or pocket flashlight seems as effective as a "transilluminator."[2]

If on a clinical basis a patient has either a high or low probability of having sinusitis, X-ray examination adds little.[2] Before the age of 6 years only the maxillary and ethmoid sinuses are sufficiently developed to be seen consistently on radiographs. In chronic or recurrent cases of sinusitis, CT is the most commonly used imagining modality, although XR imaging can help to establish the extent of sinus disease.[1]

In both adults and children, *Haemophilus influenzae* and *Streptococcus pneumoniae* account for about 70% of cases of bacterial sinusitis. In children most of the remaining cases are due to *Branhamella (Moraxella) catarrhalis*.[2] In adults other etiological agents include *Staphylococcus aureus,* Group A streptococcus, *pseudomonas aeruginosa,* anaerobes, and gram-negative enteric organisms.[1,2]

Antibiotics are considered the mainstay of treatment for sinusitis but may not always be necessary. Randomized placebo-controlled trials of amoxicillin and amoxicillin-clavulanate in patients with clinically diagnosed sinusitis found no significant treatment difference between groups at 10 days.[3,4] However, a systematic review did find limited evidence that a 7 to 10 day course of amoxicillin is effective in treating acute maxillary sinusitis, but recommended that clinicians should weigh the moderate benefits of antibiotic treatment against the potential for adverse effects.[5]

As with adults, the effectiveness of antimicrobial therapy for sinusitis in children has mixed results with some recent trials showing no effect[6] but the systematic review of placebo-controlled RCTs found that, in children with rhinosinusitis, 10 days of antibiotics (including amoxicillin +/– clavulanic acid, trimethoprim/sulfamethoxazole, and erythromycin) reduced the probability of persistent symptoms (the benefits appear to be modest and around eight children must be treated in order to achieve one additional cure).[7] Most colds are complicated by viral sinusitis. If therapy is required, the first-line antibiotics are amoxicillin 250 to 500 mg po q8h (20 to 40 mg/kg po q8h for children) or trimethoprim/sulfamethoxazole 160/800 mg po q12h(8/40 mg/kg/day in 2 divided doses for children). Second-line drugs include cefuroxime (Ceftin), Cefaclor (Ceclor), cefixime (Suprax), and clarithromycin (Biaxin).[1,2] Patients who do not show improvement within 5 to 7 days should be given a broad spectrum antibiotic such as amoxicillin-clavulanate (Augmentin, Clavulin), a quinolone (e.g., levofloxacin), or a cephalosporin.[1]

If no response is seen with broad spectrum antibiotics within 3 to 4 weeks, metronidazole (250 to 500 mg po tid-qid) or clindamycin (150 to 450 mg po tid-qid) may be considered for anaerobic coverage.[1]

Although there are no substantiating placebo-controlled trials, some adjunctive therapies that may be useful include inhaled steam or hot facial packs, saline nasal spray, oral and nasal decongestants, corticosteroid nasal sprays, and oral mucolytics (guaifenesin, bromelain).[1]

--- **REFERENCES** ---

1. Sinusitis. Kidlington, UK: First Consult, 2004. (Accessed March 13, 2004, at http://www.firstconsult.com/home/framework/fs_main.htm?msite=fs_main&)
2. Fagnan LJ: Acute sinusitis: a cost-effective approach to diagnosis and treatment, *Am Fam Physician* 58:1795-1802, 1998.
3. De Sutter AI, De Meyere MJ, Christiaens TC, et al: Does amoxicillin improve outcomes in patients with purulent rhinorrhea? A pragmatic randomized double-blind controlled trial in family practice. *J Fam Pract* 2002; 51:317-323. Reviewed in: *Clinical Evidence* 10:567-573, 2003.
4. Bucher HC, Tshudi P, Young J, et al: Effect of amoxicillin-clavulanate in clinically diagnosed acute rhinosinusitis. A placebo-controlled, double-blind, randomized trial in general practice, *Arch Intern Med* 163:1793-1798, 2003.
5. Williams JW, Aguilar C, Makela M, et al: Antibiotics for acute maxillary sinusitis (Cochrane Methodology Review). In: The Cochrane Library, 4, 2003. Chichester, UK: John Wiley. Reviewed in: *Clinical Evidence* 10:567-573, 2003.
6. Garbutt JM, Goldstein M, Gellman, et al: A randomized, placebo-controlled trial of antimicrobial treatment for children with clinically diagnosed acute sinusitis, *Pediatrics* 107:619-625, 2001.
7. Morris P, Leach A: Antibiotics for persistent nasal discharge (rhinosinusitis) in children (Cochrane Methodology Review). In *The Cochrane Library*, 4, 2003. Chichester, UK, 2003, John Wiley.

VERTIGO
(See approach to dizziness; motion sickness)

Vertigo can be caused by ear disease (peripheral vertigo) or central nervous system disease (central vertigo). Clues that vertigo is central include the presence of other central nervous symptoms or signs, spontaneous nystagmus that changes direction (in peripheral disease the direction of nystagmus is constant), and inability to walk (patients with peripheral vertigo do not like to walk, but they can). However, the symptoms and signs of inferior cerebellar infarction may be identical to those of peripheral disease.[1]

--- **REFERENCES** ---

1. Baloh RW: Vertigo, *Lancet* 352:1841-1846, 1998.

Benign Paroxysmal Positional Vertigo
Benign paroxysmal positional vertigo (BPPV) is caused by the accumulation of particles (probably otoconia) in the endolymph of the posterior semicircular canal. These appear to interfere with the free flow of endolymph and cause vertigo with head movements. The mean age of patients with BPPV is 54. The majority of cases are primary or idiopathic BPPV; the remaining 30% to 50% of cases are secondary BPPV, most commonly, as a result of head trauma. Vestibular neuronitis is the second most common cause of secondary BPPV and is implicated in up to 15% of all cases of BPPV.[1] The natural history of BPPV is one of gradual resolution over weeks or even years, with many people having remissions and exacerbations.[2]

The diagnosis of BPPV is confirmed by performing the Dix-Hallpike (Hallpike) manoeuvre. The examiner helps the patient, who is seated on the examining table, to lie rapidly back so that his or her head, which is rotated to one side by about 45 degrees, hangs down over the upper edge of the examining table by about 45 degrees. Characteristic findings in patients with BPPV are latency, adaptability, and fatigability, as well as rotary (torsional) nystagmus toward the dependent ear and the subjective sensation of vertigo. Latency refers to the fact that the patient does not experience vertigo or demonstrate nystagmus immediately after lying back on the table, but only after a latent period of a few seconds. Adaptability means that after the patient experiences 20 to 60 seconds of vertigo and nystagmus while lying back on the table, both stop spontaneously. Fatigability means that if the Hallpike manoeuvre is repeated one or more times, both vertigo and nystagmus diminish in intensity or disappear.[2] Patients with a central nervous system cause of vertigo usually do not exhibit latency, adaptability, or fatigability.

Epley's canalith repositioning procedure
In recent years head manoeuvres have been described as a means of permanently controlling the symptoms of

BPPV.[1,2] The theory is that the particles lodged in the posterior semicircular canal can be made to fall into the utricle, where they will do no further harm. The method described below is that of Epley,[3] who reported a 77% success rate after only one treatment session. The recurrence rate is about 15% per year.[2]

The Epley canalith repositioning procedure is performed as follows.[2,3] The affected ear is first determined by the Hallpike manoeuvre. It is the ear that is dependent when symptoms are produced. Each movement in the particle repositioning manoeuvre (Epley's manoeuvre) is performed rapidly and then maintained for at least 30 seconds[3] or until symptoms have subsided.[2] The initial manoeuvre is identical to the Hallpike manoeuvre. The seated patient is assisted in lying back on the examining table so that the head hangs over the edge of the table with the neck extended about 45 degrees and rotated 45 degrees toward the affected side. The physician supports the patient's head in this position while giving reassurance that the vertigo will subside. Next the head is rapidly rotated through 90 degrees to the opposite side. After remaining in this position for a short period, the patient is assisted in rolling over onto his or her side, the direction of the roll being in the direction the face was pointing in the last manoeuvre. The head rotation of 45 degrees is maintained throughout this manoeuvre so that at its completion the patient, although lying on his or her side, is looking toward the floor. After a short delay the patient is helped to a sitting position while continuing to keep the head rotated. The final manoeuvre is to rotate the head back to the straight-ahead position and flex the neck by about 20 degrees.

In cases of treatment failure the procedure may be repeated immediately. In some patients both ears are affected; in those cases only one side is treated at a time.[3]

The original studies recommended that patients try to keep the head in the vertical position for 48 hours (sleeping on the back with two or three pillows). However, a 1996 study found no benefit from this type of post-treatment protocol.[4]

Modified Epley's procedure

Radtke and associates have developed a modified Epley's procedure that patients perform three times daily at home until symptoms have resolved. The patient sits on a bed with a pillow placed so that when the patient lies down it will rest under the shoulders. The seated patient turns the head 45 degrees toward the affected side and rapidly lies down—the shoulders rest on the pillow, and the occiput on the bed. After 30 seconds the head is rapidly turned 90 degrees to the opposite side, and after another 30 seconds the patient rolls onto one side in the direction the head is pointing while maintaining the head rotation. Thus the patient ends up lying on one side with the face facing the bed. After 30 seconds the patient sits up and turns, ending up seated on the edge of the bed with the feet on the floor.[5]

Habituation exercises of Brandt and Daroff

An older home treatment for BPPV is the positional or habituation exercises of Brandt and Daroff.[2,5] The patient begins by sitting on the side of the bed with feet on the floor and the head turned 45 degrees to one side. The patient rapidly lies down on one side in the direction opposite to which he or she is looking so that the portion of the occiput behind the ear touches the mattress. The patient then sits up, turns the head so it points 45 degrees in the opposite direction, and lies down quickly on the opposite side. Every position is maintained for at least 30 seconds. Unfortunately the effects are not long lasting, but patients can restart the exercises with good effect when the vertigo returns.[6]

_____ ❧ REFERENCES ❧ _____

1. Parnes LS, Agrawal SK, Atlas J: Diagnosis and management of Benign Paroxysmal Positional Vertigo, *CMAJ* 348(11): 1027-1033, 2003.
2. Furman JM, Cass SP: Benign paroxysmal positional vertigo, *N Engl J Med* 341:1590-1596, 1999.
3. Epley JM: The canalith repositioning procedure for treatment of benign paroxysmal positional vertigo, *Otolaryngol Head Neck Surg* 107:399-404, 1992.
4. Massoud EA, Ireland DF: Post-treatment instructions in the nonsurgical management of benign paroxysmal positional vertigo, *J Otolaryngol* 25:121-125, 1996.
5. Radtke A, Neuhauser H, von Brevern M, et al: A modified Epley's procedure for self-treatment of benign positional vertigo, *Neurology* 53:1358-1360, 1999.
6. Banfield GK, Wood C, Knight J: Does vestibular habituation still have a place in the treatment of benign paroxysmal positional vertigo? *J Laryngol Otol* 114:501-505, 2000.

Ménière's Disease
(See also nausea and vomiting)

The four characteristic symptoms of Ménière's disease are episodic vertigo, fluctuating sensorineural hearing loss, tinnitus, and sense of fullness in the ear. Rarely are all these symptoms present at the onset of the disease; only in later episodes will the diagnosis become evident. Two of the major conditions to consider in the differential diagnosis are benign paroxysmal positional vertigo and vestibular neuronitis.[1]

Ménière's disease is characterized by remissions and exacerbations, and over the long term 70% of patients experience a long-term remission.[2] This fact, along with the lack of a significant number of controlled trials on treatment of the disease, has led to a huge variety of unproven management protocols. Medical regimens include limitations on the intake of salt, caffeine, alcohol, and tobacco, as well as the prescription of many classes of drugs. Medications that have been tried are the antihistamines, which include meclizine (Antivert, Bonine, Bonamine), promethazine (Phenergan), and dimenhydrinate (Dramamine, Gravol), neuroleptics, such as prochlorperazine (Compazine, Stemetil), anti-cholinergics, such as scopolamine, droperidol, and benzodiazepines, such as diazepam and clonazepam.[1-4] Some have recommended a trial of prednisone 1 mg/kg for 10 days or intravenous methylprednisolone followed by oral prednisone in the acute setting.[3] Only diuretics and betahistine (usually prescribed as 4 to 8 mg q8h) have been found to be effective in the long-term control of vertigo symptoms and none of the medical treatments stop the progression of hearing loss or alter the course of disease.[3,4]

Surgery (either conservative or destructive) should only be considered for those patients who have intractable symptoms and for whom the disease is progressing. Patients with no serviceable hearing may obtain complete relief of symptoms at the cost of total hearing loss through a complete labyrinthectomy.[1-4]

───────────── ❧ REFERENCES ❧ ─────────────

1. Knox GW, McPherson A: Meniere's disease: differential diagnosis and treatment, *Am Fam Physician* 55:1185-1190, 1997.
2. Saeed SR: Diagnosis and treatment of Ménière's disease, *BMJ* 316:368-372, 1998.
3. Sajjadi H: Medical Management of Meniere's Disease, *Otolaryngology Clinics of North America*. 35(3): 455-495, 2002.
4. daCosta SS: Meniere's Disease: Overview, epidemiology, and natural history, *Otolaryngology Clinics of North America*,35(3): 581-589, 2002.

Vestibular Neuritis

Vestibular neuritis is the syndrome of acute prolonged vertigo of peripheral origin.[1] Vestibular neuritis or vestibular neuronitis is presumed to be secondary to a viral infection. Presenting symptoms of severe vertigo, nausea, vomiting, and postural instability develop rapidly and begin to improve within a few days. Severe vertigo resolves within a week, but complete resolution of symptoms may take several weeks or even a few months.[2]

The differential diagnosis of acute onset vertigo includes many disorders. Patients with benign paroxysmal positional vertigo have brief symptoms brought on by positional changes and do not have vertigo when they are not moving. Patients with acoustic neuromas rarely have severe vertigo, and patients with Ménière's disease usually give a typical history (see previous discussion). The most important disorders to rule out in a patient with acute vertigo are brainstem or inferior cerebellar infarcts. Most patients with brainstem infarcts have other central nervous symptoms and signs, but these may be absent or subtle in cases of inferior cerebellar infarction.[2]

Three clues that help differentiate central nervous system (central) from vestibular (peripheral) lesions are the direction of nystagmus, the ability to inhibit nystagmus by fixation, and the ability of the patient to walk. With central lesions the quick component of nystagmus may change direction when the patient looks in different directions, whereas the direction of the quick component always remains the same in peripheral lesions. In peripheral lesions nystagmus is usually inhibited by fixation, whereas in central lesions it is not; this can be assessed by observing the optic disc of one eye with an ophthalmoscope while the patient alternately covers and uncovers the other eye. If pressed, patients with peripheral disease can walk, although they are unsteady and nauseated; patients with inferior cerebellar infarcts are rarely able to walk.[2]

Vertigo in young patients who do not have risk factors for cerebrovascular accident is almost always due to peripheral lesions. Older patients with risk factors for stroke who do not have obvious localizing neurological signs may have an inferior cerebellar infarct, especially if they are unable to walk. Such patients require further evaluation.[2] Two recent randomized controlled trials found that dimenhydrinate is equally as effective as droperidol and more effective than lorazepam for the treatment of acute peripheral vertigo.[1]

───────────── ❧ REFERENCES ❧ ─────────────

1. Baloh RW: Vestibular neuritis, *N Engl J Med* 348(11): 1027-1032, 2003.
2. Hotson JR, Baloh RW: Acute vestibular syndrome, *N Engl J Med* 339:680-685, 1998.

PEDIATRICS

ADOPTION

International Adoption

International adoptees should be screened for human immunodeficiency virus (HIV-1 and HIV-2), hepatitis B and C, congenital syphilis, lead poisoning, tuberculosis (by Mantoux testing), dermatological infections (scabies, lice) and parasites. HIV and hepatitis B and C screening should be repeated after 6 months.[1] Anemia is common in this population and may be due to causes rare in North America: intestinal parasites, malnutrition, malaria, and glucose-6-phosphate dehydrogenase (G6PD) deficiency. Additional screening may be performed to rule out thyroid and renal dysfunction.[2] Even if children have records of immunization from their native countries, their immunity may be inadequate; they should either be assessed for antibody levels or have repeat immunizations.[3] Vision and hearing should be assessed, and growth and development should be carefully monitored. Developmental delays are common among international adoptees and may be masked by language or cultural differences.[1,2]

_____ ✍ REFERENCES ✍ _____

1. Miller LC: Caring for internationally adopted children, *N Engl J Med* 341:1539-1540, 1999.
2. Kim J, Staat MA: Acute care issues in international adoption, *Clinical Pediatric Emergency Medicine* 5(2):130-142, 2004.
3. Miller LC, Comfort K, Kelly N: Immunization status of internationally adopted children, *Pediatrics* 108:1050-1051, 2001.

ASTHMA IN CHILDREN

(See also allergic rhinitis—environmental control; asthma)

About half of all children have one or more episodes of wheezing before the age of 3 years, usually in association with respiratory infections, but only one fourth still have wheezing episodes at the age of 6. A history of maternal asthma is associated with an increased risk of the child's continuing to wheeze at the age of 6, maternal smoking during pregnancy with an increased incidence of wheezing before the age of 3,[1,2] and exposure to passive smoke with a delayed resolution of acute asthmatic attacks.[3] Breastfeeding during the first 3 months of life is protective, resulting in lower rates of asthma in childhood.[4] The morbidity rate from asthma among poor inner city children is particularly high, almost certainly because of sensitivity and continued exposure to cockroaches.[5]

Between 30% and 70% of children with asthma have marked improvement or resolution of symptoms by the time they become adults. Such resolution is seen more often in patients with milder forms of the disease.[6]

Inhaled medications are the ideal way of controlling asthma in both children and adults. The delivery of these medications to the respiratory tract is increased with the use of a spacer device. As with adults, inhaled corticosteroids are indicated for moderate-to-severe asthma.

When initiated early in asthma attacks, inhaled medications have been shown to reduce hospital admissions.[7] A meta-analysis showed that moderate doses of the inhaled steroid beclomethasone significantly decreased linear growth velocity of children with mild-to-moderate asthma, with a smaller effect for fluticasone.[8] The average decrease, calculated through meta-analysis, was −1.54 cm per year (95% CI −1.15 cm, −1.94 cm). Some evidence shows that children "catch up" after reducing dosage later in life, but trials have not been ongoing long enough to fully prove the evidence.[9] For children for whom the use of medications is believed to be short lived, or the diagnosis uncertain (as can be the case in the first episode of wheeze that presents during peak bronchiolitis seasons), oral medications can be trialed. The first choice of an oral agent is usually a β_2-adrenergic agonist such as metaproterenol (Alupent), which has the generic name orciprenaline in Canada. Common side effects include hyperactivity, nausea, and vomiting.

Wheezing in association with upper respiratory infections is probably a separate entity from atopic asthma, and in this situation, inhaled corticosteroids may be ineffective.[10] Some authors have claimed that persistent cough may be the only symptom of asthma in children (cough variant asthma), while others question the existence of such a syndrome. Labelling cough alone as asthma is one reason that the reported incidence of asthma has been increasing.[11] The pathways for cough and bronchoconstriction are different, and a common trigger such as an upper respiratory tract infection may affect both. In some asthmatic children, coughing overshadows wheezing, which may be missed, but most children with cough but no associated wheezing or dyspnea do not have asthma. A randomized, placebo controlled trial of albuterol or inhaled corticosteroids for children with cough failed to show any benefit.[12] When the diagnosis of asthma is unclear, a short trial of asthma medications may be indicated in some children, but no evidence supports a prolonged course of inhaled corticosteroids.[11]

In children with chronic persistent symptoms who have a suboptimal response to low-to-moderate doses of inhaled corticosteroids or who are poorly adherent to this therapy, orally administered leukotriene receptor antagonists, including montelukast, pranlukast, and zafirlukast, have proven benefits as add-on therapy to allow tapering of corticosteroid dose and reduction in beta agonist use.[13]

Asthma is discussed in detail in the Respirology section.

❧ REFERENCES ❧

1. Martinez FD, Wright AL, Taussig LM, et al: Asthma and wheezing in the first six years of life, *N Engl J Med* 332: 133-138, 1995.
2. Cook DG, Strachan DP: Health effects of passive smoking-10: summary of effects of parental smoking on the respiratory health of children and implications for research, *Thorax* 54: 357-366, 1999.
3. Abulhosn RS, Morray BH, Llewellyn CE, et al: Passive smoke exposure impairs recovery after hospitalization for acute asthma, *Arch Pediatr Adolesc Med* 151:135-139, 1997.
4. Gdalevich M, Mimouni D, Mimouni M: Breast-feeding and the risk of bronchial asthma in childhood: a systematic review with meta-analysis of prospective studies, *J Pediatr* 139:261-266, 2001.
5. Rosenstreich D, Kattan M, Baker D, et al: The role of cockroach allergy and exposure to cockroach allergen in causing morbidity among inner-city children with asthma, *N Engl J Med* 336:1356-1363, 1997.
6. O'Connor GT, Weiss ST, Speizer FE: The epidemiology of asthma. In Gershwin ME, ed: *Bronchial asthma,* ed 2, Orlando, Fl, 1986, Grune & Stratton.
7. Edmonds ML, Camargo CA Jr, Pollack CV Jr: The effectiveness of inhaled corticosteroids in the emergency department treatment of acute asthma: a meta-analysis, *Ann Emerg Med* 40:145-154, 2002.
8. Sharek P, Bergman DA: The effect of inhaled steriods on the linear growth of children with asthma: a meta-analysis, *Pediatrics* 106: E8, 2000.
9. Sharek PJ, Bergman DA, Ducharme F: Beclomethasone for asthma in children: effects on linear growth (Cochrane Review). In: *The Cochrane Library,* issue 4, Chichester, UK, 2003, John Wiley.
10. Doull IJ, Lampe FC, Smith S, et al: Effect of inhaled corticosteroids on episodes of wheezing associated with viral infection in school age children: randomised double blind placebo controlled trial, *BMJ* 315:858-862, 1997.
11. Chang AB: Isolated cough: probably not asthma, *Arch Dis Child* 80:211-213, 1999.
12. Chang AB, Phelan PD, Carlin JB, et al: A randomized, placebo controlled trial of inhaled salbutamol and beclomethasone for recurrent cough, *Arch Dis Child* 79: 6-11, 1998.
13. Warner JO: The role of leukotriene receptor antagonists in the treatment of chronic asthma in childhood, *Allergy* 56(S66): 22-29, 2001.

ATTENTION DEFICIT/HYPERACTIVITY DISORDER
(See also antisocial personality disorder; conduct disorder; fetal alcohol effects; Tourette's syndrome)

Epidemiology

Between 3% and 7% of children in North America are diagnosed as having attention deficit/hyperactivity disorder (ADHD), and boys are more often affected than girls.[1] The actual number of affected girls is probably higher than is generally reported because fewer girls than boys with ADHD have oppositional or conduct disorder and therefore fewer are brought to medical attention. Even when physicians do see girls, the diagnosis of ADHD may be missed because it is often overshadowed by comorbid conditions such as anxiety disorders, mood disorders, or substance abuse.[2]

A family history of ADHD is common; 30% of first-degree relatives of children with ADHD also have the condition. The increased risk for siblings is fivefold for boys and threefold for girls.[3] A family history of conversion disorder, sociopathy, and alcoholism may also be elicited.

Common comorbid conditions of ADHD are learning disabilities (25% to 35% of children); oppositional disorder and conduct disorders in boys; and anxiety disorders, mood disorders, and substance abuse in girls. Children with ADHD are at increased risk for antisocial personality disorder or drug abuse disorder when they reach adulthood.[4]

Despite parental beliefs, a 1995 meta-analysis found no correlation between sugar intake and childhood hyperactivity or cognitive functioning.[5]

The diagnosis of ADHD is based on clinical history. The text-revised fourth edition of the *Diagnostic and Statistical Manual of Mental Disorders (DSM IV-TR)* divides the symptoms into the two major categories of inattention and hyperactivity/impulsivity. Each category contains nine sets of symptoms, and the diagnosis is made if the child has six of the listed symptoms in either category, has had symptoms before the age of 7 years, has symptoms in two or more settings (such as school and home), and suffers impairment in social, academic, or occupational functioning because of the symptoms. The following are examples of symptoms associated with inattention:

- Fails to pay attention to detail at school and makes careless mistakes
- Has difficulty sustaining attention when playing or performing tasks
- May not seem to listen when spoken to directly
- Is often distracted

Examples of symptoms of hyperactivity/impulsivity include:

- Often squirms in chair or fidgets with hands or feet
- Often runs or climbs excessively
- Often talks excessively
- May have difficulty waiting his or her turn
- Often blurts out an answer before a question is completed

Children with ADHD may not display any symptoms in the physician's office, so short periods of observation are not sufficient to rule out the diagnosis. To obtain a diagnostic history, the practitioner generally has to question a number of observers from different settings using questionnaires such as the Connors Parent Rating Scales and the Connors Teacher Rating Scales. Although ADHD may be diagnosed in preschool children, the validity of making the diagnoses in this age group is uncertain.[6] The conditions most commonly misdiagnosed as ADHD are depression and anxiety disorders. In general, ADHD begins at an earlier age and has an unremitting course, whereas mood and anxiety disorders tend to present at a somewhat older age and have episodic courses.[7]

Not all children "outgrow" ADHD; about half continue to experience symptoms in adulthood. Recognizing the disorder may be particularly difficult in adults if it was not identified in childhood. Presenting problems in adults usually involve difficulties in work or school performance, inattention, or hyperactivity, which often manifests as "restlessness" with increasing age.[8] The diagnostic criteria for adult ADHD requires that the symptoms started by age 7 and were persistently present thereafter.

Specific target outcomes should be set to guide management such as improvement in school performance or particular behaviours. A well-designed comparison of behavioural therapy, medical management, and combined medication and behavioural therapy for children with ADHD found that after 24 months, medical management alone was superior to behaviour therapy alone. However, the addition of behaviour therapy to medical management showed advantages, especially in dually co-morbid children who had both internalizing (depression and/or anxiety) and disruptive behaviour disorders (conduct and/or oppositional-defiant).[10]

Behaviour therapy strategies include individual psychotherapy, behaviour modifications such as rewards and punishments for particular behaviours, parenting classes, parent support groups, school involvement, and education about ADHD/ADD.[12]

Pharmacotherapy choices consist of 4 major classes: psychostimulants, antidepressants, central alpha agonists, and selective norepinephrine reuptake inhibitors (SNRIs).[13]

The medication of first choice for ADHD is methylphenidate (Ritalin, Methylin – orally every 4 hours at 1.0 to 2.0 mg/kg per day). If giving a noon dose at school is difficult, slow release formulations of methylphenidate (Concerta, Metadate CD, Ritalin LA – orally twice daily at 1.0 to 2.0 mg/kg per day) or mixed methylphenidate/D-amphetimine (Adderall – orally twice daily at 0.5 to 1.5 mg/kg per day) may be administered instead. Dextroamphetamine (Dexedrine, Dextrostat – orally every 4 hours at 0.3 to 1.0 m/kg per day) is as effective as methylphenidate. Some children respond only to methylphenidate, and others only to dextroamphetamine.[14] Treatment with stimulants has been shown to improve not only abnormal behaviours of ADHD, but also self-esteem and cognitive, social, and family function, thereby supporting the importance of treating ADHD patients beyond school or work hours to include evenings, weekends, and vacations.[13] Evidence does not support the notion that children will abuse their medications in the case of proper diagnosis and monitoring. The most common side effects of stimulant medications are sleep disturbances and decreased appetite leading to poor weight gain, or weight loss.

It is estimated that at least 30% of individuals with ADHD will not respond to stimulant medication. Other drugs that have been used for the treatment of ADHD are pemoline (Cylert), tricyclic antidepressants (Tofranil, Norpramin), clonidine (Catapres), and guanfacine (Tenex). Pemoline can cause toxic hepatitis, and deaths have been reported from the use of the tricyclic antidepressants clonidine and guanfacine in children.

Bupropion (Wellbutrin) has a safer side-effect profile, and has been used in adults, but its efficacy in pediatric ADHD is not as well documented.[15]

Atomoxetine (Strattera) is the newest treatment for ADHD, and it appears to be a safe and effective non-stimulant alternative for ADHD treatment in children and adults. Unlike methylphenidate and D-amphetamine, which act primarily by blocking the reuptake of dopamine, atomoxetine is a selective norepinephrine reuptake inhibitor. Double-blind, randomized control trials to date show atomoxetine to be well tolerated and associated with less sleep disturbance and appetite suppression than the psychostimluant class.

Adult ADHD is treated similarly to pediatric ADHD. Adult behavioural therapy includes cognitive behavioural therapy, support groups, and education about the disorder. First-line medications include methylphenidate (5 to 10 mg orally twice daily initially, titrated up to a maximum of 80 mg per day) and dextroamphetamine (5 mg orally once daily initially, titrated up to a maximum of 40 mg per day.) Second-line medications include desipramine (50 mg orally every day initially, titrated up to 200 mg per d) and bupropion (100 mg orally every day in the morning, never exceeding 150 mg twice daily due to the risk of seizure with more than 300 mg per day).[16] The adult response rate to pharmacotherapy is less than in children and adolescents. This may reflect the uncertainties of diagnosis, comorbidity, uncertain dosage, non-compliance, or poorly developed measures of responsiveness.[17,18]

Research into the treatment of ADHD in preschoolers is limited.

──────────── **≋ REFERENCES ≋** ────────────

1. American Psychiatric Association: *Diagnostic and Statistical Manual of Mental Disorders: DSM-IV-TR,* ed 4, Washington, DC, 2000, The Association.
2. Biederman J, Faraone SV, Mick E, et al: Clinical correlates of ADHD in females: findings from a large group of girls ascertained from pediatric and psychiatric referral sources, *J Am Acad Child Adolesc Psychiatry* 38:966-975, 1999.
3. Taylor ME: Evaluation and management of attention-deficit hyperactivity disorder, *Am Fam Physician* 55:887-901, 1997.
4. Mannuzza S, Klein RG: Long-term prognosis in attention-deficit/hyperactivity disorder, *Child Adolesc Psychiatr Clin N Am* 9(3):711-726, 2000.
5. Wolraich ML, Wilson DB, White W: The effect of sugar on behavior or cognition in children: a meta-analysis, *JAMA* 274:1617-1621, 1995.
6. Blackman JA: Attention-deficit/hyperactivity disorder in preschoolers. Does it exist and should we treat it? *Pediatr Clin North Am,* 46(5):1011-1025, 1999.
7. Zametkin AJ: Attention-deficit disorder: born to be hyperactive? *JAMA* 273:1871-1874, 1995.
8. Wender PH, Wolf LE, Wasserstein J: Adults with ADHD: an overview, *Ann N Y Acad Sci* 931:1-16, 2001.
9. Wolraich ML, Wilson DB, White W: The effect of sugar on behavior or cognition in children: a meta-analysis, *JAMA* 274:1617-1621, 1995.
10. MTA Cooperative Group: National Institute of Mental Health Multimodal Treatment Study of ADHD follow-up: 24-month outcomes of treatment strategies for attention-deficit/hyperactivity disorder, *Pediatrics* 113(4):754-761, 2004.
11. Wilens TE, Biederman J, Spencer TJ: Attention deficit/hyperactivity disorder across the lifespan, *Annu Rev Med* 53:113-31, 2002.
12. Pary R, Lewis S, Matuschka PR, et al: Attention-deficit/hyperactivity disorder: an update, *South Med J* 95(7):743-749, Jul 2002.
13. Biederman J, Spencer T, Wilens T: Evidence-based pharmacotherapy for attention-deficit hyperactivity disorder, *Int J Neuropsychopharm* 7:77-97, 2004.
14. Elia J, Ambrosini PJ, Rapoport JL: Treatment of attention-deficit-hyperactivity disorder, *N Engl J Med* 340:780-788, 1999.
15. Spencer TJ, Biederman J, Wilens TE, et al: Novel treatments for attention-deficit/hyperactivity disorder in children, *J Clin Psychiatry* 12:16-22, 2002.
16. Weiss M, Murray C: Assessment and management of attention-deficit hyperactivity disorder in adults, *Can Med Assoc J* 168(6):715-722, 2003.
17. Toon B: Attention deficit hyperactivity disorder in adulthood, *J Neurol Neurosurg Psychiatry* 75:523-525, 2004.
18. Wilens TE, Spencer TJ: The stimulants revisited, *Child Adolesc Psychiatr Clin North Am* 9:573-603, 2000.

BREASTFEEDING

(See also breast implants; diarrhea and dehydration in infants; formulas; neonatal jaundice; obesity in childhood)

The American Academy of Pediatrics and WHO recommend exclusive breastfeeding as the ideal nutrition during the first 6 months of life and state that no other solids or liquids are required during this period. Breastfeeding should continue for at least a year, (2 years recommended by the WHO), but iron-enriched solids should be added in the second 6 months of life.[1]

In the first 6 months of life, breastfed babies have lower rates of cough, wheeze, diarrhea, and otitis media and fewer sick baby visits than do non-breastfed or only occasionally breastfed infants.[2] Exclusive breastfeeding for the first 4 months of life has also been associated with a decreased incidence of asthma at 6 years of age.[3]

Presently, over 75% of Canadian women initiate breastfeeding, but 22% of those that start discontinue within 3 months.[4] Physicians should encourage both parents to accept breastfeeding[5] because there is clear evidence that professional breastfeeding support by nurses, lactation consultants, and peer breastfeeding support persons positively influences both initiation and duration of breastfeeding by 2 months compared with usual care.[6]

Written materials have not shown to be helpful in promoting initiation or duration of breastfeeding.[4]

Breastfeeding success is also facilitated by early maternal/infant contact after birth, delaying of unnecessary procedures (vitamin K and erythromycin administration), rooming in practices, delayed use of pacifiers and bottles, and early unrestricted feeding practices.[7]

The following are signs of successful breastfeeding in the neonate[8]:

- Eight to ten feedings a day
- Audible swallowing
- Six to eight wet diapers a day after 4 days of age
- Three to five bowel movements a day
- Less than 7% of birth weight loss and no continued loss after day 3
- Birth weight regained by 2 weeks

It is difficult to say with certainty that a nursing mother may safely take a given drug, but a large number of drugs are usually compatible with breastfeeding. The American Academy of Pediatrics, in their 2001 policy statement, have categorized drugs as follows: Table I is titled *Cytotoxic Drugs that May Interfere with Cellular Metabolism of the Nursing Infant* and includes cyclophosphamide, cyclosporine, doxyrubicin, and methotrexate. Table II is *Drugs of Abuse for Which Adverse Effects on the Infant During Breastfeeding Have Been Reported* and includes amphetamines, cocaine, heroin, marijuana, and phencyclidine. Smoking, which was previously on this list, has been removed pending more data on its effects. Nicotine is present in human milk at 1.5 to 3 times that of plasma concentrations and does lead to decreased milk production and weight gain in the infant as well as the effects of exposure to smoke. Studies suggest that breastfed babies of smoking mothers have fewer respiratory illnesses than bottle-fed infants.[9] Radioactive diagnostic and therapeutic agents comprise Table III and mandate temporary cessation of breastfeeding. Psychotropic drugs have been listed in Table IV, which is titled *Drugs for Which the Effect on Nursing Infants is Unknown but May be of Concern*. Although there are no reported effects with benzodiazepines and most antidepressants, they remain on the list. Fluoxetine has been associated with colic, irritability, feeding and sleeping problems, and poor weight gain. Some authors suggest that if a nursing mother requires antidepressants and continues to breastfeed, serum levels of the drug be measured in infants under 10 weeks of age once a maternal therapeutic dose of the drug has been reached. Measurement of serum levels in infants over 10 weeks is needed only if they display symptoms.[10] Chlorpromazine and haloperidol are associated with developmental delays.[9] Table V is titled *Drugs That have Been Associated with Significant Effects on Some Nursing Infants and Should be Given to Nursing Mothers With Caution,* and includes beta blockers, lithium, salicylates, ergotamine, bromocriptine, and phenobarbitol. Silicone breast implants are not a contraindication to nursing.[11]

In some cases, breastfeeding simply does not work, and the mother should not be made to feel guilty about this.[12]

REFERENCES

1. American Academy of Pediatrics Work Group on Breastfeeding: breastfeeding and the use of human milk, *Pediatrics* 100:1035-1039, 1997.
2. Raisler J, Alexander C, O'Campo P: Breast-feeding and infant illness: a dose-response relationship? *Am J Public Health* 89: 25-30, 1999.
3. Oddy WH, Holt PG, Sly PD, et al: Association between breastfeeding and asthma in 6-year-old children: findings of a prospective birth cohort study, *BMJ* 319:815-819, 1999.
4. Palda V, Guise J, Wathen N, with the Canadian Task Force on Preventative Health Care: Interventions to promote breast-feeding: applying the evidence in clinical practice, *Can Med Assoc J* 170(6):976-978, 16 Mar 2004.
5. Sharma M, Petosa R: Impact of expectant fathers in breast-feeding decisions, *J Am Diet Assoc* 97:1311-1313, 1997.
6. Sikorski J, Renfrew MJ, Pindorra S, et al: Support for breastfeeding mothers. In: *The Cochrane Library,* updated November 2001. (Cochrane Collaboration, 2004.)
7. International Lactation Consultants Association: Evidence-based guidelines for breastfeeding management during the first fourteen days, April, 1999, U.S. Maternal Child Health Bureau.
8. Spencer JP: Practical nutrition for the healthy term infant, *Am Fam Physician* 54:138-144, 1996.
9. Policy Statement: American Academy of Pediatrics, Committee on Drugs: The transfer of drugs and other chemicals into human milk, *Pediatrics* 108(3):776-789, September 2001.
10. Wisner KL, Perel JM, Findling RL: Antidepressant treatment during breast-feeding, *Am J Psychiatry* 153:1132-1137, 1996.
11. Koren G, Ito S: Do silicone breast implants affect breastfeeding? *Can Fam Physician* 44:2641-2642, 1998.
12. Bennison J: Breast feeding does not always work, *BMJ* 315:754, 1997.

BRONCHIOLITIS

Bronchiolitis is the most common lower respiratory tract infection in children less than 12 months old and is usually caused by the respiratory syncytial virus (RSV). The peak age is 2 to 6 months, although the condition occurs in children up to 2 years of age. It is more common in premature infants and those from lower socio-economic environments. There may be a history of atopy in the parents or eczema in the older infant. After a 3-day incubation period, upper respiratory tract symptoms, including rhinorrhea, nasal obstruction, and cough occur. Fine inspiratory crackles may be heard early, becoming coarser during recovery, and an expiratory wheeze is often present. The child can be tachypneic (more than 60 breaths per minute) and febrile. Between 2 and 3 days after the onset of symptoms, respiratory distress may develop. The treatment of uncomplicated bronchiolitis (respiratory rate less than 80, limited respiratory distress) is usually symptomatic but lacks quality evidence to guide therapy.[1] An interesting qualitative paper by Kai in the *British Medical Journal*[2] reflected the confusion that many parents have when they seek care for their acutely ill preschool children. These include variation in practice, with some caregivers prescribing antibiotics and some not, and the clinician declaring that they "hear nothing concerning in the chest" (lower respiratory tract), whereas the parents can clearly hear the rattle of upper respiratory tract congestion. Better understanding of parents' concerns and the causes of the concerns may promote more effective communication between health professionals and parents.[2]

Differentiating between mild (able to feed, little or no respiratory distress, good O_2 saturation), moderate (some respiratory distress/nasal flaring/chest wall retraction, some shortness of breath with feeding, some apnea) and severe (unable to feed, marked respiratory distress/chest wall retraction/nasal flaring and grunting, hypoxemic with prolonged apnea or cyanosis in some patients) bronchiolitis may be helpful. Infants with respiratory distress should be hospitalized and given oxygen. Bronchodilators have shown modest short-term benefit.[3] Some evidence exists to suggest that nebulized epinephrine may be favourable to salbutamol among outpatients; however, epinephrine has not been found to be useful among hospital inpatients.[4] Systemic or nebulized corticosteroids are not indicated except in children with asthma.[5,6]

≋ REFERENCES ≋

1. Fitzgerald DA, Kilham HA: Bronchiolitis: assessment and evidence-based management, *Med J Aust* 180:399-404, 2004
2. Kai J: What worries parents when their preschool children are acutely ill, and why: a qualitative study, *BMJ* 313:983-986, 1996.
3. Kellner JD, Ohlsson A, Gadomski AM, et al: Bronchodilators for bronchiolitis (Cochrane Review). In: *The Cochrane Library,* issue 1, Chichester, UK, 2004, John Wiley. (Last update July, 1998.)
4. Hartling L, Wiebe N, Russel K, et al: Epinephrine for bronchiolitis (Cochrane Review). Cochrane Acute Respiratory Infections Group. In: *The Cochrane Library*, issue 1, Chichester, UK, 2004, John Wiley. (Last update Sept, 2003.)
5. Cade A, Brownlee KG, Conway SP: Randomised placebo-controlled trial of nebulised corticosteroids in acute respiratory syncytial viral bronchiolitis, *Arch Dis Child* 82:126-130, 2000.
6. Bulow SM, Nir M, Levin E: Prednisolone treatment for respiratory syncytial virus infection: a randomized controlled trial of 147 infants, *Pediatrics* 104:e77, 1999.

BULLYING

Bullying in schools is common, and both bullies and those who are bullied have increased rates of psychological and psychosomatic symptoms. Children who are bullied have been reported to be at greater risk for bed wetting, sleep problems, school phobias, depression, suicidal ideation, and psychosomatic symptoms such as abdominal pain and headaches.[1-3] The victims' symptoms resemble those associated with victims of child abuse.[3] Bullies also commonly have psychosomatic symptoms[1] and, like those they bully, are at increased risk of depression and suicide.[2]

≋ REFERENCES ≋

1. Forero R, McLellan L, Rissel C, et al: Bullying behaviour and psychosocial health among school students in New South Wales, Australia: cross sectional survey, *BMJ* 319:344-348, 1999.
2. Kaltiala-Heino R, Rimpelä M, Marttunen M, et al: Bullying, depression, and suicidal ideation in Finnish adolescents: school survey, *BMJ* 319:348-351, 1999.
3. Fekkes M, Pijpers FIM, Verloove-Vanhorick SP: Bullying behaviour and associations with psychosomatic complaints and depression in victims, *J Pediatr* 144(1):17-22, 2004.

CIRCUMCISION AND DISORDERS OF THE FORESKIN
(See also circumcision, female; urinary tract infections in children)

The prevalence of circumcision varies widely in the developed world. Twenty-five percent of men worldwide are circumcised for cultural, religious, medical or parental choice reasons. In the United States, the rate is greater than 60%, while the rate in Canada and the United Kingdom is 48% and 24%, respectively.[1] Purported medical reasons for circumcision include a decreased risk of urinary tract infections, phimosis, paraphimosis, balanitis, sexually transmitted diseases, and penile cancer.

Substantial evidence shows that newborn circumcision decreases the incidence of urinary tract infections during the first year of life, especially in the first 3 months (0.11% vs 1.12%).[2,3] Wiswell[4] estimated that 99 newborn circumcisions would have to be performed to prevent one urinary tract infection. It is recommended that newborn males who have known abnormalities of the urinary tract (hydronephrosis, vesicoureteral reflux) should be circumcised to decrease the risk of developing a UTI.

Circumcision prevents phimosis and paraphimosis, but since these conditions are neither frequent nor serious, they hardly merit preventive surgical intervention.

Pathological phimosis is an absolute indication for circumcision but is rare, with an estimated incidence of only 4:10,000 boys per year.[5] In contrast, physiological phimosis, which results from the normal embryological fusion of the foreskin to the glans, is present in over 95% of newborn boys. Over the years the foreskin gradually separates from the glans, allowing the prepuce to be retracted in 20% of males by 6 months, 50% by 1 year, 90% by 3 years, and 99% by 17 years.[6]

For most cases of physiological phimosis, the only intervention required of physicians is parental reassurance. Forceful retraction of the foreskin is contraindicated, but once retraction can be accomplished with ease, the foreskin should be pulled back when bathing so the glans can be washed. Ballooning of the foreskin while urinating is common in children with physiological phimosis; the urine is partially diverted under the foreskin but drains freely, and the condition is inconsequential.[7] Pharmacological treatment of physiological phimosis consists of unrolling the foreskin once a day for a total of 4 to 6 weeks so that 0.05% betamethasone can be applied topically to the portions of the foreskin and glans that have been exposed and speed resolution.[8]

Paraphimosis is a fixed retraction of the foreskin; treatment is manual reduction, often under anesthesia. Because paraphimosis rarely recurs, a single episode is not an indication for circumcision.[7]

Most cases of mild balanitis respond to topical cleansing, although more advanced cases may require oral antibiotics. Recurrent balanitis is one indication for using topical steroids to hasten the resolution of physiological phimosis.[7]

Evidence suggests that circumcision is somewhat protective in the transmission of sexually transmitted diseases. There appears to be a modest reduction of risk in the transmission of HIV in circumcised men. This risk reduction is greatest in circumcised men at high risk for the disease.[9] Although the risk of penile cancer is less in the circumcised than the uncircumcised, cancer of the penis is so rare that the association has little clinical import.[8] The most common recognized risk factor for penile cancer identified through case control studies is phimosis.[10] There is inadequate information to recommend circumcision as a public health measure in Canada to prevent the diseases.[11]

Circumcision has been claimed to lead to a decrease in sexual satisfaction in adult life; data on this topic are sparse, but one observational study failed to confirm the hypothesis.[12]

Neonatal circumcision without anesthesia is painful.[13-15] Circumcisions done without the benefit of analgesia results in short- and long-term changes in infant behaviour.[16] Three modalities of anesthesia are in common use: a 5% eutectic mixture of the local anesthetics lidocaine and prilocaine (EMLA cream) applied to the penis under an occlusive dressing 60 to 90 minutes before the procedure, a dorsal penile nerve block (DPNB), and a subcutaneous circumferential ring block at the midshaft of the penis.[13] A comparison of 30% topical lidocaine, 5% lidocaine/prilocaine (EMLA cream), and placebo found both topical anesthetics to be superior to placebo and found EMLA cream to be superior to lidocaine cream.[14] On the other hand, a comparative evaluation of EMLA cream, dorsal penile nerve block, and penile ring block found ring block to be the most effective procedure and topical EMLA cream the least.[15,16] None of the agents have been shown to totally ameliorate pain for all infants undergoing a circumcision. It is interesting to note that the Mogen clamp has been associated with less pain, presumably because the procedure takes less time, compared with circumcisions performed with a Gomco clamp.[16] However, there is some evidence that circumcisions performed by Mogen result in higher proportion of post-procedure UTIs compared with those done by a physician. This may be due to urinary retention caused by the pressure dressing employed in a circumcision done with a Mogen clamp.[3] It is recommended that at least two methods of analgesia be employed when performing a circumcision (e.g., DPNB and sucrose-dipped pacifier).

The complication rates of neonatal circumcision are usually considered to be on the order of 0.2% to 0.6%. Most are minor episodes of bleeding or local infection.[17]

Contraindications to newborn circumcision include prematurity, blood dyscrasias or a family history of a bleeding disorder, or penile abnormalities (e.g., hypospadias or penoscrotal fusion).[18]

Should routine circumcision be recommended? The American Academy of Pediatrics and the Canadian Pediatric Society concur that existing scientific evidence demonstrates potential medical benefits of newborn male circumcision; however, these data are not sufficient to recommend routine neonatal circumcision. Parents should be given accurate and unbiased information and provided an opportunity to discuss the decision. It is legitimate for parents to take into consideration cultural, religious, and ethnic traditions.[11,13]

◢ REFERENCES ◣

1. Kaufman MW, Clark JY, Castro CL: Neonatal circumcision: benefits, risks and family teaching, *Am J Matern Child Nurs* 26(4):197-201, 2001.
2. Wiswell TE, Smith FR, Bass JW: Decreased incidence of urinary tract infections in circumcised male infants, *Pediatrics* 32:130-134, 1985.
3. Harel L, Straussberg R, Jackson S, et al: Influence of circumcision technique on frequency of urinary tract infections in neonates, *Pediatr Infect Dis J* 21(9):879-880, 2002.
4. Wiswell TE, Miller GM, Gelston HM Jr, et al: Effect of circumcision status on periurethral bacterial flora during the first year of life, *J Pediatr* 113 442-446, 1988.

5. Shankar KR, Rickwood AM: The incidence of phimosis in boys, *BJU Int* 84:101-102, 1999.
6. Oster J: Further fate of the foreskin: incidence of preputial adhesions, phimosis and smegma among Danish schoolboys, *Arch Dis Child* 43:200-203, 1968.
7. Simpson ET, Barraclough P: The management of the paediatric foreskin, *Aust Fam Physician* 27:381-383, 1998.
8. Dewan PA, Tieu HC, Chieng BS: Phimosis: is circumcision necessary? *J Paediatr Child Health* 32:285-289, 1996.
9. Updegrove KK: An evidence-based approach to male circumcision: what do we know? *J Midwifery Women Health* 46(6) 415-422, 2001.
10. Task Force on Circumcision: Circumcision policy statement, *Pediatrics* 103:686-693, 1999.
11. Fetus and Newborn Committee, Canadian Paediatric Society: Neonatal circumcision revisited, *Can Med Assoc J* 154:769-780, 1996.
12. Laumann EO, Masi CM, Zuckerman EW: Circumcision in the United States: prevalence, prophylactic effects, and sexual practice, *JAMA* 277:1052-1057, 1997.
13. American Academy of Pediatrics Task Force on Circumcision: Circumcision policy statement, *Pediatrics* 103:686-693, 1999.
14. Woodman PJ: Topical lidocaine-prilocaine versus lidocaine for neonatal circumcision: a randomized controlled trial, *Obstet Gynecol* 93:775-779, 1999.
15. Lander J, Brady-Fryer B, Metcalfe JB, et al: Comparison of ring block, dorsal penile nerve block, and topical anesthesia for neonatal circumcision: a randomized controlled trial, *JAMA* 278:2157-2162, 1997.
16. Taddio A: Pain management for neonatal circumcision, *Paediatric Drugs* 3(2) 101-111, 2001.
17. Tran PT, Giacomantonio M: Routine neonatal circumcision? *Can Fam Physician* 42:2201-2204, 1996.
18. Lerman S, Liao J: Neonatal Circumcision, *Pediatr Clin North Am* 48(6)1539-1557, 2001.

COLIC

(See also formulas)

The classic definition of colic is excessive crying that occurs in the first 3 months of an otherwise healthy infant's life, lasts longer than 3 hours a day, takes place on more than 3 days a week, and is longer than 3 weeks in duration. A more practical definition is excessive crying in a healthy, thriving infant. Colic occurs as frequently in breastfed as in bottle-fed babies and almost always resolves by 4 months.[1] It is one of the most frequent complaints brought to physicians in the first 3 months of an infant's life.[2] It is associated with significant maternal anxiety and emotional lability[3] and has been shown to trigger abuse and even death in infants.[4]

Symptoms

Crying in colicky babies varies a great deal from day to day, is typically paroxysmal, and, older literature to the contrary, occurs at any time of day. During these episodes the babies are almost impossible to soothe, but in the intervals they are settled and normal.[5,5a]

How much do normal infants cry? In 1962, Brazelton[6] reported on 80 normal infants. The median daily crying time was 1¾ hours in the second week of life, 2¾ hours at 6 weeks, and less than 1 hour by the 12th week.

Etiology

The etiology of colic is unknown. Some of the major hypotheses are that it results from a gastrointestinal disturbance, that it reflects suboptimal parent-child interactions, that it is a variant of normal, and that it consists of a variety of different conditions that at present cannot be distinguished.[1] Barr, in 1998, proposed that colic is best viewed as a clinical manifestation of normal emotional development and that the crying does not signify harm for the child.[7] Organic disease accounts for less than 5% of cases of colic but must be ruled out. Conditions that can cause excessive crying and should be considered are intussusception, testicular torsion, incarcerated hernia, and child abuse.[7] Parental reassurance is often overlooked in the treatment of colic; thus, it is important to elicit the parent's view, any unusual events, feeding patterns, and a picture of the home environment. It can be reassuring to show improvements in weight and height.[8]

Management

A 1998 systematic review of infantile colic assessed behavioural, dietary, and pharmacological interventions.[1]

Behaviour

Overresponse to and overstimulation of crying infants probably does more harm than good. The physician should inform the parents that colic is a self-limited condition and nothing they have done or are doing causes it. Parents need reassurance that their baby is not in pain and will not suffer long-term emotional consequences from the crying. When infants cry, they should be checked for hunger or for wet or dirty diapers. If neither of these is the cause of crying, parents should avoid exhausting themselves with prolonged carrying or holding of the infant and should try to find someone else to share in the caring. Parents should be given this advice not because an infant can become "spoiled" but to help them avoid caregiver burnout and possible child abuse. No reliable evidence supports use of infant carriers, vibration devices, or recordings of car sounds.[1]

Diet

For over 40 years a debate has raged over the value of eliminating cow's milk from the diet of infants with colic and substituting lactose-free, soy, or protein hydrolysate formulas. A systematic review concluded that substituting a protein hydrolysate formula is often beneficial, but that no substantial evidence supports soy, lactose-free, or fibre-enriched formulas.[1] There is no compelling evidence to suggest that breastfeeding causes more or less colic and that a breastfeeding mother should change her diet in any way. However, based on preliminary data, the Canadian Pediatric Society concludes that mothers may consider eliminating cow's milk from the diet and refrain from ingesting certain allergenic substances such as caffeine, chocolate, eggs, and nuts for a trial period to determine if symptoms improve.[9]

Herbal teas, including extracts of chamomile, fennel, balm mint, licorice, and vervain in a sucrose solution was more effective in decreasing parent-rated symptoms of colic, but the methodology made it difficult to draw many conclusions from this trial.[10]

The literature reviewing dietary therapy in the treatment of colic is limited by quality and difficult to interpret because of a large placebo effect, and the majority of cases resolve, regardless, within 3 months. Maternal diets can be difficult to control.[9]

Medications

Dicyclomine (Bentyl, Bentylol) has been proved effective but is not recommended because of rare but potentially serious adverse effects. For this reason, the manufacturer has withdrawn its use in children under 6 months of age. There is no evidence that simethicone has value.[1]

Other

A collaborative, randomized controlled trial carried out by pediatricians and chiropractors concluded that spinal manipulation was no more effective than placebo in the treatment of colic.[11] Likewise, there is no evidence that cranial osteopathy confers any benefit. Infant massage showed no benefit over the use of a crib vibrator, but the trial was small and may have lacked power.

─────────── ⚔ REFERENCES ⚖ ───────────

1. Lucassen PL, Assendelft WJ, van Eijk JT, et al: Effectiveness of treatments for infantile colic: systematic review, *BMJ* 316:1563-1569, 1998.
2. Wolke D, Meyer R: Excessive infant crying: a controlled study of mothers helping mothers, *Pediatrics* 94:322-332, 1994.
3. Miller AR, Barr RG, Eaton WO: Crying and motor behaviour of six-week-old infants and post-partum maternal mood, *Pediatrics* 92:551-558, 1993.
4. Barr RG: Colic. In Walker WA, Durie PR, Hamilton JR, et al, eds: *Pediatric gastrointestinal disease: pathophysiology, diagnosis, and management.* 2nd ed. St Louis: Mosby 241-250, 1996.
5. Forsythe BW, Leventhal JM, McCarthy PL: Mothers' perceptions of problems of feeding and crying behaviours, *Am J Disease Child* 139:269-272, 1985.
5a. Lehtonen LA, Rautava PT: Infantile colic: natural history and treatment, *Curr Probl Pediatr* 26(3):79-85, 1996.
6. Brazelton TB: Crying in infancy, *Pediatrics* 29:579, 1962.
7. Barr RG: Colic and crying syndromes in infants, *Pediatrics* 102(5):1282-1286, 1998.
8. Gatrad AR, Sheikh A: Persistent crying in babies, *BMJ* 328:330, 2004.
9. Nutrition Committee, Canadian Pediatric Society: Dietary manipulations for infantile colic, *Pediatr Child Health* 8(7):449-452, 2003.
10. Weizman Z, Alkrinawi S, Goldfarb D, et al: Herbal teas for infantile colic, *J Pediatr* 123:670-671, 1993.
11. Olafsdottr E, Forshei S, Markestad T: Randomized control trial of infantile colic treated with chiropractic spinal manipulation, *Arch Dis Child* 84:138-141, 2001.

CONDUCT DISORDER
(See also antisocial personality disorder; attention deficit/hyperactivity disorder; fetal alcohol effects)

Conduct disorder is the most common psychiatric disorder of childhood, with a prevalence between 1.5% and 3.4% of children and adolescents.[1] The ratio of boys to girls has usually been quoted as 3:1,[2] but the gender gap closes by mid-adolescence.[3] Gender-specific behaviours include violence and aggression in boys and shoplifting and prostitution in girls.[1] About 40% of 6- to 8-year-olds in whom conduct disorder is diagnosed become adolescent delinquents, and as adults they are at high risk for antisocial personality disorder, substance abuse, and participation in criminal activities.[2] Common childhood co-morbidities associated with conduct disorder include mood and anxiety disorders, substance abuse, and ADHD.[1,3] Youths with comorbid ADHD have earlier onset and more severe, more persistent conduct disorder.[1,3] There is little evidence for psychopharmacological treatment of conduct disorder with the exception of stimulants in children with coexisting ADHD.[4] Although genetics are significant in the development of conduct disorder, poor parenting, child abuse, and neglect are important risk factors. Family and parental training programs are central to treatment and have been shown to reduce re-arrest rates.[2,4]

Poor school performance, reading problems, weak social skills, and peer influence are childhood risk factors for conduct disorder. Prenatal and early developmental exposure to toxins, including maternal smoking during pregnancy, may be additional risk factors.[4]

─────────── ⚔ REFERENCES ⚖ ───────────

1. Steiner H, Dunne JE, Ayres W, et al: Practice parameters for the assessment and treatment of children and adolescents with conduct disorder, *J Am Acad Child Adolesc Psychiatry* 36: 122S-139S, 1997.
2. Scott S: Aggressive behaviour in childhood, *BMJ* 316: 202-206, 1998.
3. Loeber R, Burke JD, Lahey BB, et al: Oppositional defiant and conduct disorder: a review of the past ten years,

part I, *J Am Acad Child Adolesc Psychiatry,* 39:1468-1484, 2000.

4. Burke JD, Loeber R, Birmaher B: Oppositional defiant and conduct disorder: a review of the past ten years, part II, *J Am Acad Child Adolesc Psychiatry,* 41:1275-1293, 2002.

CROUP

Croup is characterized by a barking cough, a hoarse voice, and stridor and is usually caused by a virus, generally parainfluenza virus. Traditional treatment is exposure to humidified air (mist tents or a running shower in a closed bathroom), but no good studies have documented the efficacy of these approaches.[1] All children with croup who demonstrate respiratory difficulties should be treated with glucocorticoids.[2] Nebulized budesonide (2 mg) or oral or IM dexamethasone (0.15 to 0.6 mg/kg)[3] are all effective therapies that start having an effect on symptoms as early as 5 hours after treatment.[4-6] These trials have been conducted in the ER or in-patient ward setting, not family practice, but they all decrease repeat visits for medical treatment.[2] An outpatient trial showed effectiveness for patients with mild croup used oral dexamethasone 0.15 mg/kg. This trial used a validated scoring system for severity that just looked at stridor and chest retractions (mild for none, moderate when only with crying or exertion, or severe when at rest).[7] Oral dexamethasone is preferred because of its ease of administration and lower cost. It may need to be repeated daily for 2 to 4 days. Budesonide can be given at 6- to 8-hour dosing.[2] L-Epinephrine (5 mL of 1:1000) or racemic epinephrine (0.5 ml) should be considered for children with moderate or severe distress.[2]

⋙ REFERENCES ⋘

1. Jaffe DM: The treatment of croup with glucocorticoids (editorial), *N Engl J Med* 339:553-555, 1998.
2. Klassen TP: Croup. A current perspective, *Pediatr Clin of North Am* 46:1167-1178, 1999.
3. Geelhoed GC, Macdonald WB: Oral dexamethasone in the treatment of croup: 0.13 mg/kg versus 0.3 mg/kg versus 0.6 mg/kg, *Pediatr Pulmonol* 20:362-368, 1995.
4. Ausejo M, Saenz A, Pham B, et al: The effectiveness of glucocorticoids in treating croup: meta-analysis, *BMJ* 319:595-600, 1999.
5. Johnson DW, Jacobson S, Edney PC, et al: A comparison of nebulized budesonide, intramuscular dexamethasone, and placebo for moderately severe croup, *N Engl J Med* 339:498-503, 1998.
6. Geelhoed GC, Macdonald WB: Oral and inhaled steroids in croup: a randomized, placebo-controlled trial, *Pediatr Pulmonol* 20:355-361, 1995.
7. Geelhoed GC, Turner J, Macdonald WB: Efficacy of a small single dose of oral dexamethasone for outpatient croup, *BMJ* 313:140-142, 1996.

DIAPER RASH

Diaper rash, or *diaper dermatitis* are descriptive terms for dermatitis occurring in the diaper area. The two most common causes are irritant diaper dermatitis and *Candida* dermatitis. Irritant diaper dermatitis tends to spare the inguinal creases and is accentuated on surfaces such as the lower abdomen, buttocks, thighs, and genitalia. *Candida* dermatitis almost always involves the inguinal creases, and usually the infant has red plaques with white scales and satellite lesions.[1,2] The cause of irritant diaper dermatitis is primarily contact with moisture from urine. Contributing factors are fecal enzymes and irritant chemicals.[1,2] While these two conditions are responsible for the majority of diaper rash cases, a complete differential diagnosis should be reviewed when a diaper rash fails to respond to standard therapy.

The goal in treating diaper dermatitis is to keep the area clean and dry. Three methods should be considered: diapers, skin care, and medical treatment. Disposable super-absorbent diapers should be used rather than cloth diapers; this will keep the skin dry and maintain normal pH values.[3] In addition, diapers should contain a soft layer next to the skin and should be changed as soon as possible after soiling.[3] Gentle (to avoid frictional irritation) cleansing of the skin should be carried out using an oil-in-water lotion after the diaper has been soiled; a water repellent moisturizer (Vaseline or zinc-based barrier cream) should then be applied.[4] The baby should be bathed in a bath oil (rather than soap) at least once a day; twice-daily baths are recommended while the rash persists.[4] In cases of *Candida* dermatitis, topical antifungal agents such as nystatin (Mycostatin), clotrimazole (Canesten), or miconazole (Monistat Derm Cream) should be gently rubbed into the area several times a day, and treatment should be continued for at least 7 days after the rash has cleared.[1] A low-potency corticosteroid such as 1% hydrocortisone applied four times a day may help alleviate symptoms in more severe cases,[1,2] but is not a necessary component of treatment.[1] Parents should be instructed to apply antifungal and corticosteroid creams before applying barrier creams.[1]

⋙ REFERENCES ⋘

1. Ipp M: Pediatric dermatology: recognizing, treating hat's serious, *Patient Care Can* 7:20-32, 1996.
2. Sires UI, Mallory SB: Diaper dermatitis: how to treat and prevent, *Postgrad Med* 98:79-84, 1995.
3. Campbell R, Seymour JL, Stone LC, et al: Clinical studies with disposable diapers containing absorbent gelling materials: evaluation of effects on infant skin condition, *J Am Acad Dermatol* 17: 978-987, 1987.
4. Atherton DJ: The aetiology and management of irritant diaper dermatitis, *J Euro Acad Dermatol Venere* 15(suppl 1): 1-4, 2001.

DIARRHEA AND DEHYDRATION IN INFANTS
(See also breastfeeding; formulas; tropical medicine)

Diarrhea and dehydration are common problems in the pediatric population and require careful history and physical examination to exclude systemic causes, malabsorption, enteropathies, or serious infectious processes. In Canada and the United States, about half of all cases of diarrhea in infants are caused by rotavirus.

The management principles for rehydration in infants with diarrhea, based on recommendations by the Canadian Pediatric Society[1,2] and the American Academy of Pediatrics, include the following:

1. Children with mild diarrhea and no dehydration do not require glucose-electrolyte solutions and may be given a regular diet including milk.
2. Oral rehydration therapy is the initial treatment of choice for children with mild or moderate dehydration.

Two types of glucose-electrolyte solutions are used for oral rehydration therapy. The first type includes Rehydralyte and the WHO/UNICEF oral rehydration salts (ORS) with osmolalities of 310 and sodium contents of 75 and 90 mmol/L respectively, best suited for rehydration. Although more studies are needed, use of the high sodium WHO/UNICEF ORS may induce hypernatremia.[1] Also, some evidence suggests that hypo-osmolar ORS may decrease the amount and duration of diarrhea in comparison with the WHO/UNICEF ORS.[1] The second type of ORS, which contain 45 to 50 mmol/L of sodium and have osmolalites of 200 to 275, includes Infalyte, Pedialyte, Pediatric Electrolyte, and Naturalyte. These solutions are best suited for maintenance therapy but may be used for rehydration in otherwise healthy children with mild-to-moderate dehydration.

Chicken broth, soft drinks, apple juice, and sports beverages (such as Gatorade) should not be used. Chicken broth contains too much sodium and no glucose, and the others contain too much glucose and inadequate salt. Evidence increasingly shows that cereal-based solutions containing complex rather than simple carbohydrates are effective and will likely soon be available in North America.

For mild dehydration, 50 ml/kg of ORS should be given over a 4-hour period plus replacement of continuing losses. An additional 10 ml/kg should be given after each stool.

For moderate dehydration, 100 ml/kg of ORS should be given over a 4-hour period plus replacement of continuing losses. An additional 10 ml/kg should be given after each stool.

For severe dehydration, IV fluids are indicated. IV fluids may also be required for moderate dehydration in children with comorbidities such as diabetes and congenital adrenal hyperplasia, or in children who can-not retain orally administered fluids due to persistent vomiting.

For less severe vomiting in children, small amounts of ORS should be given at frequent intervals. Every 1 to 2 minutes the child should be given 5 ml (1 tsp) of solution. As rehydration occurs and vomiting diminishes, larger amounts may be given at less frequent intervals. Syringes are useful to facilitate oral intake.

Once rehydration is achieved, other fluids, including milk, and, if age appropriate, solid foods should be added. Breastfeeding should be continued throughout the course of illness. While breastfeeding may not prevent infection by rotavirus, it has been shown to diminish the severity of illness.[4]

Early refeeding with an age-appropriate diet is encouraged, and rather than exacerbating diarrhea, it appears to reduce stool output. The majority of children tolerate full-strength milk and have no need for lactose-free formulations. A 1994 meta-analysis found that except for infants with severe dehydration, there was no benefit in switching to a lactose-free formula or in diluting the formula.[5] Analysis of the literature has shown no adverse effects from the early introduction of solids[6] and no advantage to using the BRAT diet of bananas, rice, applesauce, and toast.[7] Foods that appear to be tolerated best include complex carbohydrates such as bread, potatoes, rice, lean meats, yogurt, fruits, and vegetables. Fatty foods and high-sucrose foods, such as fruit juices, should be avoided.

It is important to educate parents on assessing signs of dehydration and warn them that their child may need to be reassessed if the diarrhea is worsening in frequency or amount, becomes bloody, or the child develops abdominal pain or other new symptoms.

With regard to medications, antidiarrheals are not recommmended in the management of diarrhea in children due to a poor risk-benefit ratio. There have been some studies on a new antisecretory drug, racecadotril, that may eventually become widely available as a safe adjuvant therapy for diarrhea in children.[8] Antibiotics are usually not indicated except for severe bacterial diarrhea. As for future management, the focus may shift to prevention with a newer and safer vaccine for rotavirus.[9]

--- ✹ **REFERENCES** ✺ ---

1. Canadian Pediatric Society, Nutrition Committee: Treatment of diarrheal disease, *Paediatrics Child Health* 8(7):455-458, 2003.
2. Canadian Paediatric Society, Nutrition Committee: Oral rehydration therapy and early refeeding in the management of childhood gastroenteritis, *Can J Ped* 1:160-4, 1994.
3. American Academy of Pediatrics: The Management of acute gastroenteritis in young children, *Pediatrics* 97: 424-435, 1996.

4. Newburg DS, Peterson JA, Ruiz-Palacios GM, et al: Role of human-milk lactadherin in protection against symptomatic rotavirus infection, *Lancet* 351:1160-1164, 1998.
5. Brown KH, Peerson JM, Fontaine O: Use of non-human milks in the dietary management of young children with acute diarrhea: a meta-analysis of clinical trials, *Pediatrics* 93:17-27, 1994.
6. Brown KH: Dietary management of acute childhood diarrhea: optimal timing of feeding and appropriate use of milks and mixed diets, *J Pediatr* 118:S92-S98, 1991.
7. Meyers A: Modern management of acute diarrhea and dehydration in children, *Am Fam Physician* 51:1103-1115, 1995.
8. Cézard JP: Efficacy and tolerability of racecadotril in acute diarrhea in children, *Gastroenterology* 120(4):799-805, 2001.
9. Offit PA: The future of rotavirus vaccines, *Semin Pediatr Infect Dis* 13(3):190-57, 2002.

ENURESIS

Enuresis is failure to achieve bladder control by age 5.[1,2] Enuresis is primary (no period of continence) in 90% of cases and secondary (reversion to incontinence after an extended period of dryness) in 10%. Secondary incontinence is often associated with psychological stress. Daytime incontinence is rare and needs a more thorough investigation than nocturnal enuresis.[2]

The overall incidence of primary nocturnal enuresis is about 15% to 20% among 5-year-olds, 5% to 7% among 10-year-olds, and 2% to 4% among 12- to 14-year-olds. The spontaneous remission rate is 15% per year.[2] Boys are affected twice as often as girls. Enuresis may be familial; if one parent was affected, the incidence among the offspring is 40%, and if both parents were affected, the incidence is 70%.[1,2]

If by history and physical examination (including a careful neurological examination) no abnormalities are detected other than nocturnal enuresis, the only investigation required is a urinalysis, which should include specific gravity as a screen for diabetes insipidus. Urine culture is necessary only if symptoms suggest a urinary tract infection.[1]

The usual initial intervention is motivational therapy. Parents and the child are informed about the nature of the condition and are told that neither parents nor child is responsible for its development, but that with concerted effort, improvement may occur. Charts of dry and wet nights are set up, and rewards are given for each night the child is dry. Within a year, about 25% of children achieve complete resolution, which is somewhat better than the spontaneous resolution rate of 15%. Another 70% of children improve. If motivational therapy is unsuccessful, behavioural conditioning is usually attempted with use of an alarm system, which may be a sound device or a vibratory device.[1] Alarm systems are triggered by sensor pads that detect moisture. Older systems use a pad on which the child sleeps, whereas newer ones use a small Velcro pad that is attached to the child's undergarments.[3] Cendron[1] recommends using alarm systems only for children 7 years old or older. Alarm systems should be continued until the child has been consistently dry for a 3-week period. The reported success rate is 70%, but the relapse rate is 20% to 30%.[1]

Most children can be retrained by following the original alarm program. Two drugs commonly used for enuresis are imipramine (Tofranil) and desmopressin (DDAVP). Imipramine is usually first given as 25 mg 1 hour before bedtime. This may be increased to 50 mg for children ages 7 to 12 and 75 mg for older children. Treatment is usually continued for 3 to 6 months, after which time the child is gradually weaned from the drug. The long-term cure rate is about 25%. The usual initial dose of desmopressin (DDAVP) is 20 fg (1 spray in each nostril), or 0.2 mg in oral tablets 1 hour before bedtime. After 2 weeks the dose can be increased to 40 fg (0.4 mg orally) or, for children over the age of 12, to 60 fg (0.6 mg orally). When used for long-term control, treatment should be continued for 3 to 6 months and then reduced by 10-fg increments per month. DDAVP may also be used intermittently for special occasions such as sleepovers or camping trips.[1]

⊿ REFERENCES ⊾

1. Cendron M: Primary nocturnal enuresis, *Am Fam Physician* 59: 1205-1214, 1999.
2. Ullom-Minnich MR: Diagnosis and management of nocturnal enuresis, *Am Fam Physician* 54:2259-2266, 1996.
3. Tietjen DN, Husmann DA: Nocturnal enuresis: a guide to evaluation and treatment, *Mayo Clin Proc* 71:857-862, 1996.
4. Community Paediatrics Committee, Canadian Paediatric Society: Enuresis, *Paediatrics Child Health* 2(6):419-421, 1997.

FRAGILE X SYNDROME

The Fragile X syndrome (FXS) is the most common heritable cause of mental retardation. It is a sex-linked disorder, with an incidence of 1:3500 to 8900 affected males and 1:4000 to 12,000 affected females.[1] The incidence of premutation female carriers is in the order of 1:250 to 500.[1] Males are affected more severely than females, with 80% having an IQ less than 75. They have great difficulty at school, and exhibit impulsivity, inattention, and distraction. Many are unable to live independently as adults. The 20% of males who are unaffected are transmitting males who will pass the gene on to all daughters. Females may have minor learning disabilities, with one third meeting criteria for mental retardation. One third of children with FXS meet the diagnostic criteria for autism.[2] Men are at risk for early onset dementia and ataxia. Stimulants, antidepressants, and antipsychotics are helpful for behavioural disturbances in FXS.[3] Screening programs have been recommended so that women who are carriers can decide whether to have prenatal testing if they become pregnant.[4,5]

❧ REFERENCES ☙

1. Crawford DC, Acuna JM, Sherman SL: FMR1 and the fragile X syndrome: human genome epidemiology, *Rev Genetics Med* 3(5):359-371, 2001.
2. Rogers SJ, Wehner DE, Hegerman R: The behavioural phenotype in fragile X syndrome, idiopathic autism, and other developmental disorders, *Development Behav Peds* 22(6):406-417, 2001.
3. Berry-Kravis E, Potanos K: Psychopharmacology in fragile X syndrome—present and future, *Ment Retard Dev Disabil Res Rev* 10(1):42-48, 2004.
4. Song FJ, Barton P, Sleightholme V, et al: Screening for fragile X syndrome: a literature review and modelling study, *Health Technol Assess* 7(16):1-106, 2003.
5. Oostra BA, Willemsen R: Diagnostic tests for fragile X syndrome, *Expert Rev Mol Diagn* 1(2):226-232 , 2001.

FEBRILE SEIZURES
(See also fever in children; seizures)

Febrile seizures occur in 2% to 4% of children worldwide. Children with simple febrile seizures do not have increased rates of serious bacterial illness when compared with similar-age children who present with a fever and no seizure.[1,2] They do, however, have a slightly increased risk for epilepsy.[3-6] The background risk for epilepsy in the general population of children is 1.4%, and among children with simple febrile seizures, it is about 2.4%. However, the relatively small subgroup of children with "complex" febrile seizures (defined as focal, lasting more than 15 minutes, or recurring during the same febrile illness) are at higher risk for seizure disorders.[3,4] In one study the rate was 6% to 8% among children with only one "complex" feature, 17% to 22% among those with two, and 49% among those with three.[3]

The evidence suggests that the risk of recurrent febrile seizures is increased for children with a family history of febrile seizures, children who were younger when they had their first febrile seizure (less than 12 months old), children who first seized at lower temperatures (less than 40°C), children with a shorter duration of fever before the seizure (less than 24 hours), and possibly for children who exhibited complex features with their first febrile seizure.[7-9]

Vaccinations such as MMR and DPT are associated with transient increased risks of febrile seizures, with MMR causing 25 to 34 additional febrile seizures per 100,000 immunized children, and whole cell pertussis increasing the risk by 5 to 9 per 100,000 without increasing the long-term rate of developing epilepsy.[10,11] Since switching to the acellular pertussis vaccine in Canada, a 79% decrease occurred for pertussis vaccine–related hospital admissions for febrile seizures.[12]

With regard to treatment, one study randomized children with a history of febrile seizures to treatment during any subsequent febrile episodes with one of the following: acetaminophen, diazepam, acetaminophen plus diazepam, or placebo. The recurrence rate of febrile seizures was identical in all groups.[13]

At 10 years of age, children who had experienced either simple or "complex" febrile seizures in the early years of life demonstrated intellectual functioning, academic progress, and behaviour equivalent to that of children without a history of febrile seizures.[14]

❧ REFERENCES ☙

1. Trainor JL, Hampers LC, Krug SE, et al: Children with first-time simple febrile seizures are at low risk of serious bacterial illness, *Acad Emerg Med* 8:781–787, 2001.
2. Chamberlain JM, Gorman RL: Occult bacteremia in children with simple febrile seizures, *Am J Dis Child* 142:1073–1076,1988.
3. Annegars JF, Hauser WA, Shirts SB, et al: Factors prognostic of unprovoked seizures after febrile convulsions, *N Engl J Med* 316:493-498, 1987.
4. Verity CM, Golding J: Risk of epilepsy after febrile convulsions: a national cohort study, *BMJ* 303:1373-1376, 1991.
5. Shinnar S, Berg AT, Moshe SL, et al: The risk of seizure recurrence after a first unprovoked afebrile seizure in childhood—an extended follow-up, *Pediatrics* 98:216-225, 1996.
6. Verity CM, Greenwood R, Golding J: Long-term intellectual and behavioral outcomes of children with febrile convulsions, *N Engl J Med* 338:1723-1728, 1998.
7. Offringa M, Bossuyt PM, Lubsen J, et al: Risk factors for seizure recurrence in children with febrile seizures: A pooled analysis of individual patient data from five studies, *J Pediatr* 124:574–584, 1994.
8. Berg AT, Shinnar S, Hauser WA, et al: Predictors of recurrent febrile seizures: a meta-analytic review, *J Pediatr* 116:329–337, 1990.
9. Berg AT, Shinnar S, Hauser WA, et al: A prospective study of recurrent febrile seizures, *N Engl J Med* 327:1122–1127, 1992.
10. Davis RL, Barlow W: Placing the risk of seizures with pediatric vaccines in a clinical context, *Paediatr Drugs* 5(11):717-722, 2003.
11. Vestergaard H, Hviid A, Madsen KM, et al: MMR vaccine and febrile seizures: evaluation of susceptible subgroups and long-term prognosis, *JAMA* 292(3):351-357, 2004.
12. LeSaux N, Barrowman NJ, et al (IMPACT): Decrease in hospital admissions for febrile seizures and reports of hypotonic-hyporesponsive episodes presenting to hospital emergency departments since switching to acellular pertussis vaccine in Canada, a report from IMPACT. *Pediatrics.* 112(5):e348, 2003. Available from: http://pediatrics. aappublications.org/cgi/content/full/112/5/e348
13. Uhari M: Effect of acetaminophen and of low intermittent doses of diazepam on prevention of recurrences of febrile seizures, *J Pediatr* 126:991-995, 1995.

14. Robinson RJ: Febrile convulsions: further reassuring news about prognosis (editorial), *BMJ* 303:1345-1346, 1991.

FEVER IN CHILDREN
(See also febrile seizures; fever; urinalysis)

Various types of thermometers and the ability of parents to determine whether their children are febrile are discussed in the Fever section.

Fever is defined as rectal or tympanic temperature of 38° C or higher, higher than 37.5° C orally, or 37.3° C axillary.[1] Fever is a relatively harmless but effective immunological defense mechanism. No correlation between the severity of the fever and the etiology of the illness has been demonstrated.[2] The Canadian Pediatric Society recommends that rectal temperatures be used as definitive measurements until the age of 2, although axillary temperatures can be used to screen for fever. From 2 to 5 years, rectal is still most accurate, but tympanic or axillary temperatures may be used. For children older than age 5, oral temperatures are recommended, although tympanic and axillary are alternatives.[1]

Antipyretics

Antipyretics act by lowering the raised temperature set point that the infection has altered. The standard symptomatic treatment of fever in children has been acetaminophen (Tempra), approximately 50 mg/kg per day in 4 divided doses or 15 mg/kg/dose every 4 to 6 hours. A double-blind study of febrile children under 12 years of age that compared ibuprofen (Advil, Motrin) 20 mg/kg per day with acetaminophen (Tempra, Tylenol) 50 mg/kg per day found no difference in efficacy or adverse effects.[3]

When acetaminophen is prescribed for children, it is important to remember that drops are more concentrated than syrups and that various strengths of both chewable and regular tablets are available.

Response to antipyretics has not been shown to distinguish between serious and uncomplicated illness, nor does the use of antipyretics prolong the illness or negatively affect the outcome.[2]

Sponging

The primary purpose for intervening when a child has a fever is to increase the child's comfort. This consideration should be weighed against any harm that might result from intervening. Sponging is rarely if ever indicated except when temperatures exceed 40° to 41° C. If sponging is to be done, a single oral dose of an antipyretic should be given first and the sponging fluid should be lukewarm (neutral to the touch). Cold water or alcohol should never be used. Cold water causes shivering and raises body temperature, and alcohol may be inhaled and cause hypoglycemia and coma.[4] Although a few small studies have shown that tepid sponging after antipyretic administration leads to lower temperatures at 1 hour post,[5] there is a lack of evidence to support the routine use of sponging.[6]

Fever Without Source

The common practice for fever without source in children under 3 months of age has been to do a complete workup for sepsis and to treat the child with antibiotics pending culture results. In some cases this may not be necessary.[7-10] The main reason for an aggressive approach to this problem was that before mass immunization for *Haemophilus influenzae,* meningitis developed in 5% to 10% of children who had fever without source. At present, *Streptococcus pneumoniae* is the causative organism in the majority of fever-without-source cases that are found to be bacteremic. This bacterium rarely causes meningitis in young infants, and most cases resolve without treatment.[7,8] Baraff and associates[7] suggest the following management protocols for children with rectal temperatures of 38° C (100.4° F) or higher and no clinically evident focus of infection.

Infants under 28 days

All infants under 28 days of age, with or without a toxic appearance, should be admitted to the hospital and have a complete workup for sepsis, including blood, urine, and cerebrospinal fluid cultures. Most cases are treated with parenteral antibiotics pending culture results. For selected "low-risk" infants (criteria listed below) who do not appear toxic, acceptable management would be the same sepsis workup with careful observation but no antibiotic therapy pending culture results.

Infants 28 to 90 days

A variety of approaches may be taken for infants between the ages of 28 and 90 days. If infants appear toxic, they should be admitted to the hospital, have a complete sepsis workup, including blood, urine, and cerebrospinal fluid cultures, and be treated with parenteral antibiotics pending culture results.

Two options exist for the management of fever in "low-risk" infants in this age range. (Low risk is defined as previously healthy, non-toxic, no evidence of focal infection [excluding otitis media], white blood cell count of 5000 to 15,000/mm³ [5 to 15 × 10⁹/L], fewer than 1500 band cells/mm³ [1.5 × 10⁹/L], normal urinalysis findings, and if diarrhea is present, fewer than 5 white blood cells [per high-power field] in stool.) Both approaches may be accomplished on an outpatient basis provided the parents are reliable and close follow-up can be ensured.

Protocol 1 is a sepsis workup, including blood, urine, and cerebrospinal fluid cultures. Ceftriaxone 50 mg/kg (maximum 1 g) IM is given stat, and follow-up takes place within 24 hours. At follow-up, a second dose of ceftriaxone may be given.

Protocol 2 involves no sepsis workup other than a urine culture, no antibiotics (unless needed to treat otitis media), careful observation by parents, and physician follow-up within 24 hours.

Children age 3 to 36 months

Toxic-appearing children should be admitted to the hospital, have a complete sepsis workup, including blood, urine, and cerebrospinal fluid cultures, and be treated with parenteral antibiotics pending culture results.

The management of previously healthy, non–toxic-appearing children age 3 to 36 months depends on the rectal temperature. If it is below 39° C (102.2° F), no diagnostic tests or antibiotics are needed. The child should be treated as an outpatient with acetaminophen 15 mg/kg/dose every 4 hours and should be reassessed if the fever persists for more than 48 hours or if the clinical condition deteriorates. If the temperature is 39° C (102° F) or higher, management may in most cases be on an outpatient basis after the following workup:

- Urine culture for boys under 6 months of age and girls under 2 years of age or for any child who has a positive urine dipstick test for leukocyte esterase or nitrites. Urine dipsticks may be negative in up to 20% of young children with urinary tract infections, which is why culture is recommended for all young children regardless of the dipstick results.
- Stool cultures if stool contains blood and mucus or more than 5 white blood cells per high-power field.
- Chest X-ray examination if respiratory symptoms are present.
- Blood cultures for all children in this category or for those with a white blood cell count of 15,000/mm³ (15 × 10⁹/L) or higher.
- Antibiotics either for all children in this category or for those with a white blood cell count of 15,000/mm³ (15 × 10⁹/L) or higher.
- Acetaminophen 15 mg/kg per dose every 4 hours.
- Follow-up in 24 to 48 hours.

A chest X-ray examination in febrile children under 2 years of age who do not have physical signs of pulmonary infection has generally not proved valuable. However, a 1999 paper reported the presence of occult pneumonia (as interpreted by radiologists) in 19% of children age 5 years or less who had temperatures of 39° C (102° F) or higher, white blood cell counts of 20,000/mm³ or higher, and no abnormal lung findings on examination.[11] Whether detection of these cases has clinical significance is uncertain because most would probably have resolved without treatment, and the few that did not could be identified and treated with a close follow-up protocol.[12]

◗ REFERENCES ◗

1. Temperature measurement in paediatrics. Reference No. CP00-01.Community Pediatrics Committee, 2002, Canadian Pediatric Society.
2. The Drug Therapy and Hazardous Substances Subcommittee, CPS: Acetaminophen and ibuprofen in the management of fever and mild to moderate pain in children, Canadian Pediatric Society Statement, May 14, 2003, *Pediatr Child Health* 3(4): 1998.
3. McIntyre J, Hull D: Comparing efficacy and tolerability of ibuprofen and paracetamol in fever, *Arch Dis Child* 74: 164-167, 1996.
4. Impicciatore P, Pandolfini C, Casella N, et al: Reliability of health information for the public on the World Wide Web: systematic survey of advice on managing fever in children at home, *BMJ* 314:1875-1881, 1997.
5. Meremikwu M, Oyo-Ita A: Physical methods for treating fever in children (Cochrane Review), revised Jan 25, 2003, in The Cochrane Library Issue 2, Chichester, 2004, UK:John Wiley and Sons, Ltd.
6. Watts R, Robertson J, Thomas G: Nursing management of fever in children: a systematic review, Int J Nurs Pract. 9(1):S1-S8, 2003.
7. Baraff LJ: Management of fever without source in infants and children., *Ann Emerg Med* 36(6):602-614, 2000.
8. Long SS: Antibiotic therapy in febrile children: "best-laid schemes," *J Pediatr* 124:585-588, 1994.
9. Daaleman TP: Fever without source in infants and young children, *Am Fam Physician* 54:2503-2512, 1996.
10. Jaskiewicz JA, McCarthy CA, Richardson AC, et al: Febrile infants at low risk for serious bacterial infection—an appraisal of the Rochester criteria and implications for management, *Pediatrics* 94:390-396, 1994.
11. Bachur R, Perry H, Harper MB: Occult pneumonias: empiric chest radiographs in febrile children with leukocytosis, *Ann Emerg Med* 33:166-173, 1999.
12. Green SM, Rothrock SG: Evaluation styles for well-appearing febrile children: are you a "risk-minimizer" or a "test-minimizer"? (editorial), *Ann Emerg Med* 33:211-214, 1999.

FORMULAS

(See also breastfeeding; colic; diarrhea and dehydration in infants)

Infant formulas have as their bases cow's milk, soy, or protein hydrolysates (Table 63). The last named are the most expensive. Almost all formulas come with or without iron fortification, and almost all are available as ready-to-feed (the most expensive), as liquid concentrates that require dilution, and as powders that require reconstitution (the least expensive).[1] Bottle-fed infants should receive iron-fortified formulas from birth; otherwise, they are at risk for iron deficiency anemia.[1,2] (The iron is not required to prevent iron deficiency until 4 to 6 months, but because parents rarely change the formulas begun in the neonatal period, iron-fortified formulas should be used from the beginning of bottle feeding.) Although iron deficiency anemia has been claimed to be associated with developmental disadvantage, iron supplementation of bottle-fed infants in developed countries does not appear to improve developmental status.[3] The Canadian Task Force on Preventive Health Care gives iron-fortified formulas a "B" rating,[2] and the U.S. Preventive Services Task Force gives them a "C."[4]

Most cows milk–based formulas contain lactose (some are produced as lactose free), whereas soy-based formulas and protein hydrolysates do not. Traditionally, infants with diarrhea were switched to non-lactose-containing formulas or to formulas diluted with water. A 1994 meta-analysis of 29 randomized trials found that if infants with severe dehydration were excluded, no benefit was achieved by switching to soy-based formulas or protein hydrolysates or by diluting formulas with water. (See discussion of diarrhea and dehydration in infants.)[5]

Whether infantile colic responds to protein hydrolysates is controversial. (See discussion of colic.) The Nutrition Committee of the Canadian Pediatric Society found level A evidence to support a trial of hypoallergenic formulas in the treatment of colic. Although they state that there is level B evidence that soy formula may have beneficial effects, level A evidence cautions against its use because is an important allergen in infancy.[8] Infants at high risk for allergies and food intolerance develop fewer infant and childhood allergies from the use of hydolyzed formulas compared with cow's milk-based products, although it is uncertain whether this benefit persists beyond age 5.[9]

Table 63 Selected Examples of Infant Formulas

Formula	Manufacturer and comments
Milk-Based Formulas	
Bonamil	Wyeth, casein dominant
Carnation Goodstart	Carnation, partial protein hydrolysate
Enfamil, Enfalac	Mead Johnson, whey-dominant protein
Lactofree, Enfalac Lactose Free	Mead Johnson, lactose free
SMA	Wyeth, whey dominant
Similac	Ross
Similac LF	Ross, lactose free
Soy-Based Formulas	
Enfalac Soy	Mead Johnson, contains sucrose
Prosobee	Mead Johnson, does not contain sucrose
Gerber Soy Formula	Gerber
Isomil	Ross
Nursoy	Wyeth
Soyalac	Nutricia–Loma Linda
Protein Hydrolysates	
Alimentum	Ross
Nutramigen	Mead Johnson

Breastfeeding mothers interested in formula supplementation should be made aware that the introduction of regular formula feeds to breastfeeding infants has been shown to reduce the frequency and suckling duration of breastfeeding, regardless of when the formula feeds are introduced.[10]

REFERENCES

1. Spencer JP: Practical nutrition for the healthy term infant, *Am Fam Physician* 54:138-144, 1996.
2. Canadian Task Force on the Periodic Health Examination: *Clinical preventive health care,* Ottawa, 1994, Canadian Communication Group, pp 244-255.
3. Morley R, Abbott R, Fairweather-Tait S, et al: Iron fortified follow on formula from 9 to 18 months improves iron status but not development or growth: a randomised trial, *Arch Dis Child* 81:247-252, 1999.
4. U.S. Preventive Services Task Force: *Guide to clinical preventive services,* ed 2, Baltimore, 1996, Williams & Wilkins, pp 231-246.
5. Brown KH, Peerson JM, Fontaine O: Use of nonhuman milks in the dietary management of young children with acute diarrhea: a meta-analysis of clinical trials, *Pediatrics* 93:17-27, 1994.
6. American Academy of Pediatrics, Committee on Nutrition: Hypoallergenic infant formulas, *Pediatrics* 83:1068-1069, 1989.
7. Hill DJ, Hudson IL, Sheffield LJ, et al: A low allergen diet is a significant intervention in infantile colic: results of a community-based study, *J Allergy Clin Immunol* 96: 886-892, 1995.
8. Canadian Paediatric Society, Nutrition Committee: Dietary manipulations for infantile colic, *Pediatr Child Health* 8(7) 449-452, 2003.
9. Osborn DA, Sinn J: Formulas containing hydrolysed protein for prevention of allergy and food intolerance in infants, Updated May 5, 2003 (Cochrane Review). In: *The Cochrane Library*, issue 3, Chichester, UK, 2004, John Wiley.
10. Hornell A, Hofvander Y, Kylberg E: Solids and formula: association with pattern and duration of breastfeeding, *Pediatrics* 107(3):E38 1 Mar, 2001.

GROWTH HORMONE

Numerous studies, now including a placebo-controlled study, have demonstrated the positive effect of GH treatment on final height in short normal children.[1] Studies suggest that short-term height gains can range from none to approximately 0.7 SD over 1 year.[1] One long-term U.S. multicentre study reported an increased adult height of about 9 cm in boys and 6 cm in girls compared with the heights achieved by untreated children in other studies.[2] Although treated individuals may be taller than non-treated individuals, they are still relatively short when compared with peers of normal stature.[1]

When given for the treatment of growth hormone (GH) deficiency, GH therapy is effective with an average increase of 8 to 10 cm per year for the first year.[3,4] Response wanes each year, but growth velocity continues at faster than pretreatment rates.[3,4] Daily subcutaneous (SC) injections of GH are more effective than 3 times per week at the same dose.[3] Long-acting depot preparation designed for monthly or bimonthly SC injection is also effective.[4] In patients starting treatment in early to mid-puberty, the addition of a gonadotropin-releasing hormone agonist therapy to GH appears to increase final height.[5,6] The psychological effect of serial injections compared with the benefits remains difficult to judge for some individuals and families.

◢ REFERENCES ◣

1. Bryant J, Cave C, Milne R: Recombinant growth hormone for idiopathic short stature in children and adolescents, *Cochrane Database of Systematic Reviews* (4):CD004440, 2003.
2. Hintz R, Attie K, Baptista J, et al: Effect of growth hormone treatment on adult height of children with idiopathic short stature, *N Engl J Med* 340:502-507, 1999.
3. de Muinck Keizer-Schrama SM, Rikken B, Wynne HJ, et al: Dose-response study of biosynthetic human growth hormone (GH) in GH-deficient children: effects on auxological and biochemical parameters. Dutch Growth Hormone Working Group, *J Clin Endocrinol Metab* 74:898, 1992.
4. Reiter EO, Attie KM, Moshang T Jr, et al: A multicenter study of the efficacy and safety of sustained release GH in the treatment of naive pediatric patients with GH deficiency, *J Clin Endocrinol Metab* 86:4700, 2001.
5. Mericq MV, Eggers M, Avila A, et al: Near final height in pubertal growth hormone (GH)-deficient patients treated with GH alone or in combination with luteinizing hormone-releasing hormone analog: results of a prospective, randomized trial, *J Clin Endocrinol Metab* 85:569, 2000.
6. Saggese G, Federico G, Barsanti S, et al: The effect of administering gonadotropin-releasing hormone agonist with recombinant-human growth hormone (GH) on the final height of girls with isolated GH deficiency: results from a controlled study, *J Clin Endocrinol Metab* 86:1900, 2001.

INTUSSUSCEPTION

Intussusception occurs most frequently between the ages of 5 and 9 months. Males tend to be affected more often than females. Patients typically present with the sudden onset of severe, colicky abdominal pain and crying, with episodes occurring approximately every 15 minutes. Emesis, fever, and lethargy may be present.[1] The classic triad of vomiting, abdominal pain, and bloody ("red currant jelly") diarrhea is seen in less than one third of patients. Ultrasonography is an excellent imaging study with sensitivity and specificity approaching 100%[2] for detecting intussusception.

◢ REFERENCES ◣

1. Winslow BT, Westfall JM, Nicholas RA: Intussusception, *Am Fam Physician* 54:213-217, 1996.
2. Daneman A, Alton D: Intussusception: issues and controversies related to diagnosis and reduction, *Radiol Clin North Am* 34: 743, 1996.

LABIAL FUSION

Labial fusion is usually seen in girls between the ages of 3 months and 4 years. It results from denudation of the squamous epithelium of the labia minora, which is usually caused by a chemical or infectious vulvitis. Intense itching and scratching from the vulvitis can result in labial fusion secondary to superficial trauma. Fusion begins at the posterior fourchette and progresses anteriorly toward the clitoris; in more advanced cases some degree of urinary obstruction may predispose the child to urinary tract infection. Treatment consists of the nightly application of small amounts of estrogen cream (Premarin) to the fused area. Applications are continued until the adhesions lyse, which usually occurs within 2 weeks. This is an off-label indication for topical estrogen cream. Once the labia have separated, an ointment such as Vaseline should be applied to them for at least a month to prevent readhesion.[1,2]

◢ REFERENCES ◣

1. Leung AK, Robson WL, Wong B: Labial fusion, *Paediatr Child Health* 1:216-218, 1996.
2. Prepubescent vulvovaginitis—Diagnosis. Elsevier, 2004. (Accessed April 16, 2004 at http://www.firstconsult.com/home/framework/fs_main.htm?msite=fs_main&)

LEAD POISONING

In October 1991, the U.S. Centers for Disease Control and Prevention (CDC) redefined lead poisoning by lowering acceptable blood lead levels to 10 μg/dL (0.48 μmol/L). The CDC and American Academy of Pediatrics' previous guidelines had recommended universal lead level screening for children younger than 6 years of age. Revised guidelines, however, only recommend blood test screening for children who reside in communities where 27% or more of the housing was built before 1950, or where more than 12% of children have documented blood lead levels of 10 μg/dL or higher. Blood test screening is also recommended for children who live in communities for which this type of data is unavailable.

Risk questionnaires can be considered to screen all other children. Such questionnaires determine whether children live in (or regularly visit) houses or child care facilities built before 1950, or houses or child care facilities built before 1978, but renovated in the past 6 months, or whether children have siblings or playmates who have, or have had, lead poisoning. A positive or ambiguous response to any of these questions mandates blood lead level assessment.[1] Since blood levels only reflect excess environmental absorption, it may be useful to additionally measure erythrocyte protoporphyrin levels to gauge the adverse metabolic effects of such absorption.[2]

The use of vinyl mini-blinds, a newly discovered source of lead poisoning, remains an issue. Until relatively recently, lead was used as a stabilizing agent in the manufacturing process of these blinds, and as they aged, lead dust accumulated on the surface of the blinds.[3] If families with small children are unable to leave homes known to be contaminated with lead, a moderately effective alternative is regular, intensive house-cleaning, particularly wet-mopping of all floors, damp-sponging of walls and other surfaces, and high-efficiency particle-accumulating vacuuming.[4]

Importantly, published evidence suggests that lead levels lower than 10 μg/dL (0.48 μmol/L) may decrease IQ levels.[5] An association between elevated lead levels and increased incidence of dental caries has also been reported.[6]

❧ REFERENCES ❧

1. American Academy of Pediatrics Committee on Environmental Health: Screening for elevated blood lead levels, *Pediatrics* 101:1072-1078, 1998.
2. Piomelli S: Childhood lead poisoning, *Pediatr Clin North Am* 49(6):1285-1304, vii, 2002.
3. Norman EH, Hertz-Picciotto I, Salmen DA, et al: Childhood lead poisoning and vinyl miniblind exposure, *Arch Pediatr Adolesc Med* 151:1033-1037, 1997.
4. Rhoads GG, Ettinger AS, Weisel CP, et al: The effect of dust lead control on blood lead in toddlers: a randomized trial, *Pediatrics* 103:551-555, 1999.
5. Matte TD: Reducing blood lead levels: benefits and strategies (editorial), *JAMA* 281:2340-2342, 1999.
6. Moss ME, Lanphear BP, Auinger P: Association of dental caries and blood lead levels, *JAMA* 281:2294-2298, 1999.

NEONATAL JAUNDICE
(See also breastfeeding)

Unconjugated hyperbilirubinemia, or physiological jaundice, of the newborn is extremely common. It is more frequent and more severe in premature, Asian, and breast-fed infants. The unconjugated bilirubin tends to peak about the fourth day of life and then gradually declines over several weeks. The difference between normal, full-term breast-fed and bottle-fed babies is that in most studies, both the peaks and the duration of jaundice tend to be higher in the breast-fed babies.[1,2]

Gartner[2] has marshaled considerable evidence that the initial hyperbilirubinemia of the breast-fed infant is a form of starvation jaundice, and that when feeding is started early and given frequently, the bilirubin peaks of breast-fed infants are not higher than those of bottle-fed babies. He has suggested that although bottle-fed babies may thrive on six feedings a day, breast-fed infants probably require 10 in the early days and weeks of life. According to him, breast-fed babies should not be given glucose and water supplementation because this decreases their milk intake.

The differential diagnosis of physiological jaundice must consider a wide variety of conditions, including extrahepatic and intrahepatic biliary obstructions, liver disease, various metabolic abnormalities, hemolytic disorders, large hematomas, sepsis, hypothyroidism, and bowel obstruction.[1]

Not all jaundiced babies need extensive investigation. The Canadian Paediatric Society recommends that all babies who are being considered for phototherapy have a complete blood cell count and smear, measurement of conjugated and unconjugated bilirubin, blood grouping with antibody testing, and further tests such as measurement of glucose-6-phosphate dehydrogenase for those whose ethnicity (Asian, African, or Mediterranean descent) puts them at risk of glucose-6-phosphate deficiency.[3] Visual assessment of neonatal jaundice is unreliable and inaccurate.[4]

No national or international consensus has defined a threshold level of bilirubin that would mandate phototherapy for term infants without additional risk factors.[3] The 2004 recommendations of the American Academy of Pediatrics are that phototherapy be instituted in term infants age 25 to 48 hours when the bilirubin is 15 mg/dL (260 μmol/L) or higher, in those age 49 to 72 hours when it is 18 mg/dL (310 μmol/L) or higher, and in those over the age of 72 hours when it is 20 mg/dL (340 μmol/L) or higher.[5] The Canadian Paediatric Society takes a more cautious approach and advises starting phototherapy in infants age 24 hours if the bilirubin is 10 mg/dL (170 μmol/L) or higher, in infants age 48 hours if it is 15 mg/dL (260 μmol/L) or higher, and in those age 72 hours if it is 18 mg/dL (310 μmol/L) or higher.[3] Infants at increased risk for kernicterus (gestational age under 37 weeks and birth weight less than 2500 g, hemolysis, jaundice at less than 24 hours of age, sepsis, and need for resuscitation at birth) should receive phototherapy at lower levels of bilirubin than are indicated for healthy term infants.[3]

Serum bilirubin usually decreases by 2.5 to 3 mg/dL per day and 1 to 2 mg/dL in first 4 to 6 hours of phototherapy. Bilirubin level should be followed every 12 hours. Phototherapy should be discontinued when the bilirubin reaches levels of about 13 mg/dL. Bilirubin levels should be rechecked again 12 hours after discontinuation, to assess for recurrence.

Even though breastfeeding is associated with higher bilirubin levels than bottle feeding, breastfeeding is not contraindicated during phototherapy. However, the babies should be well hydrated, because dehydration may raise bilirubin levels and phototherapy itself may aggravate dehydration.[3]

---------------- **❧ REFERENCES ❧** ----------------

1. Lasker MR, Holzman IR: Neonatal jaundice: when to treat, when to watch and wait, *Postgrad Med* 99:187-193, 197-198, 1996.
2. Gartner LM: On the question of the relationship between breastfeeding and jaundice in the first 5 days of life, *Semin Perinatol* 18:502-509, 1994.
3. Fetus and Newborn Committee of the Canadian Paediatric Society: Approach to the management of hyperbilirubinemia in term newborn infants: a joint statement with the College of Family Physicians of Canada, *Paediatr Child Health* 4:161-164, 1999.
4. Moyer VA, Ahn C, Sneed S: Accuracy of clinical judgment in neonatal jaundice, *Arch Pediatr Adolesc Med* 154:391-394, 2000.
5. American Academy of Pediatrics Subcommittee on Hyperbilirubinemia: Management of hyperbilirubinemia in the newborn infant 35 or more weeks of gestation, Pediatrics 114(1):297-316, 2004.

OBESITY IN CHILDREN

(See also cholesterol-lowering studies in children; epidemiology of obesity)

Obesity in children has been increasing worldwide.[1,2] Body mass index (BMI) between the 85th and 95th percentile for age and sex is considered at risk for overweight and BMI at or above the 95th percentile is considered overweight or obese.[3] In the United States, 15.3% of 6- to 11-year-olds and 15.5% of 12- to 19-year-olds are at or above the previously established 95th percentile for BMI.[4] As with adults, obesity in childhood can lead to hypertension, dyslipidemia, hyperinsulinemia, sleep apnea, and psychological distress. Type 2 diabetes, once unknown in adolescence, is becoming highly prevalent in some young populations.[5] Obesity in the teenage years, particularly if marked, is a risk factor for adult obesity. The risk is even greater if one or both parents are obese.[6]

Both genetic and environmental factors are clearly important in determining childhood obesity. A twin study of children confirmed the powerful influence of genetics in determining the percentage of body fat,[7] and a cross-sectional study of German children ages 5 to 6 years found that the prevalence of obesity was less in those who had been breast fed than in those who had not.[8]

A lifestyle characterized by inactivity also clearly contributes to the increasing prevalence of obesity in children.[2] One fourth of U.S. children watch 4 or more hours of television daily, and two thirds watch at least 2 hours a day. These figures are exclusive of time spent playing video games, watching videos, or working or playing on the computer. Excessive TV watching correlates with increased BMI, and it is hypothesized that children are less physically active and ingest extra calories while watching TV.[9,10] However, whether the excessive weight in these individuals is caused by prolonged TV watching or whether overweight children tend to watch more TV is unknown.[11] One small prospective randomized trial of third- and fourth-grade students found a slight decrease in BMI in those who had limits set on their television, videotape, and video game time.[12] Dietary factors associated with obesity include over-consumption of sugar-sweetened beverages, increase in the intake of energy-dense foods, increased portion sizes, and a rise in the consumption of fast food.[2]

Is there any point instituting preventive interventions for children at high risk? In the absence of good data, common sense dictates that all children, not just obese ones, be encouraged to be physically active (with strict limitation of TV time) and eat a balanced diet.

The U.S. Preventive Services Task Force gives a "B" recommendation for the periodic measurement of height and weight of children and adults.[13] The Canadian Task Force on Preventive Health Care gives these strategies a "C" recommendation. The Canadian Task Force also gives a "C" recommendation to exercise and to family-based nutrition and exercise counselling as a means of controlling obesity in children, and it gives a "D" to very low-calorie diets in preadolescents.[10]

---------------- **❧ REFERENCES ❧** ----------------

1. Troiano RP, Flegal KM, Kuczmarski RJ, et al: Overweight prevalence and trends for children and adolescents: the National Health and Nutrition Examination Surveys, 1963-91, *Arch Pediatr Adolesc Med* 149:1085-1091, 1995.
2. Ebbeling CB, Pawlak DB, Ludwig DS: Childhood obesity: public health crisis, common sense cure, *Lancet* 360:473-482, 2002.
3. American Academy of Pediatrics: Prevention of pediatric overweight and obesity, *Pediatrics* 112(2):424-430, 2003.
4. Ogden CL, Flegal KM, Carroll MD, et al: Prevalence and trends in overweight among U.S. children and adolescents 1999-2000, *JAMA* 288;1728-1732, 2002.
5. Fagot-Campagna A, Pettitt DJ, Engelgau MM, et al: Type 2 diabetes among North American children and adolescence: an epidemiologic review and a public health perspective, *J Pediatr* 136:664-672, 2000.
6. Whitaker RC, Wright JA, Pepe MS, et al: Predicting obesity in young adulthood from childhood and parental obesity, *N Engl J Med* 337:869-873, 1997.
7. Faith MS, Pietrobelli A, Nunez C, et al: Evidence for independent genetic influences on fat mass and body mass index in a pediatric twin sample, *Pediatrics* 104:61-67, 1999.
8. von Kries R, Koletzko B, Sauerwald T, et al: Breast feeding and obesity: cross sectional study, *BMJ* 319:147-150, 1999.
9. Andersen RE, Crespo CJ, Bartlett SJ, et al: Relationship of physical activity and television watching with body weight and level of fatness among children: results from the Third

National Health and Nutrition Examination Survey, *JAMA* 279:938-942, 1998.

10. Canadian Task Force on the Periodic Health Examination: Periodic health examination, 1994 update. I. Obesity in childhood, *Can Med Assoc J* 150:871-879, 1994.

11. Robinson TN: Does television cause childhood obesity? (editorial), *JAMA* 279:959-960, 1998.

12. Robinson TN: Reducing children's television viewing to prevent obesity: a randomized controlled trial, *JAMA* 282:1561-1567, 1999.

13. U.S. Preventive Services Task Force: *Guide to clinical preventive services,* ed 2, Baltimore, 1996, Williams & Wilkins, 219-229.

PARENTING AND BEHAVIOURAL PROBLEMS

Behavioural Problems in Children

Emotional and behavioural problems in children are common presenting problems in family practice. Evidence suggests that adult mental health problems have their origins in infancy and childhood, and that poor parenting practices can result in significant consequences for individual and family health for a lifetime.[1,2]

In addition, evidence from a range of studies suggests that maternal psychosocial health can have significant effects on the mother-infant relationship, and that this in turn can have consequences for both the short- and long-term psychosocial health of the child.[3]

Parents frequently have concerns about their child's behaviour, and present those concerns to the family physician. In one study, 90% of mothers of preschool-age children had at least mild concerns about their child's behaviour, with problems of discipline and behaviour management constituting the majority of concerns.[4] A recent survey listed the top five parenting concerns as education (39%), health (12%), safety (8%), drugs (7%), and making time for kids (7%).[5] More than 50% of parents of preschoolers reported difficulties with their children arguing, demanding attention, and being disobedient. Other concerns for mothers were discipline, childhood illness, impatience with "the terrible two's and three's," lack of time for herself and child, and whether or not the child should attend nursery school.[6] In contrast, fathers ranked discipline, childhood illness, and time for myself and my child. Discipline was the primary concern of both mothers and fathers whether or not they were first-time parents or had two or more children.[5]

Many factors affect a child's behaviour, including temperament and attachment.[7] Temperament is a major influence and describes the "hard wiring" in each child that determines the child's response to new experiences. It includes activity level, regularity in biological functioning, approach or withdrawal to a new situation, adaptability to change in routine, level of sensory threshold, mood, intensity of response, persistence/attention span, and distractibility.[8] The child's temperament is important to recognize because it contributes to parent-child interactions by making children respond to parental caregiving with differing styles. When there is a poor fit or incompatible interaction with the caregiving environment, the child is predisposed to a variety of clinical problems.[8] In addition, a child's temperament may affect parents both as to how they feel about themselves as persons and how they function as parents. The 60% of children classified as "easy" almost never present their parents with serious behavioural problems except in quite extraordinary circumstances. The 15% who are "difficult" provide most of the work for professionals. The 10% who are classified as "slow to warm up" need very specific interactions to help them cope with their environment, such as warnings and rehearsals, which some parents and teachers work out for themselves. Parents appreciate the normalization of some of their child's behaviour as characteristic of temperament and not due to particular parenting deficits. Explanations can then lead to appropriate planning to best meet their child's particular needs.

Attachment is the act of sharing information and learning from each other.[9] Many childhood behavioural disorders reflect distortions of the normal developmental process of attachment, which forms over the first year of life. The parents' role is to learn to respond to the baby's cues, to let him or her take the lead; and the baby's role is to signal a change in the steps, to let his or her parents know what he or she needs. The quality of attachment is critical to a child's normal development and is a template for subsequent relationships. Problems with attachment may be reflected in the child's ability to tolerate separation, or may reflect degrees of insecurity. "Disorganized" patterns of attachment, which develop from inconsistent and chaotic parenting, have the strongest links to concurrent and subsequent psychopathology. Clinical disorders of attachment have been demonstrated to arise under conditions of social deprivation, such as institutionalization and maltreatment. An emotionally withdrawn/inhibited pattern and an indiscriminate/disinhibited pattern both have been described. Some distortions of attachment may later be indicated by separation anxiety, night-waking, somatoform behaviours, attention-seeking behaviours, and conduct disorders.

Sibling attachment is often a concern to parents. Most older siblings accept the newborn without difficulty but may need additional support, attention, and recognition to help make the transition as smooth as possible. Some brief regression in behaviours may be noted but should resolve fairly quickly when normalized as part of the transition process.

Parenting

Responsive, nurturing parenting is the key to optimal early childhood development; it allows the young brain to develop in a way that is less aggressive and more emotionally stable, social, and empathic.[10] Good parenting involves an understanding of child behaviour, the development of interpersonal skills, an awareness of the parent's own needs, and establishment of realistic expectations.[11] Many factors influence parenting, such as the parent's own upbringing and family of origin, the parent's health, and the parent's economic status.

Physicians have many opportunities for contact with parents about child behavioural problems. Opportunities typically occur during the course of an office visit for a well baby check-up or an illness. The traditional approach is one of anticipatory guidance using a checklist approach to cover the important developmental milestones.[3] This approach has limitations because it does not place the child's development in context, and it can place inappropriate expectations on the physician to be the expert parent. A shared-expertise approach to parenting problems may foster better problem solving by the physician and the parents, as well as other caregivers. Fostering empathy—the ability to identify with another person's feelings—can serve as an antidote to aggression in children and is crucial to good parenting.[10] The physician's most important task is to support the parents being in charge of their child's overall health care.[7]

Cultural factors in parenting are important to consider. A review of child-rearing practices in various cultures indicates that a great variety of actions on the part of parents produce satisfactory results in socializing children.[12] Culture and ethnicity determine, to a large extent, how child rearing practices are viewed and are topics that should enter into any discussion with a patient.

Mothers and fathers provide key engagement in infancy with touch and sound. Research indicates that fathers who are highly involved with their newborns have a positive effect of their child's development.[13] In one study, fathers regularly talked with and played with, soothed, fed, and changed their babies during the first month of life. At age 1, their children scored significantly higher on developmental tests of motor skills, pattern identification, word recognition, and problem-solving than those children who hadn't enjoyed the same paternal attention. While many men feel excluded from the birth and attachment process, the best situation appears to be when the father is emotionally supportive of the mother and baby. Parenting educational groups appear to have a beneficial effect on parenting and childhood behavioural problems.[14]

Discipline

The question of how to appropriately discipline a child is commonly asked of family physicians, who need to have some knowledge in this area. Discipline problems require evaluation of children, parents, and parent-child relationships, including assessment of child development and evaluation of parenting skills and stressors.[15,16] The use of physical punishment is dealt with in many coun-

tries' criminal legislations. The Canadian Paediatric Society has spoken out against this type of discipline backed by evidence that physical punishment, including spanking, doesn't improve the psychosocial development of children. In fact, growing evidence shows that such practices may be detrimental, or may escalate physical and emotional abuse.[17]

Good discipline includes creating an atmosphere of quiet firmness, clarity, and conscientiousness, while using reasoning. Bad discipline involves punishment that is unduly harsh and inappropriate, and is often associated with verbal ridicule, physical punishment, and attacks on the child's integrity.[18] To be effective, discipline needs to be given by an adult with an effective bond with the child, consistent, perceived as fair by the child, developmentally appropriate, and . ultimately leading to self-discipline. Goals of effective discipline are to protect the child from danger, to help the child learn self-discipline and develop a healthy conscience and internal sense of responsibility and control, and to instill values. Effective discipline strategies include time-outs, time-in, rewards, reasoning, or "away from the moment" discussions.

When parents feel stuck in their attempts to resolve their child-related difficulties, parents often turn to their family physician for advice and counsel.[13,16] Most often, advice can be given in the form of normalizing behaviour by emphasizing the psychodevelopmental stages and educating parents as to the appropriate behaviour of their child. When possible, the physician should meet with both parents, the child (or children), and other important child caretakers. The physician's most important job is to help parents identify their own strengths and utilize those strengths in addressing the problem they are having with their child. While physicians can empower parents to explore solutions for their own situation according to their own experience, beliefs, culture and religious values, it is usually wise not to give parents specific advice on how to raise their children. Physicians have a tendency to be problem solvers in an office setting, and this style may not be appropriate when dealing with parenting issues.

Single Parents

Mothers are aware that their own emotional health has consequences for their children. Although many mothers experience lack in their social support systems, many are reluctant to discuss parenting stress and depressive symptoms with their child's physician because of mistrust and fear of judgment. Mothers are, however, generally receptive to the idea of open communication with their physicians or other caregivers and are interested in receiving supportive written communication about these issues. Growing up in a single-parent family has disadvantages to the health of the child. Lack of household resources plays a major part in increased risks. However, even when a wide range of demographic and socio-economic circumstances are included in multivariate models, children of single parents still have increased risks of mortality, severe morbidity, and injury.[19]

--------------- ✒ REFERENCES ✒ ---------------

1. Vitacco MJ, Neumann CS, Ramos V, et al: Ineffective parenting: a precursor to psychopathic traits and delinquency in Hispanic females, *Ann NY Acad Sci* 1008:300-303, Dec 2003.
2. Barlow J, Coren E: Parent-training programmes for improving maternal psychosocial health (Cochrane review). In: *The Cochrane Library*, issue 1, Chichester, UK, 2004, John Wiley.
3. McDaniel S, Thomas LC, Seaburn DS: When parents get stuck. In: *Family-oriented primary care: a manual for medical providers*, NY, 1990, Springer.
4. MacKenzie S, Evers S: Identifying concerns of parents of young children, *Can Fam Physician* 32:1281-1284, 1986.
5. Lavigne JV, Binns HJ, Christoffel KK, et al: Behavioral and emotional problems among preschool children in pediatric primary care:prevalence and pediatricians' recognition, *Pediatrics* 91:649-656, 1993.
6. Campbell SB: Behavior problems in pre-school children: a review of recent research, *J Child Psychol Psychiat* 36(1):113-149, 1995.
7. Watson WJ, Watson L: Effective parenting strategies in office practice. In Watson WJ, McCaffrey M, eds: *Working with families: case-based modules on common problems in family medicine,* Toronto, 2003, UTPrint.
8. Carey WB, McDevitt SC: *Coping with children's temperament: a guide for professionals,* New York, 1995, Basic Books.
9. Zeanah CH, Keyes A, Settles L: Attachment relationship experiences and childhood psychopathology, *Ann N Y Acad Sci* 1008:22-30, Dec 2003.
10. Gordon M: Roots of empathy: responsive parenting, caring societies, *Keio J Med* 52(4):236-243, Dec 2003.
11. Gottman J: *Raising an emotionally intelligent child: the heart of parenting,* New York, 1997, Simon and Schuster.
12. McDermott D: Parenting and ethnicity. In Fine M, Lee S, eds: *Handbook of diversity in parent education,* New York, 2001, Academic Press.
13. Watson WJ, Watson L, Wetzel W, et al: The transition to parenthood: what about fathers? *Can Fam Physician* 41:307-312, 1995.
14. Bradley SJ, Jadaa DA, Brody J, et al: Brief psychoeducational parenting program: an evaluation and one-year follow-up, *J Am Acad Child Adolesc Psychiatry* 42(10):1171-1178, Oct 2003.
15. Murphy T, Oberlin LH: *The angry child: regaining control when your child is out of control,* New York, 2001, Random House.
16. Coloroso B: *Kids are worth it: giving your child the gift of inner discipline,* Toronto, 1994, Sommerville House.
17. Walker CR, Longstaffe S, Aziz K: Punishment or discipline? Children and youth are persons, not property, *Paediatr Child Health* 9(1):7-10, Jan 2004.
18. Tidmarsh L: If I shouldn't spank, what should I do? Behavioral techniques for disciplining children, *Can Fam Physician* 46:1119-1123, 2002.
19. Weitoff GR, Hjern A, Haglund B, et al: Mortality, severe morbidity, and injury in children living with single parents in Sweden: a population-based study, *Lancet* 361(9354):289-295, Jan 2003.

PEDIATRIC EXANTHEMS
Pityriasis Rosea
Etiology
Unknown, but may be infectious.

Diagnosis
At least half of patients have a prodromal illness consistent with a viral URTI. A herald patch appears, usually on the trunk, 2 to 10 cm, ovoid, erythematous, and slightly raised with a collarette of scale around the perimeter. The lesion cannot be distinguished from eczema and no fungal elements are seen on potassium hydroxide (KOH) preparations. Days to weeks after the herald patch, crops of smaller lesions, 5 to 10 mm in size, develop across the trunk and extremities (less common). They follow Langer's lines ("Christmas tree" pattern on back). Lesions can be itchy. Rash can worsen before eventual resolution. The rash usually lasts 5 weeks and is resolved in 8 weeks in 80% of patients. Recurrence is rare.

Differential diagnosis
Differential diagnoses include secondary syphilis, nummular eczema, tinea coporis, pityriasis lichenoides, guttate psoriasis, viral exanthem, lichen planus, and medication reaction.

Treatment. The goal is to control pruritus. Zinc oxide, calamine lotion, topical steroids, oral antihistamines, or oral steroids can all be used (level C evidence). Level B evidence is supportive of erythromycin or ultraviolet radiation treatment. Advise patients to return for reassessment if the rash lasts longer than 3 months.

Varicella in Children
(See also varicella; varicella vaccines)
Etiology
Varicella zoster virus.

Diagnosis
The patient experiences one to three days prodrome of fever and respiratory symptoms. Pruritic rash develops in crops of red macules. These soon become vesicles surrounded by erythema. New crops stop forming after 5 to 7 days.

Complications
Complications may include secondary bacterial infections, such as impetigo, abscess, cellulites, necrotizing

fasciitis, and sepsis. Pneumonia, hepatitis, encephalitis, and cerebellar ataxia also can occur. Neonates born to mothers who develop varicella from 5 days before to 2 days after delivery are at high risk and should be given varicella zoster immune globulin (VZIG) and followed closely.

Treatment

In otherwise healthy children, acyclovir (Zovirax) is of questionable value. Defervescence may occur 1 to 2 days earlier than in untreated patients, and there may be fewer skin lesions. However, there are variable results in trials, and treatment does not appear to decrease the rate of transmission of the infection, reduce complications, or cause less scarring.[1] Immunization against varicella is discussed in the section on varicella vaccines.

⚐ REFERENCES ⚐

1. Klassen TP, Belseck EM, Wiebe N, et al: Acyclovir for treating varicella in otherwise healthy children and adolescents (Cochrane Review). In: *The Cochrane Library*, issue 4, Chichester, UK, 2003, John Wiley.

Erythema Infectiosum (Fifth Disease or "Slapped-Cheek" Disease)
(See also infectious diseases in pregnancy)

Etiology
Human parvovirus B19.

Diagnosis

Clinical manifestations begin with non-specific symptoms, including headache, mild fever, and gastrointestinal symptoms. After a few days, the typical pruritic rash appears on the cheeks, causing a "slapped-cheek" appearance. Between 1 and 4 days later a lacy maculopapular rash may develop on the trunk and extremities; this rash tends to wax and wane and lasts 1 to 3 weeks. Infection is likely spread by respiratory secretions, but by the time the rash has appeared, the child can no longer spread infection. Most individuals who are positive serologically for parvovirus B19 have no recollection of having had symptomatic disease.[1]

Pregnancy

Infection of pregnant women with parvovirus B19 infection may cause a non-immune form of hydrops fetalis. (See discussion of infectious diseases in pregnancy.) In some cases, particularly in adult women, infection causes arthralgias or arthritis. In most instances, joint symptoms resolve spontaneously in 1 to 3 weeks, but in about one fifth of cases, symptoms persist for months or even years.[1]

⚐ REFERENCES ⚐

1. Sabella C, Goldfarb J: Parvovirus B19 infections, *Am Fam Physician* 60:1455-1460, 1999.

Roseola Infantum (Exanthem Subitum)
Etiology
Roseola is usually caused by human herpesvirus type 6 (HHV-6).

Diagnosis

Roseola infantum is primarily a childhood illness characterized by 3 to 5 days of fever, with a maculopapular rash occurring at or near defervescence. The typical rash appears in only about 10% of infected infants. Infected children can also have mild upper respiratory symptoms and cervical lymphadenopathy. The peak age of infection is 6 to 12 months, but can occur earlier. The incubation period is 7 to 17 days with a mean of 10 days.

Complications

Roseola is complicated by febrile seizures about 10% of the time. The causative agent, HHV-6, is estimated to cause about one third of all febrile seizures.

Reactivation disease. Like all herpes viruses, HHV-6 lives dormant in previously infected persons, but reactivation is usually asymptomatic or causes a mild febrile illness.

Differential diagnosis

Similar symptoms may be caused by human herpesvirus 7 (HHV-7; peak age 26 months), enterovirus, and parvovirus.

Treatment
Usual course of illness is benign and self-limited.

⚐ REFERENCES ⚐

1. Young Stoekle M: The spectrum of Human Herpesvirus 6 infection: from Roseola Infantum to adult disease, *Ann Rev Med* 51:423-430, 2000.

Hand-Foot-and-Mouth Disease

Hand-foot-and-mouth disease is caused by coxsackievirus A16. Outbreaks tend to occur in the late summer and fall. Vesicles in the mouth are usually the initial manifestation, followed by vesicles surrounded by erythema on the hands and feet. The buttocks may also be involved, and some children have fever. Lesions resolve in 3 to 7 days; treatment is symptomatic.[1]

⚐ REFERENCES ⚐

1. Adams SP: Dermacase: hand-foot-and-mouth disease, *Can Fam Physician* 44:985-993, 1998.

Measles

Etiology

Measles virus.

Diagnosis

Measles is an infection characterized by rash, fever, cough, and runny nose or red eyes. In developed countries the incidence of measles in immunocompetent individuals is very low, but in developing countries, the disease is common.

Complications

Frequent complications of measles infection are pneumonia, stridor, dehydration, corneal clouding, and mouth ulcers.

Immunization

In children who have been vaccinated and subsequently contract measles, the vaccine strongly protects against death. Immunization should take place after 12 months of age due to poor seroconversion rates in younger infants.

Treatment

Vitamin A deficiency is a recognized risk factor for severe measles. WHO recommends administration of an oral dose of 200,000 IU (or 100,000 IU in infants) of vitamin A per day for 2 days to children with measles in areas where vitamin A deficiency may be present, as well as antibiotics (controversial), oxygen, fluids, and good nutrition.

≈ REFERENCES ≈

1. Duke Trevor, Mgone CS: Measles: not just another viral exanthem, *Lancet* 361(9359):763, 2003.
2. D'Souza RM, D'Souza R: Vitamin A for treating measles in children (Cochrane Review). In: *The Cochrane Library,* issue 4, Chichester, UK, 2003, John Wiley.

PEDIATRIC HEART MURMURS

(See also congenital health disease)

General Approach

Murmurs in the pediatric patient are relatively common and are the most frequent reason for outpatient referral to pediatric cardiology practices.[1] More than half of the murmurs referred for evaluation have been found functional.[2] Given the potential cardiac disease underlying a heart murmur, the diagnosis is a source of concern not only for the primary care physician but also the parents, who often have preconceptions regarding a murmur's severity and prognosis.[3] Developing an approach to pediatric murmurs that distinguishes functional from pathological murmurs streamlines the referral process.

Cardiac pathology should be suspected in infants with a history of feeding intolerance, failure to thrive, unexplained respiratory symptoms, or cyanosis. In older children, chest pain (particularly with exercise), syncope, exercise intolerance, or a family history of sudden death at a young age should prompt suspicion.[1,4]

The physical examination should include the general state of the child, specifically detailing colour, respiratory effort, and any dysmorphic features.[1] Ventricular "lifts" may be evidence of an underlying cardiac abnormality involving increased ventricular stroke volume, such as an atrial septal defect, a ventricular septal defect, or a patent ductus arteriosus. Other explanations for increased precordial activity include anxiety, anemia, and hyperthyroidism.[4] Pulmonary stenosis may cause a thrill at the upper left sternal border, whereas the thrill resulting from aortic stenosis is frequently palpable in the suprasternal notch. Coarctation of the aorta is characterized by a discrepancy in pulse intensity or a delay in time between the brachial and femoral pulses.

Table 64 contains a list of murmurs best heard at different areas of the precordium. In addition to listening for the first (S_1) and second (S_2) heart sounds, it is also important to auscultate for the presence of additional heart sounds (S_3 or S_4).[1]

First heart sound

An inaudible S_1 indicates that another sound is obscuring the closure sound of the mitral and tricuspid valves, such as ventricular septal defects, atrioventricular valve regurgitation, patent ductus arteriosus, and occasionally severe pulmonary valve stenosis. These murmurs are holosystolic. If, on the other hand, S_1 is audible but appears to have two components, the patient has an "ejection click," or an asynchronous closure of the mitral and tricuspid valves. Clicks have different identifying characteristics depending on their origin; for example, pulmonic valve clicks vary with respiration, whereas aortic valve clicks do not.[4]

Table 64 Listening Areas for Common Pediatric Heart Murmurs

Area	Murmur
Upper R sternal border	Aortic stenosis, venous hum
Upper L sternal border	Pulmonary stenosis, atrial septal defect, patent ductus arteriosus
Lower L sternal border	Still's murmur, ventricular septal defect, tricuspid valve regurgitation, hypertrophic cardiomyopathy
Apex	Mitral regurgitation

Second heart sound

The second heart sound (S_2) is caused by the closure of the aortic and pulmonic valves. S_2 may split into aortic (A_2) and pulmonic (P_2) components upon inspiration as more blood is drawn into the right ventricle, prolonging ejection. Therefore, an atrial septal defect should result in a widely split and fixed second heart sound.

Systolic murmurs

Systolic murmurs may be functional (e.g., Still's murmur) or may be the result of ventricular septal defects, atrioventricular valve regurgitation, or patent ductus arteriosus. Any systolic murmur louder than grade 3 out of 6 (i.e., loud but not accompanied by a thrill) is considered pathological.[4,5]

Diastolic murmurs

"Venous hums" are caused by the flow of venous blood from the head and neck into the thorax. They are best heard in diastole, continuously while the child is seated. Venous hums disappear when the child is lying supine, when the child's head is turned, or when light pressure is applied over the jugular vein. Venous hums are not pathological; therefore, pediatric cardiology referral is not required. All other diastolic murmurs are pathological and require referral.[4,6]

Pathologic Versus Functional Murmurs

Table 65 provides a list of characteristics that increase the likelihood of cardiac pathology. Table 66 compares the physical examination findings in functional murmurs versus the murmur of atrial septal defect, a pathological murmur often confused for a functional murmur.[4] Two important characteristics that aid the clinician in differentiating pathological from functional murmurs are the "character" of the murmur and changes in the murmur with position.[1,5] Although somewhat subjective, murmurs that sound "harsh," "blowing," or "whooping" tend to be pathological, whereas "musical" or "vibratory" murmurs tend to be functional. Furthermore, the inten-sity of most pathological murmurs increases or does not change significantly with standing.[1,5,7] Still's murmur, the most frequently encountered functional pediatric murmur, is a systolic murmur believed to originate in the aortic root and has a "vibratory" or "musical" quality that decreases in intensity when the patient stands.[8]

─────────────── ≈ REFERENCES ≈ ───────────────

1. Lubabatu A, Bockoven JR, Pickoff AS, et al: Pediatric cardiology update: office-based practice of pediatric cardiology for the primary care provider, *Curr Probl Pediatr Adolesc Health Care* 33:318-347, 2003.
2. McCrindle BW, Shaffer KM, Kan JS, et al.: Factors prompting referral for cardiology evaluation of heart murmurs in children [letter], *Arch Pediatr Adolesc Med* 149:1277-1279, 1995.
3. McCrindle BW, Shaffer KM, Kan JS, et al: An evaluation of parental concerns and misconceptions about heart murmurs, *Clin Pediatr* 34:25-31, 1995.
4. McConnell ME, Adkins SB, Hannon DW: Heart murmurs in pediatric patients: when do you refer? *Am Fam Physician* 60:558-565, 1999.

Table 65 Features that Increase the Likelihood of Cardiac Pathology

• Chest pain	• Family history of Marfan Syndrome or sudden death in young family members
• Malformation syndrome (e.g., Down)	• Increased precordial activity
• Decreased femoral pulses	• Abnormal S_2
• Clicks	• Loud murmur
• Increased intensity of murmur when patient stands	• Harsh murmur

Adapted from McConnell ME, Adkins SB, Hannon DW: Heart murmurs in pediatric patients: when do you refer? *Am Fam Physician* 60:558-565, 1999; and Pelech AN: The cardiac murmur: when to refer? *Pediatr Clin North Am* 45:107-122, 1998.

Table 66 A Comparison of Physical Findings in Functional (Innocent) Heart Murmurs and Atrial Septal Defects

Finding	Innocent Murmur	Atrial Septal Defect
Precordial activity	Normal	Increased
S1	Normal	Normal
S2	Splits with inspiration	Widely split and fixed
Systolic murmur (supine)	Possibly "vibratory" at lower left sternal border	"Flow" at upper left sternal border
Systolic murmur (standing)	Decreased in intensity	Does not change
Diastolic murmur	Venous hum	"Rumble" across tricuspid valve area

5. Rosenthal A: How to distinguish between innocent and pathologic murmurs in childhood, *Pediatr Clin North Am* 31:1229-1240, 1984.

6. Pelech AN: The cardiac murmur: when to refer? *Pediatr Clin North Am* 45:107-122, 1998.

7. McCrindle BW, Shaffer KM, Kan JS, et al: Cardinal clinical signs in the differentiation of heart murmurs in children, *Arch Pediatr Adolesc Med* 150:169-174, 1996.

8. Behrman RE, Kliegman RM: *Nelson essentials of pediatrics,* ed 4, Philadelphia, 2002, WB Saunders, 560.

PERVASIVE DEVELOPMENTAL DISORDERS

Autism, Asperger's syndrome, childhood disintegrative disorder, and Rett's syndrome are all conditions that fit into the category of pervasive developmental disorders. Affected children have deficits in one or more areas, including reciprocal social interaction, verbal and non-verbal communication, and imaginative play. Their interests and activities are usually markedly restricted.[1] From a conservative analysis of existing data, the prevalence of autism spectrum disorder is reported at 27.5/10,000. This is comprised of a prevalence of 10/10,000 for autism, 15/10,000 for pervasive developmental disorder–not otherwise specified (PDD-NOS), and 2.5/10,000 for Asperger's syndrome.[2] Autism is four times more frequent in boys than in girls. The classic image of an autistic child sitting alone compulsively rocking represents only a small percentage of affected individuals. There is a wide spectrum of autism. Autistic children have difficulty with social interactions, and inadequate eye contact is an important clinical sign. Some autistic children display acceptable initial eye contact but tend not to maintain it. Autistic children rarely have close friends, since their interests are limited and often considered "odd" or "weird" by others. Although some affected children are mute, others have excellent vocabularies. However, they tend to indulge in monologues about whatever interests them and have great difficulty sustaining a give-and-take conversation.[1]

The prognosis for autistic children has not been fully defined. A 2004 Canadian Paediatric Society review of the evidence regarding the effectiveness of early intervention for children with autism states that "autism is a lifelong neurobehavioural disorder that requires a specialized approach to treatment. The quality of the studies on educational treatment programs for children with autism is suboptimal. However, the studies do show a trend toward showing a positive outcome from intervention. There is no evidence to support adopting a single autism treatment program as the gold standard."[3] Unfortunately, desperate parents often latch onto questionable regimens.[1] A single IV injection of secretin is of no value.[4]

In 1998, Wakefield and colleagues published a report in which the administration of measles-mumps-rubella (MMR) vaccine to young children was hypothesized to precipitate chronic inflammatory bowel disease that could lead to autism.[5] Further analysis of this data showed many methodological flaws such as small numbers of children studied, selection bias from a highly specialized gastroenterology clinic, recall bias of the timing of symptom onset by parents, and the lack of a control group. Since then a number of studies that addressed whether the hypothesized association between MMR and autism has scientific merit have been published and have not found a causal link. The National Board of Health and National Public Health Institute of Finland[3] reviewed 14 years of data collected on adverse events related to MMR vaccination of 1.8 million children (involving approximately 3 million vaccine doses) and did not find a single case similar to those described by Wakefield. Similar results have been found in other populations and in time trend analyses. The evidence does not suggest a causal association between MMR vaccination and autism.[6-9] Many people consider Asperger's syndrome to represent the highest functioning level of autism. Patients have normal cognition and language but tend to talk pedantically about their own esoteric interests. Patients with childhood disintegrative disorder develop normally until the age of 2 and then regress to acquire the characteristics of autistic children.

Rett's syndrome affects only girls. They display severe neurodevelopmental delay and pathognomonic hand-wringing. Deceleration of head growth is part of the syndrome.[1]

❧ REFERENCES ❧

1. Gara L, Goldfarb C: The autistic child: what can you do? *Can J Diagn* 16(2):147-155, 1999.

2. Fombonne E: Epidemiological surveys of autism and other pervasive developmental disorder: an update, *J Autism Dev Disord* 33:365-382, 2003.

3. Early interventions for Autism, *Pediatr Child Health* 9(4):267-270, 2004.

4. Sandler AD, Sutton KA, DeWeese J, et al: Lack of benefit of a single dose of synthetic human secretin in the treatment of autism and pervasive developmental disorder, *N Engl J Med* 341:1801-1806, 1999.

5. Wakefield AJ, Murch SH, Anthony A, et al: Ileal-lymphoid-nodular hyperplasia, non-specific colitis, and pervasive developmental disorder in children, *Lancet* 351:637-641, 1998.

6. Peltola H, Patja A, Leinikki P, et al: No evidence for measles, mumps, and rubella vaccine-associated inflammatory bowel disease or autism in a 14-year prospective study, *Lancet* 351:1327-1328, 1998.

7. Taylor B, Miller E, Farrington CP, et al: Autism and measles, mumps, and rubella vaccine: No epidemiological evidence for a causal association, *Lancet* 353:2026-2029, 1999.

8. Kaye JA, del Mar Melero-Montes M, Jick H: Mumps, measles, and rubella vaccine and the incidence of autism recorded by general practitioners: a time trend analysis, *BMJ* 322:460-463, 2001.

9. DeStefano F, Thompson WW: MMR vaccination and autism: is there a link? *Expert Opin Drug Saf* 1:115-120, 2002.

PNEUMONIA IN CHILDREN
(See also pneumonia)

The incidence of pneumonia in North American children is highest before age 5 and then decreases. Risk factors include prematurity, low birth weight, cystic fibrosis, malnutrition, low socio-economic status, passive exposure to smoke, cardiopulmonary and neurological disease, immunodeficiency, and attendance at daycare.[1,2]

Clinical signs of pneumonia in young children can be deceptive and broad, ranging from mild, non-specific symptoms of emesis, cough, malaise, headache, and chest and abdominal pain to severe respiratory distress. Most studies consider tachypnea to be an important sign.[1,2] WHO recommends diagnosis of pneumonia using clinical signs such as tachypnea (respiratory rate greater than 50 per minute in infants younger than 1 year of age and greater than 40 per minute in children older than 1 year of age), retractions, or cyanosis.[1]

Ideally, respiratory rate should be measured for 1 minute or for two 30-second periods when the child is awake and not crying. Intercostal, subcostal, or suprasternal notch retraction suggests more severe disease. Other suggestive signs are accessory muscle use, wheezing, nasal flaring and grunting, hypothermia, irritability, and poor feeding in neonates.[1] Depending on respiratory rates alone will lead to a failure of diagnosis in a number of cases and overdiagnosis in considerably more because sensitivity and specificity are not ideal. However, pneumonia can be excluded with confidence if the child lacks all the following signs: respiratory distress, tachypnea, crackles, and decreased breath sounds.[1,2]

The causative organisms of pneumonia in children are inferred largely from factors such as age, season, and clinical characteristics. *Streptococcus pneumoniae* causes most cases of pediatric bacterial pneumonia, and respiratory syncytial virus (RSV) is the most common viral cause. Viral infections predominate in children under 2 years old and become less common with increasing age. While *S. pneumoniae* is the most common bacterial pathogen in children less than 4 years of age, *Mycoplasma pneumoniae* and *Chlamydia pneumoniae* are more common in children over 5 years of age, particularly in adolescents; however, *Chylamidia trachomatis* is the most common cause of infection in the 4- to 11-week age group. Less common causes of bacterial pneumonia to consider include *Staphylococcus aureus*, *Moraxella catarrhalis*, *Haemophilus influenzae* (type b, encapsulated types other than b, and non-typable), Group A and B streptococci, *Mycobacterium tuberculosis*, and *Bordetella pertussis*, depending on the clinical picture. *S. aureus* is a cause of severe pneumonia, necessitating admission to an intensive care unit in all age groups.[3]

Management varies with age and severity of infection. Children should be admitted to hospital if they are under the age of 6 months, if they appear toxic or in severe respiratory distress, if they are vomiting/dehydrated, immunocompromised, non-responsive to oral antibiotics, or if parents are non-compliant.[1,2] The recommended antibiotics for outpatient treatment of pneumonia in children, as outlined by a Canadian Consensus Panel of Paediatric Infectious Disease specialists and a microbiologist, are[2]:

- For children 3 months to 5 years: amoxicillin 40 mg/kg per day in 3 divided doses for 7 to 10 days, or azithromycin 10 mg/kg on first day, then 5 mg/kg per day for 4 days, or clarithromycin (Biaxin) 15 mg/kg per day in 2 divided doses for 7 to 10 days.
- For children 5 to 16 years: azithromycin 10 mg/kg (max 500 mg) first day, then 5 mg/kg per day for 4 days, or clarithromycin (Biaxin) 15 mg/kg per day in 2 divided doses, or erythromycin 40 mg/kg per day in 4 divided doses, both for 7 to 10 days.

Antiviral therapy with Ribavirin 6 mg (20 mg/mL) via small-particle aerosol generator for 3 to 7 days) or Rimantadine (5 mg/kg per day orally, not to exceed 150 mg or 100 mg orally twice daily for children 10 years of age or older) must be started within 24 to 30 hours of onset of illness, especially in patients with influenza pneumonia. Chest X-rays should be considered in children with respiratory distress, or children less than 5 years of age with high fevers and white blood cell counts of an uncertain source, or when pneumonia is prolonged and unresponsive to antimicrobials. Pulse oximetry should be used in children with tachypnea or clinical hypoxemia.[1,2]

───────────── ❧ **REFERENCES** ❧ ─────────────

1. Lichenstein R, Suggs AH, Campbell J: Pediatric pneumonia, *Emerg Med Clin North Am* 21(2):437-451, 2003.

2. The diagnosis and management of community acquired pneumonia: pediatric, Jan 2002, Alberta Clinical Practice Guidelines Program (Accessed May 3, 2004, at http://mdm.ca/cpgsnew/cpgs/search/english/results.asp).

3. Jadavji T, Law B, Lebel MG, et al: A practical guide for the diagnosis and treatment of pediatric pneumonia, *Can Med Assoc J* 156(suppl):S703-S711, 1997.

PRETERM INFANTS

A follow-up study of surviving premature infants weighing less than 750 g at birth found that these children were at high risk for neurobehavioural dysfunction and poor school performance.[1] The rate of mental retardation (intelligence quotient below 70) was 21% versus 2% in the control group of full-term children, the rate of cerebral palsy was 9% versus none, and the rate of severe visual disability was 25.5% versus 2%. Children weighing between 750 and 1499 g at birth also had higher disability rates in all categories but to a lesser degree than the children under 750 g at birth.[1]

In regard to long-term outcome, an increased incidence of neurocognitive and behavioural dysfunction in school-age children and adolescents who were born preterm has been documented. An Australian regional cohort study examined preterm infants (less than 1 kg at birth or gestational age less than 28 weeks) born in the 1990s and demonstrated that the normal birth weight controls possessed superior general intellectual abilities compared with preterm infants by 8 years of age. The preterm subjects were not progressing as well in school and were more likely to have learning disabilities in reading, spelling, and arithmetic. Furthermore, they were reported by teachers and parents to have fewer adaptive skills, more attention problems, hyperactivity, somatic complaints, atypical behaviours, and less well-developed social skills.[2] A meta-analysis of 15 case studies also demonstrates that preterm infants are more likely to be enrolled in special needs classes when compared with their term counterparts.[3] A Canadian study of adolescents who had been extremely low-birth-weight infants (less than 1000 g) found that these children had significantly more limitations in the areas of cognition, sensation, and self-care and experienced more pain than was the case with control subjects.[4] Despite lifestyle and health limitations, the majority of individuals born preterm viewed their quality of life as quite satisfactory in adolescence and early adulthood.[5]

Being the mother of a very low-birth-weight child increases psychological stress as measured at 1 month regardless of whether the child is labelled as having a high risk of neurodevelopmental impairment. When the child is 2 years of age, mothers of very low-birth-weight children at high risk of impairment had an increased incidence of depression, but by the time the child was 3 years, psychological distress was no greater in these mothers than in mothers of term babies.[6]

❧ REFERENCES ❧

1. Hack M, Taylor G, Klein N, et al: School-age outcomes in children with birth weights under 750g, *N Engl J Med* 331:753-759, 1994.

2. Anderson P, Doyle LW, and the Victorian Infant Collaborative Study Group: Neurobehavioral outcomes of school-age children born extremely low birth weight or very pre-term in the 1990s, *JAMA* 289:3264-3272, 2003.
3. Bhutta AT, Cleves MA, Casey PH, et al: Cognitive behavioral outcomes of school-aged children who were born preterm, *JAMA* 288:728-737, 2002.
4. Saigal S, Feeny D, Rosenbaum P, et al: Self-perceived health status and health-related quality of life of extremely low-birth-weight-infants at adolescence, *JAMA* 276:453-459, 1996.
5. Cooke RWI: Health, lifestyle, and quality of life for young adults born very preterm, *Arch Dis Childhood* 89(3):201-206, 2004.
6. Singer LT, Salvator A, Guo S, et al: Paternal psychological distress and parenting stress after the birth of a very low-birth-weight infant, *JAMA* 281:799-805, 1999.

PYLORIC STENOSIS

Hypertrophic pyloric stenosis usually presents as postprandial, projectile, non-bilious vomiting in infants under 3 months of age. The child often demands to be refed shortly after vomiting. Three times as many boys as girls are affected, and the condition is more common in first-born children.[1]

Classic clinical signs are visible gastric peristalsis and a palpable "olive" in the right upper quadrant. The sensitivity of these signs has decreased in recent years, probably because of earlier referral and therefore less fully developed lesions. In one study, clinical diagnosis was possible in only about half the cases. If an olive is palpable, imaging studies are unnecessary.[1]

Aspiration of gastric contents with a number 8 feeding tube after a fast of 90 minutes may be used as an initial investigative technique when no olive is palpable. Over 90% of infants with pyloric stenosis will have an aspirate volume equal to or greater than 5 mL.[1]

Ultrasound and upper gastrointestinal X-ray series are the standard imaging techniques for diagnosis. If an initial ultrasound fails to demonstrate pyloric stenosis, an upper gastrointestinal series is needed.[1] Labwork may show a hypochloremic, metabolic alkalosis, depending on the duration of vomiting. Definitive treatment is a surgical pyloromyotomy.

❧ REFERENCES ❧

1. Mandell GA, Wolfson PJ, Adkins S, et al: Cost-effective imaging approach to the nonbilious vomiting infant, *Pediatrics* 103:1198-1202, 1999.

REYE'S SYNDROME

Reye's syndrome was first described in Australia in 1963. The major abnormalities are a fatty liver and encephalopathy. The condition usually develops within 3 weeks after the onset of a viral illness (often varicella, upper respiratory tract infection, or gastroenteritis), and the major clinical manifestations are mental status changes, which can rapidly progress to coma or death. Any suspicion warrants transfer to an emergency department. Laboratory tests usually show elevations of alanine aminotransferase (ALT), aspartate aminotransferase (AST), and ammonia levels. Although the median age for Reye's syndrome is 6 years, the disease has been reported in infants under 1 year of age and in adolescents as old as 17 years.[1]

Literature continues to support a clear association between Reye's syndrome and Aspirin use.[2] A major public health campaign warning parents about the dangers of Aspirin in children was mounted, and as a result the incidence of Reye's syndrome dropped dramatically. Because Reye's syndrome is now rare, children with encephalopathy and evidence of liver dysfunction should be investigated for inborn metabolic disorders, because some of these can mimic Reye's syndrome.[1]

✑ REFERENCES ✑

1. Belay ED, Bresee JS, Holman RC, et al: Reye's syndrome in the United States from 1981 through 1997, *N Engl J Med* 340:1377-1382, 1999.
2. Waller P, Suvarna R: Is aspirin a cause of Reye's syndrome? *Drug Safety* 27(1):71-73, 2004.

STUTTERING

Stuttering, as defined by WHO, is "a disorder in the rhythm of speech in which the individual knows precisely what he or she wishes to say, but at the same time may have difficulty saying it because of an involuntary repetition, prolongation, or cessation of sound."[1] Stuttering occurs in 3% to 5% of preschool-age children and is three to four times more common in boys than girls.[2] During infancy and in preschool-age children, distinguishing between stuttering and dysfluency may be difficult, because dysfluency is a normal part of development. Normal preschool dysfluency commonly involves repetitions of whole words or phrases, whereas stuttering is more often characterized by repetition of syllables and parts of words, and sound prolongations.[3,4]

In about 80% of cases, stuttering resolves spontaneously by age 16. Consultation with a speech therapist is indicated if the child is over 4 years of age, has had consistent stuttering for at least 3 months, and manifests struggling behaviour while stuttering. Some of the important therapeutic techniques are to avoid criticizing the child and to encourage slow speaking. Parents can model this by speaking or reading slowly to their children.[2] Physicians should also assess for co-occurring speech disorders, language disorders, and non-speech disorders such as learning disabilities, literacy disorders, attention deficit disorder, social anxiety, and depression.[4,5]

✑ REFERENCES ✑

1. *The International classification of diseases*, 9th revision, clinical modification: ICD.9.CM. 9th rev. Ann Arbor, Mich.: Commission on Professional and Hospital Activities, 1978.
2. Lawrence M, Barclay DM III: Stuttering: a brief review, *Am Fam Physician*, 57:2175-2178, 1998.
3. Leung AK, Robson WL: Stuttering, *Clin Pediatrics* 29: 498-502, 1990.
4. Costa D, Kroll R: Stuttering: an update for physicians, *Can Med Assoc J* 162(13):1849-1855, 2000.
5. Blood GW, Ridenour VJ, Qualls CD, et al: Co-occurring disorders in children who stutter, *J Commun Disord* 36(6):427-448, Nov-Dec 2003.

SUDDEN INFANT DEATH SYNDROME

Sudden infant death syndrome (SIDS) is defined as the sudden death of an infant under 1 year of age, which remains unexplained after a thorough case investigation, including performance of a complete autopsy, examination of the death scene, and review of the clinical history. Since the "Back to Sleep" campaign was begun in 1992, the incidence of SIDS in the USA has decreased by about 50%. Unfortunately, SIDS remains the most common cause of unexplained infant death in the Western world.[1]

Specific risk factors for SIDS that may be modified though education by health care professionals (and others) include prone sleeping, maternal smoking (both during pregnancy and after birth) and overheating.[2] Concurrent education about unsafe sleeping conditions (i.e., soft bedding [waterbeds, sofas], sleeping with potentially obstructive materials [stuffed toys, pillows, large bulky coverings]) would be beneficial to prevent possible airway obstruction.[3] Despite not having a full understanding of the specific cause of SIDS at this time, further reduction of SIDS will best be achieved by parent education about these potential risk factors.

Death of a sibling with SIDS has not been identified as a specific risk factor for subsequent children. Home cardiorespiratory monitoring has been shown to be ineffective in preventing SIDS death.[4]

✑ REFERENCES ✑

1. Byard RW, Krous HF: Sudden infant death syndrome: overview and update, *Perspect Pediatr Pathol* 6:112-127, 2003.
2. Daley KC: Update on sudden infant death syndrome, *Curr Opin Pediatr* 16:227-232, 2004.
3. Committee on Fetus and Newborn: Apnea, sudden infant death syndrome and home monitoring, *Pediatrics* 111: 914-917, 2003.
4. American Academy of Pediatrics Task Force on Infant Sleep Position and Sudden Infant Death Syndrome: Changing concepts of sudden infant death syndrome: implications for infant sleeping environment and sleep position, *Pediatrics* 107(4):809, 2001.

URINARY TRACT INFECTIONS IN CHILDREN

(See also circumcision, male; labial fusion; urinary tract infections)

From 2 months to 2 years of age, urinary tract infections (UTIs) are twice as frequent in girls as boys.[1] About 8% of girls and 2% of boys have a UTI during childhood, and in 5% to 15% of these cases, renal scarring develops. Renal scarring is associated with an increased incidence of recurrent pyelonephritis in adulthood, poor renal growth, hypertension, and end-stage renal failure.[2] Renal scarring as a complication of UTI is most common before 1 year of age and is rare in children over the age of 5. Whether vesicoureteral reflux causes renal scarring is uncertain.[3] Any sick child with fever without source for more than 1 or 2 days, particularly those under 2 years of age, should be checked for UTI.[4]

Urine culture is necessary to make a diagnosis of UTIs in children. Dipstick results for nitrites and leukocyte esterases are insufficiently sensitive, with a combined false-negative rate of up to 20%.[5] Almost 50% of children with culture-proven UTIs have negative nitrates because of their increased frequency of voiding.[4] False positives for the two indicators range between 2% and 40%.[4] Urinary tract infection is defined as a pure bacterial growth of more than 10^5 colony-forming units per millilitre in voided or clean-catch urine or the presence of any pathogens in suprapubic aspirates. Counts lower than 10^5 are clinically significant in boys and in catheter-obtained specimens. Although bag specimens have an extremely low false-negative rate (approaching 0), they have a false-positive rate from 85% to 99%. Therefore, if the child has a negative bag specimen and doesn't appear toxic, you can be reassured a UTI is not present. If the specimen is positive, it should be confirmed with a catheter or suprapubic sample.[4]

Acute infections should be treated for 7 to 10 days; some retrospective studies have concluded that immediate empirical treatment results in less renal scarring than does delayed treatment.[2] The American Academy of Pediatrics (AAP) 1999 Practice Parameter Guidelines suggest initial IV antibiotic treatment for any child who appears toxic. Even children ages 2 to 24 months can be treated orally if they appear well and have good follow-up.[1]

Diagnostic imaging procedures commonly used to detect vesicoureteral reflux or obstructive lesions in children with UTIs are ultrasonography, radionucleotide cystogram (RNC), and voiding cystourethrography (VCUG). No consensus exists as to which children should be investigated, mainly because no published randomized trials deal with the issue. The last AAP consensus conference graded the evidence for radiological investigations as "fair." Most literature recommends investigating all children under the age of 5 with renal ultrasound and either VCUG or RNC and those over age 5 with ultrasound only, although other options include investigating all children regardless of age,[1] males at any age, and those with UTI before toilet training or with their second UTI.[5]

Delays in performance of imaging can be safely addressed by providing interim prophylactic antibiotic coverage.

Degrees of vesicoureteral reflux are categorized from I (mild) to V (severe). For lesser degrees of reflux, the outcome is as good with medical therapy as with surgery.[2] First-line treatment for most cases of reflux is antibiotic prophylaxis, usually with nitrofurantoin 1 to 2 mg/kg once daily or trimethoprim/sulfamethoxazole (trimethoprim 2 to 4 mg/kg) once daily. Annual cystograms are obtained, and antibiotics are usually discontinued when the reflux has resolved. If break-through UTIs occur, surgical correction of the reflux may be indicated.[5]

❧ REFERENCES ❧

1. American Academy of Pediatrics. Committee on Quality Improvement. Subcommittee on Urinary Tract Infection: Practice parameters: the diagnosis, treatment, and evaluation of the initial urinary tract in febrile infants and young children (published erratum appears in *Pediatrics* 103[5 Pt 1:1052], 1999.) *Pediatrics* 104 (4 Pt 1):843-852, 1999.
2. Larcombe J: Urinary tract infection in children, *BMJ* 319:1173-1175, 1999.
3. Ahmed SM, Swedlund SK: Evaluation and treatment of urinary tract infections in children, *Am Fam Physician* 57: 1573-1580, 1998.
4. White CT, Matsell DG: Children's UTIs in the new millennium, *Can Fam Physician* 47:1603-1608, 2001.
5. Ross JH, Kay R: Pediatric urinary tract infection and reflux, *Am Fam Physician* 59:1472-1478, 1999.

WELL-BABY CARE

Primary care providers are in the optimal position to provide general health maintenance, developmental screening, and anticipatory guidance for infants, children, and their families. Recent literature has confirmed the years before the age of 3 as a critical period for development of skills leading to optimal adult capacity.[1] A complex interaction exists between genes and early experiences, which directly affects how the brain is hard-wired, including the number of cells and connections the brain develops.[2,3] The early brain has been shown to be vulnerable to environmental influences that have a decisive effect on later health and well being.[1] Although this is an evolving area of research that requires considerable time to fully elucidate effective practice, interventions during these early years that help parents to facilitate their childrens' development, such as early childhood stimulation and parent support programs, have shown impressive long-term benefits ranging from higher rates of completion of post-secondary education to less cost to the reliance on social and justice systems services, and even IQ potential.[4,5]

Numerous protocols for well-baby care have been published. One that is well organized, relevant, easy to use, and evidence based is the *Rourke Baby Record: Evidence-Based Infant/Child Health Maintenance Guide.*[6,7] The Nipissing District Developmental Screen is a comprehensive developmental screening tool that can be completed in minutes by a parent or clinic nurse. It is designed to identify delays in eight areas of development and offers activities to parents to facilitate their child's development.[8]

❧ REFERENCES ❧

1. McCain M, Mustard F: Early years study: reversing the real brain drain, Toronto, 1999, Ontario Children's Secretariat.
2. Shore R: *Rethinking the brain,* New York, 1997, Families and Work Institute, 20.
3. Carnegie Corporation of New York: *Starting points: meeting the needs of our youngest children,* New York, 1994, The Corporation, 7-8.
4. Schweinhart L, Barnes H, Weikart D: Significant Benefits: The High/Scope Perry Preschool Study Through Age 27. Monographs of the High Scope Educational Research Foundation Number 10, 1993.
5. Campbell F, Ramey C: Effects of early intervention on intellectual and academic achievement: a follow up study of children from low-income families, *Child Development* 65:684-698, 1994.
6. Panagiotou L, Rourke LL, Rourke JT, et al: Evidence-based well-baby care. 1. Overview of the next generation of the Rourke Baby Record, *Can Fam Physician* 44:558-567, 1998.
7. Panagiotou L, Rourke LL, Rourke JT, et al: Evidence-based will-baby care. 2. Education and advice section of the next generation of the Rourke Baby Record, *Can Fam Physician* 44: 568-572, 1998.
8. Nipissing District Developmental Screen Inc, revised 2002. Access this and other early childhood resources at http://www.beststart.org/resources/hlthy_chld_dev/. Accessed August 3, 2004.

FAILURE TO THRIVE

Failure to thrive (FTT) in children under age 3 is usually of mixed etiology with both organic and non-organic contributors. Well-controlled trials indicate that these children are at risk for short stature, behavioural problems, and developmental delay.[1]

Diagnosis and Assessment

History should include feeding, development, and psychosocial and family history.[1] Observing the interaction between the caregiver and the child can reveal responsiveness and ability to recognize the child's cues. Appropriate and accurate monitoring of growth over time is necessary, with published standards available for reference.[2] FTT is reflected by serial measurements showing an unexpected drop in weight-for-age of 2 major percentile lines.[1,2] Body weight less than or equal to 89% of ideal, weight-for-length/-stature less than third percentile or, for children over 2 years of age, BMI-for-age less than fifth percentile can also indicate an underweight or wasting child.[2] Routine investigations may be warranted and can include CBC, BUN, creatinine, electrolytes, albumin, calcium, phosphorus, alkaline phosphatase, urinalysis and culture, and Mantoux test.[4]

Management

Any potential underlying cause should first be corrected. All children with FTT need a high-calorie diet for catch-up growth, calculated at 150% of their recommended daily caloric intake based on their expected weight.[1] There is mixed evidence on the benefit of zinc supplementation in reducing the energy cost of weight gain during catch-up growth.[1] Education of the caregiver is also important to ensure proper social and nurturing techniques. Children should be followed up at least monthly until catch-up growth is evident.[1] Most children with FTT can be treated as outpatients. Some randomized controlled trial evidence exists that home health visitor intervention is beneficial to growth and cognition.[5,6] Hospitalization is only necessary in case of suspected child abuse or neglect, serious malnutrition, and failure of outpatient management.[1]

❧ REFERENCES ❧

1. Krugman SD, Dubowitz H: Failure to thrive, *Am Fam Physician* 68(5):879-884, 2003.
2. Schlenker J, Raja S, for Dieticians of Canada, Canadian Pediatric Society, The College of Family Physicians of Canada, Community Health Nurses Association of Canada: The use of growth charts for assessing and monitoring growth in Canadian infants and children, *J Dietet Pract Res* 65(1):22–32, 2004.
3. Corbett SS, Drewett RF: To what extent is failure to thrive in infancy associated with poorer cognitive development? A review and metaanalysis, *J Child Psychol Psychiatry* 45(3): 641-654, 2004.
4. Shah MD: Failure to thrive in children, *J Clin Gastroenterol* 35(5):371-374, 2002.
5. Wright CM, Callum J, Birks E, et al: Effect of community based management in failure to thrive: a randomised control trial, *BMJ* 317:571-574, 1998.
6. Black MM, Dubowitz H, Hutcheson J, et al: A randomized clinical trial of home intervention for children with failure to thrive, *Pediatrics* 95(6):807-814, 1995.

RESPIROLOGY

Topics covered in this section

Asthma
Bronchitis, Acute
Chronic Cough
COPD: Chronic Bronchitis, Emphysema
Lung Cancer
Pneumonia
Pulmonary Fibrosis
Sarcoidosis
Sleep Apnea
Spirometry

ASTHMA
Epidemiology

Asthma is a chronic inflammatory disease of the airways affecting 14 million to 15 million persons in the United States. It is the most common chronic disease of childhood, affecting an estimated 4.8 million American children.[1,2]

People with asthma collectively have more than 100 million days of restricted activity and 470,000 hospitalizations annually. More than 5,000 people die of asthma annually. Asthma hospitalization rates have been highest among blacks and children, while death rates for asthma were consistently highest among blacks age 15 to 24 years.[3] These rates have increased or remained stable over the past decade. (All data are from the United States.[4])

General Principles

Asthma is characterized by paroxysmal or persistent symptoms such as dyspnea, chest tightness, wheezing, sputum production and cough, associated with variable airflow limitation and a variable degree of hyperresponsiveness of airways to endogenous or exogenous stimuli.[5]

Inflammation and its resultant effects on airway structure are considered to be the main mechanisms leading to the development and maintenance of asthma; therefore, the main thrust of asthma therapy is to limit exposure to triggering factors and to reduce the inflammatory process by using anti-inflammatory agents. If needed, therapies to maintain optimal airway calibre and to control symptoms may be added to ensure acceptable asthma control and to improve quality of life. This requires tailored individualized therapy to maximize outcomes.

‍ REFERENCES ‍

1. Adams PF, Marano MA: *Current Estimates from the National Health Interview Survey, 1994.* Hyattsville, MD, 1995, National Center for Health Statistics, Public Health Service, Department of Health and Human Services (US). Vital and Health Statistics Series 10, Number 193. DHHS Publication PHS 96-1521.
2. Centers for Disease Control and Prevention: Asthma-United States, 1989-1992, *Morb Mortal Wkly Rep* 43:952-955, 1995.
3. Centers for Disease Control and Prevention: Asthma mortality and hospitalization among children and young adults—United States, 1990-1993, *Morb Mortal Wkly Rep* 45:350-353, 1996.
4. National Heart, Lung, and Blood Institute, National Institutes of Health. National Asthma Education and Prevention Program Expert Panel Report 2: *Guidelines for the Diagnosis and Management of Asthma.* Bethesda, MD, 1997, National Institutes of Health; .Pub. No. 97-4051.
5. Boulet P, Becker A, Bérubé D, et al: Summary of recommendations from the Canadian Asthma Consensus Report, 1999, *Can Med Assoc J* 161: S1-S12, 1999.

Causation

Asthma often begins in childhood, and when it does, it is frequently (but not only) found in association with atopy. Atopy is the genetic susceptibility to produce IgE directed toward common environmental allergens, such as animal proteins, pollens, moulds, or house dust mites. IgE antibodies, mast cells, and possibly other airway cells (e.g., lymphocytes) are sensitized and become activated when they encounter specific antigens, which activate the allergic cascade. Among infants and young children who have wheezing with viral infections, allergy or family history of allergy is the factor that is most strongly associated with continuing asthma through childhood.[1]

Although asthma begins most frequently in childhood and adolescence, it can develop at any time. Adult-onset asthma can occur in a variety of situations. In adult-onset asthma, allergens may continue to play an important role. However, in some adults who develop asthma, IgE antibodies to allergens or a family history of asthma are not detected. These individuals often have coexisting sinusitis, nasal polyps, and sensitivity to Aspirin or related non-steroidal anti-inflammatory drugs. Gastroesophageal reflux is another cause of adult asthma. Current studies are looking into the currently unclear role of infectious agents in adult asthma and into the role of antibiotics in therapy.

‍ REFERENCE ‍

1. Castro-Rodriguez JA, Holberg CJ, Wright AL, et al: A clinical index to define risk of asthma in young children with recurrent wheezing, *Am J Resp Crit Care Med* 162(4 Pt. 1): 1403-1406, 2000.

Diagnosis

The clinician trying to establish a diagnosis of asthma should determine that:

1. Episodic symptoms of airflow obstruction are present.
2. Airflow obstruction is at least partially reversible.
3. Alternative diagnoses are excluded.

A careful medical history including family history, physical examination, objective measurements of lung function via peak flow measurements or preferably spirometry, and additional tests will provide the information needed to ensure a correct diagnosis of asthma. Asthma is a variable disease, and if spirometry or pulmonary function testing are normal, challenge testing can be done to define hyper-responsive airways. Objective measurements are preferable to avoid mislabelling patients. In the very young (patients under age 6) or those unable to undergo these measurements, history and physical examination are currently the best tools physicians have. Allergy testing should be considered to assess environmental triggers and allow environmental control as part of the treatment plan.[1] Investigational diagnostic studies include exhaled nitrous oxide and hypertonic saline inhalation with study of the expectorated sputum.[2] (See the section on Spirometry to outline the diagnostic procedures in more detail.)

Objective measures include[3]:

- *Spirometry:* A 12% (preferably 15%) or greater (at least 180 mL) improvement in FEV_1 from the baseline 15 minutes after use of an inhaled short-acting β_2-agonist, a 20% (250 mL) improvement after 10 to 14 days of inhaled glucocorticosteroid or ingested prednisone when symptoms are stable, or a 20% (250 mL) or greater "spontaneous variability" is considered significant (level IV).
- *Peak expiratory flow:* When spirometry and methacholine testing are unavailable, variable airflow obstruction (i.e., ideally 20% or greater diurnal variability) can be documented by home-measured PEF (level II), although this measure is not as sensitive or reliable as FEV_1.
- *Airway hyper-responsiveness:* Measurement of airway responsiveness to methacholine in specialized pulmonary function laboratories may help to diagnose asthma (level III).

⚛ REFERENCES ⚛

1. Green RH, Brightling CE: Asthma exacerbation and sputum eosinophil counts. A randomized control trial, *Lancet* 360: 1715-1721, 2002.
2. Bates CA, Silkoff PE: Exaled nitric oxid in asthma: from bench to bedside, *J Allergy Clin Immunol* 111:256-262, 2003.
3. Boulet LP, Bait TR, Becker A, et al: Asthma Guidelines Update, *Can Respir J* 8(suppl A): 5A-27A, 2001.

Severity vs. Control

Control of asthma can be assessed based on the parameters as per the Canadian Guidelines (Table 67).

Table 67 Parameters for Control of Asthma

Parameter	Frequency or Value
Daytime symptoms	< 4 days/week
Night-time symptoms	< 1 night/week
Physical activity	Normal
Exacerbations	Mild, infrequent
Absence from work or school	None
Need for short-acting β_2-agonist	< 4 doses/week*
FEV_1 or PEF	> 85% of personal best, ideally 90%
PEF diurnal variation†	< 15% of diurnal variation

FEV_1, Forced expiratory volume in 1 second; PEF, peak expiratory flow obtained with a portable peak flow meter.
*May use 1 dose/day for prevention of exercise-induced symptoms.
†Diurnal variation is calculated by subtracting the lowest PEF from the highest and dividing by the highest PEF multiplied by 100.
This information was originally published in *Can Respir J* 11 (Suppl A):9A-18A, 2004. Reprinted with permission.

Severity can be assessed based on the exacerbation history, the medications required to control the asthma in the treated patient, and the patient's lung function.

The initial measure of the severity of asthma in a patient is based on the frequency and duration of respiratory symptoms and the degree of airflow limitation. Once asthma is well controlled, one of the best ways to judge severity is to determine the level of treatment needed to maintain acceptable control (see above). Indications of severity also include a prior near-fatal episode (loss of consciousness, need for intubation), recent admission to hospital or a visit to the emergency department, and recent use of systemic corticosteroids. Asthma severity may vary over time; it may also decrease after anti-inflammatory therapy and with age, especially in children. When control of asthma has been maintained for several weeks or months, an attempt should be made to reduce medication within the boundaries of acceptable control.[1]

Environment

Common triggers include:

- Atopy: Familial
- Allergy: House dust-mite allergens, pets (cat dander), pollens, mould spores, cockroaches
- Infections: Viral upper respiratory tract infections
- Cold air: Triggers asthma by cooling of airways
- Smoking: Cigarette smoke in environment
- Atmospheric pollution: Build-up of sulfur dioxide, ozone, nitrogen dioxide
- Climate: Changing climatic conditions (thunderstorms)
- Emotions: Emotional factors and psychological stress
- Medication: Beta blockers, aspirin anaphylaxis

Table 68   Asthma Severity, Symptoms, and Treatment

Asthma Severity	Symptoms	Treatment Required
Very mild	Mild–infrequent	None, or inhaled short-acting β_2-agonist rarely
Mild	Well-controlled	Short-acting β_2-agonist (occasionally) and low-dose inhaled glucocorticosteroid*
Moderate	Well-controlled	Short-acting β_2-agonist and low to moderate doses of inhaled glucocorticosteroid with or without additional therapy
Severe	Well-controlled	Short-acting β_2-agonist and high doses of inhaled glucocorticosteroid and additional therapy
Very severe	May be controlled or not well-controlled	Short-acting β_2-agonist and high doses of inhaled glucocorticosteroid and additional therapy and oral glucocorticosteroid

This information was originally published in *Can Respir J* 11 (Suppl A):9A-18A, 2004. Reprinted with permission.

- Occupational asthma: Chemicals (latex), allergens from grain, red cedar, isocyanates, and others
- Food and drink: Food allergies (peanut), food additives

The first step of treatment is to modify the environment to reduce the exposure to triggers. Smoking cessation is obvious; second-hand smoke may be more subtle. Pet removal is usually resisted. Prevention of house dust mite and mould need changes such as humidity in the home environment.

Pharmacology

Appropriate pharmacology is a continuum of asthma management (Figure 3).[2] Severity of asthma is ideally assessed by medication required to maintain asthma control. Environmental control and education should be instituted for all asthma patients. Very mild asthma is treated with short-acting β_2-agonists, taken as needed. If β_2-agonists are needed more than 3 times per week (excluding 1 dose per day before exercise), then inhaled glucocorticosteroids should be added at the minimum daily dose required to control the asthma. If asthma is not adequately controlled by moderate doses (500 to 1000 μg per day of beclomethasone or equivalent), additional therapy, including long-acting β_2-agonists, leukotriene antagonists or, less often, other medications, should be considered. Severe asthma may require additional treatment with prednisone. The NHLBI model[2] is similar, but also includes a model of stepped care and more rigid advice of desired medications at each level of control (see Table 68).

Relievers are best represented by the short-acting β_2-agonists. These quick-acting bronchodilators are used to relieve acute asthma symptoms as "rescue" therapy. Inhaled ipratropium bromide is less effective but is occasionally used as a reliever medication in patients intolerant of short-acting β_2-agonists or as adjunctive therapy in acute moderate-to-severe asthma.

Controllers (or preventers) include anti-inflammatory medications, such as inhaled (and oral) glucocorticos-

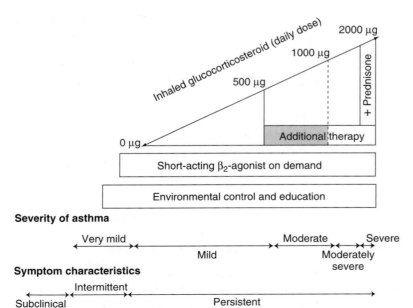

Figure 3 Model of Asthma Management. (This information was originally published in *Can Respir J* 11(Suppl A): 9A-18A, 2004. Reprinted with permission.)

teroids (ICS), leukotriene receptor antagonists (LTRAs), and antiallergic or "non-steroidal" inhaled agents, such as cromoglycate and nedocromil. These agents are generally taken regularly to control asthma, although some patients, such as those with seasonal asthma, may need them only intermittently.

ICS are the most effective agents in this category and are considered the first-line anti-inflammatory therapy.[3] LTRAs as the initial anti-inflammatory treatment remains controversial to some, but LTRAs can certainly be used for this purpose in patients who will not or cannot use glucocorticosteroids or in those people with very positive response to the LTRA in which ICS can be weaned off.[4] When ICS are insufficient, control of asthma symptoms may be achieved using additional therapy, such as the long-acting inhaled β_2-agonists salmeterol and formoterol or the LTRAs zafirlukast and montelukast, as adjuncts. (Zileuton is another option in the United States, but is unavailable in Canada.) These agents should be considered after the environment is reviewed, the inhaler technique is corrected, and compliance is ensured. In a few patients, there may be a role for other bronchodilators such as theophylline and ipratropium, but these do not have anti-inflammatory effects. Some evidence shows that theophylline may have immunomodulatory effects, but the clinical significance of this remains to be demonstrated.

Asthma drugs are preferably inhaled, because this route minimizes systemic absorption and thus, improves the ratio of the therapeutic benefit to the potential side effects. The patient must have repeated instruction on how to use the inhaled medication. LTRAs have good safety and tolerance profiles and are taken orally, which may help certain patients comply with treatment.

Asthma medications should be used at the lowest dose and frequency required to maintain acceptable asthma control; they should not be used as a substitute for proper control of the environment. Asthma medications are considered to be safe over many years when used appropriately. Long-term use of bronchial anti-inflammatory agents has not resulted in any clinically significant reduction in their efficacy (i.e., tolerance does not occur).[2]

⚓ REFERENCES ⚓

1. Cockcroft DW, Swystun VA: Asthma control versus asthma severity, *J Allergy Clin Immunol* 98:1016-1018, 1998.
2. Lemiere C, Bai T, Balter M, et al: Adult Asthma Consensus Guidelines Update 2003, *Can Respir J* 11(Suppl A):9A-18A, 2004.
3. British Thoracic Society: Scottish Intercollegiate Guidelines Network. British guidelines on the management of asthma, *Thorax* 58(suppl 1):il-94, 2003.
4. Ducharme FM: Inhaled corticorticosteroids versus leukotriene receptor antagonists as a single agent in asthma treatment. Systemic view of current evidence, *BMJ* 326:621, 2003.

Devices[1]

- Metered Dose Inhalers (MDIs) that use hydrofluoroalkane propellant are recommended over those using chlorofluorocarbons (level IV).
- Health care professionals must teach correct inhaler technique when devices are prescribed and dispensed (level I).
- Patients' method of using their inhalation device must be reassessed and reinforced periodically (level II).
- Asthma control should be reassessed when changing an aerosol device (level IV).
- Wet nebulizers for home use are rarely indicated in the management of asthma at any age (level III).
- A trial of wet nebulization in infants and children at home may be appropriate if an MDI with a spacer is not effective (level IV).
- When spacers are used, conversion from a mask to a mouthpiece is strongly encouraged as soon as the age and the co-operation of the child permit (level II).

⚓ REFERENCES ⚓

1. Boulet LP, Bai TR, Becker A, et al: What is new since the last (1999) Canadian Asthma Consensus Guidelines? *Can Respir J* 8 (Suppl A):5A-27A, 2001

Delivery Systems for Inhaled Medications

Types of delivery systems

Delivery systems for inhaled medications used for outpatients are generally divided into two major categories: MDIs with propellants, and dry powder inhalers (inspiratory flow–generated aerosols). If the patient cannot generate an adequate airflow, the latter devices are ineffective.[1]

Although traditional practice is to use nebulizers to deliver β_2-agonists to hospitalized patients and young children, the supervised use of MDIs with spacer devices has proved as effective in the emergency setting as nebulizer therapy for both adults[2] and children.[3]

Metered dose inhalers. When MDIs are used, the open-mouth technique is said to be more effective than the closed-mouth technique. The open-mouth technique is performed as follows[4]:

1. Remove the cap of the MDI.
2. Shake the MDI several times.
3. Hold the MDI vertically about 2.5 to 5 cm (1 to 2 inches) from the open mouth.
4. Tilt the head slightly backward.
5. Exhale normally (not a forced or maximum exhalation).
6. Breathe in at a moderate rate, and activate the MDI in the middle of inspiration.
7. Hold the breath for 10 seconds or more.

Whether a chlorofluorocarbon (CFC) MDI is full or empty can be determined by placing it in a bowl of water. If it sinks, it is full, and if it floats sideways, it is empty.[4]

Not all patients are able to use MDIs correctly. In a study of elderly subjects with a mean age of 70, only about half used the devices properly 1 week after an extensive instructional session. Major determinants of failure have been shown to be cognitive impairments and weak hand strength.[5] These problems may be overcome with the use of spacers.

Spacers. Spacers or aerochambers are designed to be used with MDIs. Large particles are precipitated out in the chamber, slightly higher effective doses reach the lungs, and much less drug is deposited in the oropharynx and therefore is swallowed and absorbed systemically, which will hopefully decrease both local and systemic effects of inhaled corticosteroids (ICS). MDIs connected to spacers require less coordination to use than MDIs alone, so they are particularly helpful for children, elderly, the disabled, and the uncoordinated. Proper use of spacers requires that the MDI be activated only once for each inhalation and that the inhalation be started as soon as possible after the activation.[6] Spacers for very young children and infants come with masks that are applied to the child's face. Many studies have demonstrated that the delivery of bronchodilators by MDIs with spacers is at least as effective for young children with acute asthma as are small-volume nebulizers.[7]

Commercial spacers are expensive. Homemade spacers may be created by inserting an MDI into the bottom of a polystyrene cup, with the open end pressed against the child's face to act as a face mask, or by inserting an MDI into the bottom of a soft drink bottle, with the neck of the bottle held in the mouth and the lips creating a seal. A comparison of these two types of homemade devices and a commercial spacer in the treatment of acute asthma found that the commercial and soft drink bottle spacers were both effective, while only a small benefit was achieved with the cup. A 500-ml soft drink bottle was used in this study. The bottom was cut out with a hot wire moulded to the exact shape of the mouthpiece of the MDI, and the MDI was immediately inserted and sealed in place with glue. Before use the bottle was primed with 15 activations of the MDI to decrease the electrostatic charge on its inner surface. (Rinsing the bottle with detergent and allowing it to air dry is equally effective.)[8]

Turbuhalers. The dose of medication from a Turbuhaler is made accessible by turning the bottom of the device, which loads the medication, onto a small spoon inside the device. The basic way of using a dry powder inhaler is as follows[4]:

1. Prepare the dose.
2. Expire fully (forced or maximum expiration).
3. Close the mouth tightly around the mouthpiece.
4. Inhale fully and rapidly.
5. Ensure that the air intake valves are not covered.

The inhalation technique with a Turbuhaler differs from that of the MDI, in which expiration is not forced and inspiration is at a moderate rate. The patient using a Turbuhaler will not feel the medication going into the airways, as is usually the case with MDIs. Children over the age of 6 years can easily learn to use Turbuhalers.[9]

Concentration of drugs reaching the lungs

Reports of concentrations of medications reaching the lungs from various delivery systems vary among references. All figures indicate that use of an MDI plus an aerochamber or use of a Turbuhaler leads to a greater concentration of medication deposition in the lungs than does an MDI alone. One report showed that a Turbuhaler delivers about twice as much steroid to the lungs as do standard MDIs.[10] Another study found that with a Turbuhaler, a normal inhalation resulted in almost twice as much pulmonary delivery as did a slow inhalation.[11] Recently there has been a switching of the propellants used in metered-dose inhalers from chlorofluorocarbons (CFCs) to hydrofluoroalkanes (HFAs) to help rescue the depleting ozone layer. There may be some differences in distribution of some of the HFA-propelled ICS compared with the CFC propelled ones.

_____ ➽ REFERENCES ✍ _____

1. Fong PM, Sinclair D: Inhalation devices for asthma, *Can Fam Physician* 39:2377-2382, 1993.
2. Turner MO, Patel A, Ginsburg S, et al: Bronchodilator delivery in acute airflow obstruction: a meta-analysis, *Arch Intern Med* 1736-1744, 1997.
3. Kelly HW, Murphy S: Beta-adrenergic agonists for acute, severe asthma, *Ann Pharmacother* 26:81-91, 1992.
4. Szefler SJ, Chambers CV: *Diagnosis and management of asthma,* Kansas City, MO, 1995, American Academy of Family Physicians.
5. Gray SL, Williams DM, Pulliam CC, et al: Characteristics predicting incorrect metered-dose inhaler technique in older subjects, *Arch Intern Med* 156:948-988, 1996.
6. O'Callaghan C, Barry P: Spacer devices in the treatment of asthma: amount of drug delivered to the patient can vary greatly (editorial), *BMJ* 314:1061-1062, 1997.
7. Amirav I, Newhouse MT: Metered-dose inhaler accessory devices in acute asthma, *Arch Pediatr Adolesc Med* 151:876-882, 1997.
8. Zar HJ, Brown G, Donson H, et al: Home-made spacers for bronchodilator therapy in children with acute asthma: a randomised trial, *Lancet* 354:979-982, 1999.
9. De Boeck K, Alifier M, Warnier G: Is the correct use of a dry powder inhaler (Turbohaler) age dependent? *J Allergy Clin Immunol* 103:763-767, 1999.
10. Thorsson L, Edsbäcker S, Conradson TB: Lung deposition of budesonide from Turbuhaler is twice that from a pressurized metered-dose inhaler P-MDI, *Eur Respir J* 7:1839-1844, 1994.

11. Borgstrom L, Bondesson E, Moren F, et al: Lung deposition of budesonide inhaled via Turbuhaler: a comparison with terbutaline sulphate in normal subjects, *Eur Respir J* 7:69-73, 1994.

Immunotherapy

Immunotherapy for asthma is controversial, although it has been used for over 70 years.[1] One study showed minimal benefits for seasonal allergic asthma to ragweed as measured by skin test sensitivity, bronchoconstrictor response to ragweed, and peak expiratory flow and reduction of medications in the first year, but this was not sustained during the second year.[2] Few asthmatic patients are allergic to only one allergen; many are allergic to house dust mites, cat dander, moulds, and cockroaches, and there is little evidence that immunotherapy with these agents has any value.[1] A double-blind, placebo-controlled trial of multiple-allergen immunotherapy in children with moderate-to-severe year-round asthma demonstrated no beneficial effect after at least 18 months of therapy.[3] Meta-analyses have concluded that there may be some benefit but that because of the adverse effects, the benefits may not outweigh the harm.[4,5]

◢ REFERENCES ◣

1. Barnes PJ: Is immunotherapy for asthma worthwhile? (editorial), *N Engl J Med* 334:531-532, 1996.
2. Creticos PS, Reed CE, Norman PS, et al: Ragweed immunotherapy in adult asthma, *N Engl J Med* 334:501-506, 1996.
3. Adkinson NF Jr, Eggleston PA, Eney D, et al: A controlled trial of immunotherapy for asthma in allergic children, *N Engl J Med* 336:324-331, 1997.
4. Abramson MJ, Puy RM, Weiner JM: Is allergen immunotherapy effective in asthma? A meta-analysis of randomized controlled trials, *Am J Respir Crit Care Med* 151:969-974. 1995.
5. Sigman K, Mazer B: Immunotherapy for childhood asthma: is there a rationale for its use? *Ann Allergy Asthma Immunol* 76: 299-305, 1996.

Special Situations

Asthma in the elderly[1]

- A diagnosis of asthma should be more widely considered in elderly patients with dyspnea, wheezing, or nocturnal cough (level III).
- Investigation to determine exposure to environmental and other asthma-inducing factors in elderly patients with recent-onset asthma should include a careful review of medications including self-prescribed acetylsalicylic acid (ASA) and other drugs with asthma-inducing potential (level II).
- Special care should be taken to allow elderly patients with asthma to choose an inhaler device with which they are comfortable and competent (level III).

- Measures should be taken to prevent osteoporosis in elderly patients with asthma who require prolonged treatment with oral corticosteroid (level I).
- Elderly patients with asthma require careful follow-up because they have an increased risk of exacerbations, which may be related to impaired perception of their disease severity (level II).

◢ REFERENCES ◣

1. National Heart, Lung, and Blood Institute, National Institutes of Health: National Asthma Education and Prevention Program Expert Panel Report 2: *Guidelines for the diagnosis and management of asthma,* Bethesda, MD, 1997, National Institutes of Health. Pub. No. 97-4051.

Asthma in pregnancy

During pregnancy, the severity of asthma often changes, and patients require close follow-up and adjustment of medications. Overall the rule of thirds is useful; $\frac{1}{3}$ get worse, $\frac{1}{3}$ get better, and $\frac{1}{3}$ stay the same. The use of inhaled asthma medications is not associated with any known adverse effects on the fetus, but uncontrolled asthma poses a substantial risk to both the mother and fetus.

The first step of therapy is avoidance of allergic and non-allergic triggering factors, just as it would be in the non-pregnant patient. The patient should be informed about the background risk of drugs in pregnancy in the general population. It should be made clear that, although relatively few medications have been proved harmful during pregnancy, no asthma or allergy medication can be considered to be proved safe. The possible consequences for the mother and fetus of inadequately controlled asthma, including the impact on maternal and fetal morbidity and mortality, must be emphasized. Medication choices and the rationale for the treatment plan should be discussed; they should emphasize that the treatment is considered to entail less risk than the uncontrolled illness that could result in its absence (level II).

Treatment should take the same stepped approach as in the non-pregnant patient and may include inhaled β_2-agonists, inhaled corticosteroids, ipratropium bromide, cromolyn, and systemic glucocorticosteroids. Theophylline may increase nausea and reflux and is less desirable. There is significantly less information about the effects of the long-acting β_2-agonists and the leukotriene inhibitors, and there is less clinical experience with these drugs than with other classes of drugs. These drugs should be used only for patients whose asthma cannot be controlled using the more studied therapies.

The use of systemic glucocorticosteroids for severe asthma, especially for prolonged periods, may be associated with a greater risk of pre-eclampsia, antepartum or postpartum hemorrhage, low birth weight, preterm birth, and hyperbilirubinemia. Patients requiring systemic gluco-corticosteroid therapy should be considered to be in a higher-risk pregnancy (level II). Physicians should address all of the patient's questions and obtain and document the patient's concurrence with the therapeutic decisions.

Emergency management of asthma[2]

The management of exacerbations of asthma requires rapid access to facilities and personnel capable of delivering the medication appropriately, defining the severity of the asthma episode objectively, ensuring appropriate monitoring of oxygen delivery, and instituting safe referral and disposition. Bronchodilators should be titrated using clinical and objective measurements, and systemic glucocorticosteroids should be given to almost all patients who require a visit to the emergency department because of exacerbation of asthma. In addition to relief of symptoms and improvement in objective measures of airflow, a detailed review of risk factors for severe asthma is needed, and an educational intervention should be offered.

Assessment

- A structured management plan should be used to treat patients with asthma in the emergency department (level III).
- The severity of airflow limitation should be determined objectively using spirometry (the preferred method), PEF measures, or both, before and after bronchodilator therapy (level III), unless the patient is too young (< 6 years), unco-operative or moribund. These measurements should not postpone necessary treatment (level IV).
- The arterial oxygen saturation in (S_aO_2) should be measured before and after treatment (level III).

Drug therapy in the emergency department

- Supplemental oxygen should be used in treating patients with acute asthma to maintain S_aO_2 greater than 94% (level IV).
- Short-acting β_2-agonists should be considered the primary class of medication for the management of exacerbations. It should be administered by inhalation and titrated using objective and clinical measures of airflow obstruction as guides (level I).
- The choice of delivery device (MDI with spacer, wet nebulization, dry powder) will depend on the need for expedient treatment, availability of staff, and the individual patient of any age (level I).
- The use of an MDI with a chamber (valved spacer device) is preferred over the use of a wet nebulizer for patients of all ages at all levels of severity (level I).
- All patients treated in the emergency department for an acute episode of asthma should be considered candidates for systemic glucocorticosteroid therapy (oral or intravenous) and receive it as soon as possible (level I).

- An anticholinergic drug should be added to β_2-agonist therapy for severe acute asthma and β-blocker–induced bronchospasm and may also help in cases of moderate acute asthma (level I).
- Aminophylline is not usually recommended for use as a bronchodilator in patients of any age during the first 4 hours of asthma management in the emergency department (level I).

Management of refractory cases

- Epinephrine (intramuscular or intravenous), salbutamol (intravenous) and inhaled anesthetics are recommended as alternatives to conventional therapy in unresponsive cases of life-threatening asthma (level II).
- Intravenous magnesium sulfate (level I) and heliox (level III) may be useful in addition to usual therapy for refractory asthma.
- Ketamine and succinylcholine are recommended for rapid-sequence intubation in cases of life-threatening asthma (level I).
- Intubation should be performed by physicians experienced in this procedure (level IV).

Discharge treatment plan and follow-up care

- Consideration for discharge should be based on results of spirometry (percent of previous best, or percent of predicted or absolute value) and assessment of clinical risk factors for relapse (level III).
  - Patients with a pre-treatment FEV_1 or PEF below 25% of previous best level or the predicted value (i.e., FEV_1 below 1.0 L or PEF below 100 L/min) usually require admission to hospital.
  - Patients with a post-treatment FEV_1 or PEF below 40% of previous best level or the predicted value (i.e., FEV_1 below 1.6 L or PEF below 200 L/min) usually require admission to hospital.
  - Patients with a post-treatment FEV_1 or PEF between 40% and 60% of previous best level or predicted value (i.e., FEV_1 equal to 1.6-2.1 L or PEF equal to 200 to 300 L/min) are possible candidates for discharge.
  - Patients with a post-treatment FEV_1 or PEF above 60% of previous best level or predicted value (i.e., FEV_1 above 2.1 L or PEF above 300 L/min) are likely candidates for discharge.
- Adults discharged from the emergency department who require glucocorticosteroid therapy should be given 30 to 60 mg per day of prednisone orally (or equivalent) for 7 to 14 days. No tapering is required over this period (level I). Children should receive 1 to 2 mg/kg a day of prednisone or equivalent (up to a maximum of 50 mg) for 3 to 5 days (level I).
- Inhaled glucocorticosteroids are an integral component of asthma therapy and should be prescribed for almost all patients at discharge, including those receiving oral glucocorticosteroids (level I).

• A treatment plan and clear instructions for follow-up should be given to patients discharged from the emergency department. Patients with high-risk factors, poor lung function, or indications of chronic poor control should be referred to an asthma education clinic (level IV).

Exercise-induced asthma

Exercise-induced asthma is present in almost every patient who has asthma. The author's opinion is that exercise is a trigger in patients with poorly controlled asthma in most of these cases, and exercise symptoms should trigger more aggressive management of the underlying asthma with regular doses of inhaled corticosteroids.[1] True exercise-induced bronchoconstriction (EIB) is less common. These patients do not have established asthma and do not get exacerbations with upper respiratory tract infections (URIs), etc. Factors likely to aggravate the condition are intense exercise, low temperature, and low humidity.[1] For symptoms to occur, exercise must be maintained for more than 2 minutes.[2]

In patients with EIB, symptoms usually develop shortly after they stop exercising. Spontaneous recovery is usually complete within half an hour to an hour.[2] A few individuals experience a late response, with symptoms developing 6 to 10 hours after exercise.[3]

An interesting feature of exercise-induced asthma is that a preliminary bout of mild-to-moderate exercise decreases the degree of bronchoconstriction during subsequent strenuous exercise (tachyphylaxis). This protective effect lasts for about 40 minutes and can be used therapeutically by athletes if they make a point of doing moderate warm-up exercises before participating in strenuous exercise. The warm-up should last 15 to 30 minutes and be followed by a 15-minute rest before vigorous exercise.[3]

Aside from warm-up exercises, management of exercise-induced asthma usually involves taking an inhaled β_2-adrenergic agonist, cromolyn, or nedocromil sodium 10 to 15 minutes before the exercise. For many patients, these regimens offer incomplete protection against asthma.[1] Alternatives that may offer significant improvements are the use of long-acting β_2-agonists[4,5] or a leukotriene-receptor antagonist.[6,7] A trial of montelukast (Singulair) 10 mg once daily at bedtime in patients with exercise-induced asthma found that many experienced significant improvement and that this effect persisted for the full 3 months of the study.[6]

⋑ REFERENCES ⋐

1. Hansen-Flaschen J, Schotland H: New treatments for exercise-induced asthma (editorial), *N Engl J Med* 339:192-193, 1998.
2. McFadden ER Jr, Gilbert IA: Exercise-induced asthma, *N Engl J Med* 330:1362-1367, 1994.
3. D'Urzo AD: Exercise-induced asthma: what family physicians should do, *Can Fam Physician* 41:1900-1906, 1995.
4. Nelson J, Strauss L, Skowronski M, et al: Effect of long-term salmeterol treatment on exercise-induced asthma, *N Engl J Med* 339:141-146, 1998.
5. Blake K, Pearlman DS, Scott C, et al: Prevention of exercise-induced bronchospasm in pediatric asthma patients: a comparison of salmeterol powder and albuterol, *Ann Allergy Asthma Immunol* 82:205-211, 1999.
6. Leff JA, Busse WW, Pearlman D, et al: Montelukast, a leukotriene-receptor antagonist, for the treatment of mild asthma and exercise-induced bronchoconstrictio, *N Engl J Med* 339:147-152, 1998.
7. Drazen J, Israel E, O'Byrne PM: Treatment of asthma with drugs modifying the leukotriene pathway, *N Engl J Med* 340: 197-206, 1999.

Comorbidities that Influence Asthma Treatment
Gastroesophageal reflux disease

According to studies from a few centers, gastroesophageal reflux disease (GERD) may cause asthma, probably through reflex bronchoconstriction precipitated by esophageal irritation from refluxed gastric contents or by vagal stimulation directly.[1-5] In many of these cases, GERD is asymptomatic and can be diagnosed only with tests such as 24-hour esophageal pH monitoring.[1] Harding and associates[2] state that treatment with dietary and positional modifications and proton pump inhibitors given twice daily in full dosage for 3 months (shorter treatment duration may be ineffective) causes improvement in most patients with proven GERD and asthma.[2]

⋑ REFERENCES ⋐

1. Irwin RS, Curley FJ, French CL: Difficult-to-control asthma: contributing factors and outcome of a systematic management protocol, *Chest* 103:1662-1669, 1993.
2. Harding SM, Richter JE, Guzzo MR, et al: Asthma and gastroesophageal reflux: acid suppressive therapy improves asthma outcome, *Am J Med* 100:395-405, 1996.
3. Harding SM, Richter JE: The role of gastroesophageal reflux in chronic cough and asthma, *Chest* 111:1389-1402, 1997.
4. Vandenplas Y: Asthma and gastroesophageal reflux, *J Pediatr Gastroenterol Nutr* 24:89-99, 1997.
5. Field S, Sutherland LR: Does medical antireflux therapy improve asthma in asthmatics with gastroesophageal re-flux? A critical review of the literature, *Chest* 114:275-283, 1998.

Aspirin sensitivity

Adult patients with asthma should be questioned regarding precipitation of bronchoconstriction by Aspirin and other non-steroidal anti-inflammatory drugs. If they have experienced a reaction to any of these drugs, they should be informed of the potential for all these drugs to precipitate severe and even fatal exacerbations. Adult patients with severe persistent asthma or nasal polyps should be counselled regarding the risk of using these drugs.

Sulfite sensitivity

Patients who have asthma symptoms associated with eating processed potatoes, shrimp, or dried fruit or with drinking beer or wine should avoid these products.[1]

Beta Blockers

Non-selective beta blockers, including those in ophthalmological preparations, can cause asthma symptoms and should be avoided by asthma patients,[2,3] although cardioselective beta blockers, such as betaxolol, may be tolerated.[4]

──────────── ❧ REFERENCES ❦ ────────────

1. Taylor SL, Bush RK, Selner JC, et al: Sensitivity to sulfited foods among sulfite-sensitive subjects with asthma, *J Allergy Clin Immunol* 81(6):1159-1167, Jun 1988.
2. Odeh M, Oliven A, Bassan H: Timolol eyedrop-induced fatal bronchospasm in an asthmatic patient, *J Fam Pract* 32(1):97-98, Jan 1991.
3. Schoene RB, Abuan T, Ward RL, et al: Effects of topical betaxolol, timolol, and placebo on pulmonary function in asthmatic bronchitis, *Am J Ophthalmol* 97(1):86-92, Jan 1984.
4. Dunn TL, Gerber MJ, Shen AS, et al: The effect of topical ophthalmic instillation of timolol and betaxolol on lung function in asthmatic subjects, *Am Rev Respir Dis* 133(2):264-268, Feb 1986.

Monitoring and Action Plans

Patients with asthma need to be taught how to monitor their asthma. This can be based on symptoms, β_2 use, or home peak flow readings. Physicians also need to have objective measurements of control. Again, these are based on symptom control, need of rescue medication, exacerbation history, and optimization of lung function.

An individualized action plan in concert with patient education (by either physician or preferably, when available, asthma educators) has been shown to make a difference in rates of exacerbations.[1] An example of an Asthma Action Plan can be found on the Internet at http://www.AsthmaActionPlan.com (accessed November 18, 2004).

──────────── ❧ REFERENCES ❦ ────────────

1. Gibson PG, Powell H, Coughlan J, et al: Self-management education and regular practitioner review for adults with asthma (Cochrane Review), *Cochrane Database Syst Rev,* 2003, (1):CD001117.

BRONCHITIS, ACUTE

Diagnosis

Acute bronchitis is an acute inflammation of the lower respiratory tract. It is the most common respiratory infection presenting in the primary care setting and takes one of two forms. The first affects a previously healthy patient and is usually viral in origin. The second is an acute exacerbation of chronic obstructive pulmonary disease (COPD) and may be viral or bacterial in origin.[1] This section will deal with the first form only.

Bronchitis is usually self-limiting and lasts from a few days to a few weeks.

Signs and symptoms include a prodrome of URI symptoms consisting of mild coryza (sore throat, cough, fever, runny eyes and nose), followed by cough (either productive or non-productive), and often signs of airway obstruction, including nocturnal cough and wheezing. The cough occurs in 85% of patients within 2 days of the illness. The cough is usually gone in 2 weeks but lasts longer in 26% of patients and may continue for 6 to 8 weeks.[2] Sputum colour and thickness, a useful sign in acute exacerbation COPD, is irrelevant in management of acute bronchitis.

Etiology

The vast majority of cases are caused by viruses. The common viruses are as follows: in patients under 1 year of age, respiratory syncytial virus (RSV), parainfluenza virus, and coronavirus; in patients 1 to 10 years of age, parainfluenza virus, enterovirus, RSV, and rhinovirus; and in patients greater than age 10, influenza virus, RSV, and adenovirus.[3]

Rarer causes include bacteria, yeast/fungi, and environmental triggers.

Management

Antibiotics are used in 65% to 85% of patients with acute bronchitis.[4, 5] There have been several studies looking at this practice, with mixed results. A meta-analysis of 8 randomized trials found that duration of cough and sputum production was decreased by half a day. Although statistically significant, it is likely not clinically significant. (Some patients may argue otherwise.)[1] In all studies, patients consistently show improvement when not treated with antibiotics. A recent randomized controlled trial comparing azithromycin for 5 days versus vitamin C in acute bronchitis showed no difference.[5] Previous trials of vitamin C indicate that it is likely ineffective, and a recent trial of vitamin E in the elderly actually worsened outcomes.[6] Most guidelines do not suggest treatment with antibiotics unless a bacterial superinfection or pneumonia is strongly suspected (rales, temperature over 38.5°, pulse higher than 100 bpm, decreased breath sounds, and absence of asthma).[7] When this is the case, treatment is per pneumonia guidelines.[1] Systematic reviews in adults and children suggest there is limited evidence to support the routine use of over-the-counter (OTC) cough remedies to manage acute cough, but symptomatic treatment may help patients feel better.[8] Short-acting bronchodilators may be helpful in patients with wheeze.[9] Patients with coloured sputum and cough often expect antibiotics, despite the fact that the vast majority will not benefit. This expectation is diminishing, but delayed prescriptions may help with patients who are difficult to manage.[10]

─────────────── ⅏ **REFERENCES** ⅏ ───────────────

1. Knutson D, Braun C: Diagnosis and management of acute bronchitis, *Am Fam Physician* 65:2039-2044, 2002.
2. Chesnutt MS, Prendergast TJ: *Current medical diagnosis and treatment, 2002*, ed 41, New York, 2002, McGraw Hill, 269-362.
3. Marrie TJ: Acute bronchitis and community acquired pneumonia. In: *Fishman's pulmonary diseases and disorders*, ed 3, New York, 1998, McGraw Hill, 1985-1995.
4. Gonzales R, Steiner JF, Sande MA: Antibiotic prescribing for colds, upper respiratory tract infections, and bronchitis by ambulatory care physicians, *JAMA* 278:901-904, 1997.
5. Evans AT, Husain S, Durairaj L, et al: Azithromycin for acute bronchitis: a randomised, double-blind, controlled trial, *Lancet* 359:1648-1654, 2002.
6. Graat JM, Schouten EG, Kok FJ: Effect of daily vitamin E and multivitamin-mineral supplementation on acute respiratory tract infections in elderly persons. A randomized controlled trial, *JAMA* 288:715-721, 2002.
7. Heckerling PS, Tape TG, Wigton RS: Clinical prediction rule for pulmonary infiltrates, *Ann Intern Med* 113:640-647, 1990.
8. Schroeder K, Fahey T: Over-the-counter medications for acute cough in children and adults in ambulatory settings (Cochrane Review). In: *The Cochrane Library*, issue 4, 2003.
9. Smucny JJ, Flynn CA, Becker LA, et al: Are beta-2 agonists effective treatment for acute bronchitis or acute cough in patients without underlying pulmonary disease? *J Fam Pract* 945-951, 2001.
10. Dowell J, Pitkethy M, Bailn J, et al: A randomized controlled trial of delayed antibiotic prescribing as a strategy for managing uncomplicated respiratory tract infection, *Br J Gen Pract* 51:200-205, 2001.

CHRONIC COUGH

It has been reported that chronic cough is the fifth most common complaint seen in the primary care setting.[1] Cough lasting more than 3 weeks has been described to be chronic.[2]

Recently, Irwin and Madison[3] proposed that the period be increased to 8 weeks. It is important to note that the duration of the cough is an important diagnostic feature. This text uses the definition of chronic cough as cough lasting more than 8 weeks.

Importance of Cough

Cough is an important respiratory defense mechanism, and is responsible for clearing excessive secretions, fluids, or foreign material from the airway.[4] Despite this beneficial role, excessive coughing can cause multisystem problems. Common complications, such as anxiety, fatigue, insomnia, myalgia, dysphonia, perspiring, and urinary incontinence, often force patients to seek medical help.

Differential Diagnosis

In most cases, chronic cough can be attributed to postnasal drip syndrome (PNDS), asthma, GERD, or some combination of these in immunocompetent, nonsmoking patients who have normal results on chest radiographs and who do not take angiotensin-converting enzyme (ACE) inhibitors.[2] Although a careful history and physical examination are helpful, they are not sufficient to diagnose the cause of chronic cough. Furthermore, the features and timing of chronic cough are also of little diagnostic value in the majority of patients.[5] Additional investigations and responses to a trial of empiric therapy based on the most likely etiology are essential. Initial investigations should include a chest X-ray, which can detect diseases such as bronchitis, COPD, neoplasm, and intestinal lung disease.[6] Evidence of these diseases should prompt appropriate treatment and referral. Additional investigations, including a methacholine challenge test, sinus radiography, and an esophageal pH probe, may prove helpful.[3]

Optimizing therapy by adding treatments for concomitant causes of chronic cough might be required for some patients. Repeated failure of therapy or combination therapy should prompt referral to an appropriate specialist.

Postnasal drip syndrome

PNDS is the most common cause of chronic cough. It occurs most often after a viral upper respiratory tract infection, such as that caused by respiratory syncytial or Para influenza viruses and sometimes by *Chlamydia pneumoniae* (TWAR strain), *Mycoplasma* or *Bordetella pertussis*.[2] Other important causes of PNDS include perennial rhinitis; rhinitis as a consequence of seasonal allergens, irritants, drugs and vasomotor responses; and chronic sinusitis.[2]

Patients with PNDS often report a sensation of tickling or a constant drip in the back of the throat. Throat clearing, rhinorrhea, nasal congestion, and hoarseness are the other symptoms of PNDS; some patients with PNDS have no symptoms.[3] Symptoms may be triggered by exposure to allergens, irritants, or drugs. Onset of watery rhinorrhea associated with changes in temperature implies vasomotor rhinitis. X-rays of sinuses showing air-fluid levels, opacifications, or mucosal thickening (greater than 6 mm) are diagnostic of chronic sinusitis.[2]

Treatment for post-infectious, perennial, and vasomotor rhinitis includes a first-generation antihistamine, such as dexbropheniramine, in combination with the pseudoephedrine decongestant.[7]

A cough, if caused by PNDS, usually improves within a few days to 2 weeks after therapy begins. Lack of improvement suggests that an inappropriate antihistamine was used or that there are other concomitant causes of cough.

Insomnia, tachycardia, anxiety, hypertension, palpitation, diminished micturition, increased intraocular pressure, dry eyes, and a dry mouth are all potential side effects of first generation antihistamines. Ipratropium bromide is useful for treatment of perennial and vasomotor rhinitis.[2]

Managing allergic rhinitis should begin with allergy testing to identify environmental triggers. This should occur early in the management of allergic rhinitis. Newer, non-sedating antihistamines such as loratadine are effective.[3] Steroids, sodium cromoglycate, or intranasal antihistamines such as azelastine are also successful treatments for allergic rhinitis.[2]

Treatment of chronic sinusitis should include a combination of antibiotic, anti-inflammatory, and decongestant therapy.[2] A 3-week course of antibiotic therapy is often required to treat common pathogens.

Asthma

Cough, wheezing, dyspnea, and chest tightness are common clinical manifestations of asthma. In up to 57% of asthma cases, cough is the only presenting symptom (cough variant asthma) and is often associated with normal lung function.[8] The high prevalence of asthma in patients of all ages should prompt physicians to entertain this diagnosis as a cause of chronic cough.

Airway hyper-responsiveness[9] and reversible airflow obstruction[10] can establish a diagnosis of asthma. Since reversible airflow obstruction is uncommon in patients with cough-variant asthma, measurement of airway hyper-responsiveness is required. A metacholine challenge test has a positive predictive value up to 88% and negative predictive value of 100%.[2,3] A diagnosis may be confirmed when the cough resolves after a trial of therapy.

Canadian consensus guidelines for asthma include use of a β-agonist to relieve symptoms immediately and an inhaled corticosteroid (with or without oral corticosteroid, depending on severity) to control inflammation.[11] β-Agonist therapy provides only transitory relief from chronic cough. Most patients with chronic cough are relieved completely in 6 to 8 weeks[2,3] with a β-agonist plus either inhaled corticosteroid[12] or a combination of inhaled and oral corticosteroid.[13] Steroid therapy withdrawal should be considered when the cough resolves.

Gastroesophageal reflux disease

Reflux of acidic stomach contents into the esophagus is common in most people.[14] GERD is diagnosed when this reflux produces symptoms or when complications arise. Transient loss of tone in the lower esophageal sphincter is the probable mechanism.[15] GERD-induced cough can exacerbate loss of tone in the lower esophageal sphincter and perpetuate the cycle of more reflux, irritation, inflammation, and coughing.[15] The clinical presentation of GERD is variable, and in up to 75% of cases, the sole presenting symptom is chronic cough.

Macroaspiration is another mechanism of GERD-induced chronic cough. Low pH in the distal esophagus can induce a persistent cough and symptoms of asthma even without aspiration.[2]

Management of GERD involves a trial of antireflux therapy. Preventive measures include weight reduction, smoking cessation, and a diet low in acidic foods or foods that reduce the tone of the lower esoplageal sphincter.[2] A combination of a proton pump inhibitor and a prokinetic agent relieves GERD-induced cough in most cases, although full recovery might not be evident for as long as 6 months.[7] For resistant cases, a pH probe should be used to assess the efficacy of treatment or to evaluate the need for fundoplication.[2] Physicians should also consider treating other potential causes of chronic cough that could exacerbate the reflux-cough cycle.[16]

In conclusion, most cases of chronic cough are caused by PNDS, asthma, GERD, or some combination of these common conditions. Although cough is a protective respiratory clearance reflex, for many adults it may represent a severe and prolonged health complaint. A systematic approach to diagnosis of chronic cough can reduce much of its morbidity for most of those who suffer from it.

─────────────── ◈ **REFERENCES** ◈ ───────────────

1. Braman SS, Corrao WM: Chronic cough; diagnosis and treatment, *Prim Care Clin Office Pract* 12(2);217-225, 1985.
2. Irwin RS, Boulet L-P, Cloutier MM, et al: Managing cough as a defense mechanism and as a symptom: a consensus panel report of the American College of Chest Physicians, *Chest* 114 (Suppl 2):133-81S, 1998.
3. Irwin RS, Madison JM: The diagnosis and treatment of cough, *N Engl J Med* 343: 1725-1721, 2000.
4. McCool FD, Leith DE: Pathophysiology of cough, *Clin Chest Med* 2:189-195, 1987.
5. Mello CJ, Irwin RS, Curley FJ: Predictive values of the character, timing, and complications of chronic cough in diagnosing its cause, *Arch Intern Med* 156:997-1003, 1996.
6. D'Urzo AD, Jugovic P: Chronic cough: three most common causes, *Can Fam Physician* 48:1311-1316, 2002.
7. Pratter MR, Bartter T, Akers S, et al: An algorithmic approach to chronic cough, *Ann Intern Med* 119:977-983, 1993.

8. Johnson D, Osborne LM: Cough variant asthma: a review of the clinical literature, *J Asthma* 28:85-90, 1991.

9. Cockcroft DW, Berscheid BA, Murdock KY: Unimodal distribution of bronchial responsiveness to inhaled histamine in a random human population, *Chest* 83:751-754, 1983.

10. American Thoracic Society: Lung function testing: selection of reference values and interpretation strategies, *Am Rev Resp Dis* 144:1202-1218, 1991.

11. Boulet LP, Becker A, Berube D, et al: Canadian Asthma Consensus Report, 1999, Canadian Asthma Consensus Group, *Can Med Assoc J* 161(11 supp):S1-61, 1999.

12. Cheriyan S, Greenberger PA, Patterson R: Outcome of cough variant asthma treated with inhaled steroids, *Ann Allergy* 73:478-480, 1994.

13. Doan T, Patterson R, Greenberger PA: Cough variant asthma: usefulness of a diagnostic therapeutic trial with prednisone, *Ann Allergy* 69:505-509, 1992.

14. Mittal RK, McCallum RW: Characteristics of transient lower esophageal sphincter relaxation in humans, *Am J Physiol* 252(5 pt 1):G636-641, 1987.

15. Richter JE, Castell DO: Gastroesophageal reflux: pathogenesis, diagnosis, and therapy, *Ann Intern Med* 97:93-103, 1982.

16. McGravey LP: Which investigations are the most useful in the diagnosis of chronic cough? *Thorax* 59(4):342-346, 2004.

COPD: CHRONIC BRONCHITIS, EMPHYSEMA
Chronic Obstructive Pulmonary Disease

(See also asthma; bronchitis, acute)

COPD is a chronic, slowly progressive disease characterized by airway obstruction that is largely fixed but may be partially reversible by bronchodilator or other therapy. COPD encompasses both chronic bronchitis and emphysema, which are now thought to be variants of the same basic disorder. It also includes some cases of chronic asthma.[1]

Spirometry is required to confirm the diagnosis of COPD.

1. The forced expiratory volume in 1 second (FEV_1) is less than 80% of the predicted value before *and* after a single dose of inhaled bronchodilator (i.e., not fully reversible).
2. The FEV_1/FVC (forced vital capacity) ratio is less than 70%.

Some patients may have a mild (normal FEV_1 but reduced FEV_1/FVC ratio) or moderate airflow limitation (both FEV_1 and FEV_1/FVC ratio somewhat reduced) that could indicate early COPD that will become more obvious over time with serial testing (e.g., every 12 months). Other diagnoses may be aided by enhanced testing such as bronchodilator reversibility testing (asthma), chest X-ray (TB, CHF, bronchiectasis), ECG (ischemia), and α_1 antitrypsin screening for patients with a strong family history of COPD presenting before the age of 45.[2,3]

Epidemiology

Smoking is the major risk factor for COPD and accounts for 80% to 90% of cases, although clinically significant COPD develops in only 15% of smokers. α_1-antitrypsin deficiency accounts for less than 1% of cases.[2]

Management of stable chronic obstructive pulmonary disease

Stopping smoking is the prime therapeutic intervention for COPD, even when the disease is advanced. Loss of pulmonary function is not restored when smoking is discontinued, but the age-related decline in FEV_1 is significantly reduced.[4]

Although none of the existing medications modifies the long-term decline in lung function associated with COPD, treatment can help symptoms and improve function. Inhaled bronchodilators (short-acting β-agonists such as albuterol (Salbutamol, Proventil, Ventolin) or inhaled anticholinergics such as ipratropium bromide (Atrovent) give symptomatic relief, and failure of pulmonary function testing to show a bronchodilator response does not mean the patient will not respond clinically.[2,4] Long-acting bronchodilators (e.g., formoterol twice daily, tiotropium once daily, salmeterol twice daily) are more effective and convenient but also more expensive. Combining drugs with different mechanisms and durations of action may increase the degree of bronchodilation for equivalent or lesser side effects. This has become more convenient recently with combination puffers (Fenoterol/Ipratropium 200/80 [MDI], Salbutamol/Ipratropium 75/15 [MDI]). Theophylline is effective in COPD, but due to its potential toxicity, inhaled bronchodilators are preferred when available. Inhaled corticosteroids can play a role for patients with severe COPD (i.e., FEV over 50% and over 3 exacerbations a year), but concerns about negative consequences of long-term use have resulted in guidelines generally recommending against chronic treatment.

Use of the brochodilators is generally in a step-wise fashion depending on symptoms. Use is as needed for mild symptoms (FEV_1 60% to 79% of predicted), with a second bronchodilator added for more moderate dyspnea (FEV_1 40% to 59% of predicted, and finally adding a long-acting β_2-agonist with a corticosteroid (e.g., formoterol/budesonide [Symbicort], salmeterol/fluticasone [Advair]). Cough has a significant protective role in COPD; therefore, cough suppressants are contraindicated in stable COPD.[3]

Respiratory rehabilitation for patients with COPD is defined as an exercise training program of at least 4 weeks' duration. A meta-analysis of 14 studies of this intervention concluded that it reduced the amount of dyspnea and improved the patients' abilities to cope with the disease.[5]

Home oxygen therapy has proved useful for selected patients with advanced COPD. Criteria for this therapy are that the patient be clinically stable and have a resting arterial partial pressure of oxygen (PaO_2) of 55 mm Hg or less or of 60 mm Hg or less if there is tissue hypoxia as manifested by bilateral ankle edema, polycythemia or cor pulmonale, and a hematocrit less than 56.[6] In properly selected patients, home oxygen therapy decreases mortality, secondary polycythemia, and pulmonary hypertension and improves neuropsychological functioning. Home oxygen therapy should be continuous for at least 15 hours a day, usually with an oxygen concentrator set at a flow of 2 to 4 L per minute and delivery by nasal prongs.[4]

Selected patients with emphysema benefit from bilateral lung reduction surgery, which can be accomplished through a thoracoscopic approach. Lung function and dyspnea improve immediately, and according to a 2-year follow-up study, mortality is lower than in patients having unilateral lung reduction surgery.[1]

Management of exacerbations

Sustained worsening of dyspnea, increase in sputum volume, and purulence represent an exacerbation and typically occur two to three times per year in patients with COPD.[7] Chest X-ray examination is not necessary for patients who are well enough to be managed at home and who respond to treatment, but it should be part of the initial workup for patients admitted to the hospital.

First-line treatment for the outpatient management of exacerbations of COPD is to add β-agonists or anticholinergics to the usual therapeutic regimen and maximize doses as outlined above. Addition of oral prednisone is often required (typically 10 days at a dose of 25 to 50 mg per day).[3] Patients with clinical signs of airway infection may benefit from antibiotic treatment, although viral infection likely accounts for 25% to 50% of cases.[6] Simple cases can use amoxicillin, doxycycline, trimethoprim/sulfamethoxazole, second- or third-generation cephalosporins or a macrolide. Second line is a β-lactamase inhibitor (Augmentin, Clavulin) or a fluoroquinolone, which can also be used as first line for complicated cases (e.g., in patients over the age of 65, or who have an FEV_1 less than 50%, or who have four or more exacerbations annually, or who have comorbid medical illnesses such as congestive heart failure, diabetes, chronic renal failure, or chronic liver disease. Finally, annual influenza vaccination can reduce morbidity and mortality from influenza by 50%.[3] Most, but not all, guidelines recommend the pneumococcal vaccine.[1]

❧ REFERENCES ❧

1. O'Donnell DE, Aaron S, Bourbeau J, et al: Canadian Thoracic Society recommendations for the management of chronic obstructive pulmonary disease—2003, *Can Respir J* 10(suppl A):11A-65A, 2003.

2. Friedman M, Serby CW, Menjoge SS, et al: Pharmacoeconomic evaluation of a combination of ipratropium plus albuterol compared with ipratropium alone and albuterol alone in COPD, *Chest* 115:635-641, 1999.

3. *Pocket Guide to COPD Management and Prevention.* Summary of patient care information for primary health care professionals. (Updated July 2004), Global Intitiative for Chronic Obstructive Pulmonary Disease; accessed Aug 2004 at www.goldcopd.com

4. Campbell S: For COPD a combination of ipratropium bromide and albuterol sulfate is more effective than albuterol base, *Arch Intern Med* 159:156-160, 1999.

5. Serna DL, Brenner M, Osann KE, et al: Survival after unilateral versus bilateral lung volume reduction surgery for emphysema, *J Thorac Cardiovasc Surg* 118:1101-1109, 1999.

6. Davies L, Angus RM, Calverley PM: Oral corticosteroids in patients admitted to hospital with exacerbations of chronic obstructive pulmonary disease: a prospective randomised controlled trial, *Lancet* 354:465-460, 1999.

7. Snow V, Lascher S, Mottur-Pilson C: The evidence base for acute exacerbations of COPD: clinical practice guideline Part 1. *Chest* 119(4):1185-1189, 2001.

LUNG CANCER

The two main categories of lung cancer are small cell lung cancer, accounting for one fourth of all cases, and non–small cell lung cancer, constituting the remainder. Non–small cell lung cancers are squamous cell carcinomas, adenocarcinomas, and large cell carcinomas.[1]

More than 80% of primary lung malignancies are associated with and probably caused by cigarette smoking. Smoking cessation reduces the risk of developing primary lung cancer, the rate falling to that of non-smokers within 10 to 15 years of quitting. Potential carcinogens in tobacco smoke include aromatic hydrocarbons, nitrosamines, nitrosonormiatine, polarium, and arsenic. Passive smoking, especially if exposure is prolonged and heavy, may account for a proportion of lung cancers in lifelong non-smokers. High levels of pollution, radiation (especially radon exposure) and asbestos exposure will also increase the risk, especially in smokers. Cooks, firefighters, and chemists may also have an increased risk of developing primary lung malignancies, presumably as a result of frequently inhaling carcinogens, especially if they also smoke. Heavy or prolonged exposure to industrial agents such as coal dust, ionizing radiation, asbestos, nickel, uranium, vinyl chloride, chromium, formaldehyde, and arsenic have also been implicated as a cause of primary lung malignancies.[2]

The overall prognosis of the disease is abysmal; about 90% of patients are dead within a year of the diagnosis.[2]

Presentation

Respiratory symptoms include cough, dyspnea, hemoptysis, or slow-to-resolve pneumonia, and are seen in about

30% of cases of primary lung malignancies. Generalized symptoms include weight loss, anorexia, fatigue, chest pain, bony pain, muscle weakness, and neurological symptoms.

Rarer symptoms, which occur in 12% to 20% of cases of primary lung malignancies, include dysphagia, hoarse or husky voice (from recurrent laryngeal nerve involvement), superior vena cava syndrome (headache, nausea, dizziness, visual changes, syncope, respiratory distress), and Eaton-Lambert syndrome (proximal myopathies that cause weakness). Endocrine manifestations, which occur in 12% to 20% of cases of primary lung malignancies, present with hypercalcemia (renal colic, constipation, abdominal pains), ectopic adrenocorticotropic hormone (ACTH) secretion, and diabetes insipidus, which is an inappropriate secretion of antidiuretic hormone leading to delirium and lethargy.

Metastatic spread of primary lung malignancies is likely to cause tracheal obstruction with stridor and dyspnea, dysphagia, hoarseness, Horner's syndrome, superior vena cava syndrome, pleural effusions, or even frank respiratory failure.

Staging

Staging of primary lung malignancies determines its management and prognosis. Non–small cell lung cancer is staged using the tumour, nodes, and metastases (TNM) classification (Table 69).

Examples of Stage definition and estimated 5-year survival rate (%) are as follows:

> T1-2, N0, M0 55%-75%
> T1-2, N1, M0 25%-50%

Diagnosis

A chest roentgenogram showing an isolated pulmonary nodule is one method of presentation of lung cancer. About two thirds of such nodules are benign (usually granulomas or hamartomas). Malignancy is more likely if the lesion is large, spiculated, in the upper lobe, and, if the patient is older, smokes, or has a past history of cancer.[3]

Computed tomography (CT) scanning can be helpful for diagnosis and is often necessary to evaluate mediastinal or pleural spread of suspected tumours and to assess intrathoracic lymph node involvement. CT is recommended as a staging procedure for patients with non–small cell carcinoma.

Magnetic resonance imaging (MRI) is of some value in assisting staging and mediastinal spread. Bronchsocopy with washings and lung biopsy are needed for tissue histology to decide treatment options. If the patient is too unwell to undergo either of these surgical procedures, then a repeat chest X-ray examination or CT to assess growth can help reassure benign conditions, over time.

Table 69   Staging of Lung Cancers

Tumour (T):
- T1: Tumour < 3 cm diameter
- T2: Tumour < 3 cm diameter has associated atelectasis-obstructive pneumonitis extending to the hilar region
- T3: Tumour with direct extension into the chest wall, diaphragm, mediastinal pleura or pericardium
- T4: Tumour invades the mediastinum or the presence of malignant pleural effusions

Regional lymph nodes (N):
- N0: No nodes involved
- N1: Metastasis to peribronchial or ipsilateral hilar nodes
- N2: Metastasis to ipsilateral mediastinal or subcarinal nodes
- N3: Metastasis to contralateral hilar or mediastinal nodes or to any supraclavicular or scalene nodes

Distant metastasis (M):
- M0: No known distant metastasis
- M1: Distant metastasis present

Small cell cancer is staged as follows:
- Limited stage disease: tumour confined to the one side of the chest and regional lymph nodes (mediastinal, contralateral hilar, and usually ipsilateral supraclavicular). Partly this stage relates to whether the tumour can be encompassed within a radiation port
- Extensive stage disease: defined as disease extending beyond the limited stage

Treatment

Surgery is considered the treatment of choice for patients with non–small cell lung cancer who can undergo an operation, but fewer than 20% of patients have operable disease, and of these, fewer than 50% will survive 5 years.[4] Coexisting lung disease can limit available options. With COPD, as a rough guide, if a lobectomy is being considered, patients should have an FEV_1 of greater than 1.5 L, and if a pneumonectomy is being considered, patients should have an FEV_1 of greater than 2.0 L, providing there is no interstitial lung disease or unexpected disability due to breathlessness. Cardiovascular disease will also affect perioperative mortality, although a recent coronary procedure in the absence of a myocardial infarct is not a limiting factor.

In a very few instances, patients with localized disease may be cured by radiation therapy. Overall, the 5-year survival rate for non–small cell cancer of the lung is less than 10%.[1] Chemotherapy can increase the median survival of patients with non–small cell lung cancer by 1.5 to 3 months but at the cost of considerable toxicity.[5]

Photodynamic therapy is advocated for the treatment of non–small cell cancer in patients unable to tolerate surgery or radiotherapy. Multiple other complementary therapies are being tried; however, none are licensed, none have been shown to be efficacious, and no formal clinical trials have been published.[5]

A new group founded in 1996 and based in Denver, Colorado, led by Tom Petty called Lung Cancer Frontiers, provides information about the newest techniques in treatment, which can be found at their site http://www.lungcancerfrontiers.org. Some new endobronchial treatments for early cancers are quite encouraging.

Screening

The prognosis of lung cancer is poor due to its aggressive course with early metastases, short incubation period, and lack of early presentation. Screening is thus an attractive proposition, but does it work? The value of chest X-ray examination or sputum cytology as a screening tool to detect lung cancer in smokers was the basis of a number of reports in the 1980s and early 1990s. Although 5-year survival rates were increased, long-term mortality was not affected. The U.S. Preventive Services Task Force gives both chest X-ray and sputum cytology screening a "D" recommendation.[6] The Canadian Task Force on Preventive Health Care gives chest X-ray screening a "D" and sputum cytology an "E"[7] recommendation. Unfortunately, closure of controversial issues is rarely permanent, and studies suggesting that chest X-ray screening of smokers is efficacious continue to appear. A 1998 Finnish study reported the 5-year survival of patients with lung cancer detected by a single screening X-ray study to be 19%, compared with 10% for control subjects with lung cancer who were not screened.[8]

Chest X-rays will only show masses that have attained a certain size; if malignant, they have usually metastasized, thus limiting the effectiveness of chest X-rays. Spiral CT scans are more specific and accurate than chest X-ray in the early diagnosis of primary lung malignancies. But, to be effective, scans would need to be taken frequently (every 6 to 12 months). This would be prohibitively expensive and cause problems with administering. The risks from the radiation of the annual or twice-yearly CT scans would be considerable, and may lead to an increase in incidence and mortality from primary lung malignancies. Spiral CT scanning and positron emission tomography (PET) scans serially have also been looked at for screening with less enthusiastic results.[9] Autofluorescence bronchospcopy is another technique being studied for more central airway lesions, but is still in its infancy.[10]

_____ ༔ **REFERENCES** ༖ _____

1. Simmonds P: Managing patients with lung cancer (editorial), *BMJ* 319:527-528, 1999.
2. Sethi T: Lung cancer, *BMJ* 314:652-655, 1997.
3. Swensen SJ, Silverstein MC, Ilstrup DM, et al: The probability of malignancy in solitary pulmonary nodules: application to small radiologically indeterminate nodules, *Arch Intern Med* 157:849-855, 1997.
4. Silvestri G, Pritchard R, Welch HG: Preferences for chemotherapy in patients with advanced non-small cell lung cancer: descriptive study based on scripted interviews, *BMJ* 317:771-775, 1998.
5. Non-Small Cell Cancer Collaborative Study Group: Chemotherapy for non-small cell lung cancer (Cochrane Review). In: *The Cochrane Library*, issue 1, Oxford, 2001, Update Software.
6. U.S. Preventive Services Task Force: *Guide to clinical preventive services*, ed 2, Baltimore, 1996, Williams & Wilkins, 135-139.
7. Canadian Task Force on the Periodic Health Examination: *Canadian guide to clinical preventive health care*, Ottawa, 1994, Canada Communication Group, 779-786.
8. Salomaa E-R, Liippo K, Taylor P, et al: Prognosis of patients with lung cancer found in a single chest radiograph screening, *Chest* 114:1514-1518, 1998.
9. Pastorino U, Bellomi M, Landoni C, et al: Early lung-cancer detection with spiral CT and positron emission tomography in heavy smokers: 2-year results, *Lancet* 362:593-597, 2003.
10. Soria JC, Johnson BE, Chevalier TL: Imatinib in small cell lung cancer, *Lung Cancer* 41S49-S53, 2003.

PNEUMONIA

Diagnosis

Pneumonia is an acute infection of the lung parenchyma caused by a variety of pathogens including bacteria, atypical organisms, and viruses.[1] The common causes of community-acquired pneumonia (CAP) are bacteria (*Staphylococcus pnuemoniae* 23% to 50%, *Haemophilus influenza* 3% to 10%, *Staphylococcus aureus* 3.5%, *Meningococcus catarrhalis* 1% to 3%), atypical organisms (*Meningococcus pnuemoniae* 2% to 37%, *Chlamydia pneumoniae* 5% to 17%, *Legionella pneumoniae*), and viruses (Influenza A and B, Parainfluenza 1, 2, and 3, RSV, and Epstein-Barr virus).[1] Treatment is based on this pathogen profile because there are no accurate means to differentiate between these organisms clinically.[2,3]

Diagnosis is based on clinical suspicion in the setting of two or more cardinal symptoms (i.e., temperature higher than 37.8° C, pulse greater than 100, decreased breath sounds, presence of rales, respiratory rate greater than 20) and should be confirmed by chest X-ray (demonstrating consolidation).[4] Treatment may be started with negative chest X-ray findings if the clinical suspicion is high. A negative chest X-ray, however, usually suggests an alternate diagnosis.[1] Treatment may be warranted in patients with few clinical signs and a negative chest X-ray if they have COPD, asthma, are smokers, are immunosuppressed, or are elderly. Other investigations including white blood cell count, arterial blood gases, sputum gram stain, and sputum/blood cultures are not useful in making the diagnosis or choosing therapy.[3] As a result, the treatment of CAP is essentially empirical.[1,5] Sputum cultures are obtainable in 66% of patients; however, 25% are infected with organisms not easily cultured, and false positive and negative rates are high.[5] Sputum cultures may be useful to diagnose rare infections such as Histoplasmosis, *Pneumocystis carinii,* and *Meningococcus tuberculosis.* Gram stains have been shown to be useful in patients admitted to hospital.[6]

Prognosis

Management of the patient with pneumonia, including drug choice and in-patient versus outpatient management, can be aided by use of a clinical prediction rule.[1,7] Such a scoring system determines a Risk Class Level based on age, comorbidities, and physical and lab findings. One such score, the Pneumonia Severity Index (PSI), has been proposed by Fine et al using 19 independent risk factors (Table 70).[7]

Patients with 71 to 90 points generally can be treated as outpatients. Exceptions include patients with impaired cognitive function, those unable to maintain hydration, those unable to perform activities of daily living (ADL), and those that are hypoxic. Thoracentesis should be considered in those with a pleural effusion. Patients with PSI scores greater than 91 are at significant increased risk, and hospitalization should be considered.[1,7]

Management

Antibiotic choice depends on patient characteristics and the decision to treat as an in-patient or outpatient.[1,4]

Macrolides, specifically the newer generation ones (azithromycin, clarithromycin, and telithromycin), are first line for most young healthy patients.[1,4] Erythromycin use is limited be tolerability issues. This antibiotic class covers *S. pnuemoniae, H. influenza,* and the atypical organisms. Macrolide (except telithromycin) resistance is lower but parallel to penicillin resistance for *S. pnuemoniae* and *H. influenza.* Even for most species of penicillin-resistant *S. pnuemoniae,* the minimal inhibitory concentrations (MICs) are low enough that penicillin should be effective.[1,8] Tetracyclines and/or trimethoprim-sulfamethoxazole are also acceptable alternatives.[1]

Broader spectrum antibiotics may be indicated for patients in older age groups (over age 65) or those with comorbid illnesses. These patients are at risk for infections due to oral anaerobes, gram-negative rods, *S. aureus,* and Legionella.[1,4,8]

Respiratory quinolones (levofloxacin, moxifloxacin, gatifloxacin) are first choice for patients who have recently been on an antibiotic, on steroids, or who have COPD of moderate severity.[1] Alternative choices for such patients include a combination of amoxicillin/clavulanate with a macrolide or a second generation

cephalosporin (cefaclor, cefuroxime axetil, cefprozil) with a macrolide.[1,4,8]

Ciprofloxacin is used in patients with severe COPD or others at risk for *Pseudomonas* infection.[1]

In the case of suspected macroaspiration (alcoholism), the use of amoxicillin/clavulanate is preferred.[1]

For patients intolerant of macrolides or other first-line drugs, respiratory quinolones are recommended.[1]

Patient Education

In addition to antibiotics, patient education is important. Patients should finish the entire course of antibiotics. Symptomatic relief can be achieved with oral hydration, acetaminophen, or NSAIDs, as well as other over-the-counter preparations.[1]

Criteria for follow-up include difficulty breathing, worsening cough, worsening or onset of rigors, persistent fever (greater than 48 hours) or side effects to medication.[1] Improvement generally occurs in about 48 hours. Return to work is generally reasonable 48 hours after resolution of fever and improvement in cough.[1]

Repeat chest X-ray should be obtained at 6 to 8 weeks post-treatment in smokers and patients older than age 40.[1]

Table 70   Independent Risk Factors for Scoring the Pneumonia Severity Index (PSI)

Risk Factors	Score
Demographic Factors	
Age: Males	Age in years
Females	Age in years
Nursing home residents	+ 10
Co-morbid Illnesses	
Neoplastic disease	+ 30
Liver disease	+ 20
Heart Failure	+ 10
Cerebrovascular disease	+ 10
Renal disease	+ 10
Physical Examination	
Altered mental status	+ 20
Resp rate > 30/min	+ 20
Sys BP < 90	+ 20
Temp < 35 or > 40	+ 15
Pulse > 125/ min	+ 10
Lab Findings	
pH < 7.35	+ 30
BUN > 11 mmol/L	+ 20
Sodium < 130 mEq/L	+ 20
Glucose > 14 mmol/L	+ 10
Hgb < 90	+ 10
$pO_2 < 60$ (O_2 sat < 90%)	+ 10
Pleural effusion	+ 10

From Fine MF, Auble TE, Yealy DM, et al: A prediction rule to identify low risk patient with community acquired pneumonia *N Engl J Med* 336:243-250, 1997. Copyright © 1997 Massachusetts Medical Society. All rights reserved.

❧ REFERENCES ❧

1. Kish MA, Gill M, Nomo-Ongolo S, et al. *Community acquired pneumonia in adults, ICSI Health Care Guideline.* 5th ed. Bloomington, MN, 2003, Institute for Clinical Systems Improvement (ICSI).

2. Metlay JP, Kapoor WN, Fine MJ: Does this patient have community acquired pneumonia? Diagnosing pneumonia by history and physical examination, *JAMA* 278:1440-1445, 1997.

3. Kauppinen MT, Laehde S, Syrjaelae H: Roentgenographic findings of pneumonia caused by *Chlamydia pneumoniae*: a comparison with *S. pneumoniae Arch Intern Med* 156:1851-1856, 1996.

4. Bartlett JG, Dowell SF, Mandell LA, et al: Practice guidelines for the management of community acquired pneumonia in adults, *Clin Infect Dis* 31:347-382, 2000.

5. Antoniou M, Grossman RF: Etiological diagnosis of pneumonia: a goal worth pursuing? *Can J Infec Dis* 6:281-283, 1995.

6. Watanakunakorn C, Bailey TA: Adult bacteremic pneumococcal pneumonia in a community teaching hospital, 1992-1996: a detailed analysis of 108 cases, *Arch Intern Med* 157:1965-1971, 1997.

7. Fine MF, Auble TE, Yealy DM, et al: A prediction rule to identify low risk patients with community acquired pneumonia, *N Engl J Med* 336:243-250,1997.

8. Heffelfinger JD, Dowell BF, et al: Management of CAP in the era of pneumococcal resistance: a report from the drug resistant *S. pneumonia* therapeutic working group, *Arch Intern Med* 160: 1399-408, 2000.

PULMONARY FIBROSIS

Pathophysiology

Pulmonary fibrosis is thought to be the end result of an abnormal tissue repair process in a number of chronic inflammatory lung diseases.[1] Normally, after initial tissue injury, epithelial cells migrate, proliferate, and differentiate in order to repair the damaged area, and then apoptose. Activated cells release a number of counterbalancing mediators and growth factors that promote or prevent cell proliferation and stimulate or inhibit connective tissue production. It has recently been hypothesized that abnormal repair mechanisms are related to ongoing oxidative stress, when oxidants are inhaled or produced by chronically activated and accumulated inflammatory cells in the lung.[1]

Preceding Chronic Pulmonary Inflammatory Conditions

Pulmonary fibrosis can result from primary lung injury, or as a significant part of a multi-organ process, such as in collagen vascular diseases (e.g., rheumatoid arthritis, lupus erythematosus, Sjögren's syndrome). Primary lung injury may be initiated by inhalation of inorganic dusts such as silica, asbestos, and coal, primarily in the blasting, renovation, and mining industries, and such injury is termed *pneumoconiosis*.[2] Inspiration of organic dusts,

cotton or grains by farmers, micro-organisms by occupants of buildings with poorly maintained ventilation systems, antigenic bird droppings by bird hobbyists, or chemical aerosols by plastics manufacturers (diisocyanates) or metalworkers (trimetallic anhydride), can also initiate pulmonary inflammation, classified as *hypersensitivity pneumonitis*.[3] The primary injury can also be initiated by exposure to ionizing radiation, or by ingestion of various drugs, which are thought to induce intracellular oxidative stress, including HMG-CoA reductase inhibitors, methotrexate, gold, β-adrenergic blockers, and antibiotics such as minocycline and sulphasalazine.[3] Many cases of pulmonary fibrosis are of unknown origin and so are termed *idiopathic*.[4]

Clinical Presentation

The quantity of particles or antigens inhaled and the frequency of exposure are key influences on clinical manifestations,[3] although nature of the substance plays a role,[5] and as yet undefined susceptibility factors are suspected because of variations in disease incidence in similarly exposed populations. Acute presentation with fever, chills, malaise, cough, and dyspnea may occur within 4 to 6 hours of episodic or heavy exposure to organic dusts or aerosols, clear on removal from exposure, and recur on re-exposure. However, with repeated or prolonged low-level exposure to antigenic substances, there is a more insidious subacute presentation with dry cough and increasing shortness of breath on exertion, sometimes accompanied by anorexia, weight loss, and easy fatigability.[3] When the exposure is to inorganic dusts, such as asbestos or silica, onset is insidious, and there may be an asymptomatic period for as long as 30 years after initial exposure. However, the latency period may be shortened by high-intensity exposures or cigarette smoking.[2]

Diagnosis

Once pulmonary fibrosis is established, no matter what the origin of the preceding chronic inflammatory lung disease, physical and laboratory findings are similar. Bibasilar inspiratory crackles can be heard, and clubbing may be present if the disease is prolonged. Spirometry reveals a restrictive pattern, with reduced lung volumes, diffusion capacity, and lung compliance. Arterial oxygenation is diminished, and is exacerbated by exercise. Chest X-ray may be normal for as many as 10% of those with pulmonary fibrosis, and high resolution CT may be necessary to reveal, initially, a fuzzy, ground glass appearance in the midlung zones, progressing to diffuse reticular opacities in the lower lung fields. Eventually, small cystic lesions (honeycombing) may appear. Routine laboratory tests are often not helpful, but commonly erythrocyte sedimentation rate (ESR) and serum gamma globulin are elevated if hypersensitivity pneumonitis is the prodrome.[3] ANA and rheumatoid factor may be positive, even though no collagen vascular disease is evident. In selected patients, culture of bronchoalveolar lavage fluid and analysis of its cells may help narrow the differential diagnoses. If immunosuppressive therapy, with its potential complications, is contemplated, definitive diagnosis is required, and open lung biopsy may be necessary if transbronchial biopsy yields an insufficient sample.[6]

Prevention and Management

When inciting agents for chronic lung inflammation are recognized early, and exposure is avoided, the progression to pulmonary fibrosis is curtailed. Hence, it is extremely important for physicians to take detailed exposure histories.[3] One can use the CH2OPD2 mnemonic (Community, Home, Hobby, Occupation, Personal, Diet, Drugs)[7] to help organize exposure history taking, and download exposure history tools, to be given to the patient to complete at home and then reviewed at the next appointment.[8] The patient and/or employer will likely need education in methods to avoid inciting agents. Occupational physicians, industrial hygienists, and certified home inspectors from Canada Mortgage and Housing Corporation can assist. The more complete the avoidance of antigenic substances, the better the resolution of the chronic lung inflammation.[3,9]

During severe acute episodes of hypersensitivity pneumonitis, besides antigen avoidance, corticosteroids equivalent to prednisone 1mg/kg per day may offer rapid clinical improvement, followed by gradual radiographic clearing over several weeks, and return of pulmonary function to baseline. Then prednisone may be tapered over the next 4 weeks.[3]

In pulmonary fibrosis of any origin, oxygen supplementation helps relieve hypoxemia. Prednisone has been used empirically at 1 mg/kg per day for 3 months, followed by re-evaluation of clinical and radiographic findings. Unfortunately, less than 30% show objective response.[4] Cytotoxic drugs, usually cyclophosphamide or azathioprine, have been tried if corticosteroids have not stopped fibrotic progression or are not tolerated, but recent studies have revealed significant side effects, and have not shown efficacy.[4] Lung transplantation has been successful for patients with end-stage pulmonary fibrosis.[6]

Prognosis

When lung fibrosis is idiopathic, the clinical course is progressive, with gradual deterioration to end-stage respiratory insufficiency or death within 3 to 8 years.[4] However, chronic lung inflammation secondary to identifiable precipitating agents is potentially reversible with avoidance of these agents, preventing progression to irreversible fibrosis. It is therefore critical that physicians respond to patient reports of chronic cough and dyspnea with comprehensive exposure history and recommendation for avoidance of harmful or potentially harmful exposures. Recommendation for smoking cessation is particularly relevant with concomitant inorganic dust exposure, given the increased risk for lung cancer. Preventive measures are also important, given that a recent study revealed that patients with pulmonary fibrosis had four times the amount of extensive coronary artery disease compared with patients with non-fibrotic lung disease.[10]

❧ REFERENCES ❧

1. Mastruzzo C, Crimi N, Vancheri C: Role of oxidative stress in pulmonary fibrosis, *Monaldi Arch Chest Dis* 57:173-176, 2002.
2. Greenberg MI, ed: *Occupational, industrial, and environmental toxicology*, St. Louis, 1997, Mosby, 256-260.
3. Wild LG, Lopez M: Hypersensitivity pneumonitis: a comprehensive review, *J Invest Allergol Clin Immunol* 11(1):3-15, 2001.
4. Zisman DA, Lynch JP III, Toews GB, et al: Cyclophosphamide in the treatment of idiopathic pulmonary fibrosis, *Chest* 117:1619-1626, 2000.
5. Hubbs AF, Minhas NS, Jones W, et al: Comparative pulmonary toxicity of 6 abrasive blasting agents, *Toxicol Sciences* 61:135-143, 2001.
6. Beers Mark H, Berkow R, eds: *The Merck manual of diagnosis and therapy*, ed 17, Whitehouse Station, NJ, 1999, Merck Research Laboratories, 635-637.
7. Marshall L, Weir E, Abelsohn A, et al: Identifying and managing adverse environmental health effects: 1. taking an exposure history, *Can Med Assoc J* 166(8):1049-1055, 16 Apr 2002.
8. 1 Ontario College of Family Physicians. *www.ocfp.ca* → Communications → Publications → Scroll down to Environment and Health → Taking an Exposure History.
9. Jacobs RL, Andrews CP: Hypersensitivity pneumonia-nonspecific interstitial pneumonia/fibrosis histopathological presentation: a study in diagnosis and long-term management, *Ann Allergy Asthma Immunol* 90:265-270, Feb 2003.
10. Kizer JR, Zisman DA, Blumenthal NP, et al: Association between pulmonary fibrosis and coronary artery disease, *Arch Intern Med* 164(5):551-556, 8 Mar 2004.

SARCOIDOSIS

Classification and Epidemiology

Sarcoidosis is a multisystem granulomatous disorder of unclear etiology characterized pathologically by the presence of non-caseating granulomas. It has a wide-spectrum clinical presentation and can mimic several other diseases. Onset may be acute or insidious, the latter being more serious because of progressive damage, through fibrosis, to one or more organs. The cause remains unclear, although mounting evidence suggests a combination of an environmental trigger with genetic predisposition; cases cluster within some employment groups, and the disease is more common in siblings than in spouses. An infective trigger seems likely with some form of mycobacterium being the prime suspect.

Sarcoidosis is a worldwide disease affecting both sexes, but with a female preponderance, in all races and at all ages. It is more common and more aggressive in blacks than in whites and most frequently occurs in persons under the age of 40.[1] In the United States, the annual incidence has been estimated at 35.5 per 100,000 among African Americans and 10.9 per 100,000 among Caucasians.[2]

Presentation

Sarcoidosis can present with the involvement of many tissues because the symptoms depend on the organ involved. Half of all patients present with chronic respiratory symptoms only. The more common presenting symptoms are cough, breathlessness on exertion, chest pain, fatigue, fever, anorexia, weight loss, skin rashes, swelling and stiffness of joints, nasal discharge or stuffiness, gritty or dry eyes with misty vision, and dry mouth.[2-4]

In the skin, sarcoidosis presents commonly as erythema nodosum. Small mobile, non-tender lymph nodes are found in up to 30% of cases; common sites are anterior triangle of the neck, supraclavicular fossae, axillae, and inguinal regions. In the heart, arrhythmias or congestive heart failure may be the presenting feature.

Acute cases present with arthralgia and stiffness of large joints. Chronic cases can show swelling of soft tissues around small joints with accompanying stiffness, but usually no deformity and very rarely in a monoarticular presentation. A common presentation is with that of an acute arthritis in the form of Löfgren's syndrome-characterized by triad of acute onset (days to weeks) polyarthritis, hilar adenopathy, and erythema nodosum. Fever and articular manifestations (most commonly bilateral ankles) can also be present. Löfgren's syndrome has the best prognosis of any of the variants of sarcoidosis.[5]

The spleen may be just palpable in mild cases, but a large spleen may be a sign of long-standing sarcoidosis. It is usually accompanied by hepatic enlargement, which may lead to thrombocytopenic purpura and signs of hepatic failure. Uveitis needs urgent treatment to prevent blindness. Bell's palsy from facial nerve damage is the most common manifestation if the nervous system is involved.

The respiratory tree is commonly[6] affected also, and lung involvement is present in greater than 90% of cases. In the upper respiratory tree, mucosal thickening in the nose and epistaxis is usually a sign of long-standing sarcoidosis. The lungs can present with cough or shortness of breath. Pulmonary function tests may show a restrictive deficit. Most commonly the diagnosis is made incidentally with hilar adenopathy on chest X-ray. Pleural effusions may also be found with pleural involvement. CT of the chest may detect changes not seen on chest X-ray. Ground glass opacities in areas separate from fibrosis is a finding felt to show acute alveolitis that may be amenable to therapy. (Usually stage 4 is less amenable per se.)

Five stages of X-ray findings in sarcoidosis are described:

Stage 0 being a normal result (5% to 10%).

Stage 1: Bilateral hilar lymphadenopathy (40% to 50%)

Stage 2: Bilateral hilar lymphadenopathy with parenchymal infiltration (25% to 30%)

Stage 3: Parenchymal infiltration without hilar lymphadenopathy (15% to 20%)

Stage 4: Advanced fibrosis with evidence of honeycombing, hilar retraction, bullae, cysts, and emphysema (less than 1%)

Diagnosis

No specific laboratory investigations are used for sarcoidosis. The serum level of angiotensin-converting enzyme (ACE) may be elevated, but this finding has little diagnostic value because it is non-specific; the Kveim-Siltzbach test is of historical interest only.[1] Other findings can include anemia, elevated ESR, hypergammaglobulinemia, elevated alkaline phosphatase, and eosinophilia.

Hypercalcemia is another presenting symptom in 2% to 10% of patients, which reflects abnormalities in calcitriol production. Abnormal renal function may result from undetected hypercalcemia causing renal stones or renal failure. Serum ACE may reflect disease activity.

Bronchoscopy with transbronchial and endobronchial biopsy is the procedure of choice, with a sensitivity of 90% when 4 to 5 samples are taken.[7]

Treatment[1,8]

- Systemic corticosteroids suppress granulomas and may speed up resolution in acute cases, but such cases often resolve spontaneously.
- Systemic corticosteroids also reduce symptoms and slow disease progression in chronic cases, but there is no proof that they prevent the development of fibrosis.
- Corticosteroid-sparing therapies (e.g., methotrexate, azathioprine) can be useful if high steroid doses are needed to maintain clinical improvement. They can also be useful in patients who do not respond to corticosteroids.
- Antitumour necrosis factor[9] medications (e.g., etanercept, infliximab, and possibly pentoxyfylline) are useful to decrease systemic inflammation.
- NSAIDs reduce pain from erythema nodosum or joint involvement and any associated fever; selective cyclooxygenase-2 (COX-2) inhibitors can be used in patients with a history of gastroesophageal reflux, peptic ulcer, or gastritis.

- Topical corticosteroid therapy may be all that is required in mild cases of erythema nodosum.
- Ophthalmic corticosteroids can be used to treat uveitis; they quickly reduce pain and blurred vision but require comfort in the diagnosis and need specialist follow-up.

Prognosis

Among patients with only hilar adenopathy, the disease remits spontaneously in 60% to 80% of cases. For patients with hilar adenopathy plus pulmonary infiltrates, spontaneous remission occurs in 50% to 60% of cases, whereas if there are only pulmonary infiltrates without hilar adenopathy, spontaneous remission is seen in less than 30% of cases. The prognosis is worse in patients over age 40, blacks, and those whose symptoms last longer than 6 months.[1]

Of those treated with corticosteroids (up to 50%), the vast majority stabilize or improve. Relapse occurs in 16% to 74% after reduction or cessation of therapy. Between 10% and 20% of patients have permanent disability from either pulmonary or extrapulmonary disease. Deaths are reported as being between 1% and 5% of cases and occur from pulmonary, neurological, or cardiac involvement.[10]

✍ REFERENCES ✍

1. Newman LS, Rose CS, Maier LA: Sarcoidosis, *N Engl J Med* 336:1224-1234, 1997.
2. Statement on Sarcoidosis; A joint statement of the American Thoracic Society, the European Respiratory Society (ERS) and the World Association of Sarcoidosis and Other Granulomatous Disorders (WASOG), *Am J Respir Crit Care Med* 160:736-755, 1999.
3. Morey SS: Practice Guidelines: American Thoracic Society issues a consensus statement of sarcoidosis, *Am Fam Physician* 61:553-554, 2000.
4. Belfer MH, Stevens RW: Sarcoidosis: a primary care review, *Am Fam Physician* 58:2041-2050, 1998.
5. Gran JT, Bohmer E: Acute sarcoid arthritis: a favourable outcome? A retrospective survey of 49 patients with review of the literature, *Scand J Rheumatol* 25:70-73, 1996.
6. James DG: Descriptive definition and historic aspects of sarcoidosis, *Clin Chest Med* 18:663-679, 1997.
7. Gilman MJ, Wang KP: Transbropnchial lung biopsy in sarcoidosis. An approach to determine the optimal number of biopsies, *Am Rev Resp Dis* 122:721-724, 1980.
8. Johns CJ, Michele TM: The clinical management of sarcoidosis. A 50-year experience at the Johns Hopkins Hospital, *Medicine* 78:65-111, 1999.
9. Yee AM, Pochapin MB: Treatment of complicated sarcoidosis with infliximab anti-tumor necrosis factor-alpha therapy, *Ann Intern Med* 135:27-31, 2001.
10. Gottlieb JE, Israel HL, Steiner RM, et al: Outcome in sarcoidosis. The relationship of relapse to corticosteroid therapy, *Chest* 111:623-631, 1997.

SLEEP APNEA

Sleep apnea syndromes are comprised of obstructive (absent flow with normal effort), central (absence of respiratory effort and flow), and mixed. The most common and significant syndrome is the obstructive sleep apnea-hypopnea syndrome (OSA), on which this discussion will focus. It is one of the most poorly recognized entities in general practice.[1]

OSA is typified by repetitive airway obstruction during sleep, and spans the spectrum from loud snoring to lack of airflow through the airway.

Sleep architecture is typically disrupted with frequent arousals, oxygen desaturations, and carbon dioxide retention. Often noted are significant excessive daytime sleepiness (EDS), with impaired cognitive functions (concentration, attention, memory, etc.), mood changes (depression), and impaired work and ADL performance. Excessive adrenergic stimulation in addition to other pathophysiological causes increase the occurrence of hypertension and other cardiac pathology (congestive heart failure and myocardial ischemia), with a significantly increased mortality risk.[2-4]

The most common causes of OSA are obesity (body mass index [BMI] greater than 30), adenotonsillar hypertrophy, craniofacial anomalies (macroglossia, retrognathia), and congenital diseases (e.g., cerebral palsy, Down syndrome, hemifacial micorosomia, and Pierre Robin syndrome).[1,5,6]

Other predisposing factors include type 2 diabetes mellitus, alcohol and sedative/hypnotic/muscle relaxant use, age over 40, and menopause.

Significant epidemiological trends are an overall prevalence of 2% to 15% of the adult population (more common than asthma and diabetes). Thirty percent of middle-age adults have sleep-disordered breathing, 2% of children have OSA, and among snorers, 20% have sleep apnea. A strong familial predisposition has also been found. Male to female ratio is 7 to 10:1. An increased incidence is also seen in African, Asian, and European races (mostly due to obesity in western and developed countries). An increased prevalence is also noted in pregnancy during 2nd and 3rd trimesters.[8]

Significant complications are noted in patients untreated for OSA and those poorly compliant with treatment recommendations. These complications include frequent falls and injuries, motor vehicle accidents, hypertension, myocardial ischemia, dysrhythmias, pulmonary hypertension, stroke, and death.[8,9]

Diagnosis

The most common presenting signs and symptoms are increased BMI, hypertension, large neck size (over 43 cm or 17 in), leg edema (in severe cases), impaired cognitive performance, in addition to snoring with or without witnessed choking (apnea episodes) by the bed partner. Patients also note non-refreshing sleep with early morning dry mouth, sore throat, and headaches, excessive sleepiness during the day, and enuresis in children or nocturia in adults.

Proper diagnosis of sleep apnea includes a detailed specific sleep history (that may include an Epworth Sleepiness Scale questionnaire) that reviews the points above, targeted physical examination, specific laboratory investigations (e.g., CBC and thyroid functions) and specialized sleep studies (polysomnography [PSG], multiple sleep latency test [MSLT], and maintenance of wakefulness test [MWT]). PSG is considered the gold standard for diagnosis.[10] It is typically performed overnight in a sleep lab, and includes continuous monitoring of EEG, EMG (legs and chin), EOG (electrooculography for eye movements, such as during the REM cycle), ECG, airflow, oximetry, and respiratory effort, and snoring and body position. The gathered data is scored and interpreted, looking at the number of respiratory events (apneas and hypopneas) per hour combined with degree of oxygen desaturations and sleep fragmentation.

MSLT involves similar recordings but is conducted during the day with four to five 20-minute naps to measure speed of sleep onset and presence of REM sleep during the naps, which assists in measuring degree of daytime sleepiness and helps with diagnosing narcolepsy.

Treatment

Treatment options include lifestyle changes and weight loss, nasal continuous positive airway pressure (CPAP), dental (oral appliances, which are typically better for snoring +/– mild apnea) and surgical (e.g., tonsillectomy and adenoidectomy, laser-assisted uvuloplasty [LAUP]), uvulopalatopharyngoplasty (UPPP), various facial reconstructive procedures, and lastly, tracheostomy. Medications are rarely used.[4,11-16]

Nasal CPAP is considered the gold standard for treatment, and is the most effective and commonly used method. Significant efforts may be required for proper counselling and education of patients and family to improve compliance rates. In many cases of significant OSA, patients experience a rapid improvement in symptoms and overall quality of life, in addition to improved cardiovascular health (e.g., with decreased hypertension, congestive heart failure, and ischemic events). Continuous follow-up with periodic sleep evaluations are typically undertaken, in addition to support for lifestyle modifications and risk factor assessment.

There is a significant increased risk for long-term mortality with OSA, especially if complicated by other cardiovascular conditions, poor compliance, and lack of lifestyle modifications.

❧ REFERENCES ❧

1. Flemons WW: Clinical practice. Obstructive sleep apnea, *N Engl J Med* 347:498-504, 2002.
2. Nieto FJ, Young TB, Lind BK, et al: Association of sleep-disordered breathing, sleep apnea, and hypertension in a large community-based study. Sleep Heart Health Study, *JAMA* 283:1829-1836, 2000.
3. Kaneko Y, Floras JS, Usui K, et al: Cardiovascular effects of continuous positive airway pressure in patients with heart failure and obstructive sleep apnea, *N Engl J Med* 348:1233-1241, 2003.
4. Silverberg DS, Iaina A, Okensberg A: Treating obstructive sleep apnea improves essential hypertension and quality of life, *Am Fam Physician* 65:229-236, 2002.
5. Victor LD: Obstructive sleep apnea, *Am Fam Physician* 15:2279-2286, 1999.
6. Hensley M, Ray C: Sleep apnoea, *Clin Evidence* 10:1958-1974, 2003.
7. American Academy of Pediatrics: Clinical practice guideline: diagnosis and management of childhood obstructive sleep apnea syndrome, *Pediatrics* 109:704-712, 2002. Available at the National Guideline Clearinghouse.
8. Flemons WW: Clinical practice. Obstructive sleep apnea, *N Engl J Med* 347:498-504, 2002.
9. Bridgman SA, Dunn KM, Ducharme F: Surgery for obstructive sleep apnoea (Cochrane Review). In: The Cochrane Library, issue 1, Chichester, UK, 2004, John Wiley.
10. American Academy of Sleep Medicine: Practice parameters for the indications for polysomnography and related procedures, *Sleep* 20:406-422, 1997.
11. Lojander J, Maasilta P, Partinen M, et al: Nasal-CPAP, surgery, and conservative management for treatment of obstructive sleep apnea syndrome: a randomized study, *Chest* 110:114-119,1996.
12. Schmidt-Nowara W, Lowe A, Wiegand L, et al: Oral appliances for the treatment of snoring and obstructive sleep apnea: a review, *Sleep* 18:501–510, 1995.
13. Bridgman SA, Dunn KM, Ducharme F: Surgery for obstructive sleep apnoea (Cochrane Review). In: *The Cochrane Library,* issue 1, Chichester, UK, 2004, John Wiley.
14. Gotsopoulous H, Chen C, Qian J, et al: Oral appliance therapy improves symptoms in obstructive sleep apnea: a randomized, controlled trial, *Am J Respir Crit Care Med* 166:743-748, 2002. Reviewed in: *Clin Evid*ence 10:1958-1974, 2003.
15. Walker-Engstrom ML, Wilhelmsson B, Tegelberg A, et al: Quality of life assessment of treatment with dental appliance or UPPP in patients with mild to moderate obstructive sleep apnoea. A prospective randomized 1-year follow-up study, *J Sleep Res* 9:303-308, 2000. Reviewed in: *Clin Evidence* 10:1958-1974, 2003.

16. White J, Cates C, Wright J: Continuous positive airways pressure for obstructive sleep apnoea (Cochrane Review). In *The Cochrane Library*, issue 1, Chichester, UK, 2004, John Wiley.

SPIROMETRY

Spirometry is a test performed in the office or hospital that measures airflow of the lungs. It is also known as *pulmonary function testing*.

Spirometry enables a clinician to formulate a differential diagnosis by distinguishing between airflow obstruction and restriction. Common obstructive airflow conditions include asthma and COPD.

Common restrictive airflow conditions include interstitial lung diseases, chest wall abnormalities, or respiratory muscle weakness.

The majority of abnormalities are obstructive airflow conditions. There are three key measurements of expiratory airflow, as follows:

FEV_1: The volume of airflow in the first second of effort; it usually measures the degree of obstruction.

FVC: The volume of airflow after a maximal inspiration and maximal expiration (over 6 seconds); it usually measures the degree of restriction.

FEV_1/FVC Ratio: The percentage of lung volume that is expired in the first second of effort by the patient; this ratio establishes whether there is an obstructive defect.

There are typically two flow curves: volume/time and flow/volume, which can have patterns suggestive of airway obstruction or restriction.

Improvement of greater than 12% and greater than 200 cc in the FEV_1 after a dose of inhaled bronchodilator indicates reversible airway obstruction, which is asthma by definition.

Urgent action is required if FEV_1 is less than 50% of predicted and FEV_1/FVC is less than 70%, an indication of severe obstruction.

FVC less than 50% of predicted indicates severe restriction.

Either of these results requires further investigations with arterial blood gases, chest X-ray/CT scan, and full pulmonary function tests including lung volumes and carbon monoxide diffusion capacity.

Consider referral if:

- there is a mixture of both restrictive and obstructive airflow abnormalities that need to be sorted out
- the patient's symptoms are not in keeping with the degree of abnormality, (such as moderate-to-severe dyspnea with only minor spirometry abnormalities)
- spirometry reveals severe abnormalities (FEV_1 less than 50% and/or FVC less than 50% of predicted)

✦ REFERENCES ✦

1. O'Donnell D, et al: Canadian Thoracic Society recommendations for the management of chronic obstructive pulmonary disease, *Can Resp J* 11(suppl B):1B-58B, July/Aug 2004.
2. Boulet L, et al: Canadian asthma consensus report, 1999, *Can Med Assoc J* 161(suppl 11):S1-S62, 30 Nov 1999.
3. Ferguson G, et al: Office spirometry for lung health assessment in adults: a consensus statement from the National Lung Health Education Program, *Chest* 117:1146-1161, 2000.
4. Barreiro T, et al: An approach to interpreting spirometry, *Am Fam Physician* 69(5):1107-1114, .

(See also anticoagulants; Behçet's syndrome; hemochromatosis; lyme disease; non-steroidal anti-inflammatory drugs; non-steroidal anti-inflammatory drug gastropathy; rubella immunization; Sjögren's syndrome; systemic lupus erythematosus; transient synovitis)

Topics covered in this section

Connective Tissue Diseases
Fibromyalgia
Gout
Leg Cramps
Muscle Relaxants
Osteoarthritis
Paget's Disease
Palindromic Rheumatism
Polymyalgia Rheumatica
Reflex Sympathetic Dystrophy
Rheumatoid Arthritis
Septic Arthritis
Seronegative Spondyloarthropathies

CONNECTIVE TISSUE DISEASES

(See also arthritis; biliary cirrhosis; polymyalgia rheumatica; rheumatology; erythrocyte sedimentation rate; thrombophlebitis)

Classification

The following disorders are usually included in the classification of connective tissue disorders[1]:

- CREST syndrome (calcinosis, Raynaud's phenomenon, esophageal dysfunction, sclerodactyly, and telangiectasia)
- Dermatomyositis
- Mixed connective tissue disease
- Overlap syndromes
- Polymyositis
- Progressive systemic sclerosis (scleroderma)
- Rheumatoid arthritis
- Sjögren's syndrome
- Systemic lupus erythematosus (SLE)
- Vasculitis

In some ways, listing vasculitis as a separate entity is artificial because vasculitis is an element of many "connective tissue diseases," such as rheumatoid arthritis, Sjögren's syndrome, and SLE.

Laboratory Investigations

Many laboratory investigations are available for patients with suspected connective tissue disorders. For the family physician, a complete blood count (CBC) and urinalysis are probably the two most important tests. Ordering an erythrocyte sedimentation rate (ESR) can be helpful because a normal ESR is rare in the presence of active polymyositis or vasculitis. However, false positives are common. (See erythrocyte sedimentation rate.)[1]

Other useful tests are creatine phosphokinase if polymyositis or dermatomyositis is suspected, rheumatoid factor if rheumatoid arthritis, Sjögren's syndrome, SLE, vasculitis, or dermatomyositis is being considered, thyroid-stimulating hormone (TSH) to rule out thyroid disease that may be associated with myalgias, myositis, and muscle weakness, and antinuclear antibody (ANA) for any of the connective tissue diseases.[1]

A negative ANA virtually rules out a diagnosis of SLE. When the ANA titre is positive, the accompanying pattern result can indicate scleroderma or SLE.[2] False-positive results are common with ANA tests, especially in the elderly. In one study the positive predictive value in 1010 patients was only 11% for both lupus and other rheumatic diseases.[3] Antineutrophil cytoplasmic autoantibodies (ANCA) are found in the blood of about 90% of patients with Wegener's granulomatosis or microscopic polyangiitis and 70% of those with the Churg-Strauss syndrome.[4]

C-reactive protein, LE cell preparation, and complement (C3, C4) levels are rarely helpful to diagnose connective tissue disease.[2] For help with diagnosing SLE, further tests can include anti-dsDNA and extractable nuclear antigens (i.e., Anti-SM, Anti-Ro, Anti-La) when the ANA is positive.[2]

❧ REFERENCES ❧

1. Moore PM, Pope J: Investigating connective tissue disease. I. An overview, *Can J CME* 6:39-49, 1994.
2. Shojania K: Rheumotology: 2. What laboratory tests are needed? *Can Med Assoc J* 162(8):1157-1163, 2000.
3. Slater CA, Davis RB, Shmerling RH: Antinuclear antibody testing: a study of clinical utility, *Arch Intern Med* 156: 1421-1425, 1996.
4. Jennette JC, Falk RJ: Small-vessel vasculitis, *N Engl J Med* 337:1512-1523, 1997.

Sjögren's Syndrome

Sjögren's syndrome is a chronic inflammatory autoimmune disease. It causes lymphocytic infiltration and occasionally destruction of exocrine glands; mostly salivary, lacrimal, and occasionally pancreas. Major symptoms include dry eyes and dry mouth, but these in themselves are non-specific and may be due to a variety of conditions, including drugs with anticholinergic side effects.[1] Diagnostic criteria differ between a positive minor salivary gland biopsy or a positive serum autoantibody assay for Ro (SS-A) and La (SS-B) autoantibodies.[2] In most patients, ESR is elevated and ANA and rheumatoid factor (RF) are present. It is most common between ages 50 and 80, and 90% of cases are female.[3] Patients with Sjögren's syndrome are at increased risk for developing non-Hodgkin's B-cell lymphoma.[4] Sjögren's syndrome is classified into primary and secondary forms. The primary form may involve only the salivary and lacrimal glands or may be associated with a small vessel vasculitis causing nephritis, cutaneous rashes, or pulmonary lesions. The secondary forms are usually associated with rheumatoid arthritis, SLE, scleroderma, polymyositis, or biliary cirrhosis.

Treatment is aimed at the symptoms and to prevent complications. For dry eyes, eye lubricants with no preservatives, such as oral pilocarpine, are used. For dry mouth, sugarless lemon drops, oral pilocarpine or cevimeline are used.[5] Non-steroidal anti-inflammatory drugs (NSAIDs) and hydroxycloroquine may be used for musculoskeletal symptoms. Lifestyle changes are very important and include improving oral hygiene, stopping smoking, avoiding dry and windy weather, and avoiding sugary foods.[6]

⚜ REFERENCES ⚜

1. Noble J, Greene HL, et al, editors: *Textbook of primary care medicine,* ed 3, St. Louis, 2001, Mosby, p.1307.
2. Brasington RD Jr, Kahl LE, Ranganathan P, et al: 14. Immunologic rheumatic disorders, *J Allergy Clin Immunol* 111(2 suppl):S593-S601, 2003.
3. Ruddy S, Harris ED Jr, Sledge CB, et al, editors: *Kelley's textbook of rheumatology,* ed 6, Philadelphia, 2001, W B Saunders.
4. Zufferey P, Meyer OC, Grossin M, et al: Primary Sjogren's syndrome (SS) and malignant lymphoma: a retrospective cohort study of SS patients, *Scand J Rheumatol* 24:342, 1995.
5. Fox R, Pentrone J, Condemi R, et al: Randomized, placebo-controlled trial of SNI-2011, a novel M3 muscarinic receptor agonist, for the treatment of Sjogren's syndrome, *Arthritis Rheum* 41(suppl):S288, 1998.
6. Mahoney EJ, Spiegel JH: Sjögren's disease, *Otolaryngol Clin North Am* 36(4): 733-745, 2003.

Systemic Lupus Erythematosus

Systemic Lupus Erythematosus (SLE) is a chronic multisystem disease with multiple flares and remissions. The criteria for diagnosis tends to include four or more of the following: malar rash, discoid rash, photosensitivity, oral ulcers, arthritis, serositis, renal disorder, neurological disorder, hematological disorder, immunological disorder, and ANA.[1] Arthritis is the most common clinical manifestation of SLE, and tendinitis is also common. The arthritis tends to be oligoarticular and migratory, and pain is disproportionate to any signs of inflammation. Arthritis in SLE does not involve the spine. Small joints of the hand are affected in 95% of cases, but deformities such as those seen in rheumatoid arthritis are rare.[2,3] Dermatitis is the second most common clinical feature of SLE, but the classic malar butterfly erythema is present in only one third of patients.[3] Clinically significant renal disease occurs in 40% to 75% of cases.[2]

The prevalence of SLE is generally stated to be about 40 per 100,000 in Europe and North America.[4] More than 80% of cases occur in women during the childbearing years, and in this population the prevalence rate is close to 1:1000.[2]

Patients with SLE are at risk for premature atherosclerosis.[4] Additionally, patients with lupus are at increased risk for the antiphospholipid-antibody syndrome, which is characterized by arterial and venous thrombosis, thrombocytopenia, and recurrent fetal loss.[1] (See discussion of thrombophlebitis.)

A variety of treatments are used for SLE, depending on the organ systems involved and the severity of the disease. Most joint inflammation is managed with NSAIDs, but care must be taken that these do not aggravate renal disease. Hydroxychloroquine (Plaquenil) may be used for some patients. Cutaneous manifestations are dealt with primarily by strict sun blocking and occasionally, use of topical glucocorticoids. Renal manifestations are treated with drugs, such as azathioprine (Imuran), cyclophosphamide (Cytoxan), or corticosteroids.[5] Lupus patients with the antiphospholipid antibody syndrome are given warfarin except during pregnancy. (See discussion of antiphospholipid antibody syndrome.)[6] It is important to monitor for flare-ups, infections, and complications.

⚜ REFERENCES ⚜

1. Brasington RD Jr, Kahl LE, Ranganathan P, et al: 14. Immunologic rheumatic disorders, *J Allergy Clin Immunol* 111(2 suppl): S593-601, 2003.
2. Rakel RE, editor: *Textbook of family practice,* ed 6, Philadelphia, 2002, W B Saunders, p. 978.
3. Ruddy S, Harris ED Jr, Sledge CB, et al, editors: *Kelley's textbook of rheumatology,* ed 6, Philadelphia, 2001, W B Saunders, p. 1110.
4. Goldman L, Bennett JC: *Cecil textbook of medicine,* ed 21, Philadelphia, 2000, W B Saunders, p. 1509-1517.
5. Hejaili FF, Moist LM, Clark WF: Treatment of lupus nephritis, *Drugs* 63:257-274, 2003.
6. Petri M: Treatment of systemic lupus erythematosus: an update, *Am Fam Physician* 57:2753-2760, 1998.

Vasculitis

Vasculitis can be divided into large vessel vasculitis, which includes giant cell arteritis and Takayasu's arteritis; medium-sized vessel arteritis, which includes polyarteritis nodosa and Kawasaki disease; and small vessel vasculitis, which includes cutaneous leukocytoclastic angiitis (hypersensitivity vasculitis), Behçet's syndrome, Henoch-Schönlein purpura, Goodpasture's syndrome, serum sickness, and the three entities usually associated with ANCA in the blood, namely Wegener's granulomatosis, Churg-Strauss syndrome, and microscopic polyangiitis.[1]

The dividing line between small and medium-sized arteries is not always well defined, and some of the listed disorders are not strictly limited to vessels of a particular size. Giant cell and Takayasu's arteritides are always limited to large vessels; hypersensitivity vasculitis, Henoch-Schönlein purpura, and the vasculitis of cryoglobulinemia are limited to small vessels; the remainder may affect both medium-sized and small vessels.[2]

Giant-cell or temporal arteritis

Giant-cell arteritis, formerly called *temporal arteritis,* is primarily a disease of elderly white persons. A recent meta-analysis that examined sensitivity and specificity of signs and symptoms, using temporal artery biopsy as a gold standard, confirmed that most signs and symptoms (headaches, jaw claudication, weight loss, malaise, and fever) are non-specific.[2] Jaw claudication and diplopia had some sensitivity but were only encountered 10% to 30% of the time. About 15% of patients seek treatment for fever of unknown origin. Visual symptoms, which can include partial or complete visual loss, diplopia, and ptosis, are less common but are important harbingers of complete vision loss. Between one fourth and one half of the patients have symptoms of polymyalgia rheumatica. An association between giant-cell arteritis and the later development of thoracic aneurysms has been described.[3]

The diagnosis of giant cell arteritis is usually confirmed by temporal artery biopsy, although other cranial arteries may be chosen as the biopsy site. If the biopsy cannot be performed before the start of steroid therapy, it may still be done within the next 2 weeks with reasonable expectation of showing positive results if the patient actually has the disease.[3]

Treatment of giant cell arteritis is prednisone, usually starting with 40 to 60 mg per day. In most cases the daily dose may be decreased by about 10 mg after 2 weeks and by another 10 mg 2 weeks later. Thereafter it may be lowered by a maximum of 10% every 1 to 2 weeks, depending on symptoms and the sedimentation rate or C-reactive protein levels. As the dose of prednisone decreases, the frequency and magnitude of further decrements diminish. Prognosis is excellent and life expectancy is normal.[4] Bone-saving measures should be taken, and many patients can be weaned from prednisone within 2 years.[5]

Takayasu's arteritis

Takayasu's arteritis, or pulseless disease, involves inflammation and stenosis of large and intermediate-size arteries, especially in the region of the aortic arch. Most affected are women in their teens or early twenties.[2]

Polyarteritis nodosa

Polyarteritis nodosa is a vasculitic disorder characterized by a necrotizing inflammation of the media of small and medium-size arteries, with inflammatory cell infiltration. Vascular lesions are segmental and tend to involve bifurcations of arteries. Clinical features include peripheral neuropathy, mononeuritis multiplex and skin lesions (palpable purpura, livedo reticularis, necrotic ulcers, digital infarcts). Organ infarction may occur; cardiac, peripheral nerve, skin, and gastrointestinal (GI) involvement are most frequent. Many patients present with fever, malaise, anorexia and weight loss.

Diagnosis requires the patient to have three of the following ten criteria:
1. Weight loss greater than 4 kg
2. Livedo reticularis
3. Testicular pain or tenderness
4. Myalgias, weakness, or leg tenderness
5. Mononeuropathy or polyneuropathy
6. Diastolic blood pressure greater than 90 mmHg
7. Elevated blood urea nitrogen or creatinine
8. Hepatitis B virus
9. Arteriographic abnormality
10. Biopsy of small or medium artery containing histological evidence of vasculitis[6]

Although polyarteritis nodosa is usually idiopathic, it may be associated with cryoglobulinemia, hairy cell leukemia, rheumatoid arthritis, Sjögren's syndrome, or hepatitis B.[2] Treatment for polyarteritis nodosa is high-dose prednisone, and second-line treatment is cyclophosphamide.

Kawasaki disease

The highest incidence of Kawasaki disease is in Asians, and the vast majority of cases are in children under age 5.

The following clinical manifestations are needed to make the diagnosis[7]: Fever of at least 5 days' duration plus at least four of the other five findings:
1. Changes in the extremities (erythema and edema of hands and feet in the acute phase and desquamation of fingertips in the convalescent phase)
2. Polymorphous rash over the body
3. Non-exudative bilateral conjunctival injection that usually involves the bulbar conjunctiva
4. Changes in lips and oral cavity (fissuring and erythema of lips, erythema of pharynx and oral mucosa, strawberry tongue)
5. Cervical adenopathy with at least one lymph node 1.5 cm or greater in diameter[8]

In patients with fever, the diagnosis can be based on fewer criteria if echocardiography or angiography demonstrates coronary artery disease.[7]

The most serious sequelae of the disease are cardiac and include myocarditis and pericarditis during the acute phase of the illness and, more importantly, coronary artery aneurysms and thrombosis in the later stages.

Long-term sequelae are diminished by adequate treatment. Recommended therapy is a single IV infusion of immune globulin 2 g/kg plus high-dose Aspirin (80 to 100 mg/kg per day). To maximize prevention of coronary artery abnormalities and decrease the duration of fever, IV immunoglobulin should be given within the first 10 days of the illness. High-dose Aspirin should be given at the same time as IV immunoglobulin and continued until several days after defervescence. The Aspirin dosage can then be reduced to 3 to 5 mg/kg as a single daily dose until the platelet count and ESR return to normal. If coronary artery abnormalities are detected, low-dose Aspirin therapy should be continued indefinitely.[7]

Cutaneous leukocytoclastic angiitis

Cutaneous leukocytoclastic angiitis, or hypersensitivity vasculitis, is a small vessel angiitis that affects primarily the skin of the lower legs and is manifested as palpable purpura and sometimes focal areas of necrosis. The word *leukocytoclastic* refers to the fact that on histological examination, the nuclei of white blood cells infiltrating the dermis are found to be broken up. The condition can be idiopathic, drug induced (in about 10% of cases), or rarely a manifestation of a systemic vasculitis. If no clinical evidence of systemic disease is found and possible provoking drugs have been discontinued, the condition resolves spontaneously over several weeks or months. Symptomatic treatment with antihistamines or topical corticosteroids is sufficient in most cases, although a few patients with severe disease require oral steroids.[1]

Behçet's syndrome

Behçet's syndrome is common in the eastern Mediterranean (particularly Turkey, Iran, and Saudi Arabia), China, Korea, and Japan. It is rare in Western countries. Small vessel vasculitis results in a varied clinical picture. Recurrent oral ulceration is the most common initial symptom and is present in almost all cases; recurrent genital ulcers are also common. Other clinical manifestations include ocular inflammation, arthritis, dermatitis, and GI and central nervous system symptoms.[6] The disease follows a relapsing and remitting course; treatment is mainly symptomatic.

Henoch-Schönlein purpura

Henoch-Schönlein purpura is a small vessel vasculitis of children that is characterized by IgA immune complexes in the vessels. It often follows an upper respiratory tract infection or other minor illness, although no specific etiology has been identified. The peak age is 5 years, and common manifestations are purpura, arthralgias, colicky abdominal pain, GI bleeding, and nephritis. The rash is typically on the lower extremities and buttocks, begins as erythematous papules, and progresses to palpable purpura. Renal involvement is the most serious complication, and is more likely if the rash persists or there is hematochezia. All children with Henoch-Schönlein purpura should have their urine analyzed on several occasions during the stages of the disease. The prognosis is excellent, and in most cases no specific treatment is required. Follow-up for Henoch-Schönlein purpura without renal impairment should include an annual urinalysis for several years. If renal involvement is present, follow-up involves an annual urinalysis for life.[9] Less than 1% of cases progress to end-stage renal failure, and the optimal management of this subgroup is uncertain.[1]

There are no specific drug treatments for Henoch-Schoenlein purpura; however, simple analgesics (acetaminophen) or NSAIDs, such as ibuprofen, are recommended as first-line therapy for relief of pain and inflammation, but they should be used with caution if there is active upper GI bleeding or possible renal impairment.

Systemic corticosteroids have been advocated for more severe abdominal or joint pains, or painful angioedema. They may mask further acute abdominal complications or cause or worsen GI bleeding.

Churg-Strauss syndrome

The Churg-Strauss syndrome is a vasculitis with numerous eosinophils in the inflammatory infiltrate. The vasculitis mainly affects the small arteries of the lung. Initial symptoms are those of allergic rhinitis and asthma, but after a few years or even several decades, symptoms related to vasculitis such as eosinophilic (Loeffler's) pneumonia develop. Gastroenteritis, myocarditis, neuropathy, and in some cases nephritis may also be present. Almost all patients have eosinophilia, and 70% have ANCA.[1] A number of cases of Churg-Strauss syndrome have been reported in asthmatic patients taking leukotriene inhibitors such as zafirlukast (Accolate) or montelukast (Singulair) for the treatment of asthma. Because the leukotriene inhibitors improved asthma control, the treating physicians withdrew corticosteroids, an action that appears to have unmasked pre-existing Churg-Strauss syndrome.[10]

Wegener's granulomatosis

Wegener's granulomatosis is a rare disease that inflames the blood vessels (vasculitis). It can affect any organ but typically consists of necrotizing granulomatous inflammation of the upper and lower respiratory tracts, as well as inflammation of the glomeruli (glomerulonephritis). About 20% of patients have evidence of glomerulonephritis at presentation, but as the disease evolves, this condition develops in about 80%. The typical clinical presentation is persistent inflammation of the nasal passages or sinuses in conjunction with fever, malaise, and migratory arthritis. ANCA is found in 90% of cases.

For diagnosis, two of the following four criteria must be present:
1. Nasal or oral inflammation
2. Abnormal chest X-ray (nodules, fixed infiltrates or cavities)

3. Urinary sediment (greater than 5 red blood cells per high power field or red cell casts)
4. Granulomatous inflammation on biopsy[11]

Therapy for Wegener's granulomatosis generally includes corticosteroids and cyclophosphamide, which produce remission in over 90% of cases.

Microscopic polyangiitis

Microscopic polyangiitis is a necrotizing arteritis of mainly small arteries. Some authors consider it to be a variant of Wegener's granulomatosis,[1] whereas others describe it as a variant of polyarteritis nodosa.[2]

─────────── ◢ REFERENCES ◣ ───────────

1. Jennette JC, Falk RJ: Small-vessel vasculitis, *N Engl J Med* 337:1512-1523, 1997.
2. Smetana GW, Shmerling RH: Does this patient have Temporal Arteritis? *JAMA* 287:92-101, 2002.
3. Weyand CM, Gorozny JJ: Giant-cell arteritis and polymyalgia rheumatica, *Ann Intern Med* 139:505-515, 2003.
4. Roane DW, Griger DR: An approach to diagnosis and initial management of systemic vasculitis, *Am Fam Physician* 60: 1421-1430, 1999.
5. Hunder GG: Giant cell arteritis and polymyalgia rheumatica, *Med Clin North Am* 81:195-219, 1997.
6. Sakane T, Takeno M, Suzuki N, et al: Behçet's disease, *N Engl J Med* 341:1284-1291, 1999.
7. Taubert KA: Epidemiology of Kawasaki disease in the United States and worldwide, *Prog Pediatr Cardiol* 6:181-185, 1997.
8. Lightfoot RW Jr, Michel BA, Bloch DA, et al: 1990 Criteria for the classification of polyarteritis nodosa, *Arthritis Rheum* 33:1088-1093, 1990.
9. Saulsbury FT: Henoch-Schoenlein purpura in children, *Medicine* 78:395-409, 1999.
10. D'Cruz DP, Barnes NC, Lockwood CM: Difficult asthma or Churg-Strauss syndrome? (editorial), *BMJ* 318:475-476, 1999.
11. Leavitt RY, Fauci AS, Bloch DA, et al: The American College of Rheumatology 1990 criteria for the classification of Wegener's granulomatosis, *Arthritis Rheum* 33:1101-1107, 1990.

FIBROMYALGIA

(See also chronic fatigue syndrome; irritable bowel disease; multiple chemical sensitivities)

In 1990, the report of the Multicenter Criteria Committee of the American College of Rheumatology outlined the following consensus criteria for fibromyalgia (FM)[1]:

1. History of bilateral widespread pain involving the upper and lower body and axial regions. (The axial regions are defined as the cervical, thoracic, or lumbar spine and the anterior chest.)
2. Duration of more than 3 months.
3. The report of pain by the patient in at least 11 out of 18 tender point sites (palpated with the approximate force of 4 kg, enough to blanch the nailbed, using the

thumb, or first and/or second finger). These points are bilateral and include the following:

- Suboccipital muscle insertion
- Anterior aspect of the intertransverse spaces at C 5-7
- Medial portion of supraspinatus muscles above spines of scapulae
- Midpoint of upper border of trapezius muscles
- Second costochondral junctions
- 2 cm distal to the lateral epicondyles
- Upper outer buttocks
- Prominence of the greater trochanters
- Medial fat pad of knees proximal to joint line

Patients meeting the above criteria also report a variety of other symptoms including sleep disturbances, fatigue, headache, depression, anxiety, numbness and swollen feeling, irritable bowel, and cognitive changes such as difficulty concentrating and remembering.[2]

The diagnostic approach to patients with suspected FM begins with trying to rule out other diseases such as acute or chronic viral, bacterial, fungal or parasitic infections; cancer; connective tissue diseases; endocrine/metabolic disorders; heavy metal poisoning; immune deficiencies; neurological disorders; nutritional disorders; primary psychiatric disorders; sleep apnea; and substance abuse. Initial laboratory investigations are CBC, blood urea nitrogen (BUN), creatinine, liver enzymes, serum calcium, T4, and TSH. Further testing depends on clinical and exposure histories and physical examination.[2] Exposure history-taking may be aided using the mnemonic CH2OPD2 (Community, Home and Hobby, Occupation, Personal, Diet and Drugs) and downloadable exposure history forms (*www.ocfp.ca*, Communications, Publications, scroll to Environment and Health and Taking an Exposure History).[3] The intensity of symptoms can be rated using a simple 0-10 measurement.[2]

FM, chronic fatigue syndrome (CFS), and multiple chemical sensitivities (MCS) are noted to have considerable overlap in symptoms and epidemiology.[4] These three conditions occur predominantly in middle-age women.[4, 5] The prevalence of FM is 0.5% to 1.2% worldwide, and 3.4% among U.S. women.[5] FM occurs much more frequently in patients with chronic diseases, especially connective tissue diseases, than in the general population.[6] Patients with a 6- to 8-year history of FM showed markedly abnormal measures of pain, global severity, fatigue, sleep disturbance, anxiety, depression, and health status.[7]

The precise etiologic factors and pathophysiological mechanisms remain elusive. Important clues from research suggest that lack of stage 4 restorative sleep, hyperactivity of the hypothalamic-pituitary axis, and exposure to stress leading to elevated oxidants can play a role in symptom production in FM, CFS, and MCS.[8-10]

Given the mechanistic uncertainties, it may be useful to view these conditions as multifactorial with a failure of adaptation, whereby each patient's maximum tolerance for combined stressors, no matter what their source, has been exceeded.[11] In one study, a patient-centred approach (including establishment of the diagnosis, empathic education of the patient and family, mutual discussion of treatment options) by doctors using a prompt card improved outcome in symptoms and function when compared with usual treatment.[12] To maximize the patient's sense of control, the physician can ask for input as to what factors could be contributing to the patient's total body burden, and what factors could most easily and quickly be reduced. Another option is to suggest that the patient may gradually "grow" health by planting and nurturing the appropriate SEEDS of health (Sleep, Exercise, Environment, Diet, and Support).[11]

Restorative sleep is critical in helping to relieve symptoms; therefore, education about sleep hygiene (quiet, darkened room, relaxation exercises or tapes, same retiring and arising times) is important, with addition of low-dose antidepressants or hypnotics if necessary.[11] A meta-analysis of 16 randomized, placebo-controlled trials of tricyclic antidepressants (e.g. 25 to 50 mg amitriptylene every night), selective serotonin reuptake inhibitors (SSRIs) (e.g., fluoxetine 20 mg daily), and S-adenosylmethionine (200 to 800 mg daily) in fibromyalgia patients revealed improved sleep, fatigue, pain, and well-being, but not tender points.[13] A 1996 crossover study compared 25 mg amitriptylene daily, 20 mg fluoxetine daily, a combination of the two antidepressants, and placebo, each given over a 4- to 6-week period. All of the regimens that included antidepressants led to improvement compared with placebo, but the combination of amitriptyline and fluoxetine worked best.[14] NSAIDs and corticosteroids are ineffective.[15]

While exercising beyond tolerance exacerbates the illness, a Cochrane Review of 16 trials involving 724 participants with fibromyalgia revealed that supervised aerobic training improved physical capacity and reduced symptoms. Strength training may also have benefits on some FM symptoms.[16] Physical therapy modalities such as acupuncture, biofeedback, and transcutaneous electrical nerve stimulation (TENS), as well as trigger point injections, may be somewhat helpful, based on small observational studies.[17] Encouraging decreased exposure to environmental contaminants through cleaner air, food, and water, improving nutrition, and maximizing medical, family, social, spiritual, and self-support are all practical, empirically helpful therapeutic adjuncts.[11]

❧ REFERENCES ❧

1. Wolfe F, Smythe HA, Yunus MB, et al: The American College of Rheumatology 1990 criteria for the classification of fibromyalgia: report of the multicenter criteria committee, *Arthritis Rheum* 33:160-172, 1990.

2. Yunus MB: A comprehensive medical evaluation of patients with fibromyalgia syndrome, *Rheum Dis Clin North Am* 28(2):201-217, 2002.

3. Marshall L, Weir E, Abelsohn A, et al: Identifying and managing adverse environmental health effects: 1. Taking an exposure history, *Can Med Assoc J* 166(8):1049-1055, 16 Apr 2002.

4. Buchwald D, Garrity D: Comparison of patients with chronic fatigue syndrome, fibromyalgia, and multiple chemical sensitivities, *Arch Intern Med* 154:2049-2053, 1994.

5. Wolfe F, Ross K, Anderson J, et al: The prevalence and characteristics of fibromyalgia in the general population, *Arthritis Rheum* 38(1):19-28, 1995.

6. Ang Dennis, Wilke WS: Diagnosis, etiology, and therapy of fibromyalgia, *Comp Ther* 25 (4):221-227, 1999.

7. Wolfe F, Anderson J, Harkness D, et al: Health status and disease severity in fibromyalgia, *Arthritis Rheum* 40(9):1571-1579, Sept 1997.

8. Neeck G, Crofford LJ: Neuroendocrine perturbations in fibromyalgia and chronic fatigue syndrome, *Rheum Dis Clin North Am* 26(4):989-1002 2000.

9. Buskila D, Press J: Neuroendocrine mechanisms in fibromyalgia-chronic fatigue, *Best Pract Res Clin Rheumatol* 15(5):747-758, 2001.

10. Pall ML, Satterlee JD: Elevated nitric oxide/peroxynitrite mechanism for the common etiology of multiple chemical sensitivity, chronic fatigue syndrome, and posttraumatic stress disorder, *Ann NY Acad Sciences* 933:323-329, 2001.

11. Marshall LM, Bested A, Bray RI: Tools to treat chronic fatigue syndrome, fibromyalgia, and multiple chemical sensitivity, *Can J CME* 56-65, Jan 2004.

12. Alamo MM, Moral RR, Perula de Torres LA: Evaluation of a patient-centred approach in generalized musculoskeletal chronic pain/fibromyalgia patients in primary care, *Patient Ed Counselling* 48:23-31, 2002.

13. O'Malley PG, Balden E, Tomkins G, et al: Treatment of fibromyalgia with antidepressants, *J Gen Intern Med* 15:659-666, Sep 2000.

14. Goldenberg D, Mayskiy M, Mossey C, et al: A randomized, double-blind crossover trial of fluoxetine and amitriptyline in the treatment of fibromyalgia, *Arthritis Rheum* 39:1852-1859, 1996.

15. Goldenberg DL: Fibromyalgia syndrome a decade later: what have we learned? *Arch Intern Med* 159:777-785, 1999.

16. Busch A, Schacter CL, Peloso PM, et al: Exercise for treating fibromyalgia syndrome (Cochrane Review). In: *The Cochrane Library*, issue 4, Chichester, UK, 2002, John Wiley.

17. Offenbacher M, Stucki G: Physical therapy in the treatment of fibromyalgia, *Scand J Rheumatol* 29(suppl 113):78-85, 2000.

GOUT

With gout, the most frequently affected joints are the first metatarsophalangeal joints, ankles, midfoot joints, and knees. Put another way, gout usually involves the joints of the lower extremities, excluding the hips.[1-3] The wrists and fingers are also sometimes involved.[2] An initial attack usually comes on suddenly and involves only one joint.[1-3] Subsequent attacks may be polyarticular.[2] Males are affected more often than females, and gout is almost unheard of in premenopausal women.[2] Gout is definitively diagnosed by negative birefringent crystals on synovial fluid analysis, but 10% to 15% of cases will have negative fluid.[4] The most important diagnosis to exclude is septic arthritis, which often has systemic findings such as fever as well as predisposing factors.

An acute attack of gout may be precipitated by minor trauma, systemic illnesses, surgery, or anything causing a rapid rise in the uric acid level (either by increasing uric acid or decreasing excretion).[5] The risk of gout increases with increasing levels of serum urate, but gout can occur with normal serum urate. The risk is 5% per year for persons with a urate level of 535 μmol/L. Normal is 120 to 420 μmol/L.[1] There is no clinical indication for treating asymptomatic hyperuricemia, but it would seem advisable to identify, and if possible modify, known causes of this condition such as myeloproliferative disorders, low-dose salicylates, thiazides, loop diuretics, excessive alcohol consumption, high-purine diets, and obesity.[1,2] Common foods with high purine content are all meats (including organ meats), gravies, meat extracts, seafood, yeast, yeast extracts, beer, other alcoholic beverages, asparagus, beans, cauliflower, lentils, mushrooms, oatmeal, peas, and spinach.[1] Asymptomatic hyperuricemia does not need to be treated.

The drugs of choice for acute gout are NSAIDs. The agent used most frequently is indomethacin (Indocin, Indocid) in doses of 150 to 300 mg per day (usually 50 mg three times daily or four times daily) with gradual reduction of the dose as symptoms resolve.[1-3] Other NSAIDs such as naproxen, ketoprofen, and ibuprofen have also been used starting with maximum doses and tapering as symptoms resolve.[2,3] Some degree of pain relief usually occurs within 2 to 4 hours if the drug is started reasonably soon after the onset of symptoms. Alternatives to NSAIDs are oral prednisone starting at 30 to 50 mg per day (0.5 mg/kg) and tapering gradually over 7 to 10 days as long as septic arthritis is excluded. If only one joint is involved, intra-articular injection of steroid can be used.[4] Colchicine has been shown to be effective compared with placebo and is best used if it is started within 24 hours[4]; it is ineffective if started after 5 days. The initial dose is 0.5 to 1 mg, and this is followed by 0.5 or 0.6 mg every 1 to 2 hours until the patient has diarrhea or abdominal cramps or until a total of 6 to 8 mg has been administered.[1-3] Pain relief usually begins after an interval of 12 to 18 hours if the drug has been started reasonably soon after the onset of symptoms.[1,3] A few patients with recurrent episodes of gout are able to abort acute attacks if they recognize the initial symptoms and immediately take 1 to 1.2 mg of colchicine.[3]

Long-term prophylaxis with colchicine (0.6 mg orally twice daily) will prevent attacks in over 80% of patients and may be used as the sole preventive therapy in patients with recurrent attacks who have no tophi and only modest elevations of serum uric acid (less than 9.0 mg/dl). However, long-term oral colchicine can cause neuromyopathy, especially in those with renal insufficiency. If a patient with recurrent attacks is hyperuricemic or has tophi, urate-lowering drugs (allopurinol [Zyloprim] or probenecid) should also be used. Allopurinol and other drugs that lower serum uric acid may precipitate acute attacks of gout, a risk that may be decreased by starting with low doses (allopurinol 50 to 100 mg per day, increasing weekly up to 300 mg per day in most cases but up to 600 mg per day[5] or even 800 mg per day[3] in a few), by avoiding use of these drugs until several weeks since the last acute attack, and by giving prophylactic medications such as low-dose colchicine (0.5 to 1 mg per day) before and concurrently with the allopurinol. Adverse effects of allopurinol are seen in 20% of patients, and half of these require discontinuation of the medication. The most common side effects are skin rash, GI distress, diarrhea, and headache. Lifelong treatment is often needed, and the goal is to maintain the uric acid level below 6 mg/dl (360 μmol/L) unless there are tophi, in which case the target is less than 5 mg/dl (300 μmol/L).[1,6]

Most cases of gout will resolve in 7 days, but reoccurrence is common, increasing in frequency with increasing serum uric acid levels.[4] If frequent attacks occur, or gout is untreated, chronic tophaceous gout can result, with deposition of tophi in the skin and destruction of affected joints.[2]

Pyrophosphate Arthropathy/Pseudogout

Pyrophosphate arthropathy (chondrocalcinosis, calcium pyrophosphate deposition disease [CPPD]) is also called *pseudogout* if the onset of the illness is acute and mimics gout. It is caused by the intra-articular precipitation of pyrophosphate dihydrate crystals. CPPD is usually a disease of the elderly, and the most commonly affected joint is the knee. Other joints that are commonly inflamed are the wrist, elbow, shoulder, ankle, and metacarpophalangeal joints. The disease may have an acute onset (pseudogout), affecting one or two joints. The onset of the acute disease is not quite as dramatic as that of gout but requires 2 hours to 3 days for the pain to reach maximum intensity.[7] As with gout, acute episodes of CPPD may be precipitated by minor trauma, surgery, or systemic illness.[5] A more common presentation of CPPD is that of chronic arthritis involving several joints and thus mimicking osteoarthritis.[5]

Acute CPPD can usually be controlled by NSAIDs. Other therapeutic modalities are IV colchicine (1 to 2 mg as a single dose IV on day 1 and 0.5 mg every 6 hours IV on day 2 and sometimes day 3), oral colchicine (which is not as reliably effective as the IV route), aspiration of the joint without steroid instillation (to remove the crystals), and aspiration of the joint with steroid injection. For recurrent attacks, prophylactic colchicine 0.6 mg twice daily is effective.[7]

≈ REFERENCES ≈

1. Emmerson BT: The management of gout, *N Engl J Med* 334:445-451, 1996.
2. Harris MD, Siegel LB, Alloway FA: Gout and hyperuricemia, *Am Fam Physician* 59:925-934, 1999.
3. Schumacher HR Jr: Crystal-induced arthritis: an overview, *Am J Med* 100(suppl 2A):46S-52S, 1996.
4. Ahern MJ, Reid C, Gordon TP, et al: Does colchicine work? The results of the first controlled study in acute gout, *Aust N Z J Med* 17:301-304. Reviewed in: *Clin Evidence* 10:1238-1246, 2003.
5. Joseph J, McGrath H: Gout or "pseudogout": how to differentiate crystal-induced arthropathies, *Geriatrics* 50:33-39, 1995.
6. Mahowald ML, American College of Rheumatology Guideline: Overview of the evaluation and management of gout and hyperuricemia, *Rheumatol Musculoskeletal Med Primary Care* 1:4, [Accessed June 26, 2005] Available from: URL: http://www.rheumatology.org/publications/primary care/number4/hrh0021498.asp?aud=mem
7. Handy JR: Pyrophosphate arthropathy in the knees of elderly persons, *Arch Intern Med* 156:2426-2432, 1996.

LEG CRAMPS

Leg cramps are defined as painful involuntary muscle contractions that occur at rest and resolve spontaneously. Patients over age 50 and women (sex ratio 3:2) are affected more often than anyone else.[1] Leg cramps are a common and usually benign condition, but they can be associated with metabolic (i.e., hyponatremia, hypocalcemia, hypomagnesemia, diabetes, thyroid or renal disease), neurological, and peripheral vascular diseases. Certain drugs such as calcium channel blockers, diuretics, and selective estrogen receptor modulators can precipitate leg cramps.[1] The cause of most leg cramps is idiopathic, and further tests are only necessary if the history and physical examinations indicate an underlying cause.

Until recently, only quinine has shown efficacy in treating nocturnal leg cramps, but the benefits must be weighed against the risks. Quinine ingestion has been associated with rash, ear damage, thromboctopenia, hepatitis, and visual problems including blindness and fatal hypersensitivity.[1,2] Because of these risks, in 1995 the American Food and Drug Administration banned the use of over-the-counter quinine-based products for muscle cramps. While some studies have concluded that quinine is no more effective than placebo for controlling nocturnal leg cramps, others have shown some benefit.[1] One small, non-blinded evaluation from England found quinine to be more effective than going to bed with three corks tied in a sock (an interesting control group).[3] In a meta-analysis of eight randomized, double-blind, placebo-controlled trials (four published and four unpublished), Man-Son-Hing et al[4] found that quinine sulfate (range 200 mg to 325 mg per day) was effective for reducing the number of nocturnal leg cramps by 21% compared with placebo. Given the adverse effect rate, (e.g., tinnitus) the authors recommended that non-pharmacological therapy (see below) be tried before a trial of quinine.[4] The effect of the quinine was cumulative, so a 4-week trial should be given before deciding whether the drug is beneficial.

In one study of 102 patients, hydroquinine 300 mg (a derivative of quinine) was found to reduce leg cramps by more than 50% in 65% of the study participants versus 19% in the placebo group.[5] Vitamin B complex has also been shown to be effective in a small placebo-controlled trial.[6] In a randomized, double-blind, placebo-controlled trial in 60 hemodialysis patients, muscle cramps were reduced with vitamin E (400 IU) by 54%, vitamin C (500 mg) by 61%, and the combination of the two by 97% over placebo with 7%.[7] A 2002 Cochrane Review of prevention and treatment of leg cramps in pregnancy showed no evidence for the use of calcium or multivitamins and some benefit for magnesium lactate or citrate 5 mmol/L in the morning and 10 mmol/L in the evening.[8] Magnesium was not shown to be statistically beneficial in two randomized, crossover, placebo-controlled trials in non-pregnant patients.[2,9]

Several non-pharmacological treatments of leg cramps have been recommended. Daniell[10] reported successful prevention of cramps in 44 patients who performed stretching exercises three times a day. While barefoot, patients stood 2 to 3 feet from a wall, placed their hands on the wall keeping their heels on the ground, and leaned forward for 10 seconds to the point that they felt the stretch in their calf muscles. The manoeuvre was repeated once after a 5-second rest. Another recommendation is to place a pillow at the bottom of the bed to keep the feet dorsiflexed; if cramps still occur, patients should passively dorsiflex the ankle and massage the calf.[1]

≈ REFERENCES ≈

1. Kanaan N, Sawaya R: Nocturnal leg cramps. Clinically mysterious and painful—but manageable, *Geriatrics* 56(6):34, 39-42, 2001.
2. Frusso R, Zarate M, Augustovski F, et al: Magnesium for the treatment of nocturnal leg cramps: a crossover randomized trial, *J Fam Pract* 48(11):868-71, 1999.
3. Maule B: Nocturnal cramp: quinine versus folklore, *Practitioner* 234:420-421, 1990.
4. Man-Son-Hing M, Wells G, Lau A: Quinine for nocturnal leg cramps: a meta-analysis including unpublished data, *J Gen Intern Med* 13(9):600-606, 1998.
5. Jansen PH, Veenhuizen KC, Wesseling AI, et al: Randomised controlled trial of hydroquinine in muscle cramps, *Lancet* 349(9051):528-532, 1997.

6. Chan P, Huang TY, Chen YJ, et al: Randomized, double-blind, placebo-controlled study of the safety and efficacy of vitamin B complex in the treatment of nocturnal leg cramps in elderly patients with hypertension, *J Clin Pharmacol* 38(12):1151-1154, 1998.

7. Khajehdehi P, Mojerlou M, Behzadi S, et al: A randomized, double-blind, placebo-controlled trial of supplementary vitamins E, C and their combination for treatment of haemodialysis cramps, *Nephrol Dialysis Transplant* 16(7):1448-1451, 2001.

8. Young GL, Jewell D: Interventions for leg cramps in pregnancy. *Cochrane Database of Systematic Reviews* (1):CD000121, 2002.

9. Roffe C, Sills S, Crome P, et al: Randomised, cross-over, placebo controlled trial of magnesium citrate in the treatment of chronic persistent leg cramps, *Med Science Monitor* 8(5):CR326-30, 2002.

10. Daniell HW: Simple cure for nocturnal leg cramps (letter), *N Engl J Med* 301:216, 1979.

MUSCLE RELAXANTS

Recent reviews have found that muscle relaxants are beneficial versus placebo for acute low back pain, but further trials need to be done to compare them with NSAIDS. The side effects of dependency, drowsiness, and dizziness need to be taken into consideration when prescribing these drugs.[1,2] Some of the drugs available in this class are listed in Table 71.

◢ REFERENCES ◣

1. van Tulder MW, Touray T, Furlan AD, et al: Muscle relaxants for non-specific low-back pain. (Cochrane Review) In: *The Cochrane Library*, issue 2, Chichester, UK, 2004, John Wiley.

2. van Tulder MW, Koes B: Low back pain and sciatica (acute), *Clin Evidence* 10:1343-1358, 2003.

OSTEOARTHRITIS

(See also non-steroidal anti-inflammatory drugs; non-steroidal anti-inflammatory drug gastropathy; prescribing habits and the elderly)

Epidemiology

Osteoarthritis (OA) is the most common chronic disabling condition, increasing with age and affecting females more frequently than males.[1] Generally, OA is thought to affect more than 10% to 12% of the population. Prevalence is relatively low below the age of 50, but rises precipitously with advancing age. Almost all persons over 65 years old show signs of OA based on radiographic criteria, but only 33% of the same group will have symptomatic OA. Given the population distribution, it has its highest population impact among people of working age. Risk factors for OA include obesity and previous joint injury. Sporting activities may be associated with the development of hip OA, but the evidence for this is weak.[2,3] An occupational history of heavy lifting has also been reported to be associated with an increased risk of OA of the hip, and agricultural work appears to confer risk for OA.[4,5]

Clinical Presentation

Joints frequently and rarely involved by OA are listed in Table 72.

Prognosis

Mild OA in elderly patients rarely progresses to severe joint damage; severity of symptoms correlates more with depression and isolation than with degree of joint damage.[6] Osteoarthritis of the hands usually does not impair function except when the thumb joints are involved.[1]

Management

Management of OA centres on pain control and improving function. Simple measures for those with hip pain include splitting or evenly distributing heavy loads. Physical activity is important because the health of cartilage depends on normal loads being applied to joints.[1] A 2003 systematic review concluded that land-based therapeutic exercise reduced pain and improved function for people with knee OA.[8] Individual and group-based

Table 71 Muscle Relaxants

Drugs	Usual doses
Chlorzoxazone (Paraflex, Parafon Forte DSC)	250-500 mg tid-qid
Chlorzoxazone + acetaminophen (Parafon Forte)	1-2 tablets tid-qid
Chlorzoxazone + acetaminophen + codeine (Parafon Forte C8)	1-2 tablets tid-qid
Cyclobenzaprine HCl (Flexeril)	10 mg tid po
Methocarbamol (Robaxin)	1-2 g tid-qid
Methocarbamol + acetaminophen (Robaxacet)	1-2 tablets tid-qid
Methocarbamol + acetaminophen + codeine (Robaxacet-8)	1-2 tablets tid-qid
Orphenadrine citrate (Norflex)	100 mg bid
Orphenadrine HCl (Disipal)	0 mg tid

Table 72   Joint Involvement in Osteoarthritis

Frequently Involved	Rarely Involved
Upper Extremity	
Distal interphalangeal joints of fingers (Heberden's nodes)	Metacarpophalangeal joints of fingers
Proximal interphalangeal joints of fingers (Bouchard's nodes)	Wrists
First carpometacarpal joints	Elbows
Acromioclavicular joints	Glenohumeral joints
Lower Extremity	
Hips	
Knees	
First metatarsophalangeal joints	Ankles (unless previous trauma)
Spine	
Cervical spine	Thoracic spine
Lumbar spine	

exercise had similar effects. Psychosocial issues augmenting the perception of pain should be identified and treated.[6] Health education for self-management, given through programs like the Arthritis Self-Management Program, appears to be effective in improving arthritis symptoms and function.[9]

One set of evidence-based prescribing guidelines recommends starting with acetaminophen 4 g/day and, if that does not adequately control pain, substituting ibuprofen (Advil, Motrin) 1.2 g/day. If pain relief is still inadequate, acetaminophen 4 g/day may be added to the ibuprofen, or the dose of ibuprofen may be doubled to 2.4 g/day. If pain still persists, other NSAIDs may be tried.[10] Compared with acetaminophen, NSAIDs appear to provide superior pain relief, but not better functional improvement, for moderate and severe OA.[11]

Combining analgesia with codeine can enhance short-term analgesia but with adverse effects. Intra-articular corticosteroid injections provide short-term relief of pain[12] and can be safely given in primary care. Hyaluronic acid and its hylan derivatives have been available for treatment of joint injection in Europe for many years, in Canada since 1992, and in the United States since 1997. Intra-articular hyaluronic acid injections (Synvisc and Hyalgan) have mixed effectiveness data,[13] the size of the therapeutic effect is small,[14] and this modality is expensive. Topical capsaicin applied 3 to 4 times daily may have modest benefit in a few patients, but trials are few and not well done, and many patients cannot tolerate the burning sensation.

Glucosamine and chondroitin have been shown in a few short-term controlled trials to relieve pain and increase range of motion in patients with OA.[15] Meta-analysis confirms this, but analysis of the trials shows publication bias (only positive trials being published).[16] In doses of 500 mg orally three times daily, it is about equivalent to 400 mg of ibuprofen three times daily. However, it can take a month to work. The product is available over the counter, but in North America, purity and concentrations are not regulated.[17]

Joint replacement is highly effective and cost-effective for relief of pain and improving function for patients with advanced OA. Referral for surgery is indicated after a reasonable trial of conservative management. Women and people with low socio-economic status have higher prevalence of severe OA, but receive proportionately fewer hip and knee replacements. More attention to informational needs and referral is needed for these groups.[18,19]

❧ REFERENCES ❧

1. Sack KE: Osteoarthritis: a continuing challenge. *West J Med* 163:579-586, 1995.
2. Cooper C, Inskip H, Croft P, et al: Individual risk factors for hip osteoarthritis: obesity, hip injury, and physical activity. *Am J Epidemiol* 147:516-522, 1998.
3. Lievense AM, Bierma-Zeinstra SM, Verhagen AP, et al: Influence of sporting activities on the development of osteoarthritis of the hip: a systematic review, *Arthritis Rheum* 49:228-236, 2003.
4. Coggon D, Kellingray S, Inskip H, et al: Osteoarthritis of the hip and occupational lifting, *Am J Epidemiol* 147:523-528, 1998.
5. Kirkhorn S, Greenlee RT, Reeser JC: The epidemiology of agriculture-related osteoarthritis and its impact on occupational disability, *West Med J* 102:38-44, 2003.
6. Dieppe P: Osteoarthritis: time to shift the paradigm (editorial), *Brit Med J* 318:1299-1300, 1999.
7. Reference deleted in pages.
8. Fransen M, McConnell S, Bell M: Exercise for osteoarthritis of the hip or knee (Cochrane Collaboration). In: *The Cochrane Library,* Issue 4, Chichester, UK, 2003, John Wiley.
9. Lorig K, Mazonson P, Holman H: Evidence suggesting that health education for self-management in patients with chronic arthritis has sustained health benefits while reducing health care costs, *Arthritis Rheum* 36:439-446, 1993.
10. Eccles M, Freemantle N, Mason J (North of England Non-Steroidal Anti-Inflammatory Drug Guideline

Development Group): North of England evidence based guideline development project: summary guideline for non-steroidal anti-inflammatory drugs versus basic analgesia in treating the pain of degenerative arthritis, *Brit Med J* 317:526-530, 1998.

11. Towheed TE, Judd MJ, Hochberg MC, et al: Acetaminophen for osteoarthritis (Cochrane Review). In: *The Cochrane Library,* issue 1, Chichester, UK, 2004, John Wiley.

12. Godwin M, Dawes M: Intra-articular steroid injections for painful knees. Systematic review with meta-analysis, *Can Fam Physician* 50:241-248, 2004.

13. Felson DT, Anderson JJ: Hyaluronate sodium injections for osteoarthritis: hope, hype, and hard truths, *Arch Intern Med* 162:245-247, 2002.

14. Lo GH, LaValley M, McAlindon T, et al: Intra-articular hyaluronic acid in treatment of knee osteoarthritis, *JAMA* 290:3115-3121, 2003.

15. Towheed TE, Anastassiades TP, Shea B, et al: Glucosamine therapy for treating osteoarthritis (Cochrane Review). In: *The Cochrane Library,* issue 1, Chichester, UK, 2004, John Wiley.

16. McAlindon TE, LaValley MP, Gulin JP, et al: Glucosamine and chondroitin for treatment of osteoarthritis. A systematic quality assessment and meta-analysis, *JAMA* 283:1469-1475, 2000.

17. Glucosamine for osteoarthritis, *Med Lett* 39:91-92, 1997.

18. Hawker GA, Wright JG, Coyte PC, et al: Differences between men and women in the rate of use of hip and knee arthroplasty, *N Engl J Med* 342:1016-1022, 2000.

19. Hawker GA, Wright JG, Glazier RH, et al: The effect of education and income on need and willingness to undergo total joint arthroplasty, *Arthritis Rheum* 46:3331-3339, 2002.

PAGET'S DISEASE

Paget's disease is a localized metabolic bone condition. It is caused by excessive breakdown of bone followed by formation of abnormal, weak bone. The disease will progress within a given bone but may rarely present in a new site after diagnosis. Sites of predilection are the axial skeleton, long bones, and skull. The vast majority of lesions are asymptomatic. Although the individual lesions of Paget's disease may cause pain and deformity, many of the symptoms result from complications of the disease. These include enlargement of the skull, hearing loss, bowing of long bones, pain from secondary osteoarthritis or fractures, osteosarcoma (in less than 1% of cases), and neurological deficits from entrapment of nerves or compression of the spinal cord. Paget's disease is common in Europe and North America. The cause is unknown. Its prevalence increases with age and is very rare in persons under the age of 40. The serum alkaline phosphatase level is usually but not always elevated. X-ray films tend to show patchy lytic and sclerotic changes and bone enlargement. Bone scans are the investigative procedure of choice.[1]

Treatment is indicated for patients with symptoms or for asymptomatic patients at risk of complications such as hearing loss (lesions at base of skull), spinal cord compression (lesions in vertebrae), and osteoarthritis or fractures (lesions in long bones).[1] NSAIDs are used to treat the pain, whereas bisphosphonates and calcitonin work by decreasing osteoclastic activity. In many cases the drug of choice is alendronate (Fosamax) in oral doses of 40 mg per day. Alternatives are etidronate (Didrocal), calcitonin (Calcimar, Miacalcin),[1] pamidronate (Aredia), risedronate (Actonel), and tiludronate.[2]

➣ REFERENCES ➣

1. Delmas PD, Meunier PJ: The management of Paget's disease of bone, *N Engl J Med* 336:558-566, 1997.

2. Risedronate for Paget's disease of bone, *Med Lett* 40:87-88, 1998.

PALINDROMIC RHEUMATISM

Palindromic rheumatism consists of recurrent attacks of arthritis (swelling, pain, and erythema) that usually involve one or only a few joints. Patients can be quite incapacitated during the attacks, but once an attack resolves, they are asymptomatic, with no evidence of residual joint damage. The natural course of palindromic rheumatism is variable. Some patients have lasting remissions, while others have recurrent attacks. By 6 years, a little over one fourth of patients will have rheumatoid arthritis and 5% will have developed lupus or other connective tissue diseases. Those at greatest risk of progression to connective tissue diseases are women with a positive rheumatoid factor and involvement of hand joints.[1] Antimalarials were shown to decrease the risk of progression to further diseases by more than one half in one retrospective analysis.[2]

➣ REFERENCES ➣

1. Gonzalez-Lopez L, Gamez-Nava JI, Jhangri GS, et al: Prognostic factors for the development of rheumatoid arthritis and other connective tissue diseases in patients with palindromic rheumatism, *J Rheumatol* 26:540-545, 1999.

2. Gonzalez-Lopez L, Gamez-Nava JI, Jhangri G, et al: Decreased progression to rheumatoid arthritis or other connective tissue diseases in patients with palindromic rheumatism treated with antimalarials, *J Rheumatol* 27(1):41-46, Jan 2000.

POLYMYALGIA RHEUMATICA

(See also giant cell arteritis; erythrocyte sedimentation rate)

The onset of polymyalgia rheumatica can be indolent or sudden. In most cases, aching and stiffness of proximal limb muscles, especially the shoulder girdle, are prominent symptoms. Morning stiffness and gelling after activities, as well as malaise, fever, and fatigue, are also common. The patient may have pain, especially at night, that makes getting out of bed or into and out of the bathtub difficult. Transient synovitis of joints may occur. Elevated sedimentation rates and a mild normocytic anemia are common findings; slight elevation of liver function tests may also occur.[1] It is important to realize that in one fifth of patients, the sedimentation rate is normal (30 mm per hour or less).[2]

If biopsy specimens of temporal artery are obtained from patients with polymyalgia rheumatica, many of them will be found to have histological evidence of temporal arteritis. However, this finding is a poor predictor for the development of clinical temporal arteritis. Furthermore, temporal arteritis develops later in a number of patients with negative biopsies. Fortunately, severe sequelae, such as vision loss, are rarely if ever the initial manifestation of temporal arteritis. Therefore temporal artery biopsies should be reserved for patients with suggestive symptoms or signs such as jaw claudication, headaches, visual changes, or tender temporal arteries.[3]

The differential diagnosis of polymyalgia rheumatica includes FM, paraneoplastic syndromes, endocarditis, hypothyroid myopathy, polymyositis, SLE, monoclonal gammopathies, and rheumatoid arthritis, particularly if it is seronegative. Investigations that may clarify the diagnosis are urinalysis (looking for hematuria), creatine kinase, rheumatoid factor, ANA, thyroid-stimulating hormone, and serum and urine electrophoresis.[1]

An important diagnostic test for polymyalgia rheumatica is a response within 24 to 48 hours to low-dose steroids such as prednisone 10 mg per day. A few other conditions, most commonly seronegative rheumatoid arthritis, respond in the same way.[3]

The usual treatment of polymyalgia rheumatica is corticosteroids.[1,3] The initial dose, which is titrated to a level that gives complete symptom relief and ESR normalization, is usually prednisone 10 to 20 mg per day.[4] This is decreased every 2 to 4 weeks by 2.5 mg until a daily dose of 10 mg is achieved, and thereafter tapering continues by 1-mg decrements every 2 to 4 weeks until a maintenance dose of 5 to 7.5 mg is achieved. Total duration of treatment varies from 2 to 15 years. Between one fourth and one half of patients have a relapse after discontinuation of treatment.[3] Relapse should be treated with a return to the initial dosage.[4] Mild symptoms may be successfully managed with NSAIDs.[1] Adverse effects from both NSAIDs and corticosteroids are common and are dose related. Minimal doses should be used.[5]

Patients with polymyalgia rheumatica who have sedimentation rates lower than 40 mm per hour tend to have a milder clinical course. Fever, anemia, and weight loss are less common than in patients with higher sedimentation rates.[6]

──────────── ⚹ **REFERENCES** ⚹ ────────────

1. Hunder GG: Giant cell arteritis and polymyalgia rheumatica, *Med Clin North Am* 81:195-219, 1997.

2. Helfgott SM, Kieval RI: Polymyalgia rheumatica in patients with a normal erythrocyte sedimentation rate, *Arthritis Rheum* 39:304-307, 1996.
3. Brooks RC, McGee SR: Diagnostic dilemmas in polymyalgia rheumatica, *Arch Intern Med* 157:162-168, 1997.
4. Meskimen S, Cook T, Blake R: Management of giant cell arteritis and polymyalgia rheumatica, *Am Fam Physician* 61:2061-2068, 2073, 2000.
5. Gabriel SE, Sunku J, Salvarani C, et al: Adverse outcomes of anti-inflammatory therapy among patients with polymyalgia rheumatica, *Arthritis Rheum* 40:1873-1878, 1997.
6. González-Gay MA, Rodriguez-Valverde V, Blanco R, et al: Polymyalgia rheumatica without significantly increased erythrocyte sedimentation rate–a more benign syndrome, *Arch Intern Med* 157:317-320, 1997.

REFLEX SYMPATHETIC DYSTROPHY

COMPLEX regional pain syndrome (CRPS) type I, formerly known as reflex sympathetic dystrophy (RSD), and CRPS type II, formerly known as causalgia, are debilitating pain syndromes that have been recognized for more than a century.[1] They are usually precipitated by trauma, but the severity of the trauma does not correlate with the incidence of reflex sympathetic dystrophy. Women are more commonly affected than men and white persons more than other races. Patients should have at least one symptom[2] in each of the following general categories: sensory (hyperesthesia = increased sensitivity to a sensory stimulation), vasomotor (temperature abnormalities or skin colour abnormalities), sudomotor–fluid balance (edema or sweating abnormalities), or motor (decreased range of movement, weakness, tremor, or neglect); and at least one sign within two or more of the following categories[3]: sensory (allodynia or hyperalgesia), vasomotor (objective temperature abnormalities or skin colour abnormalities), sudomotor–fluid balance (objective edema or sweating abnormalities), or motor (objective decreased range of motion, weakness, tremor, or neglect).[1] Symptoms occur more often in the lower than upper extremity. The cardinal symptom is pain, which is accompanied by tenderness of the affected limb. Some patients cannot tolerate light touch as occurs with bed clothing. In the early stages, patients may have edema; later, dystrophic changes are found with smooth, shiny skin and mottling and coolness of the extremity. Ultimately, the treatment goal is pain relief, functional recovery, and psychological improvement. No one therapeutic modality achieves this goal in all patients, and a scientifically proven cure for CRPS does not exist. The cornerstone of treatment is pain management and physiotherapy. Some patients require sympathetic blockade or even a sympathectomy. Drugs that may be useful aside from analgesics include COX-2 non-steroidal medications, low-dose amitriptyline (25 mg three times daily or 50 mg nightly); and either phenytoin (100 mg three times daily) or gabapentin (starting at 100 mg three times daily), or a calcium channel blocker (e.g., amlodipine 5 mg every day). Implantable neuromodulators *and* IV bisphosphonates are currently being evaluated.[1]

──────────────── **≥ REFERENCES ≤** ────────────────

1. Raja SN: Complex regional pain syndrome I (reflex sympathetic dystrophy), *Anesthesiology* 96(5):1254-1260, 1 May 2002.
2. Drake WT, Anderson K: Reflex sympathetic dystrophy: what are the signs? *Can J Diagn* 12:67-81, 1995.
3. Teasdall R: Complex regional pain syndrome (reflex sympathetic dystrophy), *Clin Sports Med* 23(1):145, Jan 2004.

RHEUMATOID ARTHRITIS

(See also non-steroidal anti-inflammatory drugs; non-steroidal anti-inflammatory drug gastropathy; palindromic rheumatism)

Three times more women than men have rheumatoid arthritis (RA), but among the elderly the ratio evens out.[1] Some studies have shown an association between smoking and RA.[2] According to the American Rheumatism Association, a diagnosis of rheumatoid arthritis can be made if the patient has four or more of the following findings[3]:

- Morning stiffness for 1 hour or more persisting for at least 6 weeks
- Soft tissue swelling (arthritis) in three or more locations for at least 6 weeks; the swelling has to be documented by a physician
- Swelling of the wrist, metacarpophalangeal joints, or proximal interphalangeal joints for at least 6 weeks
- Symmetrical joint involvement for at least 6 weeks
- Rheumatoid nodules
- Presence of rheumatoid factor
- X-ray examination findings consistent with rheumatoid arthritis (erosion or osteopenia of wrist or hand joints)

It is now believed that "disease-modifying" drugs should be started as early as possible when RA is diagnosed. (See later discussion.) To achieve this goal, primary care physicians must make the diagnosis without delay and, when indicated, arrange appropriate referral.[4]

Non-Steroidal Anti-Inflammatory Drugs

Until recently, NSAIDs were considered the first-line drugs for RA, with no one drug superior to another. The protocol for using NSAIDs involves starting with one and continuing it for 10 to 14 days before deciding whether it is effective. If the initial drug fails to control symptoms after a 10- to 14-day trial, another NSAID is chosen, and the process is continued until several different NSAIDs have been tried.[5] NSAIDs such as celecoxib (Celebrex), and Valdecoxib (Bextra), which selectively inhibit cyclooxygenase 2 (COX-2), are commonly used. Rofecoxib (Vioxx) has been removed from the market due to an increased risk of cardiac events.[6]

Disease-Modifying Drugs

Traditional "disease-modifying" drugs for RA include methotrexate (Rheumatrex), sulfasalazine (Azulfidine), hydroxychloroquine (Plaquenil), azathioprine (Imuran), cyclosporine (Sandimmune), gold salts (Myochrysine, Solganal), and penicillamine (Cuprimine, Depen). Newer biological drugs are the pyrimidine synthesis inhibitor leflunomide (Arava) and the tumour necrosis factor (TNF) inhibitors etanercept (Enbrel) and infliximab (Remicade), which have been shown to improve severity of rheumatoid arthritis to a significant extent, although there is some concern that TNF blockade may increase the risk of infection and cancer, particularly lymphoproliferative malignancies.[7,8] The rationale for using disease-modifying drugs is to alter the basic pathological processes responsible for the inflammation, and through this mechanism, to prevent deformities and disabilities. Evidence to date suggests that if treatment is started early, this goal can be achieved provided that patients continue to take their medications.[10,11] If medications are discontinued, relapses are frequent.[10]

No disease-modifying drug has been definitively shown to have more beneficial effects than another, but at present methotrexate and hydroxychloroquine are preferred for single-drug therapy by most North American rheumatologists,[12] while the most popular drug in Great Britain is sulfasalazine.[13] Growing evidence shows that combinations of disease-modifying drugs are more effective than single agents from this class.[10]

Several long-term studies of patients taking disease-modifying drugs have shown a high rate of discontinuation of the medications because of toxic side effects or perceived lack of beneficial effect.[14,15] Among all these drugs, methotrexate appears to have the lowest discontinuation rate.[15] In one 5-year study of methotrexate in RA, 36% of patients discontinued the medication, 7% because of adverse effects and 7% because of lack of efficacy. However, in the same study, more than two thirds of the patients showed a marked clinical improvement.[14] Mucosal and GI side effects of methotrexate can be reduced by regular folate supplementation.[16]

When methotrexate is used, it is usually given in small weekly doses in the range of 7.5 to 25 mg. Methotrexate may be given orally or parenterally. The parenteral route is preferred for doses over 20 mg weekly for patients who cannot tolerate oral medications because of GI side effects, and for patients who have not responded to orally administered methotrexate.[14] Most disease-modifying agents and all of the new biological drugs require routine monitoring for adverse effects.

Minocycline (Minocin) may be beneficial in the treatment of early seropositive RA. In one double-blind, placebo-controlled trial, patients who had received 100 mg of minocycline twice daily for 3 to 6 months had a much higher remission rate when assessed 4 years later than did those who were given placebos.[17]

Corticosteroids

Corticosteroids in combination with disease-modifying agents were shown in one study to decrease erosion rates,[18] and they also improve symptoms.[18,19] Whether these benefits outweigh potential adverse effects is uncertain.[10]

Multidisciplinary Team

Effective high-quality treatment of early RA is multifaceted and involves the GP, rheumatologist, physiotherapist, occupational therapist, nurse specialist, dietitian, podiatrist, pharmacist, and social worker.[15]

◣ REFERENCES ◢

1. Akil M, Amos RS: Rheumatoid arthritis. I. Clinical features and diagnosis, *BMJ* 310:587-590, 1995.
2. Karlson EW, Lee IM, Cook NR, et al: A retrospective cohort study of cigarette smoking and risk of rheumatoid arthritis in female health professionals, *Arthritis Rheum* 42:910-917, 1999.
3. Arnett FC, Edworthy SM, Bloch DA, et al: The American Rheumatism Association 1987 revised criteria for the classification of rheumatoid arthritis, *Arthritis Rheum* 31:315-324, 1988.
4. Weinblatt ME: Rheumatoid arthritis: treat now not later (editorial), *Ann Intern Med* 124:773-774, 1998.
5. Grondin C: L'arthrite rhumatoïde: approche thérapeutique, *Can Fam Physician* 36:487-490, 499, 1990.
6. Juni P, Nartey L, Reichenbach S, et al: Risk of cardiovascular events and rofecoxib: cumulative meta-analysis, *Lancet* 5 Nov 2004.
7. Blumenauer B, Judd M, Cranney A, et al: Infliximab for the treatment of rheumatoid arthritis (Cochrane Review). In: *The Cochrane Library*, issue 2, Chichester, UK, 2004, John Wiley.
8. Management of early rheumatoid arthritis: a national clinical guideline. Edinburgh (Scotland): Scottish Intercollegiate Guidelines Network (SIGN), 2000.
9. Reference deleted in pages.
10. Brooks P: Rheumatology, *BMJ* 316:1810-1812, 1998.
11. Strand V, Tugwell P, Bombardier C, et al: Function and health-related quality of life: results from a randomized controlled trial of leflunomide versus methotrexate or placebo in patients with active rheumatoid arthritis, *Arthritis Rheum* 42:1870-1878, 1999.
12. Drugs for rheumatoid arthritis, *Med Lett* 36:101-106, 1994.
13. Emery P: Therapeutic approaches for early rheumatoid arthritis. How early? How aggressive? *Br J Rheumatol* 34(suppl 2):87-90, 1995.
14. Weinblatt ME, Kaplan H, Germain BF, et al: Methotrexate in rheumatoid arthritis: a five-year prospective multicenter study, *Arthritis Rheum* 37:1492-1498, 1994.
15. Pincus T: Long-term outcomes in rheumatoid arthritis, *Br J Rheumatol* 34(suppl 2):59-73, 1995.
16. Oritz Z, Shea B, Suarez-Almazor ME, et al: The efficiency of folic acid and folinic acid in reducing methotrexate gastro-intestinal toxicity in rheumatoid arthritis: a meta-analysis of randomized controlled trials, *J Rheumatol* 24:36-43, 1998.
17. O'Dell JR, Paulsen G, Haire CE, et al: Treatment of early seropositive rheumatoid arthritis with minocycline: four-year folllowup of a double-blind, placebo-controlled trial, *Arthritis Rheum* 42:1691-1695, 1999.
18. Kirwan JR (Arthritis and Rheumatism Council Low-Dose Glucocorticoid Study Group): The effect of glucocorticoids on joint destruction in rheumatoid arthritis, *N Engl J Med* 333:142-146, 1995.
19. Boers M, Verhoeven AC, Markusse HM, et al: Randomised comparison of combined step-down prednisolone, methotrexate and sulphasalazine with sulphasalazine alone in early rheumatoid arthritis, *Lancet* 350:309-318, 1997.

SEPTIC ARTHRITIS

Septic arthritis (SA) has a prevalence of 2 to 10 cases per 100,000 in the general population and is somewhat higher in children.[1] The two major classes of SA are gonococcal and non-gonococcal. *Staphylococcus aureus* is the most common cause of SA in all age groups, while *Neisseria gonorrhoeae* is the most frequent pathogen (75%) among younger sexually active individuals. *Streptococcus viridans, Streptococcus pneumoniae,* and group B streptococci account for 20% of cases and aerobic gram-negative rods for another 20% to 25%.[2] Suspected or diagnosed SA requires immediate referral to the emergency department. The pathogenesis of SA is usually from hematogenous inoculation, but it also may develop by contiguous spread from an adjacent cellulitis or via a penetrating wound. Previously damaged joints, especially in RA, are the most susceptible to infection. Prosthetic joint infections may be a consequence of local infection, such as intraoperative contamination (60% to 80% of cases), or from a bacteremia (20% to 40% of cases).[3]

Early diagnosis is difficult. In adults, the most important historical feature is the existence of underlying joint disease, especially RA. The classic triad consists of fever (40% to 60% of cases), pain (75% of cases), and impaired range of motion. These symptoms may evolve over a few days to a few weeks. The most commonly involved joint is the knee (50% of cases), followed by the hip (20%), and shoulder (8%).[4] The most consistent sign is pain with passive motion. The patient generally will hold the joint in the position that maximizes intracapsular volume. For a hip, these positions are flexion, abduction, and external rotation, and for a knee, the position is a moderate flexion.[5]

The pattern of joint involvement is an important diagnostic feature. Eighty-five to ninety percent of non-gonococcal arthritis cases are monoarticular. If the disease affects more than one joint, then *S. aureus* most commonly is implicated. Polyarticular arthritis usually is observed in gonococcal disease, various viral infections, Lyme disease, reactive arthritis, and a variety of non-infectious processes.[6]

Distinguishing transient synovitis from septic arthritis is an area of particular concern in children. Four independent variables that have been found useful as clinical predictors for SA are as follows: history of fever, non–weight bearing, ESR higher than 40 mm per hour, and WBC count higher than 12,000/mL. The incidence of SA is 0.2% for no predictors, 3.0% for one, 40.0% for two, 93.1% for three, and 99.6% for all four.[7] In a series of 95 children with SA, one third were afebrile at presentation. Absence of fever should not sway the clinician from the diagnosis.[8]

Culture of the synovial fluid or of synovial tissue itself is the only definitive method of diagnosing infective arthritis. If microscopy demonstrates no crystals, treat the patient for presumed infection even if the Gram stain findings are negative. (Sensitivity of Gram stain is less than 60%.) If the patient does not improve significantly after a few days, the affected joint must be re-aspirated. Most septic joints have a white count greater than 50,000, with more than 75% polymorphonuclear leukocytes. However, a variety of sterile inflammatory processes may exhibit the same cellular profile.

Plain X-ray films are not sensitive to early findings. MRI is preferred because of its greater ability to image soft tissue. Radionuclide scintigraphy (i.e., technetium Tc 99m, gallium Ga 67, indium In 111 leukocyte scans) is extremely sensitive but extremely non-specific. Ultrasonography may be used to diagnose effusions in chronically distorted joints (secondary to trauma or rheumatoid arthritis) and guide the aspiration.[9,10]

Medical management of infective arthritis focuses on adequate and timely drainage of the infected synovial fluid, administration of appropriate parenteral antimicrobial therapy, and immobilization of the joint to control pain.[11] Fifty percent of patients with SA have significant morbidity and mortality after infection.[1,12] Predictors of poor outcome include age older than 60 years, infection of the hip or shoulder joints, underlying rheumatoid arthritis, positive findings on synovial fluid cultures after 7 days of appropriate therapy, and delay of 7 days or more in instituting therapy.[13]

─────────────── ❧ **REFERENCES** ❧ ───────────────

1. Pioro MH, Mandell BF: Septic arthritis, *Rheum Dis Clin North Am* 23(2):239-258, May 1997.
2. van der Heijden IM, Wilbrink B, Vije AE: Detection of bacterial DNA in serial synovial samples obtained during antibiotic treatment from patients with septic arthritis, *Arthritis Rheum* 42(10):2198-2203, 1999.
3. Kaandorp CJ, Dinant HJ, van de Laar MA, et al: Incidence and sources of native and prosthetic joint infection: a community based prospective survey, *Ann Rheum Dis* 56(8):470-475, 1997.
4. Pioro MH, Mandell BF: Septic arthritis, *Rheum Dis Clin North Am* 23(2):239-258, 1997.
5. Siva C, Velazquez C, Mody A, et al: Diagnosing acute monoarthritis in adults: a practical approach for the family physician, *Am Fam Physician* 68:83-90, 2003.
6. Smith JW, Piercy EA: Infectious arthritis, *Clin Infect Dis* 20(2):225-230, 1995.
7. Kocher MS, Zurakowski D, Kasser JR: Differentiating between septic arthritis and transient synovitis of the hip in children: an evidence-based clinical prediction algorithm, *J Bone Joint Surg Am* 81(12):1662-1670, 1999.
8. Simon RR, Koenigsknecht SJ: Transient synovitis. In: *Emergency orthopedics: the extremities,* 89-90, 404-406, New York, 2001, McGraw-Hill.
9. Greenspan A, Tehranzadeh J: Imaging of infectious arthritis, *Radiol Clin North Am* 39(2):267-276, 2001.
10. Lee SK, Suh KJ, Kim YW, et al: Septic arthritis versus transient synovitis at MR imaging: preliminary assessment with signal intensity alterations in bone marrow, *Radiology* 211(2):459-465, 1999.
11. Broy SB, Schmid FR: A comparison of medical drainage (needle aspiration) and surgical drainage (arthrotomy or arthroscopy) in the initial treatment of infected joints, *Clin Rheum Dis* 12(2):501-522, 1986.
12. Kaandorp CJ, Krijnen P, Moens HJ, et al: The outcome of bacterial arthritis: a prospective community-based study, *Arthritis Rheum* 40(5):884-892, 1997.
13. McGuire NM, Kauffman CA: Septic arthritis in the elderly, *J Am Geriatr Soc* 33(3):170-174, 1985.

SERONEGATIVE SPONDYLOARTHROPATHIES
(See also sexually transmitted diseases)

The seronegative spondyloarthropathies are a group of inflammatory arthritides that are rheumatoid factor and ANA negative and that have a much greater frequency in HLA-B27-positive persons. Conditions included in this category are ankylosing spondylitis, psoriatic arthritis, Reiter's syndrome, and arthritis associated with inflammatory bowel disease.[1] Undifferentiated spondyloarthropathy and juvenile spondyloarthropathy are newer additions to the classification. Frequent clinical findings in patients with seronegative spondyloarthropathies are involvement of the back and the sacroiliac joints, involvement of only a few peripheral joints, most often in an asymmetrical pattern in the lower extremities, and inflammatory reactions involving the sites of attachments of ligaments and tendons to bones (enthesopathy) such as plantar fasciitis and Achilles tendonitis. Extra-articular manifestations are common with the seronegative spondyloarthropathies. Iritis or other inflammatory eye conditions may be seen in all of them, skin lesions in psoriatic arthritis and Reiter's syndrome, and urethritis in Reiter's syndrome even when precipitated by a dysenteric syndrome.[1]

Ankylosing Spondylitis
Archaic synonyms for ankylosing spondylitis (AS) are rheumatoid spondylitis and Marie-Strumpell disease. Males are affected three times more often than females.

Approximately 5% of patients who visit their primary care physician for low back pain have AS.[2] The following findings suggest this diagnosis[3,4]:

- Insidious onset
- Onset before age 40
- Pain for more than 3 months
- Morning stiffness longer than 30 minutes
- Pain relief with activity
- Pain forcing the patient from bed
- History of psoriasis, Reiter's disease, uveitis, or colitis
- Chest expansion of less than 2 inches
- Peripheral joint disease

The classic physical findings of ankylosing spondylitis are a positive Schober's test, a positive occiput-to-wall test, and decreased chest expansion (less than 5 to 6 cm or 2 inches). Schober's test is performed as follows. With the patient standing vertically, the end of a measuring tape is placed over the spinous processes at the level of the posterior superior iliac spines and stretched proximally along the spine. A mark is placed on the skin at the 10-cm level. With the end of the tape kept in place, the patient is asked to flex as fully forward as possible. The distance to the skin mark is measured. Normally it is about 15 cm because of flexion of the lumbar spine. In patients with ankylosing spondylitis it is less because most or all flexion takes place at the hips.

In the occiput-to-wall test the patient stands with heels against the wall and tries to press the occiput against the wall. Many patients with ankylosing spondylitis cannot do this because of fixed flexion deformity of the spine.

Unfortunately, the defining signs are not usually present in the early stages of the disease. Testing for HLA-B27 is not usually helpful. If the clinical picture is convincing, this study is unnecessary (10% of patients with the disease are HLA-B27 negative), and if the diagnosis is unlikely on a clinical basis, the presence of a positive HLA-B27 adds little useful information.[1] An X-ray is often useful to show bilateral sacroiliitis, and lumbar films may reveal changes characteristic of AS. However, its use in patients under the age of 21 may not be reliable until the skeletal system matures. A fat-suppressed MRI helps detect early changes in the sacroiliac joint when X-rays are still negative and the diagnosis is in question.[2]

First-line treatment includes NSAIDs and physiotherapy. The anti-TNFs etanercept and infliximab have been shown in randomized controlled trials to be helpful in AS and are recommended after two NSAIDs have failed.[2]

Physicians should continue to look for ocular and cardiac complications such as uveitis and aortic regurgitation. They also need to be aware of the increased risk of cervical fractures, osteoporosis, and respiratory diffi-culty in these individuals.[5] The prognosis is variable, but those without treatment and continued physiotherapy are more likely to develop immobility and respiratory complications.

Reiter's Syndrome

Reiter's syndrome may be initiated by either urethritis, usually chlamydial in origin, or a dysentery-like syndrome caused by a variety of organisms, including *Shigella, Salmonella, Campylobacter,* and *Yersinia.* The post-venereal form of Reiter's syndrome affects about five to nine times as many men as women, whereas the post-dysentery form affects the sexes equally. The classic triad is urethritis, conjunctivitis, and arthritis, usually appearing in that order, but only one third of patients have all three entities. Symptoms of urethritis usually develop 2 to 4 weeks after either sexual exposure or a diarrheal illness. Ocular symptoms are reported in about half the cases and are usually the result of a short-lived mild conjunctivitis; some patients have iritis, uveitis, or keratitis. Patients presenting with symptoms suggestive of uveitis, such as severe eye pain, blurred vision, conjunctivitis, or photophobia should be referred to an ophthalmologist. Arthritis develops last. The most frequently affected joints are the knees, ankles, and toes ("sausage" digits). Asymmetrical oligoarthritis is the rule. In half the patients the spine or sacroiliac joints are involved. Enthesopathy, circinate balanitis of the penis, and keratoderma blennorrhagicum of the palms and soles are common. Investigations to consider include vaginal or penile culture, stool cultures, and/or X-rays of infected joints.

Standard treatment is NSAIDs for symptom relief and antibiotics if active chlamydial infection is still present. (See discussion of sexually transmitted diseases.)[1,6,7] Low-dose prednisone is usually not helpful. Disease-modifying antirheumatic drugs (DMARDs) can be considered in patients with refractory arthritis. Antibiotics are not beneficial for Reiter's syndrome that results from enteric infections.[7] About half of the patients have a prolonged course or recurrences over months or years, but only a few have functional disability.[1,6]

Psoriatic Arthritis

Psoriatic arthritis occurs in over 10% of people with psoriasis.[5] In 85% of patients with psoriatic arthritis, skin lesions develop before the arthritis. In some patients, skin stigmata of psoriasis may not be obvious at first glance; patients may have pitting of nails, onycholysis, scalp lesions, and/or lesions between the buttocks or in the umbilicus. The arthritis is usually asymmetrical and involves only a few joints. Dactylitis of a toe or finger is characteristic of psoriatic arthritis or Reiter's syndrome.[1]

Treatment options include methotrexate, cyclosporine, sulfasalazine, and the new anti-TNFs such as entanercept and infliximab.[8]

Enteropathic Arthropathies

Thirty-nine percent of patients with inflammatory bowel disease have enteropathic arthropathy, and a further 18% have asymptomatic sacroiliitis.[5] Larger joints of the lower extremities are usually involved, and the activity of the arthritis tends to parallel that of the bowel disease.[1] The anti-TNFs entanercept and infliximab have also been used in this case with the added benefit of often helping the bowel disease.

❧ REFERENCES ❧

1. Osial TA Jr, Cash JM, Eisenbeis CH Jr: Arthritis-associated syndromes, *Primary Care* 20:857-882, 1993.
2. Maksymowych WP: Ankylosing spondylitis. Not just another pain in the back, *Can Fam Physician* 50:257-262, Feb 2004.
3. Calin A, Porta J, Fries JF, et al: Clinical history as a screening test for ankylosing spondylitis, *JAMA* 237:2613-2614, 1977.
4. Calin A, Kaye B, Sternberg M, et al: The prevalence and nature of back pain in an industrial complex: a questionnaire and radiographic and HLA analysis, *Spine* 5:201-205, 1980.
5. Khan MA: Update on spondyloarthropathies, *Ann Intern Med* 136(12):896-907, 2002 Jun 18.
6. Kirchner JT: Reiter's syndrome: a possibility in patients with reactive arthritis, *Postgrad Med* 97:111-112, 115-117, 121-122, 1995.
7. Barth WF, Segal K: Reactive arthritis (Reiter's syndrome), *Am Fam Physician* 60:499-503, 1999.
8. Gottlieb AB: Psoriatic arthritis: a guide for dermatology nurses, *Dermatol Nurs* 15(2):107-10, 113-8; quiz 119, Apr 2003.

SPORTS MEDICINE, EXERCISE, AND INJURIES

(See also anticoagulants; dentistry)

Topics covered in this section

APPROACH TO SOFT TISSUE INJURIES

Soft tissue describes the muscle, tendon, ligament, bursa, or capsule of a joint, but most commonly, soft tissue injuries involve the muscle or tendon. Soft tissue injuries arise from an acute injury, an overuse injury, or an acute on chronic musculoskeletal (MSK) condition and occur when the demand outstrips the supply. *Strain* is a term used to describe micro to gross tears to a muscle or tendon, while a *sprain* is used to describe the same damage to a ligament or a joint. *Enthesopathy* describes an inflammatory condition in which the tendon inserts into the bone. Strains and sprains are graded first, second, and third degree based on physical examination. With each degree is greater looseness, and laxity. First degree has the best prognosis and the fastest recovery. With a third-degree strain, surgery is likely necessary for full recovery. Most soft tissue injuries can be treated conservatively, but occasionally surgical consultation is required.

Acute MSK Injuries

Soft tissue injury treatment can be summarized with the acronym *P.R.I.C.E.*[1]

*P*rotect the structure from further aggravation; i.e., use of crutches, a cane, a splint, a sling, or a cast.
*R*est it, but do not necessarily immobilize it. The extent of the injury will determine the degree of immobilization.[2]
*I*cing for 15 minutes at a time, with a thin towel between the ice and the affected structure (to avoid frostbite), three to four times per day is suggested. Icing has been shown to reduce edema and pain and shorten recovery time if used within 48 hours for ankle sprains,[3] but the evidence is weak for other injuries.[4] Cold gel applica-
tion significantly reduced pain over placebo in a randomized trial of sports injuries.[5]
*C*ompression will help avoid any significant swelling.
*E*levating the area, if possible, will help as well.

Non-steroidal anti-inflammatory drugs (NSAIDs) can be added. These medications have been proven to decrease recovery time and pain in ankle sprains, though one is not more effective than another.[3] The role of physical rehabilitation is very important, right from the outset, to enter the patient into the *Five Stages of Rehabilitation*. Acute on chronic injuries are treated very similarly to acute injuries, with special attention directed toward any underlying scar tissue or adhesions that have developed, causing interference with normal functioning of the structure or joint. The above principles of treatment can be applied to a whole spectrum of soft tissue injuries, such as rotator cuff tendonopathy, biceps/triceps tendonopathy, tennis elbow, golfer's elbow, Achilles tendonopathy, patella tendonopathy, hamstring strain, quadriceps strain or contusion, trochanteric bursitis of the hip, and plantar fasciitis.

Five Stages of Rehabilitation

There are five stages of rehabilitation[6] that therapists such as a registered physiotherapist (R.P.T.), chiropractor (D.C.), osteopath (D.O.), kinesiologist (BSc.Kin), certified athletic therapist (C.A.T.), or registered massage therapist (R.M.T.) should follow:

- Stage I is simply to control the pain, swelling, and stiffness of the injured area.
- Stage II involves working on re-establishing the range of motion of the affected area/joint (through stretching), and some light strengthening exercises.
- Stage III involves further range of motion (more aggressively), and more advanced strengthening exercises.
- Stage IV involves performing more sport/occupational specific exercises (preparing the individuals for their return).
- Stage V involves working on the patient's overall cardio-respiratory fitness, and further strengthening exercises.

Once an individual has achieved at least 90% of his or her normal functioning, then the individual is ready to enter into a stepwise return to his or her work/activity/sport. Passive modalities, such as ultrasound, interferential current, laser therapy, muscle stimulation, and others, should be used as an adjunct only, and not as the principle mode of treatment.

Radiological Investigations

The most commonly used radiological investigations are X-ray examinations, soft-issue ultrasounds (US), bone scans, computed tomography (CT) scans, bone densitometry, and magnetic resonance imaging (MRI) scans.

X-rays are used mostly for assessing the status of the bones and joints. Soft tissue structures are not well seen on X-ray films. US is good at delineating soft tissue structures. In particular, it is commonly used for rotator cuff pathology in the shoulder, Achilles tendonopathies, tennis elbow, plantar fasciitis, and patella tendonopathy. Bone scans are used for ruling out stress fractures, enthesopathies, tumours, and osteochondral lesions of a joint. Bone densitometry is used to assess bone density in relation to stress fractures or soft fractures (fractures that occur with little force). CT scans are used more for the view of the spine, depth of bony injury, and the extent of osteochondral injury. MRI scans are used to detail the soft tissue in the joint and disc pathology of the spine. Performing arthrograms in conjunction with an MRI will help to delineate some articular structures better (i.e., the labrum in the shoulder) than MRI alone. One systematic review of diagnostic tests for shoulder pain found MRI and US to be equally effective in detecting full-thickness tears, but suggested that US might be better at detecting partial-thickness tears.[7] Tumours are imaged well with both CT and MRI. Consider a tumour if the pain is out of proportion to the overt pathology, and if there is a lot of nighttime pain.[8]

────────── ❧ **REFERENCES** ❧ ──────────

1. Winston H: What's your game plan? Sports injuries, *Can J Diagnosis* 21(2):78-82, Feb 2004.
2. Jarvinen TA, Kaariainen M, Jarvinen M, et al: Muscle strain injuries, *Curr Opin Rheumatol* 12(2):155-61, Mar 2000.
3. NHS Centre for Reviews and Dissemination: Treatment modalities for soft tissue injuries of the ankle, *Database of abstracts of reviews of effectiveness,* issue 2, Document No. 123379, Accession No. 951779 31011997, York, UK, 2004.
4. Bleakley C, McDonough S, MacAuley D: The use of ice in the treatment of acute soft-tissue injury: a systematic review of randomized controlled trials, *Am J Sports Med* 32(1):251-261, Jan-Feb 2004.
5. Airaksinen OV, Kyrklund N, Latvala K, et al: Efficacy of cold gel for soft tissue injuries: a prospective randomized double-blinded trial, *Am J Sports Med* 31(5):680-684, Sep-Oct, 2003.
6. Vad V, Hong HM, Zazzali M, et al: Exercise recommendations in athletes with early osteoarthritis of the knee, *Sports Med* 32(11):729-739, 2002.
7. Dinnes J, Loveman E, McIntyre L, et al: The effectiveness of diagnostic tests for the assessment of shoulder pain due to soft tissue disorders: a systematic review, *Health Technol Assess* 7(29):iii, 1-166, 2003.
8. Slipman CW, Patel RK, Botwin K, et al: Epidemiology of spine tumors presenting to musculoskeletal physiatrists, *Arch Phys Med Rehabil* 84(4):492-495, Apr 2003.

CONCUSSION

In 2001 in Vienna, Austria, the Concussion in Sport Group (CISG) created the following definition: "Concussion is defined as a complex pathophysiological process affecting the brain, induced by traumatic biomechanical forces."[1] A concussion may be caused by either a direct blow to the head, or indirectly (without direct impact), causing sufficient biomechanical forces to injure the brain. Most concussions occur rapidly, with the short-lived neurological impairment resolving spontaneously. The majority of neuroimaging studies of concussed individuals are grossly normal.[1] That is the reason the emphasis of injury is on functional changes, not structural changes. No gold standard exists for concussion grading scales.

Many concussions are unwitnessed. An individual may or may not have suffered loss of consciousness. To determine prognosis, it is necessary to seek information from all available sources, though information from teammates and/or coaches can be unreliable.[2] Attention and memory have been shown to be most sensitive in determining the extent of concussion.[1] The Maddocks questions[3] and the Standardized Assessment of Concussion (SAC)[4] can be used for the acute neuropsychological evaluation of the concussed individual. This is a practical and effective means of evaluating the degree of concussion on the sideline.

Signs and Symptoms of Acute Concussion

The following are various signs and symptoms that indicate an individual has suffered a head injury. There are cognitive features, typical symptoms, and physical signs. Cognitive changes involve abnormalities in mental status exhibited by the athlete, such as being unaware of all facets of the competition (the period of play, opposition, or score of the game), confusion, amnesic tendency, experiencing a loss of consciousness, and being disoriented to person, place, and time. Typical symptoms seen are headache, dizziness, nausea, imbalanced feeling, feeling "dinged" or "dazed," seeing flashing lights, and experiencing tinnitus and/or diplopia. A lingering symptom of fatigue and sleep disturbance indicates that complete recovery has not been achieved. The physical signs are loss of or impaired consciousness, vomiting, concussive seizure, imbalance, poor coordination or concentration, slurred speech, generalized slowness in mentation, inappropriate emotions or behaviour, change in personality, and sleepiness during inappropriate times.[1]

Neuroimaging with CT or MRI should be saved for those patients in whom there is suspicion of a structural lesion (i.e., focal neurological deficit, seizure activity, persistent loss of consciousness, or prolonged clinical symptomatology).[1] The Canadian Academy of Sports Medicine's (CASM) guideline for management of concussion[5] states that when an athlete shows any signs or symptoms of a concussion:

1. The player should not be allowed to return to play in the current game or practice.
2. The player should not be left alone, and regular monitoring for deterioration is essential.
3. The player should be medically evaluated following the injury serially in time.
4. Return to play must follow a medically supervised, stepwise process.
5. "When in doubt, sit them out."

Before commencing a rehabilitation program, the patient must be completely asymptomatic and have a normal neurological and cognitive exam. There is a movement away from sitting an athlete out for a predetermined period of time. The CASM Return to Play Protocol[5] allows an individualized to progress based on symptoms, not time.

1. No activity, complete rest. Once asymptomatic, proceed to level 2.
2. Light aerobic exercise in the form of walking, stationary cycling.
3. Sport-specific training (e.g., skating in hockey, running in football).
4. Non-contact training drills.
5. Full-contact training after medical clearance.
6. Game play.

If any post-concussion symptoms return at any of these levels, the athlete is forced to return to the previous level until those symptoms have cleared. It is important to be aware of the Second Impact Syndrome (SIS), which is a phenomenon that is believed to occur if an athlete returns to play prior to complete recovery. The brain will swell uncontrollably and cause herniation inferiorly.[6] While evidence of its true existence is weak,[7] currently one should err on the side of caution. A valuable resource for information on concussion is at http://www.concussionsafety.com.

─────────────── **❧ REFERENCES ❧** ───────────────

1. Aubry M, Cantu R, Dvorak J, et al: Summary and agreement statement of the 1st International Symposium on Concussion in Sport, Vienna 2001, *Clin J Sport Med* 12: 6-11, 2002.
2. McCrory PR, Berkovic SF: Second impact syndrome, *Neurology* 50(3):677-683, 1998.
3. Maddocks DL, Dicker GD, Saling MM: The assessment of orientation following concussion in athletes, *Clin J Sport Med* 5(1):32-35, 1995.
4. McCrea M, Kelly J, Randolph C, et al: Standardised assessment of concussion (SAC):on site mental status evaluation of the athlete, *J Head Trauma Rehabil* 13:27–36, 1998.
5. Anonymous: Guidelines for assessment and management of sport-related concussion. Canadian Academy of Sport Medicine Concussion Committee, *Clin J Sport Med* 10(3):209-211, Jul 2000.
6. Bowen AP: Second impact syndrome: a rare, catastrophic, preventable complication of concussion in young athletes, *J Emerg Nurs* 29(3):287-289, Jun 2003.
7. McCrory P: Does second impact syndrome exist? *Clin J Sport Med* 11(3):144-149, Jul 2001.

CERVICAL SPINE

(See also functional somatic syndromes)

Whiplash Injury

Whiplash injury is characterized by neck, head, and upper thoracic pain, often in association with minor cognitive changes, dizziness, tinnitus, and blurred vision. Women are more often affected than men. The pathogenesis of symptoms is uncertain, but facet joint injury may be responsible for the pain in many cases.[1] A Swiss prospective study of outcome found that 56% of patients had recovered by 3 months, 69% by 6 months, and 76% by 12 months.[2] Risk factors for a more prolonged course include severe initial symptoms, rotated or inclined head position at the time of injury, being unprepared for the injury, and being in a stationary automobile that is struck from the rear.[1]

Whether litigation plays a role in prolonging recovery is uncertain. Most claims that this is the case come from studies of patients in tertiary referral centers who have prolonged pain, and such patients constitute a small proportion of those suffering whiplash injury. That patients with prolonged pain have psychological disturbances is unquestionable, but a number of studies have found that psychological symptoms resolve once the pain is relieved.[1] The possibility that compensation is a factor in prolonging symptoms is suggested by a Lithuanian prospective study of rear-end automobile collisions. In Lithuania, few drivers are insured, and the population is unaware that whiplash can cause chronic pain and disability. In this study, half of those involved in accidents suffered acute neck or head pain, but after 3 weeks all patients were asymptomatic.[3] Chronic whiplash injury seems to be more of a cultural than a biomechanical phenomenon; in other European countries such as Germany and Greece, where drivers are insured and have access to litigation if they so desire, chronic pain and even short-term disability are extremely rare after whiplash injuries.[4] Barsky[5] classifies it as a functional somatic syndrome. (See discussion of functional somatic syndromes.)

Radiological studies of the cervical spine taken at the time of the accident are generally unremarkable or reveal evidence of pre-existing degenerative changes. As a rule, radiological investigations are of limited value in diagnosis and prognosis of whiplash injuries. In a prospective study of 100 patients with whiplash injury, no abnormality on neurological examination was shown, and normal plain radiographs and MRI performed within 3 weeks of injury did not reveal clinically significant abnormalities.[6] CT scanning and MRI imaging should be reserved for ruling out more serious surgical anatomical injuries. The only means currently available of validly pinpointing a cervical source as the "pain generator" are controlled diagnostic nerve blocks, and only the C2-3 facet joint has been systematically studied.[7,8]

No good evidence-based trials of treatment of whiplash injury have been published, so management decisions must be based on expert opinion.[1] A 2003 Cochrane Review also cited the weak evidence but concluded that "rest makes rusty." In other words, rest and immobilization using collars are not recommended for the treatment of whiplash, while active interventions, such as advice to "maintain usual activities" might be effective in whiplash patients.[9]

Carette[10] emphasizes the importance of a conservative approach focused on the maintenance of function. Although analgesic or anti-inflammatory drugs are useful in the early stages, the use of a collar is counterproductive if continued for more than a few days. Patients should be encouraged to partake in a home exercise program aimed at mobilizing the injured areas, and be reassured that this will not aggravate the condition. Intra-articular injections of corticosteroids into cervical zygapophyseal joints have not been shown to be valuable.[10] Freund and Schwartz conducted a study on the use of Botox in whiplash injury and reported that patients experienced improved pain and range of motion (ROM) scores that were statistically significant at 4 weeks compared with placebo.[11]

≈ REFERENCES ≈

1. Teasell RW, Shapiro AP: Whiplash injuries: an update, *Pain Res Manag* 3:81-90, 1998.

2. Radanov BP, Di Stefano G, Schnidrig A, et al: Role of psychosocial stress in recovery from common whiplash, *Lancet* 328: 712-715, 1991.

3. Obelieniene D, Schrader H, Bovim G, et al: Pain after whiplash: a prospective controlled inception cohort study, *J Neurol Neurosurg Psychiatry* 66:279-283, 1999.

4. Ferrari R: Whiplash cultures (letter), *Can Med Assoc J* 161:368, 1999.

5. Barsky AJ, Borus JF: Functional somatic syndromes, *Ann Intern Med* 130:910-921, 1999.

6. Ronnen HR, Dekorte PJ, Brink PR, et al: Acute whiplash injury—is there a role for MR imaging: prospective study of 100 patients, *Radiology* 201:93-96, 1996.

7. Bogduk, N, Marsland, A: On the concept of third occipital headache, *J Neurol Neurosurg Psychiatry* 49:775-780, 1986.

8. Lord SM, Barnsley L, Wallis BJ, et al: Third occipital headache: a prevalence study, *J Neurol Neurosurg Psychiatry* 57:1187-1190, 1994.

9. Verhagen AP, Peeters GG, de Bie RA, et al: Conservative treatment for whiplash (Cochrane Review). In: *The Cochrane Library,* issue 4, Chichester, UK, 2003, John Wiley.

10. Carette S: Whiplash injury and chronic neck pain (editorial), *N Engl Med J* 330:1083-1084, 1994.

11. Freund BJ, Schwartz M: Treatment of chronic cervical-associated headache with Botulinum toxin A: a pilot study, *Headache* 40:231-236, 2000.

SCOLIOSIS

The degree of scoliosis is measured by obtaining a standing posteroanterior X-ray of the full spine and calculating the Cobb angle. The angle is measured at the intersection of one line perpendicular from the top of the vertebrae at the start of the curve and the other perpendicular to a line along the bottom of the end vertebrae. Using a definition of 10 degrees or more, 2% of adolescent population is estimated to have idiopathic scoliosis.[1] Curvatures less than 30 degrees tend to have minimal lifetime progression, 40 to 50 degrees progress 10 to 15 degrees over time, and curvatures over 50 degrees can continue to develop at 1 to 2 degrees a year.[1] Interestingly, patients do not exhibit clinically significant respiratory symptoms with idiopathic scoliosis until their curves are 60 to 100 degrees, and there is no difference in the prevalence of back pain or mortality among patients with untreated adolescent idiopathic scoliosis and the general population.[1] Atypical cases such as incidence under the age of 8, rapid curve progression of more than 1 degree per month, an unusual curve pattern such as left thoracic curve, neurological deficit, or pain require an MRI and further investigation.[1] Patients with curvatures greater than 45 degrees in adolescents and 50 degrees in adults can be considered surgical candidates.[1]

One long-term study found that 22 years later, the degree of progression of scoliosis in surgically treated patients (3.5 degrees) was significantly lower then brace therapy (7.9). Surgical candidates had more severe scoliosis, with a pre-treatment average curvature of 62 degrees, an end-of-treatment correction to 33 degrees, and a measurement at the time of the study of 36.5 degrees. The corresponding figures for brace patients were 33 degrees, 30 degrees, and 38 degrees respectively.[2] Brace therapy was superior to electrical stimulation, which was equal to the control in preventing progression in a separate 4-year study of patients with curvatures between 25 and 35 degrees.[3] Studies suggest there is minimal symptomatic relief to bracing curves less than 60 degrees.[1] There is some evidence that resistance exercises prevent progression and diminish the curvature,[4] and that aerobic exercise improves lung function.[5] There is much controversy around the subject of screening for asymptomatic scoliosis. A Rochester, Minnesota, school scoliosis screening program found that to identify one child requiring treatment, 448 children had to be screened and 20 had to have further medical assessments.[6] The U.S. Preventive Services Task Force has recently reviewed their position on adolescent scoliosis screening and now give it a "D" recommendation (previously was "C"). Their rational is that clinically significant scoliosis is likely to be detected by other means, and screen-detected scoliosis is less likely to require any intervention.[7] In contrast, such organizations as the American Academy of Pediatrics and the American Academy of Orthopaedic

Surgeons advocate screening, and 26 U.S. states have enacted compulsory scoliosis screening laws.[1] British and Canadian authorities do not recommend adolescent screening.[8]

❧ REFERENCES ❧

1. Greiner KA: Adolescent idiopathic scoliosis: radiologic decision-making, *Am Fam Physician* 65(9):1817-1822, 1 May 2002.
2. Danielsson AJ, Nachemson AL: Radiologic findings and curve progression 22 years after treatment for adolescent idiopathic scoliosis: comparison of brace and surgical treatment with matching control group of straight individuals, *Spine* 26(5):516-525, 1 Mar 2001.
3. Nachemson AL, Peterson LE: Effectiveness of treatment with a brace in girls who have adolescent idiopathic scoliosis. A prospective, controlled study based on data from the Brace Study of the Scoliosis Research Society, *J Bone Joint Surg (Am)* 77(6):815-822, Jun 1995.
4. Mooney V, Brigham A: The role of measured resistance exercises in adolescent scoliosis, *Orthopedics* 26(2):167-171; discussion 171, Feb 2003.
5. Athanasopoulos S, Paxinos T, Tsafantakis E, et al: The effect of aerobic training in girls with idiopathic scoliosis, *Scand J Med Science Sports* 9(1):36-40, Feb 1999.
6. Yawn BP, Yawn RA, Hodge D, et al: A population-based study of school scoliosis screening, *JAMA* 282:1427-1432, 1999.
7. U.S. Preventive Services Task Force Screening for Adolescent Idiopathic Scoliosis 2004: Accessed at http://www.ahrq.gov/clinic/uspstf/uspsaisc.htm on June 17, 2004.
8. Canadian Task Force on the Periodic Health Examination: *Clinical preventive health care,* Ottawa, 1994, Canadian Communication Group, 345-354.

LUMBAR SPINE
Low Back Pain

(See also ankylosing spondylitis; detrimental effects of smoking; investigations; muscle relaxants)

Epidemiology

In developed countries the lifetime risk of low back pain (LBP) is about 75%. In the vast majority of cases the disorder is self-limited, but it recurs in 40% to 80% of patients. The highest prevalence rate is in those ages 45 to 64. Frequent lifting of heavy objects and twisting are important risk factors. Being sedentary, driving a motor vehicle for prolonged periods, and smoking are also associated with an increased risk of LBP. The likelihood in family medicine that patients with LBP have underlying systemic or visceral disease is low. Figures vary but range from about 0.05% to 0.1% for neoplasms and about half that for infectious disorders.[1]

Diagnosis

In about 85% of cases of LBP, a definite pathophysiological diagnosis (substantive diagnosis) cannot be made.[2]

Inflammatory back pain (ankylosing spondylitis) is a rare but important cause of LBP in those under age 40. The first step in assessing back pain is to rule out "red flags"[3]:

- Systemic signs suggesting cancer or infection (unexplained weight loss, sustained fever, age over 50, history of cancer)
- Signs suggestive of acute cauda equina syndrome (loss of bowel or bladder control, saddle anesthesia)
- High impact injury (e.g., car accident, a bad fall)

Imaging

X-ray examination, MRI, or CT scans should not be ordered for most patients with LBP unless there are "red flags" as described above.[3-5] A study comparing MRIs with X-rays in acute LBP showed no benefit.[6] The conundrum is that while there is no improvement in clinical outcome, patients are more satisfied when radiology is employed and hypothetically may ambulate more and sooner, which is therapeutic.[4,5] CTs and MRIs tend to be utilized with red flags or when sciatica or spinal stenosis are unresolving or atypical but carry with them the danger of negative labelling. Disk bulging or disk protrusions are extremely common in individuals without back pain. In one MRI study of the lumbar spine in persons age 20 to 80 (mean 42) with no back pain, 52% of the subjects had a bulge in at least one level, 27% had a protrusion, and 1% had an extrusion.[7]

Prognosis

Seventy percent of acute LBP will improve within 2 weeks, and 90% will improve within approximately 4 weeks.[8] The vast majority of patients return to work within 6 weeks.[2] A 1998 British primary care study confirmed that 90% of patients with LBP stopped consulting their physicians after 3 months, but follow-up assessment of these patients found that after 1 year, only 25% had completely recovered in terms of pain and disability.[9]

Only 1% of patients with acute LBP require surgery, most being patients who have proven disk protrusion with nerve root irritation unresponsive to conservative therapy. Of patients with proven disk protrusions causing neurological symptoms, only 5% to 10% require surgery.[2] When surgery is undertaken for patients with proven sciatica and disk herniation, 90% have good results at 1 year compared with 60% among those followed conservatively. However, after 10 years of follow-up, results are similar in the two groups, with about one third having persistent motor or sensory abnormalities. Thus the prime indication for surgery (aside from the acute cauda equina syndrome) is immediate pain relief.[10] Patients with LBP and fibromyalgia have a poor prognosis.[11] Reigo et al found that tenderness of the trapezius and scolisis was predictive of more time taken off work.[12]

Management

Optimal management of LBP remains controversial. Waddell[2] summed up the nihilistic view of many when he stated that for the vast majority of patients, there is no evidence that any form of treatment is better than time and placebo effect. Although bedrest was formerly an integral aspect of treatment, evidence shows that it has no value for non-specific LBP.[13] The value of physiotherapy for acute LBP also remains uncertain; several studies have not proven its effectiveness.[14,15] Another trial showed that when physiotherapy, aerobics, and muscle reconditioning were compared, all significantly reduced pain at 1 year, but no one modality was superior.[16]

A systematic review of randomized controlled trials of treatment modalities for acute (less than 6 weeks' duration) and chronic (longer than 12 weeks' duration) non-specific LBP came to the following conclusions.[13] Evidence indicates that for acute LBP, NSAIDs and analgesics are equally effective and that no one NSAID is better than another. Muscle relaxants are also effective. Massage therapy has been proven to reduce pain.[17] Little evidence supports the use of manipulation or traction, and no evidence supports back schools, transcutaneous electrical nerve stimulation (TENS), or behaviour therapy for acute LBP. For chronic back pain there is good evidence supporting exercise programs and moderate evidence that NSAIDs are effective, although no one NSAID is better than another. Antidepressants reduce pain but not function and have added side effects.[18] Evidence for beneficial effects from analgesics and muscle relaxants is limited. Manipulation and back schools are clearly better than no treatment, and limited evidence suggests that they are superior to other treatment modalities. A cognitive-behavioural–oriented physiotherapy program appears beneficial,[19] and a multidisciplinary bio-psycho-social rehabilitation program seems to work better than a less coordinated approach.[20] No good evidence supports TENS, behaviour therapy, traction, or acupuncture. While epidural steroid injections are better than placebo treatments, they offer no advantage over other therapeutic modalities.

The value of bedrest for patients with nerve root compression (sciatica) has been a subject of controversy. Most practitioners advocate bedrest for at least a few days. A randomized trial of 2 weeks of bedrest compared with "being up and about whenever possible" demonstrated no benefit from bedrest.[21] Given time, a herniated nucleus pulposus shrinks; in a prospective MRI study, substantial shrinkage was found in 36% of patients at 6 weeks and in 60% of patients at 6 months after presentation.[22]

An observational study from North Carolina found that for patients with LBP who did not require surgery, the times to functional recovery, return to work, and complete recovery were identical for patients treated by primary care physicians, orthopedic surgeons, and chiropractors. The cost of care was highest for orthopedic surgeons and chiropractors (the latter because of multiple visits) and least for primary care physicians. However, patient satisfaction was greatest when patients were treated by chiropractors.[23]

Patients with root compression who do not respond to conservative therapy may be treated with a number of specific interventions. Some of the newer ones are laser disk decompression, nucleus replacement, and microlumbar diskectomy, a procedure that may be done on an outpatient basis. A new surgical technique for mechanical back pain is intradiscal electrothermal therapy, where the posterior annulus is heated to 90° C.[24]

Prevention

A Cochrane Review looking at prevention of back pain in healthy subjects by either educational programs, lumbar supports, exercises, ergonomics, or risk factor modification found only exercising was an effective intervention for prevention.[25]

❧ REFERENCES ❧

1. Deyo RA, Diehl AK: Lumbar spine films in primary care: current use and the effects of selective ordering criteria, *J Gen Intern Med* 1:20-25, 1986.
2. Waddell G: A new clinical model for the treatment of low-back pain (1987 Volvo Award in Clinical Sciences), *Spine* 12:632-644, 1987.
3. Health Care Guideline: Adult Low Back Pain Institute for Clinical Systems Improvement (2002). Accessed at http://gacguidelines.ca/article.pl?sid=02/07/03/2022215 on June 17, 2004.
4. Gillan MG, Gilbert FJ, Andrew JE, et al, Scottish Back Trial Group: Influence of imaging on clinical decision making in the treatment of lower back pain, *Radiology* 220(2):393-399, Aug 2001.
5. Kendrick D, Fielding K, Bentley E, et al: Radiography of the lumbar spine in primary care patients with low back pain: randomised controlled trial, *BMJ* 322(7283):400-405, Feb 17 2001.
6. Jarvik JG, Hollingworth W, Martin B, et al: Rapid magnetic resonance imaging vs radiographs for patients with low back pain. A randomized controlled trial, *JAMA* 289:2810-2818, 2003.
7. Jensen MC, Brant-Zawadzki MN, Obuchowski N, et al: Magnetic resonance imaging of the lumbar spine in people without back pain, *N Engl J Med* 331:69-73, 1994.
8. Pengel LHM, Herbert RD, Maher CG, et al: Acute low back pain: systematic review of its prognosis, *BMJ* 327; 323-328, 2003.
9. Croft PR, Macfarlane GJ, Papageorgiou AC, et al: Outcome of low back pain in general practice: a prospective study, *BMJ* 316:1356-1359, 1998.
10. Gibson JN, Grant IC, Waddell G: Surgery for lumbar disc prolapse (Cochrane Back Group). *Cochrane Database of Systematic Reviews*. 2, 2005. [Accessed June 27, 2005]

Available from: URL: http://www.mrw.interscience.wiley.com/cochrane/clsysrev/articles/CD001350/frame.html

11. Thomas E, Silman AJ, Croft PR, et al: Predicting who develops chronic low back pain in primary care: a prospective study, *BMJ* 318:1662-1667, 1999.

12. Reigo T, Tropp H, Timpka T: Clinical findings in a population with back pain. Relation to one-year outcome and long-term sick leave, *Scand J Prim Health Care* 18(4):208-214, Dec 2000.

13. Van Tulder MW, Koes BW, Bouter LM: Conservative treatment of acute and chronic nonspecific low back pain: a systematic review of randomized controlled trials of the most common interventions, *Spine* 22:2128-2156, 1997.

14. Faas A, van Eijk JT, Chavannes AW, et al: A randomized trial of exercise therapy in patients with acute low back pain: efficacy on sickness absence, *Spine* 20:941-947, 1995.

15. Chiropractic manipulation and McKenzie physiotherapy were not effective for low back pain *ACP J Club* 130:42 April, 1999. 16. Mannion AF, Muntener M, Taimela S, et al: Comparison of three active therapies for chronic low back pain: results of a randomized clinical trial with one-year follow-up, *Rheumatology* 40(7):772-778, Jul 2001.

17. Preyde M: Effectiveness of massage therapy for subacute low-back pain: a randomized controlled trial, *Can Med Assoc J* 162(13):1815-1820, 27 Jun 2000.

18. Salerno SM, Browning R, Jackson JL: The effect of antidepressant treatment on chronic back pain: a meta-analysis, *Arch Intern Med* 162(1):19-24, 14 Jan 2002.

19. Moffett JK, Torgerson D, Bell-Syer S, et al: Randomised controlled trial of exercise for low back pain: clinical outcomes, costs, and preferences, *BMJ* 319:279-283, 1999.

20. Guzman J, Esmail R, Karjalainen K, et al: Multidisciplinary bio-psycho-social rehabilitation for chronic low back pain, *Cochrane Database of Systematic Reviews.* (1):CD000963, 2002.

21. Vroomen PC, de Krom MC, Wilmink JT, et al: Lack of effectiveness of bed rest for sciatica, *N Engl J Med* 340:418-423, 1999.

22. Modic MT, Ross JS, Obuchowski NA, et al: Contrast-enhanced MR imaging in acute lumbar radiculopathy: a pilot study of the natural history, *Radiology* 195:323-324, 1995.

23. Carey TS, Garrett J, Jackman A, et al: The outcomes and costs of care for acute low back pain among patients seen by primary care practitioners, chiropractors, and orthopedic surgeons, *N Engl J Med* 333:913-917, 1995.

24. Deen HG, Fenton DS, Lamer TJ: Minimally invasive procedures for disorders of the lumbar spine, *Mayo Clin Proceed* 78(10):1249-1256, Oct 2003.

25. Linton SJ, van Tulder MW: Preventive interventions for back and neck pain problems: what is the evidence? *Spine* 26(7):778-787, 1 Apr 2001.

SHOULDER

(See also investigations)

Dislocation

Always assess the neurovascular status pre- and post-reduction, especially of the axillary nerve, which supplies sensation and motor coordination in the deltoid area. One easy way to reduce an anterior dislocation without using anesthesia is to have the patient lie on his or her stomach and allow the arm to hang. The patient can hold 5 to 10 pounds of weight, or gentle downward traction can be applied. This step alone can reduce the shoulder, but if not, locate the inferior tip of the scapula and push it medially (toward the spine). This is known as the *scapular rotation method*.

In one prospective study from the University of California, Hendey et al evaluated the utility of pre- and post-reduction X-rays in 104 patients with suspected shoulder dislocations.[1] If X-rays had not been ordered in patients with recurrent dislocations with atraumatic mechanisms, and if post-reduction films skipped in patients with first and/or traumatic dislocations without fracture (assuming physicians were confident in their assessments), about half of the films would have been avoided without missing a fracture or persistent dislocation. These findings suggest that a significant number of X-rays can be avoided in a subset of patients with suspected shoulder dislocations if the physician is confident in his or her clinical assessments.[1]

In a Swedish prospective study of 247 anterior dislocations, the patients were assigned at random to three forms of initial treatment post-reduction: immobilization for 3 to 4 weeks by binding the arm to the torso, sling for pain relief that was discontinued when the patient was comfortable, and immobilization for various durations. The rate of recurrent dislocations was unrelated to the initial treatment[2]; therefore, dislocations can be treated with sling immobilization until the patient is comfortable.

Age appears to be the only predictor of recurrence, with the highest rates for those between 21 and 30 years of age.[3]

Kirkley evaluated early (within 4 weeks) arthroscopic stabilization followed by immobilization for 3 weeks versus non-operative care with immobilization for 3 weeks.[4] She found that early stabilization in these first-time dislocators reduced recurrence rates to only 16% versus 47% in the non-surgical group. Also, patient satisfaction scales achieved 86% versus 70% respectively.[4] This is mirrored in other studies and indicates a trend toward early repair of first-time anterior dislocators. Active physiotherapy directed toward restoring ROM and strength is recommended but has not been shown to decrease recurrence rates. Passive, modality-based therapy is not recommended.

Imaging Studies of the Shoulder
Treat the patient, not the test!

MRI of the dominant asymptomatic shoulder of subjects over 60 years of age found 28% had complete rotator cuff tears and 26% had partial tears. Figures for those between the ages of 40 and 60 were 4% and 24%.[5]

Teefry compared preoperative US with findings on arthroscopy and determined that US was 96% sensitive for detecting full-thickness tears but only 60% sensitive for partial-thickness tears. Magnetic resonance arthrography is more useful for evaluating partial-thickness rotator cuff and biceps tears as well as labral pathology.[6] Order these only if you think the results will change your management.

Rotator Cuff Dysfunction

Shoulder impingement syndrome is a group of symptoms identified by but not limited to painful abduction greater than 90 degrees and abnormal Hawkins and Neers impingement tests. (For the Hawkins test, the shoulder should be forward flexed 90 degrees. Internally rotate the shoulder and determine if pain is elicited in the subacromial space. For the Neers test, passively move the shoulder into full forward flexion to 180 degrees and see if pain is reproduced.)

A 2003 Systematic Review of the management of Shoulder Impingement Syndrome showed that the studies with the best methodological designs demonstrate only limited evidence supporting the efficacy of therapeutic exercise (TE) and manual therapy.[7] TE consists of a comprehensive, progressive group of stretching and strengthening exercises for the scapulothoracic and rotator cuff muscles. More methodologically sound studies are needed to further evaluate these two interventions.[7]

Generally, current recommendations support 6 months of a TE program followed by a cortisone injection trial before referral for surgical consideration. Passive physiotherapy is not recommended. Patients who present with an acute full-thickness rotator cuff tear should be referred immediately for surgical consultation.

Frozen Shoulder

A study of patients with frozen shoulder (adhesive capsulitis) compared corticosteroid injections given by family physicians (mean of 2.2 per patient) with physiotherapy. After 7 weeks, those receiving corticosteroids did much better, but by 26 and 52 weeks, little difference was found between the groups.[8] This fits with the fact that the first two phases of frozen shoulder are the more painful. Early subacromial or intra-articular injection is an effective tool for pain management but has not been shown to change the natural history of this self-resolving disease. Tell patients that the problem will eventually resolve but on average lasts 14 months. Patients can be referred for surgical consultation and possible capsular mobilization or release after this time.

A self-administered home rehabilitation program (taught by a physiotherapist) is an effective way to maintain ROM and strength. Physiotherapy has not been found to be effective in either pain management or restoration of ROM.

≥ REFERENCES ≤

1. Hendey GW, et al: Necessity of radiographs in the emergency department management of shoulder dislocations, *Ann Emerg Med* 36(2):108, Aug 2000.
2. Hovelius L, Augustini BG, Fredin H, et al: Primary anterior dislocation of the shoulder in young patients–a ten-year prospective study, *J Bone Joint Surg Am* 78A:1677-1684, 1996.
3. Kralinger FS, et al: Predicting recurrence of shoulder dislocation, *Am J Sports Med* 30:116-120, 2002.
4. Kirkley A, et al: Prospective randomized clinical trial comparing the effectiveness of immediate arthroscopic stabilization vs. immobilization and rehabilitation in first traumatic dislocations of the shoulder, *Arthroscopy* 15(5):507-514, 1999.
5. Sher JS, Uribe JW, Posada A, et al: Abnormal findings on magnetic resonance images of asymptomatic shoulders, *J Bone Joint Surg Am* 77A:10-15, 1995.
6. Teefey SA, et al: Ultrasonography of the rotator cuff: a comparison of ultrasonographic and arthroscopic findings in one hundred consecutive cases, *J Bone Joint Surg Am* 82:498-504, 2000.
7. Desmeules F, et al: Therapeutic exercise and orthopaedic manual therapy for shoulder impingement syndrome: a systematic review, *Clin J Sport Med* 13(3):176-181, 2003.
8. Van der Windt DA, Koes BW, Devillé W, et al: Effectiveness of corticosteroid injections versus physiotherapy for treatment of painful stiff shoulder in primary care: randomised trial, *BMJ* 317:1292-1296, 1998.

ELBOW

Thrower's Elbow

The extreme valgus stresses on the elbow in throwing athletes can lead to injuries of the ulnar collateral ligament, the ulnar nerve, or the origin of the flexor musculature, including medial epicondylitis. Management may be conservative, including omission of the offending activity for 3 to 6 weeks.[1] Occasionally, surgery to repair the ulnar collateral ligament (UCL) or ulnar nerve transposition may be required.

Supracondylar Fractures

Supracondylar fractures are the most common elbow fractures of children that require surgery, with most cases occurring between the ages of 5 and 8. They usually result from a fall onto the outstretched hand.[2] Neurovascular damage is an important complication. Closed reduction and casting can give good results, particularly in minimally displaced fractures.[3] However, poor reduction of more displaced fractures may result in cubitus varus. Better results may be achieved with either open reduction internal fixation (ORIF) or open or closed reduction and percutaneous pinning.[4,5]

Tennis Elbow/Golfer's Elbow

In tennis elbow, pain and tenderness are located over the lateral epicondyle of the humerus, and pain occurs with resisted extension of the wrist, middle finger, or both. In golfer's elbow, the pain is over the medial epicondyle, and pain occurs with resisted wrist flexion and pronation. In more than 95% of patients, tennis elbow has nothing to do with tennis.[6] In most young persons it is caused by participation in sports, and in older persons, by occupation.[7] Some studies support the use of various physiotherapy modalities in the treatment of lateral epicondylitis (LE),[8] including the use of a tennis elbow band.[9] Consideration should also be given to occupational assessment and treatment, such as safer computer ergonomics. A recent Cochrane Review found that topical NSAIDs, oral NSAIDs, or steroid injection provided short-term relief, but long-term evidence of effect was lacking.[10] There is also some evidence to support the use of extracorporeal shock wave therapy in treating LE.[11] Failing all conservative therapy, surgical release of the common extensor origin may help reduce pain and restore function.

Radial Head Fracture

These fractures usually occur from a fall on an outstretched arm.[1] Minimally displaced (1 to 2 mm) radial head fractures may be treated conservatively (i.e., sling, then early active ROM as soon as is tolerated). However, better results may be obtained with ORIF in fractures with greater displacement.[12]

❧ REFERENCES ❧

1. Onieal ME: Common wrist and elbow injuries in primary care, *Lippincotts Prim Care Pract* 3(4):441-450, Jul-Aug 1999.
2. Turra S, Santini S, Zandonadi A, et al: Supracondylar fractures of the humerus in children. A comparison between non-surgical treatment and minimum synthesis, *Chir Organi Mov* 80(3):293-299, Jul-Aug 1995.
3. Shoaib M, Hussain A, Kamran H, et al: Outcome of closed reduction and casting in displaced supracondylar fracture of humerus in children, *J Ayub Med Coll Abbottabad* 15(4):23-25, Oct-Dec 2003.
4. de Buys Roessingh AS, Reinberg O: Open or closed pinning for distal humerus fractures in children? *Swiss Surg* 9(2): 76-81, 2003.
5. France J, Strong M: Deformity and function in supracondylar fractures of the humerus in children variously treated by closed reduction and splinting, traction, and percutaneous pinning, *J Pediatr Orthop* 12(4):494-498, Jul-Aug 1992.
6. Chop WM Jr: Tennis elbow, *Postgrad Med* 86:301-304, 307-308, 1989.
7. Gellman H: Tennis elbow (lateral epicondylitis), *Orthop Clin North Am* 23:75-82, 1992.
8. Trudel D, Duley J, Zastrow I, et al: Rehabilitation for patients with lateral epicondylitis: a systematic review, *J Hand Ther* 17(2):243-266, Apr-Jun 2004.
9. Borkholder CD, Hill VA, Fess EE: The efficacy of splinting for lateral epicondylitis: a systematic review, *J Hand Ther* 17(2):181-199, Apr-Jun 2004.
10. Green S, Buchbinder R, Barnsley L, et al: Non-steroidal anti-inflammatory drugs (NSAIDs) for treating lateral elbow pain in adults (Cochrane Musculoskeletal Group). *Cochrane Database of Systematic Reviews*. 2, 2005. [Accessed June 27, 2005] Available from: URL: http://www.mrw.interscience.wiley.com/cochrane/clsysrev/articles/CD003686/frame.html
11. Rompe JD, Decking J, Schoellner C, et al: Repetitive low-energy shock wave treatment for chronic lateral epicondylitis in tennis players, *Am J Sports Med* 32(3):734-743, Apr 2004.
12. Geel CW, Palmer AK, Ruedi T, et al: Internal fixation of proximal radial head fractures, *J Orthop Trauma* 4(3):270-274, 1990.

HAND INJURIES

Phalangeal Fractures

Among all fractures to the hand, fractures of the proximal phalanx are the most common. Particular attention should be paid to note angulation and rotational deformities. Angulation is most likely to be volar because the tension of the extrinsic flexors of the finger is much stronger than the extensors. Rotational deformity will vary.

Reduction of the fracture will usually be successful with a digital block and placement of the metacarpophalangeal (MCP) joint of the affected finger in flexion to decrease intrinsic pull. A splint is usually adequate for maintenance of the reduction, but if the fracture is spiral or oblique, a better choice is a gutter type of splint.

Open reduction is indicated for comminution, bone loss, or significant displacement.[1]

Boxer's Fracture

Treatment of boxer's fracture (fracture of the neck of the fourth or fifth metacarpal) varies among surgeons. Unless the angulation of the distal fragment is greater than 45 degrees or there is a rotational deformity causing "scissoring" of the fingers, reduction is usually unnecessary. It may be necessary to apply a gutter type of splint for a fracture of the fifth metacarpal; however, fixation may not be necessary for a fracture of the fourth metacarpal because it is buttressed on both sides by normal metacarpals; pain can be relieved with a tensor bandage.[2]

Scaphoid Fractures

Scaphoid fractures usually occur with a fall on the outstretched hand, with the wrist in dorsiflexion. The classic sign is "snuff-box" tenderness. The radial styloid acts as a fulcrum upon which the scaphoid is stressed. It is usually divided into four classes: proximal pole, waist, distal one third, or distal tubercle. Because the blood supply to the bone flows from distal to proximal, the more proximal the fracture the more likely bone may necrose.

The fracture is also described as either stable (nondisplaced with minimal comminution) or unstable (displaced with comminution) in order to determine therapy. If the fracture is stable, the thumb should be immobilized in a thumb spica cast for an average of 12 weeks. If it is unstable, ORIF is required. If this fracture is suspected, but the X-ray is negative, immobilize the hand and have X-rays repeated in 2 weeks' time.[3]

Dislocations

The most common dislocation in the hand is a dislocation of the proximal interphalangeal (PIP) joint. This joint is most vulnerable because of its greater mobility. Most dislocations are dorsal.

The PIP joint is most mobile in flexion where it is limited only by the extensor mechanism and soft tissues. The collateral ligaments limit lateral motion, while the volar plate limits extension. Dislocations will injure at least one of these structures.

Reduction of a dorsal dislocation is easily done with in-line traction. Volar dislocations may be troublesome because soft tissue entrapment may occur, and this may require open reduction. Buddy tape or a simple aluminum splint is sufficient to maintain the reduction. However, many times, the dislocation will be reduced on-site either by the patient, or a team trainer; therefore, the physician must examine the joint closely. When examining the joint, always check for hyperextension (volar plate injury), dorsal slip (boutonniere deformity), or lateral laxity of greater than 20 degrees. X-rays should always be taken to assess for articular surface congruence. Abnormal examination or an abnormal X-ray may require surgical consultation.[4]

Skier's Thumb

Skier's or gamekeeper's thumb is a laxity of the ulnar collateral ligament of the metacarpophalangeal ligament of the thumb. The latter name comes from repetitive strain when killing snared small game by forcefully hyperextending their heads using the thumb and forefinger. At present most injuries to this ligament take place as a result of forced abduction during sports injuries, particularly the skier who combines high speeds with an abducted thumb because of pole grip. If the patient has a complete tear of the ligament, surgical repair is indicated, because in at least 50% of cases the proximal end is trapped in such a way that healing cannot take place.[5]

It is important to distinguish ligamentous tears from avulsion fractures. Before stress is placed on the ligament, X-ray examination should be performed; if a small avulsion fracture is found and the displacement is less than 5 mm, conservative treatment with a short-arm or even glove-type spica cast for 4 to 6 weeks will suffice. If the gap is greater than 5 mm or the fragment

involves more than 25% of the joint surface, surgical repair is indicated.[5]

If no fracture is seen on the X-ray film, the joint should be stressed for the assessment of a complete ligamentous tear. This manoeuvre should not be performed if the patient has an avulsion fracture, because it may cause displacement of the fragment. The ligament is at maximum tension when the metacarpophalangeal joint is fully flexed, so that is the correct position for stressing. If the degree of angulation exceeds 30 degrees, or if it is 15 degrees more than on the unaffected side, surgical consultation is indicated. In many cases, local anesthesia is necessary so the physician can adequately stress the joint.[5]

──────── ✍ REFERENCES ✍ ────────

1. Hoffman DF, Schaffer TC: Management of common finger injuries, *Am Fam Physician* 43(5):1594-1607, May 1991.
2. Ford MH: What's best for "boxer's fracture," *Patient Care Can* 7:15, 1996.
3. Calandra JJ, Goldner RD, Hardaker WT Jr: Scaphoid fractures assessment and treatment, *Orthopedics* 15(8):931-937, Aug 1992.
4. Bach AW: Finger joint injuries in active patients, *Phys Sports Med* 27(3): 89-91, 96-97, 101-104, 1999.
5. Richard JR: Gamekeeper's thumb: ulnar collateral ligament injury, *Am Fam Physician* 53:1775-1780, 1996.

HIP

(See also apophyseal injuries, foot; apophyseal injuries, knee; geriatrics; osteoarthritis; osteoporosis; septic arthritis; stress fractures)

Apophyseal Injuries

Apophyseal injuries occur in the region of the hip and are most likely to be seen in young athletes between 15 and 18 years of age. Apophysitis of the anterior superior iliac spine (at the origin of the sartorius muscle), the ischial tuberosity (hamstrings), and the iliac crest (gluteus medius, external obliques, tensor fascia lata, latissimus dorsi and gluteus maximus muscles) are the most likely sites to be involved.[1] Diagnosis is usually suggested by the gradual onset of localized pain and tenderness in the involved region and focal tenderness over these areas.[2] X-rays are normal in patients with apophysitis, but may show widening of the physis in those complicated by the presence of an avulsion fracture. Rest, ice, and NSAIDs are usually effective, and symptoms usually resolve in 4 to 6 weeks.[3]

Developmental Dysplasia of the Hip

Developmental dysplasia of the hip (DDH) is the terminology currently preferred over *congenital dislocation of the hip* because it is more inclusive and includes poorly developed acetabula without true dislocation. The single biggest risk factor is a family history of the condition; other risk factors are female sex, breech presentations, and foot deformities. Standard screening techniques for detecting hip dysplasia are the Ortolani test, which relocates a displaced hip, and Barlow test, which attempts to dislocate the hip. When done properly, these tests have relatively good sensitivity.[4]

Although in most affected infants the problem resolves spontaneously in the first several months of life, persistent DDH may result in chronic pain, gait abnormalities, and degenerative arthritis.[4] Treatment of hip dysplasia has included abduction splinting such as the Pavlik Harness or Abduction Pillows, although there are risks of treatment, including avascular necrosis, and true effectiveness is unknown.[4]

Hip Fractures

Many but not all of the risk factors for hip fracture parallel those for osteoporosis. Current alcohol use is a risk factor for hip fracture,[5] as are long- and short-acting benzodiazepines.[6] High rates of prescription medication use also correlate with hip fractures.[6,7] A prospective multicentre U.S. study of hip fractures in white women found that most had multiple risk factors; weight gain after the age of 25 was protective.[8] Moderate levels of walking or other leisure activities were associated with a 50% reduction in the risk of hip fracture in post-menopausal women.[9] External hip protectors have also been shown to reduce fractures in some studies,[10] although there is debate as to their efficacy.[11] Prevention and treatment of osteoporosis is also very important in prevention of hip fractures.

The type of surgery selected for hip fractures depends on a number of variables. Non-displaced femoral neck fractures in patients over age 70 or even displaced fractures in those under age 70 may be treated with internal fixation. The rate of non-union and femoral head necrosis in displaced femoral neck fractures in patients over age 70 is high, and such fractures are usually treated with a prosthesis. Intertrochanteric fractures are usually managed by internal fixation.[12]

Mortality rates after hip fractures are reported to be between 14% and 36%. Between 50% and 65% of patients regain their previous ambulatory status, 10% to 15% can ambulate only in the home, and 20% become non-ambulatory. Recovery of ambulation is more likely among patients who are male, non-demented, and relatively young.[12] In many cases, mortality associated with hip fractures appears to be due to serious underlying conditions that in themselves contribute to the fractures.

The long-term results of hip prostheses are excellent even after 20 years.[13,14] One of the original problems with hip arthroplasty was aseptic loosening of the femoral component, but with advances in cementing techniques, this is now a rare complication.[14]

Transient Synovitis

Transient synovitis of the hip (TSH) is the most common cause of hip pain in children ages 3 to 10 years. It affects males twice as often as females. TSH is often found in a child with an acute or gradual onset of limp with unilateral hip, knee, or thigh pain. Fever may be present, and symptoms are bilateral in approximately 5% of cases. The affected hip is usually held in a flexed, abducted, and externally rotated position, and pain is usually elicited with internal rotation.[15] The most important differential diagnosis is septic arthritis. Clues to septic arthritis are severe hip pain and spasm. Some studies have shown that if fever and elevated erythrocyte sedimentation rate (ESR) is present, septic arthritis is more likely, although these symptoms can also be present in TSH.[15] Patients with TSH can be treated with rest and NSAIDs and usually improve spontaneously within a week to 10 days, but should be watched closely. Other joints may also be affected by transient synovitis; after the hip, the knee is the most frequently involved joint.[16]

❧ REFERENCES ❧

1. Christopher NC, Congeni J: Orthopedic emergencies: overuse injuries in the pediatric athlete: evaluation, initial management, and strategies for prevention, Clin Pediatr Emerg Med 3(2):118-128, Jun 2002.
2. Scopp JM: The assessment of athletic hip injury, Clin Sports Med 20(4):647-659, 1 Oct 2001.
3. Peck DM: Apophyseal injuries in the young athlete, Am Fam Physician 51:1891-1895, 1995.
4. Patel H: Preventive health care, 2001 update: screening and management of developmental dysplasia of the hip in newborns; Canadian Task Force on Preventive Health Care, Can Med Assoc J 164(12):1669-1677, 12 Jun 2001.
5. Grisso JA, Kelsey JL, Strom BL, et al: Risk factors for hip fracture in black women, N Engl J Med 330:1555-1559, 1994.
6. Gerings RM, Stricker BH, de Boer A, et al: Benzodiazepines and the risk of falling leading to femur fractures: dosage more important than elimination halflife, Arch Intern Med 155:1801-1807, 1995.
7. Davidson W, Molloy DW, Bédard M: Physician characteristics and prescribing for elderly people in New Brunswick: relation to patient outcomes, Can Med Assoc J 152:1227-1234, 1995.
8. Cummings SR, Nevitt MC, Browner WS, et al: Risk factors for hip fracture in white women, N Engl J Med 332:767-773, 1995.
9. Gregg E, Galuska D: Walking was associated with a reduced risk of hip fracture in postmenopausal women, 5(3): 2003.
10. Melton LJ: External hip protectors reduce hip fractures in the elderly, Evid Healthcare 5(3):69, Sep 2001.
11. Bhandar M: Do hip protectors help prevent hip fractures? Can Med Assoc J 169(3):215, 2003.
12. Zuckerman JD: Hip fracture, N Engl J Med 334:1519-1525, 1996.

13. Schulte KR, Callaghan JJ, Kelley SS, et al: The outcome of Charnley total hip arthroplasty with cement after a minimum twenty-year follow-up: the results of one surgeon, *J Bone Joint Surgery (Am)* 75:961-975, 1993.
14. Mulroy RD, Harris WH: The effect of improved cementing techniques on component loosening in total hip replacement, *J Bone Joint Surg (Br)* 72:757-760, 1990.
15. Kim MK: *The limping child, CPEM* 3(2):129-137, Jun 2002.
16. Hart JJ: Transient synovitis of the hip in children, *Am Fam Physician* 54:1587-1591, 1996.

KNEE

(See also ankle trauma; apophyseal injuries, foot; apophyseal injuries, hip; foot trauma; osteoarthritis)

Knee Trauma

Clinical decision rules for ordering knee X-ray studies after trauma (Ottawa knee rules) are any of the following[1]:

- Age greater than 55
- Inability to walk four consecutive steps immediately after injury or in the emergency room (two steps on each limb)
- Inability to flex 90 degrees
- Isolated tenderness over the head of the fibula
- Isolated tenderness over the patella (no tenderness of bone elsewhere on knee)

Use of these rules was 100% sensitive for detecting fractures and had the potential for decreasing the number of X-rays by 28%.[1]

Meniscal Tears

Meniscal tears can be diagnosed with a history of a valgus force or twisting injury such as may be seen in football, basketball, or ice hockey. Patients often present with a knee swelling, clicking, locking, giving way, or pain along the medial joint line. Physical examination can demonstrate an effusion in addition to either a positive McMurray's or Apley's sign.[2] Unfortunately, a recent meta-analysis revealed that none of the manoeuvres (McMurray, joint line tenderness, joint effusion, Apley compression test) was terribly accurate. The McMurray test was somewhat helpful at ruling in meniscal injury when positive, but was not helpful when negative.[3] Definitive diagnosis is either by MRI or arthroscopy, and the treatment is either by arthroscopic repair or excision.

Ligament Injuries

Posterior cruciate and lateral collateral ligament injuries are less common than injuries to the medial collateral ligament and the anterior cruciate ligament. Again, the mechanisms and presentation are similar to that encountered in meniscal injuries. Medial collateral injuries are best diagnosed by applying a valgus stress to the knee.

A positive is when the movement is excessive compared with the other knee. There would also be point tenderness at the origin of the collateral ligament and/or at the insertion. Anterior cruciate ligament injuries can be diagnosed by either an anterior drawer sign, a lachman sign, or a pivot-shift test.[4] Treatment for isolated collateral ligament injuries is usually immobilization for 6 weeks, whereas anterior curciate ligament injuries may be placed in a sport brace or undergo arthroscopic ligament repair.

Isolated Non-Traumatic Effusions

It is important to keep in mind that isolated non-traumatic effusions of the knee may be due to various different disease states. Osteoarthritis, gout, and psuedogout may be treated with medications, but a septic arthritis (a warm, red, and extremely painful knee joint) would require urgent aspiration for diagnosis and culture as well as treatment with IV antibiotics.

Patellofemoral Pain Syndrome

The patellofemoral pain syndrome is characterized by retropatellar pain and often crepitus, which are brought on by such activities as squatting or going up and down stairs. Adolescents and young adults are most frequently affected. Although the condition has been reported to be more common in individuals with malalignment of the knee-extensor mechanism, trauma, overuse, immobilization, and excessive weight gain, the etiology is unknown. Some patients have demonstrable chondromalacia on arthroscopy but most do not, and many patients with chondromalacia have no pain. The treatment of choice is intensive quadriceps stretching and strengthening exercises. After such a program, two thirds of patients become symptom free within 6 months and maintain this improvement for at least 7 years.[5] Often, custom orthotics to treat forefoot pronation may be of use in chronic patellofemoral pain syndrome.[4] Pain and tenderness inferior to the patella and on the patellar tendon is known as *patellar tendonitis* or "jumper's knee," which can be treated in the same manner.

Osgood-Schlatter Disease

Osgood-Schlatter disease of the tibial tuberosity is the best-known apophyseal disorder in the knee region. A similar phenomenon about the inferior patella is called the *Sindig-Larsen-Johansson syndrome*.[6] These conditions are also sometimes referred to as *traction apophysitis*. The specific etiology of these diseases is unknown, but they are clearly exacerbated by activity with repetitive jumping and pivoting, especially when combined with tight hip flexors, quadriceps, and hamstring muscle groups. This combination is most seen in growing young people between 10 and 18 years of age.

Treatment is rest, ice, strengthening, and possibly orthotics in major pronators.

⚖ REFERENCES ⚖

1. Stiell IG, Greenberg GH, Wells GA, et al: Prospective validation of a decision rule for the use of radiography in acute knee injuries, *JAMA* 275:611-615, 1996.
2. Mellion M, Walsh W, Shelton G: *The team physician's handbook,* Philadelphia, 1990, Hanley and Belfus.
3. Scholten RJ, Deville WL, Opstelten W, et al: The accuracy of physical diagnostic tests for assessing meniscal lesions of the knee, *J Fam Pract* 50:938-944, 2001.
4. Mellion M: *Office management of sports injuries and athletic problems,* Philadelphia, 1988, Henley and Belfus.
5. Kannus P, Natri A, Paakkala T, et al: An outcome study of chronic patellofemoral pain syndrome: seven-year follow-up of patients in a randomized, controlled trial, *J Bone Joint Surg (Am)* 81:355-363, 1999.
6. Peck DM: Apophyseal injuries in the young athlete, *Am Fam Physician* 51:1891-1895, 1995.

ANKLE

The most common injury to the ankle is the "ankle sprain." Most ankle sprains are caused by a forced inversion of the ankle. Inversion can result from stepping on an uneven surface while walking or running. In sports, it usually occurs by landing on someone's foot after jumping. Sports that involve jumping, such as basketball and volleyball, put the athlete at higher risk for sprains. Racquet sports can also cause sprains because of the sudden changes in direction required for the game. The most common ligament to be injured is the anterior talofibular ligament at the lateral side of the joint.[1] The deltoid ligament on the medial side of the ankle joint can be injured in the more severe sprains because it gets pinched during forced inversion. It is important to verify that the Achilles tendon is intact. A ruptured Achilles tendon can be mistaken for a "sprained ankle"[2] and needs to be specifically tested so as not to miss the diagnosis. To test for Achilles tendon integrity, squeeze the gastrocnemius muscle and look for plantar flexion (Thompsons sign), and palpate the tendon too looking for a defect.

Less than 15% of ankle sprains that present to the emergency department have a fracture.[3] To look for a fracture of the ankle, palpate for tenderness over the medial and lateral malleoli, the cuboid and navicular bones, and the base of the fifth metatarsal. Also, palpate for tenderness over the fibular head because it is sometimes fractured during forced inversion.[1] The Ottawa Ankle Rules help assess the need for X-rays of "sprained ankles." The rules state that you should order X-rays if there is pain in the region of either malleolus plus one of the following[4]:

1. Inability to bear weight both immediately after the injury and for four steps in the emergency department

2. Bone tenderness at the tip of either malleolus or over the posterior tibia or fibula in the regions 6 cm proximal to the tips of the malleoli

In a recent systematic review of 15 studies applying these rules to the ankle, the sensitivity was 98% and specificity was 40%.[3]

When treating ankle sprains, try to avoid crutches. Delayed weight bearing in ligamentous injuries can lead to serious delay of recovery and can even promote the debilitating complication of complex regional pain syndrome (reflex sympathetic dystrophy).[5] The initial treatment is the standard PRICE (protection, rest, ice, compression, and elevation). Some studies have demonstrated the best results from no support and minimal bandaging, with early physiotherapy having the same results but higher patient satisfaction.[6] To allow for early weight bearing, the patient can be put in a functional ankle brace that allows for plantar and dorsiflexion but prevents the ankle from inverting. The mainstay of rehabilitation of ankle ligamentous injuries is the retraining of proprioception (balance). Ankle injuries decrease the patient's proprioception, which puts them at a much higher risk for re-injury. Many patients with inversion ankle injuries report having had a similar injury in the not too distant past.[1] Up to 20% of patients will have ankle instability after a lateral inversion injury. A U.S. population survey found that 6 to 18 months after an ankle sprain, 40% of patients reported at least one moderate-to-severe symptom that interfered with long walks, jumping, or pivoting. Few patients had participated in physiotherapy-type rehabilitation programs, which may be one reason for the prolonged duration of symptoms.[7] There is good evidence to support that ankle sprains can be prevented by wearing semi-rigid orthoses or air-cast braces in high-risk sports.[8]

⚖ REFERENCES ⚖

1. Childs S: Acute ankle injury, *Lippincotts Prim Care Pract* 3(4):428-437; quiz 438-440, Jul-Aug 1999.
2. Mazzone MF, McCue T: Common conditions of the Achilles tendon, *Am Fam Physician* 65:1805-1810, 2002.
3. Bachmann LM, Kolb E, Koller MT, et al: Accuracy of Ottawa ankle rules to exclude fractures of the ankle and midfoot: systematic review, *BMJ* 326(7386):417, Feb 22, 2003.
4. Stiell I: Ottawa ankle rules, *Can Fam Physician* 42:478-480, 1996.
5. Mutch P, Grossman VG: A 22-year-old woman with exquisite burning pain 4 weeks after an ankle sprain, *J Emerg Nurs* 27(3):234-237, Jun 2001.
6. Wilson S, Cooke M: Double bandaging of sprained ankles, *BMJ* 317(7174):1722-1723, 19-26 Dec 1998.
7. Braun BL: Effects of ankle sprain in a general clinic population 6 to 18 months after medical evaluation, *Arch Family Med* 8: 143-148, 1999.
8. Handoll HH, Rowe BH, Quinn KM, et al: Interventions for preventing ankle ligament injuries (Cochrane Musculoskeletal Injuries Group). *Cochrane Database of Systematic Reviews,* 2, 2004.

FOOT

Plantar Fasciitis

The plantar fascia is a fibrous aponeurosis, which runs from the medial calcaneus forward to form the longitudinal foot arch. It supports this arch and provides dynamic shock absorption. Plantar fasciitis is a common cause of heel pain in adults, which occurs when there is collagen degeneration at the origin of the plantar fascia. Often, the patient experiences maximal pain on their first steps in the morning, and the pain lessens as the patient warms up. This is often mis-named "heel spurs." These bony osteophytes on the anterior calcaneus occur in up to 25% of the general asymptomatic population and do not occur in many symptomatic individuals. Clinically, there is a point of maximal tenderness at the anteromedial aspect of the calcaneus. This condition is usually self-limiting and lasts 6 to 18 months. However, early treatment is thought to shorten the duration of symptoms. Treatment includes relative rest, stretching, strengthening the intrinsic muscles of the foot, ice, arch supports or orthotics, night splints, anti-inflammatory agents, and if conservative management fails, corticosteroid injections or surgical release of the plantar fascia.[1]

Tendinopathies

Frequently, Achilles tendon disorders cause posterior heel pain. Posterior tibial tendon dysfunction commonly causes painful acquired flatfoot deformity. Peroneal tendinopathies can cause persistent lateral ankle pain and instability. Ultrasound and MRI are helpful in delineating the degree of injury.[2]

Sprains

A midfoot (Lisfranc) strain occurs when the Lisfranc ligament, which runs obliquely from the medial cuneiform to the second metatarsal (MT) base, is injured. Diastasis of the first to second MT joint can occur following a crushing trauma or violent motor vehicle accident. In severe injuries, the base of the second MT may avulse. If there is no diastasis, this can be treated by a non–weight-bearing cast for 4 to 6 weeks. Diastasis greater than 2 mm may require operative treatment.[3]

Turf toe is a sprain of the first metatarsalphalangeal (MTP) joint, occurring when the first MTP is forced into hyperextension. Patients with the less severe sprains may return to sports participation with taping; more severe sprains may require brief periods of cast immobilization.[3]

Foot Fractures

The Ottawa Ankle Rules have been established to assist in determining which patients with foot trauma require X-rays. A foot X-ray series is only required if the patient has some pain in the midfoot *and* bone tenderness at the base of the fifth MT *or* bone tenderness at the navicular *or* an inability to bear weight both immediately and in the emergency department.[4] A recent review of 10 studies of the Ottawa Ankle Rules found a pooled sensitivity of 99% for foot fractures and specificity of 38%. The application of these rules missed less than 2% of fractures in most of the studies.[5] The specificity is even lower in children; therefore, these rules cannot be as readily applied to patients younger than 18 years.[6] The rules may not be reliable in instances in which patient assessment is difficult: intoxication, head injury, multiple painful injuries, or diminished sensation due to neurological deficit. Patients should always be instructed to seek follow-up if pain or ability to bear weight has not improved in 5 to 7 days.

Fifth MT fractures may be divided into three types:
1. Avulsion of the tuberosity
2. Jones fracture (distal to the tuberosity but proximal to the metaphyseal-diaphyseal junction)
3. Diaphyseal stress fracture

The first is the most common and is usually caused when an acute inversion injury avulses the peroneus brevis tendon from the tuberosity of the fifth MT. This usually resolves after a short period of immobilization. The latter two types require 6 to 10 weeks of non-weight-bearing rest and may require surgical fixation.[2,3]

A stress fracture can be defined as a partial or complete bone fracture that results from repeated stress lower than the stress required to fracture the bone in a single loading.[3] Specific sports will frequently have different sites of stress fractures: for example, the navicular in track athletes, and the metatarsal bones in dancers. Non-critical stress fractures in the foot include the second, third, and fourth metatarsals and may be treated with relative rest and possibly short periods of immobilization. Critical foot stress fractures include the talus, navicular, fifth MT and sesamoids and may require more aggressive immobilization or surgery due to a higher rate of non-union.[2]

Freiberg's Disease

Freiberg's disease is an osteochondritis of bone involving the distal portion of one of the metatarsals. It is seen most often in girls between the ages of 12 and 15. Two thirds of the cases involve the second MT, most of the remainder the third, and about 5% of cases involve the fourth MT. Patients have pain, swelling, and tenderness, and the X-ray picture is typical. Treatment involves metatarsal pads or orthotics to decrease weight bearing on the area.[7]

Sever's Disease

Sever's disease is a traction apophysitis of the posterior calcaneus and is thus similar to Osgood-Schlatter disease of the knee. The disease usually affects girls between the ages of 8 and 10 and boys between 10 and 12 years. The patients complain of unilateral or bilateral heel pain that comes after weight bearing and often after starting a new sport. They usually have no pain on arising in the morning, and the pain, when present, is relieved by rest. On examination there may be tenderness both over the posterior insertion of the Achilles tendon to the calcaneus and along the medial and lateral borders of the calcaneus near its posterior border, which is the line of junction of the posterior epiphysis of the calcaneus and the body of the calcaneus. The manoeuvre that reveals this pain is called the *squeeze test*. Initial treatment is ice, rest, and heel lifts. These treatments are followed by heel cord, calf, and hamstring stretching exercises, as well as ankle dorsiflexion strengthening exercises. Sever's disease is not associated with long-term sequelae.[8]

◢ REFERENCES ◣

1. Young CC: Treatment of plantar fasciitis, *Am Fam Physician* 63(3):467-474, 477-478, 1 Feb 2001.
2. Wilder R: Overuse injuries: tendinopathies, stress fractures, compartment syndrome, and shin splints, *Clin Sports Med* 23(1):55, Jan 2004.
3. Title CI: Traumatic foot and ankle injuries in the athlete, *Orthop Clin North Am* 33(3):587-598, Jul 2002.
4. Stiell IG, Greenberg GH, McKnight RD, et al: Decision rules for the use of radiography in acute ankle injuries: refinement and prospective validation, *JAMA* 269:1127-1132, 1993.
5. Bachmann LM, Kolb E, Koller MT, et al: Accuracy of Ottawa ankle rules to exclude fractures of the ankle and mid-foot: systematic review *BMJ* 326(7386):417, 22 Feb 2003.
6. Clark KD, Tanner S: Evaluation of the Ottawa ankle rules in children, *Pediatr Emerg Care* 19(2):73-78, Apr 2003.
7. Griffin LY: Common sports injuries of the foot and ankle seen in children and adolescents, *Orthop Clin North Am* 25:83-93, 1994.
8. Madden CC, Mellion MB: Sever's disease and other causes of heel pain in adolescents, *Am Fam Physician* 54:1995-2000, 1996.

STRESS FRACTURES

Most stress fractures occur in the lower extremities, most commonly at the necks of the second and third MTs.[1] They generally occur as a result of a repetitive use injury that exceeds the intrinsic ability of the bone to repair itself.[2] In athletes, the tibia and tarsal bones head the list, followed by the MTs and shaft of the femur. Any portion of the tibia may be involved, while most stress fractures of the femur involve the upper shaft, with a small percentage occurring in the femoral neck.[3] Women are more likely to develop stress fractures than are men, and an incidence of 49% has been reported in oligomenorrheic runners.[3] A change in exercise pattern or training often precedes the onset of symptoms by a few weeks.[1] Stress fractures are rare in children.[4] Stress fractures can result

from participation in many activities and sports, especially those requiring running and jumping.

Pain is the complaint of patients with stress fractures. Initially, pain arises after physical activity or late during the activity, but as the condition worsens, it begins earlier. There may be some swelling, but point tenderness is the most common physical finding. The usual symptom of a femoral neck stress fracture is groin pain with exercise. Physical examination may reveal pain or limitation of motion on internal rotation of the hip. Making the correct diagnosis and obtaining appropriate consultations are important because of the high rate of progression to complete femoral neck fractures.[3] X-rays usually fail to reveal the lesions early in the course of the disease and are often normal even after several weeks or months. Repeat X-rays obtained during the convalescent phase reveal the fracture in approximately 50% of cases. The gold standard for making a specific diagnosis is the bone scan, which can be positive within a few days of the onset of symptoms; however, the specificity of this test is relatively low.[1] MRI can also be useful.[2]

Management of stress fractures involves rest, pain control, and exercises to prevent deconditioning. These are followed by gradual reintroduction of the causative exercise activity.[1] Pneumatic casts may be helpful in allowing for mobility and earlier resumption of activity.[5] A Cochrane Review involving four trials suggested that the use of shock-absorbing insoles may prevent stress fractures and stress reactions of the lower extremities.[5]

◢ REFERENCES ◣

1. Monteleone GP Jr: Stress fractures in the athlete, *Orthop Clin North Am* 26:423-432, 1995.
2. Sanderlin BW: Common stress fractures, *Am Fam Physician* 68(8):1527-1532, 2003.
3. Boden BP, Speer KP: Femoral stress fractures, *Clin Sports Med* 16:307-317, 1997.
4. Griffin LY: Common sports injuries of the foot and ankle seen in children and adolescents, *Orthop Clin North Am* 25:83-93, 1994.
5. Gillespie WJ, Grant I: Interventions for preventing and treating stress fractures and stress reactions of bone of the lower limbs in young adults (Cochrane Review). In: *The Cochrane Library*, issue 2, Chichester, UK, 2004, John Wiley.

EXERCISE

Exercise Guidelines

Traditional exercise prescriptions

Exercise should be prescribed and monitored as any intervention with appropriate screening, dosage, and instructions to the patient. The Par Q Readiness screening form is a user-friendly patient tool that is available from the Health Canada Physical Activity Unit at http://www.hc-sc.gc.ca/hppb/fitness/questionnaire.html.

Target heart rates can be used as general guidance:

Healthy individuals	70%-85% of 220 – Age
Cardiovascular-compromised individuals	50%-70% of 220 – Age

The exercise prescription for healthy adults is:

Frequency	3-5 times a week
Intensity	Sweat on your Brow, Talk Test or Heart Rate at 70% of 220–Age.
Time	30-60 minutes
Type	Aerobic

Some of the major recommendations of the 1996 NIH Consensus Conference on exercise are as follows[1]:

1. Children and adults should attempt to accumulate 30 minutes of moderate-intensity exercise on most and preferably all days of the week.
2. Several brief bouts of moderate activity are beneficial.
3. Types of exercise that are classified as moderate activity include many occupational functions or activities of daily living, as well as leisure-time activity: brisk walking, cycling, swimming, home repair, and yard work.

Persons already meeting these recommendations may gain further benefits through more exercise.

Exercise reduces all-cause mortality and cardiovascular mortality in patients with known cardiovascular disease. Patients with these conditions should participate in appropriately prescribed and supervised exercise training programs.

≈ REFERENCES ≈

1. Physical activity and cardiovascular health: NIH Consensus Development Panel on Physical Activity and Cardiovascular Health, *JAMA* 276:241-246, 1996.

Epidemiology of Physical Activity

Physical Activity is studied by many national governments as an indicator of health. The Canadian Fitness and Lifestyle Research Institute (*www.cflri.ca*) produces comparison statistics on all sectors of the population. The January 2004 twenty-year trend survey concluded that although Canadians are more active now than 20 years ago, two thirds still do not accumulate the recommended 60 minutes a day or 10,000 steps per day.[1] The numbers are similar for the United States, with more than 60% of adults not achieving the recommended amounts of physical activity. Inactivity increases with age and is more common among women and those with lower income and less education.[2] In Britain, the average annual walking distance has decreased by 22% in the last third of the twentieth century, largely because of increased car travel; one fourth of all car trips are shorter than 3.2 km (2 miles). In 1972, 12% of children were driven to school; by 1994, the figure was 23%.[3]

≈ REFERENCES ≈

1. Canadian Fitness and Lifestyle Research Institute: Twenty year trends of physical activity among Canadian adults. (Accessed on May 13, 2004 at http://www.cflri.ca/cflri/news/2004/0401b_1.html).
2. Physical Activity and Health, A Report of the Surgeon General United States (Accessed on May 13, 2004 at http://www.cdc.gov/nccdphp/sgr/ataglan.htm).
3. Roberts I: Reducing road traffic: would improve quality of life as well as preventing injury (editorial), *BMJ* 316:242-243, 1998.

Aerobic Exercise Equivalencies

(See also nutrition)

The energy consumed by aerobic exercise depends on the individual's weight and the type of exercise. Compared with brisk walking (7.5 km/h) (4.5 mi/h), swimming at 20 metres (or yards) per minute consumes one third less energy, bicycling at 21 km/h (13 mi/h) one third more, and cross-country skiing or jogging at 13 km/h (8 mi/h) a little more than twice as much.[1] In a study using healthy volunteers on six pieces of indoor exercise equipment, the most energy was expended with the treadmill and the least with the Airdyne and cycle.[2] The use of a pedometer is an inexpensive, accurate manner of assessing one's physical activity levels, including the estimated output of caloric energy.[3]

≈ REFERENCES ≈

1. An amble a day, *Consum Rep* 58(7):421, July 1993.
2. Zeni AI, Hoffman MD, Clifford PS: Energy expenditure with indoor exercise machines, *JAMA* 275:1424-1427, 1996.
3. Tudor-Locke C, Williams JE, Reis JP, et al: Utility of pedometers for assessing physical activity; construct validity, *Sports Med* 34(5):281-291, 2004.

Benefits of Exercise

Exercise as a protection against all-cause mortality

A study of both sexes by Blair and associates[1] with a mean follow-up period of 8.4 years found that moderate fitness as measured by maximal exercise testing was associated with decreased mortality regardless of whether the individuals were healthy, smokers, obese, hypercholesterolemic, or hypertensive or had strong family histories of coronary artery disease. The Harvard Alumni Study has also shown that an increase in physical activity reduces mortality.[2] The degree of benefit correlated with the total increase in energy expenditure per week.[2] A more recent report from the Harvard Alumni Study concluded that vigorous activities, but not non-vigorous activities, were associated with longevity. It is important to realize that the term "vigorous" included not only running, jogging, swimming laps, playing tennis, and shovelling snow, but also brisk walking. The Iowa Women's Health Study documented decreased mortality in post-menopausal women participating in moderate activity,[3] and the Framingham Study found that current or recent physical activity decreased mortality rates in both men and women.[4] Observational studies such as those discussed above clearly show that people who exercise have decreased mortality rates. This difference is not due merely to the fact that healthy people are more likely to exercise; studies have shown that even small improvements in physical fitness over time decrease the risk of death.[5] Physically active people have been shown to have a decreased rate of all-cancer mortality. The incidence of colon, breast, and perhaps prostate cancer are decreased in more active people when compared with their sedentary peers, which may be mediated by effect on natural immunity and antioxidant defenses.[6]

❧ REFERENCES ❧

1. Blair SN, Kampert JB, Kohl HW III, et al: Influences of cardiorespiratory fitness and other precursors on cardiovascular disease and all-cause mortality in men and women, *JAMA* 276:205-210, 1996.
2. Paffenbarger RS Jr, Kampert JB, Lee I-M, et al: Changes in physical activity and other lifeway patterns influencing longevity, *Med Sci Sports Exerc* 26:857-865, 1994.
3. Kushi LH, Fee RM, Folsom AR, et al: Physical activity and mortality in postmenopausal women, *JAMA* 277:1287-1292, 1997.
4. Sherman SE, D'Agostino RB, Silbershatz H, et al: Comparison of past versus recent physical activity in the prevention of premature death and coronary artery disease, *Am Heart J* 138:900-907, 1999.
5. Erikssen G, Liestøl K, Bjørnholt J, et al: Changes in physical fitness and changes in mortality, *Lancet* 352:759-762, 1998.
6. Friedenreich CM, Orenstein MR: Physical activity and cancer prevention: etiological evidence and biological mechanisms, *J Nutr* 132(11 suppl):3456s-3464s, Nov 2002.

Exercise as a protection against coronary artery disease

Protection against coronary artery disease is probably the most important health gain from exercise programs. Numerous studies have demonstrated this benefit in the prevention of both first-time events[1-4] and recurrences of myocardial infarction.[5] Results of the Harvard Alumni Study indicate that the quantitative benefit of exercise in reducing coronary artery mortality is as great as avoiding obesity, achieving good blood pressure control, or stopping smoking.[2]

A recent review of the literature in *Canadian Family Physician* concluded that moderate physical activity such as brisk walking for 30 to 60 minutes a day on most days of the week is associated with significant reduction in the incidence and mortality of cardiovascular disease.[6] Although most exercise plans involve structured programs, lifestyle counselling leading to individualized programs has been found equally effective over the short term in reducing such risk factors as lipid levels and blood pressure. Some of the innovations that were developed include wearing a headset with a long cord while walking about during conference calls, scheduling 10-minute walking breaks at regular intervals throughout the day, or walking briskly around play areas while supervising children.[7]

Relatively few studies have evaluated the cardioprotective effects of exercise in women; those that have been done showed a significant decrease in the risk of coronary events.[3,8] For example, the Nurses' Health Study found that 3 hours of brisk walking per week was as beneficial as more vigorous exercise and led to a 30% to 40% reduction in the risk of coronary events, compared with sedentary women.[8] Few studies have evaluated the effect of exercise in smokers, but a Swedish prospective study found that vigorous physical activity decreased cardiovascular mortality in smokers by almost 40%.[9]

❧ REFERENCES ❧

1. Hakim AA, Petrovitch H, Burchfiel CM, et al: Effects of walking on mortality among nonsmoking retired men, *N Engl J Med* 338:94-99, 1998.
2. Paffenbarger RS Jr, Hyde RT, Wing AL, et al: The association of changes in physical-activity level and other lifestyle characteristics with mortality among men, *N Engl J Med* 328:538-545, 1993.
3. Kushi LH, Fee RM, Folsom AR, et al: Physical activity and mortality in postmenopausal women, *JAMA* 277:1287-1292, 1997.
4. Wannamethee SG, Shaper AG, Walker M: Changes in physical activity, mortality, and incidence of coronary heart disease in older men, *Lancet* 351:1603-1608, 1998.
5. Oldridge NB, Guyatt GH, Fischer ME, et al: Cardiac rehabilitation after myocardial infarction: combined experience of randomized clinical trials, *JAMA* 260:945-950, 1988.
6. Haennel RG, Lemire F: Physical activity to prevent cardiovascular disease, *Can Fam Physician* 48:65-71, Jan 2002.
7. Dunn AL, Marcus BH, Kampert JB, et al: Reduction in cardiovascular disease risk factors: 6-month results from Project Active, *Prev Med* 26:883-892, 1997.
8. Manson JE, Hu FB, Rich-Edwards JW, et al: A prospective study of walking as compared with vigorous exercise in the prevention of coronary artery disease in women, *N Engl J Med* 341:650-658, 1999.
9. Hedblad B, Ogren M, Isacsson SO, et al: Reduced cardiovascular mortality risk in male smokers who are physically active: results from a 25-year follow-up of the Prospective Population Study Men Born in 1914, *Arch Intern Med* 157:893-899, 1997.

Exercise as a protection against stroke

Two prospective observational studies published in 1999 documented a decreased risk of stroke in men over age 40 or 45 who exercised.[1,2] The Physicians' Health Study assessed only exercise that was vigorous enough to "work up a sweat," and found that those who exercised the most at baseline had the lowest risk of both ischemic and hemorrhagic strokes.[1] An Icelandic study found that moderate exercise such as walking and swimming was associated with a decreased risk of ischemic strokes.[2]

REFERENCES

1. Lee I-M, Hennekens CH, Berger K, et al: Exercise and risk of stroke in male physicians, *Stroke* 30:1-6, 1999.
2. Agnarsson U, Thorgeirsson G, Sigvaldason H, et al: Effects of leisure-time physical activity and ventilatory function on risk for stroke in men: the Reykjavík Study, *Ann Intern Med* 130: 987-990, 1999.

Exercise as a protection against hypertension

The 2003 Recommendations for the Management of Hypertension include exercise as an adjunct therapy requiring 50 to 60 minutes of moderate physical activity at a frequency of 3 to 4 times a week.[1]

REFERENCES

1. Canadian Hypertension Society: 2003 Recommendations for the Management of Hypertension, *www.gacguidelines.ca*

Exercise as a protection against type 2 diabetes mellitus

A follow-up study of male alumni from the University of Pennsylvania found a significant protective effect of exercise against the development of type 2 diabetes.[1] The incidence was much lower in the most physically active compared with the least active, and a significant difference remained even after correction for obesity. The greatest protection was noted for men at highest risk for the disease because of obesity, hypertension, and a family history of diabetes.[1] Aside from a decrease in the level of obesity, the mechanism of protection is probably an increased insulin sensitivity induced by the exercise.[2] Recent randomized controlled trials in patients with impaired glucose tolerance have shown that activity (25 minutes a day, 6 days a week) combined with decreased saturated fat intake, weight loss of 5% to 7%, and increased fibre intake, can delay and possibly prevent the development of diabetes by 42% to 58%.[3]

REFERENCES

1. Helmrich SP, Ragland DR, Leung RW, et al: Physical activity and reduced occurrence of non-insulin-dependent diabetes mellitus, *N Engl J Med* 325:147-152, 1991.
2. Horton ES: Exercise and decreased risk of NIDDM (editorial), *N Engl J Med* 325:196-198, 1991.
3. Harris SB, Petrella RJ, Leadbetter W: Lifestyle interventions for type 2 diabetes: relevance for clinical practice, *Can Fam Physician* 49:1618-1625, 2003.

Exercise as a protection against osteoporosis

The Canadian Consensus on Osteoporosis recommends that adequate daily exercise is a component of healthy bone maintainance.[1] Impact and weight resistance exercise have both been found to decrease bone loss in pre-menopausal and post-menopausal women in various studies. Impact exercise includes some form of running, skipping, jumping, or aerobics. Walking is not enough to induce bone density advancement.[2] General conditioning such as walking, tai chi, and strengthening have been shown to be effective fall prevention.[1] Exercise is important during adolescence, when both boys and girls are building their peak bone density.[3] In both men and women, excessive physical activity can be detrimental to bone health.[4,5]

REFERENCES

1. Society of Obstetricians and Gynecologists of Canada: Canadian Consensus on Osteoporosis, 2003, *Can Fam Physician* 49:487, Apr 2003.
2. Osteoporosis Society of Canada (2002):Clinical practice guidelines for the diagnosis and management of osteoporosis in Canada, *Can Med Assoc J* 167(10 suppl): Nov 2002.
3. Petit MA, MacKay HA, MacKelvie KJ et al: A randomized school-based jumping intervention confers site and maturity benefits on bone structural properties in girls, *J Bone Mineral Res* 17:834-844, 2002.
4. Bilanin JE, Blanchard MS, Russek-Cohen E: Lower vertebral bone density in male long distance runners, *Med Sci Sports and Exer* 21:66-70, 1989.
5. National Institute of Health. Osteoporosis prevention, diagnosis, and therapy [NIH Consensus Statement, 2000]. NIH Consensus Development Conference on Osteoporosis Prevention, Diagnosis, and Therapy; Mar 27-29, 2000(1):1-45

Exercise as a protection against colon cancer

In a review of epidemiological studies, the data clearly indicates that physically active men and women have a 30% to 40% reduction in their risk of developing colon cancer as compared with their inactive counterparts.[1]

A possible explanation of this finding is that exercise decreases intestinal transit time and so diminishes exposure of the colonic mucosa to fecal carcinogens.

REFERENCES

1. Lee IM: Physical activity and cancer prevention, *Med Sci Sport Exer* 35(11):1823-1827, Nov 2003.

Exercise as a protection against anxiety and depression

Evidence supports the role of exercise as a protective factor against or therapeutic agent for anxiety and depression.[1-4]

REFERENCES

1. King AC, Taylor CB, Haskell WL, et al: Influence of regular aerobic exercise on psychological health, *Health Psychol* 8:305-324, 1989.
2. Taylor CB, Sallis JF, Needle R: The relationship of physical activity and exercise to mental health, *Public Health Rep* 100:195-201, 1995.

3. Martinsen EW: Physical activity and depression: clinical experience, *Acta Psychiatr Scand* 377(suppl):23-27, 1994.

4. Byrne A, Byrne DG: The effect of exercise on depression, anxiety and other mood states: a review, *J Psychosom Res* 37:565-574, 1993.

Exercise in the Elderly
(See also geriatrics)

In a study on physical activity and 10-year mortality rates, men ages 64 to 84 who participated in moderate exercise such as walking or bicycling for 20 minutes a day, three times a week, were found to have lower all-cause and cardiovascular mortality than more sedentary control subjects.[1]

A study from the Hebrew Rehabilitation Center for the Aged in Roslindale, Massachusetts, has demonstrated a dramatic effect of resistance exercises in improving the mobility of the very elderly. The patients who were evaluated were residents of a nursing home. All were over 70 years of age, 38% were over 90 years of age, and the mean age was 87. The resisted exercise group underwent a regimen of high-intensity progressive resistance training of the hip and knee extensors lasting 45 minutes, three times a week, for 10 weeks. Muscle strength and mass increased significantly, but more important, the exercise intervention increased the habitual gait velocity, improved the ability to climb stairs, and produced an overall increase in physical activity. The authors postulated that the failure of some other studies to show benefits in nursing home residents given endurance training (in contrast to resistance training) was because the patients had insufficient muscle strength to benefit from it.[2]

For the ambulatory elderly, Shephard[3] recommends endurance exercises plus eight to ten repetitions or resistance exercises twice a week for each set of major muscle groups. The degree of resistance should be enough to induce slight fatigue by the tenth repetition. The goal of such exercises is to maintain lean muscle mass.

≥ REFERENCES ≤

1. Bijnen FC, Caspersen CJ, Feskens EJ, et al: Physical activity and 10-year mortality from cardiovascular diseases and all causes: the Zutphen Elderly Study, *Arch Intern Med* 158:1499-1505, 1998.

2. Fiatarone MA, O'Neill EF, Ryan ND, et al: Exercise training and nutritional supplementation for physical frailty in very elderly people, *N Engl J Med* 330:1769-1775, 1994.

3. Shephard RJ: Physical activity, fitness and cardiovascular health: a brief counselling guide for older patients, *Can Med Assoc J* 151:557-561, 1994.

Risks of Exercise
(See also benefits of exercise; cardiac arrest; cardiopulmonary resuscitation; diarrhea and hematochezia in runners; exercise-induced hematuria; female athletes; pre-participation medical examinations; urinalysis-blood)

Although exercise is clearly beneficial, it does entail a number of risks, the most common of which are probably musculoskeletal problems. These are most likely to occur with high-intensity exercise.[1] Other important adverse effects in women come about when weight loss from the exercise is of such degree as to induce amenorrhea. This is associated with osteoporosis and an increased risk of infertility.[1] Cultural pressures on women athletes may also foster the so-called female athlete triad of disordered eating, amenorrhea, and osteoporosis.[2]

The relative risk of myocardial infarction during vigorous exercise (6 METS [metabolic equivalents of oxygen consumption]) is increased in sedentary individuals but not in physically active ones.[3,4] About 5% of myocardial infarctions are associated with heavy exercise. The mechanism is uncertain. Platelets are activated with exercise in sedentary individuals but not in those who are regularly physically active. Regular exercise increases the endogenous fibrinolytic system.[3] Vigorous exercise also alters mechanical forces on coronary arteries and may lead to plaque rupture.[4]

The risk of having cardiac events during exercise is 10 times greater in individuals with cardiovascular disease than in those without it. Therefore screening for cardiovascular disease before an exercise program is often recommended. Risk can be assessed by a short self-administered questionnaire such as the Revised Physical Activity Readiness Questionnaire (PAR-Q). If the answers to the questionnaire fail to raise any concern, no limitations to physical activity are needed; in all other cases further medical evaluation is indicated. For patients with heart disease, exercise prescriptions are based on a combination of clinical findings and the results of exercise tests. In general, patients are advised to monitor their heart rates and not to exceed the levels at which abnormalities were detected during the exercise tests.[5]

≥ REFERENCES ≤

1. Manson JE, Lee I-M: Exercise for women–how much pain for optimal gain? (editorial), *N Engl J Med* 334:1325-1327, 1996.

2. Nattiv A, Agostini R, Drinkwater B, et al: The female athlete triad: the inter-relatedness of disordered eating, amenorrhea, and osteoporosis, *Clin Sports Med* 13:405-418, 1994.

3. Curfman G: Is exercise beneficial—or hazardous—to your heart? (editorial), *N Engl J Med* 329:730-731, 1993.

4. Giri S, Thompson PD, Kiernan FJ, et al: Clinical and angiographic characteristics of exertion-related acute myocardial infarction, *JAMA* 282:1731-1736, 1999.

5. Balady GJ, Chaitman B, Driscoll D, et al (American Heart Association/American College of Sports Medicine): Recommendations for cardiovascular screening, staffing, and emergency policies at health/fitness facilities, *Circulation* 97:2283-2293, 1998.

UROLOGY

BLADDER AND URETHRA
Acute Urinary Retention

Acute urinary retention is caused by urethral obstruction, damage to the spine or peripheral nerves, or distention of the bladder by other causes. Factors associated with acute urinary retention include alcohol consumption; medications such as sedatives, antipsychotics, anticholinergics, antihistamines, and analgesics; prolonged delay in urination; long periods of inactivity or bedrest; excessive exposure to cold temperatures; spinal cord injury/nerve damage; complications of surgery and anesthesia; urinary system obstruction (e.g., benign prostatic hyperplasia [BPH], kidney stones); and urinary tract infection.[1]

Elderly men are at greatest risk because of BPH; the chance of suffering acute retention within 5 years is 1 in 10 for men in their seventies and 1 in 3 for men in their eighties. The immediate management of acute urinary retention in elderly men is catheterization. After a variable period of catheterization, some men may be able to void spontaneously, although the recurrence rate of acute retention is reported to be 50% within a week and 68% within a year. Ability to void after removal of the catheter is more likely if the catheter has been left in place for a week and if the man has taken an α-adrenergic blocker (such as terazosin [Hytrin]) while catheterized.[2] Acute urinary retention in younger people or women of any age requires careful investigation.

≈ REFERENCES ≈

1. Acute Urinary Retention from Urology Channel. (Accessed on April 29, 2004 at http://www.urologychannel.com/emergencies/index.shtml#acute).
2. Emberton M, Anson K: Acute urinary retention in men: an age-old problem, *BMJ* 318:921-925, 1999.

Bladder Cancer
(See also hematuria; urinalysis)

Bladder cancer is the fourth most common cancer in men and is associated with carcinogens in the urine. The two major risk factors are cigarette smoking, which contributes to more than 50% of cases (smoking cigars or pipes also increases the risk), and occupational carcinogen exposure. Other risk factors include age, male sex, chronic cystitis or stones, diet high in saturated fat, genetic factors, parasitic infections, and exposure to second-hand smoke, drugs and herbs, and radiation.[1] A prospective epidemiological study of male health professionals found that a high intake of fluids was associated with a decreased risk of bladder cancer.[2] In addition, infections, dysuria, workplace reactions, and several genetic factors contribute to risk. The primary symptoms of bladder cancer are painless gross or microscopic hematuria, urinary frequency, and dysuria.[3]

Diagnosis is usually based on flexible cystoscopy and biopsy. In 80% of cases, the tumour is confined to the mucosa (superficial tumours), while 20% are invasive. The prognosis of superficial tumours is excellent. They are usually treated with transurethral resection followed by the instillation of chemotherapeutic drugs or bacille Calmette Guerin (BCG) into the bladder. Adjuvant therapy prolongs disease-free intervals but does not prevent invasion. Invasive tumours are highly malignant and are generally treated with cystectomy, often with adjuvant chemotherapy or radiation therapy. The 5-year survival with invasive tumours is 50%.[3]

≈ REFERENCES ≈

1. What You Need To Know About™ Bladder Cancer, NIH Publication No. 01-1559, 2002.
2. Michaud DS, Spiegelman D, Clinton SK, et al: Fluid intake and the risk of bladder cancer in men, *N Engl J Med* 340:1390-1397, 1999.
3. van der Meijden AP: Bladder cancer, *BMJ* 317:1366-1369, 1998.

Catheters, Urethral
(See also urinalysis; bacteriuria and pyuria in the elderly; urinary tract infections)

Permanent indwelling Silastic catheters are usually changed every 3 to 12 weeks. Bacteriuria develops in virtually all patients with long-term urinary catheters,[1,2] but despite this, changing the catheter almost never leads to sepsis.[1] Complications associated with long-term indwelling catheters include obstruction by encrustations, bladder and kidney stones, pyelonephritis, renal failure, bacteremia, and bladder cancer.[2,3] Options to long-term urethral catheterization are intermittent self-catheterization, which can be performed with a clean but non-sterile technique, suprapubic catheterization,[4] and condom catheters. Intermittent self-catheterization is effective and has few adverse effects. Condom catheters have on rare occasion been responsible for penile ulceration, necrosis, and gangrene,[2] but the major concern about these devices stems from a report that the incidence of urinary tract infections (UTIs) was greater in patients using condom catheters than in those with indwelling catheters.[5] The validity of this report has been questioned in large part because the diagnosis of UTIs was based on cultures, and unless special precautions are taken, cultures of urine obtained from condom devices are likely to have a high false-positive rate because of the growth of organisms on the penile skin.[3] Earlier studies of men in nursing homes found that the incidence of clinical UTIs was 2.5 times greater in those with indwelling catheters than in control subjects using condom catheters.[6]

The Canadian Task Force on Preventive Health Care gives an "E" rating to screening and treatment of asymptomatic bacteriuria in patients with indwelling catheters.[7]

◁ REFERENCES ▷

1. Bregenzer T, Frei R, Widmer AF, et al: Low risk of bacteremia during catheter replacement in patients with long-term urinary catheters, *Arch Intern Med* 157:521-525, 1997.
2. Stickler DJ, Zimakoff J: Complications of urinary tract infections associated with devices used for long-term bladder management, *J Hosp Infect* 28:177-194, 1994.
3. Warren JW: Urethral catheters, condom catheters, and nosocomial urinary tract infections (editorial), *Infect Control Hosp Epidemiol* 17:212-214, 1996.
4. Cravens DD, Zweig S: Urinary catheter management: *Am Fam Physician* 61(2):369-376, 2000.
5. Zimakoff J, Stickler DJ, Pontoppidan B, et al: Bladder management and urinary tract infections in Danish hospitals, nursing homes and home care: a national prevalence study, *Infect Control Hosp Epidemiol* 17:215-221, 1996.
6. Ouslander JG, Greengold B, Chen S: Complications of chronic indwelling urinary catheters among male nursing home patients: a prospective study, *J Urol* 138:1191-1195, 1987.
7. Canadian Task Force on the Periodic Health Examination: *Canadian guide to clinical preventive health care,* Ottawa, 1994, Canada Communication Group, 966-967.

Interstitial Cystitis

Interstitial cystitis is a disease of unknown etiology and uncertain management. It usually affects middle-age women and is characterized by urinary frequency (more than eight times during the day and twice at night), urgency, and perineal, suprapubic, or pelvic pain that is relieved in part by voiding. The diagnosis of interstitial cystitis is a diagnosis of exclusion. There are no specific findings on bladder biopsy.[1,2] There is very little evidence to guide treatment except for conservative supportive therapy with therapy trials including diet modification and oral treatment with pentosan polysulfate (Elmiron) 100 mg twice daily, amitriptyline, or hydroxyzine. Some patients go on to intravesical treatments with heparin-like medications, dimethyl sulfoxide, or BCG.[2-4]

◁ REFERENCES ▷

1. Keller MS, McCarthy DO, Neider RS: Measurement of symptoms of interstitial cystitis: a pilot study, *Urol Clin North Am* 21:67-71, 1994.
2. Thompson AC, Christmas TJ: Interstitial cystitis—an update, *Br J Urol* 78:813-820, 1996.
3. Wein AJ, Hanno P: Introduction: Interstitial cystitis: an update of the current information, *Urology* 49(5A, suppl1):1, 1997.
4. Nickel JC: Interstitial cystitis, *Can Fam Physician* 46(12):2430-2434, 2437-2440, Dec 2000.

INCONTINENCE

(See also geriatrics)

Classification

Urinary incontinence may be classified as transient or persistent.[1]

Transient urinary incontinence

Acute or transient incontinence is caused by a new, treatable medical condition. In a survey of Canadian family physicians, less than half (46.0%, 284/617) indicated that they clearly understood incontinence, and just 37.9% (232/612) had an organized plan for incontinence problems.[2]

The following are important causes of transient incontinence[1]:

1. Delirium
2. Urinary tract infections (not asymptomatic bacteriuria)
3. Atrophic urethritis and vaginitis
4. Medications, especially polypharmacy (sedatives, hypnotics, anticholinergics such as antipsychotics and tricyclic antidepressants, narcotics, α-adrenergic antagonists, dihydropyridine calcium channel blockers, diuretics)
5. Excess urine output (such as from diabetes)
6. Restricted mobility
7. Fecal impaction

A useful mnemonic device to remember the acute causes is "DIAPPERS": *D*elirium, *I*nfection, *A*trophic, *P*sychological, *P*olypharmacy, *E*ndocrine, *R*estricted, and *S*tool.

Persistent urinary incontinence

The two most common causes of persistent urinary incontinence are stress incontinence and detrusor overactivity (detrusor instability, detrusor hyperreactivity, urge incontinence).[2] Although overflow incontinence accounts for only 5% to 10% of cases of urinary incontinence, it should be ruled out in all cases.[1,3]

Stress incontinence. Stress incontinence is one of the major forms of incontinence in women, and its diagnosis can often be made with reasonable certainty on the basis of the history.[1] If the patient is mentally competent and denies that incontinence occurs instantaneously with a stress manoeuvre, the diagnosis of stress incontinence can be ruled out with 90% certainty.[1] An important aggravating factor in some cases of stress incontinence is the treatment of hypertension with α-adrenergic blockers such as terazosin (Hytrin), doxazosin (Cardura), labetalol (Trandate), methyldopa (Aldomet), and clonidine (Catapres). These drugs, now uncommonly used with women, inhibit the α-adrenergic receptors of the internal sphincter, which stimulate the sphincter's closure. If possible they should be discontinued.[3]

Specific management of stress incontinence may involve behavioural techniques, pharmacological agents, or a combination of the two. A standard behavioural technique is pelvic muscle-strengthening exercises, an approach first described by Kegel in 1948. A 1999 study of women with stress incontinence compared a group that performed pelvic muscle exercises three times a day with a non-exercising control group. Each exercise session consisted of near-maximum contraction of the pelvic muscles held for 6 to 8 seconds and repeated up to 12 times with 6 seconds of rest between contractions. Marked improvement in incontinence was observed in the exercising group.[4] A report on elderly women with stress incontinence found that 75% became continent when they followed this procedure.[5] Contracting the pelvic floor muscles beginning 1 second before coughing has also been reported effective when studied in a clinic setting.[6] Reassurance is important as it can take over 6 weeks for effect.

First-line pharmacological treatment for stress incontinence is probably estrogen, both topical and oral.[3] These should be given in the usual doses for hormonal replacement therapy, and, when indicated, progestins should be added. Beneficial effects may be delayed for several weeks. Estrogen acts by thickening the mucosa of the urethra and trigone and also seems to increase the sensitivity and numbers of α-adrenergic receptors, which supply and cause contraction of the internal urethral sphincter.[3] Topical application of estrogen also appears to be effective when applied regularly to the area.

However, beneficial effects have not been found in all studies. A randomized, double-blind, placebo-controlled study found no improvement when a group of postmenopausal women with stress incontinence, detrusor instability, or both were treated with equine estrogens (Premarin) 0.625 mg and medroxyprogesterone (Provera) 10 mg given cyclically over 3 months.[7] One needs to make the patient aware of the relevant risks and benefits of using HRT.

Detrusor overactivity. Detrusor overactivity or urge incontinence is characterized by the sudden onset of an intense desire to void or even a sudden gush of urine unrelated to a stress manoeuvre without any urge to void.[1] It is a common problem in the elderly and is caused by failure of cortical centres to inhibit detrusor activity or by spontaneous premature contractions of the detrusor muscle. Exacerbating factors are excessive caffeine intake, β-blockers (β-adrenergic stimulation inhibits the detrusor muscle), and sedatives.[3]

Bladder training is the usual initial therapeutic intervention for patients with detrusor overactivity.[1,8] The intervals between periods of incontinence are recorded, and the patient is instructed to void before that interval ends. For example, if incontinence occurs after 3 hours, the patient should void after 2 hours and consciously suppress any voiding urges during those first 2 hours. After this routine is established and the incontinence is controlled, the intervals between voidings are gradually lengthened.[1] An alternative that proved effective in one study was teaching patients to contract the pelvic muscles voluntarily without contracting the abdominal muscles whenever they had the urge to urinate. The program consisted of an initial session of anorectal biofeedback, three follow-up sessions with trained nurse practitioners, and a series of pelvic muscle contraction exercises done three times daily at home.[9]

Pharmacotherapy for detrusor overactivity may be tried if behavioural approaches and removal of exacerbating factors fail. Commonly used drugs are those with antimuscarinic activity that lead to relaxation of the detrusor muscle.[1,3] When these drugs are used, care should be taken not to induce urinary retention.[3] Oxybutynin (Ditropan) is one of the most commonly used drugs. Although the usual recommended dose is 5 mg two or three times a day, many patients respond to 2.5 mg at bedtime, and at that dosage, patients have fewer adverse effects. Maximum benefit may not be observed for several weeks.[8]

Some other antimuscarinic drugs and their usual doses are flavoxate (Urispas) 200 mg two to four times daily, tolterodine (Detrol) 1 to 2 mg twice daily, Unidet 4 mg per day, dicyclomine (Bentyl, Bentylol) 10 to 30 mg four times daily, propantheline (Pro-Banthine) 15 to 30 mg four times daily, and imipramine (Tofranil) and desipramine (Norpramin, Pertofrane) in low doses, usually 10 to 25 mg. Occasionally, Minirin (desmopressin acetate) may be useful for patients with nocturia and/or bedtime incontinence.[10]

Eradicating bacteriuria in incontinent nursing home residents did not improve the degree of incontinence.[11]

Overflow incontinence. Overflow incontinence may be due to obstructive lesions, neurological disorders such as multiple sclerosis, or diabetic neuropathy with denervation of the detrusor muscle, or to the secondary effects of medications such as the tricyclic antidepressants. (The anticholinergic actions inhibit detrusor muscle contraction.)[1] Thus, abdominal assessment for a distended bladder is an essential part of the examination of a patient complaining of incontinence. The presence of a distended bladder points to overflow incontinence, although the absence of this finding does not rule it out.

Pharmacotherapy for inadequate detrusor muscle function is not very effective, but the cholinergic drug bethanechol (Urecholine) 10 to 25 mg twice daily or four times daily may be tried. Adverse effects include diarrhea and abdominal cramps, bradycardia, hypotension, and bronchospasm.[1]

Together with an adequate neurological assessment, rectal and vaginal examinations, urinalysis, residual urine test, and perhaps an ultrasound, most causes of incontinence can be assessed and managed by the primary care physician. Consultation can be considered for uncertain diagnosis, non-response, surgery (e.g., for an enlarged prostate or a suspicion of cancer) and those patients requiring urodynamic evaluation.

≫ REFERENCES ≪

1. Resnick NM: An 89-year-old woman with urinary incontinence, *JAMA* 276:1832-1840, 1996.
2. Swanson G, Skelly J, Hutchison B, et al: Urinary incontinence in Canada: a national survey of family physicians' knowledge, attitudes, and practices, *Can Fam Physician* 48:86-92, 2002.
3. Mold JW: Pharmacotherapy of urinary incontinence, *Am Fam Physician* 54:673-680, 1996.
4. Bø K, Talseth T, Holme I: Single blind, randomised controlled trial of pelvic floor exercises, electrical stimulation, vaginal cones, and no treatment in management of genuine stress incontinence in women, *BMJ* 318:487-493, 1999.
5. Norton PA, Baker JE: Postural changes can reduce leakage in women with stress urinary incontinence, *Obstet Gynecol* 84: 770-774, 1994.
6. Miller JM, Ashton-Miller JA, DeLancey JO: A pelvic muscle precontraction can reduce cough-related urine loss in selected women with mild SUI, *J Am Geriatr Soc* 46:870-874, 1998.
7. Fantl JA, Bump RC, Robinson D, et al (Continence Program for Women Research Group): Efficacy of estrogen supplementation in the treatment of urinary incontinence, *Obstet Gynecol* 88: 745-749, 1996.
8. Resnick NM: Improving treatment of urinary incontinence (editorial), *JAMA* 280:2034-2035, 1998.
9. Burio KL, Locher JL, Goode PS, et al: Behavioral vs drug treatment for urge urinary incontinence in older women: a randomized controlled trial, *JAMA* 280:1995-2000, 1998.
10. Rembratt A, Norgaard JP, Andersson KE: Desmopressin in elderly patients with nocturia: short-term safety and effects on urine output, sleep and voiding patterns, *BJU Int* 91(7):642-646, May 2003.
11. Ouslander JG, Schapira M, Schnelle JF, et al: Does eradicating bacteriuria affect the severity of chronic urinary incontinence in nursing home residents? *Ann Intern Med* 122:749-754, 1995.

INFERTILITY, MALE
(See also infertility, female; vasovasostomy)

An estimated 15% of couples have fertility problems. The problem rests exclusively with the male in 30% of cases and partly with the male in another 20%. Unfortunately, the causes of the male abnormalities usually remain unknown even after a thorough workup.[1]

Factors believed to adversely affect spermatogenesis include medications (cimetidine, sulfasalazine, nitrofurantoin, tetracyclines, colchicine), illicit drugs (marijuana, cocaine, anabolic steroids), cryptorchidism, cigarette smoking, and excessive heat exposure from hot tubs.[1,2]

Varicoceles are present in about one fourth of men seeking help for infertility. Whether varicoceles are etiologically related to infertility is unknown, and if treating them provides any benefit, it is minimal after the age of 30. Although infertile men should avoid soaking in a hot tub, which can raise scrotal temperatures, saunas and hot showers are not contraindicated.[2] Wearing briefs rather than boxer shorts does not alter scrotal temperatures, and there is no evidence that switching to boxer shorts increases fertility.[3]

Infection is a rare cause of male infertility even though considerable literature supports such a relationship.[1] Nevertheless, the patient should be tested for *Chlamydia trachomatis,* usually with a fresh urine sample.[2] Enquiring about a history of mumps may be useful. Antisperm antibodies may be associated with male infertility, but the role of corticosteroid treatment under these circumstances is controversial.[4]

Semen analysis is the major investigation of the male in cases of infertility. The normal values given by the World Health Organization (20 million or more sperm/mL[3] and 60% progressive motility) are derived from population studies of normal and infertile men. They are not applicable to individual men, since good fertility has been documented with motile sperm counts even lower than 1 million/mL[3].[2] A minimum of two semen should be analyzed to confirm any abnormalities.

When infertility is related to sperm dysfunction in the male, the intracytoplasmic injection of a single sperm or spermatid into the ovum is used in many centres. (See discussion of female infertility.) If the ejaculate contains no sperm, sperm may be obtained from the testes. Needle aspiration results in a retrieval rate of about 10%, whereas open testicular biopsy (which can be done with the patient under local anesthesia) has a retrieval rate of around 50%.[5] Pre-operative genetic screening of men with non-obstructive azoospermia may be desirable; one study in which screening was done found genetic abnormalities in 17%.[6]

Intracytoplasmic sperm injection (ICSI) was first reported in 1992, so no long-term studies of children conceived by this technique are available. One trial comparing children conceived naturally or by in vitro fertilization (IVF) with those conceived by ICSI at 1 year of age found no differences in major congenital anomalies among the groups, although a greater number of children conceived by ICSI had lower scores on a mental development index than in the other two groups.[7] A subsequent study of 17-month-old children found no clinically significant differences in mental development between ICSI-conceived children and naturally conceived control subjects.[8]

✎ REFERENCES ✎

1. Howards SS: Treatment of male infertility, *N Engl J Med* 332:312-317, 1995.
2. Hargreave TB, Mills JA: Investigating and managing infertility in general practice, *BMJ* 316:1438-1441, 1998.
3. Munkelwitz R, Gilbert BR: Are boxer shorts really better? A critical analysis of the role of underwear type in male subfertility, *J Urol* 160:1329-1333, 1998.
4. Haas GG Jr: Antisperm antibodies in infertile men, *JAMA* 275:885, 1996.
5. Silber SJ: The cure and proliferation of male infertility (editorial), *J Urol* 160:2072-2073, 1998.
6. Rucker GB, Mielnik A, King P, et al: Preoperative screening for genetic abnormalities in men with nonobstructive azoospermia before testicular sperm extraction, *J Urol* 160:2068-2071, 1998.
7. Bowen JR, Gibson FL, Leslie GI, et al: Medical and developmental outcome at 1 year for children conceived by intracytoplasmic sperm injection, *Lancet* 351:1529-1534, 1998.
8. Sutcliffe AG, Taylor B, Thornton S, et al: Children born after intracytoplasmic sperm injection: population control study, *BMJ* 318:704-705, 1999.

PENIS
Erectile Dysfunction

Erectile dysfunction (ED) is the persistent inability to obtain and/or maintain an erection satisfactory for sexual activity.[1] Estimates of rates of erectile dysfunction are less precise, but to put in personal terms, the Health Professionals Follow-Up Study revealed ED rates of 12% in men younger than 59 years, 22% in men ages 60 to 69, and 30% in men over age 70.[2] Other reviews suggest that ED affects 52% of men ages 40 to 70 years.[3] Epidemiological evidence links well-recognized risk factors for coronary artery disease (CAD), such as obesity, hypertension, hypercholesterolemia with erectile dysfunction, and some evidence even suggests that ED can be a sentinel event for CAD in asymptomatic men.[4,5] Diabetes can double the risk of ED. Additionally, many medications can affect sexual and erectile function, and it

may be useful to the practitioner to start with medications that affect the brain, such as antidepressants, and the heart, such as antihypertensives.

To step back for a moment, it is always helpful to consider the bigger picture of sexual health. While most men consider intercourse paramount to sexual intimacy, some would disagree, and many couples have certainly found different strategies to satisfy. Also, many factors affect erectile function, including relationships, anxiety, aging, mood, and self-efficacy.

Testing of erectile function includes ultrasound, the nocturnal penile tumescence test, and injecting papaverine. However, these have been used less recently with the advent of the phosphodiesterase inhibitors, because clinicians often trial these medications as beginning of the work-up. Although practical, one has to be sure that the sexual health problem could be solved with simple relationship or sexual health counselling. Delineating the phases of sexual response can be a good starting point. A helpful mnemonic is DAO, where D is desire, A is arousal, and O stands for orgasm. Men seem to be troubled mostly by arousal (and premature ejaculation), whereas females can struggle more with achieving orgasm. Trouble in any of these areas is typically linked with desire issues. Discussion regarding the sexual response and where the key problem is located can be diagnostic and therapeutic.

Treatment

An often overlooked treatment for ED is lifestyle counselling. Men who initiated physical activity in midlife in the Massachusetts Male Aging Study had a 70% reduced ED rate compared with their sedentary peers.[6] A 2004 randomized controlled trial of 110 obese Italian men with erectile dysfunction showed that they were able to cure this problem about one third of the time by making lifestyle changes and reducing weight.[7] Although still required by some, the use of intracavernosal and transurethral alprostadil (Muse), penile prostheses, and vacuum constriction devices, has been mostly replaced by the advent of oral PDE5 inhibitors (sildenafil, tadalafil, vardenafil).

[handwritten: Cavernosal]

PDE5 inhibitors [handwritten: Phosphodiesterase type 5 inhibitor]

There are now three choices of PDE5 inhibitors, and they are chiefly separated by their half-life. These include sildenafil (Viagra), tadalafil (Cialis), and vardenafil (Levitra). They have all shown to be significantly better than placebo but there have been no comparative trials. These agents can all be used in patients with cardiac disease *except* those taking nitrates. There is a degree of risk to activity in all patients with a cardiac history, and sexual activity is no different. PDE5 inhibitors are primarily metabolized by the cytochrome P450 3A4 system. It should be stressed to the patient that these agents do not

[handwritten: Used c nitro, hypotension + death.]

directly cause erections but instead require sexual stimulation. In general, the lowest possible dose that does the job is the objective, but there is a dose response curve, so that men who do not have success at lower doses can go to higher doses. Lower doses are wise in patients with compromised hepatic or renal function.[8]

Sildenafil (Viagra) (25 to 100 mg) has the most experience, and time to sexual activity is approximately 60 minutes; however, clinical results have been reported from 30 minutes to 4 to 6 hours. Doses taken with food are delayed. Tadalafil (Cialis) (10 to 25 mg) has a longer half-life, and erectile support can be expected to last from 30 minutes to 24 hours. This can theoretically lead to more spontaneity. It is unaffected by food, and dosage adjustments are not necessary in the elderly. Vardenafil (Levitra) (5 to 20 mg) can be typically taken 25 to 60 minutes before planned sexual activity with some data suggesting effectiveness in the 15- to 120-minute window. High-fat meals will delay absorption. All of these medications are expensive. Headache, flushing, and dyspepsia are the most common side effects of the PDE5 inhibitors.[8] *Nasal congestion ↓BP*

Other drugs that are postulated to improve outcomes include apomorphine (Uprima), testosterone, and trazadone, but they have less evidence of effectiveness. Apomorphine is a morphine derivative that has structural similarities to dopamine. Sublingual 2-mg and 3-mg doses are fast acting and moderately effective in the treatment of ED. Higher doses are associated with increased side effects similar to the PDE5s. Apomorphine has not been evaluated in men with spinal cord injuries, multiple sclerosis, prostatectomy, and pelvic surgery. Efficacy in men with diabetes has not been established.[9] Testosterone has some supportive evidence, but a systematic review revealed only small numbers and concerns about methodology.[10] Trazadone may be useful in men with erectile dysfunction of psychogenic etiology, but the evidence is quite weak at this point. A systematic review found trials that used 50 mg daily in one trial, and 150 to 200 mg daily in the other four. The review revealed methodological flaws in the small trials-to-date and therefore could not make a conclusive statement.[11]

⩗ REFERENCES ⩗

1. Kaye JA, Jick H: Incidence of erectile dysfunction and characteristics of patients before and after the introduction of sildenafil in the United Kingdom: cross sectional study with comparison patients, *BMJ* 326:424-425, 2003.
2. Bacon CG, Mittleman MA, Kawachi I: Sexual function in men older than 50 years of age: results from the Health Professionals Follow-Up Study, *Ann Intern Med* 139:161-168, 2003.
3. Jackson G, Betteridge J, Dean J, et al: A systematic approach to erectile dysfunction in the cardiovascular patient: a consensus statement-update 2002, *Int J Clin Pract* 56(9):663-671, 2002.
4. Saigal CS: Obesity and erectile dysfunction: common problems, common solutions? *JAMA* 294:3011-3012, 2004.
5. Fung MM, Bettencourt R, Barrett-Connor E: Heart disease risk factors predict erectile dysfunction 25 years later, *J Am Coll Cardiol* 43:1405-1411, 2004.
6. Derby CA, Mohr BA, Goldstein I, et al: Modifiable risk factors and erectile dysfunction: can lifestyle changes modify risk? *Urology* 56:302-306, 2000.
7. Esposito K, Giugliano F, Di Palo C, et al: Effect of lifestyle changes on erectile dysfunction in obese men, *JAMA* 291:2978-2984, 2004.
8. Montorsi F, Salonia A, Deho' F, et al: Pharmacological managment of erectile dysfunction, *BJU Int* 91(5):446-454, 2003.
9. Dula E, Bukofzer S, Perdok R, et A: Double-blind, crossover comparison of 3 mg Apomorphine SL with placebo and with 4 mg Apormorphine SL in male erectile dysfunction, *Eur Urol* 39:558-564, 2001.
10. Jain P, et al: Testosterone supplementation for erectile dysfunction: results of a meta-analysis, *J Urology* 164:371-375, 2000.
11. HA Fink, et al: Trazodone for erectile dysfunction: a systematic review and meta-analysis, *BJU Int* 92:441-446, 2003.

Paraphimosis

Paraphimosis is the inability of the retracted foreskin to return to its resting position. It is a urological emergency. Medical therapy involves reassuring the patient, reducing the preputial edema, and restoring the prepuce to its original position and condition. Several methods can reduce the penile swelling. Wrap the penis in plastic and apply ice packs or wrap with compressive elastic dressings[1]; apply topical anesthetic minutes to 1 hour in advance (2% lidocaine gel, 5% lidocaine ointment, 2.5% prilocaine or 2.5% lidocaine cream) before direct circumferential manual compression.[1,2] Another method is to reduce swelling by osmosis with granulated sugar.[3] (Apply granulated sugar to the surface of the edematous prepuce and cover it with a condom or a finger of a rubber glove.) Swelling may also be reduced with hyaluronidase injections. (Use a tuberculin syringe and inject 1 mL of hyaluronidase [150 U/cc Wydase] directly into several sites of the edematous prepuce.[3]) If a Foley catheter is present, remove it until the paraphimosis is resolved.[1]

Pearly Penile Papules (Hirsutoid Papillomatosis)

Pearly penile papules are normal anatomical structures found around the corona of the penis in up to 20% of young men. They are smooth, whitish elevations and are said to be more common in blacks and in the uncircumcised. Treatment is reassurance.

Peyronie's Disease

Peyronie's disease is a disorder of unknown etiology characterized by a curvature of the penis caused by inelastic scar or plaque formation. The incidence is increased in patients with Dupuytren's contracture. Some patients cannot perform vaginal penetration because of the penile curvature or because of distal flaccidity. Pain and tenderness in the region of the plaque may be the presenting symptoms. The condition resolves spontaneously in 20% to 50% of patients. Local corticosteroid injections are sometimes helpful, but in more intractable cases, surgery is necessary.[4]

------------------------ ◿ **REFERENCES** ◿ ------------------------

1. Choe JM, Kim H: Paraphymosis, 2004. (Accessed April 28, 2004 emedicine.com/med/topic2874/htm).
2. Olson C: Emergency treatment of paraphimosis, *Can Fam Physician* 44:1253, 1998.
3. Cahill D, Rane A: Reduction of paraphimosis with granulated sugar, *BJU Int* 83(3):362, Feb 1999.
4. Fitkin J, Ho GT: Peyronie's disease: current management, *Am Fam Physician* 60:549-554, 1999.

PROSTATE
Benign Prostatic Hyperplasia
(See also an approach to complementary and alternative medicine)

Definition
BPH is a condition of obstructive and irritative urinary symptoms. The prevalence is rare under age 40, 50% at age 50, and 80% at age 80.

Symptoms
The major symptoms of BPH are found in the American Urological Association questionnaire, which was developed to give a quantitative estimate of symptomatic distress.[1] The questionnaire can be filled in by the patient and is very useful to administer. The seven symptoms of significance are as follows:

Obstructive symptoms:
1. Decrease in force and/or caliber of urinary stream
2. Urinary hesitancy
3. Post-micturition dribble
4. Sensation of incomplete voiding
5. Overflow incontinence
6. Acute or chronic retention of urine—acute retention of urine is of sudden onset and is usually painful; chronic retention develops gradually and tends to be painless

Irritative symptoms:
1. Frequency
2. Urgency
3. Urge incontinence
4. Nocturia

Other symptoms:
1. Hematuria
2. Symptoms of obstructive uropathy with decrease in renal function (tiredness, anorexia, nausea, malaise)

Watchful waiting
The simplest form of treatment is no treatment. A review of five studies on the natural history of moderately symptomatic BPH concluded that over time, 40% of the men improve, 45% have no change in symptoms, and 15% deteriorate.[2] A recent collaborative study from nine U.S. centres compared transurethral resection with watchful waiting for 800 men with benign prostatic hypertrophy. At the end of 3 years, 24% of those who were in the watchful waiting group underwent surgery.[3]

Medical treatment
α_1-Adrenergic blocking agents relieve the symptoms of BPH by relaxing the smooth muscles within the prostate. Four such agents that have been used for this purpose are terazosin (Hytrin), doxazosin (Cardura), prazosin (Minipress), and tamsulosin (Flomax). Most of the studies to date have involved terazosin, which improved urine flow rates and symptoms in 50% to 70% of patients. Tamsulosin works directly on the bladder, which should theoretically reduce untoward effects of α-blockade, but this has not translated to fewer episodes of falls in trials.[4] The usual dosages of these agents are terazosin 5 to 10 mg at bedtime, doxazosin 4 to 8 mg at night, and tamsulosin 0.4 to 0.8 mg once daily. BPH can wax and wane so some patients may prefer to modify their doses based on symptoms.

Finasteride (Proscar) inhibits 5-α-reductase, an intracellular enzyme that metabolizes testosterone into the more potent dihydrotestosterone. Use of this drug (usual dose is 5 mg daily) causes atrophy of the prostate.[5] Finasteride is more effective than placebo, but only a small number of treated patients benefit.[5,6] In one 4-year double-blind, randomized, placebo-controlled trial, 80 men had to be treated for 1 year to prevent one man from requiring surgery, and 100 men had to be treated for 1 year to prevent one man from having urinary retention.[6] Side effects, which include impotence and breast tenderness, are relatively infrequent.[5]

A 1996 Veterans Administration study compared placebo with finasteride (Proscar), terazosin (Hytrin), and a combination of terazosin and finasteride. Finasteride was no more effective than placebo, terazosin resulted in significant symptom relief, and the addition of finasteride to terazosin gave no additional benefit.[4] Although finasteride was ineffective in this study, it was effective in two previous randomized controlled studies,[7,8] as well as in at least one subsequent study.[9] This may have been because the subjects had much larger prostates than was the case in the Veterans Administration trial. Relatively small prostates may respond to the muscle relaxation of an α_1-adrenergic antagonist such as terazosin, whereas larger prostates may respond only if epithelial elements are caused to atrophy through the use of a 5-α-reductase drug such as finasteride.[9,10] A more recent trial randomized finasteride and doxasozin together versus placebo or either drug alone in clinical progression of BPH. After 4 years, the combination therapy seemed to work best. However, there are some concerns that finasteride may be associated with increased risk of high-grade prostate cancer. Combination therapy with finasteride and doxazosin for at least 4 years reduces the risk of clinical progression of BPH.[5] However, long-term use of finasteride is also associated with an increased risk of high-grade prostate cancer.[6] Until this risk is better elucidated, combination therapy should be limited to patients who have larger prostates (greater than 40 mL) and are interested in more vigilant assessment for prostate cancer.

Surgical treatment

The standard surgical treatment of benign prostatic hyperplasia is transurethral resection. For patients with moderate-to-severe symptoms, immediate results are excellent.[2,3] However, 20% to 25% of patients do not have long-term satisfactory outcomes, and the re-operation rate in men followed for 10 or more years is 15% to 20%. Reported complications of surgery include retrograde ejaculation in about three fourths of the patients, impotence in 5% to 10%, some degree of urinary incontinence in 2% to 4%, post-operative urinary tract infections in 5% to 10%, and blood transfusions in 5% to 10%.[2] In one study of men who were sexually active both before and after transurethral prostatic resections, half reported absent or altered orgasm.[11] Because of the potential complications of surgery, and because there is now good evidence that BPH is not always a progressive disease, watchful waiting is a reasonable therapeutic option for many patients with mild or moderate symptoms. (See section on watchful waiting below.)[3] Aside from transurethral and retropubic prostatectomy, a surgical option for treating BPH is a transurethral incision of the prostate. This is a relatively simple intervention that is effective in many instances. It is used particularly for men with small prostate glands, for those who want to avoid retrograde ejaculation, and for those who are debilitated and therefore not good candidates for more extensive procedures. Another option for some patients is a permanently indwelling prostatic stent. Procedures under development include microwave and laser therapies.[2] Transurethral microwave thermotherapy can be given using topical urethral anesthesia. In one study comparing this procedure with oral terazosin (Hytrin), greater improvement was seen in the terazosin patients at 6 weeks, but the microwave-treated patients had better outcomes at 6 and 12 months.[12]

Alternative medical treatment

A systematic review concluded that saw palmetto extracts (Permixon) were more effective in improving urinary symptoms in patients with BPH than placebo and as effective as finasteride. Long-term benefits and benefit relative to α blockers have not been evaluated.[8] Pygeum, an herbal product derived from the bark of the African prune tree (*Pygeum africanum*), has been used in Europe for 30 years to treat symptoms of benign prostatic hypertrophy. A meta-analysis of 18 studies comparing the herb with placebo in men with symptomatic benign prostatic hypertrophy showed benefit.[13] No benefit was seen in acupuncture therapy.[14] The usual concerns about standardized doses for herbal therapies remain.

Prevention

Data from the Health Professionals Follow-up Study found that moderate exercise such as walking decreased the risk of symptoms associated with BPH.[10]

◢ REFERENCES ◣

1. Barry MJ, Fowler FJ Jr, O'Leary MP, et al (Measurement Committee of the American Urological Association): The American Urological Association symptom index for benign prostatic hyperplasia, *J Urol* 148:1549-1557, 1992.
2. Oesterling JE: Benign prostatic hyperplasia: medical and minimally invasive treatment options, *N Engl J Med* 332:99-109, 1995.
3. Wasson JH, Reda DJ, Bruskewitz RC, et al: A comparison of transurethral surgery with watchful waiting for moderate symptoms of benign prostatic hyperplasia, *N Engl J Med* 332: 75-79, 1995.
4. Lepor H, Williford WO, Barry MJ, et al: The efficacy of terazosin, finasteride, or both in benign prostatic hyperplasia, *N Engl J Med* 335:533-539, 1996.
5. McConnell JD, et al (The Medical Therapy of Prostatic Symptoms [MTOPS] Research Group): The long-term effect of doxazosin, finasteride, and combination therapy on the clinical progression of benign prostatic hyperplasia, *N Engl J Med* 349:2387-2398, 18 Dec 2003.
6. Thompson IM, et al: The influence of finasteride on the development of prostate cancer, *N Engl J Med* 349:215-224, 17 Jul 2003.
7. Nickel JC, Fradet Y, Boake RC, et al: Efficacy and safety of finasteride therapy for benign prostatic hyperplasia: results of a 2-year randomized controlled trial (the PROSPECT Study), *Can Med Assoc J* 155:1251-1259, 1996.
8. Wilt TJ, Ishani A, Stark G, et al: Saw palmetto extracts for treatment of benign prostatic hyperplasia, *JAMA* 280:1604-1609, 1998.
9. McConnell JD, Bruskewitz R, Walsh P, et al: The effect of finasteride on the risk of acute urinary retention and the need for surgical treatment among men with benign prostatic hyperplasia, *N Engl J Med* 338:557-563, 1998.
10. Platz EA, Kawachi I, Rimm EB, et al: Physical activity and benign prostatic hyperplasia, *Arch Intern Med* 158:2349-2356, 1998.
11. Dunsmuir WD, Emberton M, Neal DE (Steering Group of the National Prostatectomy Audit): There is significant sexual dissatisfaction following TURP, *Br J Urol* 77:161A, 1996.

12. Djavan R, Roehrborn CG, Shariat S, et al: Prospective randomized comparison of high-energy transurethral microwave thermotherapy versus α-blocker treatment of patients with benign prostatic hyperplasia, *J Urol* 161:139-143, 1999.

13. Ishani A, MacDonald R, Nelson D, et al: Pygeum africanum for the treatment of patients with benign prostatic hyperplasia: a systematic review and quantitative meta-analysis, *Am J Med* 109:654-664, 2000.

14. Johnstone PAS, Bloom TL, Niemtzow RC, et al: A prospective, randomized pilot trial of acupuncture of the kidney-bladder distinct meridian for lower urinary tract symptoms, *J Urol* 169:1037-1039, 2003.

Prostate Cancer

(See also prevention; screening; vasectomy)

Epidemiology

(See also BRCA1 and BRCA2 mutations; prostate-specific antigen; screening; vasectomy)

Prostate cancer is the second most common cause of cancer-related death in men, after lung cancer.[1] The current lifetime risk of diagnosis is 12%[2] to 16.7%.[3] Twenty to 25% of men with prostate cancer die of their disease. The incidence of prostate cancer has been increasing since the 1970's due to prostate-specific antigen (PSA) screening and incidental detection of cancer following transurethral resection of the prostate (TURP) surgery.[4]

A consequence of increased screening has been a sharp increase in the rate of radical prostatectomies.[5]

Mortality rates for prostate cancer vary. Mortality from this cancer for African American men is twice that of white men[6], while mortality for Hispanics is 35% lower, and for Asians, 40% lower.[7]

Known risk factors for prostate cancer include family history and race (Table 73).[8]

A rare form, "hereditary prostate cancer," accounts for 43% of prostate cancers diagnosed before 55 years of age. This form appears to have a dominant mode of inheritance with high penetrance.[9] These tumours tend to be high grade and more advanced at diagnosis than non-hereditary prostate cancers.[10] Hereditary prostate cancer accounts for less than 10% of families with a family history of prostate cancer.[11] In a few cases, hereditary prostate cancer may be related to a BRCA1 or BRCA2 mutation. (See discussion of BRCA1 and BRCA2 mutations in the section on breast cancer.)

Table 73   Risk Factors for Prostate Cancer

Risk factor	Relative risk
Family History	
First-degree relative	
• One relative	2.2
• Two relatives	4.9
• Three or more	10.9
Second-degree relative	
• Paternal or maternal	1.7
First- and second-degree relative	8.8
High-fat Diet	1.7
African-American	1.4

From Greiver M: PSA screening for prostate cancer. *Educational module. Practice Based Learning Programs.* The Foundation for Medical Practice Education, 10(2): 1-13, 2002. Reprinted with permission.

❧ REFERENCES ❧

1. U.S. Task Force on Preventive Health Services: *Screening for Prostate Cancer: Recommendations and Rationale. December 2002,* Agency for Healthcare Research and Quality, Rockville, MD. Available http://www.ahrq.gov/clinic/3rduspstf/prostatescr/prostaterr.htm. Accessed March 6, 2004.

2. National Cancer Institute of Canada: Canadian Cancer Statistics 2001, Toronto, 2001, The Institute.

3. American Cancer Society: *Cancer facts & figures, 2003,* Atlanta, 2003, The Society.

4. Levy IG, Iscoe NA, Klotz LH: Prostate cancer: 1. The descriptive epidemiology in Canada, *Can Med Assoc J* 159:509-13

5. Olsson CA, Goluboff ET: Detection and treatment of prostate cancer: perspective of the urologist, *J Urol* 152:1695-1699, 1994.

6. Harris RP, Lohr KN: Screening for prostate cancer: an update of the evidence for the U.S. Preventive Services Task Force, *Ann Intern Med* 137:917-929, 2002.

7. National Cancer Institute: Surveillance, Epidemiology, and End Results (SEER) Program Public-Use Data (1973-1998). Available at: http://seer.cancer.gov. Accessed March 01, 2004.

8. Greiver M: Screening for prostate cancer: Practice based small group educational module, *Found Med Pract Ed* 10(2): Feb 2002.

9. McLellan DL, Norman RW: Hereditary aspects of prostate cancer, *Can Med Assoc J* 153:895-900, 1995.

10. Grönberg H, Isaacs SD, Smith JR, et al: Characteristics of prostate cancer in families potentially linked to the hereditary prostate cancer 1 (HPC1) locus, *JAMA* 278:1251-1255, 1997.

11. Grönberg H, Wiklund F, Damber J-E: Age specific risks of familial prostate carcinoma: a basis for screening recommendations in high risk populations, *Cancer* 86:477-483, 1999.

Staging and histological grading

Prostate cancer is staged using the TNM system outlined in Table 74. Tumour histology is graded using the Gleason score, as shown in Table 75.

Chemoprevention of Prostate Cancer

A recent randomized controlled trial reported a 25% reduction of the risk of prostate cancer after 7 years of therapy with 5 mg of finasteride.[1] However, there was a 1.7-fold increase in the risk of high-grade tumour (Gleason score 7 to 10) when cancer did develop (6.4% versus 5.1% of participants). Additionally, there was a greater rate of sexual side effects on finasteride.

Urology

Urology **473**

Table 74   TNM Classification of Prostate Cancer (Tumour Only)

Classification	Description
T1	Clinically inapparent; not palpable or visible on imaging
T1a	Incidental histological finding ≤5% of tissue resected
T1b	Incidental histological finding >5% of tissue resected
T1c	Identified by blind biopsy done because of elevated prostate-specific antigen
T2	Palpable; confined to the prostate
T2a	Involves half a lobe or less
T2b	Involves more than half a lobe but not both lobes
T2c	Involves both lobes
T3	Extends through prostate capsule
T4	Fixed or invades structures other than seminal vesicles

Table 75   Histological Grading of Prostate Cancer

Degree of differentiation	Gleason score
Well differentiated	2-4
Moderately differentiated	5-7
Poorly differentiated	8-10

Men who consider chemoprevention need to weigh the decrease in the rate of prostate cancer against the increase in high-grade cancer and the side effects. The final effect on morbidity and mortality is unknown at present.

Other agents that could potentially prevent prostate cancer include selenium, vitamin E, vitamin D, other 5-α-reductase inhibitors, cyclooxygenase-2 inhibitors, lycopene, and green tea.[2] These will need to be tested in well-designed trials before being recommended.

────────────── ◢ REFERENCES ◣ ──────────────
1. Thompson IM, Goodman PJ, Tangen CM, et al: The influence of finasteride on the development of prostate cancer, *N Engl J Med* 349:215-224, 2003.
2. Klein EA, Thompson IM: Update on chemoprevention of prostate cancer, *Curr Opin Urol* 14:143-149, 2004.

Screening
(See also informed consent; prevention; radical prostatectomy; screening;)

Screening for cancer of the prostate is a controversial topic because we don't know if screening decreases mortality.[1] Screening manoeuvres can include digital rectal examination (DRE) and PSA, or a combination of the two. The U.S. Preventive Services Task Force reviewed prostate cancer screening in 2002, and assigned it an "I" rating (insufficient evidence).[1] No organization currently recommends mass screening; the American Cancer Society, American Urological Association, and American College of Physicians recommend that men be informed of the risks and benefits of screening, so that they can make their own decision.[2-4] Men with life expectancies of less than 10 years should not be screened.

Digital rectal examination
DRE is the traditional method of screening for prostate cancer. However, DRE cannot reach the anterior aspect of the prostate, and will thus miss over 40% of cancers.[5]

Prostate-specific antigen
PSA is a newer screening method that became widely available in North America in the mid-1980s. In the United States in 1988, 1.2% of men had undergone PSA testing, whereas by 1994, 40% had undergone the test.[6] Despite the increasing use of this test for screening, evidence of reduced mortality is still lacking. A single trial[7] found decreased risk of death in screened men; however, experts have criticized the study design and analysis.[8] We will likely know the answer once the results of two large, well-designed, randomized controlled trials are available, probably between 2005 and 2008. (Those trials are the Prostate, Lung, Colon and Ovary Screening trial, and the European Randomized Study of Screening for Prostate Cancer.)

Causes of elevated PSA other than prostate cancer can include BPH, prostatitis, urinary retention, cystoscopy, and prostate surgery. PSA testing should be deferred for 2 months after resolution of reversible conditions. DRE does not affect PSA,[9] but ejaculation can cause a transient elevation; testing should be deferred for 2 days after ejaculation.[10] Drugs such as finasteride (Proscar) decrease PSA levels; PSA should be multiplied by 2 for men on this drug.[11]

A variety of methods for increasing the specificity of PSA determinations are under active investigation. These include PSA velocity, which is a measurement of the rate of change of PSA over time, age-specific PSA ranges, and PSA density, which correlates prostatic gland volume as determined by ultrasound with PSA levels. None of these tools has been sufficiently evaluated to merit general clinical application.[9]

The cutoff value for further investigation of an elevated PSA is controversial. A common threshold is 4 ng/mL; however, values from 3.0 to 10 ng/mL have been proposed. Trans-rectal ultrasound (TRUS) with biopsy is recommended for a PSA of 4.0 or greater.[12] For men with a PSA between 4.0 and 10, measuring the free PSA may help to avoid some biopsies. A free PSA to total PSA ratio of 23.4 or greater decreases the probability of cancer to 8%[13], and some men may opt to avoid biopsy. See Figure 4 for a suggested care map.[14]

If screened, 10% to 15% of men will have a PSA above 4 ng/mL requiring further investigation.[15] The number of men with "positive" PSA tests who actually have cancer (positive predictive value) is low, ranging from 8% to

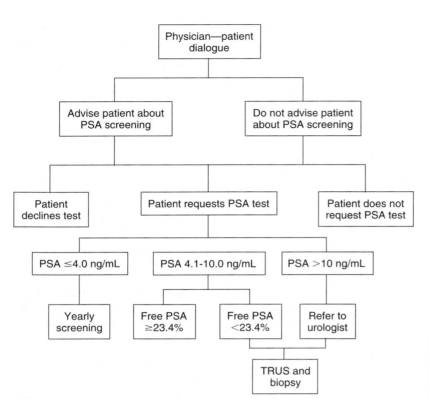

Figure 4. Suggested care map for PSA screening. (From Greiver M, Rosen N: *CMAJ* 162:789-790, 2000. Copyright © 2000 Canadian Medical Association. Reprinted with permission.)

33%.[16] This means that many men will undergo an unnecessary TRUS and biopsy with the accompanying risks of pain, hematuria, hemospermia, and infection (1% to 6% without prophylactic antibiotics) as well as emotional stress.[17,18] A rare complication is acute urinary retention.[17]

The fact that PSA screening results in a "stage shift" to less advanced tumours does not necessarily mean that treatment will improve mortality. Small tumours are merely surrogate endpoints for decreased mortality, and apparent short-term beneficial results of treatment may be spurious because of lead-time bias and length bias (see section on prevention). Treatment for prostate cancer can cause erectile dysfunction and incontinence, without necessarily decreasing mortality for men whose cancer was discovered through screening.

A normal PSA does not guarantee one does not have prostate cancer. In one series of men with PSA levels of 2.6 to 4.0 ng/mL and normal prostate examinations, 22% were found to have prostate cancer when subjected to biopsy.[13]

The recommended age range for patients at average risk who choose PSA is age 50 and up.[1,19,20] Screening should be stopped at age 70, or if life expectancy is less than 10 years. In spite of this recommendation, screening of elderly men for PSA is widespread in the United States.[21] A recent survey of U.S. primary care physicians found that PSA screening was ordered routinely for 65% of men ages 70 to 74, 58% of men ages 75 to 79, and 53% of men age 80 or over.[21] About one third of all radical prostatectomies are performed in men over the age of 70.[22]

Whether PSA screening is more beneficial for high-risk groups such as African Americans or men with strong family histories is unknown.

Combining PSA and DRE improved sensitivity, specificity, and positive predictive value (PPV) (Table 76).[23] For those reasons, if the patient chooses screening, both should be used.

--- **≥ REFERENCES ≥** ---

1. U.S. Task Force on Preventive Health Services: *Screening for Prostate Cancer: Recommendations and Rationale. December 2002,* Agency for Healthcare Research and Quality, Rockville, MD. (Accessed April 29, 2004 at http://www. ahrq.gov/clinic/3rduspstf/prostatescr/prostaterr.htm).

Table 76   Results of PSA, DRE, and Combined PSA/DRE Screenings for Prostate Cancer

	Abnormal PSA	Abnormal DRE	Combined
Sensitivity	35%	27%	38%
Specificity	75%	33%	92%
PPV	28%	18%	56%

From Crawford ED, Leewansagtong S, Goktas S, et al: *Prostate* 38(4):296-302, 1999.

2. American Cancer Society: Guidelines for the early detection of cancer: update of early detection guidelines for prostate, colorectal, and endometrial cancers. Also: Update 2001—testing for early lung cancer detection, *CA Cancer J Clin* 51(1):38-75, Jan-Feb 2001.

3. American College of Physicians: Clinical guideline. 3. Screening for prostate cancer, *Ann Intern Med* 126:480-484, 1997.

4. American Urological Association (AUA): Prostate-specific antigen (PSA) best practice policy, *Oncology* 14(2):267-272, Feb 2000.

5. Harris RP, Lohr KN, Beck R, et al: *Screening for Prostate Cancer.* Systematic Evidence Review No. 16 (Prepared by the Research Triangle Institute—University of North Carolina Evidence-based Practice Center under Contract No. 290-97-0011). Agency for Healthcare Research and Quality, Rockville, MD. (December 2001. Available on the AHRQ web site at: http://www.ahrq.gov/clinic/serfiles.htm).

6. Hankey BF, Feuer EJ, Clegg LX, et al: Cancer surveillance series: interpreting trends in prostate cancer. I. Evidence of the effects of screening in recent prostate cancer incidence, mortality, and survival rates, *J Natl Cancer Inst* 91:1017-1024, 1999.

7. Labrie F, Candas B, Dupont A, et al: Screening decreases prostate cancer death: first analysis of the 1988 Quebec Prospective Randomized Controlled Trial, *Prostate* 38:83-91, 1999.

8. Barry MJ: Clinical practice: prostate specific antigen testing for early diagnosis of prostate cancer, *N Engl J Med* 344(18):1373-1377, 2001.

9. Coley CM, Barry MJ, Fleming C, et al: Clinical guideline. 1. Early detection of prostate cancer. 1. Prior probability and effectiveness of tests, *Ann Intern Med* 126:394-406, 1997.

10. Tchetgen M-B, Song JT, Strawderman M, et al: Ejaculation increases the serum prostate-specific antigen concentration, *Urology* 47:511-516, 1996.

11. Andriole GL, Guess HA, Epstein JI, et al: Treatment with finasteride preserves usefulness of prostate-specific antigen in the detection of prostate cancer: results of a randomized, double-blind, placebo-controlled clinical trial. PLESS Study Group: Proscar Long-term Efficacy and Safety Study, *Urology* 52(2):195-201, Aug 1998.

12. Karakiewicz PI, Aprikian AG: Prostate cancer. 5. Diagnostic tools for early detection, *Can Med Assoc J* 159:1139-1146, 1998.

13. Catalona WJ, Smith DS, Wolfert RL, et al: Evaluation of percentage of free serum prostate-specific antigen to improve specificity of prostate cancer screening, *JAMA* 274:1214-1220, 1995.

14. Greiver M, Rosen N: PSA screening: a view from the front lines, *Can Med Assoc J* 162:789-790, 2000.

15. Smith DS, Catalona WJ, Herschman JD: Longitudinal screening for prostate cancer with prostate-specific antigen, *JAMA* 276:1309-1315, 1996.

16. Feightner JW: The early detection and treatment of prostate cancer: the perspective of the Canadian Task Force on the Periodic Health Examination, *J Urol* 152:1682-1684, 1994.

17. Webb JA, Shanmuganathan K, McLean A: Complications of ultrasound-guided transperineal prostate biopsy: a prospective study, *Br J Urol* 72:775-777, 1993.

18. Gustafsson, Norming U, Nyman CR, et al: Complications following combined transrectal aspiration and core biopsy of the prostate, *Scand J Urol Nephrol* 24:249-251, 1990.

19. Von Eschenbach A, Ho R, Murphy GP, et al: American Cancer Society guideline for the early detection of prostate cancer: update 1997, *CA Cancer J Clin* 47:261-264, 1997.

20. American Urological Association: Early detection of prostate cancer and use of transrectal ultrasound. In *American Urological Association 1992 policy statement book,* vol 4, Baltimore, MD, 1992, The Association, 20.

21. Fowler FJ, Bin L, Collins MM, et al: Prostate cancer screening and beliefs about treatment efficacy: a national survey of primary care physicians and urologists, *Am J Med* 104:526-532, 1998.

22. Murphy GP, Mettlin C, Menck H, et al: National patterns of prostate cancer treatment by radical prostatectomy: results of a survey by the American College of Surgeons Commission on Cancer, *J Urol* 152:1817-1819, 1994.

23. Crawford ED, Leewansagtong S, Goktas S, et al: Efficiency of prostate specific antigen and digital rectal examination in screening, using 4.0 ng/ml and age-specific reference range as a cutoff for abnormal values, *Prostate*, 38(4):296-302, 1999.

Management of clinically localized prostate cancer
(See also prostate-specific antigen)

Risk stratification. Risk stratification should be done prior to choosing a therapy. Stratification combines the PSA level, the Tumour stage (see Table 74) and the Gleason score (see Table 75).[1] Online and downloadable nomograms are available at http://www.mskcc.org/mskcc/html/10088.cfm

Therapeutic options. The standard treatment options for patients with clinically localized prostate cancer (no metastases and no spread beyond the capsule) include radical prostatectomy, external beam radiation therapy, brachytherapy through computer-optimized transperineal implantation of radioactive material into the prostate, and watchful waiting.[2]

Radical prostatectomy. A recent study compared watchful waiting with prostatectomies in patients with low-risk prostate cancer (T1b, T1c, or T2). After 6.2 years, the risk of metastatic disease was 13.4% in the prostatectomy group, compared with 27.3% in the watchful waiting group, and the risk of dying of prostate cancer was 4.6%, compared with 8.9%. Total mortality was not significantly reduced (20% versus 28%).[3] Only 5% of men in this study had their cancer detected through screening, and thus the study does not resolve the screening question.

Adverse effects of prostatectomies can include erectile dysfunction (80% versus 45% for watchful waiting), and urinary incontinence (49% versus 21%).[4]

Radiation therapy. A 1998 report that compared external beam radiation therapy, radical prostatectomy, and brachytherapy for localized prostate cancer concluded that after 5 years, the three modalities were equally effective for low-risk patients (low Gleason scores, relatively low PSA levels, and less advanced staging), whereas for patients at higher risk, brachytherapy was less effective than external beam radiation or radical prostatectomy.[5] A subsequent report of a 10-year follow-up of men who received brachytherapy for prostate cancer was more encouraging. The overall survival was 65%, and 64% of patients were clinically and biochemically free of disease at 10 years; 2% of patients had died of prostate cancer, and only 6% had metastases. The results of brachytherapy reported in this study are comparable to the published results of radical prostatectomy.[6]

About one fourth of patients undergoing external beam radiation therapy have genitourinary symptoms such as frequency, urgency, dysuria, and nocturia during the initial 2 months of therapy, and close to half have gastrointestinal symptoms such as tenesmus and diarrhea. These symptoms usually resolve within a few weeks. The most common long-term sequela is impotence, which affects about 50% of men. A dry ejaculate is common in those who remain potent. Long-term rectal or genitourinary symptoms are relatively infrequent. Brachytherapy has fewer adverse effects. The rate of impotence is low; a number of patients may have late urinary tract or gastrointestinal symptoms.[7]

Watchful waiting. Men with well-differentiated tumours (low Gleason scores, in the range of 2 to 5) do well, and few die of prostate cancer even after follow-up periods of 10 to 15 years, whereas the majority of men who have the most undifferentiated tumours (Gleason scores of 8 to 10) die of prostate cancer. Watchful waiting may be appropriate for men with low-risk cancers, and those with shorter life expectancies.

Because several treatment modalities have been found to be equivalent,[2] patients with localized prostate cancer and their physicians must base therapeutic decisions on overall health status, life expectancy, quality of life, and patient preference.

--- **REFERENCES** ---

1. Lukka H, Warde P, Pickles T, et al: Controversies in prostate cancer radiotherapy: consensus development, *Can J Urol* 8(4):1314-1422, 2001.
2. Chodak GW: Comparing treatments for localized prostate cancer—persisting uncertainty (editorial), *JAMA* 280:1008-1010, 1998.
3. Holmberg L, Bill-Axelson A, Helgesen F, et al: A randomized trial comparing radical prostatectomy with watchful waiting in early prostate cancer, *N Engl J Med* 347:781-789, 2002.
4. Steineck G, Helgesen F, Adolfsson J, et al: Quality of life after radical prostatectomy or watchful waiting, *N Engl J Med* 347:790-796, 2002.
5. D'Amico AV, Whittington R, Malkowicz B, et al: Biochemical outcome after radical prostatectomy, external beam radiation therapy, or interstitial radiation therapy for clinically localized prostate cancer, *JAMA* 280:969-974, 1998.
6. Ragde H, Elgamal A, Snow PB, et al: Ten-year disease free survival after transperineal sonography-guided iodine-125 brachytherapy with or without 45-gray external beam irradiation in the treatment of patients with clinically localized, low to high Gleason grade prostate carcinoma, *Cancer* 83:989-1001, 1998.
7. Warde P, Catton C, Gospodarowicz MK: Prostate cancer. 7. Radiation therapy for localized disease, *Can Med Assoc J* 159: 1381-1388, 1998.

Advanced Prostate Cancer

Locally advanced cancer extending beyond the capsule, stage T3 or T4, without metastases, should be treated with androgen ablation. About 80% of patients with metastatic prostate cancer respond to androgen ablation, and the median disease-free survival is 2 to 3 years. Rising PSA levels predate clinical recurrence by 6 to 12 months.[1]

Major adverse effects of androgen ablation are loss of libido and potency, hot flashes, gynecomastia, fatigue, and after many years of use, loss of muscle mass, osteoporosis, adverse lipid profiles, glucose intolerance, and perhaps depression and irritability.[1]

Castration is as effective as any pharmacological method of androgen ablation and generally has fewer adverse physical effects. The bulk of evidence has not shown that adding pharmacological androgen ablation to castration (to suppress adrenal androgens) gives additional benefit.[1]

Several classes of pharmacological agents may be used to induce androgen ablation. Luteinizing hormone-releasing hormone (LH-RH) agonists that suppress the hypothalamic release of LH-RH include goserelin (Zoladex), leuprolide (Lupron), and buserelin (Suprefact). They are given by injection at 1- to 3-month intervals. Antiandrogens compete with androgens for androgen receptors on cell membranes and are divided into two classes: non-steroidal antiandrogens such as flutamide (Eulexin, Euflex), nilutamide (Nilandron, Anandron), and bicalutamide (Casodex), and steroidal antiandrogens such as cyproterone acetate (Androcur) and megestrol (Megace). Steroidal antiandrogens control hot flashes.[1] LH-RH agonists cause an initial rise in LH and testosterone lasting about 2 weeks—the so-called *flare phenomenon*. This reaction can be blocked by giving non-steroidal antiandrogens or cyproterone acetate.[1]

Clinical trials are currently evaluating the feasibility of intermittent androgen ablation. If survival is as good as that achieved with continuous treatment, quality of life may be better because adverse effects such as impotence dissipate during the months when no treatment is given.[1]

Patients treated with goserelin (Zoladex) in addition to radiotherapy had increased rates of survival at 5 years compared with radiotherapy alone (79% versus 62%).[2]

Chemotherapy is ineffective in prolonging life in patients with hormone-refractory prostate cancer. However, mitoxantrone (Novantrone) combined with prednisone gives pain relief to a number of patients. The role of bisphosphonates in controlling symptoms from bone metastases is being evaluated.

❧ REFERENCES ❧

1. Gleave ME, Bruchovsky N, Moore MJ, et al: Prostate cancer. 9. Treatment of advanced disease, *Can Med Assoc J* 160:225-232, 1999.
2. Bolla M, Gonzalez D, Warde P, et al: Improved survival in patients with locally advanced prostate cancer treated with radiotherapy and goserelin, *N Engl J Med* 337:295-300, 1997.

Prostatitis

The classification for prostatitis developed by the National Institutes of Health is as follows[1]:
1. Acute bacterial prostatitis
2. Chronic bacterial prostatitis
3. Chronic prostatitis/chronic pelvic pain syndrome
   - Inflammatory
   - Non-inflammatory
4. Asymptomatic inflammatory prostatitis

Acute bacterial prostatitis is the least common of the four types but also the easiest to diagnose and treat effectively.[2] It usually affects younger men and is caused by *Escherichia coli* in 80% of cases and other gram-negative rods or enterococci in most other instances. Patients are clinically ill with fever, malaise, and low back or perineal pain. The prostate is enlarged, very tender, and warm. It should not be massaged. Urinalysis shows leukocytes, and urine culture is usually positive for the organism. Treatment is administration of fluoroquinolones such as ciprofloxacin, trimethoprim-sulfamethoxazole, or doxycycline for 4 to 6 weeks.[3]

Chronic bacterial prostatitis, also relatively uncommon, begins as acute prostatitis, but an underlying defect in the prostate becomes a focal point for bacterial persistence.[2] It is a disease of elderly men and is usually manifested as recurring UTIs, often with suprapubic, perineal, low back, or testicular pain. The prostate may or may not be tender. White blood cells and lipid-laden macrophages are found in the prostatic secretions, and cultures of prostatic secretions and voided urine after prostatic massage are positive for bacteria. Treatment is usually with a fluoroquinolone or sometimes doxycycline for 3 to 4 months.[3]

Chronic prostatitis/chronic pelvic pain syndrome is the most common but least understood form of prostatitis. It is found in men of any age, its symptoms come and go, and it may be inflammatory or non-inflammatory.[2] Chronic pain in the perineum, scrotum, penis, pelvis, or lower back is often associated with urinary urgency, noc-turia, weak stream, dribbling, dysuria, and sexual dysfunction such as painful ejaculations, post-ejaculatory pain, and hematospermia. The prostate may or may not be tender.[3]

In the inflammatory form of chronic prostatitis/chronic pelvic pain syndrome, white blood cells and lipid-laden macrophages are found in prostatic secretions, but cultures of these secretions and urine voided after prostatic massage are negative. No treatment modality has proved to be effective. A trial of doxycycline, minocycline, or erythromycin for at least 6 weeks is often given in case *Chlamydia trachomatis* or *Ureaplasma urealyticum* is the cause of the condition.[3] Patients with non-inflammatory chronic prostatitis/chronic pelvic pain syndrome have similar symptoms and signs to those of patients with the inflammatory form, but no white blood cells or macrophages are found in prostatic secretions.[1,3] Treatments that have been tried include α-adrenergic blockers such as terazosin (Hytrin), non-steroidal anti-inflammatory drugs (NSAIDs), diazepam, hot sitz baths, avoidance of spicy foods or excessive alcohol, and even transurethral microwave thermotherapy.[3] Such a smorgasbord of therapeutic recommendations is clear evidence that no treatment has been shown to be effective. Having said this, a 2003 trial using terazosin (Hytrin) (1 mg initially, titrated to 5 mg daily) showed significant effect at 14 weeks.[4]

Asymptomatic inflammatory prostatitis is the classification used for asymptomatic patients who for one reason or another have a prostatic biopsy and are found on histological examination to have "prostatitis."[1]

❧ REFERENCES ❧

1. Krieger JN, Nyberg L Jr, Nickel JC: NIH consensus definition and classification of prostatitis (letter), *JAMA* 282:236-237, 1999.
2. National Kidney and Urological Diseases Information Clearinghouse (NKUDIC): http://kidney.niddk.nih.gov/kudiseases/pubs/prostatitis/2004
3. Roberts RO, Lieber MM, Bostwick DG, et al: A review of clinical and pathological prostatitis syndromes, *Urology* 49:809-821, 1997.
4. Cheah PY, Liong ML, Yuen KH, et al: Terazosin therapy for chronic prostatitis/chronic pelvic pain syndrome: a randomized, placebo controlled trial, *J Urology* 169:592-596, 2003.

RENAL CELL CARCINOMA

Renal cell carcinomas (RCCs) account for 80% to 85% of all primary renal neoplasms, and represent 2% of all cancers. RCC is twice as likely to occur in men as in women. Risk factors include cigarette smoking, obesity, hypertension, unopposed estrogen, and occupational exposure to petroleum products. The peak incidence of RCC is in people over age 50, with the highest incidence occurring in Scandinavia and North America.[1]

RCC manifests itself with many different presentations, anything from asymptomatic to a variety of paraneoplastic syndromes. For this reason it is often described as the "internist's tumour." The classic triad used to describe RCC, although together only arising in 10% of cases, includes hematuria (in 50% to 60% of patients), flank pain (in 40%), and a palpable abdominal/flank renal mass (in 30% to 40%).[1] Systemic or paraneoplastic syndromes include: fever, cachexia, amyloidosis, anemia, hepatic dysfunction, hormonal abnormalities, erythrocytosis, thrombocytosis, hypercalcemia, and polymyalgia-like syndrome.[2] Because most RCC's are usually asymptomatic, the diagnosis is often delayed until the disease is advanced. However, with the widespread use of CT and ultrasound for other indications, there has been an increased detection of RCC as an incidental finding. As such, when suspecting RCC, diagnostic investigation would include an ultrasound and CT.

Treatment is surgical with an overall cure rate of 58%. An occasional patient in whom a solitary metastasis develops after nephrectomy is cured by surgical removal of the metastasis. Chemotherapy has little value.[1]

--- ❧ REFERENCES ❧ ---

1. Motzer RJ, Bander NH, Nanus DM: Renal-cell carcinoma, *N Engl J Med* 335:865-875, 1996.
2. Atkins MB, Garnick MB: Clinical manifestations and evaluation of renal cell carcinoma. In Rose BD, ed: *UpToDate*, Wellesley, MA, 2004, UpToDate.

RENAL COLIC
Epidemiology

The lifetime incidence of nephrolithiasis in the United States is 15% for men and 7% for women. The incidence increases with age, peaking at 65. Half of all patients who have experienced a bout of renal colic will have a subsequent episode within 10 years.[1]

Diet

High calcium intake is not associated with an increased risk of kidney stones. In fact, the reverse may be true. As calcium intake is reduced, oxalate absorption increases, leading to hyperoxaluria and the formation of calcium oxalate stones.[1]

Meat protein intake is associated with increased oxalate excretion in one third of people.[2]

Diagnostic Imaging

Although excretory urography has been the gold standard for diagnosing ureteral calculi, unenhanced helical computed tomography (helical CT) is faster, safer, and more accurate. It has the additional advantage of detecting many non-urological causes of abdominal or flank pain.[1,3]

Hematuria in the Diagnosis of Renal Colic

In a study of patients proved by helical CT to have ureteral stones, 26% had no red blood cells on urine microscopy and 34% had negative results with urinary dipsticks. On the other hand, 40% of patients with symptoms of renal colic and microscopic hematuria did not have urolithiasis; non-urinary tract disorders associated with hematuria included torsion of ovarian masses, appendicitis, and diverticulitis.[3]

Investigations

Recommended investigations for patients with a first episode of nephrolithiasis are ultrasonography or CT, urinalysis, stone analysis (if the stone can be recovered), and measurements of blood urea nitrogen and creatinine, electrolytes, uric acid, calcium, and phosphate. If the calcium level is elevated or in the high-normal range, the parathyroid hormone level should be measured. Analyses of 24-hour urine collections are usually reserved for patients with recurrent stones.[1]

Natural History of Ureteral Calculi

Most ureteral stones pass spontaneously, especially if they are small and in the distal ureter. One prospective study found that the average time for stone passage was 8.2 days for stones 2 mm or smaller, 12.2 days for 2- to 4-mm stones, and 22.1 days for stones greater than 4 mm. Some 2- to 4-mm stones took 40 days to pass. Degree of pain was unrelated to time of passage.[4]

Urgent urological intervention (direct vision ureteroscopy or shock wave lithotripsy) is necessary if the stone is greater than 6 mm or if the patient has renal failure, a solitary kidney, urinary obstruction, or a significant urinary infection.[5] Delayed intervention is indicated when pain cannot be adequately controlled,[4,5] the patient is unwilling to wait any longer,[4] or the stone fails to pass after 2 months.[5]

Non-Pharmacological Treatment

A 2003 study took the simple route and asked whether local active warming with a heating blanket to the lower abdomen and back is effective in reducing the pain, anxiety, and nausea caused by renal colic secondary to urolithiasis. All 74 patients in the active warming group reported a 50% or more pain decrease compared with almost no change in pain scores reported by patients in the passive warming group.[6]

Non-Steroidal Anti-Inflammatory Drugs in the Treatment of Renal Colic

In Europe, parenteral NSAIDs are frequently used to relieve the pain of acute renal colic.[7,8] The drugs most frequently used are diclofenac (Voltaren) and indomethacin (Indocid). A meta-analysis of randomized controlled studies in which these drugs were administered parenterally showed them to have excellent analgesic effects compared with placebo, and to be equal to or better than analgesics.[7] The only NSAID available for parental use in North America is ketorolac (Toradol), and in one study, 90 mg of ketorolac administered intramuscularly was as effective as 100 mg of meperidine intramuscularly.[8] A British study found that a 100-mg rectal suppository of diclofenac was more effective than 100 mg of meperidine plus 12.5 mg of prochlorperazine (Compazine, Stemetil) intramuscularly.[9]

Alpha Blockers in the Treatment of Renal Colic

Alpha blockers have been shown to dilate the distal ureters. In one study with 102 patients, 80.4% of patients receiving tamulosin 0.4 mg once daily passed their stone within 7 days compared with 62.8% of those receiving placebo.[10]

Prevention of Recurrent Nephrolithiasis

The most important way to prevent recurrent stones is a high fluid (preferably water) intake. Patients should drink 2.5 to 3 L per day (more in hot weather or if exercising) and should drink 8 to 12 oz before bedtime to counter urine concentration during sleep. For patients with recurrent stone formation, pharmacotherapy is tailored to biochemical abnormalities detected by 24-hour urine collections. Thiazides are commonly used to decrease urinary calcium excretion and are often combined with potassium citrate 20 to 30 mEq twice daily. Potassium citrate not only counters hypokalemia, but also increases urinary citrate levels, which helps prevent the formation of both calcium and uric acid stones.[1]

◣ REFERENCES ◢

1. Goldfarb DS, Coe FL: Prevention of recurrent nephrolithiasis, *Am Fam Physician* 60:2269-2276, 1999.
2. Quan-Vinh N, et al: Sensitivity to meat protein intake and hyperoxaluria in idiopathic calcium stone formers, *Kidney Int* 59:2273-2281, 2001.
3. Bove P, Kaplan D, Dalrymple N, et al: Reexamining the value of hematuria testing in patients with acute flank pain, *J Urol* 162:685-687, 1999.
4. Miller OF, Kane CJ: Time to stone passage for observed ureteral calculi: a guide for patient education, *J Urol* 162:688-691, 1999.
5. Preminger GM: Editorial comment on Miller OF, Kane CJ: Time to stone passage for observed ureteral calculi: a guide for patient education, *J Urol* 162:690-691, 1999.
6. Kober A, Dobrovits M, Djavan, et al: Local active warming: an effective treatment for pain, anxiety and nausea caused by renal colic, *J Urol* 170:741-744, 2003.
7. Labrecque M, Dostaler L-P, Rousselle R, et al: Efficacy of nonsteroidal anti-inflammatory drugs in the treatment of acute renal colic, *Arch Intern Med* 154:1381-1387, 1994.
8. Oosterlinck W, Philp NH, Charig C, et al: A double-blind single dose comparison of intramuscular ketorolac tromethamine and pethidine in the treatment of renal colic, *J Clin Pharmacol* 30:336-341, 1990.
9. Thompson JF, Pike JM, Chumas PD, et al: Rectal diclofenac compared with pethidine injection in acute renal colic, *BMJ* 299:1140-1141, 1989.
10. Cervenakov I et al: Speedy elimination of ureterolithiasis in lower part of ureters with alpha 1-blocker – Tamsulosin, *Int Urol Nephrol* 34:25-29, 2002.

TESTES

Testicular Masses (in the Adult)

Patients may present either with a painful, or a painless, scrotal swelling. The presentation and characteristics of the swelling will help the clinician arrive at a diagnosis.

Painful swellings include: epididymitis, testicular torsion, orchitis, hematocele, and a strangulated indirect hernia.

- **Epididymitis** is the most common cause of painful swelling of the testis in post-pubertal males. Presentation is usually a gradual development of scrotal pain radiating to the flank, associated with fever, irritative voiding symptoms, and possibly urethral discharge. Examination reveals an enlarged and indurated epididymis. Because the etiology is often an ascending infection, investigations should include a urinalysis, urine C&S, and/or urethral discharge Gram stain for gonorrhea or chlamydial infection. Treatment is dependent on whether the etiology is more consistent with a urinary tract infection, or an infection with *Neisseria gonorrhoeae* and *Chlamydia trachomatis*.[1]

- **Testicular torsion** occurs due to an anatomical deformity known as the "bell-clapper" deformity, which allows the spermatic cord to twist, resulting in the occlusion of testicular blood flow. Precipitating factors usually include either trauma or vigorous exercise. The presentation is usually of a young male with acute onset; severe, unilateral scrotal pain; and/or nausea and vomiting. Scrotal edema and erythema are typically present. On examination, the affected testis is extremely tender, firm, may appear retracted upward, and the epididymis may be anterior rather than its natural posterior position. If torsion is suspected, immediate referral should be made to a urologist. Colour Doppler ultrasound can be used if the diagnosis is uncertain. Treatment is detorsion, and bilateral orchiplexy.[1,2]

  If surgical consultation is unavailable, an attempt may be made to detort the testis manually. The direction of rotation in torsion is usually toward the midline, so the physician corrects the rotation by sitting on the examining table at the patient's feet, grasping the affected testis, and rotating it from the inside toward the outside (right testis counterclockwise and left testis clockwise).[1,3]

- **Acute orchitis** may have a similar presentation as epididymitis: sudden onset of testicular pain, fever, nausea and vomiting. Etiology is mainly pyogenic bacteria or viruses. Treatment is usually conservative with bedrest, scrotal support, local ice therapy, and analgesics. If the source is bacterial, then antibiotics can be prescribed.[1]

- **Hematocele** is associated with trauma, and is a bleed into the tunica vaginalis. Treatment is with ice packs, analgesics, and surgical repair.
- **Strangulated inguinal hernia** should be considered if the testes can be palpated as separate from the hernia, and if a cough impulse is transmitted. Transillumination test is negative to distinguish from a hydrocele. Treatment is surgical.

  Painless swellings include hydrocele, varicocele, and spermatocele. Testicular cancer (discussed separately below) is also included in this group.

- **Hydrocele** is a collection of fluid within the tunica vaginalis. It presents as a painless scrotal swelling that transilluminates. A scrotal ultrasound should be done because hydroceles may present alongside a testicular neoplasm. No treatment is required unless complications are present, including hemorrhage into the hydrocele sac following trauma, bulky mass compromising testicular blood flow, or severe pain.[1,2]
- **Varicocele** is an abnormal dilation of the veins in the pampiniform plexus resulting from incompetent veins in testicular veins. It is present in up to 20% of all males. It is usually asymptomatic, but can present with a heavy, dragging sensation of the testes after walking or standing. It predominantly occurs on the left side. On examination, the tortuosity of the veins can be palpated, and has been described as a "bag of worms." Varicoceles have been associated with infertility, but not all patients with varicoceles are infertile. Treatment consists of surgical ligation of the testicular vein above the inguinal ligament. Indications for treatment are infertility or symptoms.[1,2]
- **Spermatocele** presents as a painless cystic mass that is palpable as separate from the testes, and transilluminates. Aspiration of the mass reveals dead sperm. Treatment is usually conservative.

Testicular cancer

(See also clinical practice guidelines; prevention; screening)

Testicular tumours are uncommon, but are the most common malignant disease in men between the ages of 29 and 34 years.[1] Ninety-five percent of testicular tumours are germ cell tumours. The two major types of germ cell tumours are seminomas and non-seminomatous germ cell tumours (embryonal carcinoma, yolk cell carcinoma, teratoma, and choriocarcinoma).[4] The initial investigation of a suspected testicular mass is ultrasound, and if it indicates a mass within the testes, the diagnosis is cancer until proven otherwise.[5] Both seminomas and non-seminomatous germ cell tumours may cause elevations of human chorionic gonadotropin levels, whereas only non-seminomatous germ cell tumours increase alpha-fetoprotein.[4,5]

The overall cure rate for all germ cell tumours is greater than 90%. Most cases of seminomas are treated with orchiectomy plus retroperitoneal and pelvic lymph node irradiation, whereas non-seminomatous germ cell tumours are usually treated with orchiectomy with or without pelvic lymph node resection. Recurrences or widespread disease can usually be cured by chemotherapy, although the prognosis is considerably worse if there are hepatic, cerebral, or osseous metastases.[4] A protocol for high-risk non-seminomatous germ cell tumours that appears to have excellent results is orchiectomy plus immediate administration of two courses of adjuvant chemotherapy.[6]

Widely variable recommendations have been proposed for testicular examination as a means of cancer screening. Some of these are listed in Table 77.[7]

────────────────── ⊋ REFERENCES ⊱ ──────────────────

1. Junnila J, Lassen P: Testicular masses, *Am Fam Physician* 57: 685-692, 1998.
2. Eyre RC: Evaluation of scrotal pathology. In Rose BD, ed: *UpToDate*, Wellesley, MA, 2004, UpToDate.
3. Leduc C: La douleur scrotale aiguë: un cas de torsion testiculaire, *L'Omnipraticien* 3(2):9-16, 1999.
4. Bosl GJ, Motzer RJ: Testicular germ-cell cancer, *N Engl J Med* 337:242-259, 1997.
5. Kinkade S: Testicular cancer, *Am Fam Physician* 59:2539-2544, 1999.
6. Böhlen D, Borner M, Sonntag RW, et al: Long-term results following adjuvant chemotherapy in patients with clinical stage I testicular nonseminomatous malignant germ cell tumors with high risk factors, *J Urol* 161:1148-1152, 1999.
7. US Public Health Service: Cancer detection in adults by physical examination, *Am Fam Physician* 51:871-885, 1995.

Table 77 Recommendations for Testicular Examinations by Physicians

Authority	Recommendations
Canadian Task Force on Preventive Health Care	Only if history of cryptorchidism, infertility, atrophic testes, or ambiguous genitalia
U.S. Preventive Services Task Force	Ages 13-39 only if history of cryptorchidism, orchiopexy, or testicular atrophy
National Cancer Institute	Routine as part of periodic health examination
American Cancer Society	Every 3 years from 20-39 and thereafter annually
American Urological Association	Regularly starting at age 15
American Academy of Family Physicians	Ages 13-18 if history of cryptorchidism, orchiopexy, or testicular atrophy; as part of periodic health examination ages 19-39

URINARY TRACT INFECTIONS

(See also catheters; hormone replacement therapy; interstitial cystitis; prostatitis; urinalysis; urinary tract infections in children)

Classification

The following are the major categories of urinary tract infection (UTI)[1]:
Uncomplicated
1. Cystitis in young women,
2. Recurrent cystitis in young women
3. Pyelonephritis in young women
Complicated
1. Persistent or recurrent infections
2. Infections in men
3. Catheter related
4. Asymptomatic bacteriuria

Diagnosis

Diagnosis is made primarily by history. In women with dysuria and frequency, in the absence of vaginitis, the diagnosis is UTI 80% of the time.[2] A recent diagnostic study conducted at four family medicine clinics at the University of Toronto with 231 women found that four factors accounted for about 79% of UTIs[3]:
1. Burning or discomfort on voiding
2. Seeking care within 1 day of onset of symptoms
3. Detectable leukocytes in urine
4. Detectable nitrite in urine

Patients with two of these risk factors had a 63% risk of having a UTI. Those with three factors had an 84% risk, and those with all four factors had a 100% risk. In contrast, patients with one risk factor had a 28% risk, and those with none of the four risk factors had a 16% risk. The symptom of frequency is notably absent. This pattern suggests that when patients have two or more of these risk factors, they're likely to have a true UTI. However, this rule has yet to be tested in another independent population.

Dipsticks and Cultures

(See also urinalysis)

Leukocyte esterase dipsticks have sensitivities of 75% to 96%. Nitrites, when positive, are very suggestive of a UTI, but are often absent. This is because the reaction depends on the conversion of nitrates to nitrites by bacteria, but some fairly common organisms such as *Staphylococcus saprophyticus* do not have this capacity. As a result, the sensitivity of the test is rather low, but its specificity is high.[1]

Pyuria should also be tested for if a UTI is suspected. Testing for pyuria and nitrites in women with classic symptoms of UTI reduces unnecessary antibiotic use, and more women with a confirmed UTI receive immediate antibiotics.[3]

A urine culture is *not* indicated in the vast majority of UTIs.[2] In the past, urine cultures producing fewer than 100,000 colony-forming units (CFUs) of bacteria per millilitre of urine were not considered diagnostic of UTI. New data suggest that the presence of as few as 100 CFUs/mL correlates well with uncomplicated cystitis in symptomatic women. Many laboratories do not report such low values, but in most instances this is academic because cultures are not required for the diagnosis or treatment of uncomplicated UTIs in young women. Consider urine culture only in recurrent UTI or in the presence of complicating factors.[2] Patients with complicated UTIs and women with uncomplicated pyelonephritis generally have more than 100,000 CFUs/mL.[1,3]

Risk Factors for Urinary Tract Infections

Commonly stated risk factors for uncomplicated UTIs in young women include the following[1,4]:
1. Sexual intercourse
2. Diaphragm use
3. Spermicide use (including spermicide-coated condoms)
4. History of recurrent UTIs
5. Delayed post-coital micturition

A prospective study of sexually active young women failed to find any protective effect of post-coital voiding, but the frequency of UTIs increased with the frequency of coitus and the frequency of diaphragm use.[4] Both the diaphragm and spermicides are thought to foster colonization of the periurethral area with coliform bacteria.[1]

Treatment of Uncomplicated Cystitis in Women

Between 80% and 90% of uncomplicated UTIs are caused by *Escherichia coli*, 10% to 20% by coagulase-negative *S. saprophyticus,* and less than 5% by other organisms. Although many of the common organisms are resistant to ampicillin or sulfonamides, the vast majority are sensitive to trimethoprim-sulfamethoxazole and fluoroquinolones.[1]

The treatment of choice for most uncomplicated UTIs in women is a 3-day course of oral trimethoprim-sulfamethoxazole (Bactrim, Septra).

Second-line treatment options include a 3-day course of one of the fluoroquinolones, a 3-day course of trimethoprim, a 7-day course of nitrofurantoin, amoxicillin, first generation cephalosporin, or a single dose of fosfomycin (Monurol).[2] (Note: Fluoroquinolones are contraindicated in pregnancy.)

Cultures are only indicated for recurrent infections, and in these cases, the antibacterials of choice are usually fluoroquinolones, amoxicillin/clavulanic acid, or third-generation cephalosporins. Amoxicillin alone is usually not a drug of first choice because many organisms are resistant to it.[1,5] Resistance is growing with trimethoprim-sulfamethoxazole, and some authorities caution that if your local resistance rates are above 20%, you could consider other therapy. Single-dose treatments are effective for many women, but with the exception of fosfomycin, they are not generally recommended because of a relatively high risk of recurrence within 6 weeks.[1]

Some of the suggested treatment regimens for uncomplicated UTIs are listed in Table 78.

Phenazopyridine (Pyridium) is an azo dye that was first marketed in the United States in 1914 as a urinary antiseptic. It is not effective in this role but continues to be prescribed as a urinary analgesic. There are no good studies supporting this indication, and since antibiotics give rapid relief of symptoms and phenazopyridine can cause methemoglobinemia, its use has little justification.[6]

Prophylaxis of Uncomplicated Urinary Tract Infections in Women

Recurrent UTIs are defined as more than three infections documented by urine cultures in 1 year. A variety of acceptable antibiotic prophylactic regimens can be used for this condition in women[1]:

1. Prescription of repeated 3-day treatment regimens so the patient can treat herself at the onset of symptoms.
2. Continuous prophylaxis for a 6-month period using drugs such as a single daily dose of trimethoprim-sulfamethoxazole 40/200 mg (1/2 regular strength tablet), trimethoprim 100 mg, nitrofurantoin 50 to 100 mg, or norfloxacin 200 mg.
3. If UTIs are related to intercourse, antibiotics such as trimethoprim-sulfamethoxazole 40/200 mg (1/2 regular strength tablet) should be taken immediately after intercourse.

An Israeli study found that intravaginal estriol was effective in preventing recurrent UTIs in post-menopausal women. Estrogens facilitate the colonization of lactobacilli in the vagina, which lowers the vaginal pH and inhibits the growth of coliform bacteria.[7] Estriol is not absorbed systemically. It is not available in Canada or the United States.

A study of elderly women found that those who drank 300 mL of cranberry juice daily had a decreased incidence of bacteriuria with pyuria compared with control subjects given placebo.[8] However, whether drinking cranberry or blueberry juice will prevent UTIs in young women is unknown.[9]

Pyelonephritis in Young Women

E. coli is the cause of most cases of uncomplicated pyelonephritis in young women, and in about one third of cases, the organism is resistant to ampicillin, amoxicillin, and first-generation cephalosporins. If a patient with pyelonephritis is not toxic and can tolerate oral medications, she may be treated as an outpatient for 10 to 14 days with trimethoprim-sulfamethoxazole or a fluoroquinolone.[1,8] Examples include trimethoprim-sulfamethoxazole 160 mg/800 mg (DS) every 12 hours, ciprofloxacin 500 mg every 12 hours, ofloxacin 200 to 300 mg every 12 hours, and norfloxacin 400 mg every 12 hours.[10]

Complicated Urinary Tract Infections

Complicated UTIs are due to anatomical, functional, or pharmacological factors that lead to persistent or recurrent infections. Obstruction is a common cause. *E. coli* is responsible for less than one third of complicated UTIs, and therapy is usually with a fluoroquinolone or a third-generation cephalosporin administered for at least 10 to 14 days.[1]

Urinary Tract Infections in Men

Initial (uncomplicated) UTIs in men are commonly due to obstruction, instrumentation, or prostatitis. Usual treatment is trimethoprim-sulfamethoxazole or a fluoroquinolone for at least 7 days; if prostatitis is present, treatment may have to be continued for 6 to 12 weeks. (See discussion of prostatitis.) Urological workup is indicated for elderly men and for men of any age with clinical evidence of pyelonephritis. In otherwise healthy young men with symptoms of cystitis, only a culture is required.[1]

Catheter-Related Urinary Tract Infections

Long-term catheterization is always associated with bacteriuria, and no effective means of preventing this have been devised. Antibiotic treatment of asymptomatic bacteriuria in patients with long-term catheters is rarely indicated. If patients are symptomatic, they are usually treated with fluoroquinolones for 10 to 14 days.[1]

Bacteriuria and Pyuria in the Elderly

Asymptomatic bacteriuria and asymptomatic pyuria are common findings in elderly women. In a prospective observational study from Boston, 61 women from a long-care institution or community housing sites submitted monthly clean-catch urine specimens for a 6-month period; 28% of patients had at least one sample showing

Table 78 Pharmacotherapy for Uncomplicated Urinary Tract Infections

Drugs	Usual doses
Trimethoprim-sulfamethoxazole (Bactrim, Septra)	160-800 mg (1 DS tablet) bid × 3 days
Ciprofloxacin (Cipro)	100 mg bid × 3 days
Norfloxacin (Noroxin)	400 mg bid × 3 days
Ofloxacin (Floxin)	200 mg bid × 3 days
Fosfomycin (Monurol)	3 grams as a single dose
Amoxicillin	250 mg tid × 3 days
Nitrofurantoin (Macrobid)	100 mg bid × 7 days

bacteriuria alone, while bacteriuria with pyuria was found in at least one sample from 26% of patients. Bacteriuria with symptoms occurred in only 10% of patients. Spontaneous clearance of both bacteriuria and pyuria was common. For patients with symptoms, the sensitivity of urine dipstick (leukocyte esterase) and microscopic examination for bacteria and white cells was 80% or better, and the negative predictive value of these tests approached 100%.[11]

The Canadian Task Force on Preventive Health Care has concluded that no evidence has shown that the treatment of asymptomatic bacteriuria in the elderly is beneficial. It gives "E" ratings for screening elderly institutionalized men and women and persons of either sex with indwelling catheters; a "D" rating to screening of ambulatory elderly men; and a "C" rating to screening of ambulatory elderly women.[12] The U.S. Preventive Services Task Force also gives an "E" rating to screening for bacteriuria in institutionalized elderly patients and a "C" rating to such screening in ambulatory elderly women.[13]

❧ REFERENCES ❧

1. Orenstein R, Wong ES: Urinary tract infections in adults, *Am Fam Physician* 59:1225-1234, 1999.
2. University of Michigan Health System (1999): *Urinary tract infection: adult women with uncomplicated UTI: guidelines for clinical care*, Ann Arbor MI, 1999, The University.
3. McIsaac W, Low D, Biringer A, et al: The impact of empirical management of acute cystitis on unnecessary antibiotic use, *Arch Intern Med* 162:600-605, 2002.
4. Hooton TM, Scholes D, Hughes JP, et al: A prospective study of risk factors for symptomatic urinary tract infection in young women, *N Engl J Med* 335:468-474, 1996.
5. The choice of antibacterial drugs, *Med Lett* 40:33-42, 1998.
6. Zelenitsky SA, Zhanel GG: Phenazopyridine in urinary tract infections, *Ann Pharmacother* 30:866-868, 1996.
7. Raz R, Stamm WE: A controlled trial of intravaginal estriol in postmenopausal women with recurrent urinary tract infections, *N Engl J Med* 329:753-756, 1993.
8. Avorn J, Monane M, Gurwitz JH, et al: Reduction of bacteriuria and pyuria after ingestion of cranberry juice, *JAMA* 271: 751-754, 1994.
9. Ronald A: Sex and urinary tract infections (editorial), *N Engl J Med* 335:511-512, 1996.
10. Stamm WE, Hooton TM: Management of urinary tract infections in adults, *N Engl J Med* 329:1328-1334, 1993.
11. Monane M, Gurwitz JH, Lipsitz LA, et al: Epidemiologic and diagnostic aspects of bacteriuria: a longitudinal study in older women, *J Am Geriatr Soc* 43:618-622, 1995.
12. Canadian Task Force on the Periodic Health Examination: *Canadian guide to clinical preventive health care*, Ottawa, 1994, Canada Communication Group. 966-967.
13. U.S. Preventive Services Task Force: *Guide to clinical preventive services*, ed 2, Baltimore, 1996, Williams & Wilkins, 347-359.

VASECTOMY

(See also infertility, male; tubal sterilization)

Vasectomy and Prostate Cancer

While a number of publications have reported a positive association between vasectomy and prostate cancer, a systematic review of the literature concluded that such reports are rife with methodological problems and that there is no evidence that vasectomy increases the risk of prostate cancer.[1]

Vasectomy Methods

There are several methods of disrupting the vas, but one of the newest techniques is the No-Scalpel Vasectomy (NSV). This method was devised in China around 1974 and introduced to North America in 1986.[2] "No-scalpel" is slightly misleading, because a hole is made in the skin, but it is not made with a scalpel. NSV delivers the vas through an opening in the skin with the least trauma possible. The complication rate (bleeding, infection, pain, swelling) is about 10% of the more traditional method, which uses a scalpel to expose the vas.

There are many methods of actually treating the vas, such as cutting, tying, clipping, folding over, burying, or cauterizing. One study of 2,500 patients demonstrated a statistically significant reduction in reconnection when intraluminal cautery and fascial interposition (enclosing the upper cut end within its sheath by suture or clip) were used together.[3] Recovery time is shorter with NSV, and often men are comfortable enough to return to a physically inactive job the next day. Men can anticipate some mild aching, but this is usually controlled with an athletic support, ice, acetaminophen and/or an NSAID. Post-operative patients are advised to continue contraception for at least 20 to 30 ejaculations in order for sperm stored above the vasectomy site to be cleared. In the active healing phase, it is possible for a microscopic channel to form in the scar tissue and reconnect the upper and lower vas sections, accounting for a failure rate of 1/1200.[2] Two semen analyses (preferably analyzed within 1 hour of production) are highly recommended at least 10 weeks post-vasectomy to confirm azospermia. The main long-term complication of chronic aching or pain occurs in 1% to 2% of men.[2]

❧ REFERENCES ❧

1. Bernal-Delgado E, Latour-Pérez J, Pradas-Arnal F, et al: The association between vasectomy and prostate cancer: a systematic review of the literature, *Fertil Steril* 70:191-200, 1998.
2. Pfenninger JL, Tuggy ML, Denniston GC, et al: No-scalpel vasectomy. First Consult (Accessed April 28, 2004 at http://www.firstconsult.com/home/framework/fs_main.htm?msite=fs_main&).
3. Clenney TC, Higgins JC: Vasectomy techniques, *Am Fam Physician* 60:137-152, 1999.

VASOVASOTOMY

A review of close to 1500 microsurgical procedures to reverse vasectomies found that if the procedure was performed within 3 years of vasectomy, the patency rate was 97% and the pregnancy rate 76%. If the procedure was performed 15 years after the vasectomy, the patency rate was 71% and the pregnancy rate 30%.[1]

A second important factor was the microsurgical experience level of the surgeon. Lastly, the presence of sperm and the quality of the fluid from the proximal vas is predictive of surgical success.[1]

❧ REFERENCES ❧

1. Belker AM, Thomas AJ Jr, Fuchs EF, et al: Results of 1,469 microsurgical vasectomy reversals by the Vasovasostomy Study Group, *J Urol* 145:505-511, 1991.

WOMEN'S HEALTH: BREAST DISEASES

Topics covered in this section

Benign Breast Conditions
Breast Cancer

BENIGN BREAST CONDITIONS
Management of a Breast Lump
Non-Palpable lump

Management of non-palpable lumps picked up on mammography or ultrasound should be guided by the radiologist's recommendations. Ultrasound or stereotactically (mammographically) guided fine needle aspiration or core biopsy may be required for definitive diagnosis.

Palpable lump

Further investigation is required in this instance. The quickest way to determine if the lump is cystic or solid is by performing fine needle aspiration biopsy.[1] If the lesion proves to be a cyst, the fluid aspirated is not bloody; if on palpation the breast lump has completely disappeared, the specimen does not have to be sent for cytological analysis. If the fluid is bloody, the lump does not completely disappear, or it recurs, surgical consultation is indicated.[1] If the lump proves to be solid, the patient should be referred to a surgeon. For women 35 and older a mammogram should be performed and those less than 35 years old should have an ultrasound to better assess the characteristics of the solid lesion.

≈ REFERENCES ≈

1. Heisey R, Mahoney L, Watson B: Management of palpable breast lumps. Consensus guideline for physicians, *Can Fam Physician* 45:1849-1854, 1999.

Breast Implants

(See also breastfeeding; functional somatic syndromes; multiple chemical sensitivities)

A meta-analysis of 20 studies done in 2000 showed no evidence of an association between breast implants in general, or silicone breast implants specifically, and any connective tissue or autoimmune disease.[1] Breast augmentation does reduce the sensitivity of screening mammograms; despite the lower accuracy of mammograms in women with implants, those who develop cancer do not appear to present at a more advanced stage.[2]

≈ REFERENCES ≈

1. Janowsky EC, Kupper LL, Hulka BS: Meta-analyses of the relation between silicone breast implants and the risk of connective-tissue diseases, *N Engl J Med* 342(11):781-790, 2000.

2. Miglioetti DL, Rutter CM, Geller BM, et al: Effect of breast augmentation on the accuracy of mammography cancer characteristics, *JAMA* 291(4):442-450, 2004.

Breast Pain

(See also an approach to complementary and alternative medicines)

Mastalgia should be categorized as cyclical pre-menstrual breast pain, non-cyclic breast pain, or extramammary pain. Two thirds of women with mastalgia have cyclical pain. Many women with breast pain worry that this is a symptom of cancer. Reassurance after a careful examination is often the only therapy required. If a breast lump is found, management should proceed as described above. The risk of cancer in a woman who presents with breast pain as her only symptom is extremely low.[1] In a woman 35 or older with new onset breast pain, a mammogram should also be considered. Vitamin E and caffeine reduction have been tested in controlled trials and found to be no better than placebo.[2] A diet high in fibre and low in fat may decrease breast pain.[2] Evening primrose oil, an extract of the seeds of the evening primrose, contains gamma linolenic acid, linolenic acid, and vitamin E and it has been promoted as beneficial for a wide variety of ailments, including breast pain. In a recent randomized trial it was shown to offer no clear benefit over control oils or fish oils in the treatment of mastalgia.[3]

Three drugs that have been used for cyclical breast pain are bromocriptine (Parlodel), danazol (Cyclomen) and tamoxifen.[1]

Fewer than 10% of women have severe and prolonged enough breast pain to warrant treatment with bromocriptine or danazol. Bromocriptine is usually started as a single daily dose of 1.25 mg and is increased by 2.5 mg every 2 to 4 weeks as necessary MFE. The usual dosage for mastalgia is 2.5 mg twice per day. The initial dosage of danazol is 100 to 150 mg twice per day with reduction to about 100 mg per day once symptoms are controlled MFE. Therapy with danazol is usually continued for 6 to 9 months. Both bromocriptine and danazol have significant side effects. The major one for bromocriptine is nausea. For danazol the adverse effects are related to the medication's androgenic effects and include weight gain, fluid retention, fatigue, a decrease in breast size, hirsutism, atrophic vaginitis, hot flashes, acne, greasy skin, depression, and hoarse voice. All except hoarseness are said to be reversible when the medication is discontinued. Tamoxifen has also been used starting at 10 mg per day MFE. It tends to have fewer side effects. Any of these medications should be reassessed after 3 months of use.

Women with chest wall pain only can be treated with non-steroidal anti-inflammatory drugs (NSAIDs).

❧ REFERENCES ❧

1. Smith RL, Pruthi S, Fitzpatrick LA: Evaluation and management of breast pain, *Mayo Clin Proc* 79:353-372, 2004.
2. Fentiman IS: Management of breast pain. In JR Harris et al, editors: *Diseases of the breast,* ed 2, Philadelphia, 2000, Lippincott, Williams and Wilkins, pp 57-61.
3. Blommers J, de Lange-De Klerk ES, Kuik DJ et al: Evening primrose oil and fish oil for severe chronic mastalgia: a randomized double-blind controlled trial, *Am J Obstet Gynecol* 187:1389-1394, 2002.

BREAST CANCER

Epidemiology of Breast Cancer

(See also ductal carcinoma in situ)

Widely published figures from The Canadian Cancer Society state that a woman's lifetime risk of breast cancer is 1 in 9.[1] In the United States the equivalent figure is 1 in 8.[2] Such figures are deceptive for three main reasons.[2,3]

Lifetime risk figures apply only to the relatively few women who live to a ripe old age. When life table analyses are performed, a different picture emerges. For example, the lifetime risk of breast cancer is 1 in 625 for a woman between 30 and 34 years of age, 1 in 18 for a 50 year old, and 1 in 13 for a 75 year old.[3] Another useful way of evaluating breast cancer risk is to determine the probability that the disease will develop within the next decade. This risk is higher in older than in younger women, but no matter what the age, it is never greater than 1 in 32.[1] Chemoprevention strategies often use a woman's risk of breast cancer over a 5-year period to help direct treatment. A breast cancer risk assessment tool based on the Gail Model can be accessed at http://bcra.nci.nih.gov/brc/.

Mortality from breast cancer is much lower than incidence, in part because of improved treatment, and in part because many of the cases diagnosed with mammography, such as ductal carcinoma in situ, are relatively innocuous (see below). The probability of a woman dying of breast cancer is 1:2873 by age 34, 1:136 by age 54, and 1:39 by age 75. Overall, 70% of women treated for breast cancer are still alive 10 years later.[3]

Many people interpret lifetime risk figures to mean that breast cancer is a greater health risk than other potentially preventable diseases such as coronary artery disease and lung cancer, both of which kill many more women than does breast cancer.[2,3] In part this is due to the fact that cancer (all types) is the leading cause of potential years of life lost and because of the relatively young age of death for some women with breast cancer. Nevertheless potential years of life lost in Canada is greater for lung cancer in women.[4] In terms of overall mortality, if a cohort of 1000 women is followed for 85 years from the time of birth, 33 will have died of breast cancer and 203 will have died of cardiovascular disease. No matter what age bracket is considered, breast cancer never accounts for more than 20% of deaths.[2]

❧ REFERENCES ❧

1. Canadian Cancer Society/National Cancer Institute of Canada: Probability of developing/dying from cancer. In: Canadian Cancer Statistics 2005, Toronto, 2005, Canadian Cancer Society/National Cancer Institute of Canada, pp. 56-58. [Accessed June 20, 2005] Available from: URL: http://www.cancer.ca/ccs/internet/standard/0,3172_14291_langId-en,00.html.
2. Phillips KA, Glendon G, Knight JA: Putting the risk of breast cancer in perspective, *N Engl J Med* 340:141-144, 1999.
3. Bunker JP, Houghton J, Baum M: Putting the risk of breast cancer in perspective, *BMJ* 317:1307-1309, 1998.
4. Canadian Cancer Society/National Cancer Institute of Canada: Potential years of life lost due to cancer. In: Canadian Cancer Statistics 2005. Toronto, 2005, Canadian Cancer Society/National Cancer Institute of Canada, pp. 58-60. [Accessed June 20, 2005] Available from: URL: http://www.cancer.ca/ccs/internet/standard/0,3172_14291_langId-en,00.html.

Risk Factors and Primary Prevention

(See also hormone replacement therapy; oral contraceptives)

Table 79 lists some of the established and probable risk factors for breast cancer.[1-18]

The incidence of breast cancer increases progressively with age.[1,2] However, the rate of increase slows at the time of the menopause, presumably because of estrogen withdrawal (see below).

After increasing age, the next most significant risk factor for breast cancer is a family history of the disease.[1,2] A small proportion of women with a strong family history have identifiable genetic mutations in the BRCA1 or BRCA2 genes.[2,3] Hereditary breast cancer is discussed in the next section.

Women with a history of benign breast disease with proliferative epithelial patterns[2,4] or fibroadenomas[4] have a slightly increased risk of breast cancer that varies according to the degree of histological atypia.[4]

A rare but important risk factor for breast cancer is previous radiation exposure such as that used in the treatment of childhood Hodgkin's disease.[5]

Changes in the hormonal milieu appear to affect breast cancer risk. Early menarche and late first pregnancies increase the risk slightly,[1,2] as does failure to breast-feed.[6] The menopause is protective, and thus the incidence of breast cancer in pre-menopausal women is higher than that of post-menopausal women of equivalent age. The earlier the onset of menopause, whether natural or surgically induced, the greater the protective effect. Hormone replacement therapy is associated with clinically important increases in incidence and mortality rate[7-9] from breast cancer (see discussion of hormone replacement therapy—adverse effects). Women with high bone density[10] and obese post-menopausal women[1,11,12] have increased rates of breast cancer; in both cases higher estrogen levels probably account for the findings. Paradoxically, obesity is associated with a decreased risk of pre-menopausal breast cancer, probably because obese women have higher rates of anovulation.[12]

Alcohol is a risk factor for breast cancer, probably due to the effect of alcohol on increasing endogenous estrogen levels. In a pooled analysis of 53 studies the risk of breast cancer increased linearly with increasing alcohol use, with the relative risk increasing by 7.1% for each drink consumed per day.[13] There are data to suggest that recent drinking is more important than patterns early in life.[14] Advising women to decrease alcohol intake to no more than one drink per day could reduce breast cancer risk while still allowing for the positive cardiovascular benefits. High-fat diets have been suggested as a risk factor, but this has not been substantiated.[15] Further data from the Nurses' Health Study indicated that pre-menopausal women who ate five or more servings of fruit or vegetables each day had a decreased risk of breast cancer.[16]

Both active and passive smoking have been associated with an increased risk of breast cancer although the data are not conclusive because alcohol use has been a significant confounder.[13] An epidemiological study of over 25,000 Norwegian women reported that regular exercise was associated with a decreased risk of breast cancer.[17] Prospective data from the Women's Health Initiative Cohort study suggested that increased physical activity in post-menopausal women is associated with a reduced likelihood of breast cancer. Brisk walking for 1.25 to 2.5 hours per week resulted in an 18% decreased risk.[18]

Table 79   Breast Cancer Risk Factors

Well-Documented Risk Factors
Increasing age[1,2]
Family history of breast cancer or genetic mutations[1,2]
Geographic location (West versus Asia)[1]
History of proliferative breast dysplasia[2-4]
History of fibroadenoma[4]
Radiation[1,5]
Menarche before age 12[1,2]
First pregnancy over age 30[1,2]
Failure to breast-feed[6*]
Delayed menopause[1,2]
Hormone replacement therapy for 5 years or more[7-9]
Elevated bone density[10]
Increased post-menopausal body mass index[11-12]
Increased mammographic breast density[19]
Alcohol[13,14]

Possible Risk Factors
Current oral contraceptive use[21]
Diet[15,16]
Smoking[13]
Sedentary lifestyle[17,18]

*Elevated risk reported only for breast cancer developing in pre-menopausal women.

High mammographic density is associated with increasing risk of breast cancer.[19] There is no association between antiperspirant use and breast cancer. History of induced abortion is not associated with increased risk.[20]

⊰ REFERENCES ⊱

1. McPherson K, Steel CM, Dixon JM: Breast cancer—epidemiology, risk factors, and genetics, *BMJ* 309:1003-1006, 1994.
2. Gail MG, Costantino J, Bryant J, et al: Weighing the risks and benefits of tamoxifen treatment for preventing breast cancer, *J Natl Cancer Inst* 91:1829-46, 1999.
3. Warner E, Heisey RE, Goel V, et al: Hereditary breast cancer: risk assessment of patients with a family history of breast cancer, *Can Fam Physician* 45:104-112, 1999.
4. Fitzgibbons PL, Henson DE, Hutter RV: Benign breast changes and the risk for subsequent breast cancer—an update of the 1985 consensus statement, *Arch Path Lab Med* 122:1053-1055, 1998.
5. Bhatia S, Robison LL, Oberlin O, et al: Breast cancer and other second neoplasms after childhood Hodgkin's disease, *N Engl J Med* 334:745-751, 1996.
6. Furberg H, Newman B, Moorman P, et al: Lactation and breast cancer risk, *Int J Epidemiol* 28:396-402, 1999.
7. Beral V, with the Million Women Study Collaborators: Breast cancer and hormone-replacement therapy in the million women study, *Lancet* 362(9382):419-427, 2003.
8. Chlebowski RT, Hendrix SL, Langer RD, et al: Influence of estrogen plus progestin on breast cancer and mammography in healthy postmenopausal women: the Women's Health Initiative randomized trial, *JAMA* 289(24):3243-3253, 2003.
9. Grodstein F, Stampfer MJ, Colditz A, et al: Postmenopausal hormone therapy and mortality, *N Engl J Med* 336:1769-1775, 1997.
10. Zhang Y, Kiel DP, Kreger BE, et al: Bone mass and the risk of breast cancer among postmenopausal women, *N Engl J Med* 336:611-617, 1997.
11. Endogenous Hormones and Breast Cancer Collaborative Group: Body mass index, serum hormones, and breast cancer risk in postmenopausal women, *J Natl Cancer Inst* 95:1218, 2003.
12. Huang Z, Hankinson SE, Colditz GA, et al: Dual effects of weight and weight gain on breast cancer risk, *JAMA* 278:1407-1411, 1997.
13. Hamajima N, Hirose K, Tajima K, et al: Alcohol, tobacco and breast cancer-collaborative reanalysis of individual data from 53 epidemiological studies, including 58,515 women with breast cancer and 95,067 women without the disease, *Br J Cancer* 87:1234-1245, 2002.
14. Reichman ME, Judd JT, Longcope C, et al: Effects of alcohol consumption on plasma and urinary hormone concentrations in premenopausal women, *J Natl Cancer Inst* 85:722-727, 1993.
15. Holmes MD, Hunter DJ, Colditz GA, et al: Association of dietary intake of fat and fatty acids with risk of breast cancer, *JAMA* 281:914-920, 1999.
16. Zhang S, Hunter DJ, Forman MR, et al: Dietary carotenoids and vitamins A, C, and E and risk of breast cancer, *J Natl Cancer Inst* 91:547-556, 1999.

17. Thune I, Brenn T, Lund E, et al: Physical activity and the risk of breast cancer, *N Engl J Med* 336:1269-1275, 1997.

18. McTiernan A, Kooperberg C, White E, et al: Recreational physical activity and the risk of breast cancer in post-menopausal women: the Women's Health Initiative cohort study, *JAMA* 290:1331-1336, 2003.

19. Boyd N, Dite I, Stone J, et al: Heritability of mammographic density, a risk factor for breast cancer, *N Engl J Med* 347:886-94, 2002.

20. Beral V, Bull D, Doll R, et al: Breast cancer and abortion: collaborative reanalysis of data from 53 epidemiological studies, including 83,000 women with breast cancer from 16 countries, *Lancet* 363(9414):1007-1016, 2004.

21. Collaborative Group on Hormonal Factors in Breast Cancer: Breast cancer and hormonal contraceptives: collaborative reanalysis of individual data on 53,297 women with and 100,239 women without breast cancer from 54 epidemiological studies, *Lancet* 347:1713-1727, 1996.

Family History of Breast Cancer
(See also informed consent; prevention; screening)

BRCA1 and BRCA2 mutations

While most breast cancers occur sporadically in families for unknown reasons, in a minority of cases (5% to 10% overall), a strong hereditary factor can be identified. Germline mutations in BRCA1 and BRCA2 are known to be associated with significantly increased susceptibility to both breast and ovarian cancers and are inherited in an autosomal dominant fashion.[1] The frequency of mutations in BRCA1 and 2 is about 1 in 500 in the general population and 1 in 40 in those individuals of Ashkenazi Jewish descent.[2]

Presence of a BRCA mutation in women confers a risk of developing breast cancer of up to 85%. Ovarian cancer risk is up to 50% in carriers of BRCA1 mutations and up to 25% with BRCA2. In men, BRCA1 mutations increase prostate, breast, and pancreatic cancer risk. BRCA2 mutations increase the risk of breast, prostate, pancreatic, and stomach cancer, as well as melanoma.[3] Carriers affected with breast cancer have a 40% risk of contralateral breast cancer within 10 years.[4]

Recommendations for breast cancer screening in female carriers include yearly mammography starting at age 25 to 30, twice yearly clinical breast examination and monthly breast self-examination. Addition of annual breast MRI and ultrasound appears to increase sensitivity, but studies are still ongoing.[5] Bilateral prophylactic mastectomy, including removal of the nipple-areolar complex, reduces the risk of breast cancer by 90%.[6] Chemoprevention is an evolving area (see below). Regular physical activity has been shown to reduce the risk of breast cancer in the general population, but specific data for mutation carriers is not available. Prophylactic pre-menopausal oophorectomy reduces the risk of breast cancer by up to 50%.[7]

Ovarian surveillance with transvaginal pelvic ultrasound and Ca125 is recommended every 6 to 12 months beginning at age 30. Because this screening has limited sensitivity and specificity, prophylactic removal of the ovaries and fallopian tubes should be considered after age 35 to reduce the risk of breast, ovarian, and fallopian tube cancer.[6] Hormone therapy does not appear to negate the reduction in breast cancer risk when used up to the average age of menopause.

Formal genetic counselling to evaluate the likelihood of a BRCA mutation and to facilitate genetic testing if appropriate is recommended for any woman with a personal or family history suggestive of hereditary breast cancer. Pertinent family history may be either maternal or paternal but should be on the same side of the family. If genetic testing is undertaken, it normally starts with the highest-risk *affected* individual in the family. Suggestive history includes

1. Multiple cases of breast cancer (particularly if diagnosed before age 50) and/or ovarian, fallopian tube, or peritoneal cancer in the family
2. Breast cancer diagnosed before age 35
3. A family member with both breast and ovarian cancer
4. Breast and/or ovarian cancer in Jewish families
5. A family member with bilateral breast cancer—especially with at least one diagnosis before age 50
6. A family member with serous ovarian cancer
7. Male breast cancer in the family
8. Known BRCA1 or BRCA2 mutation in the family

When a BRCA1 or 2 mutation is identified in a family, other family members may have predictive testing. If testing is negative, then this family member is considered to be at population risk of cancer. If no BRCA1 or 2 mutation can be found in the family, the results are considered uninformative because they do not provide an explanation for the family history. This may be a false negative result, because testing does not identify 100% of BRCA1 and 2 mutations, or it may be due to an as yet unidentified gene, common environmental factors, or chance. No reassurance can be given about risk in this situation.

The benefits and harms of screening for mutations in BRCA1 and 2 remain unclear, because long-term outcomes of screening and risk-reducing strategies have not yet been determined. Nonetheless, the potential benefits of the current approaches include less aggressive treatment of cancer if found at an earlier stage and improved survival. Harms include increased anxiety and possible insurance implications. Genetic counselling should be offered to anyone with a significant family history to allow informed decisions to be made.[8]

Selective estrogen receptor modulators for high-risk women

An approach that has generated a great deal of controversy is the use of tamoxifen, a selective estrogen receptor modulator (SERM), for the primary prevention of breast cancer in women at increased risk. The National Surgical Adjuvant Breast and Bowel Project (NSABP) in the United States enrolled women over age 60, as well as younger women who had a strong family history of breast cancer or who had had a history of breast biopsies showing atypical hyperplasia or lobular carcinoma in situ. Their BRCA status was not determined. The women were treated with either tamoxifen (20 mg per day) or a placebo. The study was stopped prematurely after about 4 years because the group taking tamoxifen had a 49% relative reduction in invasive breast cancer (70 women had to be treated for 5 years to prevent one invasive cancer) and a 50% relative reduction in ductal carcinoma in situ. Whether this intervention can prevent death from breast cancer and how long tamoxifen can be given safely are unknown. In the NSABP study a small but significant increase in early stage endometrial carcinoma and thromboembolic disease (stroke, pulmonary embolism, and deep vein thrombosis) occurred in the tamoxifen-treated group. Three patients in the tamoxifen group died from pulmonary embolisms, whereas none in the placebo group died from this cause.[9] Other trials have had conflicting results. A recent meta-analysis of tamoxifen trials showed that, overall, tamoxifen reduced the incidence of breast cancer by 38%.[10] Based on these results the FDA has approved the use of tamoxifen for the reduction of breast cancer risk in women at increased risk for the disease. A joint guideline from the Canadian Task Force on Preventive Health Care and the Canadian Breast Cancer Initiative's Steering Committee on Clinical Practice Guidelines for the Care and Treatment of Breast Cancer supports counselling women at higher risk of breast cancer (Gail index greater than 1.66% at 5 years) on the potential benefits and harms of breast cancer prevention with tamoxifen (Grade B recommendation).[11] It suggests that as the five-year risk of breast cancer increases above 5% and the benefits outweigh the harms, a woman may choose to take tamoxifen. The recommended duration of use is 5 years.

A trial of another SERM, raloxifene (Evista), for osteoporosis in post-menopausal women reported a 76% decrease in incidence of breast cancer and no increase in endometrial cancer, but a small increased incidence of thrombophlebitis and pulmonary embolism.[12] The long-term harm/benefit ratio of raloxifene in the prevention of breast cancer or breast cancer mortality has not been established, and the drug should probably be limited to clinical trial settings.[13] Aromatase inhibitors (anastra-zole, exemestane) are being investigated as alternatives to tamoxifen in breast cancer prevention.[14] These drugs to not appear to cause endometrial carcinoma but may cause osteoporosis. There is also early evidence that regular use of Aspirin or NSAIDs may be effective as chemoprevention agents for breast cancer.[15]

❧ REFERENCES ❧

1. Petrucelli N, Daly MB, Burke W, et al: BRCA1 and BRCA2 hereditary breast/ovarian cancer [gene review] 3 Sep 2004 [accessed June 20, 2005]. Available from: URL: http://geneclinics.org/servlet/access?id=8888891&key=nXf NQ-wDNciIR&gry=INSERTGRY&fcn=y&fw=eTVF &filename=/profiles/brca1/index.html

2. National Cancer Institute: Genetics of breast and ovarian cancer (PDQ) → Major genes→ Models for prediction of the likelihood of a BRCA1 or BRCA2 mutation→ Population estimates of the likelihood of having a BRCA1 or BRCA2 mutation [last modified: April 21, 2005] [accessed: June 20, 2005]. Available from: URL: http://www.cancer.gov/cancertopics/pdq/genetics/breast-and-ovarian/HealthProfessional/page2#Section_110

3. Liede A, Karlan B, Narod S: Cancer risks for male carriers of germline mutations in BRCA1 or BRCA2: a review of the literature, J Clin Oncol 22:735-742, 2004.

4. Metcalfe K, et al: Contralateral breast cancer in BRCA1 and BRCA2 mutation carriers, Journal of Clinical Oncology 22:2328-2335, 2004.

5. Warner E, Plewes DB, Shumak RS, et al: Comparison of breast magnetic resonance imaging, mammography, and ultrasound for surveillance of women at high risk for hereditary breast cancer, J Clin Oncol 19:3524-3531, 2001.

6. Rebbeck T, et al: Bilateral prophylactic mastectomy reduces breast cancer risk in BRCA1 and BRCA2 mutation carriers: the PROSE study group, Journal of Clinical Oncology 22: 1-8, 2004.

7. Rebbeck T, Lynch H, Neuhausen SL, et al: Prophylactic oophorectomy in carriers of BRCA1 or BRCA2 mutations, N Engl J Med 346(21):1616-1622, 2002.

8. Robson M: Clinical considerations in the management of individuals at risk for hereditary breast and ovarian cancer, Cancer Control 9(6):457-465, 2002

9. Fischer B, Costantino JP, Wickerham DL, et al: Tamoxifen for prevention of breast cancer: report of the National Surgical Adjuvant Breast and Bowel Project P-1 Study, J Natl Cancer Inst 90:1371-1388, 1998.

10. Cuzick J, Powles T, Veronisi U, et al: Overview of the main outcomes in breast cancer prevention trials, Lancet 361: 296-300, 2003.

11. Levine M, Moutquin JM, Walton R, et al: A joint guideline from the Canadian Task Force on Preventive Health Care and the Canadian Breast Cancer Initiative's Steering Committee on clinical practice guidelines for the care and treatment of breast cancer, CMAJ 164:1681-1690, 2001.

12. Cummings SR, Eckert S, Krueger KA, et al: The effect of raloxifene on risk of breast cancer in postmenopausal women: results from the MORE randomized trial, JAMA 281:2189-2197, 1999.

13. Chlebowski RT, Collyar DE, Somerfield MR, et al (American Society of Clinical Oncology Working Group on Breast Cancer Risk Reduction Strategies): Tamoxifen and raloxifene, *J Clin Oncol* 17:1939-1955, 1999.

14. Goss PE, Strasser-Weippl K: Prevention strategies with aromatase inhibitors, *Clin Cancer Res* 10: 372s-379s, 2004.

15. Terry MB, Gammon MD, Zhang FF, et al: Association of frequency and duration of aspirin use and hormone receptor status with breast cancer risk, *JAMA* 291:2433-2440, 2004.

Breast Cancer Screening Strategies

Breast self-examination

(See also breast examination by health professionals; mammography; prevention; screening)

There is no convincing evidence that breast self-examination is beneficial,[1-6] and such examination may even be detrimental.[1] Breast self-examination reveals many benign lesions, leading to anxiety and possibly surgery.[1]

A Finnish cohort study reported a benefit from breast self-examination.[2] Two case-control trials of this procedure (one from Canada and one from the United States) found a slight decrease in death or advanced disease among the relatively few women in the programs who practiced proficient self-examination but not among those who were not proficient.[3,4] Proficiency in the Canadian study was defined as a combination of visual inspection, use of the fingerpads for palpation, and palpation with the three middle fingers. In this study each woman was seen annually and counselled on performing breast self-examination by specially trained nurses.[3] One year after the first visit about a third of the women were deemed proficient at breast self-examination, and after 4 years (and four training sessions) about two thirds were proficient.[5] The final results of the only satisfactory randomized prospective trial of breast self-examination published to date showed no reduction in breast cancer mortality after 10 years.[6]

Based on a review by Baxter and colleagues,[7] the Canadian Task Force on the Periodic Health Exam changed its recommendation from "C" to "D" regarding breast self-examination. The U.S. Preventive Services Task Force[8] still gives breast self-examination a "C" recommendation. The Canadian Cancer Society continues to recommend regular breast self-examination.[9] Although it may not prevent breast cancer deaths, BSE may allow women to feel more in control of their health.

--- ◼ REFERENCES ◼ ---

1. Kosters JP. Gotzsche PC: Regular self-examination or clinical examination for early detection of breast cancer, Cochrane Breast Cancer Group *Cochrane Database of Systematic Reviews, 2, 2004.*

2. Gastrin G, Miller AB, To T, et al: Incidence and mortality from breast cancer in the Mama Program for breast screening in Finland 1973-86, *Cancer* 73:2168-2174, 1994.

3. Harvey BJ, Miller AB, Baines CJ, et al: Effect of breast self-examination techniques on the risk of death from breast cancer, *CMAJ* 157:1205-1212, 1997.

4. Newcomb PA, Weiss NS, Storer BA, et al: Breast self-examination in relation to the occurrence of advanced breast cancer, *J Natl Cancer Inst* 83:260-265, 1991.

5. Harvey BJ, Miller AB, Baines CJ, et al: Breast self-examination techniques (response to letter), *CMAJ* 158:870, 1998.

6. Thomas D, Gao D, Ray R, et al: Randomized trial of breast self-examination in Shanghai: final results, *J Natl Cancer Inst* 94:1445-1457, 2002.

7. Baxter N, with the Canadian Task Force on Preventive Health Care: Preventive health care, 2001 update: should women be routinely taught breast self-examination to screen for breast cancer? *CMAJ* 164(13):1837-1846, 2001.

8. U.S. Preventive Services Task Force: *Guide to clinical preventive services,* ed 2, Baltimore, 1996, Williams & Wilkins, pp 73-87.

9. Canadian Cancer Society: Early detection and screening for breast cancer [Accessed May 22, 2005]. Available from: URL: http://www.cancer.ca/ccs/internet/standard/0,3182, 3172_10175_74544430_langId-en,00.html

Breast examinations by health professionals

(See also breast self-examination; mammography)

Only one series of investigations, the Canadian National Breast Screening Studies (NBSS), has compared physical examination alone with mammography plus physical examination (in almost all cases, physical examination was performed by trained nurses). All other mammographic studies have compared mammography plus physical examination against no systematic examination. After 11 to 16 years of follow-up in the NBSS, no decrease in death rates was found in the mammography plus physical examination cohorts compared with the physical examination only cohorts.[1,2] The results of these studies suggest that a careful CBE may be as effective as mammography in preventing cancer deaths. There is, however, an increase in breast biopsies in women who undergo regular clinical breast exams.[3] Guidelines vary as to when physicians should perform breast examinations for cancer detection. The Canadian Task Force on Preventive Health Care gives a "D" recommendation to physician breast examination of women 40 to 49 years of age but an "A" recommendation to performing clinical breast exam in conjunction with mammography every 1 to 2 years in women 50 to 69 years of age.[4] CBE, although not proven to reduce deaths from breast cancer, allows the physician an opportunity to emphasize the importance of preventive health.

--- ◼ REFERENCES ◼ ---

1. Miller AB, To T, Baines CJ, et al: The Canadian National Breast Screening Study-1: breast cancer mortality after 11 to 16 years of follow-up. A randomized screening trial of mammography in women age 40-49 years, *Ann Intern Med* 137:305-12, 2002.

2. Miller AB, To T, Baines CJ, et al: Canadian National Breast Screening Study-2:13 Breast cancer detection and 13-year results of a randomized trial in women 50-59 years, *J Natl Cancer Inst* 92:1490-1499, 2002.

3. Elmore JG, Barton MB, Moceri VM, et al: Ten-year risk of false positive screening mammograms and clinical breast examinations, *N Engl J Med* 338:1089-1096, 1998.

4. Morrison BJ: Screening for breast cancer: summary table of recommendations (Canadian Task Force on Preventive Health Care). [Accessed May 22, 2005]. Available from: URL: http://www.ctfphc.org/Tables/Ch65tab.htm

Mammography

(See also breast examinations by health professionals; breast - self-examination; informed consent; prevention; screening)

As a screening tool, mammography can detect tumours years before they are clinically palpable, allowing less extensive therapeutic interventions in many cases and an overall better prognosis. Because breast cancer has a relatively long natural history it may take years before reductions in mortality are documented due to mammography screening. Screening mammography in the 50-to 69-year-old woman has received widespread acceptance as an effective public health strategy to reduce deaths from breast cancer. The evidence is not as compelling in women under 50 years of age, and there is not much data for women over 70 years of age.[1] False positive results occur in about 11% of mammograms on average.[1] False negative rates are as high as 25% in women 40 to 49 years of age.[2] The following provides a summary of published trials and discussion of findings and ongoing controversies.

REFERENCES

1. Fletcher SW, Elmore JG: Mammographic screening for breast cancer, *N Engl J Med* 348:1672-80, 2003.

2. National Institutes of Health Consensus Development Panel: National Institutes of Health Consensus Development Conference Statement: Breast cancer screening for women ages 40-49, *J Natl Cancer Inst* 89:1015-1026, 1997.

Intervals between Mammographic Screenings

(See also controversies and uncertainties about mammographic screening; efficacy of mammography)

The intervals between mammographic screenings usually vary between 1 and 3 years The lead time for tumour growth is 2.4 years in the 40- to 59-year-old age group versus 3.7 years in the 50 to 59 year olds.[1] As such, if the decision is made to screen a woman in her forties it would seem that the screening interval should be less than 2 years to achieve adequate reduction in mortality. However, the United States Preventive Services Task Force's meta-analyses of recent mammographic trials found annual mammography no more effective than biennial mammography even this group of younger women.[2]

REFERENCES

1. Duffy SW, Day NE, Tabar L, et al: Markov models of breast tumour progression: some age-specific results, *J Natl Cancer Inst Monogr* 22:93-97, 1997.

2. Humphrey L, Helfand M, Chan B, et al: Breast cancer screening: a summary of the evidence for the U.S. Preventive Services Task Force, *Ann Intern Med* 137:347-360, 2002.

Overview of Mammography Trials and Meta-Analyses

(See also controversies and uncertainties about mammography screening; evidence-based medicine; surrogate outcomes)

The major randomized controlled trials of mammographic screening are listed below. These trials are referenced in almost every article discussing the efficacy of mammography and may cause confusion as they have somewhat conflicting results

Health Insurance Plan of Greater New York (HIP)[1]	United States
Two-County (Kopparberg and Ostergotland)[2,3]	Sweden
Malmö[4]	Sweden
Stockholm[5]	Sweden
Gothenburg[6]	Sweden
Edinburgh[7,8]	United Kingdom
National Breast Screening Study–1 (NBSS-1)[9,10]	Canada
National Breast Screening Study–2 (NBSS-2)[11,12]	Canada

There continues to be discussion about the efficacy of mammography as a screening tool and knowledge of these trials is helpful in understanding the debate.

A number of meta-analyses have also been performed. A much criticized Cochrane Review by Gotsche and Olsen questioned the efficacy of mammography.[13] The most recent is by the United States Preventive Services Task Force (USPSTF) published in 2002.[14] It concluded that mammography screening results in an estimated 30% reduced risk of mortality from breast cancer in women between the ages of 50 to 74 and a 15% reduction in mortality in women 40 to 49 years of age. The task force did not find annual mammography more effective than biennial screening.

REFERENCES

1. Shapiro S: *Periodic screening for breast cancer: the Health Insurance Plan Project and its sequelae, 1963-1986,* Baltimore, 1988, Johns Hopkins University Press.

2. Tabar L, Fagerberg G, Chen H, et al: Efficacy of breast cancer screening by age: new results from the Swedish Two-County trial, *Cancer* 75:2507-2517, 1995.

3. TaberL, Vitak B, Chen HH, et al: Beyond randomized controlled trials: organized screening substantially reduces breast carcinoma mortality, *Cancer* 91: 1724-1731, 2001.

4. Andersson I, Aspegren K, Janzon L, et al: Mammographic screening and mortality from breast cancer: the Malmö Mammographic Screening trial, *BMJ* 297:943-948, 1988.

5. Frisell J, Lidbrink E, Hellstrom L, et al: Follow-up after 11 years: update of mortality results in the Stockholm mammographic screening trial, *Breast Cancer Res Treat* 45:263-270, 1997.

6. Bjurstam N, Bjorneld L, Duffy SW, et al: The Gothenburg breast screening trial: first results on mortality, incidence, and mode of detection for women ages 39-49 years at randomization, *Cancer* 80:2091-2099, 1997.

7. Roberts MM, Alexander FE, Anderson TJ, et al: Edinburgh trial of screening for breast cancer: mortality at seven years, *Lancet* 335:241-246, 1990.

8. Alexander FE, Anderson TJ, Brown HK, et al: 14 Years of follow-up from the Edinburgh randomized trial of breast-cancer screening, *Lancet* 353:1903-1908, 1999.

9. Miller AB, Baines CJ, To T, et al: Canadian National Breast Screening Study-1: breast cancer detection and death rates among women aged 40 to 49 years, *CMAJ* 147:1459-1476, 1992.

10. Miller AB, To T, Baines CJ, et al: The Canadian National Breast Screening Study-1: breast cancer mortality after 11 to 16 years of follow-up: a randomized screening trial of mammography in women age 40-49 years, *Ann Intern Med* 137:305-312, 2002.

11. Miller AB, Baines CJ, To T, et al: Canadian National Breast Screening Study-2: breast cancer detection and death rates among women aged 50 to 59 years, *CMAJ* 147:1477-1488, 1992.

12. Miller AB, To T, Baines CJ, et al: Canadian National Breast Screening Study-2: breast cancer detection and 13-year results of a randomized trial in women 50-59 years, *J Natl Cancer Inst* 92:1490-1499, 2000.

13. Olsen O, Gotzsche PC: Cochrane review on screening for breast cancer with mammography, *Lancet* 358:1340-1342, 2001.

14. Preventive Services Task Force: Screening for breast cancer: recommendations and rationale, *Ann Intern Med* 137:344-346, 2002.

Mammography in Women Aged 40 to 49 years. Whether screening mammography for women less than 50 years of age is beneficial remains controversial.[1] Only two trials have demonstrated statistically significant decreases in mortality for women in this age group and the validity of these findings has been questioned. Mammography is less sensitive in women younger than 50. In one study, the sensitivity of mammography in women older than 50 who were followed for 25 months was 87.5%. It was only 71.4% in women less than 50 who were followed for the same length of time.[2] In 1995 three meta-analyses of randomized mammography trials in women less than 50 years of age were published. The first reviewed seven randomized trials involving 160,000 women and found no benefit from the intervention.[3] The second concluded that there was a trend toward decreased mortality after 10 to 12 years of follow-up, but in the opinion of the authors, even if this trend were to be verified with time and further studies, screening beginning at 50 years of age would probably achieve the same benefit.[4] In con-

trast, the third 1995 meta-analysis, that of Smart and associates,[5] concluded that the previous reports were erroneous and that mammographic screening indeed produced a statistically significant decrease in mortality in this age group, provided the Canadian National Breast Screening Study-1 (NBSS-1) was excluded.

The NBSS-1 program that Smart and co-workers chose to exclude from their meta-analysis showed an increase in breast cancer mortality at 7 years of follow-up in the screened group compared with the control group.[6] A number of workers have criticized the randomization process of this study,[5,7] but a careful review by two eminent outside epidemiologists failed to find fault with the randomization.[8]

One of the most controversial studies of mammography for women in their forties is the Gothenburg study published in 1997. It reported a 45% relative reduction of mortality (the absolute reduction is on the order of 0.13%) in this age group.[9] Some epidemiologists question the effectiveness of the randomization process and therefore treat the results with skepticism (see controversies and uncertainties about mammographic screening).[10]

Long-term follow-up results of the Edinburgh breast-screening project showed that women who entered the program between ages 45 and 49 and continued in it after age 50 had slight benefit; the number of women who were screened only between ages 45 and 49 was small, and the results were "equivocal."[11]

A comprehensive analysis of the controversies surrounding mammographic screening of women in their forties was published by Antman and Shea[12] in *JAMA* in April 1999. The most recent meta-analysis (USPSTF) found a small benefit in this age group.[13]

The decision to screen or not to screen in this age group should probably be made on an individual basis. If a woman wants screening she should be offered it after being advised of the increased likelihood of false positives in her age group. If she has significant risk factors (see risk factor section) screening may be recommended.

Women 50 to 69 Years of Age. Most of the trials have shown a statistically significant decrease in mortality for women aged 50 to 64 or 69 with mammography screening and that benefit seems to persist with time. There was, however, no decrease in mortality in the NBSS-2 study of Canadian women aged 50 to 59 at entry who had mammography with CBE compared with CBE alone even at 13 year follow-up.[14] In their review of all published trials by Gøtzsche and Olsen in the *Lancet* in 2000, the authors claimed that "screening for breast cancer with mammography is unjustified."[15] They based this stand on their assessment of the randomization processes of the various major trials; according to their calculations the randomization process was flawed in all trials but the two that showed no benefit (Malmö and Canadian; see previous discussion of trials). There was great criticism of this review and in an update of the Swedish trials of almost

250,000 women that was published in 2002, an overall reduction in breast cancer mortality of 21% was found in the screened group at a median follow-up of 15 years.[16] The 2002 meta-analysis by the USPSTF showed a 30% reduction in mortality and strongly supported mammography in this age group.[13]

All women between the ages of 50 and 69 should be offered regular mammography screening.

Women Older than 70 Years of Age. Whether mammography decreases breast cancer mortality in women aged 70 or older is unknown because randomized trials have not included enough women in this age group to draw any meaningful conclusions. Mammography is a very sensitive tool in this age group because the breast tissue is predominately replaced by fat and easier to image. For women with comorbid medical conditions such as coronary artery disease or diabetes, the chance of dying from breast cancer is remote. Even without comorbid conditions, diagnosing and treating slowly progressive lesions such as ductal carcinoma in situ may not offer any benefit.[17] However, if a woman older than 70 is otherwise reasonably healthy and could survive a lumpectomy, screening should be considered.

✎ REFERENCES ✎

1. Fletcher SW, Elmore JG: Mammographic screening for breast cancer, *N Engl J Med* 348:1672-80, 2003.
2. Kerlikowske K, Grady D, Barclay J, et al: Effect of age, breast density, and family history on the sensitivity of first screening mammography, *JAMA* 276:33-38, 1996.
3. Glasziou PP, Woodward AJ, Mahon CM: Mammographic screening trials for women aged under 50: a quality assessment and meta-analysis, *Med J Aust* 162:625-629, 1995.
4. Kerlikowske K, Grady D, Rubin SM, et al: Efficacy of screening mammography: a meta-analysis, *JAMA* 273:149-154, 1995.
5. Smart CR, Hendrix RE, Rutledge JH, et al: Benefit of mammography screening in women ages 40-49, *Cancer* 75:1619-1626, 1995.
6. Miller AB, Baines CJ, To T, et al: Canadian National Breast Screening Study. 1. Breast cancer detection and death rates among women aged 40 to 49 years, *Can Med Assoc J* 147:1459-1476, 1992.
7. Leitch AM: Controversies in breast cancer screening, *Cancer* 76(suppl 10):2064-2069, 1995.
8. Bailar JC III, MacMahon B: Randomization in the Canadian National Breast Screening Study: a review for evidence of subversion, *CMAJ* 156:193-199, 1997.
9. Bjurstam N, Bjorneld L, Duffy SW, et al: The Gothenburg Breast Screening Trial: first results on mortality, incidence, and mode of detection for women ages 39-49 years at randomization, *Cancer* 80:2091-2099, 1997.
10. Nelson NJ: The mammography consensus jury speaks out, *J Natl Cancer Inst* 89:344-47, 1997.
11. Alexander FE, Anderson TJ, Brown HK, et al: 14 years of follow-up from the Edinburgh randomized trial of breast-cancer screening, *Lancet* 353:1903-1908, 1999.
12. Antman K, Shea S: Screening mammography under age 50, *JAMA* 281:1470-1472, 1999.
13. Preventive Services Task Force: Screening for breast cancer: recommendations and rationale, *Ann Intern Med* 137:344-346, 2002.
14. Miller AB, To T, Baines CJ, et al: Canadian National Breast Screening Study-2: 13 breast cancer detection and 13-year results of a randomized trial in women 50-59 years, *J Natl Cancer Inst* 92:1490-99, 2000.
15. Gøtzsche PC, Olsen L: Is screening for breast cancer with mammography justifiable? *Lancet* 355:129-134, 2000.
16. Nystrom L, Andersson I, Bjurstam N, et al: Long-term effects of mammography screening: updated overview of the Swedish randomized trials, *Lancet* 359:909-919, 2002.
17. Smith-Bindman R, Kerlikowske K: Is there a downside to elderly women undergoing screening mammography? *J Natl Cancer Inst* 90:1322-1323, 1998 (editorial).

Adverse Effects of Mammography
(See also attitudes, physician; prevention; screening)

Psychological distress is common in women who are recalled for further investigation after a routine mammogram. Lerman and associates[1] studied women 3 months after they had undergone thorough workups for "highly suspicious" mammograms and had been found not to have cancer; 41% were worried that they had breast cancer and 17% reported decreased ability to participate fully in activities of daily life.

Concern has been raised that women who have had false-positive mammograms may be reluctant to participate in further mammographic screening programs. According to one retrospective[2] and one prospective[3] study, this did not occur; if anything, the experience reinforced the need for further screening.

Mammography is not a perfect test. The specificity of a single mammogram is 94% to 97% and the sensitivity of the initial mammogram ranges from 94% to 97%. False positives are common and occur more often in the 40 to 49 year olds, resulting in increased numbers of biopsies and patient anxiety.[4,5] One study estimated that after 10 mammograms about one half of women had a false positive result that, in 19% of women with false positives, led to needle or open biopsy.[6] The usual false-negative rate for mammograms is 10% for women 50 to 69 years of age. For women aged 40 to 49 it is as high as 25%.[7] The danger of a false-negative result is unwarranted reassurance of a patient who actually has cancer.

Open surgical breast biopsies are not innocuous. Among other things they cause pain and loss of time from work. Fortunately, most significant mammographic abnormalities can now be determined as benign or malignant by additional views or radiologically guided biopsies and do not need to progress to open surgical biopsies.

Since abnormal mammograms requiring follow-up testing often generate anxiety, it is important to know how rapidly follow-up examinations can be performed.

Early radiological intervention was shown to decrease anxiety in a study of U.S. women who had abnormal mammograms and ultimately benign pathology.[8]

Women undergoing mammography should be fully informed about the risks and benefits of screening. Women less than the age of 50 overestimate their risk of dying of breast cancer in the next 10 years twentyfold and overestimate the benefit of screening sixfold.[9] If women are not informed of the actual figures and the pros and cons of screening, they may choose to participate in a program on the basis of false assumptions and suffer adverse effects as a result.[10] Most articles on mammography downplay or avoid any discussion of the adverse effects. As Dixon[11] points out, it is the family physician, not the mammographer, who has to deal with the emotional havoc that this can induce.

The major adverse physical effect of mammography is pain. In one study about 90% of women experienced some pain, about 30% had moderately severe pain, and 5% to 15% reported severe pain.[12] Women who are concerned about pain can use ibuprofen or acetaminophen one hour before the mammogram to alleviate pain.

❧ REFERENCES ❧

1. Lerman C, Trock B, Rimer BK, et al: Psychological and behavioral implications of abnormal mammograms, *Ann Intern Med* 114:657-661, 1991.
2. Pisano ED, Earp J, Schell M, et al: Screening behavior of women after a false-positive mammogram, *Radiology* 208:245-249, 1998.
3. Burman ML, Taplin SH, Herta DF, et al: Effect of false-positive mammograms on interval breast cancer screening in a health maintenance organization, *Ann Intern Med* 131:1-6, 1999.
4. Mushlin AI, Kouides RW, Shapiro DE: Estimating the accuracy of screening mammography: a meta-analysis, *Am J Prev Med* 14:143-153, 1998.
5. Fletcher SW, Black W, Harris R, et al: Report of the International Workshop on screening for breast cancer, *J Natl Cancer Inst* 85:1644-1656, 1992.
6. Elmore JG, Barton MB, Moceri VM, et al: Ten-year risk of false positive screening mammograms and clinical breast examinations, *N Engl J Med* 338:1089-1096, 1998.
7. National Institutes of Health Consensus Development Panel: National Institutes of Health Consensus Development Conference Statement: Breast cancer screening for women ages 40-49, *J Natl Cancer Inst* 89:1015-1026, 1997.
8. Barton MB, Morley DS, Moore S, et al: Decreasing women's anxieties after abnormal mammograms: a controlled trial, *J Natl Cancer Inst* 96:529-538, 2004.
9. Black WC, Nease RF, Tosteson AN: Perceptions of breast cancer risk and screening effectiveness in women younger than 50 years of age, *J Natl Cancer Inst* 87:720-731, 1995.
10. Harris R, Leininger L: Clinical strategies for breast cancer screening: weighing and using the evidence, *Ann Intern Med* 122:539-547, 1995.
11. Dixon T: Breast screening: time for translation? *Can Fam Physician* 37:2544-2548, 1991 (editorial).
12. Kornguth PJ, Keefe FJ, Conaway MR: Pain during mammography: characteristics and relationship to demographic and medical variables, *Pain* 66:187-194, 1996.

Other Controversies about Mammographic Screening
(See also ductal carcinoma in situ; efficacy of mammographic trials; guidelines for mammographic screening; informed consent; length bias; prevention; screening)

Most of the major mammographic studies used a combination of mammography and physical examination of the breasts in the study group and no breast examinations in the control group. It is therefore uncertain how much of the decline in mortality rate in women over the age of 50 is attributable to physical examination of the breasts and how much to mammography.[1] In the Canadian National Breast Screening Studies (NBSS), which showed no decrease in mortality after up to 16 years of follow-up, physical examination and mammography were used in the study group and physical examination in the control group.[1,2] If physical examination alone is an important modality for decreasing breast cancer mortality, this may account for the failure of the NBSS to demonstrate decreased mortality in women over the age of 50 who had mammography.

Another controversial issue about mammography is the clinical importance of diagnosing ductal carcinoma in situ. Carcinoma in situ accounts for nearly half of all mammographically diagnosed breast cancers, but whether the detection and treatment of this lesion decrease mortality is unknown (see later discussion of ductal carcinoma in situ). One hypothesis is that length bias accounts for much of the observed benefit of mammography; mammography may preferentially detect tumours, such as ductal carcinoma in situ, that have very slow growth rates and little or no propensity to spread even if untreated. A report from Yale gives some support to this. The recurrence and mortality rates were lower among women with breast cancers detected by mammography than among those with cancers detected by other means even when tumours of identical TNM stages were compared.[3]

❧ REFERENCES ❧

1. Miller AB, To T, Baines CJ, et al: Canadian National Breast Screening Study-2: 13 Breast cancer detection and 13-year results of a randomized trial in women 50-59 years, *J Natl Cancer Inst* 92:1490-1499, 2000.
2. Miller AB, To T, Baines CJ, et al: The Canadian National Breast Screening Study-1: breast cancer mortality after 11 to 16 years of follow-up. A randomized screening trial of mammography in women age 40-49 years, *Ann Intern Med* 137:305-312, 2002.

3. Moody-Ayers SY, Wells CK, Feinstein AR: Does the reduced breast cancer mortality after mammography screening represent cure, early detection or discovery of relatively "benign" tumors? Robert Wood Johnson Clinical Scholars Program, 1996 National Meeting, Key Largo, FL, November 1996 (abstract).

Guidelines for Mammographic Screening

(See also breast examination by health professionals; breast self-examination; clinical practice guidelines; prevention; screening)

The recommendations of the Canadian Task Force on Preventive Health Care (2003) are that women aged 50 to 69 years have CBE and mammography every 1 to 2 years. ("A" recommendation).[1] There is insufficient evidence for or against mammography in the 40 to 49 year olds ("C" recommendation).[2] The recommendations of the U.S. Preventive Services Task Force are that women aged 40 to 70 have screening mammography every 1 to 2 years. They feel the evidence is inconclusive for CBE and BSE.[3]

The Canadian Cancer Society recommends mammography and CBE every 2 years between the ages of 50 and 69. Women younger than 50, or 70 and older, are advised to discuss their risk of breast cancer, and risks and benefits of mammography with their doctors. For recommendations of other professional bodies, see Table 80.

◢ REFERENCES ◣

1. Canadian Task Force on the Periodic Health Examination: *Canadian guide to clinical preventive health care,* Ottawa, 1994, Communication Group, pp 788-795.
2. Ringash J and the Canadian Task Force on the Periodic Health Examination: Preventive healthcare, 2001 update: screening mammography among women age 40-49 at average risk of breast cancer, *CMAJ* 164:469-476, 2001.
3. U.S. Preventive Services Task Force: *Guide to clinical preventive services,* ed 2, Baltimore, 1996, Williams & Wilkins, pp 73-87.

Table 80　Breast Cancer Screening Recommendations

Organization	Recommendation
USPSTF (2002)	Mammography every 1-2 y, age 40-70; inconclusive for CBE and BSE
AAFP (2001)	Annual mammography with CBE, age 50-69; every 1-2 y, age 40-49, if high risk
ACS, ACOG (2003)	Annual mammography starting at age 40; CBE every 1-3 y, age 20-39 and annually thereafter; BSE an option starting at age 20
NCI (2002)	Mammography every 1-2 y from age 40
AMA (2000)	Annual mammography from age 40, along with CBE
CTFPHC (2003)	Mammography and clinical exam every 1-2 y, age 50-69; recommends against BSE

AAFP, American Academy of Family Physicians; ACOG, American College of Obstetricians and Gynecologists; ACS, American Cancer Society; AMA, American Medical Association; BSE, breast self-examination; CBE, clinical breast examination; CTFPHC, Canadian Task Force on Preventive Health Care; NCI, National Cancer Institute; USPSTF, U.S. Preventive Services Task Force. Adapted from Patient Care April 2004, p. 87.

Ductal Carcinoma in Situ

(See also mammography; surrogate outcomes)

Ductal carcinoma in situ (DCIS), a form of breast cancer confined to the duct, is an important disease because it is detectable by mammography and as a result the incidence of the disorder has skyrocketed in the past decade.[1,2] In the United States in 1992, DCIS accounted for about 12% of all breast cancers that were diagnosed but comprised between 30% and 40% of those diagnosed by mammography.[1] Between 1985 and 1995, 43% of breast cancers diagnosed in women aged 40 to 49 were ductal carcinomas in situ, while for women aged 30 to 39 the percentage was 92%.[1]

DCIS is found in 6% to 18% of autopsies of women who have died due to other diseases.[1] Although it seems likely that some cases of DCIS will become invasive over a 15- to 25-year period, it is unknown which will and which will not and, by extension, whether detecting these lesions by mammography saves lives (see discussion of controversies and uncertainties about mammographic screening).[4]

A decade ago it was thought that all cases of DCIS were multicentric and therefore the usual treatment was mastectomy. It is now clear that the vast majority of cases are localized and are amenable to local resection.[5] The prognosis of DCIS is excellent with 10-year survival rates greater than 95%.[6] Most DCIS can be excised with lumpectomy alone. Three trials demonstrate the benefit of radiation therapy following lumpectomy to reduce the relative risk of local recurrence rate by about 50%.[7-9] In addition to local resection and radiation therapy, tamoxifen may be beneficial for some patients with DCIS. In one study patients with DCIS who had been taking this drug for 5 years had decreased incidence of invasive and non-invasive cancer in both the ipsilateral and contralateral breasts, but they also had increased rates of endometrial cancer and thrombophlebitis.[10]

Tamoxifen is not universally used as adjuvant therapy for women with DCIS and discussion with a medical oncologist regarding the risks and benefits is advised.[11] It is well established that axillary lymph node dissection is not indicated for patients with ductal carcinoma in situ.[2,5] However, if the DCIS is widespread, multifocal, or if a mastectomy is being performed, there may be assessment of the sentinel nodes (see Lumpectomy and axillary node sampling). Lobular carcinoma in situ is a different entity from ductal carcinoma in situ. It cannot be detected by mammography and is an incidental finding in breast biopsies performed for other reasons. It is not an anatomical precursor of breast cancer but imparts a significant increased risk for breast cancer in either breast.

❧ REFERENCES ❧

1. Ernster VL, Barclay J, Kerlikowske K, et al: Incidence of and treatment for ductal carcinoma in situ of the breast, *JAMA* 275:913-918, 1996.
2. Silverstein MJ: Ductal carcinoma in situ of the breast, *BMJ* 317:734-739, 1998.
3. Page DL, Dupont WD, Rogers LW, et al: Continued local recurrence of carcinoma 15-25 years after a diagnosis of low grade ductal carcinoma in situ of the breast treated only by biopsy, *Cancer* 76:1197-1200, 1995.
4. National Institutes of Health Consensus Development Panel: National Institutes of Health Consensus Development Conference Statement: breast cancer screening for women ages 40-49, *J Natl Cancer Inst* 89:1015-1026, 1997.
5. Page DL, Simpson JF: Ductal carcinoma in situ—the focus for prevention, screening, and breast conservation in breast cancer, *N Engl J Med* 340:1499-1500, 1999 (editorial).
6. Fisher B, Dignam J, Wolmark N, et al: Lumpectomy and radiation therapy for the treatment of intraductal breast cancer: findings from National Surgical Adjuvant Breast and Bowel Project B-17, *J Clin Oncol* 16:441-452, 1998.
7. U.K. Coordinating Committee on Cancer Research (UKCCR) Ductal Carcinoma in Situ (DCIS) Working Party: Radiotherapy and tamoxifen in women with completely excised ductal carcinoma in situ of the breast in the U.K., Australia, and New Zealand: randomized controlled trial, *Lancet* 362:95-102, 2003.
8. Fisher B, Land S, Mamounas E, et al: Prevention of invasive breast cancer in women with ductal carcinoma in situ: an update of the National Surgical Adjuvant Breast and Bowel Project Experience, *Semin Oncol* 28:400-418, 2001.
9. Julien J, Bijker N, Fentiman I, et al: Radiotherapy in breast conserving treatment for ductal carcinoma in situ: first results of EORTC randomized phase III trial 10853, *Lancet* 355:528-533, 2000.
10. Fisher B, Dignam J, Wolmark N, et al: Tamoxifen in treatment of intraductal breast cancer: National Surgical Adjuvant Breast and Bowel Project B-24 randomized controlled trial, *Lancet* 353:1993-2000, 1999.
11. Leonard GD, Swain SM: Ductal carcinoma, complexities and challenges, *J Natl Cancer Inst* 96:906-920, 2004.

Management of Breast Cancer

(See also alternative medicine; follow-up of cancer patients who have had curative treatments; hormone replacement therapy)

Prognosis and staging

The most important factor determining the prognosis of breast cancer is the presence of positive axillary nodes. The more positive nodes present, the worse the prognosis.[1,2] However, even the presence of multiple positive nodes is not necessarily an immediate death sentence; in one study the actuarial 10-year survival of women with more than 10 positive nodes was 29%.[3] If nodes are negative, tumour size is the dominant factor in determining prognosis.[1] Other factors of prognostic importance include estrogen receptor concentration and histological grade.[2]

Tumours with a lower grade and estrogen or progesterone receptor positivity have a better prognosis. Those cancers that are Her-2/neu oncogene–positive tend to have a poorer prognosis.[4] Furthermore, those tumours that overexpress Her-2/neu are more responsive to certain types of chemotherapy and hormonal therapy. Survival of women with metastatic breast cancer varies with the site of metastases. For those with bone or skin metastases it may be years, whereas for those with hepatic metastases or lymphangitic spread in the lungs it is months.[2]

❧ REFERENCES ❧

1. Berkowitz LD, Love N: Adjuvant systemic therapy for breast cancer: issues for primary care physicians, *Postgrad Med* 98:85-94, 1995.
2. Phillips DM, Balducci L: Current management of breast cancer, *Am Fam Physician* 53:657-665, 1996.
3. Walker MJ, Osborne MD, Young DC, et al: The natural history of breast cancer with more than 10 positive nodes, *Am J Surg* 169:575-579, 1995.
4. Ross JS and Fletcher JA: The HER-2/neu oncogene in breast cancer: prognostic factor, predictive factor and target for therapy, *Stem Cells* 16: 413, 1998.

Follow-up care for women with early-stage breast cancer

Blood work and diagnostic imaging as part of screening for distant disease should not be done because there is good evidence from well-designed RCTs that it does not have an impact on survival or quality of life. There is evidence from expert opinion only that annual mammography and physical examination should be performed to detect ipsilateral or contralateral cancers.[1] Most clinicians also ask about signs or symptoms of metastatic disease and side effects of adjuvant therapies.

❧ REFERENCES ❧

1. Temple LKF, Wang EEL, McLeod RS, et al: Preventive health care, 1999, update:3. Follow-up after breast cancer, *CMAJ* 161:1001-1008, 1999.

Delay in diagnosis and treatment of breast cancer

Delay in the diagnosis and treatment of breast cancer may occur at the level of the patient or her medical providers; provider delay may be due to delay in surgical consultation or to a delay in diagnostic and therapeutic interventions by the surgeons.[1] Although some studies have reported a small increase in mortality when combined patient and provider delay was 3 to 6 months,[2] a British study failed to find any evidence that provider delays of up to 3 months increased mortality.[3] A recent Canadian trial of women with stage I and II breast cancer examined wait time to radiation treatment and suggested that a delay may increase the risk of local recurrence at 5 years, although numbers were not large enough to come to a definitive conclusion.[4]

REFERENCES

1. Coates AS: Breast cancer: delays, dilemmas, and delusions, *Lancet* 353:1112-1113, 1999 (editorial).
2. Richards MA, Westcombe AM, Love SB, et al: Influence of delay on survival in patients with breast cancer: a systematic review, *Lancet* 353:1119-1126, 1999.
3. Sainsbury R, Johnston C, Haward B: Effect on survival of delays in referral of patients with breast cancer symptoms: a retrospective analysis, *Lancet* 353:1132-1135, 1999.
4. Benk V, Joseph L, et al: Effect of delay in initiating radiotherapy for patients with early stage breast cancer, *Clin Oncol (R Coll Radiol)* 16:6-11, 2004.

Lumpectomy and axillary node sampling
(See also adjuvant systemic therapy; practice patterns)

Numerous well-designed randomized prospective trials of early-stage breast cancer have shown no differences in mortality rates between local tumour resection plus radiation therapy and modified radical mastectomy.[1] Thus with few exceptions, breast-conserving surgery followed by local radiation is the treatment of choice for women with stage I or II breast cancer whether or not the tumour is centrally located and whether or not axillary lymph nodes are involved. The presence of an implant is not a contraindication to local resection.[2] Radiation therapy is usually given 5 days a week (Monday through Friday) for 5 consecutive weeks. If both radiation therapy and chemotherapy (see later discussion) are to be given, chemotherapy is generally administered first.[1]

In patients with invasive breast cancer, axillary dissection has traditionally been considered essential for staging and for assessing the need for adjuvant hormonal or chemotherapy (see later discussion of adjuvant systemic therapy).[3] However, axillary dissection may cause considerable morbidity, including lymphedema, numbness, pain, limitation of arm movement, and increased risk of infection.[4] In one study close to three fourths of women subjected to axillary node dissection experienced one or more of these symptoms even many years after the procedure.[5]

A novel surgical approach is to attempt to identify the node or nodes that receive the initial lymph drainage from the tumour (sentinel nodes). A coloured dye and/or a radioactive material is injected in the region of the tumour, and at surgery one or a very few nodes that are coloured or radioactive are selectively resected. If no tumour is found in the sentinel nodes, the chance that other nodes are involved is very small and axillary dissection can be avoided.

Accumulating evidence from several trials has validated the sentinel lymph node biopsy as an accurate method to detect the presence of metastatic disease in axillary lymph nodes.[6-8] Results from the National Surgical Adjuvant Breast and Bowel Project (NSABP) B-32 trial, comparing axillary node dissection to sentinel node biopsy, are anxiously awaited. Currently for women with clinically node negative early breast cancers, sentinel node biopsy may be offered.

Rates of local resection and of mastectomy for early stage breast cancer vary considerably among geographical regions (see discussion of practice patterns).

REFERENCES

1. Kotwall CA: Breast cancer treatment and chemoprevention, *Can Fam Physician* 45:1917-1924, 1999.
2. Margolese RG (Steering Committee on Clinical Practice Guidelines for the Care and Treatment of Breast Cancer): 3. Mastectomy or lumpectomy? The choice of operation for clinical stages I and II breast cancer, *CMAJ* 158(suppl 3):S15-S21, 1998.
3. McCready DR, Cantin J (Steering Committee on Clinical Practice Guidelines for the Care and Treatment of Breast Cancer): 4. Axillary dissection, *CMAJ* 158(suppl 3):S22-S26, 1998.
4. Warmuth MA, Bowen, Prosnitz LR, et al: Complications of axillary lymph node dissection for carcinoma of the breast: a report based on a patient survey, *Cancer* 83:1362-1368, 1998.
5. Hack TF, Katz J, Robson LS, et al: Physical and psychological morbidity after axillary lymph node dissection for breast cancer, *J Clin Oncol* 17:143-149, 1999.
6. Veronesi U, Paginelli G, Gallimberti V, et al: Sentinel-node biopsy to avoid axillary dissection in breast cancer with clinically negative lymph nodes, *Lancet* 349:1864-1867, 1997.
7. Krag D, Weaver D, Ashikaga T, et al: The sentinel node in breast cancer: a multicenter validation study, *N Engl J Med* 339: 941-946, 1998.
8. Quan, ML, McCready D, Temple WJ, et al: Biology of lymphatic metastases in breast cancer: lessons learned from sentinel node biopsy, *Ann Surg Oncol* 9:467-471, 2002.

Adjuvant systemic therapy
(See also lumpectomy and axillary node dissection)

The 2003 Ontario Guidelines suggest the following for adult patients with node-negative breast cancer:
Choice of Therapy
- **Pre-menopausal and post-menopausal women at minimal or low risk of recurrence** (less than 2 cm, well-differentiated, and all other factors favourable or less than 1 cm, intermediate grade, and all other factors favourable) should receive no adjuvant systemic treatment. They should, however, be made aware that systemic therapy is offered to women at higher risk of recurrence.
- **Pre-menopausal women** (age less than 50 years) **at moderate risk of recurrence** (1 to 3 cm and intermediate grade or 2 to 3 cm and well-differentiated) with estrogen-receptor-positive tumours should be offered tamoxifen. Chemotherapy added to tamoxifen may

provide a modest incremental benefit over tamoxifen alone. This is an ideal situation for a decision aid.

- **Pre-menopausal women** (age less than 50 years) **at high risk of recurrence** (greater than 3 cm irrespective of any other factors, or less than 1 cm with either estrogen-receptor-negative, high-grade, or lymphatic/vascular invasion) should be offered chemotherapy. There are insufficient data at the present time to recommend the addition of tamoxifen to chemotherapy in this subgroup. If the patient refuses chemotherapy and the tumour is estrogen-receptor-positive, tamoxifen may be considered. There are insufficient data to determine the risk category of a tumour less than 1 cm in diameter associated with a poor prognostic factor (e.g., grade III, estrogen-receptor-negative, lymphatic/vascular invasion).

- **Post-menopausal women** (age greater than 50 years) **at high risk of recurrence** (greater than 3 cm, or greater than 1 cm with high grade or lymphatic/vascular invasion) with estrogen-receptor-positive tumours should be offered tamoxifen plus chemotherapy. The benefits and risks of additional chemotherapy should be discussed with the patient. If the patient refuses chemotherapy, then tamoxifen alone should be considered. Post-menopausal women at high risk of recurrence and with estrogen-receptor-negative tumours should be offered chemotherapy.

- **Post-menopausal women** (age greater than 50 years) **at moderate risk of recurrence** (1 to 3 cm and intermediate grade, or 2 to 3 cm and well-differentiated) and with estrogen-receptor-positive tumours should be offered tamoxifen. Chemotherapy added to tamoxifen may provide a modest incremental benefit over tamoxifen alone. This is an ideal situation for the use of a decision aid.

Duration of Tamoxifen. Hormonal therapy should consist of oral tamoxifen 20 mg daily for 5 years.

Chemotherapy Regimen. Polychemotherapy should reasonably comprise six cycles of cyclophosphamide (oral)/methotrexate/fluorouracil or four cycles of doxorubicin/cyclophosphamide.[1]

Metastatic breast cancer
(See also osteoporosis; pain)

Recurrent breast cancer is often responsive to therapy, although treatment is rarely curative at this stage of disease. However, patients with localized breast or chest wall recurrences may be long-term survivors with appropriate therapy. Therefore, prior to treatment for recurrent or metastatic cancer, restaging to evaluate extent of disease is indicated. Cytologic or histologic documentation of recurrent or metastatic disease should be obtained whenever possible.[1a] Patients should be fully informed of all

the treatment options and should be aware of the risks and benefits associated with each of them. Full review of treatment options is beyond the scope of this book but 2004 Ontario guidelines suggest the following[2]:

- There is generally little difference in overall survival between chemotherapeutic agents in the treatment of metastatic breast cancer. Treatment in this setting should be based on clinical considerations and patient preferences, with a focus on palliation and quality of life.[3]

- Anastrozole and letrozole are modestly superior to tamoxifen (in terms of objective response rate and time to disease progression) as first-line therapy for post-menopausal women with stage IV breast cancer and are the preferred treatment option in this setting.[4]

- Tamoxifen remains an acceptable alternative.[4]

- There are insufficient data to recommend any one aromatase inhibitor over others in this setting.[4]

Second-line Therapy

- Anastrozole, letrozole, and exemestane are superior to megestrol acetate or aminoglutethimide as second-line hormonal therapy and are the preferred treatment option in this setting.[4]

- There are insufficient data to recommend any one aromatase inhibitor over others in this setting.[4]

Third- or Greater-line Therapy

- For post-menopausal women with advanced breast cancer who have been heavily pretreated with hormonal agents and chemotherapy, exemestane is an acceptable therapy.[4]

- There is no evidence that initial combination therapy with anthracyclines and taxanes in the metastatic setting provides a survival advantage over the usual sequence of treatments conventionally employed in patients with metastatic breast cancer (e.g., an anthracycline followed by a taxane followed by capecitabine).[3]

- The combination of paclitaxel (infused over 3 hours) and doxorubicin in rapid sequence should not exceed doses of doxorubicin greater than 360 mg/m^2 due to the high incidence of congestive heart failure.[3]

- Although few trials have compared weekly to three-weekly taxane therapy, the toxicities observed with weekly taxane therapy appear to be lower than those observed with the conventional three-weekly regimen. Weekly therapy could be considered for selected patients (elderly, low performance status, or women who wish to avoid some of the toxicities associated with the three-weekly taxane therapy).[3]

Patients with breast cancer who have bone metastases should be offered treatment with oral clodronate, intravenous pamidronate, or intravenous zoledronate.[5]

- An exception may be patients with a short expected survival (i.e., less than six months), who have well-controlled bone pain.[5]
- Patients who have difficulty tolerating oral medications (e.g., those with nausea/vomiting or esophagitis) should be offered intravenous pamidronate or zoledronate.[5]
- Intravenous zoledronate may be preferable to pamidronate when a shorter infusion time (15 minutes versus 2 hours, respectively) is important.[5]
- Intravenous clodronate has not been examined for its ability to reduce morbidity from bone metastases with long-term use. When clodronate is used for this purpose, the oral route is recommended.[5]

For patients with bone metastases and pain, treatment with pamidronate, zoledronate, or clodronate may be a useful adjunct to conventional measures for pain control.[5]

Bisphosphonates are not recommended to prevent bone metastases or improve survival in *women with locally advanced breast cancer or non-skeletal metastases*.[5] Current evidence is insufficient to support the use of bisphosphonates as *adjuvant therapy* to either prevent skeletal events or improve survival in *women with early-stage breast cancer*.[5]

◿ REFERENCES ◺

1. Cancer Care Ontario Evidence-Based Practice Guideline Report #1-8: Adjuvant Systemic Therapy for Node-negative Breast Cancer, May 1 2003. Available at http://www. cancercare.on.ca/pdf/pebc1-8s.pdf. Accessed Aug 2, 2004.
1a. National Cancer Institute, U.S. National Institutes of Health: Breast cancer (PDQ): treatment Stage IV, recurrent, and metastatic breast cancer [Last modified: May 20, 2005] [Accessed May 22, 2005] Available from URL: http://www. cancer.gov/cancertopics/pdq/treatment/breast/Health Professional/page8
2. Cancer Care Ontario: Breast cancer practice guidelines, metastic breast cancer, both metastatic breast cancer and non-metastatic breast cancer 2003/2004 [Accessed May 22, 2005]. Available from: URL: http://www.cancercare.on.ca/index_breastCancerGuidelines.htm
3. Verma S, Trudeau M, Pritchard K, et al: The role of taxanes in the management of metastatic breast cancer, practice guideline report #1-3, Hamilton, ON, 2003, Cancer Care Ontario. [Accessed May 22, 2005] Available from URL: http://www.cancercare.on.ca/pdf/pebc1-3f.pdf
4. Breast Cancer Disease Site Group: The role of aromatase inhibitors in the treatment of postmenopausal women with metastatic breast cancer, practice guideline report #1-5, Hamilton, ON, 2003, Cancer Care Ontario. [Accessed May 22, 2005] Available from: URL: http://www.cancercare.on.ca/pdf/pebc1-5f.pdf
5. Warr D, Johnston M, et al: Use of bisphosphonates in women with breast cancer, practice guideline report #1-11 (version 2.2002), Hamilton, ON, 2004, Cancer Care Ontario. [Accessed May 22, 2005] Available from URL: http://www.cancercare.on.ca/pdf/pebc1-11f.pdf

Hormone replacement therapy in patients with breast cancer

Hot flashes are often a greater problem for women with breast cancer than for other women because they can be precipitated or aggravated by chemotherapy that inhibits ovarian function or by the antiestrogenic effect of tamoxifen.[1] Most authorities consider estrogen replacement therapy to be contraindicated in women who have had breast cancer. No large prospective randomized controlled trials dealing with this issue have been reported.[2]

Another method of attempting to control hot flashes is the use of clonidine (Catapres, Dixarit) 0.025 mg, 2 tablets twice per day. Overall, this drug has not been very effective.[3] The antidepressant venlafaxine (Effexor) at dosages from 37.5 mg to 75 mg daily has been shown to reduce the severity of vasomotor symptoms in women with breast cancer.[4] Estring, a vaginal estrogen ring can reduce local urinary symptoms with little systemic absorption and is probably safe for women with a history of breast cancer.[5] Pending further research, most clinicians advise against the use of phytoestrogens in women with breast cancer.

◿ REFERENCES ◺

1. Carpenter JS, Andrykowski, Cordova M, et al: Hot flashes in postmenopausal women treated for breast carcinoma: prevalence, severity, correlates, management, and relation to quality of life, *Cancer* 82:1682-1691, 1998.
2. Vassilopoulou-Sellin R, Asmar L, Hortobagyi GN, et al: Estrogen replacement therapy after localized breast cancer: clinical outcome of 319 women followed prospectively, *J Clin Oncol* 17:1482-1487, 1999.
3. Goldberg RM, Loprinzi CL, O'Fallon JR, et al: Transdermal clonidine for ameliorating tamoxifen-induced hot flashes, *J Clin Oncol* 12:155-158, 1994.
4. Loprinzi CL, Kugler JW, Sloan JA, et al: Venlafaxine in management of hot flashes in survivors of breast cancer: a randomized controlled trial, *Lancet* 356: 2059-2063, 2000.
5. Pritchard KI: The role of hormone replacement therapy in women with a previous diagnosis of breast cancer and a review of possible alternatives, *Ann Oncol* 12:301-310, 2001.

Pregnancy and invasive breast cancer

No evidence has shown that women who have invasive breast cancer diagnosed during pregnancy have a worse prognosis than do non-pregnant women.[1] However, invasive breast cancer occurring in women before the age of 35 years has more aggressive biological behaviour and is associated with a worse prognosis than in older postmenopausal women past child-bearing years. Numerous studies of patients with breast cancer who subsequently became pregnant have failed to demonstrate any adverse effect of pregnancy on prognosis. At present it seems advisable for women with stage I disease (tumour 2 cm or smaller and negative nodes) or stage II disease (tumour 2 cm or greater with or without movable axillary nodes, or movable axillary nodes but no palpable tumour) to delay pregnancy for 2 years simply because most tumour recurrences occur within that time period. Women with stage III disease (any local extension of tumour, or inflammatory breast cancer, or matted or fixed axillary nodes) should probably delay pregnancy for 5 years. Those with stage IV disease (distant metastases) should avoid pregnancy.[1]

Among women who have had breast cancer the fertility rate is decreased because of chemotherapy-induced ovarian dysfunction.[1]

_____ ⚘ REFERENCES ⚘ _____

1. Averette HE, Mirhashemi R, Moffat FL: Pregnancy after breast carcinoma: the ultimate medical challenge, *Cancer* 85:2301-2304, 1999.

ABNORMAL UTERINE BLEEDING
(see oral contraceptives)

Abnormal uterine bleeding (AUB) refers to changes in duration, frequency, or amount of menstrual bleeding, or to vaginal bleeding that occurs outside the reproductive years. Dysfunctional uterine bleeding (DUB) is abnormal uterine bleeding that is not caused by a clear anatomical or pathological abnormality. DUB may be ovulatory or anovulatory.[1] Ovulatory bleeding tends to be cyclical and proceeded by molimina whereas anovulatory bleeding is irregular. Anovulatory bleeding is associated with a higher likelihood of endometrial hyperplasia.

The initial workup of AUB includes a history and physical, cervical cytology, and a complete blood count. Testing for thyroid disease and bleeding disorders should be undertaken only as clinically indicated.[2] Other investigations to consider include prolactin, progesterone day 21 to 23 (ovulatory status), FSH or LH (menopause, PCOD).[1] A transvaginal ultrasound should be done if bleeding is irregular to assess for endometrial polyps or submucous fibroids.[3] Detection of polyps or submucous fibroids can be further enhanced by transvaginal sonohysterogram.

Submucous fibroids may be the cause of abnormal bleeding; however, the vast majority of fibroids are asymptomatic. Pelvic pain with fibroids is atypical and may be caused by torsion, degeneration, or adenomyosis. Leiomyosarcoma is rare, but must be considered especially in the post-menopausal woman presenting with pain and rapidly growing fibroids.[4]

In post-menopausal women with AUB (defined as bleeding after 12 months with no menses), an endometrial thickness equal to or greater than 5 mm on transvaginal ultrasound (TVUS) is 95% sensitive (CI 92% to 97%) for detecting endometrial carcinoma, although it has a low positive predictive value for cancer, especially in women on HRT.[5] In post-menopausal women TVUS can therefore be helpful in triaging for further investigation.[3] Endometrial biopsy may not be needed in post-menopausal women with symptoms that resolve and a negative TVUS, because the probability of cancer is only 1%.[6] It is also not as helpful with bleeding in the pre-menopausal woman.[6]

Office endometrial biopsy should be considered in all women older than 40 years with AUB or in any woman at increased risk for endometrial cancer.[1] Hysteroscopic-directed sampling may be valuable and is considered more helpful than dilation and curettage (D&C) as a diagnostic procedure.[2] D&C is also a poor treatment option, because it provides no long-term decrease in bleeding.[1]

Medical Management

Non-steroidal anti-inflammatory drugs (NSAIDs) such as naproxen or mefenamic acid started with the first day of the menstrual cycle and continued for 5 days or until cessation of menses significantly reduce bleeding.[7] Antifibrinolytic agents such as tranexamic acid (Cyclokapron) at 1 g every 6 hours for the first 2 days of menstrual flow have been shown to be more effective than NSAIDs in reducing heavy menstrual flow.[7] GI side effects are dose dependant.

The combined oral contraceptive pill can decrease and regulate bleeding and, when no contraindications are present, may be used right up to the time of the menopause. There is no evidence that oral contraceptives cause benign fibroids to grow and although hormone replacement therapy may cause myoma growth in post-menopausal women, it does not seem to cause clinical symptoms.[4] Cyclic progestins have not been shown to be effective in controlling regular heavy menstrual bleeding relative to other methods, but may be helpful for women with irregular or anovulatory cycles when used as Provera (10 mg once daily for 12 to 14 days of each month).[1] Progestins may be associated with fibroid growth.[4] The levonorgestrel (Mirena) intrauterine device (IUD) delivers sustained-release levonorgestrel to the endometrium and is as effective as some surgical techniques and superior to oral progestins in reducing menstrual bleeding.[7,8]

Danazol (100 to 200 mg daily for three months) minimizes endometrial tissue, thereby reducing menstrual blood loss by up to 80%.[1,7] Androgenic side effects limit its use. Gonadotropin-releasing hormone (GnRH) agonists cause a reversible hypoestrogenic state, which may reduce bleeding in perimenopausal women. Significant side effects include hot flashes and a decrease in bone density.[1] They are helpful in reducing fibroid size pre-operatively.[4]

Surgical Management

Endometrial destruction techniques by either hystero-scopic or non-hysteroscopic (blind) techniques can be use-ful for menorrhagia. Hysteroscopic techniques result in 10% repeat ablation and 10% need for hysterectomy within the study periods examined. The newer non-hysteroscopic techniques (e.g., balloon thermoablation) are easier to per-form and appear to be safe and equally effective.[8]

Myomectomy for symptomatic fibroids is a good option in women who wish to preserve their fertility, although many will require further intervention. Uterine artery embolization is an alternative for some women with symptomatic fibroids, though long-term outcome data are not yet available.[4]

Seventy-five percent of hysterectomies done worldwide are for menorrhagia and uterine fibroids.[1] Hysterectomy provides definitive treatment for women with difficult-to-control symptoms but is associated with operative risks.

Endometrial Carcinoma

Endometrial carcinoma is primarily a disease of elderly women, although 25% of cases occur pre-menopausally and 5% of cases are reported in women under the age of 40. Abnormal uterine bleeding occurs in more than 80% of cases. Major risk factors are obesity, diabetes, and unopposed estrogen therapy or anovulatory cycles. Some increased risk is also associated with tamoxifen therapy, nulliparity, and menopause occurring after the age of 52. Smoking and taking combined oral contraceptives decrease the risk. Eighty percent of endometrial carcino-mas are adenocarcinomas and are thought to be pre-ceded by endometrial hyperplasia.

──────── ❧ REFERENCES ❧ ────────

1. SOGC clinical practice guidelines, Guidelines for the Management of Abnormal Uterine Bleeding, No. 106, August 2001.
2. Oehler MK, Rees, MCP: Menorrhagia: an update, *Acta Obstet Gynecol Scand* 82:405-422, 2003.
3. Kilbourn CL, Richards CS: Abnormal Uterine Bleeding: Diagnostic considerations, management options, *Postgrad Med* 109(1):137-150, 2001 (online).
4. SOGC Clinical Practice Guidelines, The management of uterine leiomyomas, No. 128, May 2003.
5. Smith-Bindman R, Kerlikowske K, Feldstein VA, et al: Endovaginal ultrasound to exclude endometrial cancer and other endometrial abnormalities, *JAMA* 280:1510-1517, 1998.
6. Symonds I: Ultrasound, hysteroscopy and endometrial biopsy in the investigation of endometrial cancer, *Best Pract Res Clin Obstet Gynaecol* 15(3): 381-391, 2001.
7. Lethaby A, Augood C Duckitt K: Nonsteroidal anti-inflam-matory drugs for heavy menstrual bleeding, [Systematic Review] Cochrane Menstrual Disorders and Subfertility Group, *Cochrane Database of Systematic Reviews* 1, 2004.
8. Lethaby A, Hickey M: Endometrial destruction techniques for heavy menstrual bleeding, [Systematic Review] Cochrane Menstrual Disorders and Subfertility Group, *Cochrane Database of Systematic Reviews* 1, 2004.

ABORTION (MISCARRIAGE AND THERAPEUTIC ABORTION)
(See also ectopic pregnancy)

Miscarriage

Miscarriage occurs in up to 20% of clinically recognized pregnancies; 80% occur within the first 12 weeks of gestation.[1]

Risk factors

Maternal age is an important risk factor for miscar-riage, which occurs in 40% of pregnancies in women aged 40.[2] Cigarette smoking, alcohol, high caffeine intake, and cocaine use are all associated with an increased risk.[3] In a case-controlled study of caffeine intake, risk of mis-carriage was increased in pregnant women who con-sumed more than 100 mg of caffeine per day, and it became statistically significant at a consumption of 150 to 300 mg (6 cups of coffee per day).[4] Use of NSAIDs around the time of conception may be associated with an increased rate of miscarriage.[5]

Recurrent miscarriage is the loss of three consecutive pregnancies prior to 12 weeks gestation. Women with uterine abnormalities such as fibroids or septate uterus or who carry lupus anticoagulant or anticardiolipin anti-bodies[6] (carriers of factor V Leiden) are at increased risk. There is no evidence that progesterone administration can prevent miscarriage; however, it may decrease mis-carriage rates in women with recurrent miscarriage of unknown cause.[7] It can be used vaginally (50 to 100 mg twice a day) or orally (micronized progesterone 100 mg twice a day).

Management of miscarriage

The standard treatment of incomplete miscarriage has been dilation and curettage. Recent studies suggest that in most cases this is unnecessary. Patients in these studies were in good health, hemodynamically stable, not ane-mic, and had a gestational age of less than 13 weeks and maximum anterior-posterior diameter of retained prod-ucts less than 50 mm on vaginal ultrasound. Women ran-domized to expectant management were not different from those receiving curettage in terms of pain, duration of bleeding, time off work, or future fertility. In almost all cases, pain and bleeding had stopped within 1 week.[8,9]

There is debate about the most appropriate manage-ment of missed abortion (non-viable pregnancy without spontaneous passage). Expectant management can be safely offered to women with gestational sacs less than

9 weeks size but has had disappointing success rates.[10] Medical methods using the prostaglandin analogue misoprostol to assist in expulsion of products of conception have been advocated. A dose of 800 μg given vaginally (4 tablets of 200 μg) and repeated in 24 hours may result in success in 80% to 90% of women with gestations up to 8 weeks in size.[10] In Canada and the United States, anti-D immune globulin (anti-D Ig) is recommended for all Rh-negative women who have a miscarriage, although the evidence is limited for its use in early miscarriage. Before 12 weeks, a dose of 50 to 120 μg is sufficient but a 300 μg dose should be given for pregnancies beyond 12 weeks.[11,12] Treatment should be given within 72 hours. British guidelines recommend giving anti-D Ig for any spontaneous abortion with surgical or medical intervention, any spontaneous abortion after 12 weeks, and any threatened abortion after 12 weeks.[13]

There is general agreement that anti-D Ig should be given to Rh-negative women after therapeutic abortions whether by medical or surgical methods, regardless of gestational age.[11-13]

Therapeutic Abortion

There is one abortion for every 3 to 4 live births in North America. Suction curettage is the most common method of pregnancy termination but medical methods are becoming increasingly common for early terminations.

Mifepristone-induced abortion

Mifepristone, or RU 486, is an antiprogestin drug that has been used in many parts of the world to induce abortion. It is not available in Canada. Maximum efficacy is achieved if a prostaglandin such as misoprostol (Cytotec) is given as either 400 μg orally or 800 μg intravaginally 48 hours after the administration of the mifepristone. Although used up to 63 days gestation in some countries, in the United States mifepristone is approved for use in pregnancies only up to 49 days gestation. For gestations up to 49 days the route of administration of misoprostol does not affect efficacy (92% to 98%), but from 49 to 63 days the vaginal route appears to be more effective.[14] A 200 mg dose of mifepristone is just as effective as the approved 600 mg dose,[14,15] and most clinicians use the lower (and less costly) dose. Mifepristone can also be used in very low doses for emergency contraception (see discussion of emergency contraception). Misoprostol taken during pregnancy is associated with an increased incidence of cranial, facial, and limb abnormalities in surviving infants.

Abortion induced by methotrexate plus misoprostol

Methotrexate is known to be cytotoxic to trophoblasts and is used in the treatment of trophoblastic neoplasms and ectopic pregnancies. A Canadian RCT compared it with mifepristone for abortion up to 49 days gestation.

Women randomized to receive methotrexate (50 mg/m²) followed in 4 to 6 days by 800 μg of misoprostol administered vaginally and repeated once if necessary had the same success in avoiding a surgical procedure as did women who received mifepristone and oral misoprostol (96% versus 95.9%). The abortions with methotrexate took longer to occur and the women were overall slightly more satisfied with the mifepristone abortions (88% versus 83.2%).[16]

Grief and Depression after Miscarriage and Abortion

Grief in women who have had a miscarriage may be as intense as that which follows a neonatal death. The male partners of women who abort may also have grief reactions. Miscarriage is a risk factor for major depression, especially in women who are childless, who have a past history of depression, or who have poor social supports.[17] Most women desire a follow-up physician visit after miscarriage and this provides an opportunity to assess for psychological difficulty. Women who undergo therapeutic abortion have high levels of anxiety and depression that fall after the abortion. After one month, 30% still experience emotional distress. Over the long term they are not psychologically worse than women who give birth.[18]

Risk of Breast Cancer

Claims have been made that induced abortions are associated with an increased risk of breast cancer. These have no scientific validity.[19]

❧ REFERENCES ❧
---

1. Hemminki E: Treatment of miscarriage: current practice and rationale. *Obstet Gynecol* 91:247-253, 1998.
2. Nybo Andersen AM, Wohlfahrt J, Christens P, et al: Maternal age and fetal loss: population based register linkage study. *BMJ* 320:1708, 2000.
3. Ness RB, Grisso JA, Hirschinger N et al: Cocaine and tobacco use and the risk of spontaneous abortion, *N Engl J Med* 340:333-339, 1999.
4. Cnattingius S, Signorello LB, Anneren G, et al: Caffeine intake and the risk of first-trimester spontaneous abortion, *N Engl J Med* 343:1839, 2000.
5. Li DK, Liu L, Odouli R: Exposure to non-steroidal anti-inflammatory drugs during pregnancy and risk of miscarriage: population based cohort study. *BMJ* 327:368, 2003.
6. Rey E, Kahn SR, David M, et al: Thrombophilic disorders and fetal loss: a meta-analysis. *Lancet* 361:901, 2003.
7. Oates-Whitehead RM, Haas DM, Carrier JAK: Progestogen for preventing miscarriage. Cochrane Pregnancy and Childbirth Group *Cochrane Database of Systematic Review* 2, 2004.
8. Chipchase J, James D: Randomized trial of expectant versus surgical management of spontaneous miscarriage, *Br J Obstet Gynaecol* 104:840-841, 1997.
9. Nielsen S, Hahlin M: Expectant management of first-trimester spontaneous abortion, *Lancet* 345:84-86, 1995.

10. Creinin MD, Schwartz JL, Guido RS, et al: Early pregnancy failure-current management concepts. *Obstet Gynecol Survey* 56:105-113, 2001.

11. Fung K, Fung K, Eason E, et al: Prevention of Rh alloimmunization. *JOGC* 25(9):765-73, 2003.

12. American College of Obstetricians and Gynecologists: Prevention of Rh D isoimmunization. *ACOG Practice Bulletin*, 1999.

13. Royal College of Obstetricians and Gynaecologists: Use of anti-D immunoglobulin for Rh prophylaxis (22) Clinical green-top guideline. Revised May 2002. [Accessed June 27, 2005] Available from: http://www.rcog.org.uk/index.asp?PageID=512

14. Christin-Maitre S, Bouchard P, Spitz I: Medical termination of pregnancy. *N Engl J Med* 342:946-956, 2000.

15. Kulier R, Gulmezoglu AM, Hofmeyr GJ, et al: Medical methods for first trimester abortion, Cochrane Fertility Regulation Group, *Cochrane Database of Systematic Reviews* 2, 2004.

16. Wiebe E, Dunn S, Guilbert E, et al: Comparison of abortions induced by methotrexate or mifepristone followed by misoprostol. *Obstet Gynecol* 99:813-9, 2002.

17. Athey J, Spielvogel AM: Risk factors and interventions for psychological sequelae in women after miscarriage. *Prim Care Update Ob Gyns* 7(2):64-9, 2000.

18. Bradshaw Z, Slade P: The effects of induced abortion on emotional experiences and relationships: a critical review of the literature. *Clinical Psychology Review* 23(7):929-58, 2003.

19. Beral V, Bull D, Doll R, et al (Collaborative Group on Hormonal Factors in Breast Cancer): Breast cancer and abortion: collaborative reanalysis of data from 53 epidemiological studies, including 83,000 women with breast cancer from 16 countries. *Lancet* 363(9414):1007-16, 2004.

AMENORRHEA

(See also anorexia nervosa; female athletes, polycystic ovarian syndrome)

Amenorrhea, absence of menses, is divided into primary and secondary forms.[1] Primary amenorrhea is rare and is defined as the absence of vaginal bleeding in a 14 year old with no secondary sexual characteristics or in a 16 year old with normal secondary sexual development. Primary amenorrhea is most commonly due to chromosomal abnormalities (45% of cases) or physiological delay of puberty (20%).[2] Other causes include structural abnormalities (absent uterus, imperforate hymen) and androgen insensitivity (testicular feminization).

Evaluation of primary amenorrhea should include a history and physical focused on the following:

- Stages of puberty (growth spurt, axillary/pubic hair, breast development)
- Signs and symptoms of virilization or Turner's syndrome (short stature, webbed neck, wide carrying angle)
- Family history—short stature, delayed or absent puberty

A careful genital exam noting clitoral size, hymenal opening, vagina, and cervix is also necessary. Investigations may include a karyotype and pelvic ultrasound for presence or absence of a uterus if indicated by history and physical examination.

Secondary amenorrhea is the absence of menstruation for more than 3 cycles or at least 6 months in women who previously had normal periods. The overall prevalence of secondary amenorrhea is 1% to 3%, but the rate is 3% to 5% among college students, 5% to 60% among competitive athletes, and 19% to 44% among ballet dancers.[1] The most common cause of secondary amenorrhea is pregnancy, and it must be ruled out before any further investigations are undertaken.

Other important causes for secondary amenorrhea are

1. Hypothalamic dysfunction (35%); usually functional in origin and associated with conditions such as low body mass, low body fat, poor nutrition, emotional and physiological stress, strenuous exercise, and weight loss (about 10% below ideal body weight)
2. Pituitary dysfunction (19%) includes hyperprolactinemic states, empty sella syndrome, ACTH-secreting tumours and Sheehan syndrome. Hyperprolactinemia can be secondary to a prolactinoma, hypothyroidism, or medications (e.g., metoclopramide, estrogen, antipsychotics).
3. Ovarian dysfunction (40%) includes ovarian failure and Polycystic Ovarian Syndrome (PCOS). Premature ovarian failure occurs before the age of 40 and is characterized by high follicle stimulating hormone (FSH) and low estrogen levels.
4. Uterine disorders (5%); Asherman's syndrome, a rare complication of dilation and curettage can cause amenorrhea due to intrauterine adhesions.
5. Miscellaneous (1%) conditions such as hyperandrogenic states (Cushing syndrome, adrenal hyperplasia)

The essential elements in the initial evaluation of a patient with secondary amenorrhea are as follows[1,3]:

1. History. Drugs, exercise, weight loss, psychological stress, galactorrhea, thyroid disease, gynecological surgery, hot flashes, and androgenic symptoms such as hirsutism, acne, frontal balding, and lowering of the voice
2. Physical examination. BMI, signs of thyroid disease, galactorrhea, androgen excess, or genital tract abnormalities
3. Laboratory investigations. Pregnancy test, thyroid-stimulating hormone, prolactin; if symptoms suggest that the patient is hypoestrogenic, FSH and luteinizing hormone; testosterone measurement is not needed unless the patient shows clinical evidence of androgen excess

The normal maximum prolactin (PRL) level is 20 ng/mL. If the level is elevated above 100 ng/mL (100 μg/L), a careful neurological examination and imaging of the sella turcica are indicated.[1] Transient PRL elevation may be seen secondary to stress, sleep, and sexual intercourse (greater than 50 ng/mL).

The estrogen status of a non-pregnant amenorrheic woman may be evaluated by performing a progesterone challenge test.[1,3] The patient is given 10 mg of medroxyprogesterone acetate (Provera) orally for 5 to 10 days.[3] The test is positive if any vaginal bleeding occurs within 2 to 7 days of completion of the drug course. A positive test indicates a normal "estrogenized" endometrium with an unobstructed outflow tract. A failure to bleed indicates inadequate estrogen stimulation, an unresponsive endometrium, ovarian failure, or outflow tract obstruction.[1] Most young women who fail to bleed have hypothalamic amenorrhea caused by psychological stress, excessive exercise, or excessive weight loss. In this condition the FSH level is normal or low (with primary ovarian failure it would be high).[3]

An amenorrheic woman who is hypoestrogenic has long-term risk of developing osteopenia. Benefits of estrogen replacement for bone preservation in hypothalamic amenorrhea are unclear.[4] A small prospective randomized controlled trial of amenorrheic young women found that over a 12-month period, birth control pills containing 35 μg of ethinyl estradiol increased lumbar spine density and total body bone mineral compared with control subjects receiving placebo or medroxyprogesterone.[5]

_____ ◢ **REFERENCES** ◣ _____

1. Kiningham RB, Apgar BS, Schwenk TL: Evaluation of amenorrhea, *Am Fam Physician* 53:1185-1194, 1996.
2. Ryan, K.J, editor: *Kistner's gynecology and women's health,* ed 7, St. Louis, 1999, Mosby.
3. Davis A: A 21-year-old woman with menstrual irregularity, *JAMA* 277:1308-1314, 1997.
4. Apgar, BS: Diagnosis and management of amenorrhea, *Clin Fam Practice* 4(3):643, 2002.
5. Hergenroeder AC, O'Brian Smith E, Shypailo R, et al: Bone mineral changes in young women with hypothalamic amenorrhea treated with oral contraceptives, medroxyprogesterone, or placebo over 12 months, *Am J Obstet Gynecol* 176:1017-1025, 1997.

CERVIX
Cervical Cancer and Cervical Cytology
(See also human papillomavirus; prevention; screening; sexually transmitted diseases)

Epidemiology
Cervical cancer is the eleventh most common cancer in Canadian women and is the ninth leading cause of death amongst U.S. women.[1,2] The most significant risk factor for cervical cancer is human papillomavirus (HPV). The most common high-risk oncogenic strains

are types 16, 18, 31, and 45.[3] Risk factors for HPV are early onset of sexual intercourse, multiple partners, a partner who has had multiple partners, and lower SES. Other important risk factors for cervical cancer are HIV infection and smoking. Cervical cancer may be asymptomatic; however, signs or symptoms include intermenstrual, post-coital, or post-menopausal bleeding, unusual vaginal discharge, rectal or bladder bleeding, and leg or pelvic pain.[3]

Techniques for cervical cancer screening
Cervical cancer arises from cells at the junction of the squamous and columnar epithelium of the cervix (transformation zone [TZ]). Adequate screening must include cells from this area. A systematic review of sampling devices used for obtaining cervical cytology smears by conventional cytology concluded that extended tip spatulas are superior to the traditional Ayre's spatula for collecting endocervical cells and identifying abnormal squamous cells. The combined use of the extended tip spatula and Cytobrush provides even better sampling.[4]

Newer technologies for screening utilize liquid-based cytology (LBC) and HPV-DNA testing. With LBC, the sampling brush is placed directly in a liquid fixative and suspended cells are processed to remove blood and inflammatory cells. A cleaner sample is produced for evaluation. Most studies have found LBC to be more sensitive for squamous intraepithelial neoplasia (SIL) than conventional smears (65% to 85% versus 50% to 60%, respectively) but less specific.[5] Too few reliable studies have been done to indicate the true accuracy of LBC and there are no prospective studies comparing LBC to conventional smears using health outcomes (e.g., invasive cervical cancer, costs or cost-effectiveness). As a result, the United States Preventive Services Task Force (USPSTF) currently gives LBC an "I" recommendation.[6]

Given the relationship of high-risk HPV types to cervical cancer, technologies that test for the presence of oncogenic HPV DNA (Hybrid Capture 2) have emerged. Although HPV-DNA testing alone is not indicated as a primary screening method for cervical cancer, it is valuable for management decisions if used as an adjunct to cytological technologies[6,7] (see ALTS trial in the section below on management of abnormal Pap smears). HPV-DNA cell samples are collected using an endocervical brush. This can be done as a separate test or using residual samples from LBC (termed reflex HPV testing).

Guidelines for cervical cytology screening
Randomized controlled trials demonstrating the effectiveness of cervical cytology screening have not been performed. However, since the inception of Pap screening in 1950, there has been a 75% decrease in cervical cancer mortality.

The USPSTF gives an "A" recommendation to initiating Pap smears for all women within 3 years of first sexual activity or at age 21, whichever comes first, and to performing repeat examinations at least every 3 years.[6] The American Cancer Society (ACS) recommends screening every 3 years only after age 30, after at least two normal preceding Pap smears.[5] For women over 65, the USPSTF recommends against screening if they have had adequate recent screening with normal smears and are not at high risk for cervical cancer (grade "D").[6] The Canadian Task Force on Preventive Health Care (CTF) gives a grade "B" recommendation to: initiation of screening after onset of sexual activity or at age 18 and, after two normal annual smears, screening every 3 years; screening can be discontinued at age 69, given a history of adequate recent screening.[1]

Women who have had a hysterectomy with removal of the cervix for benign disease do not need Pap smears unless there is a recent history of cervical neoplasia. In this case, screening can be discontinued after three normal consecutive vaginal vault smears.[6]

Patients having a hysterectomy for cervical dysplasia or carcinoma in situ should have follow-up vaginal vault smears at regular intervals.[1,6]

Classification of Papanicolaou smears

The Bethesda System (BS) for reporting cervical cytology was updated in 2001 and is now used throughout North America. One of the most significant changes in the new BS is the reporting of specimen adequacy. To avoid confusion associated with "Satisfactory but limited by," this terminology has been replaced with "Satisfactory" or Unsatisfactory for evaluation," with comments on presence or absence of the endocervical/TZ component and other quality indicators (e.g., blood, inflammation).[8]

Another important change is the combination of "Within normal limits" and "Benign cellular changes" into the single category "Negative for intraepithelial lesion or malignancy." Reporting now includes an interpretation of non-neoplastic findings such as organisms or reactive changes.

Important in triage for further management is the division of the ASC (atypical squamous cells) category into ASC-US (atypical squamous cells of undetermined significance) and ASC-H (atypical squamous cells, cannot exclude HSIL).

Other categories remain unchanged. LSIL (low grade squamous intraepithelial lesions) includes HPV, mild dysplasia, CIN 1; and HSIL (high grade squamous intraepithelial lesions) includes moderate/severe dysplasia, CIN (cervical intraepithelial neoplasia) 2/3 and CIS (carcinoma in situ).[8]

Management of abnormal Papanicolaou smears

An important caveat to remember is that Pap smears are screening techniques and that women with a visible abnormality that is cause for concern should be referred for colposcopy regardless of Pap smear results. Approximately 5% to 8% of Pap smears are annually reported as abnormal; less than 1% are HSIL.[9]

There is general agreement that patients with Pap smears reported as ASC-H, HSIL, atypical glandular cells (AGC), or carcinoma require immediate colposcopic evaluation.[10] Management of lesser degrees of atypia (ASC-US or LSIL) is more controversial.

ASC-US. A majority of patients with smears reported as ASC-US is normal histologically, and in most cases the cytological abnormalities revert to normal spontaneously after at least 3 months.[9] With ASC-US, there is a 5% to 17% chance of histological HSIL on cervical biopsy. With ASC-H, the risk is 24% to 94%. With any type of ASC, there is a low risk of invasive cervical cancer (0.1% to 0.2%).[10] The ASCUS/LSIL Triage Study (ALTS) for Cervical Cancer[9,11] examined the use of HPV-DNA testing in the management of ASC-US and LSIL. The study involved 5000 women with ASC-US or LSIL on Pap smear who were randomized into either immediate colposcopy, follow-up with repeat cytology or HPV testing with triage to colposcopy if HPV-positive. The ALTS showed that HPV-DNA testing had a sensitivity of 96% for detecting precancerous lesions (CIN 3) in women with ASC-US on Pap smears and had a NPV of 98%. A single repeat cytology had a sensitivity of only 44% for detecting CIN 3. In clinical practice this means that women with ASC-US smears can be tested for HPV, and if oncogenic strains are detected, they should be referred for immediate colposcopy; if no oncogenic strains are found, women can receive regular follow-up Pap smears. Thus, HPV testing is a viable option in managing women with ASC-US, because it helps identify which women require colposcopy and is likely cost-effective. It is time efficient in that liquid-based specimens allow the original Pap specimen to be tested for HPV should it show ASC-US (reflex testing).[9]

Other acceptable methods for ASC-US management include repeating the Pap smear at 4- to 6-month intervals[12] or immediate colposcopy.[7,10] If repeat Pap smears result in 2 normal smears, the patient may revert to the normal screening interval. If any smear shows ASC or higher, the patient should be referred for colposcopy.[10]

LSIL. Seventy percent of LSIL cases will spontaneously regress to normal because of regression of the underlying histological abnormalities.[7] Fifteen to thirty percent of women with LSIL have histological HSIL on biopsy.[9] The American Society for Colposcopy and Cervical Pathology recommends colposcopy for LSIL except in the case of adolescents and post-menopausal women.[10] In Canada, the recommendation is the same as for ASC-US (repeat smear every 4 to 6 months with referral for colposcopy if the abnormality persists), except in certain situations such as poor compliance or previous abnormal Pap, whereupon immediate colposcopy is suggested.[12] In the ALTS, HPV testing in women with LSIL was not found to be useful for management because 83% also tested positive for HPV.[9]

Standard treatment methods for lesions detected by colposcopy are electrocautery, cryosurgery, and loop electrosurgical excision (LEEP). A randomized trial of these three modalities found no differences in cure rates (81% to 87%), the adverse effects of infection, bleeding, and cervical stenosis (2% to 8%).[13]

Considerations in special populations

Adolescents. Although previous guidelines recommended screening with onset of sexual activity, there is evidence to show that a clinically significant lesion (such as CIS) is not likely to be detected until 3 to 5 years after exposure to HPV.[5] This rationale supports the USPSTF guidelines that recommend screening within 3 years of initiation of sexual activity. Because adolescents have high rates of active HPV infection, most of which clear over time, U.S. guidelines consider that for adolescents with LSIL it is acceptable to repeat cytology at 6 and 12 months and to refer for colposcopy if any repeat is ASC or higher (grade "C").[10]

HIV. The relative risk of developing cervical cancer is very high if a woman is HIV-positive. The CDC and USPSTF recommend two Pap smears 6 months apart following initial diagnosis of HIV. If both are negative, annual screening is considered sufficient.

HIV-positive women with ASC-US or LSIL should be referred directly for colposcopy.[14]

Post-Menopausal Women. In post-menopausal women, atrophic vaginitis can be the cause of ASC-US or LSIL. Accordingly, some groups recommend that postmenopausal women with ASC-US or LSIL with clinical or cytological evidence for atrophic changes can be initially managed with a course of twice-weekly intravaginal estrogen, followed by repeat cytology 1 week after completing the course (within 6 months). If the repeat test is negative, it must be repeated again in 4 to 6 months. If the second repeat is negative, routine screening can be resumed. If either repeat is ASC or greater, colposcopy is indicated (grade "C").[10]

Pregnancy. Use of an endocervical brush is safe in pregnancy.[4]

Invasive cervical cancer

Very early "microinvasive" cancer is usually treated with hysterectomy or in some cases cone biopsy. For more extensive but potentially curable disease, radical hysterectomy or radiation therapy give equal results.[15] Sexual dysfunction is common after treatment of cervical cancer by surgery or radiation therapy; difficulties reported included inadequate lubrication, short vagina, inadequate vaginal elasticity, and dyspareunia.[16]

Inflammation found on Papanicolaou smears

Data from British Columbia show that 52% of inadequate Pap smear samples were due to inflammatory exudates. This is a limitation of conventional Pap smears that is significantly reduced by LBC. However, a recent study has challenged this idea by showing that routine cervical cleaning with an oversized cotton swab prior to the Pap decreased the proportion of Pap smears obscured by inflammation. Thus, conventional Pap smears have the potential to be as good quality as LBC.[17]

In addition to limiting interpretation of smears, inflammation is clinically significant because it can be associated with certain infections (*Chlamydia*, *Trichomonas*, HSV, bacterial vaginosis, and *Candida*). There is also a 24% to 48% risk of underlying dysplasia in cases of severe inflammation. The Institute for Clinical Systems Improvement currently recommends clinical evaluation and treatment when initial Pap smears show evidence of severe inflammation; the Pap smear should be repeated in 6 months.[18]

─────────────── ◢ **REFERENCES** ◣ ───────────────

1. Morrison B: *Screening for Cervical Cancer*, Canadian Task Force on Preventive Health Care, 1992. Accessed May 23, 2005 at www.ctfphc.org/Full_Text/Ch73full.htm.
2. Nanda MD, et al: Accuracy of the Papanicolaou test in screening for and follow-up of cervical cytologic abnormalities: a systematic review, *Ann Intern Med* 132:810-819,2000.
3. National Cancer Institute-Division of Cancer Prevention. *Human Papillomavirus Information*, Accessed May 23, 2005 at www3.cancer.gov/prevention/alts/hpv.html.
4. Martin-Hirsch P, Jarvis G, Kitchener H et al: Collection devices for obtaining cervical cytology samples, Cochrane Gynaecological Cancer Group, *Cochrane Database of Systematic Reviews* 1, 2004.
5. Saslow D, Runowicz CD, Solomon D, et al: American Cancer Society guideline for the early detection of cervical neoplasia and cancer -*CA Cancer J Clin* 52:342-362, 2002.
6. U.S. Preventive Services Task Force: *Cervical Cancer Screening* 2003, Accessed May 23, 2005 at www.ahcpr.gov/clinic/uspstf/uspscerv.htm.
7. Ball MD, Madden MD: Update on Cervical Cancer Screening, Postgrad Med 113(2):59-64, 70, 2003 [located]
8. Solomon MD et al: The 2001 Bethesda System, *JAMA* 287:2114-2119, 2002.
9. National Cancer Institute Division of Cancer Prevention: ASCUS/LSIL triage study for cervical cancer (ALTS). Accessed May 23, 2005 at www3.cancer.gov/prevention/alts/.
10. Wright et al: 2001 Consensus Guidelines for the Management of Women with Cervical Cytological Abnormalities, *JAMA* 287:2120-2129, 2002.
11. Solomon D, Schiffman M, Tarone R: Comparison of three management strategies for patients with atypical squamous cells of undetermined significance: baseline results from a randomized trial, *J Natl Cancer Inst* 93:293-299, 2001.
12. Cancer Care Ontario, 1996, Accessed May 23, 2005 at http://www.cancercare.on.ca/index_cervicalscreening.htm.

13. Mitchell MF, Tortolero-Luna G, Cook E, et al: A randomized clinical trial of cryotherapy, laser vaporization and loop electrosurgical excision for treatment of squamous intraepithelial lesions of the cervix, *Obstet Gynecol* 92:737-744, 1998.

14. Ferenczy A, Coutlée F, Franco E, et al: Human papillomavirus and HIV co-infection and the risk of neoplasias of the lower genital tract: a review of recent developments, *CMAJ* 169(5): 431-434, 2003.

15. Cannistra SA, Niloff DIM: Cancer of the uterine cervix, *N Engl J Med* 334:1030-1038, 1996.

16. Bergmark K, Avall-Lunqvist E, Dickman PW, et al: Vaginal changes and sexuality in women with a history of cervical cancer, *N Engl J Med* 340:1383-1389, 1999.

17. Kotaska AJ, Matisic JP: Cervical cleaning improves Pap smear quality, *CMAJ* 169(7):666, 2003.

18. Anderson JM, Cullinan B, Mason C, et al: Cervical cancer screening, ed 10 [Health care guideline, Institute for Clinical Systems Improvement (ICSI)] Aug 2004 [Accessed June 27, 2005]; Available from URL: http://www.icsi.org/knowledge/detail.asp? catID=29&itemID=156

CIRCUMCISION, FEMALE

Female circumcision is practiced almost exclusively in Africa and among immigrants from Africa. Depending on the area, the prevalence rate varies from 5% to 99%. Female circumcision is practiced not only by those who espouse indigenous African religions, but also by Christians, Muslims, and Jews. It is a custom that involves all socio-economic groups.[1]

Circumcision is usually performed by lay surgeons without the use of anesthesia on girls between the ages of 4 and 10. The procedure may involve removal of the clitoris alone ("Sunna circumcision") or the clitoris along with some of the labia minora, or it may include clitorectomy plus removal of the labia minora plus incisions on the labia majora that are stitched together for near occlusion of the vaginal orifice (infibulation).[1]

─────────────── ◥ **REFERENCE** ◤ ───────────────

1. Toubia N: Female circumcision as a public health issue, *N Engl J Med* 331:712-716, 1994.

CONTRACEPTION

It is estimated that 41% of pregnancies are unplanned among women aged 35 to 39 and 51% among those aged 40 to 44.[1] A good online resource for contraception is www.sexualityandu.ca.

─────────────── ◥ **REFERENCE** ◤ ───────────────

1. Peterson HB: A 40-year-old woman considering contraception, *JAMA* 279:1651-1658, 1998.

Comparative Efficacy of Various Contraceptive Methods

Contraceptive efficacy can be calculated on the basis of theoretical or perfect-use failure rates and real-use failure rates (Table 81[1]). Theoretical effectiveness can be considerably better than real use. For example, the theoretical failure rate of the condom alone is 3% whereas in actual use it is 14%. The figures given for efficacy are generally derived from studies of young women. The efficacy of all modes is better in older women, partly because of decreasing fertility and partly because of lower frequency of intercourse.

─────────────── ◥ **REFERENCES** ◤ ───────────────

1. Black A, et al: Canadian contraception consensus. 2: Contraceptive care and access, *J Obstet Gynaecol Can* 26(2):148-153, 2004.

Natural Family Planning Methods

Calendar method

This method is suitable only for women who have fairly regular periods. It assumes that ovulation occurs somewhere between days 12 to 16 before the onset of the next menses, that sperm survive up to five days, and that the oocyte is viable for up to 24 hours.

Women should keep a diary of their menstrual periods for several months. The beginning of the fertile period is determined by subtracting 20 days from the shortest cycle, and the end of the fertile period by subtracting 10 days from the longest cycle.[1]

Basal body temperature

Women's body temperatures drop slightly at the time of ovulation followed by a subsequent rise of at least 0.5° C (measured orally after at least 6 hours of sleep)

Table 81   Contraceptive efficacy

Type of contraceptive	Theoretical pregnancy rate/year	Typical rate per year
None	85%	85%
OCP (combined)	0.1%	6-8%
Progestin only OC	0.5%	5-10%
Copper IUD	<2%	
Levonorgestrel IUD	0.09%	
Depo-provera (medroxyprogesterone acetate)	0.3%	0.3%
Male condom	3%	14%
Diaphragm, cervical cap, female condoms	6%	20%
Spermicide	6%	26%
Fertility awareness	1-9%	20%
Tubal ligation	0%	1.85% by 10 years

From Black A, et al: Canadian contraceptive consensus. Chapter 2: Contraceptive care and access. *J Obstet Gynaecol Can* 26(2):148-153, 2004 (Table 1). Reprinted with permission.

that persists until the next menses. The infertile period begins 3 days after the temperature rise.[1]

Billings or cervical mucus method

Women are taught to monitor changes in cervical mucus that occur under the influence of ovarian hormones. Infertile days of the menstrual cycle include days of menses, the subsequent days when the vagina is dry, and the interval beginning 4 days after the "peak" (clearest and most elastic) mucus until the next menstrual period.[1] Spinnbarkeit is the phenomenon observed with "peak" mucus whereby the mucus has become sufficiently elastic to allow it to be stretched out between thumb and fingers like an egg white. Samples of cervical mucus are obtained by placing the fingers in the lower vagina; touching the cervix is not necessary.[2] Use of vaginal products (e.g., medications, lubricants) and secretions from sexual arousal can cause confusion.

Symptothermal method

The symptothermal method combines the cervical mucus method and basal body temperature measurements.[1]

Coitus interruptus or "withdrawal" method

Although failure rates are high, up to 9% of sexually active women in Canada use this method of birth control.[3] Emergency contraception should be provided as a backup method to couples who use withdrawal for contraception.

Lactational amenorrhea method (LAM)

LAM is an effective temporary postpartum method of birth control. It relies on the infertility experienced by breastfeeding women caused by hormonal suppression of ovulation. The pregnancy rate over 6 months is 2% if the following conditions are met:
1. The woman's menses have not returned.
2. She is fully or nearly fully breastfeeding (i.e., only additional intake for the baby is infrequent water or juice).
3. She is less than 6 months postpartum.

Intervals between breastfeedings should not exceed 4 hours during the day and 6 hours at night.[1]

----------------- ✎ **REFERENCES** ✎ -----------------

1. Black A, et al (Society of Obstetricians and Gynaecologists of Canada): SOGC clinical practice guidelines: Canadian contraception consensus. 9 Natural family planning methods. *J Obstet Gynaecol Can* 26(4):363-368, 2004.
2. Geerling JH: Natural family planning. *Am Fam Physician* 52:1749-56, 1994.
3. Fisher W, Boroditsky R, Bridges M: The 1998 Canadian contraception study, *Can J Hum Sex* 8(3):167-173, 1999.

Patient resource:
Wechsler, T: *Taking Charge of Your Fertility: the definitive guide to natural birth control, pregnancy achievement, and reproductive health*, revised ed, New York, 2002, Quill, Harper Collins.

Barrier Contraceptives
(See also sexually transmitted diseases)

Condoms

Regular condom use decreases the transmission of all sexually transmitted diseases, including HIV. Most condoms are made of latex, but some are made of polyurethane or lambskin and are suitable for people with latex allergies. All types of condoms help to prevent pregnancy, but lambskin condoms do not protect against viral STIs such as hepatitis B, herpes, and HIV.[1] Aside from non-compliance, condom failures are usually due to breakage or slippage, and both of these events are more common among inexperienced users. Breakage is more likely if condoms are stored in a hot humid environment.

Use of oil-based lubricants or vaginal products (e.g., vaginal anti-yeast therapies) can weaken condom integrity. Other causes of failure include damage from opening the package with a sharp object or teeth, unrolling the condom before application, and using an inappropriate size. Slippage is more common if the male withdraws after losing an erection or if the condom base is not held during withdrawal.[2]

In one small survey of male college students in Georgia, slippage, breakage, or failure to use condoms throughout intercourse was reported in 13% of acts of vaginal intercourse. In a 1-month period, one third of consistent condom users and their partners were potentially exposed to STD transmission or pregnancy.[3] Another study revealed that one third of the men who experienced a condom breakage failed to inform their partners of this event.[4] Emergency contraception and STI testing should be recommended if slippage or breakage occurs.

Diaphragms

The diaphragm is used with spermicidal jelly and acts as a barrier and vehicle for spermicide. It may be inserted up to 6 hours before intercourse and should be left in place for 6 hours afterwards. For repeated intercourse within that time the diaphragm should not be removed and contraceptive jelly should be placed in the vagina before each episode.

Studies show a range of failure rates from 6% with perfect use to 20% with typical use.[1] There is debate about whether diaphragms are effective without use of a spermicide. A recent review of the sparse literature found no rigorous studies to distinguish effectiveness of the diaphragm with or without the use of spermicide and concluded that current practice of using spermicide with the diaphragm should be continued.[5]

The role of diaphragms in preventing STIs is controversial. When compared directly with condoms, they are less effective, but evidence suggests that they provide some protection. Frequent use of spermicide has however been shown to increase the risk of HIV transmission.[6] Diaphragm users have also been shown to have higher rates of bacterial vaginosis and urinary tract infections.[1]

Women using vaginal barrier methods of contraception are at an increased risk of developing toxic shock syndrome and should be aware of the danger signs of this condition.

Female condoms

The female condom (Reality) is a loose-fitting polyurethane sheath which is inserted into the vagina up to 8 hours before intercourse and is removed immediately after.[1] These condoms are intended for one time use and should not be used with the male condom as the two can adhere to one another resulting in slippage or displacement. The female condom also provides protection from STIs including HIV. A significant feature is that it is female-controlled. One of its benefits is that it may have an "empowerment effect" among women who are counselled and trained to use it.[7]

The female condom is expensive, with an average cost of $3 per condom in Canada. Research into the safety and feasibility of re-use of the condom suggest it can be washed and reused.[8]

------------------------- ❧ REFERENCES ❧ -------------------------

1. Black A, et al (Society of Obstetricians and Gynaecologists of Canada): SOGC clinical practice guidelines: Canadian contraception consensus, 8. barrier methods, *J Obstet Gynaecol Can* 26(4):348-360, 2004.
2. Spruyt A, Steiner MJ, Joanis C, et al: Identifying condom users at risk for breakage and slippage: findings from three international sites, *Am J Public Health* 88:239-244, 1998.
3. Warner L, Clay-Warner J, Boles J, et al: Assessing condom use practices: implications for evaluating method and user effectiveness, *Sex Transm Dis* 25:273-277, 1998.
4. Warner DL, Boles J, Goldsmith J: Disclosure of condom breakage to sexual partners, *JAMA* 278:291-292, 1997 (letter).
5. Cook L, Nanda K, Grimes D: Diaphragm versus diaphragm with spermicides for contraception, Cochrane Fertility Regulation Group, *Cochrane Database of Systematic Reviews* 2, 2004.
6. VanDamme L, et al: Effectiveness of COL-1492, a Nonoxynol-9 vaginal gel, on HIV-1 transmission in female sex workers: a randomized controlled trial, *Lancet* 360(9338):971-977, 2002.
7. Gollub EL: The female condom: tool for women's empowerment, *Am J Public Health* 90(9):1377-1381, 2000.
8. Potter B, Gerofi J, Pope M, et al: Structural integrity of the polyurethane female condom after multiple cycles of disinfection, washing, drying and relubrication, *Contraception* 67(1):65-72, 2003.

Spermicidal Contraceptives

Spermicides come in the form of foams, creams, gels applied with an applicator or films, sponges or ovules inserted with a finger. The active agent in most is nonoxynol-9. In general, foams and creams should be inserted no more than an hour before intercourse, and if intercourse is to be repeated, further applications are required. Manufacturers of some of the newer products such as Advantage-24 Gel claim that it can be applied up to 24 hours before intercourse, with further applications if intercourse is to be repeated. Sponges or ovules should be inserted at least 15 minutes before intercourse and should not be removed until 6 hours after intercourse. However, they should remain in place no longer than 12 hours because of the risk of toxic shock syndrome. Instructions for individual products should be followed. N-9 is not an effective microbicide and does not protect against STIs or HIV.[1] It has been shown that frequent use of N-9 by women at high risk of STIs increases the risk of HIV infection.[2] N-9 can cause vaginal irritation and epithelial damage, potentially facilitating the transmission of microbes. It is recommended that women who engage in intercourse numerous times daily should choose an alternative method of contraception.[1] Furthermore, spermicides may predispose women to urinary tract infections (see discussion of urinary tract infections).

------------------------- ❧ REFERENCES ❧ -------------------------

1. Wilkinson D, Ramjee G, Tholandi, M, et al: Nonoxynol-9 for preventing vaginal acquisition of sexually transmitted infections by women from men. Cochrane Sexually Transmitted Diseases Group, *Cochrane Database of Systematic Reviews,* 2, 2004.
2. VanDamme L, et al: Effectiveness of COL-1492, a Nonoxynol-9 vaginal gel, on HIV-1 transmission in female sex workers: a randomized controlled trial. *Lancet* 360(9338):971-977, 2002.

Intrauterine Devices

Two major variants of intrauterine devices (IUDs) are the copper IUD (Gyne T 380, Nova T, Flexi T) and the levonorgestrel-releasing IUD (Mirena/LNG-IUS).

The copper Nova-T and Flexi-T (available in Canada) and the LNG-IUS are effective for 5 years. The copper Gyne T 380 (available in the United States) is effective for 10 years. The failure rates are 1.3% for the Nova T, 0.6% for the Gyne-T 380, and 0.1% for the LNG-IUS (as effective as tubal ligation).[1,2] Whether all women should be screened for STIs prior to insertion is controversial, but screening should be done if there is any risk or there is evidence of mucopurulent cervicitis.[1] IUDs may be inserted at any time during the menstrual cycle provided pregnancy is ruled out.

The major complications of IUD insertion are infection and uterine perforation. Pelvic inflammatory disease (PID) is rare in women, who along with their partners, have monogamous relationships. If PID does occur, it is usually within the 3 to 4 weeks after insertion or it is due to acquisition of an STI and not due to the IUD. Perforation occurs at a rate of 0.6 to 1.6 instances per 1000 insertions.[1]

Copper IUDs protect against pregnancy mainly by interfering with sperm transport and motility. The LNG-IUS thickens cervical mucous, creating a barrier to sperm penetration and causes atrophic changes in the endometrium. Endometrial changes are responsible for the therapeutic effect of the LNG-IUS on dysfunctional uterine bleeding.

----------------- ⚐ **INTERNET SOURCES** ⚐ -----------------

www.sexualityandu.ca. Accessed May 23, 2005.

----------------- ⚐ **REFERENCES** ⚐ -----------------

1. Canadian Contraception Consensus: Intrauterine devices, *JOGC* 26(3):248-254, 2004.
2. Nelson AL: The intrauterine contraceptive device, *Obstet Gynecol Clin North Am* 27:723-739, 2000.

Combined Oral Contraceptives

(See also cerebrovascular accidents; dysfunctional uterine bleeding; migraines; thrombophlebitis)

Oral contraceptives (OCs) are highly effective in preventing pregnancies. The risk of pregnancy is 5 out of 100 typical OC users per year and 1 in 100 perfect OC users per year.[1]

Benefits

Oral contraceptives have a number of non-contraceptive benefits. These include control of dysfunctional uterine bleeding and dysmenorrhea,[1-3]decreased acne,[1,2] relief of hot flashes in perimenopausal women,[2] and reduced incidence of benign breast disease,[2] ovarian cysts,[2] endometrial cancer,[1-3] ovarian cancer,[1-3] ectopic pregnancy,[2] iron-deficiency anemia,[1] and possibly osteoporosis, endometriosis, and colorectal cancer.[1]

Ovarian Cancer. The risk of ovarian cancer is reduced by at least 50% among women who use oral contraceptive pills (OCPs). This benefit is achieved after taking the pill for 5 years and persists for 10 to 20 years after the pill has been discontinued. Women with a family history of ovarian cancer, or who carry the BRCA1 or BRCA2 gene can expect the same benefit from the pill.[1]

Endometrial Cancer. The older OCs with higher estrogen content reduce the risk of endometrial cancer by 60% when used for 4 or more years.[1] The benefit persists for at least 15 years after discontinuing the pill. Newer formulations, although not studied, are thought to similarly reduce risk.[1]

Adverse effects

Mild adverse effects of oral contraceptives such as breakthough bleeding, nausea, and breast tenderness are often a reason for discontinuation. Women should be informed about these "nuisance" side effects and asked to contact the physician if they become bothersome.

Cerebrovascular Accidents. A number of studies in the 1960s and 1970s of women using higher dose OCs clearly showed an increased incidence of ischemic strokes and subarachnoid hemorrhages in pill users. This was particularly marked if the women were smokers and over the age of 35. Only a few studies of the cerebrovascular complications of oral contraceptives have been published since the advent of low-dose estrogen birth control pills and the results have been conflicting. A pooled analysis of two U.S. case-control studies found no increased risk of ischemic or hemorrhagic stroke in women taking low-dose oral contraceptives even if they had additional risk factors such as age over 35, smoking, obesity, or hypertension.[4] A recent meta-analysis reported an odds ratio for stroke of 193 in users of current low dose OCs after controlling for smoking and hypertension.[5] OC users who have hypertension are at increased risk of stroke compared with users without hypertension. As a result, uncontrolled hypertensives should not be prescribed combined OCs. Migraine sufferers have also been shown to have an increased risk of stroke and the use of OCs increases that risk further.[4-6] Women who suffer migraine with aura should generally not be prescribed combined OCs (see progestin only contraception) and women with simple migraines should have other risk factors for stroke (age, smoking) considered before being prescribed OCs.

Venous Thromboembolic Events. Rates of venous thromboembolism (VTE) in OC users are 3 to 4 times higher than in non-users.[7] Users of third-generation oral contraceptives containing desogestrel (Marvelon, Ortho-Cept) or gestodene (none marketed in North America) are at slightly increased risk of VTE (adjusted odds ratio 1.7, with absolute risk of 1.5 in 10,000) compared with users of second-generation oral contraceptives containing levonorgestrel or norethindrone (Ortho 1/35, Min-Ovral, Lo-Ovral, and others).[8] Because the absolute risk is very low the clinical significance of these differences is debatable. Diane-35 (35 μg ethinyl estradiol and 2 mg cyproterone acetate) is approved in Canada as therapy for androgen excess. It also functions as a contraceptive. Users of Diane-35 have been shown to be at increased risk for VTE compared to those taking second generation OCs.[9] Treatment is advised only until 3 to 4 cycles after improvement of the skin condition.[10]

Women with thrombophilia are at much increased risk of VTE if they take oral contraceptives (see discussion of thrombophlebitis). Oral contraceptive users who are heterozygous for factor V Leiden have an eight times greater risk of thromboembolic events than non-carrier OC users and a 30 times greater risk than women who are not taking OCs. However, the absolute risk is low-one event per 350 women per year[11] (Table 82). While 5% of the Caucasian population is heterozygous for factor V Leiden, screening for thrombophilia in all women who request oral contraceptives is not recommended. More than 20,000 women would need to be screened to prevent one episode of VTE and two million women would need to be screened to prevent one death from pulmonary embolism.[12] Women with a family history of idiopathic VTE should probably be screened for thrombophilia such as homozygous factor V Leiden, protein C, protein S, and antithrombin II deficiencies prior to initiation of OCs.[13]

Myocardial Infarction. The OCs that are currently used do not appear to increase the risk of myocardial infarction (MI) in non-smoking normotensive women.[13] Women who smoke or have hypertension have been shown to have a significantly increased risk of MI when they also use the combined OC. Because risk also increases with age, the OCP is not advised for women over 35 who smoke, particularly those who smoke more than 15 cigarettes per day.[1,13] Past oral contraceptive users are not at increased risk of myocardial infarction.

An evaluation of the risks of contraceptives should be balanced against the risks associated with pregnancy. Table 83 provides estimates of excess cardiovascular and thromboembolic events and mortality due to pregnancy for various age groups. Oral contraceptive use by healthy non-smoking women is considered safe until the time of menopause.

Breast Cancer. The effect of OC use on the risk of breast cancer is still somewhat controversial. If there is an effect, it is very small. A large 1996 meta-analysis found that the relative risk for development of breast cancer among current users of the pill was 1.24 (95% CI, 1.15-1.33). No increase in risk was found for women who had stopped the pill 10 years before.[14] A recent U.S. study of 4575 women with breast cancer showed no significant association between breast cancer and current or past OC use even in women with a family history of breast cancer.[15] It is unknown whether women who carry BRCA1 or BRCA2 gene mutations are at increased risk of breast cancer with use of the OCs.[1]

Carcinoma of the Cervix. Women who take oral contraceptives and have HPV have very small increased incidence of squamous cell carcinoma and adenocarcinoma of the cervix.[16] The data suggest a promotional rather than causal effect.[1]

Total Mortality. There is no increase in mortality in women who have ever used oral contraceptives compared with women who have not, nor is there evidence that prolonged use of oral contraceptives increases mortality.[17]

Contraindications to the use of oral contraceptives

Oral contraceptives can be used safely by most women. For some women, however, the use of OCs is contraindicated or requires use with caution. Table 84 provides a summary of two guidelines on OC use and medical conditions. In addition to the conditions cited in the table, OCs should not be used in breastfeeding women earlier than 6 weeks postpartum. Blood pressure should be checked before providing OCs but no evidence has shown that routine laboratory investigations have value.[2]

Table 82   Estimates of Risk of Non-Fatal Venous Thromboembolism

Group	Estimated 1-year risk of non-fatal venous thromboembolism
Baseline (women not using OC)	1 in 20 000 to 1 in 9090
Women using OC containing levonorgestrel	1 in 6666 to 1 in 6211
Women using OC containing desogestrel†	1 in 3333
Women using any low-dose OC	1 in 3333
Women not using OC but who have factor V Leiden mutation	1 in 1754
Women using OC containing cyproterone‡	1 in 1666
Pregnant women and those post partum	1 in 1666 to 1 in 1500
Women using OC and who have factor V Leiden mutation	1 in 350

OC, Oral contraceptive.
†Based on relative risk of twice that among women using OC containing levonorgestrel.
‡Based on relative risk of 4 times that among women using OC containing levonorgestrel.
Adapted from Woolorton E: Diane 35 (cyproterone acetate): safety concerns, *CAMJ* 168(4):455-456, 2003. Copyright © 2003 Canadian Medical Association. *Reprinted with permission.*

Table 83   Age-Specific Estimates of the Excess Rates of Myocardial Infarction, Ischemic Stroke, and Venous Thromboembolism Attributable to the Use of Low-Estrogen Oral Contraceptives and Pregnancy-Related Mortality*

Variable	Age		
	20-24 yr	30-34 yr	40-44 yr
No. of excess cases of myocardial infarction and ischemic stroke attributable to oral-contraceptive use (per 100,000 woman-yr of use)†			
Among non-smokers	0.4	0.6	2
Among smokers	1	2	20
Among women with hypertension	4	7	29
No. of pregnancy-related deaths (per 100,000 live births)	10	12	45
No. of excess cases of venous thromboembolism attributable to oral-contraceptive use (per 100,000 woman-yr of use)			
With norethindrone, norethindrone acetate, levonorgestrel, or ethynodiol diacetate	6	9	12
With desogestrel or gestodene	16	23	30

*Low estrogen was defined as less than 50 µg.
†Data from Farley et al: *Contraception* 57:211-230, 1998; adapted from Petitti DB: Combination estrogen-progestin oral contraceptives, *N Engl J Med* 349(15):1443-1450, 2003. Copyright © 2003 Massachusetts Medical Society. All rights reserved.

Table 84   Summary of Guidelines for the Use of Combination Estrogen-Progestin Oral Contraceptives in Women with Characteristics that Might Increase the Risk of Adverse Effects

Variable	ACOG Guidelines	WHO Guidelines
Smoker, >35 yr of age		
<15 cigarettes/day	Risk unacceptable	Risk usually outweighs benefit
≥15 cigarettes/day	Risk unacceptable	Risk unacceptable
Hypertension		
Blood pressure controlled	Risk acceptable; no definition of blood-pressure control	Risk usually outweighs benefit if systolic blood pressure is 140-159 mm Hg and diastolic blood pressure is 90-99 mm Hg
Blood pressure uncontrolled	Risk unacceptable; no definition of uncontrolled blood pressure	Risk unacceptable if systolic blood pressure is ≥160 mm Hg or diastolic blood pressure is ≥100 mm Hg
History of stroke, ischemic heart disease, or venous thromboembolism	Risk unacceptable	Risk unacceptable
Diabetes	Risk acceptable if no other cardiovascular risk factors and no end-organ damage	Benefit outweighs risk if no end-organ damage and diabetes is of ≤20 yr duration
Hypercholesterolemia	Risk unacceptable if LDL cholesterol <160 mg/dL and no other cardiovascular risk factors	Benefit-risk ratio is dependent on the presence or absence of other cardiovascular risk factors
Multiple cardiovascular risk factors	Not addressed	Risk usually outweighs benefit or risk unacceptable, depending on risk factors
Migraine headache		
Age ≥ 35 yr	Risk usually outweighs benefit	Risk usually outweighs benefit
Focal symptoms	Risk unacceptable	Risk unacceptable
Breast cancer		
Current disease	Risk unacceptable	Risk unacceptable
Past disease, no active disease for 5 yr	Risk unacceptable	Risk usually outweighs benefit
Family history of breast or ovarian cancer	Risk acceptable	Risk acceptable

*The American College of Obstetricians and Gynecologists (ACOG) guidelines recommend the use of formulations containing less than 50 µg of ethinyl estradiol with the "lowest progestin does," without mention of the type of progestin. The World Health Organization (WHO) guidelines pertain explicitly to formulations containing 35 µg or less of ethinyl estradiol and do not mention the dose or type of progestin. To convert values for low-density lipoprotein (LDL) cholesterol to millimoles per litre, multiply by 0.02586.
Adapted from Petitti DB: Combination estrogen-progestin oral contraceptives, *N Engl J Med* 349(15):1443-1450, 2003. Copyright © 2003 Massachusetts Medical Society. All rights reserved.

Selection of product

Low-dose oral contraceptives containing estrogens (mainly ethinyl estradiol [EE] in doses varying from 20 to 50 µg) and progestins (several different types) are formulated to give either the same dose every day (monophasic) or varying doses (biphasic or triphasic). Oral contraceptives are also classified according to the type of progestin, with the newer "selective" progestins (norgestimate, desogestrel) having little or no androgenic activity.[2] A new type of progestin, drospirenone (contained in Yasmin) has a chemical structure similar to aldosterone and may be beneficial for women who have fluid retention and bloating with other OCs but the current evidence does not show a clinically meaningful difference in weight compared to other OC's. A number of the currently available oral contraceptives are listed in Table 85.

No firm rules govern selection of a pill. All the low-estrogen pills (less than 50 mcg) are safe and effective and selection should take into account the provider's judgment and the user's preference. Patients prone to acne, oily skin, hirsutism, and mood swings or premenstrual tension might benefit from selective progestin pills. Patients who experience nausea or breast tenderness may benefit from a very low dose (20 mcg EE) pill.

Starting day

Different starting days may be used. Common ones are the first day of the cycle, the fifth day of the cycle, or the first Sunday after the beginning of the cycle. Another alternative is the "Quick Start" method where the new pill user takes her first pill during the office visit after pregnancy has been ruled out (by history or urine pregnancy test). With this method, starting instructions are simple and compliance may be improved without any increase in incidence of breakthrough bleeding.[18] If the starting day is after the fifth day of the cycle, contraceptive reliability is uncertain until seven daily consecutive tablets have been taken and a back up method should be used during the first 7 days of taking the pill. Pills should be taken at the same time each day. A protocol for missed pills is given in Table 86.

Adherence

Adherence to taking oral contraceptives is poor. Only 50% to 75% of women who do not want to become pregnant and start the pill are still taking it after one year. In one survey almost half of all women on the pill missed one pill per cycle and nearly a quarter missed two or more pills per cycle.[19]

Continuous use

Oral contraceptives can be used continuously or on an extended basis rather than the usual 3 weeks of pills and 1 pill-free week cycle. A continuous regimen is useful for women who have symptoms such as menstrual migraine, dysmenorrhea, or mood swings during the pill-free week or for women who want to avoid their periods. Breakthrough bleeding is common initially but decreases over time; it is less likely when monophasic pills are used and when bleeding is not a problem on a regular 21-pill cycle.[2]

Table 85   Types of Combined Oral Contraceptives

Type	Product	EE (µg)	Progestin (µg)
Fixed dose			
EE/Desogestrel*	Marvelon, Ortho-Cept, Desogen	30	150
EE/ethynodiol diacetate	Demulen 30	30	2000
EE/levonorgestrel	Min-Ovral, Levlen, Nordette	30	150
	Alesse	20	100
EE/Norethindrone	Brevicon 0.5/35, Ortho 0.5/35	35	500
	Brevicon 1/35, Ortho 1/35	35	1000
EE/norethindrone acetate	MinEstrin	20	1000
	LoEstrin 1.5/30	30	1500
EE/norgestimate*	Cyclen	35	250
EE/norgestrel	Ovral	50	500
	Lo-Femenol, Lo-Ovral	30	300
EE/cyproterone acetate†*	Diane 35	35	2000
Biphasic			
EE/norethindrone	Synphasic	35	500/1000
Triphasic			
EE/norethindrone	Ortho 7/7/7	35	500/750/1000
EE/norgestimate*	Tri-Cyclen	35	180/215/250
EE/levonorgestrel	Triquilar, Triphasil	30/40/ 30	50/75/125

Adapted from Black A, et al: *Journal of Obstetrics & Gynaecology Canada* 26(3):220-236, 2004. Reprinted with permission.
*Selective progestins.
†Indicated for severe acne/androgen excess, not indicated solely for contraception.

Table 86   Protocol for Missed Pills

Consecutive Pills Omitted	Time of Cycle	Instructions
1	Any time	Take the missed pill as soon as possible and take the next pill at the normally scheduled time.
2	1st and 2nd week of the cycle/pills	Take 2 pills per day for 2 days then continue taking one pill per day. Use back-up contraception for the next 7 days from the time of missed pills.*
2	3rd week of cycle/pills	Discard the rest of the pack. Start a new pack immediately. Use back-up contraception for 7 days from the time of missed pills* There may be a new start day of the cycle.
3 or more	Any time	Discard the rest of the pack. Start a new pack immediately. Use back-up contraception for 7 days from the time of missed pills.* There may be a new start day of the cycle.

*Use emergency contraception if unprotected intercourse after the missed pills.
Adapted from Black A, et al: *J Obstet Gynaecol Canada* 26(3):220-236, 2004. Reprinted with permission.

Antibiotics and oral contraceptives

Rifampicin and griseofulvin have been shown to decrease the efficacy of OCs. There is no good evidence that other antibiotics affect efficacy.[20]

Discontinuing the pill in perimenopausal women

If a non-smoking perimenopausal woman is taking an oral contraceptive pill on a regular basis, how does the physician know when menopause has occurred so that the birth control pill may be discontinued? Haney[21] suggests simply stopping oral contraceptives arbitrarily at age 51 or 52. If periods do not resume within 3 months, menopause has occurred. This seems a reasonable approach considering a recent study by Bastian showing that age and the gradual cessation menses are the best indicators of menopausal status.[22] If menses do recur oral contraceptives can be restarted for another year. FSH levels during the pill-free week have been suggested in the past but are so variable that they are not felt to be helpful in this situation.[22]

❧ REFERENCES ❧

1. Petitti DB: Combination estrogen-progestin oral contraceptives, *N Engl J Med* 349(15):1443-1450, 2003.
2. Black A, et al (Society of Obstetricians and Gynaecologists of Canada): SOGC clinical practice guidelines: Canadian contraception consensus. 4: Combined hormonal contraception, *J Obstet Gynaecol Can* 26(3):220-36, 2004.
3. Peterson HB: A 40-year-old woman considering contraception, *JAMA* 279:1651-1658, 1998.
4. Schwartz SM, Pettitti DB, Siscovick DS, et al: Stroke and use of low-dose oral contraceptives in young women: a pooled analysis of two U.S. studies, *Stroke* 29:2277-2284, 1998.
5. Gillum LA, et al: Ischemic stroke risk with oral contraceptives: a meta-analysis, *JAMA* 284:72-78, 2000.
6. Chang CL, Donaghy M, Poulter N (World Health Organisation Collaborative Study of Cardiovascular Disease and Steroid Hormone Contraception): Migraine and stroke in young women: case-control study, *BMJ* 318:13-18, 1999.
7. Vandenbrouke JP, Rosing J, Bloemenkamp KW, et al: Oral contraceptives and the risk of venous thrombosis, *N Engl J Med* 344(22):1527-1535, 2001.
8. Kemmeren JM, Algra A, Grobbee DE: Third generation oral contraceptives and risk of venous thrombosis: meta-analysis, *BMJ* 323:1-9, 2001.
9. Vasilakis-Scaramozza C, Jick H: Risk of venous thromboembolism with cyproterone or levonrogestrel contraceptives, *Lancet* 38:1427-1429, 2001.
10. Wooltorton E: Diane-35 (cyproterone acetate): safety concerns, *CMAJ* 168(4):455-456, 2003.
11. Vandenbroucke JP, Koster T, Briet E, et al: Increased risk of venous thrombosis in oral-contraceptive users who are carriers of factor V Leiden mutation, *Lancet* 344:1453-1457, 1994.
12. Vandenbroucke JP, et al: Factor V Leiden: should we screen oral contraceptive users and pregnant women? *BMJ* 313:1127-1130, 1996.
13. Black A, et al (Society of Obstetricians and Gynaecologists of Canada): SOGC clinical practice guidelines: Canadian contraception consensus. 6: Special considerations, *J Obstet Gynaecol Can* 26(3):242-248, 2004.
14. Collaborative Group on Hormonal Factors in Breast Cancer: Breast cancer and hormonal contraceptives: collaborative reanalysis of individual data on 53,297 women with and 100,239 women without breast cancer from 54 epidemiological studies, *Lancet* 347:1713-1727, 1996.
15. Marchbanks PA, McDonald JA, Wilson HG, et al: Oral contraceptives and the risk for breast cancer. *N Engl J Med* 356(26):2025-2032, 2002.
16. Moreno V, Bosch FX, Munoz N, et al: Effect of oral contraceptives on risk of cervical cancer in women with human papillomavirus infection: the IARC multicentric case-control study. *Lancet* 359:1085-1092, 2002.
17. Colditz GA (Nurses' Health Study Research Group): Oral contraceptive use and mortality during 12 years of follow-up: the Nurses' Health Study, *Ann Intern Med* 120:821-826, 1994.

18. Lara-Torre E, Schroeder B: Adolescent compliance and side effects with Quick Start initiation of oral contraceptive pills, *Contraception* 66:81-5, 2002.

19. Rosenberg MJ, Waugh MS, Burnhill MS: Compliance, counseling and satisfaction with oral contraceptives: a prospective evaluation, *Fam Plan Perspect* 30:89-92, 104, 1998.

20. Dickinson BD, Altman RD, Fielsen H, et al: Drug interactions between oral contraceptives and antibiotics. *Am J Obstet Gyencol* 98(5 Pa 1):853-60, 2001.

21. Haney AF: Hormonal needs of the perimenopausal woman, *J SOGC* 15:1-8, 1993.

22. Bastian LA, Smith CM, Nanda K: Is this woman perimenopausal? *JAMA* 289:895-902, 2003.

The Contraceptive Patch

Recently Ortho Evra, a patch containing ethinyl estradiol and norelgestromin (similar to norgestimate), became available in North America. The patch is applied to the skin of the buttocks, torso, upper arm, or lower abdomen once weekly for 3 weeks followed by a patch-free week. It provides contraceptive effectiveness similar to oral contraceptives. Effectiveness appears to be decreased in women over 90 kg (198 lb).[1] Contraindications are the same as for the combined OC. Compared with OC users, patch users have higher rates of spotting and breast discomfort in the first few cycles. Adhesion of the patch is good even in hot or humid environments. Skin reactions occurred in 20% of women but only 2% discontinued use for this reason.[2]

The vaginal contraceptive ring

The NuvaRing delivers a low daily dose of ethinyl estradiol (15 μg per day) and etonogestrel, a selective progestin that is the active metabolite of desogestrel (in Marvelon, Ortho-Cept). It is available in the United States and is being considered for approval in Canada. The ring is placed in the vagina for 3 weeks and then removed for one week. Contraindications are as for the combined OC. Contraceptive effectiveness is similar to the pill with a failure rate of 0.65 pregnancies per 100 women years with typical use. Some women or their partners may be aware of the ring during intercourse but only 1% to 2.5% discontinued use due to coital problems or expulsion. Vaginal symptoms led to discontinuation in about 1% to 2%.[2]

------------------- **⇞ REFERENCES ⇞** -------------------

1. Zieman M, et al: Contraceptive efficacy and cycle control with the Ortho Evra/Evra trandermal system: the analysis of pooled data, *Fertil Steril* 77(2 suppl 2):S13-8, 2002.

2. Black A, et al (Society of Obstetricians and Gynaecologists of Canada): SOGC clinical practice guidelines: Canadian contraception consensus. Chapter 4: Combined hormonal contraception, *J Obstet Gynaecol Can* 26(3):220-236, 2004.

Emergency Contraception

There are two regimens of emergency contraceptive pills (ECPs) currently available, the Yuzpe method and the newer progestin only method. Both are safe and have no absolute contraindications except known pregnancy. The older Yuzpe method consists of 100 μg of ethinyl estradiol and 500 μg (0.5 mg) of levonorgestrel (two Ovral pills) repeated in 12 hours. Other commonly available oral contraceptives can be substituted for Ovral such as Alesse (5 tablets per dose) or 4 tablets per dose of Minovral, Levlen, Levora, Lo/Ovral, Min-Ovral, Nordette, Tri-Levlen (yellow tablets only), or Triphasil (yellow tablets only). Preven, a product containing the Yuzpe regimen with a pregnancy test is available in the United States. The progestin only method approved for use in North America (Plan B) consists of levonorgestrel at 750 μg repeated in 12 hours. ECPs are thought to work primarily by delaying or inhibiting ovulation.[1]

In randomized trials the Yuzpe and progestin only regimens have been shown to reduce the risk of pregnancy by approximately 75% and 85%, respectively with the progestin only method being associated with significantly less nausea and vomiting (5.6% versus 18.8%).[2] For these reasons, the progestin only regimen is the preferred method although its availability and cost may preclude its use in some circumstances. With the Yuzpe regimen an antiemetic such as meclizine (Bonine, Bonamine) or dimenhydrinate (Dramamine, Gravol) and an extra dose of the antiemetic should be given. A single dose of 1.5 mg of levonorgestrel, achieved by taking both tablets of the Plan B formulation at once, appears to be just as effective as the standard two-dose regimen with no increase in side effects; it also avoids the problem of a missed or vomited second dose.[3]

Although standard guidelines have stated that ECPs should be initiated with 72 hours of intercourse, recent trials have shown that both regimens continue to have some effect (although diminished) up to 120 hours.[3,4] Maximum protection occurs if they are taken within 24 hours. An analysis of emergency contraception among women using either levonorgestrel or the Yuzpe regimen found levonorgestrel prevented 95% of pregnancies up to 24 hours, 85% for 25 to 48 hours, and 58% for 49 to 72 hours. The corresponding rates for Yuzpe were 77%, 36%, and 31%, respectively.[2] Women using ECPs should be advised to use ongoing birth control and to have a pregnancy test if menses have not begun within 21 days of treatment.[5]

A practical difficulty with emergency contraception is that the pills are currently available only by prescription and this is not always easy to obtain when the need arises. A good case can be made for giving a supply of ECPs to women who want to have them.[5] In many European countries ECPs are non-prescription drugs, and in Canada Plan B should soon be available without prescription. Currently ECPs can be obtained directly from a pharmacist in some jurisdictions in North America.

Although not available in North America for this purpose, mifepristone (RU 486) a drug with antiprogestational properties has been shown even at very low doses (10 mg single dose) to be as effective as the progestin only method.[3] Insertion of a copper IUD within 5 days of presumed ovulation (up to 7 days after intercourse) is also effective.[5]

─────────────── ⩗ **REFERENCES** ⩘ ───────────────

1. Croxatto HB, Devoto L, Durand M, et al: Mechanism of action of hormonal preparations used for emergency contraception: a review of the literature, *Contraception* 63:111-21, 2001.
2. Task Force on Postovulatory Methods of Fertility Regulation: Randomized controlled trial of levonorgestrel versus the Yuzpe regimen of combined oral contraceptives for emergency contraception, *Lancet* 352:428-433, 1998.
3. von Hertzen H, Piaggio G, Din J, et al: Low dose mifepristone and two regimens of levonorgestrel for emergency contraception: a WHO multicentre randomized trial, *Lancet* 360:1803-1810, 2002.
4. Ellertson C, Evans M, Ferden S, et al: Extending the time limit for starting the Yuzpe regimen of emergency contraception to 120 hours, *Obstet Gynecol* 101:1168-1171, 2003.
5. Dunn S, et al (Clinical Practice Gynaecology and Social Sexual Issues Committees, Society of Obstetricians and Gynaecologists of Canada, SOGC): Emergency contraception, *J Obstet Gynaecol Can* 25(8):673-687, 2003.

Progestin Only Contraceptives

Progestin only oral contraceptives

Progestin only pills (POPs) containing 350 μg of norethindrone include Nor-QD and Micronor. This form of contraception is indicated when estrogen compounds are contraindicated such as in smokers over the age of 35, breastfeeding women, women with migraine with aura, a history of VTE, or women with hypertension. POPs must be taken at the same time every day (within 3 hours)[1] and are taken continuously without a pill-free interval. They are slightly less effective than estrogen/progestin OCs. Irregular vaginal bleeding is common with POPs.

Medroxyprogesterone acetate injections

Medroxyprogesterone acetate (Depo-Provera/DMPA) provides highly effective contraception with a failure rate of less than 1%.[1] The recommended dosage for contraception is 150 mg every 11 to 13 weeks injected deeply into the deltoid or gluteal muscle. Pregnancy must be ruled out, so the drug is often initiated only during the first 5 days of a normal menstrual period.

DMPA is very useful for women who have difficulty adhering to the daily OC regimen, and like progestin-only pills, it can be used in women who have contraindications to estrogen. The most commonly reported side effects of DMPA are menstrual irregularities (e.g., irregular bleeding followed by amenorrhea), headaches, weight gain, and mood changes. However, prospective trials have not demonstrated a consistent relationship between DMPA use and weight gain or mood changes.[1] Education surrounding the potential menstrual irregularities has been shown to reduce rates of discontinuation.[2]

One ongoing question has been the effect of DMPA use on bone density. While many studies have demonstrated a decrease in bone density, DMPA use has not been associated with increased risk of fracture or accelerated osteoporosis in those at risk. BMD has been shown to recover after DMPA discontinuation. BMD also seems to stabilize after the first couple years of use of DMPA with no ongoing losses.[3]

DMPA is long acting. Re-establishment of menstruation after discontinuing DMPA takes, on average, 6 to 8 months but can be up to two years. The median time to conception is 10 months following the last injection.[3]

─────────────── ⩗ **REFERENCES** ⩘ ───────────────

1. Black A, et al: Canadian contraception consensus. 5. Progestin only contraception, *JOGC* 26(3):236-238,2004.
2. Injectable Contraception, *Contraception* 47(Supp 9):777-798, 2002.
3. Westhoff C: Depot-medroxyprogesterone acetate injection (Depo-Provera): a highly effective contraceptive option with proven long-term safety, *Contraception* 68:75-87, 2003.

Sterilization
(See also vasectomy; vasovasostomy)

Tubal sterilization

On a worldwide basis the most common form of contraception is tubal sterilization. This can be accomplished using tubal coagulation, clips, rings, or salpingectomy. A transcervical procedure with hysteroscopic placement of an occlusive device (e.g., Essure) in the tube is becoming more available. Although tubal sterilization is considered a permanent method, successful reversal can occur and is highest for the clip.[1] Occlusion with the Essure device is not reversible. The overall reported incidence of poststerilization regret is low but varies widely from one country to another and from one region to another within the same country. A prospective cohort study in the United States found that 14 years after tubal sterilization, regret was expressed by 20% of women who were 30 years of age or younger at the time of the procedure and 6% of women who were over 30 years of age at the time of the procedure. Among younger women the rate of regret did not plateau but continued to increase with time.[2] Other risk factors for regret are having young children, experiencing couple discord, being sterilized at the time of C-section, or shortly after delivery, miscarriage, or abortion.[1,3]

≈ REFERENCES ≥

1. Black A, et al: Canadian contraception consensus. 10. Sterilization, *JOGC* 368-76, 2004.
2. Hillis SD, Marchbanks PA, Tylor LR, et al: Poststerilization regret: findings from the United States Collaborative Review of Sterilization, *Obstet Gynecol* 93:889-895, 1999.
3. Jamieson KJ, et al: A comparison of women's regret after vasectomy versus tubal sterilizations, *Obstet Gynecol* 99:1073-1079, 2002.

DYSMENORRHEA

Primary dysmenorrhea has a prevalence rate approaching 90%. Pain develops within hours of the onset of menstruation and peaks within the first 2 days. It may be associated with nausea, vomiting, diarrhea, and faintness. Primary dysmenorrhea usually develops 6 to 12 months after menarche and may be more frequent in those who are smokers or have a family history. Full therapeutic doses of any of the NSAIDs or COX-2 inhibitors are usually effective; if one drug does not work, another from different class should be tried. Oral contraceptives, alone or in combination with NSAIDs, are effective in approximately 80% of cases and lack of effectiveness should prompt a look for secondary causes.[1] In a randomized double-blind crossover trial, transdermal nitroglycerin at 0.1 mg per hour significantly improved pain compared to placebo but also caused significant headache.[2] For those wishing non-prescription treatment, possible alternatives include heat, exercise, high frequency TENS, or acupuncture.[1,3]

≈ REFERENCES ≥

1. Coco AS: Primary dysmenorrhea, *Am Fam Physician* 60:489-496, 1999.
2. Moya RA, Moisa CF, Morales F, et al: Transdermal glyceryl trinitrate in the management of primary dysmenorrhea, *Intl J Gynaecol Obstet* 69:113-118, 2000.
3. Akin MD, Weingand KW, Hengehold DA, et al: Continuous low level topical heat in the treatment of dysmenorrheal, *Obstet Gynecol* 97:343-349, 2001.

ECTOPIC PREGNANCY

Ectopic pregnancy is the leading cause of maternal death and serious morbidity during the first trimester of pregnancy. In the United States ectopic pregnancies account for 2% of all pregnancies and 9% of all pregnancy-related maternal deaths. Risk factors are past pelvic inflammatory disease, especially with *Chlamydia trachomatis* (odds ratio 2.0 to 7.5), tubal surgery, previous ectopic pregnancy, in vitro fertilization, induced ovulation, cigarette smoking, pregnancy in a current IUD user, diethylstilbestrol exposure, and increasing age.[1,2]

The classic triad of amenorrhea, abdominal pain, and vaginal bleeding is neither sensitive nor specific for ectopic pregnancy. Pain ranges from mild to severe, and some patients experience no pain. Similarly, abnormal vaginal bleeding ranging from scant to profuse occurs in only 50% to 80% of ectopic pregnancies. The patient may have abdominal or pelvic tenderness, peritoneal signs, cervical motion tenderness, or a palpable adnexal mass; however, absence of these findings does not exclude the diagnosis.[3]

Distinguishing between an early viable intrauterine pregnancy (IUP), a non-viable IUP, and an ectopic pregnancy can be difficult. A combination of serial quantitative β-hCG levels, transvaginal ultrasound, and selected suction and curettage can be used to make the diagnosis. Although β-hCG levels in ectopic pregnancies are usually lower than in viable pregnancies, there is no definitive level that distinguishes between the two. Declining β-hCG levels exclude a viable pregnancy but do not differentiate between a failed IUP and an ectopic pregnancy. Twenty percent of ectopic pregnancies have declining β-hCGs.[4] Although a subnormal rise in β-hCG is very common, 17% of ectopic pregnancies have normal doubling times (every 1.3 to 2 days up to 6 weeks gestation) and 15% of viable pregnancies are associated with less than a 66% increase in β-hCG over 48 hours.[5] β-hCG levels should be monitored at 48-hour intervals and results interpreted in conjunction with ultrasound examination.

Transvaginal ultrasound (TVUS) is diagnostic if an ectopic gestation is identified. It is often indeterminate at β-hCG levels less than 1000 mIU per mL because it is difficult to identify an intrauterine pregnancy below this level and an ectopic pregnancy may not be visualized. A presumptive diagnosis of ectopic pregnancy can be made on the basis of a β-hCG titre above the "discriminatory zone" of 2000 mIU per mL (level at which a gestational sac should be visualized in a normal IUP) and an empty uterus on TVUS. If a patient has persistently low β-hCG and ultrasound is non-diagnostic, distinguishing between a failed intrauterine or ectopic pregnancy may require D&C. If products of conception are obtained, an intrauterine pregnancy is confirmed. If not, then it may be necessary to use laparoscopy to confirm a diagnosis.

Management of ectopic pregnancy includes expectant, medical, or surgical options. All Rh-negative women should receive anti-D immunoglobulin. Surgical management is required if a patient is hemodynamically unstable or if conservative management fails. Salpingostomy is now favoured over salpingectomy in hopes of conserving the tube for future pregnancy, although it is less successful in eliminating all trophoblastic tissue.[6] The procedure is now generally performed laparoscopically. After surgery, serial β-hCG levels should be followed until resolution.

In patients with small or early ectopic pregnancies, medical treatment with methotrexate has been found to be equivalent to surgical therapy in terms of success rates (64% to 94%), subsequent tubal patency, and fertility following resolution of ectopic pregnancy.[3,6] Patients may experience increased abdominal pain and cramping on days 3 to 7 of therapy and this may be difficult to differentiate from tubal rupture on clinical exam.

Expectant management (following β-hCGs to a baseline of 0) should be done under the supervision of a gynecologist. Success for selected patients ranges from 47% to 82%.[7] Criteria for possible expectant management include an ectopic pregnancy less than 3 cm in diameter, β-hCG less than 1000 mIU per mL and decreasing, no fetal cardiac activity, absent or minimal pain, no signs of hemoperitoneum, and patient reliability for follow-up.

─────────── ⊰ REFERENCES ⊱ ───────────

1. ACEP Clinical Policies Committee and Clinical Policies Subcommittee on Early Pregnancy: Clinical policy: critical issues in the initial evaluation and management of patients presenting to the emergency department in early pregnancy, *Ann Emerg Med* 41:123-33, 2003.
2. Pisarska MD, Carson SA: Incidence and risk factors for ectopic pregnancy, *Clin Obstet Gynecol* 42:2-8, 1999.
3. Della-Giustina D, Denny M: Ectopic pregnancy, *Emerg Med Clin N Am* 21:565-584, 2003.
4. Letterie GS, Hibbert M: Serial serum human chorionic gonadotropin (hCG) levels in ectopic pregnancy and first trimester miscarriage, *Arch Gynecol Obstet* 263(4):168-169, 2000.
5. ACOG Committee on Practice Bulletins, Obstetrics: ACOG practice bulletin: Medical management of tubal pregnancy, *Intl J Gynecol Obstet* 65: 97-103,1999.
6. Hajenius PJ, Mol BWJ, Bossuyt PMM, et al: Interventions for tubal ectopic pregnancy (Cochrane Review), In *The Cochrane Library,* 1, 2004, Chichester, 2004, John Wiley.
7. Eisinger S: Early pregnancy bleeding: a rational approach, *Clin Family Pract* 3(2):225-249, 2001.

ENDOMETRIOSIS

Major symptoms of endometriosis are pelvic pain, dysmenorrhea, dyspareunia, backache, and infertility.

The presence of endometriotic tissues in up to 45% of reproductive age women means that its presence may not be pathological.[1] Evidence supports the use of NSAIDs as first-line management of women with dysmenorrhea. Other medical therapies for endometriosis pain target the hormonal responsiveness of endometriotic tissue. Common practice is to use oral contraceptives as first-line therapy (low-dose monophasic with use of a new pack every 21 days).[1] If pain relief with NSAIDs and oral contraceptives is not obtained within 3 to 6 months of initiating therapy, referral is indicated.[2] The definitive diagnosis of endometriosis is established by laparoscopic visualization and biopsy of lesions,[1,2] but laparoscopic confirmation of the diagnosis may not be required before initiating second-line therapy. In one study, clinical diagnosis based on history, examination, and imaging was

shown to be accurate in the vast majority of patients, all of whom were subsequently evaluated by laparoscopy.[4] At the time of laparoscopy all visible endometrial lesions should be ablated and adhesions lysed to decrease pain and increase fertility.[1,2]

Second-line therapy for 6 months of any of the following regimens, danazol (200 to 600 mg/day), Provera (20 to 30 mg/d), medroxyprogesterone acetate (150 mg q 3 months), and gonadotropin-releasing hormone analogues (GnRHas) such as leuprolide acetate (Lupron, 3.75 mg intramuscularly once a month) are equally effective in managing pain.[1,2] Gonadotrophin analogs are effective treatments but their side effects need to be balanced against their benefit. The side effect profiles are different, with danazol having more androgenic side effects and GnRHas producing more hypoestrogenic symptoms. Add-back hormone therapy to counter hypoestrogenic symptoms and bone loss is recommended with GnRHas (i.e., norethindrone acetate at 5 to 10 mg orally once per day, OR premarin at 0.625 to 1.25 mg with norethindrone acetate at 5 mg orally once per day, OR cyclic etidronate at 400 mg with OsCal at 500 mg and norethindrone acetate at 2.5 mg orally once per day).[1]

If medical management of pain fails, or if conception is desired by a woman experiencing pain, laparoscopic surgery is an effective modality for pain and may treat subfertility.[1,2,4]

─────────── ⊰ REFERENCES ⊱ ───────────

1. Winkel C: Evaluation and management of women with endometriosis, *Obstet Gynecol* 102:397-408, 2003.
2. Prentice A: Endometriosis, *BMJ* 323:93-95, 2001.
3. Ling F: Randomized controlled trial of depot leuprolide in patients with chronic pelvic pain and clinically suspected endometriosis, *Obstet Gynecol* 93:51-8, 1999.
4. Jacobson TZ, Barlow DH, Koninckx PR, et al: Laparoscopic surgery for subfertility with endometriosis (Cochrane Review), In *The Cochrane Library*, Issue 1, 2004, Chichester, 2004, John Wiley & Sons.

HUMAN PAPILLOMAVIRUS
(See also cervical cancer)

Human papillomavirus is common and can be found using highly sensitive techniques in close to 50% of normal cervixes in sexually active women.[1] Over 30 subtypes of human papillomavirus can infect the human genital tract. Subtypes 6 and 11 are most commonly associated with condylomata acuminata (anogenital warts) and are only rarely associated with invasive squamous cell carcinoma of the external genitalia.[2] Detection of subclinical condyloma by enhancing techniques such as the application of acetic acid is not indicated because treatment has not been shown to prevent the spread of infection.[2] Human papillomavirus subtypes 16 and 18 and some of the 30s, 50s, and 60s groups are associated with intraepithelial neoplasia and are thought to be onco-genic. They are etiologically necessary but not sufficient for almost all cases of cervical cancer, as well as some anal, vulvar, vaginal, penile, and oropharyngeal cancers.[2] Using HPV alone for primary cervical cancer screening is controversial. Currently, the Canadian Task Force on Preventive Health Care[3] gives this a grade "D" recom-mendation and the the U.S. Preventive Services Task Force gives it a grade "I" rating but adds that "trials are underway that should soon clarify the role of HPV test-ing in cervical cancer screening."[4] There is a role for HPV testing as an adjunct to conventional cytological screen-ing methods. Evidence from the ALTS (ASCUS/LSIL Triage Study) has shown that HPV-DNA is valuable in deciding how to manage ASC-US on cervical cytology.[5]

A number of treatment modalities are available for anogenital warts. One of the newer ones is the applica-tion three times a week of 5% Imiquimod (Aldara) cream. In one RCT this immunomodulator cleared lesions in 50% of patients who used it 3 times each week for up to 16 weeks.[6] Other modalities for HPV treatment include the topical agent podofilox (Condylox), which is available as a 0.5% solution or gel that is applied to the lesions twice per day[7]; cryotherapy; electrodessication; and surgical excision. The clearance efficacy of these methods ranges from 60% to 90%.

The latest advance in the approach to preventing cervi-cal cancer is the development of an anti-HPV vaccine. Although no vaccines are currently approved for use, trials are underway. Encouragingly, one study of HPV-16 vac-cine demonstrated protection against preinvasive disease (100%), persistent infection (100%), and transient infec-tion (91%).[8] Future directions will include developing a vaccine that can target multiple oncogenic HPV strains.

REFERENCES

1. Bauer HM, Ting Y, Greer CE, et al: Genital human papillo-mavirus infection in female university students as deter-mined by a PCR-based method *JAMA* 1991: 265;472-477
2. Center for Disease Control and Prevention: Sexually trans-mitted diseases treatment guidelines 2002. *MMWR* 2002;51(RR-6):1-80
3. Johnson K (Canadian Task Force on the Periodic Health Examination): Periodic health examination, 1995 update 1. Screening for human papillomavirus infection in asympto-matic women *Can Med Assoc J* 1995: 152;483-49
4. U.S. Preventive Services Task Force (USPSTF): Screening for cervical cancer. Website http://www.ahrq.gov/clinic/3rduspstf/cervcan/cervcanrr.htm (Accessed April 27, 2004)
5. National Cancer Institute: Division of Cancer Prevention. ASCUS/LSIL Triage Study for Cervical Cancer (ALTS) website: www3.cancer.gov/prevention/alts/
6. Berman MD: Imiquimod: a new immune response modifier for the treatment of external genital warts and other diseases in dermatology *International Journal of Dermatology* 2002: 41(Suppl 1); 7-11.
7. Tyring S, Edwards L, Cherry LK, et al: Safety and efficacy of 0.5% podofilox gel in the treatment of anogenital warts *Arch Dermatol* 1998: 134;33-38
8. Koutsky LA, et al: for the Proof of Principle Study Investigators. A controlled trial of a human papillomavirus type 16 vaccine. *N Engl J Med* 2002;347:1645-51.

INFERTILITY, FEMALE
(See also appendicitis; pelvic inflammatory disease; sexually transmitted diseases)

One definition of infertility is the inability to conceive after 1 year of adequately timed unprotected intercourse. In Canada, 8% of couples experience infertility. Approximately 60% of couples who do not use contra-ception and have regular intercourse will conceive in 6 months, 80% within 12 months, and 90% in 18 months. Consequently, women who have been trying to get preg-nant for more than 12 to 18 months should be referred to an infertility specialist.[1] A woman's age is one of the main factors determining her fertility.[2] Therefore, earlier referral is advisable for woman who are 35 years of age or older, or for those with a history of pelvic inflamma-tory disease, amenorrhea, or oligomenorrhea, or whose partners have azoospermia.[1]

Family physicians play an important role in counseling patients about ways to optimize pregnancy outcome.[2] The chance of conception in an ovulatory cycle lasts 6 days, ending on the day of ovulation.[3] Timing inter-course to coincide with ovulation causes stress and is not recommended. Intercourse two to three times a week is adequate.[4] Potentially reversible causes of decreased fecundity are smoking, marijuana, and medications such as NSAIDs.[4] There is inconsistent evidence about the impact of alcohol intake on female fertility. Weight gain or loss where the BMI is less than 20 or greater than 30 should be advised.[4]

The basic workup for infertility includes a thorough history and physical examination of both partners. Assessment of rubella immunity, folic acid supplementa-tion, Pap smear status, *Chlamydia* screening, and semen analysis should be included.[4] Investigations aim to iden-tify the main causes of infertility, including ovulatory dysfunction (15% to 25%), tubal blockage (30%), and sperm abnormalities (20%).[1] Regular 24 to 35 day menses suggest ovulation. This can be confirmed with luteal phase serum progesterone 7 days prior to menses. Prolonged use of ovulation predictor kits which detect the midcycle LH surge and basal body temperature charts is not recommended.[5] When ovulatory disorders are suspected, thyroid stimulating hormone, prolactin, gonadotrophins, and estradiol determinations are appro-priate to rule out polycystic ovarian syndrome (PCOS), premature ovarian failure, and hypothalamic amenor-rhea.[6] Androgens are indicated in the clinical setting of hirsutism.[5] In women over 35, a cycle-day-3 follicle stimulating hormone level may predict ovarian reserve.[2] However, this test currently has limited sensitivity and specificity.[4] Consider tubal blockage if there is a history of sexually transmitted disease, pelvic or abdominal surgery or endometriosis.[2]

A number of options are available for the management of infertility. For many couples the first-line approach is ovulation induction with clomiphene citrate, which minimizes the risk of multiple pregnancies. There has been recent interest in the use of insulin-lowering agents such as metformin in women with PCOS.[2] In vitro fertilization (IVF) is another option. It is expensive, time consuming, and complicated.[2] It is associated with live birth rates up to 25 % per cycle.[7] If the problem is male subfertility, intrauterine insemination may be all that is required. In cases of severe deficits in semen quality or failed IVF, intracytoplasmic sperm injection of the ovum may be used (see discussion of male infertility).[7] People who present with infertility should be offered counseling because fertility problems themselves and their investigation and treatment can cause psychological stress.[4]

➷ REFERENCES ➹

1. Belisle S: Introduction. In Belisle S, Pierson R, eds: *CFAS Consensus document for the investigation of infertility by first-line physicians,* Montreal, 2002, Canadian Fertility and Andrology Society. Available at www.cfas.ca.
2. Case AM: Infertility evaluation and management: strategies for family physicians, *Can Fam Physician* 49:1465-1472, 2003.
3. Taylor A: ABC of subfertility: extent of the problem, *BMJ* 327:434-436, 2003.
4. National Collaborating Centre for Women's and Children's Health Clinical Guideline 11: *Fertility: assessment and treatment for people with fertility problems,* London, 2004, National Institute for Clinical Excellence. Available at www.nice.org.uk.
5. Fluker M: Ovulation. In: Belisle S, Pierson R, editors, *CFAS Consensus document for the investigation of infertility by first-line physicians,* Montreal, 2002, Canadian Fertility and Andrology Society. Available at www.cfas.ca
6. American College of Obstetricians and Gynecologists: *Management of Infertility Caused by Ovulatory Dysfunction,* ACOG Practice Bulletin No.34, February 2002. Available at www.acog.org to members only.
7. Smith S, Pfeifer SM, Collins JA: Diagnosis and management of female infertility. *JAMA* 290(13):1767-1770, 2003.

MENOPAUSE

(See also abnormal uterine bleeding; endometrial carcinoma; exercise; informed consent; osteoporosis; sexual dysfunction in women)

Menopause is defined as the cessation of menses for 12 months and usually occurs in the sixth decade of a woman's life. It is preceded by a period of declining frequency of cyclic ovulation and increasing frequency of anovulatory cycles. By 45 years of age, 40% of women will have started or completed the menopause transition (32% are perimenopausal, 8% are post-menopausal), and by 50 years of age, 75% will have started or completed the menopause transition (38% perimenopausal, 37% post-menopausal). By 55 years of age, only 2% of women are pre-menopausal.[1]

The decline of ovarian estrogen production causes multiple endocrine, somatic, and physiological changes to women in this phase of their lives. Fifty to 85% of menopausal women will experience hot flashes, although only 6% experience flashes that last longer than 6 minutes. There is a cultural component because 10% to 20% of Indonesian and 10% to 25% of Chinese woman report experiencing hot flashes. Night sweats are common and can interfere with sleep. Vaginal dryness estimates range from 18% to 21%. Some studies have found an association between declining estrogen levels and urinary incontinence; others have not. The prevalence of UI is 26% to 55% in middle-aged women.[1] Menopausal women face an increased risk of chronic disease including cardiovascular disease, cancer, osteoporosis, and cognitive decline.[2] One of the major issues concerning menopause over the past decade has been the use of hormone replacement therapy (HRT). Since the publication of the Women's Health Initiative in 2002, physicians and their patients no longer feel that HRT is the first line of treatment for menopausal symptoms. Lifestyle methods of disease prevention such as exercise and discontinuation of smoking and non-hormonal therapies for menopausal symptoms are now at the forefront of treatment options. The investigation of post-menopausal bleeding is discussed in the section on abnormal uterine bleeding.

➷ REFERENCES ➹

1. Bastian LA, Smith CM, Nanda K: Is this woman perimenopausal? *JAMA* 289:895-902, 2003.
2. Nevin JE, Pharr ME: Preventive care for the menopausal woman, *Prim Care* 29:583-597, 2002.

Life-Style Changes for Disease Prevention in Menopausal Women

(See also alcohol; exercise; osteoporosis; smoking)

The lack of evidence to support the benefit of HRT as a preventive measure in menopausal women mandates increased emphasis on lifestyle measures to prevent disease.[1]

Smoking cessation is one of the most important measures that can be taken. Another is increasing physical activity. A 10-year follow-up of vigorous activity patterns in 77,743 post-menopausal women has affirmed the benefits of exercise. With each quintile increase of activity, there was a strong graded inverse association with risk of both coronary and total cardiovascular events. Importantly, the results did not vary substantially across age, race, or BMI so even heavy women demonstrated benefit.[2] Regular exercise can also improve many of the other physical changes associated with menopause including obesity, diabetes, and osteoporosis. Exercise alone, exercise plus calcium supplementation, or exercise plus hormone replacement therapy has been shown to decrease bone loss in post-menopausal women.[3,4] These issues are discussed more fully under "Osteoporosis." There is good evidence that exercise decreases the risk of colon cancer and endometrial cancer,[5-7] and that it may reduce the risk of breast cancer.[7]

❧ REFERENCES ❧

1. Wilson, MM: Menopause, *Clin Geriatr Med* 19:483-506, 2003.
2. Manson JE, et al: Walking compared with vigorous exercise for the prevention of cardiovascular events in women, *N Eng J Med* 347:716-725, 2002.
3. Aloia JF, Vaswani A, Yeh JK et al: Calcium supplementation with and without hormone replacement therapy to prevent postmenopausal bone loss, *Ann Intern Med* 120:97-103, 1994.
4. Nelson ME, Fiatarone MA, Morganti CM, et al: Effects of high-intensity strength training on multiple risk factors for osteoporotic fractures: a randomized controlled trial, *JAMA* 272:1909-1914, 1994.
5. Colditz GA, Cannuscio CC, Frazier AL: Physical activity and reduced risk of colon cancer: Implications for prevention, *Cancer Causes Control* 8:649-667, 1997.
6. Terry P, Baron JA, Weiderpass E, et al: Lifestyle and endometrial cancer risk: a cohort study from the Swedish Twin Registry, *Int J Cancer* 82:38-42, 1999.
7. Key TJ, Schatzkin A, Willett WC, et al: Diet, nutrition, and the prevention of cancer, *Public Health Nutr* 7:187, 2004.

Management of Menopausal Symptoms

(See also consensus conferences; informed consent; osteoporosis; sleep disturbances; sexual dysfunction in women; statistics; urinary tract infections)

Hormone replacement therapy may be the most effective treatment for the management of many symptoms of menopause, but its use and the duration of treatment must be discussed in the light of current knowledge and recommendations concerning the risks and benefits of HRT. Although it is useful for the short-term relief of menopausal symptoms, there is no indication for use of HRT for primary prevention.

Vasomotor symptoms

One of the initial symptoms of estrogen withdrawal is hot flashes or vasomotor symptoms. These occur in 75% of post-menopausal women and persist for longer than 5 years in 25%. Women who smoke or whose mothers suffered from hot flashes are at increased risk of having hot flashes.[1]

Until recently, first-line therapy for hot flashes was hormone replacement therapy (HRT). Such therapy is effective, resulting in a 77% reduction in the frequency of vasomotor hot flashes as well as significant reductions in symptom severity.[2] Reduction in hot flash severity is even greater when estrogen is combined with progesterone.[2] Progestins alone (megestrol acetate, 20 mg twice daily, or transdermal progesterone, 20 mg once daily) have also been shown to reduce vasomotor symptoms by 2 to 6 times more than placebo.[3,4]

Several behavioural alternatives have been suggested for the relief of menopausal symptoms. These include breathable clothing, ice packs, air conditioners, and a small fan at close proximity. Also the routine practice of relaxation techniques, yoga, biofeedback, and exercise may reduce the incidence of vasomotor symptoms as well as improve possible sleep disturbances or mood changes.[5] Smoking cessation should also be reinforced.

Some women may respond to oral or transdermal clonidine. One small RCT (30 women) found that transdermal clonidine (3.5 cm patch delivering 0.1 mg clonidine per day for 7 days) significantly reduced the number and intensity of hot flashes after 8 weeks when compared with placebo.[6] Tibolone is a synthetic tissue-specific hormonal agent with estrogenic and weak progestogenic and androgenic effects that has been used in Europe for almost 2 decades. A recent systematic review evaluating eight RCTs concluded that tibolone (2.5 mg/day)[7] significantly reduced vasomotor symptoms. However, tibolone has not yet been approved in North America because of concerns about the need to evaluate the possibility of adverse estrogenic effects.

New insights into the pathophysiology of hot flashes[8] have made antidepressants a promising class of medications for non-hormonal treatment. Venlafaxine is a novel antidepressant that inhibits both serotonin and norepinephrine reuptake. A double-blind placebo-controlled trial of 191 patients demonstrated that patients receiving 75 mg by mouth daily experienced a twofold reduction in hot flash scores (61% versus 27%) after 4 weeks when compared with placebo.[9] Early trials of SSRIs (fluoxetine, 20 mg; paroxetine, 10 to 30 mg) and gabapentin (900 mg once daily) have also been promising, and larger controlled trials are currently underway. In general, these trials did not eliminate hot flashes but reduced them from 7 a day to 3 per day.

There is limited evidence based on small placebo-controlled RCTs of short duration with inconsistent results that say isoflavone (50 to 100 mg daily) may reduce symptom severity in some women after 12 to 16 weeks.[10] Black cohosh may effective for the relief of hot flashes; however, rigorous RCTs are still unavailable. There are concerns with its long-term use given the possible estrogenic effect, and use in women with a personal history or strong family history of breast cancer remains controversial.[5,11]

Vulvar and vaginal atrophy

Aside from hot flashes, a common problem of post-menopausal women is vulvar and vaginal atrophy, which often manifests itself subjectively as a feeling of vaginal dryness, vulvar itch, decreased lubrication during sexual arousal, and dyspareunia. In addition, atrophy of the urethra and base of the bladder may lead to urinary urgency and frequency and perhaps even to urethral stenosis. These symptoms are caused by estrogen deficiency and are usually relieved by estrogen hormone replacement therapy.[12]

Water-soluble lubricating gels such as Replens may relieve vaginal dryness. This may be tried prior to starting HRT. Women should be instructed on pelvic muscle exercises and counselled to decrease caffeine intake in order to improve urinary frequency and incontinence. The vaginal route of administration of HRT provides a more rapid local response, and lower doses of estrogen are needed to achieve therapeutic response. Vaginal estrogen preparations include creams, tablets, gels, and slow-release vaginal rings. Slow-release vaginal rings have been found to be more acceptable to women than creams.[12]

Sleep disturbances

Hot flashes may cause sleep disturbances. A randomized placebo-controlled trial found that hormone replacement therapy significantly diminished sleep disturbances in post-menopausal women.[13] SSRIs may improve sleep by their effects on hot flashes. Avoiding alcohol and caffeine may also decrease hot flashes and improve sleep.[14]

Dysphoria

Whether dysphoria is a true menopausal symptom and whether estrogen treatment improves either the mood or the quality of life is unclear. A 1996 review of 46 primary research papers on the relationship of menopause to depression found little evidence supporting the menopause as a cause of depression.[15] A recent cohort study of over 400 American women found that depressive symptoms increased during transition to menopause and decreased in post-menopausal women. The authors hypothesized that the changing hormonal milieu contributes to dysphoric mood during transition to menopause.[16] SSRIs are an important treatment option for mood disturbance in menopausal women, because these provide dual treatment for hot flashes and depression.[17]

Decreased libido
(see sexual dysfunction in women)

A number of reports have suggested that androgen plus estrogen replacement therapy is effective for women with decreased libido.[18] In Canada, replacement androgen is available as an injectable testosterone-estradiol combination, Climacteron, which is given as 1 mL intramuscularly every 4 to 8 weeks with progestin given to women with an intact uterus. Andriol, an oral form of testosterone, can be given as 40 mg orally every other day together with estrogen/progestin HRT. In the United States combined estrogen and testosterone oral replacement is available as Estrotest, which is given orally in the lowest dose that will control symptoms.

◈ REFERENCES ◈

1. Staropoli DC, Flaws JA, Bush TL, et al: Predictors of menopausal hot flashes, *J Women's Health* 7:1149-1155, 1998.
2. MacLennan A, Lester S, Moore V: Oral oestrogen replacement therapy versus placebo for hot flushes (Cochrane Review), In *The Cochrane Library*, 1, 2004, Chichester, 2004, Wiley & Sons.
3. Loprinzi CL, Michalak JC, Quella SK, et al: Megesterol acetate for the prevention of hot flashes, *N Engl J Med* 331:247-352, 1994. Reviewed in *Clinical Evidence* 10:2138-2150, 2003.
4. Leonetti HB, Longo S, Anasti JN: Transdermal progesterone cream for vasomotor symptoms and postmenopausal bone loss, *Obstet Gynecol* 94:225-228, 1999. Reviewed in *Clinical Evidence* 10:2138-2150, 2003.
5. Stearnes V, et al: Hot flushes, *Lancet* 360:1851-1859, 2002.
6. Nagamani M, Kelver ME, Smith ER: Treatment of menopausal hot flashes with transdermal administration of clonidine, *Am J Obstet Gynecol* 156:561-565, 1987. Reviewed in *Clinical Evidence* 10:2138-50, 2003.
7. Modelska K, Cummings S: Tibolone for postmenopausal women: systematic review of randomized trials, *J Clin Endocrinol Metabol* 87(1):16-23, 2002.
8. Shanafetl TD, Barton D, Adjel A, et al: Pathophysiology and treatment of hot flashes, *Mayo Clin Proc* 77:1207-1218, 2002.
9. Loprinzi CL, Kugler JW, Sloan JA, et al: Venlafaxine in management of hot flashes in survivors of breast cancer: a randomized controlled trial, *Lancet* 356:2059-2063, 2000.
10. Han KK, Soares JM Jr, Haider MA, et al: Benefits of soy isoflavone therapeutic regimen on menopausal symptoms, *Obstet Gynecol* 99:289-294, 2002.
11. Kligler B: Black Cohosh, *Am Fam Physician* 68(1):114-116, 2003.
12. Suckling J, Lethaby A, Kennedy R: Local oestrogen for vaginal atrophy in postmenopausal women, Cochrane Menstrual Disorders and Subfertility Group, *Cochrane Database of Systematic Reviews*, 2, 2004.
13. Polo-Kantola P, Erkkola R, Helenius H, et al: When does estrogen replacement therapy improve sleep quality? *Am J Obstet Gynecol* 178:1002-1009, 1998.
14. National Heart, Lung and Blood Institute Working Group on Insomnia: Insomnia: assessment and management in primary care Am Fam Physician 59(11):3029-3038, 1999.
15. Nicol-Smith L: Causality, menopause, and depression: a critical review of the literature, *BMJ* 313:1229-1232, 1996.
16. Freeman EW, Sammel MD, Liu L, et al: Hormones and menopausal status as predictors of depression in women in transition to menopause, *Arch Gen Psychiatry* 61:62-70, 2004.

17. Joffe H, Soares C, Cohen L: Assessment and treatment of hot flushes and menopausal mood disturbance, *Psychiatr Clin North Am* 26:3, 2003.

18. Modelska K, Cummings S: Female sexual dysfunction in postmenopausal women: systematic review of placebo-controlled trials, *Am J Obstet Gynecol* 188:286-93, 2003.

Hormone Replacement Therapy

When considering HRT for management of menopausal symptoms, the therapeutic benefits must be weighed against the risks of treatment. The actual risks and benefits of HRT have become much more clearly known since the results of the Women's Health Initiative Trial were released in 2002.

The Women's Health Initiative (WHI)

The Women's Health Initiative is the largest preventative study ever mounted to look at healthy postmenopausal women. It began accruement in 1995 and was to run until 2008. Subset arms that specifically looked at HRT in a randomized double blind trial were the estrogen-progesterone (E/P) arm that recruited 16,608 women and the estrogen only arm that recruited 11,000 women with prior hysterectomy. Regimens used continuous oral conjugated equine estrogen (Premarin; 0.625 mg) and medroxyprogesterone (Provera; 2.5 mg) daily, or 0.625 mg Premarin daily, or placebo. The study was formulated to compare risk and benefit simultaneously in a schema that ranked major and minor events postulated to be affected by hormone replacement therapy. Invasive breast cancer and coronary heart disease were the major diseases quantified. DVT, pulmonary embolism, endometrial cancer, stroke, hip fracture, and colorectal cancer were the minor diseases. In July 2003, the E/P arm of the WHI was terminated at the 5.5-year mark when the Data and Safety Monitoring and Review Board determined that the overall risks of E/P HRT outweighed the benefits.[1] The increased risks for coronary heart disease, stroke, breast cancer, and venous thromboembolism outweighed the benefits realized with respect to decreases in colorectal cancer and hip fracture (Table 87).[1,2]

In 2004 the estrogen only arm of the WHI study was closed prematurely at the 7-year mark because it failed to show any overall benefit in the estrogen only arm. The results showed that estrogen increased the risk of stroke,

Table 87   Annual Rates of Events Prevented or Caused per 10,000 Women Taking Combined Estrogen-Progestin or Estrogen-Only Hormone Replacement Therapy (HRT) Versus Placebo

Outcome	Combined Estrogen-Progestin HRT		Estrogen-Only HRT	
	Prevented	**Caused**	**Prevented**	**Caused**
Cardiovasculare Disease Events				
Coronary artery disease events	-	7*	-	-
Stroke	-	8*	-	12†
Thromboembolism	-	18*	-	7†
Total Cardiovascular Disease Events	-	25*	-	24†
Cancer				
Breast (invasive)	-	8*	-	-
Ovarian	-	-	-	2‡
Colorectal	6*	-	-	-
Cholecystitis				
< 5 yr of therapy or placebo use	-	25§	-	-
≥ 5 yr of therapy or placebo use	-	53.5§	-	-
Fracture				
Hip	5*	-	6†	-
Vertebra	6*	-	6†	-
Other (includes wrist)	39*	-	-	-
Total	44*	-	56†	-

*Data from the Women's Health Initiative (WHI) estrogen-plus-progestin trial, in which the HRT regimen was the daily combination of oral conjugated equine estrogen (0.625 mg) and medroxyprogesterone acetate (2.5 mg).
†Data from the WHI estrogen-only trial, in which the daily estrogen-only HRT regimen was oral conjugated.
‡Data from Lacey et al: JAMA 288:334-341, 2002.
§Data from Nelson et al: JAMA 288(7):872-881, 2002.
Table adapted from Wathen CN, et al: Hormone replacement therapy for the primary prevention of chronic diseases; recommendation statement from the Canadian Task Force on Preventive Health Care, CMAJ 170:1535-1539, 2004 (Table1). Copyright © 2004 Canadian Medical Association. Reprinted with permission.

decreased the risk of hip fracture, and did not affect CHD incidence over an average of 6.8 years. There was a non-significant decrease in breast cancer risk.[3]

The E/P arm of the WHI looked at a number of quality of life issues that had also been the subject of much anecdotal reporting. Between the treatment group and the controls, there were no significant effects on general health, vitality, mental health, depressive symptoms, or sexual satisfaction. The use of estrogen plus progestin was associated with a statistically significant but small and not clinically meaningful benefit in terms of sleep disturbance, physical functioning, and bodily pain after one year. It is important to recognize that women who entered the trial were generally free of major menopausal symptoms.[4]

HRT and risk of coronary artery disease

Although it was believed for years that estrogen was protective for coronary artery disease, both the WHI and Heart and Estrogen Replacement Study (HERS) have shown that HRT with CEE and Provera does not prevent coronary events. In the WHI study the absolute excess risk of coronary events was 7 per 10,000 women per year in the E/P arm.[1] The estrogen only arm of the WHI showed no increase in coronary events in the treated group compared with placebo but also no benefit.[3] The HERS study enrolled 2763 post-menopausal women with known coronary artery disease who were randomly assigned to receive Premarin plus Provera or placebo. At follow-up averaging 4.1 years the two groups showed no difference in cardiovascular events, despite an improved lipid profile in the treated group.[5]

HRT and risk of stroke

Both combined HRT and estrogen alone increase the risk of stroke. In the WHI the hazard ratio for ischemic or hemorrhagic stroke was 1.50 (95% CI, 1.08 to 2.08) for E/P versus placebo when adjusted for adherence. Excess risk was apparent in all age groups, in all categories of baseline stroke risk, and in women with and without hypertension, prior history of cardiovascular disease, use of hormones, statins, or Aspirin.[1,3,6]

HRT and risk of thromboembolism

Women taking hormone replacement therapy have twice the risk of venous thromboembolism compared with non-users.[1,7] The increase in risk seems to be greater in the first year of use, with an odds ratio of 4.6 during the first 6 months. Women with predisposing factors such as a family history of thromboembolic disease, severe varicose veins, obesity, surgery, trauma, or prolonged bed rest, and increasing age may be particularly at risk.[7] Route of estrogen administration may have some effect on VTE risk. A recent case-control study of idiopathic VTE in post-menopausal women in France found no increased risk of VTE for women using transdermal estrogen.[8]

HRT and prevention of osteoporosis and fractures

Good evidence from the WHI and other studies demonstrates that estrogens decrease the rate of development of osteoporosis. In the combined E/P group of the WHI, 8.6% of women experienced a fracture compared with 11.1% in the placebo treated group (hazard ratio 0.76) and BMD increased. The decreased risk of fracture attributed to estrogen plus progestin appeared to be present in all subgroups of women examined. Even so, if the global model of risk to benefit is used, there was no net benefit, even in women considered to be at high risk of fracture.[9] Studies of low dose estrogen therapy (e.g., conjugated equine estrogen; 0.3 mg) are somewhat conflicting but suggest that the effect of estrogens on bone density is likely dose dependent. A recent placebo-controlled trial compared low-dose conjugated estrogens (0.3 or 0.45 mg/day) to standard dose therapy (0.625 mg), with or without progestin (medroxyprogesterone acetate, 1.5 or 2.5 mg/day), for two years in 822 healthy postmenopausal women. Spine and hip bone mineral density increased in a dose-dependent fashion in all hormone treatment groups, but not the placebo group. Bone mineral density increased more in the combined estrogen-progestin groups compared with the estrogen-alone groups.[10] Low-dose estrogen may not protect against bone loss unless adequate calcium is given.[11]

The Canadian Task Force on Preventive Health Care recommends against using HRT for the prevention of osteoporosis.[12] For women with severe osteoporosis who cannot tolerate bisphosphonates or raloxifene, HRT can be considered.[13]

HRT and cognitive functioning

There has been considerable conjecture about the role of estrogen in improving cognitive function. Recent trials have dampened the enthusiasm of those who postulate a positive effect for estrogen. In the HERS trial, cognitive function showed no difference between treated and placebo groups (average age 71 years).[14] In the WHI Memory Study of women aged 65 or older, estrogen plus progestin did not improve cognitive function when compared with placebo. Although most women receiving E/P did not experience adverse effects on cognition compared with placebo, a small increased risk of clinically meaningful cognitive decline occurred in the treated group. The increased risk would result in an additional 23 cases of dementia per 10,000 women per year.[15] Preliminary data from the estrogen only arm of the WHIMS show that participants who were on estrogen alone had a trend toward increased risk of probable dementia and/or mild cognitive impairment when compared to the women who were taking placebo.[16]

HRT and cancer

Risk of Colon Cancer. HRT appears to have a protective effect for colon cancer. A meta-analysis of 18 epidemiologic studies of post-menopausal hormone therapy and colorectal cancer, found a 20% reduction in risk of colon cancer and a 19% decrease in the risk of rectal cancer for post-menopausal women who had ever taken the hormone therapy compared with women who never used hormones.[17] The WHI confirmed the reduced risk of colon cancer in women in the E/P arm but not in the estrogen only arm of the trial.[2]

Risk of Gynecological Cancers. Long-term unopposed estrogen use, whether in the form of conjugated estrogens or estradiol, is known to increase the risk of endometrial cancer. This risk may persist for more than 5 years after estrogens are discontinued. Long-term use of estrogen and cyclical progestins is associated with a small increase in the risk for endometrial cancer, but this risk does not persist beyond 5 years after discontinuation of the hormones. Women taking estrogens plus continuous progestins have a lower risk of endometrial cancer than women not taking hormone replacement therapy.[18] Routine endometrial biopsies to rule out endometrial carcinoma before starting hormone replacement therapy are unnecessary for asymptomatic women.[19]

The long-term use of estrogen alone may be associated with an increased risk of developing ovarian cancer. In a study of over 44,000 women from the National Cancer Institutes, ever use of estrogen alone increased risk by 1.6. Increasing duration of use was significantly associated with ovarian cancer with a relative of 1.8 for 10 to 19 years of use and 3.2 for more than 20 years of use.[20]

Risk of Breast cancer. Until 1995 the existence of an association between hormone replacement therapy and breast cancer was controversial. The publication in 1995 of the Nurses' Health Study made it clear that hormone replacement therapy of more than 5 years duration is a risk factor for breast cancer. Women who were currently taking hormones and had been doing so for more than 5 years had a relative risk of acquiring breast cancer of 1.46. This risk was even greater in older women; those aged 60 to 64 who had been taking hormones for at least 5 years had a relative risk of 1.7. The mortality rate from breast cancer was also increased by a relative rate of 1.45 among women who had used hormone replacement more than 5 years.[21] Additional evidence that hormone replacement therapy increases the risk of breast cancer comes from The Million Women Trial in the United Kingdom, which showed a RR of 2.0 for current users of combined E/P hormone therapy[22] and from the E/P arm of the WHI (HR 1.24).[23] The cancers diagnosed were similar in histology and grade but were larger and were at a more advanced stage compared with those diagnosed in the placebo group.[23]

The contribution of progestins to breast cancer risk has been a subject of debate. The Million Women Trial found that the risk of breast cancer in women taking hormone replacement therapy was lower in those receiving estrogen only compared with those receiving E/P combinations.[24] Similarly the WHI estrogen alone arm showed a non-significant 23% reduction in breast cancer in the estrogen users compared with placebo.[3] While this may be due to chance, further studies are required.

Current evidence suggests that the risk of breast cancer is not increased or is only minimally increased in women who take hormone replacement therapy for 4 years or less, a view supported by the Canadian Task Force on Preventive Health Care[12] and the U.S. Preventive Services Task Force.[25] This knowledge should allow both patients and physicians to feel more comfortable about short-term hormonal replacement therapy.

◈ REFERENCES ◈

1. Writing Group for the Women's Health Initiative Investigators: Principal results from the Women's Health Initiative Randomized Controlled Trial, *JAMA* 288: 321-333, 2002.
2. Chlebowski, et al: Estrogen plus progestin and colorectal cancer in postmenopausal women, *N Engl J Med* 350: 991-1004, 2004.
3. Anderson GL, et al: Effects of conjugated equine estrogen in postmenopausal women with hysterectomy: the Women's Health Initiative randomized controlled trial, *JAMA* 291(14):1701-12, 2004.
4. Hays J, et al: Effects of estrogen and progestin on health-related quality of life issues, *N Engl J Med* 348:1839-1854, 2003.
5. Hulley S, Grady D, Bush T, et al (Heart and Estrogen/ Progestin Replacement Study Research Group): Randomized trial of estrogen plus progestin for secondary prevention of coronary heart disease in postmenopausal women, *JAMA* 280:605-613, 1998.
6. Wessertheil-Smoller S, et al: Effect of estrogen plus progestin on stroke in postmenopausal women: the Women's Health Initiative, *JAMA* 289:2717-2719, 2003.
7. Rymer J, et al: Making decisions about HRT, *BMJ* 326:322-326, 2003.
8. Scarabin PY, et al: Differential association of oral and transdermal oestrogen-replacement therapy with venous thromboembolism risk, *Lancet* 362(9382):428-432, 2003.
9. Cauley JA, et al: Effects of estrogen plus progestin on risk of fracture and bone mineral density: the Women's Health Initiative randomized trial, *JAMA* 290:1729-1738, 2003.
10. Lindsay R, et al: Effect of lower doses of conjugated equine estrogens with and without medroxyprogesterone acetate on bone in early postmenopausal women, *JAMA* 287:2668, 2002.
11. Crandall C: Low-dose estrogen therapy for menopausal women: a review of efficacy and safety, *J Women's Health* 12:723-47, 2003.
12. Wathen CN, et al: Hormone replacement therapy for the primary prevention of chronic diseases; recommendation statement from the Canadian Task Force on Preventive Health Care, *CMAJ* 170:1535-1539, 2004.
13. Cheung AM, et al: Prevention of osteoporosis and osteoporotic fractures in postmenopausal women: recommenda-

tion statement from the Canadian Task force on Preventive Health Care, *CMAJ* 170:1665-1667, 2004.

14. Grady D, et al: Effect of postmenopausal hormone therapy on cognitive function: the Heart and Estrogen/Progestin Replacement Study, *Am J Med* 113:543-548, 2002.

15. Rapp SR, et al: Effect of estrogen plus progestin on global cognitive function in postmenopausal women: the Women's Health Initiative Memory Study-a randomized controlled trial, *JAMA* 289(20):2663-2672, 2003.

16. National Heart, Lung, and Blood Institute (NHLBI): NHLBI Statement: NIH Asks participants in Women's Health Initiative Estrogen-Alone Study to stop study pills, begin follow-up phase, March 2, 2004. [Accessed June 27, 2005] Available from: URL: http://www.nhlbi.nih.gov/new/press/04-03-02.htm

17. Grodstein F, et al: Postmenopausal hormone therapy and the risk of colorectal cancer: a review and meta-analysis, *Am J Med* 106:574-582, 1999.

18. Weiderpass E, Adami HO, Baron JA, et al: Risk of endometrial cancer following estrogen replacement with and without progestins, *J Natl Cancer Ins* 91:1131-1137, 1999.

19. Korhonen MO, Symons JP, Hyde BM, et al: Histologic classification and pathologic findings for endometrial biopsy specimens obtained from 2964 perimenopausal and postmenopausal women undergoing screening for continuous hormones as replacement therapy (Chart 2 Study), *Am J Obstet Gynecol* 176:377-380, 1997.

20. Lacey JV, et al: Menopausal hormone replacement therapy and risk of ovarian cancer, *JAMA* 288:334-341, 2002.

21. Colditz GA, Hankinson SE, Hunter DJ, et al: The use of estrogens and progestins and the risk of breast cancer in postmenopausal women, *N Engl J Med* 332:1589-1593, 1995.

22. Beral V and the Million Women Study Collaborators: Breast cancer and hormone-replacement therapy in the million women study, *Lancet* 362(9382):419-427, 2003.

23. Chlebowski RT, et al: Influence of estrogen plus progestin on breast cancer and mammography in healthy postmenopausal women: the Women's Health Initiative randomized trial, *JAMA* 289(24):3243-3253, 2003.

24. Schairer C, Lubin J, Troisi R, et al: Menopausal estrogen and estrogen-progestin replacement therapy and breast cancer risk, *JAMA* 283:485-491, 2000.

25. U.S. Preventive Services Task Force: *Guide to clinical preventive services,* ed 2, Baltimore, 1996, Williams & Wilkins, pp 829-843.

Guidelines for hormone replacement therapy

Since the publication of the WHI report in 2002, several health organizations have re-evaluated their positions on hormone replacement therapy (HRT) and put forward guidelines aiding physicians to optimally counsel patients. The Society of Obstetricians and Gynecologists of Canada (SOGC) support the short-term use (up to 4 years) of continuous combined HRT for the management of moderate to severe menopausal symptoms for women with an intact uterus.[1] They recommend that a longer use of HRT should be re-evaluated on an annual basis with the patient's physician contrasting possible

harms and benefits. However, the SOGC states that continuous combined HRT regimen should *not* be recommended for all post-menopausal women.[2]

Along the same lines, both the U.S. Preventive Services Task Force (USPSTF) and the Canadian Task Force on Preventive Health Care recommend against the routine use of HRT for the prevention of chronic conditions in post-menopausal women ("D" recommendation).[3,4] The USPSTF did not evaluate the use of HRT for the symptomatic treatment of vasomotor or urogenital symptoms associated with menopause.

≥ REFERENCES ≤

1. SOGC: Short term HRT is a safe and effective option for the treatment of distressing menopausal symptoms, SOGC media release, January 13, 2004. http://www.sogc.org/SOGCnet/sogc_docs/press/releases2004/pdfs/HRT_remains_safe_Jan_12_2004.pdf. Accessed May 24, 2005.

2. SOGC: *The SOGC statement of the WHI report on estrogen and progesterone use in postmenopausal women. Appendix: revisions to recommendations,* vol. 24, no.10, Canadian Consensus Conference on Menopause and Osteoporosis, October 2002.

3. U.S. Preventive Services Task Force: Postmenopausal hormone replacement therapy for the primary prevention of chronic conditions; recommendations and rationale. *Ann Intern Med* 137:834-839, 2002.

4. Wathen CN, et al: Hormone replacement therapy for the primary prevention of chronic diseases; recommendation statement from the Canadian Task Force on Preventive Health Care, *CMAJ* 170:1535-1539, 2004.

Methods of prescribing hormone replacement

Multiple therapeutic regimens for hormone replacement therapy exist that use different routes of administration. They include oral and transdermal preparations, injectables, topical vaginal creams, and intravaginal tablets. The transdermal options are the preferred route for women with hypertriglyceridemia or impaired liver function. Vaginal creams, intravaginal tablets, and vaginal rings are mainly indicated for the symptomatic relief of atrophic vaginitis due to estrogen deficiency. Vaginal rings and tablets provide slow release of hormone that has minimal systemic absorption and minimal effect on the endometrium.

Most of the examples given below use conjugated estrogens (Premarin) or estrogen patches containing estradiol (e.g., Estraderm, Climara, Estradot) plus medroxyprogesterone acetate (Provera) simply because these are the most frequently used drugs in practice. Progestins are required only for women who have an intact uterus and are not required for women using vaginal products. Regimens given are the standard ones. Recently lower than standard doses have been advocated (e.g., 0.3 mg Premarin; 0.5 mg 17 β-estradiol tablet; or 25 μg 17 β-estradiol patch), possibly providing therapeutic benefit but with lower adverse risk. Evidence for this is currently lacking.

Table 88 lists generic and selected trade names of some of the available agents used for hormonal replacement. Methods of prescribing most of them are discussed in the text.

Continuous Estrogen and Continuous Progestin. Premarin (0.625 mg orally) is taken daily or a 50 μg estradiol patch is applied twice a week; in addition Provera (2.5 mg) is given daily. This protocol is followed continuously throughout the year. Spotting or bleeding is common in the first 6 months. In one trial 27% of women receiving continuous Provera (5 mg) and 39% of women receiving continuous Provera (2.5 mg) had breakthrough bleeding.[1] After 6 to 12 months of this regimen, many women had become completely amenorrheic.[2] Once a woman is amenorrheic, any vaginal bleeding requires evaluation. A meta-analysis of 42 studies of combined continuous estrogen-progestin use found that after 6 months of therapy, 75% or more of women were amenorrheic.[3] There are several oral and transdermal preparations that can be used to provide continuous estrogen-progestin therapy (Premplus, Prempro, Combipatch [United States], Estalis).

Continuous Estrogen and Cyclical Progestogen. The standard method of using a continuous estrogen and cyclical progestogen combination is to take Premarin (0.625 mg orally) daily or to apply a 50 μg estradiol patch twice a week throughout the year. Provera (5 or 10 mg) is taken for the first or last 10 to 14 days of each calendar month or of each 28-day cycle. The progestin withdrawal leads to bleeding in most women. A package containing 14 tablets of 0.625 mg conjugated estrogens (taken during the first 14 days) and 14 tablets of 0.625 mg conjugated estrogens combined with 5 mg medroxyprogesterone acetate (taken on days 15 to 28; Premphase) is available in the United States. In Canada, a monthly sequential patch regimen is provided by Estracomb and Estalissequi.

Estrogen-Androgen Injections and Cyclical Progestogen. Testosterone plus estradiol (Climacteron) is given as a 1-mL intramuscular injection deep in the gluteus muscles once every 4 to 8 weeks. If the woman has an intact uterus, 5 to 10 mg of Provera should be given once between days 12 to 25 of the cycle, counting the day of injection as day 1.

❧ REFERENCES ❧

1. Archer DF, Pickar JH, Bottiglioni F: Bleeding patterns in post-menopausal women taking continuous combined or sequential regimens of conjugated estrogens with medroxyprogesterone acetate, *Obstet Gynecol* 83:686-692, 1994.
2. Rosenfeld J: Update on continuous estrogen-progestin replacement therapy, *Am Fam Physician* 50:1519-1523, 1994.
3. Udoff L, Langenberg P, Adashi EY: Combined continuous hormone replacement therapy-a critical review, *Obstet Gynecol* 86:306-316, 1995.

Table 88 Selected Medications for Hormonal Replacement

Compound	Oral	Intravaginal	Transdermal
		Trade Names	
Estrogens			
• Conjugated equine estrogen	Premarin	Premarin vaginal cream	
• Synthetic conjugated estrogen	Cenestin (US)		
• Estropipate	Ogen, Ortho-est (US)		
• 17-beta-estradiol	Estrace	Estrace vaginal cream Estring Vagifem tablets	Alora (US), Climara, Estraderm, Estradot, Estrogel, Oesclim
• Dienestrol		Ortho dienestrol vaginal cream	
Progestins			
• Medroxyprogesterone acetate	Provera		
• Micronized progesterone	Prometrium		
• norethindrone	Micronor		
Combined estrogen/progestin			
• conjugated equine estrogen plus medroxyprogesterone acetate	Premplus, Prempro (US)		
• 17 β estradiol and norethindrone Estracomb			Combipatch (US), Estalis,
Combined estrogen/testosterone	Estratest (US) In Canada only product is Climacteron for IM use		

OVARIES
Ovarian Cancer

(See also breast cancer; positive predictive value; prevention; screening)

Epidemiology

Ovarian cancer is the sixth most common malignancy among women in Canada and the leading cause of death from gynecological cancers.[1,2] The lifetime risk is estimated to be 1.4%. It is primarily a disease of post-menopausal women, with median age at diagnosis between 60 and 65, and peak incidence in the seventh decade of life. In 70% of women, the disease is advanced (stage III or IV) at the time of diagnosis.

Risk factors

The most important risk factor is family history, especially if two or more first-degree relatives are affected. Other risk factors may include high body mass index during adolescence, infertility, exposure to post-menopausal hormone therapy, and talc exposure, but studies are inconsistent. The majority of women developing ovarian cancer have no known risk factors. Protective factors include the use of oral contraceptives, tubal ligation or hysterectomy, and having and breastfeeding children.[3,4]

Screening or case finding

There is insufficient evidence to suggest that screening modalities such as regular pelvic examination, transvaginal pelvic ultrasound, or CA125 alter the mortality rate of ovarian cancer. False positive results are common and may lead to anxiety and unnecessary surgery.[4,5] In women at significantly increased risk, the increased positive predictive value may justify screening with transvaginal pelvic ultrasound and CA125 every 6 to 12 months, with review of the risks and benefits. While not recommended for screening, ultrasound and CA125 may be useful to aid in evaluation of symptoms. The symptoms are often vague and include fatigue, persistent abdominal bloating, and gastrointestinal complaints, so a high index of suspicion must be maintained.

Hereditary ovarian cancer syndromes

In any woman with a personal or family history of ovarian cancer, formal genetic counselling is recommended to evaluate the likelihood of hereditary disease and facilitate genetic testing if appropriate.

The most common form of hereditary ovarian cancer is the hereditary breast/ovarian cancer syndrome associated with mutations in BRCA1 or BRCA2. These mutations are responsible for about 10% of all ovarian cancers in the general population; however, in Ashkenazi Jewish women as many as 40% may carry a mutation.[6] Ovarian cancer in mutation carriers is mostly of the papillary serous type.[7] Several studies estimate the risk of ovarian cancer by age 70 to be 16% to 44% for BRCA1 mutation carriers and 15% to 25% for those with mutations in BRCA2.[8] The mean age of onset of ovarian cancer appears to about 5 years earlier in mutation carriers than in sporadic cases, with some evidence suggesting this is more true of BRCA1 than BRCA2.

The optimal methods for screening and preventing ovarian cancer in mutation carriers have not yet been established. Oral contraceptives for 5 years or more are thought to decrease the risk, though one study has suggested that the use of higher dose pills in BRCA1 carriers under the age of 25 may be of concern regarding subsequent breast cancer risk.[9] Tubal ligation also appears to reduce the risk and should be considered once pregnancy is no longer desired. The current most effective preventive strategy is prophylactic removal of the ovaries and fallopian tubes (and generally the uterus as well), usually considered after completion of childbearing between ages 35 and 50. This appears to reduce ovarian cancer risk by at least 95%. Such surgery does not remove the risk of primary peritoneal cancer, which is histologically indistinguishable from serous ovarian cancer. Pre-menopausal removal of the ovaries also has the advantage of decreasing breast cancer risk by up to 50%, even if hormone replacement is given. For women who are not candidates for surgical prophylaxis, screening is recommended with transvaginal pelvic ultrasound and CA125 every 6 to 12 months, though there is currently no evidence that this changes outcomes.[7,10]

Another form of hereditary ovarian cancer is that associated with hereditary non-polyposis colorectal cancer (HNPCC). Women with this disorder are at increased risk of colon, ovarian, endometrial, other gastrointestinal and urinary cancers. The risk of developing ovarian cancer in this situation is about 10%.

◢ INTERNET SOURCE ◣

National Ovarian Cancer Association: www.ovarian-canada.org

◢ REFERENCES ◣

1. National Cancer Institute of Canada: Canadian Cancer Statistics 2003, Toronto, Canada, 2003. Available online at www.ncic.cancer.ca

2. Supplement on Ovarian Cancer, *Gynecol Oncol* 88, 2003 (includes key information to date, areas of uncertainty, research in progress, goals for future research).

3. National Cancer Institute: Prevention of Ovarian Cancer, Health Professional Version, 03/23/2004. Available at www.cancer.gov.

4. National Cancer Institute: Screening for Ovarian Cancer, Health Professional Version 02/30/3004. Available at www.cancer.gov.

5. Canadian Task Force on the Periodic Health Examination: *Clinical Preventive Health Care*, Ottawa, 1994, Canadian

Communication Group Publishing. Available online at www.ctfphc.org/index.html.

6. Leide A, Karlan B, Baldwin R, et al: Cancer incidence in a population of Jewish women at risk of ovarian cancer, *J Clin Oncol* 20(5):1570-1577, 2002.

7. Robson M: Clinical considerations in the management of individuals at risk for hereditary breast and ovarian cancer, *Cancer Control* 9(6):457-465, 2002.

8. www.geneclinics.org (good resource for physicians on genetic conditions). Accessed May 24, 2005.

9. Narod SA, et al: Oral contraceptives and the risk of breast cancer in BRCA1 and BRCA2 mutation carriers, *J Natl Cancer Inst* 94(23):1773-1779, 2002.

10. Pichert G, Bolliger B, Buser K, et al: Evidence-based management options for women at increased breast/ovarian cancer risk, Ann Oncol 14:9-19, 2003.

Polycystic Ovarian Syndrome

Between 5% and 10% of women in the reproductive age range are thought to have the polycystic ovarian syndrome.[1] The usual clinical manifestations are menstrual dysfunction or infertility caused by oligoovulation or anovulation, and acne and hirsutism caused by elevated testosterone levels. Serum-free testosterone levels are elevated, and in most patients ultrasound detects enlarged ovaries with multiple small peripheral follicles. Many women with this disorder, particularly if they are obese, have insulin resistance and hyperinsulinemia. Women with PCOS are at increased risk of type 2 diabetes, hyperlipidemia, cardiovascular disease, and endometrial cancer. If the diagnosis is established, screening for diabetes and hyperlipidemia is advised.[2]

Treatment of polycystic ovarian syndrome includes measures to manage symptoms and prevent long-term consequences of the metabolic abnormalities. This includes using oral contraceptives for menstrual irregularities, clomiphene citrate (Clomid) for infertility, and antiandrogens such as spironolactone (Aldactone) or cyproterone (Androcur) for hirsutism. Weight loss, which reduces insulin resistance, is an essential part of treatment for obese patients. Loss of as little as 5% of initial weight may improve metabolic abnormalities and reproductive function. Metformin has been shown to improve metabolic parameters and restore ovulation. There is only limited data on its safety in early pregnancy.[3]

────────── ☙ REFERENCES ❧ ──────────

1. Richardson MR: Current perspectives in polycycstic ovary syndrome, *Am Fam Physician* 68:697-704, 2003.

2. Schroeder B: Practice guidelines: ACOG releases guidelines on diagnosis and management of polycystic ovary syndrome, *Am Fam Physician* 67:1619-1620, 2003.

3. Lord JM, Flight IH, Norman RJ: Metformin in polycystic ovary syndrome: systematic review and meta-analysis, *BMJ* 327(7421):951-953, 2003.

PELVIC INFLAMMATORY DISEASE

Pelvic inflammatory disease refers to an ascending lower genital tract infection that leads to endometrial, tubal/ovarian, or peritoneal infection. Sexually transmitted organisms *Chlamydia trachomatis* and *Neissieria gonorrhoeae* are the main etiologic agents. Eight to ten percent of women with chlamydial or gonococcal cervicitis develop PID. Other organisms, including anaerobes, CMV, mycoplasma, and ureaplasma have also been causally implicated.[1]

The clinical diagnosis of PID is difficult and imprecise due to the variety of signs and symptoms, including asymptomatic or mild presentations. The current gold standard for diagnosis, laparoscopy, is of minimal practical value. Clinical diagnosis unfortunately has a sensitivity and specificity of only 50%.[2] Thus, the latest CDC guidelines recommend that empiric treatment of PID should be initiated in sexually active women if "the minimum criteria of adnexal tenderness or cervical motion tenderness is present and no other causes for illness can be identified."[3] Additional clinical features that support a diagnosis of PID include lower abdominal pain, dyspareunia, abnormal vaginal discharge, fever higher than 38° C, cervical infection with chlamydia or gonorrhea, and elevated ESR/CRP. Absence of positive tests for chlamydia or gonorrhea infections does not exclude a diagnosis of PID.[1] The sequelae of untreated or delayed treatment may be serious and include infertility (20%), ectopic pregnancy (10%), and chronic pelvic pain (20%).[4] The Pelvic Inflammatory Disease Evaluation and Clinical Health (PEACH) Trial randomized 831 women to in-patient intravenous antibiotics or outpatient treatment with one dose of intramuscular cefoxitin followed by oral doxycycline. There was no difference between in-patient and outpatient treatment regimens with respect to subsequent reproductive outcomes.[5] Multiple regimens for outpatient treatment are suggested and include ofloxacin (400 mg twice daily) plus metronidazole (500 mg twice daily) for 14 days, or a third-generation cephalosporin plus doxycycline (100 mg twice daily) for 14 days.[1,3] Criteria for hospitalization or parenteral treatment include pregnancy, tuboovarian abscess, inability to tolerate oral regimen, or no response to oral treatment within 72 hours. Comprehensive management includes contact tracing and treatment of any sexual partners within the past 60 days. Screening for cervical chlamydial infection in high-risk populations has been shown to reduce the incidence of PID.[6]

────────── ☙ REFERENCES ❧ ──────────

1. Royal College of Obstetricians and Gynecologists: *Management of Acute Pelvic Inflammatory Disease*, Guideline No. 32, 2003.

2. Ross J: An update on pelvic inflammatory disease, *Sex Transm Infect* 78(1):18-19, 2002.

3. Centers for Disease Control and Prevention: Pelvic Inflammatory Disease. Sexually transmitted disease treatment guidelines, *MMWR* 10;51(RR-6):48-52, 2002

4. Ross J: Pelvic inflammatory disease: extracts from clinical evidence, *BMJ* 322(7287):658-659, 2001.

5. Ness RB, Soper DE, Holley RL, et al: Effectiveness of inpatient and outpatient treatment strategies for women with pelvic inflammatory disease: results from the pelvic inflammatory disease evaluation and clinical health (PEACH) randomized trial, *Am J Obstet Gynecol* 186(5):929-937, 2002.

6. Scholes D, Stergachis A, Hedrich F, et al: Prevention of pelvic inflammatory disease by screening for cervical chlamydial infection, *N Engl J Med* 334(21):1362-1366, 1996.

PREMENSTRUAL SYNDROME
(See also depression, breast pain)

The nature or even the existence of premenstrual syndrome (PMS) has been a subject of controversy. Since over 200 symptoms of the disorder have been described in the medical literature, such uncertainty is understandable.[1] Recently more rigorous studies have shed considerable light on the issue. PMS does exist, and it is characterized by both emotional and physical symptoms that recur cyclically during the luteal phase of the menstrual cycle. Symptoms are behavioural (fatigue, insomnia, dizziness, change in sexual interest), psychological (irritability, depressed mood, anxiety), and physical (headache, breast tenderness and swelling, back pain, abdominal pain and bloating, water retention).[2]

Women with more severe affective symptoms are classified as having premenstrual dysphoric disorder (PMDD), which is thought to affect about 5% of menstruating women.[2,3] It must be distinguished from the less severe disturbances of cognition, behaviour, and mood that affect 20% to 80% of women during the premenstrual phase.[4] PMS is more common in women whose mothers were affected and in women with a history of depression.[4] To meet the criteria for the diagnosis of PMS, symptoms must be severe enough to interfere with social and occupational functioning, occur during the second half of the menstrual cycle, and remit completely at the time of menstruation. For PMDD, affective symptoms must be marked and cause severe disturbance in work or social functioning.[3,4] To confirm the diagnosis, timing of symptoms should be documented by symptom diaries over two or three cycles.[2,4-6]

Although there is little available evidence, women with mild symptoms should be advised that lifestyle changes, including healthy diet, sodium and caffeine restriction, aerobic exercise, and stress reduction may be helpful.[2] In women with moderate symptoms, treatment includes both medication and lifestyle modifications. Many therapies have been tried for PMS, and most have shown little evidence of benefit. These include vitamins, minerals, herbal remedies, diuretics, and estrogens and progesterone, including oral contraceptives.[2] For example, although the main conclusion of a 1999 systematic review of vitamin B_6 was that most of the studies evaluated were of poor quality, it appeared possible that 50 to 100 mg of vitamin B_6 daily might be helpful.[7] A 1998 multicenter randomized placebo-controlled trial of elemental calcium (600 mg twice daily) or calcium carbonate (1500 mg twice daily) for treatment of premenstrual dysphoric disorder found significant amelioration of all symptoms, including mood dysfunction, in the group taking calcium.[8] Spironolactone has been found to have some effect on improving irritability, breast tenderness, and bloating.[9] For women with moderate to severe symptoms, selective serotonin reuptake inhibitors (SSRIs) are the drugs of choice.[2,4,5] A systematic review found the SSRIs to be highly effective in treating both physical and behavioural symptoms with similar efficacy for continuous or intermittent therapy.[10] Sertraline (Zoloft) in doses of 50 to 150 mg, paroxetine (Paxil; 10 to 30 mg), fluoxetine (Prozac; 10 to 20 mg) and citalopram (Celexa; 10 to 30 mg) have all been shown to be effective. Interestingly citalopram was more effective when used only in the luteal phase than with continuous use.[11] Venlafaxine (Effexor; 50 to 200 mg daily) and clomipramine (Anafranil) have also been shown to be effective. Alprazolam (Xanax) improves symptoms of anxiety, but the danger of addiction militates against its use.[4] Danazol and GnRh analogs are effective but their cost and side effects make them third-line therapies.[4]

REFERENCES

1. Steiner M, Born L: Diagnosis and treatment of premenstrual dysphoric disorder: an update, *Int Clin Psychopharmacol* 15(suppl 3):S5-17, 2000.

2. Dickerson LM, Mazyck PJ, Hunter MH: Premenstrual syndrome, *Am Fam Physician* 67:1743-52, 2003.

3. Premenstrual dysphoric disorder. In *Diagnostic and statistical manual of mental disorder*, ed 4, DSM-IV-TR. Washington, DC, 2000, American Psychiatric Association, p 771.

4. Parry BL: A 45-year-old woman with premenstrual dysphoric disorder, *JAMA* 281:368-373, 1999.

5. Bhatia SC, Bhatia SK: Diagnosis and treatment of premenstrual dysphoric disorder, *Am Fam Physician* 66:1239-48, 2002.

6. Grady-Weliky TA: Premenstrual dysphoric disorder, *N Engl J Med* 348(5):433-438, 2003.

7. Wyatt KM, Dimmock PW, Jones PW, et al: Efficacy of vitamin B-6 in the treatment of premenstrual syndrome: systematic review, *BMJ* 318:1375-1381, 1999.

8. Thys-Jacobs S, Starkey P, Bernstein D, et al: Calcium carbonate and the premenstrual syndrome: effects on premenstrual and menstrual symptoms, *Am J Obstet Gynecol* 179:444-452, 1998.

9. Wang M, et al: Treatment of premenstrual syndrome by spironolactone: a double-blind, placebo-controlled study, *Acta Obstet Gynecol Scand* 74:803-808, 1995.

10. Wyatt KM, Dimmock PW, O'Brien PMS: Selective serotonin reuptake inhibitors for premenstrual syndrome, Cochrane Menstrual Disorders and Subfertility Group, *Cochrane Database of Systematic Reviews*, 2, 2004.

11. Wikander I, Sundblad C, Andersch B, et al: Citalopram in premenstrual dysphoria: is intermittent treatment during luteal phases more effective than continuous medication throughout the menstrual cycle? *J Clin Psychopharmacol* 18:390-398, 1998.

SEXUAL DYSFUNCTION IN WOMEN

(See sexual dysfunction in men)

Female sexual dysfunction can be subdivided into desire, arousal, orgasmic, and sexual pain disorders.[1,2] Sexual problems are highly prevalent, affecting 30% to 50% of women but are recorded in less than 2% of primary care physician encounters.[1] Causes include hormonal and medical conditions (e.g., diabetes, prolactinoma), local physical factors (gynecological), medications, psychological, and partnership factors.

Disorders of desire may be challenging to manage. They may be secondary to lifestyle factors (e.g., careers, children), medications, or other sexual dysfunction (e.g., pain or orgasmic disorder).[1] Decreased libido and sexual response in post-menopausal women may be due to depression, but in a few instances they may be related to low testosterone. If free testosterone levels are low, small replacement doses of testosterone (used with HRT) may be helpful. Trials to date have primarily been with women who have had their ovaries removed. Only a modest benefit was observed. This could be provided as monthly combined estrogen/testosterone (Climacteron). In Canada, oral testosterone undecenoate (Andriol) is available and can be given as one 40-mg capsule every second day.[3] Combined oral estrogen and testosterone products are available in the United States (Estratest).

Arousal and orgasmic disorders may be attributed to lack of sufficient stimulation. Treatment involves use of lubricants; maximizing stimulation, and minimizing inhibition, respectively.[1] Urogenital atrophy is the most common cause of arousal disorders in post-menopausal women. Estrogen replacement or local estrogen (e.g., vaginal ring) is usually effective.[1] Sildenafil has not been shown to be helpful in women.[4]

Sexual pain disorders include vaginismus and dyspareunia.[1,2] Vaginismus is caused by spasm of the levator muscles, which can be detected on pelvic examination. (Pelvic examination should not be performed if it is too anxiety-provoking or painful.) The essence of treatment is progressive muscle relaxation and vaginal dilation.[1] This includes Kegel exercises (contraction of the levators), reverse Kegel exercises (relaxation of the levators), and eventual vaginal penetration with lubricated fingers, commercial dilators, or tampons. Once the patient can accomplish these exercises effectively, she may get her partner to participate in introducing fingers with eventual penile insertion. Dyspareunia may be superficial, vaginal, or deep. Diagnosis of underlying etiology should be pursued, possibly involving surgical (laparoscopic) investigation in the case of deep dyspareunia.

❧ REFERENCES ❧

1. Phillips NA: Female sexual dysfunction: evaluation and treatment, *Am Fam Physician* 62:127-36, 141-2, 2000.
2. Maurice WL: *Sexual Medicine in Primary Care*. St. Louis, 1999, Mosby.
3. Basson R: Androgen replacement for women, *Can Fam Physician* 45:2100-2107, 1999.
4. Modelska K, Cummings S: Female sexual dysfunction in postmenopausal women: systematic review of placebo-controlled trials, *Am J of Obstet Gynecol* 188:286-93, 2003.

SEXUALLY TRANSMITTED DISEASES

(See also condoms; herpes simplex; HIV and AIDS; drugs and chemicals in pregnancy human papillomavirus; infertility, female; Papanicolaou smears; pelvic inflammatory disease; Reiter's syndrome; septic arthritis)

Gonorrhea

(Causative agent: Neisseria gonorrhoeae)

After chlamydia, gonorrhea is the next leading cause of urethritis and cervicitis in both men and women.[1] In North America, the incidence is highest in downtown urban centres among people under the age of 24. Worldwide, the rate is highest in developing countries (400 to 10,000 per 100,000). The incubation period generally ranges from 2 to 21 days. Purulent vaginal or urethral discharge may be present, but many cases individuals may remain asymptomatic, especially women. Transmission is higher from men to women than women to men. When used properly, condoms are thought to decrease transmission from 70% to 100%. Education about safer sex is still a problem, particularly among the groups at highest risk. In addition, a recent Canadian study has found that simply providing information about condom use may be ineffective unless accompanied by education about "sexual negotiation skills" related to limit-setting and dealing with partner resistance.[2] Diagnosis can be made by gram stain, culture, or where available, by urine nucleic acid amplification techniques like PCR. Table 89 summarizes the recommended treatment regimens (see notes below on pregnancy and lactation and emerging trends in resistance). A test of cure is not recommended. All patients should be treated for *Chlamydia* at the same time due to high co-infection rates (Table 90).[1,2]

Table 89   Gonorrhea Treatment*

Strategy	Drug	Dosage
1st line	**Cefixime**	400 mg PO × 1*†
2nd line	**Ceftriaxone**	125 mg IM × 1*
	Ciprofloxacin	500 mg PO × 1‡
	Ofloxacin	400 mg PO × 1‡
	Levofloxacin	250 mg PO × 1‡
	Spectinomycin	2 g PO × 1*

*Safe in pregnancy and lactation
†Cefixime was discontinued in the U.S. in 2002. While the availability of the 400 mg tablet remains limited, it is available in a suspension (100mg/5cc) as of Feb 2004.
‡Due to increasing resistance, Fluoroquinolones are *not* recommended for the treatment of gonococcal infections acquired in Hawaii, California, Asia and the Pacific, or in cases arising from men having sex with men.[1] Recent evidence suggests that resistance to Fluoroquinolones is also on the rise in Michigan, Massachusetts, NYC and Seattle.[3]

Chlamydia Infection

(Causative agent: Chlamydia trachomatis)

Chlamydia is the most common sexually transmitted disease in North America (2 to 5 times more prevalent than gonorrhea). As many as 50% of men and 70% of women can be asymptomatic, but complications can include PID, ectopic pregnancy, and infertility. For those that become symptomatic, the incubation period is usually 2 to 6 weeks but can be longer.[2] Diagnosis can be made by obtaining cervical swabs for culture, enzyme immunoassay, or detection of *Chlamydia* DNA through DNA probe or nucleic acid amplification techniques (NAAT). NAATs have very high sensitivity and specificity and are the preferred methods for screening if available. NAATs (e.g., PCR) of urine specimens are more sensitive than cervical or urethral culture (91% versus 65% for women, and 96% versus 48% for men).[4] A urine specimen may be more acceptable to patients, given the ease of the test compared to a urethral or cervical swab. The question of whether it is safe to delay Pap tests and pelvic exams in the adolescent female population has yet to be resolved.[5-7] While it might be preferable to screen all sexually active women with these manoeuvres, the perceived increase in discomfort of a bimanual and speculum exam as compared to a urine test may dissuade young patients from seeking testing at all. This is important to consider as women between the ages of 15 and 19 have the highest rates of chlamydial infection (5% to 15% prevalence). Treatment is summarized in Table 90. Patients should be advised not to have sex for a period of at least 7 days following the start of treatment.[1] *Chlamydia* is highly infectious (60% to 70% rate of transmission in one study).[8] On this basis, it is recommended that all partners within 60 days should be evaluated and treated. If the last act of sexual intercourse occurred more than 60 days prior to the appearance of symptoms

Table 90   Chlamydia Treatment*

Strategy	Drug	Dosage
1st Line	**Azithromycin**	1 gm PO × 1*
Alternative	**Doxycycline**	100 mg PO BID × 7d
2nd Line	**Erythromycin**	500 mg PO QID × 7d*
	Ofloxacin	300 mg PO BID × 7d
	Levofloxacin	500 mg PO OD × 7d
	Amoxicillin	500 mg PO TID × 7d*

*Likely safe in pregnancy and lactation

or diagnosis, the most recent sexual partner should be treated.[1,2] Reinfection with *Chlamydia* most often occurs when partners are not treated, or when the patient resumes sexual activity within a network of individuals with a high prevalence of infection. Repeat infection can substantially increase the risk of PID and other complications; health care providers should consider rescreening all women with chlamydial infection 3 to 4 months after treatment.[1] It should be noted that rescreening is distinct from early retesting to detect therapeutic failure (test of cure). As with gonorrhea, a test of cure is not recommended in the asymptomatic non-pregnant patient unless reinfection is suspected.

Prevention and Control of Gonorrhea and Chlamydia (STIs) in high risk groups

The Canadian STD Guidelines state that asymptomatic patients *most* at risk for contracting an STI include: men and women who have had two or more partners in the last six months, a history of STIs, a history of sex without a condom, and men who have sex with men. More broadly, all sexually active adults under 25 years of age are at risk of STIs and should therefore be considered for screening.[2] Both the Canadian and U.S. Task Forces on Preventive Health Services recommend screening all sexually active females younger than 25 years of age for *Chlamydia* and counselling all adolescents and adults about STD prevention.[9,10] How well are we doing? A recent survey in *Canadian Family Physician* showed that out of 805 family doctors, only 20% to 40% reported routinely asking about sexual risk behaviours during an annual physical exam.[11] There are wide discrepancies in what individuals mean by "having sex." In one survey, 59% of male and female college students from the Midwest did not consider oral-genital contact to be "having sex."[12] Risk assessments and preventive counselling must be very specific. Counselling seems to be most effective when it is individualized to the patient's specific personal risk and focuses on harm reduction strategies as opposed to abstinence.[13] Partner notification is vital to controlling the spread of STIs. Approaches to contact tracing vary from region to region, but ultimately depend on the patient disclosing his or her partners. The healthcare provider should raise the issue in a non-judgemental way and assure the patient that tracing will be handled in a confidential manner. The local Department of Public Health is a key resource in this regard.

Syphilis

Syphilis is rare in North America but recently there have been outbreaks in a number of communities. Toronto has experienced a tenfold increase in the number of syphilis cases in the last few years (30 cases in 2001 and 308 cases in 2003). This trend is also seen in other parts of Canada, the United States, and Europe. The vast majority of cases involve men, and in particular, men who have sex with men. This raises a concern around the potential increase in HIV, because approximately 30% of men with infectious syphilis are also HIV-positive.[14] Intramuscular Penicillin G (2.4 million IU) remains the standard treatment for primary, secondary, and latent infections of less than 1 year duration. In Penicillin-allergic patients doxycyline (100 mg orally twice daily) for 14 days or tetracycline (500 mg orally four times per day) for 14 days can be used as alternatives. Preliminary studies suggest that Azithromycin (2 g oral one-time dose) may also be effective.[1]

─────────── ≈ **REFERENCES** ≈ ───────────

1. CDC: Sexually transmitted diseases treatment guidelines 2002, *MMWR* 51(No. RR-6), 2002.
2. LCDC Expert Working Group on Canadian Guidelines for Sexually Transmitted Diseases: Canadian STD guidelines, Ottawa, 1998. Avilable at http://www.hc-sc.gc.ca/hpb/lcdc/publicat/std98/index.html.
3. CDC: *Sexually transmitted disease surveillance 2002 supplement: gonococcal isolate surveillance project (GISP) annual report 2002*, Atlanta, GA: U.S. Department of Health and Human Services, CDC, 2003.
4. Young H, et al: PCR testing of genital and urine specimens compared with culture for the diagnosis of chlamydial infection in men and women, *Int J STDs AIDS* 9(11):661-5, 1998.
5. National goals for the prevention and control of sexually transmitted diseases in Canada, *Canada Communicable Diseases Report* 23:S6, 1997.
6. Joffe A: Amplified DNA testing for sexually transmitted diseases: new opportunities and new questions, *Arch Pediatr Adolesc Med* 153:111-113, 1999 (editorial).
7. Shafer MB: Annual pelvic examination in the sexually active adolescent female: what are we doing and why are we doing it? *J Adolesc Health* 23:68-73, 1998.
8. Quinn TC, Gaydos C, Shepherd M, et al: Epidemiologic and microbiologic correlates of Chlamydia trachomatis infection in sexual partnerships, *JAMA* 276:1737-1742, 1996.
9. Davies HD, Wang EE (Canadian task Force on the Periodic Health Examination): Periodic Health Examination 1996 update. 2. Screening for chlamydial infection, *CMAJ* 154:1631-1644, 1996.
10. U.S. Preventive Services Task Force: *Guide to clinical preventive services,* ed 2, Baltimore, 1996, Williams & Wilkins, pp 325-334.
11. Haley N, et al: Lifestyle health risk assessment. Do recently trained family physicians do it better? *Can Fam Physician* 46:1609-16, 2000.
12. Sanders SA, Reinisch JM: Would you say you "had sex" if . . .? *JAMA* 281:275-77, 1999.
13. Kamb ML, Fishbein M, Douglas JM, et al: Efficacy of risk-reduction counseling to prevent immunodeficiency virus and sexually transmitted diseases: a randomized controlled trial, *JAMA* 280:1161-1167, 1998.
14. Toronto Public Health: *Bulletin on the incidence of infectious syphilis in Toronto.* Toronto, April 1, 2004.

VAGINITIS

(See also drugs and chemicals in pregnancy; inflammatory Papanicolaou smears; pelvic inflammatory disease)

The differential diagnosis of vaginitis should include lichen sclerosus, atrophy, and lichen simplex chronicus. Furthermore, potential causes of allergic or irritant dermatitis should be sought. However, it is thought that up to 90% of cases are secondary to bacterial vaginosis, candidiasis, and trichomonas.[1] When the etiology is infectious, symptoms may occur from the disruption of normal vaginal flora and resultant depletion of lactobacillus. Common errors in the diagnosis and management of vaginitis include not obtaining a vaginal specimen and failing to perform a speculum exam to rule out cervicitis.[2]

Bacterial Vaginosis

Bacterial vaginosis (BV) is currently the most common cause of vaginitis. BV is polymicrobial. Some of the implicated organisms include *Gardnerella vaginalis, Mycoplasma hominis,* and anaerobes.[1] Many women remain asymptomatic, in which case treatment is usually not necessary. One should consider screening and treating all positive results in women who are undergoing cesarean section, first trimester abortion, and hysterectomy.[3] Whether or not to identify and treat pregnant women with BV has long been an area of controversy. A recent Cochrane review (2004) states that the current evidence does not support screening and treating all pregnant women with asymptomatic BV to prevent preterm delivery. However, treating women with a previous history of preterm birth may reduce the risk of preterm premature rupture of membranes and low birthweight.[4] Treatment options are summarized in Table 91. There is no evidence that BV is an STD and treating partners is not recommended.[1]

Candidiasis

Candida is present in the vaginas of a quarter of all women. Many of these women will be asymptomatic

Table 91   Vaginitis Treatment

Strategy	BV	Candida	Trichomonas
1st Line	Metronidazole* 500 mg PO BID × 7d	*Intravaginal Preparations:*[†] -Clotrimazole - Miconazole *Oral Therapy:* Fluconazole 150 mg PO × 1	Metronidazole* 2 gm PO × 1
Alternatives	Clindamycin 2% cream 5 g intra-vaginally OD × 7d Clindamycin 300 mg PO BID × 7d	Gentian violet 1-2% aqueous solution apply q 3 to 4 days[‡] Boric Acid 600 mg gel capsule OD PV × 10 to 14d[§]	Metronidazole 500mg PO BID × 7d

*Although traditionally avoided in pregnant women, according to Motherisk, metronidazole has *not* been shown to be harmful in pregnancy.[2,3]
[†]These include ovules and creams and come as 1, 3, and 7d preparations.
[‡]Irritation may result if more than three applications are used.
[§]Highly effective in resistant infection, particularly when the etiologic agent is not *C. albicans.*

and, therefore, require no treatment. For those that do experience symptoms of vaginal discharge or irritation many treatment options exist (see Table 91). Partners need not be treated unless *Candida balanitis* is present.[5] If a patient is experiencing recurrent bouts of vulvovaginal candidiasis (defined as three or more episodes within a year), underlying causes should be sought. These may include uncontrolled diabetes, antibiotic use, and immunosuppression. In the majority of women, no predisposing conditions are found.[2] Treatment for such patients may include a trial of oral fluconazole (100 or 150 mg per week or per month) as prophylaxis.[5] If the patient provides a history of antibiotic use that always precipitates a yeast infection, a 3-day course of an intravaginal preparation or a single oral dose of fluconazole (150 mg orally) may be given near or at the end of the antibiotic course. There is some evidence to support the notion that yogurt containing *Lactobacillus acidophilus* may be helpful in preventing yeast infections.[6] Boric acid (300 mg) in gelatin capsules used vaginally once daily for 14 days followed by use for 5 days during the menstrual period has been shown to have comparable effectiveness to long-term monthly use of oral antifungal agents in women with recurrent vulvovaginal candidiasis.[7]

Trichomoniasis

This is the only known STI to cause vulvovaginitis. Symptoms often include copious discharge, which is frothy and yellow, pruritis, and dyspareunia. Up to half of infected individuals may be asymptomatic but should be identified because they are at risk for other STDs, including HIV. Patients *and* their partners should be treated (see Table 91).

━━━━━━━━━━━━━━━   **⋟ REFERENCES ⋞**   ━━━━━━━━━━━━━━━

1. Egan ME, Lipsky MS: Diagnosis of Vaginitis, *Am Fam Physician* 62:1095-104, 2000.
2. LCDC Expert Working Group on Canadian Guidelines for Sexually Transmitted Diseases: Canadian STD Guidelines, Ottawa, 1998. Available at http://www.hc-sc.gc.ca/hpb/lcdc/publicat/std98/index.html.
3. Society of Obstetricians and Gynaecologists of Canada: Clinical practice guidelines: committee opinion; bacterial vaginosis, *J SOGC* 19(5):528-533, 1997.
4. McDonald H, et al: Antibiotics for treating bacterial vaginosis in pregnancy (Cochrane Review), In *The Cochrane Library*, Issue 2, 2004, Chichester, 2004, Wiley & Sons.
5. CDC: Sexually transmitted diseases treatment guidelines 2002, *MMWR* 51(No. RR-6), 2002.
6. Hilton E, Isenberg HD, Alperstein P, et al: Ingestion of yogurt containing *Lactobacillus acidophilus* as prophylaxis for candidal vaginitis, *Ann Intern Med* 116:353-357, 1992.
7. Guaschino S, et al: Efficacy of maintenance therapy with topical boric acid in comparison with oral itraconazole in the treatment of recurrent vulvovaginal candidiasis, *Am J Obstet Gyencol* 184:598-602, 2001.

Topics covered in this section

Pregnancy
Disorders of Pregnancy
Episiotomy
Postpartum Depression

PREGNANCY
Pre-Pregnancy Planning

Health care providers should discuss a woman's thoughts about becoming pregnant during routine periodic health assessments. Important topics to cover are nutrition, supplementation with folic acid, substance use, and violence and abuse. All women in the preconception and early prenatal periods should receive supplements containing 0.4 to 0.8 mg of folic acid to prevent neural tube defects.[1-3] The Society of Obstetricians and Gynecologists of Canada (SOGC) also recommends that women in intermediate- to high-risk categories take 4 to 5 mg daily.[3] This is most easily done by prescribing a daily multivitamin containing adequate quantities of folic acid (see section on congenital anomalies for more information). Ask for a history of rubella and varicella infection or immunization. Titres can be checked if unsure and immunizations given preconception if needed, or postpartum if already pregnant. If a patient and her partner belong to an ethnic group whose members may carry genes for a testable genetic condition, then referral for testing is advised (i.e., Tay-Sachs, sickle cell disease). Any chronic health conditions (diabetes, asthma, hypertension, depression) should be optimized. Motherisk is a good source of information regarding the safety of medications in pregnancy.[4]

⇗ REFERENCES ⇖

1. Canadian Task Force on the Periodic Health Examination: *Canadian guide to clinical preventive health care*, Ottawa, 1994, Canada Communication Group Publishing, pp 74-81.
2. U.S. Preventive Services Task Force: *Guide to clinical preventive services,* ed 2, Baltimore, 1996, Williams & Wilkins, pp 467-483.
3. Wilson RD, et al: The use of folic acid for the prevention of neural tube defects and other congenital anomalies, *J Obstetr Gynaecol Can* 25:959-965, 2003.
4. www.motherisk.org. Accessed May 23, 2005. Motherisk. Drugs in pregnancy. [Accessed May 23, 2005] Available from: URL: http://www.motherisk.org/drugs/index.php

Prenatal Genetic Screening
Introduction

Three percent of all newborns in Canada are born with some type of congenital anomaly. Congenital anomalies are the leading cause of infant death in Canada. The birth of a child with a severe congenital anomaly represents a personal tragedy for the child and the child's family. Many of these conditions are treatable; others are not. They carry with them social, financial, and psychological burdens.[1] The scope of prenatal genetic screening has in recent years been expanded greatly by the introduction of a large number of non-invasive tests including ultrasound and serum markers. Primary care providers are now expected to provide basic counselling prior to offering prenatal testing and to be familiar with new screening and diagnostic techniques so that all options can be discussed at the appropriate time.

To determine whether there is an indication for prenatal testing, an assessment should include the medical and obstetric history of the woman as well as specific inquiry regarding ethnic background and family history in both partners for possible genetic disorders.

Counselling should be comprehensive, non-directive, in a language understood by the patient, and should include a discussion of the following:
- Available methods of prenatal diagnosis
- Risks and benefits of various techniques
- Timing of diagnostic prenatal procedures
- The conditions for which genetic testing is to be considered and current management of relevant genetic disorders
- Accuracy of prenatal results
- The option of abortion as an outcome and the patient's opinions of that option. Screening may not be indicated in cases where the woman does not want to consider pregnancy termination.

Referral to a genetic centre along with the appropriate information for in-depth counselling should be offered in cases where special genetic assessment or invasive testing is necessary.

Screening for chromosome abnormalities
Abnormalities of Chromosome Number (Aneuploidy). The most common abnormality in chromosome number is Down Syndrome (trisomy 21). The overall risk of this occurrence is 1 to 2 in 1000 in developed countries,[2] but varies according to maternal age from approximately 1 in 1500 at age 20 to 1 to 129 at age 40.[3] The second most common is trisomy 18. The risk of this is much lower (1 to 2 in 10,000) and is not age related.

The methods available for screening for these disorders have become complex, involving age, serum markers, ultrasound findings, and computer algorithms to calculate risks for the multimarker profile thus generated. The choice of the test parameters is influenced by the perceived relative importance of the detection rate and the positive rate (the number of pregnancies referred for further testing). The interpretation of findings can be affected by maternal disease (e.g., diabetes), by multiple gestation pregnancies, and by incorrect gestational age. The chance of the fetus being affected given that the result of the test is positive depends on the prior risk of those screened. Screening does not aim to make a diagnosis, but rather to ration the use of diagnostic procedures that would be too hazardous (amniocentesis, CVS, cordocentesis) and tests that would be too expensive to offer without prior selection.

Table 92 lists some of the most commonly used screening tests[4] together with the detection rate and the rate of positive tests.

A positive test indicates those who should be referred for invasive testing and is reported in the format of a risk ratio, which is dependent on the pretest likelihood of the disorder in that particular patient. The cut-off ratio is related to the risk of the diagnostic procedure. A risk reported as 1/200 means that of 200 women tested 1 will have an affected child (true positive test), and 199 will have a normal child (false positive test). The risk of miscarriage due to amniocentesis is 0.5% to 1.0% (i.e., 1 in 100 to 200).

Screening for Down syndrome should be offered to all pregnant women regardless of age ("B" recommendation, 1996; Canadian Task Force on Preventive Health Care[5] and U.S. Preventive Services Task Force[6]).

Diagnostic testing for these conditions should be offered to women at increased risk ("B" recommendation, 1994 CTFPHC). This includes the following[7]:
- Women with a positive test
- Women who will be age 35 or older at delivery

- Family history:
  a. Previous stillbirth or live birth with a chromosomal abnormality
  b. Parent with a potentially transmissible chromosome rearrangement
  c. Relatives (other than offspring) with Down syndrome or other trisomy
  d. Genetic disorders with an identifiable chromosomal marker or abnormality
  e. Carriers and affected individuals of some X-linked disorders
  f. Paternal history of therapeutic radiation
  g. Fetal anomalies detected on ultrasound

Available diagnostic tests[8]

1. *Amniocentesis.* Amniocentesis is an ultrasound-guided removal of amniotic fluid performed at 15 to 17 weeks gestation for determination of fetal karyotype, molecular and biochemical abnormalities. This test will accurately predict almost 100% of these disorders. Three to four weeks are required for results. Risk of miscarriage is an additional 0.5% to 1% above background risk of 3%, risk of infection 1 to 2 in 3000 procedures, and risk of amniotic fluid leakage, bleeding, or uterine irritability of 1% to 5%.
2. *Chorionic Villus Sampling (CVS).* CVS is an ultrasound-guided sampling of placental tissue performed at 10 to 12 weeks gestational age for the same indications as amniocentesis. Both transcervical

Table 92   Common Screening Options

Method	Components	Detection of Down Syndrome		Detection of NTD	
		Detection Rate	Positive Rate	Detection rate	Positive Rate
First trimester Screening FTS 12 weeks	NT*† Serum HCG Serum PAPP-A	About 90%	About 5%	50%	Less than 1%
Second Trimester Screening MSS 16-18 weeks	a. HCG Estriol AFP	About 75%	About 8%	80%	Less than 2%
	b. with inhibin	About 75%	About 6%	80%	Less than 2%
Integrated Screening IPS 12 weeks	a. NT PAPP-A hCG AFP Estriol	About 90%	About 4%	90%	Less than 2%
16 weeks	b. with inhibin	About 90%	About 4%	90%	Less than 2%

Adapted from Milunsky A, editor: *Genetic disorders and the fetus: diagnosis, prevention, and treatment,* ed 5, 2004, Johns Hopkins University Press, chapter 22. Reprinted with the permission of the Johns Hopkins University Press.
FTS, First Trimester Screening; *hCG,* human chorionic gonadotrophin; *MSS,* second trimester maternal serum screening; *AFP,* alpha-fetoprotein; *IPS,* integrated prenatal screening; *PAPP-A,* pregnancy-associated plasma protein.
*NT is ultrasound measurement of swelling at the back of baby's neck at 11 to 14 weeks gestational age. The normal range is less than 3 mm. The measurements must be done by designated radiologists who have been certified. Abnormal NT has been associated with aneuploidy (trisomy 21, 18, 13), congential heart disease, syndromes, diaphragmatic hernia and other defects.
†Nasal Bone calcification rates using ultrasound shows promise as an additional marker, but is not yet in use in screening programs.

and transabdominal techniques are available. The major advantage is that earlier sampling affords earlier availability of results. The main disadvantages are less accuracy due to mosaicism in the placenta or maternal contamination in the sample, and greater risk of miscarriage (1% to 2% for transabdominal and 3% to 6% for transcervical methods above background risk of 5%). In addition there may be a risk of limb or facial anomalies. Hence it is only offered when the risk of congenital problems is greater than the risk of the procedure and earlier diagnosis is imperative.

3. *Cordocentesis.* This is used for both diagnostic testing and treatment using direct fetal blood sampling.

Abnormalities of Specific Genes, Microdeletion, and Microduplication Syndromes. Many biochemical and DNA tests are now available to identify these abnormalities in a fetus. One example of such testing is FISH (fluorescence in situ hybridization). This test is a DNA probe for specific abnormalities. Recurrence risks for affected patients or for the parents of an affected child depend on the specific syndrome. Such patients should be referred for genetic counselling.

Neural tube defects

Neural tube defects (NTDs) are severe birth anomalies due to lack of neural tube closure at either the upper or lower end in the third to fourth week after conception (days 26 to 28 post-conception). They occur in Canada at a rate of approximately 1 to 2 in 1000 live births, and the rate varies with geographical location and ethnic background. They are associated with many syndromes and other congenital conditions. The spectrum of NTDs includes anencephaly (40%), spina bifida (50%),[9] encephalocoele, and multiple vertebral defects.

Pregnancies at increased risk for NTDs include[10]:

- Previously affected child—recurrence risk 2% to 5%
- First-, second-, or third-degree relative with NTD
- Women with type 1 diabetes mellitus
- Women with epilepsy taking valproic acid or carbamazepine
- Women taking folic acid antagonists aminopterin on methotrexate

Prevention of Neural Tube Defects[8]. Over a decade ago, large randomized trials in Britain demonstrated that periconception supplementation with folic acid alone or in combination with multivitamins reduced the incidence of NTDs in newborn infants. More recently there is growing epidemiological and research evidence that nutritional status and vitamin intake including folic acid have an impact in reducing congenital cardiac defects, specifically conotruncal defects, urinary tract anomalies, limb defects and orofacial cleft defects.

Folate is a general term for both the native form of the B vitamin occurring in food and the synthetic form, folic acid, which is found in supplements and fortified foods. Humans are unable to synthesize folate and are dependent on dietary sources.[1] The average daily diet contains 0.2 mg per day.

Since 1998, enriched cereal-grain products (e.g., breads, pasta, rice) produced in Canada and the United States have been supplemented to contain 0.14 mg to 0.2 mg folic acid per 100 gm. This adds 0.1 mg to dietary sources for a total of 0.3 mg per day. Most prenatal vitamins contain 1.0 mg. Supplementation with folic acid has been shown in several subsequent studies to reduce the incidence of NTDs[1] (recommendation by CTFPHC and USPSTF).

Guidelines for Folic Acid Supplementation. Supplementation should begin after discontinuation of reliable birth control (or at least 2 to 4 weeks prior to conception) and continue until 10 to 12 weeks after the last menstrual period.

- To prevent primary occurrence in low-risk pregnancies; 0.4 mg per day (risk decreases by 40% to 85%)
- To prevent recurrence or occurrence in high-risk women; 4.0 mg per day (risk reduced by 72% for women with previously affected child)

Folate supplementation in later pregnancy may also be beneficial. Studies are underway to determine if optimal levels will reduce pre-eclampsia, fetal growth restriction, and intrauterine fetal death, perhaps through regulation of homocysteine levels.

Screening for NTDs[1,11,12]

Maternal serum alpha-fetoprotein (MSAFP) is elevated in the second trimester (16 to 18 weeks) in pregnancies affected by open neural tube defects. It detects 85% to 90% of NTDs; when combined with second trimester fetal ultrasound screening, the detection rates for anencephaly and spina bifida are 100% and 95%, respectively. The most difficult NTDs to detect are either small or covered with skin. In these cases, the reliability of ultrasound and MSAFP is significantly decreased (see Table 92). ("B" recommendation by both CTFPHC and USPSTF.)

Carrier screening[7]

Screening for heterozygote or carrier state is recommended for individuals and their partners belonging to population groups known to have an increased risk (greater than 3% to 4%) for carrying certain genetic disorders. Ideally, testing and counselling should be done prior to pregnancy; otherwise prenatal testing should be offered. The most common of these abnormalities are listed here:

1. **Tay-Sachs Disease:** The carrier frequency is 1 in 30 among Ashkenazi Jews, and 1 in 14 among French Canadians in Eastern Quebec. The carrier state can be detected by measuring hexosaminidase A

activity. Other common diseases carried in the Ashkenazi population for which the carrier state can be detected are Canavan disease and familial dysautonomia. In some labs ordering "Ashkenazi Screen" will initiate testing for all three.

2. **Hemoglobinopathies:** Adult hemoglobin is made up of two alpha- and two beta-globin chains. Mutations for hemoglobinopathies are common in people whose ancestors came from areas where malaria is endemic, including Africa, the Mediterranean basin, the Middle East, the Indian subcontinent, Southeast Asia, and southern China.

3. **Thalassemia** is caused by mutations in either the alpha- or the beta-globin chains. If both partners are carriers, and the fetus is homozygous, severe hydrops can occur in the fetus (α-thalassemia) or severe anemia in the child (β-thalassemia). Women pregnant with these fetuses are at risk for serious maternal complications. An at-risk pregnant woman with an MCV greater than 80 fL and a normal ferritin should undergo hemoglobin electrophoresis. B thalassemia is diagnosed by elevated HbA2 and Hb F. α-Thalassemia can be diagnosed by a preparation for Hb H inclusion bodies or DNA testing.

4. **Sickle Cell Disease** is caused by a specific mutation of the beta-globin gene resulting in Hb S. Carriers are asymptomatic; however, homozygosity causes severe disease including septicemia, strokes in childhood, and vaso-occlusive crises causing multiple organ damage in adults. Carrier frequency is 1 in 12 in people of black African origin. Hemoglobin electrophoresis is the diagnostic test of choice as this population is also at risk for thalassemia.

5. **Cystic Fibrosis:** Carrier frequency in Caucasians is 1 in 20. DNA testing is available for relatives of cystic fibrosis patients and their partners. Carrier testing should also be offered to both parents of a fetus with an ultrasound finding of echogenic bowel, also taking into consideration their ethnic background. This requires referral to a genetics center.

❧ REFERENCES ❧

1. Preconception Health: *Folic acid for the primary prevention of neural tube defects*, Health Canada, 2002
2. Cuckle HS, Arbuzova S. Multimarker maternal serum screening for chromosomal abnormalities, chapter 22. In: Milunsky A, editor: *Genetic disorders and the fetus:diagnosis, prevention and treatment,* ed 5, Baltimore, 2004, Johns Hopkins University Press, PR Wyatt North York General Hospital (table).
3. Cuckle HS, Wald NJ, Thompson SG: Estimating a woman's risk of having a pregnancy associated with Down Syndrome using her age and serum alpha-fetoprotein level, *Br J Obstet Gynaecol* 94:387-346, 1987.
4. Cuckle H, Arbuzova S: Multi-marker maternal serum screening for chromosomal abnormalities. In: Milunsky A, editor: *Genetic disorders and the fetus: diagnosis, prevention, and treatment,* ed 5, chapter 22, Baltimore, 2004, Johns Hopkins University Press
5. Canadian Task Force on Preventive Health Care: www. ctfphc.org. Accessed May 23, 2005.Dick PT, Canadian Task Force on Preventive Health Care. Periodic health examination, 1996 update: 1. Prenatal screening for and diagnosis of Down syndrome. [Accessed May 23, 2005] Available from: URL: http://ctfphc.org/
6. U.S. Preventive Services Task Force: www.ahrq.gov/ clinic/uspstfix.htm. Accessed May 23, 2005. U.S. Preventive Services Task Force. Screening: down syndrome. 1996 [Accessed May 23, 2005] Available from: URL: http://www. ahrq.gov/clinic/uspstf/uspsdown.htm
7. Chodirker BN, Cadrin C, Davies G: Canadian guidelines for prenatal diagnosis, *J Obstet Gynaecol Can* 23(6):525-531, 2001.
8. Chodirker BN, Cadrin C, Davies G: Canadian guidelines for prenatal diagnosis, *J Obstet Gynaecol Can* 23(7):616-624, 2001.
9. McDonald S, Ferguson S, Tam L: The prevention of congenital anomalies with periconceptual folic acid supplementation, *J Obstet Gynaecol Can* 25(2):115-121, 2003.
10. Wilson D: The use of folic acid for the prevention of neural tube defects and other congenital anomalies, *J Obstet Gynaecol Can* 25(2):959-965, 203.
11. Cadrin C, Harman R: The use of ultrasound in conjunction with maternal serum screening for aneuploidy, *SOGC Clinical Practice Guidelines*, No. 17, 1997.
12. Johnson J, Summers A: Prenatal genetic screening for Down syndrome and open neural tube defects using maternal serum marker screening, *SOGC Clinical Practice Guidelines*, No.79, 1999.

Risk Assessment in Pregnancy

(See also attitudes, physician; prevention; risk analysis)

Many pregnancy risk assessment protocols have been developed. On the basis of these, 16% to 55% of pregnancies are labelled high risk, yet half of perinatal mortality and morbidity occur in "low-risk" pregnancies.[1-3] One thoughtful analyst of this subject concluded that pregnancy risk scoring has not been proved to do more good than harm.[1] Klein[4] speculated that categorizing women as being at high risk is in itself a factor leading to increased consultations and interventions and asked whether risk scoring may not actually make women sick.

❧ REFERENCES ❧

1. Hall PF: Rethinking risk, *Can Fam Physician* 40:1239-1244, 1994 (editorial).
2. Wall EM: Assessing obstetric risk: a review of obstetric risk-scoring systems, *J Fam Pract* 27:153-163, 1988.
3. Hall PF: Obstetric risk scoring: a Trojan horse, *Manitoba Med* 63:43-45, 1993.

4. Klein M: Family physician maternity care: outcomes when family physicians provide most community-based care, *Can Fam Physician* 41:546-548, 1995 (editorial).

Antenatal Care

(See also relevant topics in this section that pertain to counselling and screening throughout pregnancy)

Physicians who do not practice obstetrics will have patients who are pregnant or who want to become pregnant, and the physician should be able to give them some basic counselling.

Diagnosis of pregnancy

Signs and symptoms of pregnancy include absence of expected menses, breast tenderness and fullness, fatigue, nausea, and urinary frequency. Biochemical diagnosis of pregnancy is by detection of the beta subunit of human chorionic gonadotropin (hCG) in urine or blood. When tested in a clinical laboratory, the sensitivity and specificity for both blood and urine pregnancy tests are between 97% and 100%.[1] However, the sensitivity falls to 75% when patients test their urine at home.[2] False-negative tests are usually the result of testing too soon after ovulation.

A standard schedule of visits is as follows:

Frequency of Visits
Initial visit   8-10 weeks
Weeks 10-28   Every 4 weeks
Weeks 28-36   Every 2 weeks
Week 36-term   Every week

The minimum number of required visits and the interval between visits have not been determined,[3-5] and the frequency of prenatal visits should be based upon patient needs.

Initial visit

The initial visit comprises a complete history, physical examination, appropriate laboratory investigations, and counselling.

History. The history should include personal and demographic information, menstrual history, past obstetrical history, history of current pregnancy (bleeding, vomiting, substance use, exposure to radiation, history of infertility, occupational and environmental hazards), personal history including history of infection, family medical history, genetic history (age greater than 35 at time of delivery, family history of genetic anomalies), and availability of social supports.

Traditionally, an obstetrical risk assessment is done to help determine how a particular patient will be managed and by what provider. This is controversial. The development of pregnancy risk protocols has led to the labelling of 16% to 55% of pregnancies as high risk, yet half of the perinatal morbidity and mortality occurs in "low-risk"

pregnancies.[6-8] Risk assessments have not been proven to benefit the mother or fetus,[6] and the labelling is in itself a factor leading to increased consultations and perhaps unnecessary interventions.[9]

An estimated date of delivery can be calculated from the date of the last menstrual period by adding 7 days and then subtracting 3 months in women with 28-day cycles. Women with longer or shorter cycles should have their dates adjusted accordingly because it affects interventions for post-date pregnancies.

Physical Examination. The physical examination involves a general physical examination including weight, blood pressure, and examination of systems including a speculum and bimanual exam to assess the size of the uterus and the pelvic architecture.

Laboratory Investigations

Routine: The usual laboratory investigations are a complete blood count, ABO/Rh typing and antibody screen, rubella titre, syphilis screen, hepatitis B surface antigen, HIV counselling, and testing. Additional tests may be advised in certain populations, for example, hemoglobin electrophoresis for sickle cell and thalassemia in patients at risk.

Other initial tests: Although practice may vary, most care providers tend to routinely obtain a Papanicolaou (Pap) smear depending on past results and when the last Pap smear was done. Cervical cultures for gonorrhea and *Chlamydia* also tend to be routinely done. Currently, there are no guidelines to support these routine screens.

Urinalysis is obtained, although this practice is being questioned because the urine dipsticks that detect nitrites and leukocyte esterases are relatively insensitive and will miss 25% of cases of asymptomatic bacteriuria (ASB) in pregnant women.[10] In addition, the conventional urine dipstick test is unreliable in detecting glycosuria and the proteinuria of pre-eclampsia.[5] Urine cultures in asymptomatic pregnant women should be obtained between 12 and 16 weeks. This will identify 80% of women who will ultimately have ASB in pregnancy.[11] ASB occurs in 2% to 7% of pregnant women.[12] Detection and treatment of ASB reduce complications including acute pyelonephritis, preterm delivery, and low birth weight, which will develop in 25% to 30% of those affected. There are inadequate data to determine the optimal frequency of urine testing during pregnancy.

Counselling. Important points to cover in counselling include HIV screening, genetic screening, nausea and vomiting during pregnancy, avoidance of smoking and secondhand smoke, risks of alcohol and drug use in pregnancy, and the need to eat a balanced diet. Asking about prior varicella infection is also advised.[5] This type of counselling is best given before the patient becomes pregnant, and advice at the first prenatal visit should function as a reinforcement of what has already been said. Whether routine iron supplementation is indicated is uncertain, and both the Canadian Task Force on

Preventive Health Care[13] and the U.S. Preventive Services Task Force[14] give this a "C" recommendation. Patients, especially primiparous women, should be offered referral to prenatal classes.

Follow-up visits

Routine pregnancy monitoring includes weight, blood pressure, urinalysis, fetal activity and heart rate at each visit. Fetal heart rate can be heard at 9 to 12 weeks, although it may be difficult to hear at this early gestational age. It is now recommended that assessment for psychosocial issues during pregnancy be a standard of obstetrical care. Wilson and colleagues[15] identified 15 antenatal factors that are strongly associated with poor postpartum outcomes. Outcomes include child abuse, woman abuse, couple dysfunction, postpartum depression, and increased infant physical illness. The Antenatal Psychosocial Health Assessment (ALPHA) Form was developed to guide health care providers in the assessment of these associated factors.[16]

Uterine growth in pregnancy

The uterus has the features below at various stages of pregnancy:

Weeks	Uterine Size
6	Normal
8	Globular; slightly enlarged
12	Symphysis
20	Just below umbilicus
20-38	Ht/cm=weeks of pregnancy

Nutrition and weight gain

All pregnant women should be encouraged to eat a well-balanced diet following the guidelines recommended by respective national resources. Recommended weight gain in pregnancy for women of normal weight is 11 to 16 kg (25 to 35 lb). Underweight women should gain about 16 to 18 kg (35 to 40 lb) and obese women about 7 to 11 kg (15 to 25 lb). For normal weight women the rate of gain should be about 1.3 to 2.3 kg (3 to 5 lb) per month in the first trimester and 0.5 to 1.0 kg (1 to 2 lb) per week during the second and third trimesters.[18] Feig and Naylor[19] advise a minimal weight gain of 6.8 kg (15 lb), and for women with a normal body mass index a maximum weight gain of 11.4 kg (25 lb).[19] Monitoring maternal weight gain is unlikely to detect women who will have SGA infants or develop hypertension.[20]

Quickening

Quickening takes place at approximately 16 weeks for multiparas and at approximately 20 weeks for primiparas.

Vaginal bleeding

About one fifth of pregnant women have vaginal bleeding during the first 20 weeks of pregnancy, and about half of these go on to spontaneous abortion. In one study women who had spontaneous abortions were not at increased risk of abortion in subsequent pregnancies.[21] Recurrent spontaneous abortions, defined as three consecutive miscarriages, should be considered abnormal and referred for investigation.

Bedrest

In the United States, prescription of bedrest is almost the norm for a variety of complications of pregnancy, such as hypertension, incompetent cervix, premature labour, premature rupture of the membranes, placenta previa, and even twin pregnancies. No randomized controlled trials supporting this intervention have been published. Since bedrest is known to be associated with physical deconditioning and a variety of detrimental psychosocial effects, bedrest for these conditions may do more harm than good (see discussion of bedrest complications).[22]

❧ REFERENCES ❧

1. O'Connor RE, et al: The comparative sensitivity and specificity of serum an during HCG determinations in the ED, *Am J Emerg Med* 11:434, 1993 (letter).
2. Bastian LA, et al: Diagnostic efficiency of home pregnancy test kits: a meta-analysis, *Arch Fam Med* 7:465, 1998.
3. McDuffie RS, et al: Effect of frequency of prenatal care visits on perinatal outcome among low-risk women: a randomized controlled trial, *JAMA* 275:847, 1996.
4. www.nice.org.uk. Accessed May 23, 2005. (See Clinical guidelines→Completed guidelines and cancer service guidance→ Antenatal Care: Routine Care for the Healthy Pregnant Woman). National Institute for Clinical Excellence. Antenatal care: routine care for the healthy pregnant woman, October 2003 [Accessed May 23, 2005] Available from: URL: http://www.nice.org.uk/page.aspx?o=89893
5. www.icsi.org. Accessed May 23, 2005. (See Healthcare guidelines→Prenatal Care, Routine). Akkerman D, Kreider J, Jefferies JA, et al. Routine prenatal care [Health care guideline, Institute for Clinical Systems Improvement (ICSI)] ed 8, July 2004 [Accessed May 23, 2005] Available from: URL: http://www.icsi.org/knowledge/detail.asp?catID=29&itemID=191
6. Hall PF: Rethinking the risk, *Can Fam Physician* 40:1239-1244, 1994 (editorial).
7. Wall EM: Assessing obstetric risk: a review of obstetric risk-scoring systems, *J Fam Pract* 27:153-163, 1988.
8. Hall PF: Obstetric risk scoring: a Trojan horse, *Manitoba Med* 63:43-5, 1993.
9. Klein M: Family physician maternity care: outcomes when family physicians provide most community-based care, *Can Fam Physician* 41:546-548, 1995 (editorial).
10. Tincello DG, Richmond DH: Evaluation of bleeding before the 20th week of pregnancy: prospective study from general practice, *BMJ* 316:435-437, 1997.

11. Stenqvist K, Dahlen-Nilsson I, et al: Bacteriuria in pregnancy: frequency and risk of acquisition, *Am J Epidemiol* 129:372-379, 1989.

12. Bachman JW, et al: A study of various tests to detect asymptomatic urinary tract infections in an obstetric population, *JAMA* 270:1971-1974, 1993.

13. Canadian Task Force on the Periodic Health Examination: *Canadian guide to clinical preventive health care,* Ottawa, 1994, Canada Communication Group, pp 64-72.

14. U.S. Preventive Services Task Force: *Guide to clinical preventive services,* ed 2, Baltimore, 1996, Williams & Wilkins, pp 231-246.

15. Wilson LM, Reid AJ, Midmer DK, et al: Antenatal psychosocial risk factors associated with adverse postpartum outcomes, *CMAJ* 154(6):785-799, 1996.

16. Midmer D , Biringer A, Carroll JC, et al: *A reference guide for providers: the ALPHA form—antenatal psychosocial health assessment form,* ed 2, Toronto, 1996, University of Toronto Faculty of Medicine, Department of Family and Community Medicine.

17. Reference deleted in pages.

18. Kolasa K, Weismiller DG: Nutrition during pregnancy, *Am Fam Physician* 56:205-212, 1997.

19. Feig D, Naylor D: Eating for two: are guidelines for weight gain during pregnancy too liberal? *Lancet* 351:1054-1055, 1998.

20. Dawes MG, Grudzinskas JG: Patterns of maternal weight gain in pregnancy, *Brit J Obstet Gynecol* 98:195-201, 1991.

21. Everett C: Incidence and outcome of bleeding before the 20th week of pregnancy: prospective study from general practice, *BMJ* 315:32-34, 1997.

22. Maloni JA, Cohen AW, Kane JH: Prescription of activity restriction to treat high-risk pregnancies, *J Women's Health* 7:351-358, 1998.

Exposures in Pregnancy

(See also alopecia; breastfeeding; hypertensive disorders of pregnancy; nausea and vomiting in pregnancy)

Acid-suppressing drugs

H_2 blockers do not appear to be teratogenic with exposure during the first trimester. The best-studied drug in this class is ranitidine (Zantac). There is no evidence for adverse effects on pregnancy outcomes or neonatal health. Few studies have been done with proton pump inhibitors, but so far no evidence has been found that omeprazole (Prilosec, Losec) is associated with an increased risk of malformations.[1]

Misoprostol (Cytotec and one of the drugs in Arthrotec) should not be used because of an increased risk of Möbius syndrome (congenital facial paralysis).[2,3]

────────────── **⬩ REFERENCES ⬩** ──────────────

1. Lalkin A, Magee L, Addis A, et al: Motherisk update: acid-suppressing drugs during pregnancy, *Can Fam Physician* 43:1923-1924, 1997.

2. Koren G, Pastuszak A, Ito S: Drugs in pregnancy, *N Engl J Med* 338:1128-1137, 1998.

3. Pastusazak AL, Schüler L, Speck-Martins CE, et al: Use of misoprostol during pregnancy and Möbius syndrome in infants, *N Engl J Med* 338:1881-1885, 1998.

Alcohol

(See also attention deficit disorder; conduct disorder)

The safe level of alcohol consumption during pregnancy has not been defined and, thus, abstinence from alcohol use in pregnancy is recommended. An estimated 25% of all pregnant Canadians have some exposure to alcohol before realizing they had conceived. Two meta-analyses failed to show any adverse effects after mild social drinking (up to several drinks a week).[1] Similarly, moderate alcohol consumption before realizing that conception had occurred showed no increased risk of spontaneous abortion, stillbirth, or premature birth.[2]

However, alcohol is a documented teratogen with a spectrum of recognized defects with heavy daily drinking. Fetal alcohol syndrome (FAS) has been described as the most severe effect due to antenatal alcohol exposure. Characteristics of FAS include evidence of growth retardation, CNS abnormalities, and a characteristic pattern of facial anomalies (short palpebral fissures and abnormalities in the pre-maxillary zone).[3] Full expression of FAS has been demonstrated with chronic ingestion of at least 2 g/kg/day which is the equivalent of eight 1 oz alcohol containing drinks or eight beers.[1] The estimated incidence of FAS in the general population in Canada is between 0.5 and 3 per 1000 live births. This rate increases to 4% to 5% in heavy drinkers. Fetal alcohol spectrum disorder (FASD) refers to the wide range of adverse fetal effects of ethanol including milder and more subtle cognitive and behavioural problems.[1] The estimated incidence of FASD is 10 cases per 1000 live births with these conditions occurring in 30% to 40% of children of heavy drinkers.[1,3]

Binge drinking is defined as a minimum of five drinks per single occasion and represents a common pattern of drinking among Canadian women. In a study conducted by Motherisk, the vast majority of women reported one to three binge drinking episodes prior to finding out about their pregnancies. Results showed that temperament was different among children of women who engaged in six or more binges during pregnancy, including increased willingness to approach unknowns and increased risk-taking behaviours.[4] Cognitive outcomes and developmental milestones were unaffected by this exposure to alcohol.

The risk of drinking alcohol during breastfeeding has not been well established. Alcohol does pass into breastmilk, with infants being exposed only to a fraction of the amount ingested by the mother. Occasional drinking while nursing has not been shown to cause any overt harm to infants. In contrast, regular high doses of alcohol (greater than six drinks) during breastfeeding can affect milk flow as well as lead to impaired motor development, disturbed sleep-wake patterns, and decreased breastmilk intake, possibly explained by differences in taste and smell of breastmilk.[5] Given that a safe level of alcohol in breastmilk has not been determined, women may want to abstain from exposing their infants to alcohol in breastmilk.

❧ REFERENCES ❧

1. Koren G, Nulman I, Chudley AE, et al: Fetal alcohol spectrum disorder, *CMAJ* 169(11):1181-1185, 2001.
2. Makarechian N, Agro K, Devlin J, et al: Association between moderate alcohol consumption during pregnancy and spontaneous abortion, stillbirth and premature birth: a meta-analysis, *Can J Clin Pharmacol* 5(3):169-176, 1998.
3. Clarke M: Understanding FAS: a practical approach to prevention, diagnosis and management, *Can J CME* 13(10):67-83, 2001.
4. Nulman, I., Kennedy D, Rover J, et al: Neurodevelopment of children exposed in utero to maternal binge alcohol consumption: a prospective, controlled study, *The Motherisk Newsletter* 12:2-3, 2000.
5. Koren G: Drinking alcohol while breastfeeding: Will it harm my baby? *Can Fam Physician* 48:39-41, 2002.

Analgesics and non-steroidal anti-inflammatory drugs (NSAIDs)

The analgesic drugs of choice in pregnancy are acetaminophen and opioids, both of which are believed to be non-teratogenic.[1]

Opioids. Morphine, codeine, oxycodone, and hydromorphone belong to the opioid class, which is known for its analgesic properties. Opioids have not been associated with any minor or major congenital malformations. Heroin is an illicit opioid that has a high prevalence of dependence. Opioid dependence during pregnancy has been associated with adverse fetal outcomes due to withdrawal. It can trigger uterine contractions leading to spontaneous abortion in the first trimester, premature labour in the third trimester, and fetal distress and stillbirth at the time of delivery.[1,2] Opioid-dependent women tend to also have pregnancies complicated by intrauterine growth retardation due to the effect of the drug itself, as well as secondary to poor nutrition and inadequate prenatal care.[2] Detoxification from opioids is generally not recommended during pregnancy due to risk of spontaneous abortion.

Methadone maintenance treatment is the standard of care for opioid dependence in pregnancy. Methadone is a long-acting opioid with a half-life of 24 to 36 hours and women on methadone are less likely to experience withdrawal symptoms. As a result, methadone-maintained pregnancies tend to experience lower rates of prematurity, higher birth-weight infants, and lower infant mortality.[3,4] Methadone has not been reported to increase

congenital defects. The main risk of methadone in pregnancy is a neonatal abstinence syndrome (NAS).[2] NAS requires admission to a nursery for observation. Approximately 60% to 80% of infants experience NAS, yet few develop significant symptoms requiring morphine treatment. NAS symptoms may include irritability, sleep disturbances, sweating, diarrhea, and feeding difficulties. Severe untreated withdrawal can lead to seizures and death. No long-term consequences have been demonstrated with methadone use during pregnancy.

NSAIDs. Low-dose Aspirin (less than 3 g per day) and NSAID use is not associated with an increased risk of congenital birth defects, prematurity, or low birth weight.[5] However, there is a significant link between NSAID use and miscarriage in the first trimester.[6] It is unclear if this association is due to underlying disease. NSAIDs should not be used in the latter half of pregnancy, particularly in the third trimester, because of an increased risk of early constriction or closure of the fetal ductus arteriosus, persistent fetal pulmonary hypertension, intracranial hemorrhages, and renal toxicity in the fetus.[7,8]

❧ REFERENCES ❧

1. Behnke M, Davis EF: The consequences of prenatal substance use for the developing fetus, newborn, and young child, *Int J Addict* 28(13):1341-1391, 1993.
2. Kaltenbach K, Finnegan L: Opioid Dependence during Pregnancy: effects and management, *Obstet Gynecol Clin North Am* 25(1):139-151, 1998.
3. Chang GC, Behr HM, Kosten TR: Improving treatment outcome in pregnant opiate-dependent women, *J Subs Abuse Treat* 9:327-330, 1992.
4. Kandall SR, Jantunen M, Stein J: The methadone-maintained pregnancy, *Clin Perinatol* 26(1):173-183, 1999.
5. CLASP (Collaborative Low-dose Aspirin Study in Pregnancy) Collaborative Group: CLASP: a randomized trial of low-dose aspirin for the prevention and treatment of pre-eclampsia among 9364 pregnant women, *Lancet* 343(8898):619-629, 1994.
6. Nielsen Gl, Sorensen HT, Larsen H, et al: Risk of adverse birth outcome and miscarriage in pregnant users of nonsteroidal anti-inflammatory drugs: population-based observation study and case-control study, *BMJ* 322(7281):266-270, 2001.
7. Janssen NM, Genta MS: The effects of immunosuppressive and anti-inflammatory medications on fertility, pregnancy and lactation, *Arch Intern Med* 160(5):610-619, 2000.
8. Alano MA, Ngougmna E, Ostrea EM Jr, et al: Analysis of nonsteroidal anti-inflammatory drugs in meconium and its relation to persistent pulmonary hypertension of the newborn, *Pediatrics* 107(3):519-523, 2001.

Antibacterials agents

Beta-lactams (Penicillin and its Derivatives) Extensive use of these agents during pregnancy has demonstrated no adverse effects on the fetus or on infants.[1]

Cephalosporins are structurally related to penicillins and are produced synthetically. These antibiotics have broader spectrum of activity. Similarly, these antibiotics have not been found to cause any major birth defects.[2]

Macrolides. Macrolides include many forms of erythromycin, clarithromycin (Biaxin), and azithromycin (Zithromax). Erythromycin estolate is contraindicated in pregnancy because of drug-related hepatotoxicity. Two forms currently recommended in pregnancy include erythromycin base (E-Mycin) and erythromycin ethylsuccinate (EES).[1]

Metronidazole. There is no evidence that using metronidazole during pregnancy increases the rate of major birth defects.[3,4] The use of metronidazole during breastfeeding has not demonstrated any adverse effects on infants.[3]

Quinolones. Quinolones such as norfloxacin (Noroxin), ofloxacin (Floxin), and ciprofloxacin (Cipro) are contraindicated in children because they have been shown to cause arthropathy in the weight-bearing joints of immature animals. However, they have not been shown to cause birth defects in the limited studies that have been done in humans.[2,5,6] Fluoroquinolones are contraindicated in pregnancy and while breastfeeding because of this potential adverse effect.

Sulfonamides. Trimethoprim-sulfonamide (TMP-SMX) combinations are commonly used to treat urinary tract infections in women. Numerous studies have documented the increased risk of major malformations such as neural tube defects and cardiovascular defects associated with the use of TMP-SMX in early pregnancy because of their interference with folic acid synthesis.[7-9] In the latter part of pregnancy, sulfonamides should be avoided after 32 weeks gestation due to the potential of developing kernicterus. Acute hemolytic anemia could occur in newborns with glucose-6-phosphate dehydrogenase deficiency.[7]

Tetracyclines. All of the tetracyclines are contraindicated in pregnancy. Exposure to tetracyclines at 5 to 6 months in utero will result in staining of teeth and inhibition of bone growth.[1,2]

◁ REFERENCES ◮

1. Valerie R: Antimicrobial agents: pharmacology and clinical application in obstetric, gynecologic, and perinatal infections, *J Obstet Gynecol Neonatal Nurs* 28(6):639-648, 1999.
2. Duff, P: Antibiotic selection in obstetrics: making cost-effective choices, *Clin Obstet Gynecol* 45(1):59-72, 2002.
3. Einarson A, Ho E, Koren G: Can we use metronidazole during pregnancy and breastfeeding? Putting an end to the controversy, *Can Fam Physician* 46:1053-1054, 2000.
4. Burtin P, Taddio A, Ariburnu O, et al: Fetus-placenta-newborn: safety of metronidazole in pregnancy: a meta-analysis, *Am J Obstet Gynecol* 172(2):525-529, 1995.
5. Giamarellou H, Kolokythas E, Petrikkos G, et al: Pharmacokinetics of three newer quinolones in pregnant and lactating women, *JAMA* 87(5A):49S-51S, 1989.
6. Berkovitch M, Pastuszak A, Gazarian M, et al: Safety of the new quinolones in pregnancy, *Obstet Gynecol* 84(4):535-538, 1994.
7. Sivojelezova A, Einarson A, Shuhaiber S, et al: Trimethoprim-sulfonamide combination therapy in early pregnancy, *Can Fam Physician* 49:1085-1086, 2003.
8. Hernandez-Dias S, Werler MM, Walker AM, et al: Neural tube defects in relation to use of folic acid antagonists during pregnancy, *Am J Epidemiol* 153(10):961-968, 2001.
9. Czeisel A, Rockenbaer M, et al: The teratogenic risk of trimethoprim-sulfonamides: a population based case-control study, *Reprod Toxicol* 15:637-646, 2001.

Antiviral agents

Acyclovir. Acyclovir (Zovirax) is not approved for use in pregnant women, but no evidence has shown that it is teratogenic.[1]

◁ REFERENCES ◮

1. Drugs for sexually transmitted diseases, *Med Lett* 37:117-122, 1995.

Anticonvulsants in pregnancy
(See also seizures)

Pregnant patients with seizure disorders have an increased risk of having an infant with major congenital anomalies. The overall risk of birth defects in untreated patients is 4%, and in treated patients it is between 5% and 10% compared with a rate of 2% in the general population.[1] This risk increases with the number of antiepileptic drugs; with one antiepileptic medication, the rate is 3% but increases to 5% with two, 10% with three, and 20% with four.[2,3] A common syndrome resulting from a variety of antiepileptic drugs such as phenytoin (Dilantin), carbamazepine (Tegretol), and valproic acid (Depakene, Depakote) consists of facial dimorphism, cleft lip, cleft palate, cardiac defects, hypoplasia of the digits, and nail dysplasia.[2,3] Patients taking carbamazepine and valproic acid have an increased risk of neural tube defects. These patients should be given 4 or 5 mg of folic acid daily before and after conception, even though no studies evaluating the efficacy of such a protocol have been published.[1,4]

Antiepileptic drugs can cause a transient deficiency in vitamin K-dependent clotting factors in the neonate, with increased risk of intracerebral hemorrhage. Women should be given 10 mg of vitamin K daily during the last four weeks of pregnancy.[1,2]

Neonatal consequences of maternal valproic acid use include withdrawal symptoms (irritability, jitteriness, abnormal tone, and feeding difficulties), hyperbilirubinemia, hepatotoxicity, and intrauterine growth retardation.[4] Phenytoin is also associated with an increased risk of developmental delays such as lower intelligent quotients (IQ) and lower language development scores.[5,6]

✍ REFERENCES ✍

1. Bruni J: Examining epilepsy in pregnancy, *Canadian Journal of Diagnosis* 17(8):57-61, Aug 2000.
2. Brodie MJ, Dichter MA: Antiepileptic drugs, *N Engl J Med* 334:168-175, 1996.
3. Samrén EB, van Duijn CM, Christiaens GC, et al: Antiepileptic drug regimens and major congenital abnormalities in the offspring, *Ann Neurol* 46:739-746, 1999.
4. Koren G: Safe use of valproic acid during pregnancy, *Can Fam Physician* 45:1451-1453, 1999.
5. Koren G: In utero exposure to phenytoin or carbamazepine, *Can Fam Physician* 41:1862-1863, 1995.
6. Scolnik D, Nulman I, Rovet J, et al: Neurodevelopment of children exposed in utero to phenytoin and carbamazepine monotherapy, *JAMA* 271:767-770, 1994.

Antihistamines

Allergies occur in 20% to 30% of women of childbearing age with rhinitis being the most common diagnosis. Rhinitis may indirectly affect sleep, eating, and emotional stability. Plasma histamine levels are lower in the first trimester so allergy attacks are less likely to happen. First generation antihistamines (chlorpheniramine, diphenhydramine) may cause maternal sedation and anticholinergic effects. Second generation antihistamines such as cetirizine (Allegra), fexofenadine (Zyrtec), and loratadine (Claritin) have limited fetal safety data.[1,2] A 1997 meta-analysis of over 200,000 women who were exposed to a variety of antihistamines in the first trimester of pregnancy not only found no increase in the risk of congenital anomalies, but documented a slight decrease in risk. Possibly the use of antihistamines to control nausea and vomiting in pregnancy actually improves fetal outcomes.[3]

✍ REFERENCES ✍

1. Mazzotta P, Loebstein R, Koren G: Treating allergic rhinitis in pregnancy: safety considerations, *Drug Safety* 20(4):361-375, 1999.
2. Peggs JF, Shimp SA, Opdycke RAC: Antihistamines: the old and the new, *Am Fam Physician* 52:593-600, 1995.
3. Koren G: Antihistamines are safe during the first trimester, *Can Fam Physician* 43:33-34, 1997.

Antihypertensives

Antihypertensives are discussed in the section on hypertensive disorders of pregnancy.

Asthma medications

None of the common asthma medications, including β_2-adrenergic agonists, inhaled and oral steroids, cromolyn, and theophylline, have been shown to be teratogenic.[1,2] In one study, asthmatic patients taking oral steroids had a slightly increased incidence of pre-eclampsia,[2] but since severe asthma is associated with maternal and fetal mortality, the benefits outweigh the risks.[1,2] Unfortunately, pregnant women with acute asthma exacerbations are less likely than non-pregnant women to receive oral corticosteroids during emergency room visits and are more likely to have continuing exacerbations. Pregnancy is an indication, not a contraindication, for prescribing oral corticosteroids during an asthmatic exacerbation.[3]

✍ REFERENCES ✍

1. Bailey B, Addis A: Motherisk update: asthma during pregnancy, *Can Fam Physician* 43:1717-1718, 1997.
2. Schatz M, Zeiger RS, Harden K, et al: The safety of asthma and allergy medications during pregnancy, *J Allergy Clin Immunol* 100:301-306, 1997.
3. Cydulka RK, Emerman CL, Schreiber D, et al: Acute asthma among pregnant women presenting to the emergency department, *Am J Respir Crit Care Med* 160:887-892, 1999.

Caffeine

Caffeine metabolism changes during pregnancy with substantial delays in clearance during the second and third trimester.[1] The normal half-life of caffeine extends from a level of 2.5 to 4.5 hours to 19.5 hours later on in the pregnancy. Caffeine has also been demonstrated to cross the placenta and human fetuses have low levels of the enzymes needed to metabolize caffeine. However, the exact mechanism for causing adverse effects has not been elucidated. A meta-analysis conducted by Motherisk showed a small, statistically significant increase in the risk of spontaneous abortion and low birth weight babies in pregnant women consuming greater than 150 mg of caffeine per day (the equivalent of six cups of coffee daily).[1] Women should be counselled to maintain intake from all caffeine sources below 150 mg daily.

✍ REFERENCES ✍

1. Koren, G: Caffeine during pregnancy? In moderation, *Can Fam Physician* 46:801-803, 2000.

Chemicals

Aspartame,[1] cosmetics,[2] and hair care products[3] have not been reported to cause adverse effects in pregnancy. Pregnant women should not be exposed to mercury. Occupational exposure to mercury is increased in the amalgamation and paint production industries and in dentistry. The main dietary source is contaminated fish and seafood.[4] Organic solvents are teratogenic in experimental animals. A meta-analysis of five studies concluded that exposure to organic solvents during pregnancy increased the risk of major malformation (odds ratio 1 to 64),[5] but according to one prospective study, the increase was seen predominantly in women who reported symptoms from their exposure to solvents.[6]

⋧ REFERENCES ⋦

1. Zuber C, Librizzi RJ, Bolognese RJ: Do aspartame and video display terminals pose pregnancy risks? *Postgrad Obstet Gynecol* 9:1-5, 1989.
2. Zuber C, Hom M, Vought L, et al: Common chemical exposures in pregnancy: cosmetics, paint fumes, and cold medications, *Postgrad Obstet Gynecol* 12:1-6, 1992.
3. Koren G: Hair care during pregnancy, *Can Fam Physician* 42:625-626, 1996.
4. Moienafshari R, Bar-Oz B, Koren G: Occupational exposure to mercury: what is a safe level? *Can Fam Physician* 45:43-45, 1999.
5. McMartin KI, Koren G: Exposure to organic solvents: does it adversely affect pregnancy? *Can Fam Physician* 45:1671-1673, 1999.
6. Khattak S, K-Moghtader G, McMartin K, et al: Pregnancy outcome following gestational exposure to organic solvents: a prospective controlled study, *JAMA* 281:1106-1109, 1999.

Dermatological medications

Isotretinoin (Accutane) is teratogenic and strictly contraindicated for women who are or might become pregnant during therapy and in the month following discontinuation of the therapy.[1] Retinoic acid embryopathy includes central nervous system, cardiac, craniofacial, and thymic malformations. A Pregnancy Prevention Program for isotretinoin strongly suggests simultaneous use of two forms of contraception to reduce the likelihood of fetal exposure.[1] A small series found no adverse effects to the fetus when women used topical tretinoin during pregnancy.[2]

Retinoids are also used in the treatment of psoriasis, which occurs in 1% to 3% of the population. Oral retinoids such as etretinate (Tegison) are associated with teragenicity.[3] Topical retinoids such as tazarotene (Tazorac) avoid many of the systemic side effects; however, it may be teratogenic, so women of child-bearing age should use birth control.

⋧ REFERENCES ⋦

1. Atanackovic G, Koren G: Young women taking isotretinoin still conceive: role of physicians in preventing disaster, *Can Fam Physician* 45:289-292, 1999.
2. Shapiro L, Pastuszak A, Curto G, et al: Is topical tretinoin safe during the first trimester? *Can Fam Physician* 44:495-498, 1998.

3. Federman DG, Froelich CW, Kirsner RS: Topical psoriasis therapy, *Am Fam Physician* 59:957-962, 1999.

Dextromethorphan

Dextromethorphan use in the first trimester has not shown an increase in the rate of birth defects above the 1% to 3% baseline rate.[1]

⋧ REFERENCES ⋦

1. Einarson A, Koren G: Dextromethorphan, *Can Fam Physician* 45:2309-2310, 1999.

Psychiatric Medications

Antidepressants. Many women of childbearing age are treated for depression and require ongoing therapy during their pregnancies and into the postpartum period. Untreated depression during pregnancy has been associated with worsening of symptomatology, compromised maternal-fetal health, and impaired bonding and child care in the postpartum period.[1]

SSRIs are lipid soluble, cross into the placenta, and are excreted into breastmilk. This class of medications include fluoxetine (Prozac), sertraline (Zoloft), paroxetine (Paxil), and fluvoxamine (Luvox). Several controlled studies have studied the safety of SSRIs, especially fluoxetine (Prozac), during pregnancy and lactation. The evidence revealed no increased risk of major malformations, spontaneous abortion, stillbirth, prematurity, or low birth weight with the use of any of these medications.[2] Neonatal withdrawal syndrome has been reported repeatedly with late-trimester use of fluoxetine, sertraline, and paroxetine. These short-term symptoms include restlessness, sleep problems, and feeding problems. Therefore, it is recommended to reduce drug dosage prior to delivery in an attempt to decrease withdrawal symptoms in newborns.[1] There have also been no long-term neurobehavioural effects of in utero exposure to SSRIs.[3,4] Pregnant women who request to discontinue antidepressants should be advised about the risks of stopping their medications. This includes mood relapse with a high rate of suicidal ideation resulting in admission to the hospital. Women may also experience discontinuation symptoms if their medications are stopped abruptly.[5] Physicians should counsel women about these risks and conduct a slow taper if women opt for having a "drug-free" pregnancy.

Newer antidepressants (venlafaxine, nefazodone, bupropion) have also been studied by Motherisk. Results demonstrate no difference for several endpoints, including spontaneous abortions and major malformations.[6] This evidence supports the view that benefits of pharmacological treatment outweigh the risks of no treatment for depression in pregnancy and in the postpartum period.

Some women are still being treated with tricyclic anti-depressants (TCA) for their depressive symptoms. Similar to SSRIs, there is no evidence of teratogenicity with use of TCAs and there is no increase in the incidence of major malformations, intrauterine death, or miscarriage. However, the use of TCAs late in pregnancy is also associated with neonatal withdrawal symptoms at delivery that consist of irritability, rapid breathing, tremor, and high-pitch cry.[7] These symptoms appear to be dose-dependent and resolve within one week. No long-term effects have been noted with the use of TCAs during pregnancy.

❧ REFERENCES ❧

1. Misri S, Kostaras D: Are SSRIs safe for pregnant and breastfeeding women? *Can Fam Physician* 46:626-633, 2000.
2. Misri S, Kostaras D: The use of selective serotonin reuptake inhibitors in pregnancy and lactation: a review, *J SOGC* 21(2):120-125, 1999.
3. Nulman I, et al: Neurodevelopement of children exposed in utero to antidepressant drugs, *N Engl J Med* 336:258-262, 1997.
4. Kulin NA, Pastuszak A, Sage SR, et al: Pregnancy outcome following maternal use of the new selective serotonin reuptake inhibitors: a prospective controlled multicenter study, *JAMA* 279:609-610, 1998.
5. Einarson A, Selby P: Abrupt discontinuation of psychotropic drugs during pregnancy: fear of teratogenic risk and impact of counselling, *J Psychiatry Neurosci* 26(1):44-48, 2000.
6. Einarson A, Koren G: New antidepressants in pregnancy, *Can Fam Physician* 50:227-229, 2004.
7. Craig M, Abel K: Prescribing for psychiatric disorders in pregnancy and lactation, *Best Pract Res Clin Obstet Gynaecol* 15(6):1013-1030, 2001.

Antipsychotics. Recent literature reports that women with schizophrenia are at increased risk for poor obstetrical outcomes including preterm delivery, low birth weight, and infants that are small for gestational age. These results may be due to various factors such as alcohol and drug use and low socio-economic status.[1]

No antipsychotics have been approved for use during pregnancy and lactation. The risks of infant exposure must be balanced against the risks of untreated maternal psychosis. The use of typical antipsychotics during pregnancy has been associated with an increased risk of congenital abnormalities, neonatal toxicity, and long-term neurobehavioural problems.[2] The risk of congenital malformations is increased with exposure to low-potency phenothiazines during weeks 4 to 10 of gestation. No such effect has been documented with high-potency typical antipsychotics such as haloperidol and trifluoperizine.[2,3] There have also been case reports of extra-pyramidal side effects in newborns who had in utero exposure. Symptoms vary from excessive crying, motor restlessness, tremor, difficulty feeding, and hypertonicity. Findings from rat studies have also raised concern about possible long-term neurobehavioural effects. However, there are no human data available at the present time.[2]

Exposure to typical antipsychotic medication can also occur via breast milk. Levels of these medications have been measured at less than 1% of the maternal daily dosage. Infants followed for up to 1 year showed no abnormalities.[1]

There is limited information regarding the safety of atypical antipsychotics during pregnancy and lactation. Current case reports have found no evidence of increased congenital abnormalities. One case report cautioned regarding the risk of neonatal seizure with the use of clozapine in pregnancy.[2,3]

❧ REFERENCES ❧

1. Patton SW, Misri S, Corral MR, et al: Antipsychotic medication during pregnancy and lactation in women with schizophrenia: evaluating the risk, *Can J Psychiatry* 47(10):959-965, 2002.
2. Niki G: Psychopharmacology in pregnancy, *J Perinat Neonatal Nurs* 14(4):12-25, 2001.
3. Craig M, Abel K: Prescribing for psychiatric disorders in pregnancy and lactation, *Best Pract Res Clin Obstet Gynaecol* 15(6):1013-1030, 2001.

Benzodiazepines. There have been conflicting reports about the teratogenic effects of benzodiazepines with respect to increased risk of cleft palate or cleft lip when taken during pregnancy. A recent analysis of the literature found that pooled data from cohort studies showed no relationship between first trimester benzodiazepine use and facial clefts, whereas case control studies found a small but significant increase in both facial clefts and other major malformations.[1] If women are concerned about this risk, level II ultrasonography can be used to detect this abnormality.

❧ REFERENCES ❧

1. Dolovich LR, Addis A, Vaillancourt JM, et al: Benzodiazepine use in pregnancy and major malformations or oral cleft: meta-analysis of cohort and case-control studies, *BMJ* 317:839-843, 1998.

Lithium. Lithium exposure during the first trimester of pregnancy leads to abnormalities involving the great vessels and heart. The incidence of Ebstein anomaly is increased in patients taking lithium in the first trimester. Although the relative risk is increased tenfold to twentyfold, the condition is rare; the absolute risk is about 1 in 1000 or 0.1%.[1] Pregnant women should consider a fetal echocardiogram in addition to a level II ultrasound to rule out cardiac anomalies.

Use of lithium later in pregnancy can lead to lithium toxicity in the newborn. Presenting symptoms and signs may include cyanosis, hypotonia, bradycardia, thyroid depression with goiter, atrial flutter, cardiomegaly, hepatomegaly, and diabetes insipidus. These toxic effects disappear within 1 to 2 weeks upon renal excretion of this medication.[1,2]

REFERENCES

1. Altshuler LL, Cohen L, Szuba MP, et al: Pharmacologic management of psychiatric illness during pregnancy; dilemmas and guidelines, *Am J Psychiatry* 153:592-606, 1996.
2. Jacobson S, et al: Prospective multicentre study of pregnancy outcome after lithium exposure during first trimester, *Lancet* 339(8792):530-533, 1992.

Vitamin A supplements in pregnancy
(See also vitamin A)

In one study, the odds ratio of having a child with a congenital anomaly was 4.8 for women taking vitamin A supplements of 10,000 IU or more compared with those taking 5000 IU or less. Among women taking more than 10,000 units, about 1 in 57 had a baby with congenital malformation attributable to the vitamin. These data do not apply to β-carotene.

Smoking in pregnancy
(See also poverty)

Smoking throughout pregnancy occurs in 25% to 30% of pregnancies.[1] Approximately 80% of women try to quit or reduce smoking during pregnancy with only 23% of women maintaining their cessation over the course of the pregnancy. An additional 17% reduce by more than 5 cigarettes per day.[2] Overall, most smokers continue during pregnancy. Nicotine is not teratogenic and does not increase the risk of congenital anomalies; however, there are numerous adverse fetal and neonatal effects.

The major detrimental effects of smoking during pregnancy range from increased risk of spontaneous abortion in the first trimester to increased likelihood of prematurity and decreased birth weight in the final trimester.[3] The physiological effect of tobacco on fetal growth is a result of vasoconstrictive effects of nicotine on the uterine and umbilical arteries and the deleterious reduction of oxygen in red blood cells caused by carboxyhemoglobin.[4] Use of nicotine during the first trimester reduces a woman's ability to become pregnant in dose-dependent fashion and contributes to higher rates for early, as well as late fetal loss. Women have one and a half times greater risk of spontaneous abortion if smoking 1 to 10 cigarettes per day.[2] The incidence of low birth weight (less than 2500 g) also increases with increased cigarette consumption in a dose-dependent manner. The average birth weight of infants exposed to nicotine may be 100 to 320 g less than normal.[4] There is a 20% increase in the overall perinatal mortality rate if the mother smokes more than 20 cigarettes per day.[2] This increased rate is due to a higher incidence of abruptio placentae, placenta previa, and premature rupture of membranes in smoking mothers, as well as intrauterine growth retardation.[3]

Maternal cigarette smoking has also been shown to affect child development. However, these studies have confounding factors such as socio-economic class, parental education, and passive smoking. Correlations have been observed between smoking in pregnancy and adverse behavioural problems such as attention deficit disorder.[4] Children exposed during the prenatal period to nicotine scored lower in two subcategories of expressive language and conceptual comprehension. Although the risks of nicotine replacement therapy (NRT) during pregnancy remain unclear, the benefits outweigh the risks for pregnant women who are heavy smokers (20 cigarettes daily) and for whom all behavioural interventions have failed.[5] Thus, the nicotine patch and gum are considered safer than smoking for the pregnant woman and her fetus.

The risk of relapse to smoking is high in the postpartum period. Among women who quit smoking during pregnancy, over 60% start smoking again by 6 months postpartum. If the mother smokes fewer than 20 cigarettes a day, the risk to the baby from the nicotine in breastmilk is small. However, the risk increases above this. Smoking can decrease the quantity and quality of breastmilk by 30% and lead to feeding difficulty. Overall, the risks of not breastfeeding are greater to the baby than the risks of breastfeeding and smoking. NRT can be considered for breastfeeding women since these products pose no more problems for the breastfeeding infant than maternal smoking.[2]

Passive smoke exposure has also shown several neonatal effects such as a 2 to 5 times higher risk of sudden infant death syndrome. In addition, children of smokers have a higher risk of developing asthma, allergies, bronchitis, pneumonia, and ear infections.[6]

REFERENCES

1. Koren G: Nicotine replacement therapy during pregnancy, *Can Fam Physician* 47:1971-1972, 2001.
2. www.pregnets.com. Accessed May 23, 2005. Pregnets. Common questions. [Accessed May 23, 2005] Available from: URL: http://www.pregnets.org/mothers/questions.cfm

3. Benowitz N: Nicotine replacement therapy during pregnancy, *JAMA* 266(22):3174-3177, 1991.

4. Lambers D, Clark KE: The maternal and fetal physiologic effects of nicotine, *Seminars in Perinatology* 20(2):115-126, 1996.

5. Scalera A, Koren G: Rationale for treating pregnant smokers with nicotine patches, *Can Fam Physician* 44:1601-1603, 1998.

6. www.motherisk.org. Accessed May 23, 2005. Motherisk. Cigarette smoke and pregnancy. [Accessed May 23, 2005] Available from: URL: http://www.motherisk.org/alcohol/smoke.php3

Cocaine use in pregnancy

A Canadian study estimated the rate of cocaine exposure during pregnancy at 6%.[1] Cocaine use in pregnancy has been associated with serious fetal and neonatal health hazards including intrauterine growth retardation, placental abruption, prematurity, stillbirth, and perinatal complications.[1,2] Women using cocaine also tend to smoke more cigarettes and are more likely to experience vaginal bleeding, urinary tract infections, and test positive for hepatitis B.[3] Babies exposed in utero to cocaine also required more medical interventions at the time of delivery.[1] Cocaine has also been linked to increased motor tone and trouble settling in the neonatal period. This in turn leads to concerns about the negative effects of these neonatal behaviours on maternal-infant bonding and on caregiving abilities, especially in substance-abusing families.[4]

Despite evidence for the effect of cocaine on birth size, controversies remain regarding the persistence of these growth deficits into childhood. Several long-term studies have documented some developmental delays in cocaine-exposed babies, particularly in the area of language.[5,6] Behaviour problems have also been identified at school age especially in boys.[7] These findings persisted even after control for other exposures during pregnancy and social and home environment factors.

---------------- ◙ **REFERENCES** ◖ ----------------

1. Forman R, Klein J: Fetal exposure to cocaine in Toronto: an epidemic, *The Motherisk Newsletter* 3:1-4, 1994.

2. Eyler F, et al: Birth outcome from a prospective, matched study of prenatal crack/cocaine use: I. Interactive and dose effects on health and growth, *Pediatrics* 101(2):229-237, 1998.

3. Koren G: Cocaine use by pregnant women in Toronto, *Can Fam Physician* 42:1677-1679, 1996.

4. Eyler F, et al: Birth outcome from a prospective, matched study of prenatal crack/cocaine use: II. Interactive and dose effects on neurobehavioral assessment, *Pediatrics* 101(2):237-241, 1998.

5. Delaney-Black V, et al: Expressive language development of children exposed to cocaine prenatally: literature review and

report of a prospective cohort study, *J Commun Disord* 33(6):463-480, 2000.

6. Nulman I, et al: Neurodevelopment of adopted children exposed in utero to cocaine: the Toronto Adoption Study, *Clin Invest Med* 24(3):129-137, 2001.

7. Delaney-Black V, et al: Teacher-assessed behavior of children prenatally exposed to cocaine, *Pediatrics* 106(4):782-791, 2000.

Marijuana use in pregnancy

Prenatal marijuana exposure is prevalent especially during the first trimester with a significant number of women continuing to use marijuana throughout the entire pregnancy.[1] THC (delta-9-tetrahydrocannabinol) is the psychoactive component of marijuana and crosses the placenta, resulting in prolonged fetal exposure with regular maternal use.[1] The effects of marijuana exposure remain equivocal with not all findings replicated consistently among studies due to confounding factors such as polysubstance use and home environments.

Marijuana use has not been linked to adverse pregnancy outcomes in terms of maternal effects; however, the length of gestation may be affected especially among heavy users.[1] So far, studies are conflicted on the effect of marijuana on birth parameters such as weight, height, or head circumference. Marijuana has not been found to be teratogenic.[2]

THC is found in breastmilk and has been linked to delay in motor development of infants at one year of age.[3] Therefore, abstinence from marijuana is recommended while breastfeeding.

There is a good evidence for the effects of marijuana on neurobehavioural characteristics of the newborn. Neonates demonstrated increased tremors, exaggerated startles to minimal or no stimuli, and persistent "jitteriness" and decreased total quiet sleep at 1 month of age.

Subsequent development can also be affected by prenatal marijuana exposure. Early development and language development differences were not noted despite the fact that women who used marijuana prenatally tended to be less well-educated, of lower social class, more likely to use other substances, and less involved with their children at 24 months.[1] However, at 3 years of age, children had sleep disturbances with lower sleep efficiency and maintenance and more awake time after sleep onset.[4] A difference in child behaviour was also found at 10 years of age, with significantly increased hyperactivity, inattention, impulsivity, and delinquency among exposed children.[5]

---------------- ◙ **REFERENCES** ◖ ----------------

1. Day NL, Richardson GA: Prenatal marijuana use: epidemiology, methodologic issues and infant outcome, *Clinics in Perinatology* 18(1):77-91, 1991.

2. Kozer E, Koren G: Effects of prenatal exposure to marijuana, *Can Fam Physician* 47:263-264, 2001.
3. Astley S, Little R: Maternal marijuana use during lactation and infant development at one year, *Neurotoxicol Teratol* 12:161-168, 1990.
4. Dahl R, et al: A longitudinal study of prenatal marijuana use. Effects on sleep and arousal at age 3 years, *Arch Pediatr Adolesc Med* 149(2):145-150, 1995.
5. Goldschmidt L, Day NL, Richardson GA: Effects of prenatal marijuana exposure on child behavior problems at age 10, *Neurotoxicol Teratol* 22:325-336, 2000.

Rave drugs in pregnancy

There is a paucity of data on the effects of prenatal ecstasy exposure. The use of ecstasy during pregnancy has demonstrated no teratogenic effect, with the risk of congenital anomalies remaining at 1% to 3%.[1]

----------- ◢ REFERENCES ◣ -----------

1. McElhatton P, Bateman DN, Pughe KR, et al: Congenital anomalies after prenatal ecstasy exposure, *Lancet* 354:1441-1442, 1999.

Exercise and Pregnancy

Research literature supports the prescription of exercise during pregnancy as an effective tool for improving general emotional well-being, maintaining optimal weight, and controlling blood glucose.[1,2] The Par-Med X is a validated screening tool to assess readiness for physical activity and screen for contraindications while providing current exercise education.[3] This tool is available at www.csep.ca.

Exercise prescription

Physically active women are recommended to continue their exercise regimens in the first trimester provided that they have been on a stable exercise program for the previous 3 months and that they are not participating in a high-risk sport such as scuba diving, unpredictable contact, or altitude sports. Sedentary women and those with medical or obstetrical complications must be medically evaluated and cleared before embarking on a low-impact exercise program no earlier than the second trimester. An exercise regimen should be conducted at a frequency of 3 to 5 times per week at moderate intensity for 30 to 40 minutes. Activities such as walking, swimming, and use of aerobic gym equipment are encouraged.[4]

Adverse effects

No studies have proven that splanchnic blood flow reduction or increased heart rate during exercise has any adverse effects on the fetus. Studies of experimental animals where an elevation of body temperature to 39 or 40°C has occurred suggest an increased incidence of neural tube defects.[3] There are no prospective studies in humans to validate this concern but caution against hyperthermia is advised. No studies have proven that exercise is associated with an increase in spontaneous abortion in a low-risk pregnancy. Exercise is not associated with increased premature rupture of membranes or labour, nor is it linked to an easier or shorter labour.[4]

Contraindications

Absolute contraindications to exercise during pregnancy include restrictive cardiovascular disease, hypertension, uncontrolled diabetes, incompetent cervix, placenta previa at 26 weeks, persistent vaginal bleeding, multiple gestation at risk for premature delivery, premature labour, or ruptured membranes. Relative contraindications include severe anemia, significantly altered body weight (obese or underweight), intrauterine growth restriction, orthopedic limitations, and poorly controlled metabolic or cardiovascular disorders.[1-5]

Musculoskeletal effects

Women who exercise during pregnancy should be aware of changes in balance due to altered weight distribution and centre of gravity. Ligamentous laxity occurs with the secretion of estrogen and relaxin hormones that increase the hypermobility at key joints such as the sacroiliacs, knees, and hips. Common pregnancy-related musculoskeletal conditions include rectus diastasis, sacroiliac hypermobility, sciatica, and symphysis pubis disruption.[5]

----------- ◢ REFERENCES ◣ -----------

1. Clapp J: Exercise during pregnancy: a clinical update, *Clin Sports Med* 19(2):273-86, 2000.
2. Sempowski L, et al: Managing diabetes during pregnancy: guide for family physicians, *Can Fam Phyician* 49:761-67, 2003.
3. Davies G, Wolfe L, Mottola M, et al: Joint SOGC/CSEP clinical practice guideline: exercise and pregnancy and the postpartum period, *Can J Appl Physiol* 28(3):329-41, 2003.
4. Artal R, O'Toole M: Guidelines of the American College of Obstetricians and Gynecologists for exercise during pregnancy and the postpartum period, *Br J Sports Med* 37:6-12, 2003.
5. Ritchie JR: Orthopaedic considerations during pregnancy, *Clin Obst Gyn* 46(2):456-66, 2003.

Ultrasound in Pregnancy

(See also congenital anomalies; Down syndrome; informed consent)

Routine ultrasound is usually scheduled at 18 weeks, and a number of fetal abnormalities may be detected at this stage of gestation.[1-5] However, the sensitivity is low (17%[1] to 40%[2]) as is the positive predictive value.[5] Gestational age can be assessed and multiple pregnancies detected,[3,4] and in many cases fetal sex can be determined.[1] Studies comparing patients undergoing routine antenatal ultrasound with those having selective ultrasound (when clinically indicated) have shown that those in the routine ultrasound group had twin pregnancies accurately diagnosed in all cases, a lower frequency of induction for apparent post-term pregnancy, fewer low-weight babies, and more induced abortions for fetal abnormalities.[3,4]

Whether a single routine ultrasound screening during the second trimester of pregnancy actually improves perinatal morbidity and mortality is another question. Probably it does not, but this is still an area of heated controversy. Evidence-based reviews of numerous trials addressing this issue[4,6,7] have concluded that except in one study, the Helsinki Ultrasound Trial,[2] no decreased perinatal morbidity or mortality has been documented. The Helsinki study, which has been updated[8] since these reviews were published, reported a decrease in perinatal mortality in the screened group. The explanation was that more children with severe congenital malformation were being born and dying in the control group and the difference disappeared if the induced abortions for congenital anomalies in the screened group were categorized as deaths.[7] A South African trial that was reported in 1996 found no differences in perinatal outcome between the ultrasound screened group and the control group.[9]

The U.S. Preventive Services Task Force[6] gives a single routine mid-trimester ultrasound screening a "C" recommendation, while the Canadian Task Force on Preventive Health Care[7] gives it a "B."

First trimester ultrasound is discussed in the section on prenatal genetic screening. The use of routine ultrasound late in pregnancy (greater than 24 weeks gestational age) in low-risk populations does not offer any benefit to mother or baby.[13]

❧ REFERENCES ❧

1. Ewigman BG, Crane JP, Frigoletto FD, et al (RADIUS Study Group): Effect of prenatal ultrasound screening on perinatal outcome, *N Engl J Med* 329:821-827, 1993.
2. Saari-Kemppainen A, Karjalainen O, Ylostalo P, et al: Ultrasound screening and perinatal mortality: controlled trial of systematic one-stage screening in pregnancy; the Helsinki Ultrasound Trial, *Lancet* 336:387-391, 1990.
3. Enkin M, Keirse MJ, Renfrew M, et al, editors: *A guide to effective care in pregnancy and childbirth,* ed 2, Oxford, 1995, Oxford University Press, pp 41-42.
4. Neilson JP: Routine ultrasound in early pregnancy. In Enkin MW, Keirse MJNC, Renfrew MJ, Neilson JP, editors: *Pregnancy and childbirth module,* Cochrane Database of Systematic Reviews, Review No. 03872, June 9, 1993, Oxford, 1994, Update Software.
5. Buskens E, Grobbee DE, Frohn-Mulder IM, et al: Efficacy of routine fetal ultrasound screening for congenital heart disease in normal pregnancy, *Circulation* 94:67-72, 1996.
6. U.S. Preventive Services Task Force: *Guide to clinical preventive services,* ed 2, Baltimore, 1996, Williams & Wilkins, pp 407-417.
7. Canadian Task Force on the Periodic Health Examination: *Canadian guide to clinical preventive health care,* Ottawa, 1994, Canada Communication Group Publishing, pp 4-14.
8. Leivo T, Tuominen R, Saarikemppainen A, et al: Cost-effectiveness of one-stage ultrasound screening in pregnancy–a report from the Helsinki Ultrasound Trial, *Ultrasound Obstet Gynecol* 7:309-314, 1996.
9. Geerts LT, Brand EJ, Theron GB: Routine obstetric ultrasound examinations in South Africa–cost and effect on perinatal outcome: a prospective randomized controlled trial, *Br J Obstet Gynaecol* 103:501-507, 1996.
10. Snijders RJ, Noble P, Sebire N, et al: U.K. multicentre project on assessment of risk of trisomy 21 by maternal age and fetal nuchal-translucency thickness at 10-14 weeks of gestation, *Lancet* 352:343-346, 1998.
11. McFadyen A, Gledhill J, Whitlow B, et al: First trimester ultrasound screening: carries ethical and psychological implications, *BMJ* 317:694-695, 1998 (editorial).
12. Price BE: Scanning during pregnancy is often for doctors' benefit rather than parents', *BMJ* 318:1489, 1999 (letter).
13. Bricker L, Neilson JP: Routine ultrasound in late pregnancy (after 24 weeks gestation). (Cochrane Review), In *The Cochrane Library* Issue 3:2004. Updated Oct 1, 1999.

DISORDERS OF PREGNANCY
Gestational Diabetes
Definition

Gestational diabetes refers to carbohydrate intolerance that begins, or is first detected, during pregnancy. Gestational diabetes occurs when a woman's pancreatic function is not sufficient to overcome the insulin resistance created by the anti-insulin hormones and the increased fuel consumption necessary to provide the growing mother and fetus. The definition applies whether or not insulin is used for treatment or the condition persists postpartum. It does not exclude the possibility that the glucose intolerance may have antedated the pregnancy.[1,2] The Toronto Tri-Hospital Gestational Diabetes Project reported a prevalence of 3.8% in the study population.[3] This is in keeping with the standard quoted prevalence of 3% to 4%.[1]

Risk factors

The following are risk factors, though up to 50% of those affected have none of these factors[4]:

- First-degree relative with diabetes
- Maternal age greater than 25
- Maternal obesity
- Previous history of gestational diabetes or glucose intolerance
- Prior macrosomic infant (larger than 4 kg)
- Polyhydramnios
- Prior birth defects or stillbirths
- Ethnicity
- Previous neonatal hypoglycemia, hypocalcemia, or hyperbilirubinemia

Screening debate

The debate is not whether an abnormality of glucose metabolism exists but rather whether or not there is clinical merit in screening for it. At present, no good quality RCTs conclusively show that diagnosing and treating gestational diabetes mellitus (GDM) will lead to a reduction in negative outcomes.[5]

Macrosomia occurs in 10% to 25% of GDM pregnancies, but the majority of macrosomic infants are born to non-GDM mothers. Macrosomia is associated with shoulder dystocia although most cases occur in infants larger than 4 kg. Screening for and treating GDM has been shown to reduce the rate of fetal macrosomia, but this does not necessarily translate into a reduction in birth trauma.[6]

Conflicting evidence exists as to the effect of diagnosis and treatment of GDM on perinatal mortality, pre-eclampsia, neonatal metabolic complications, and the long-term complications of GDM on the woman and her children.[5] With regard to cesarian section, the diagnosis of GDM may act as a self-fulfilling prophecy and increase the rates in these women, most likely due to a labelling bias.[3]

Societies and associations such as The American College of Obstetricians and Gynecologists,[7] The American Diabetes Association (ADA),[8] The Canadian Diabetes Association,[9] The Fourth International Workshop Conference on Gestational Diabetes Mellitus,[10] and The Society of Obstetricians and Gynecologists of Canada (SOGC),[5] have recommended either universal or selective screening, although the SOGC's 2002 guidelines include no screening as one of the acceptable options given the evidence presented above.

Selective screening involves screening of all but low-risk women, criteria for which include maternal age greater than 25, ethnic group membership with low prevalence of diabetes (Caucasian), body mass index (BMI) less than 27, no previous history of GDM or no DM in a first-degree relative.[11] The sensitivity of this approach is 63%, with a specificity of 56%.[5] Presently, recommendations are based on expert opinion, not evidence, because the evidence for the benefits of screening, who should be screened, and how to screen varies among published guidelines. The recommendations reflect the interests of the committee publishing the guidelines; the Canadian Diabetes 2003 Clinical Practice Guidelines highlight the potential benefit of identifying those at risk of developing diabetes in the future, with focus on prevention of type 2 diabetes. Both the Canadian Task Force on Preventative Health Care and the U.S. Preventative Services Task Force give screening for GDM a "C" recommendation, concluding that there is insufficient evidence to recommend for or against screening.[12,13] The controversy will only end once a randomized double blind trial is conducted and published (in progress) that determines whether identification and management of GDM is associated with significant improvement in neonatal or maternal outcome.

If screening is offered, it is performed between 24 and 28 weeks gestational age by measuring plasma glucose level 1 hour after a 50 g glucose load given at any time of day. GDM is confirmed if the level is 10.3 mmol/L or greater. If the result is 7.8 to 10.2 mmol/L, a 75 g oral glucose tolerance test (OGTT) should be conducted because it is more acceptable to patients than the 3-hour 100 g OGTT, and it is endorsed by the WHO.[5,9]

Management

First line treatment of gestational diabetes is diet, regular moderate upper body exercise, and careful home glucose monitoring, although evidence for the optimal diet is lacking.[9] Optimal glucose levels are less than 5.3 mmol/L when fasting, less than 7.8 mmol/L one hour after a meal, and less than 6.7 mmol/L two hours afterward. If optimal glucose levels cannot be achieved by diet and exercise after two weeks, then pharmacologic therapy (i.e., insulin) must be considered. Glyburide does not appear to cross the placenta and may be effective in the management of GDM; however, its safety in pregnancy has not been shown to be comparable to that of insulin and is therefore not yet recommended for routine use.[9] Gestational diabetes is best managed by a multidisciplinary team.

Follow-up of women diagnosed with GDM involves a 2-hour PG 75 g OGTT within 6 to 12 weeks of delivery,[10] or within 6 months by other recommendations[9] because up to 50% will develop type II diabetes within 20 years. These women should be advised to exercise regularly and maintain a healthy body weight.

────────────── ❧ REFERENCES ❧ ──────────────

1. Metzger BE, Coustan DR: Summary and recommendations of the fourth international workshop-conference on gestational diabetes mellitus (The Organizing Committee). *Diabetes Care* 21(Suppl 2):161-167, 1998.

2. Report of the Expert Committee on the Diagnosis and Classification of Diabetes Mellitus. *Diabetes Care* 20:1183-1197, 1997.

3. Naylor CD, et al (Toronto Trihospital Gestational Diabetes Investigators): Caesarian delivery in relation to birth weight and gestational glucose tolerance: pathophysiology or practice style? *JAMA* 275:1165-70, 1996.

4. Greene MF: Screening for gestational diabetes mellitus, *N Engl J Med* 337:1625-26, 1997 (editorial).

5. SOGC Clinical Practice Guidelines: *Screening for Gestational Diabetes Mellitus* No 121, November 2002.

6. Sermer M, Naylor CD, Farine D, et al: The Toronto Tri-Hospital Gestational Diabetes Project. A preliminary review, *Diabetes Care* 21(Suppl 2):B33-42, 1998.

7. ACOG Practice Bulletin: *Clinical management guidelines for obstetrician-gynecologists.* Number 30, September 2001 (replaces Technical Bulletin 200, December 1994). Gestational Diabetes, *Obstet Gynecol* 98:525-38, 2001 (Medline).

8. American Diabetes Association: Gestational diabetes mellitus, *Diabetes Care* 22(Suppl 1):S74-76, 1998.

9. Canadian Diabetes Association 2003 Clinical practice guidelines for the prevention and management of diabetes in Canada, *Canadian Journal of Diabetes* 27(Suppl 2):S1-S52, Dec 2003.

10. Metzger BE, Coustan DR: Summary and recommendations of the Fourth International Workshop-Conference on gestational diabetes mellitus (The Organizing Committee), *Diabetes Care* 21(Suppl 2):B161-7, 1998.

11. Naylor CD, Sermer M, Chen MB, et al: Selective screening for gestational diabetes mellitus, *N Engl J Med* 337:159106, 1997.

12. Canadian Task Force on the Periodic Health Examination: *Clinical preventative health care*, Ottawa, 1994, Canadian Communication Group-Publishing, pp 16-23.

13. U.S. Preventative Services Task Force: *Guide to clinical preventative services*, ed 2, Baltimore, 1996, Williams and Wilkins, pp 193-208.

Group B Streptococcal Disease
(See also clinical practice guidelines; prevention; screening)

Group B *Streptococcus* (GBS) has emerged over the past three decades as the most frequent infectious cause of mortality and morbidity among newborn infants in North America and Europe. Before the implementation of preventative guidelines, neonatal GBS disease occurred in 0.2 to 5 of 1000 live births worldwide. Canadian rates ranged between 0.44 and 2.1 per 1000 live births in the early 1990s, with case fatality rates of 16.2%.[1]

GBS is spread vertically from the mother to the neonate during the birthing process. The rate of transmission from colonized women to the fetus is 50%. However, only 1% to 2% of all colonized infants will develop early-onset GBS disease (before 1 week of life). Approximately 10% to 30% of pregnant women are colonized with GBS. Culture screening of both the lower vagina and rectum late in gestation during prenatal care can detect women who are likely to be colonized with GBS at the time of delivery and are thus at higher risk of perinatal transmission of the organism. Women who have had a previously affected GBS neonate or GBS bacteriuria in the current pregnancy are also at risk of transmission.

Intrapartum chemoprophylaxis (IPC) is effective in reducing the incidence of colonization by 80% to 90%. Since the introduction of preventative strategies, early onset GBS rates have declined in North America, with rates as low as 0.25 per 1000 and case fatality rates of less than 10%. Over the past decade, the challenge has been how to best identify and manage women at risk.

Since 1992 there have been a number of guidelines issued on neonatal GBS prevention recommending either a screening-based or risk-based approach as effective methods of managing GBS. In 2001, the U.S. Centers for Disease Control conducted a multistate, retrospective cohort study that concluded that the universal screening approach (at 35 to 37 weeks gestation) was 50% more effective than the risk-based approach at preventing perinatal GBS disease. The 2002 CDC Guidelines for Prevention of Perinatal GBS Disease recommend

1. Vaginal and rectal GBS screening cultures at 35 to 37 weeks gestation for *all* pregnant women (unless patient had GBS bacteriuria during the current pregnancy or a previous infant with invasive GBS disease)

2. Intrapartum chemoprophylaxis/IPC is indicated in the following situations:
   - Previous infant with invasive GBS disease
   - GBS bacteruria during current pregnancy
   - Positive GBS screening culture during current pregnancy (unless planned cesarean section delivery in the absence of amniotic membrane rupture is performed)
   - Unknown GBS status (culture not done, incomplete, or results unknown) and any of the following:
     - Delivery before 37 weeks
     - Amniotic membrane rupture occurring 18 hours or more earlier
     - Intrapartum temperature of 38.0 degrees C or higher; (If amnionitis is suspected, broad-spectrum antibiotic therapy that includes an agent known to be active against GBS should replace GBS IPC.)

3. Intrapartum chemoprophylaxis/IPC is not indicated in the following situations:
   - Previous pregnancy with a positive GBS screening culture (unless a culture was also positive during current pregnancy)
   - Planned cesarean delivery performed in the absence of labour or membrane rupture (regardless of maternal GBS culture status)
   - Negative vaginal and rectal screening culture in late gestation during the current pregnancy, regardless of intrapartum risk factors[2]

The Canadian Task Force on Preventative Health also endorses the above guidelines, but gives the option of selective IPC to all colonized women or to only those with positive cultures and risk factors.[3] GBS-positive women who do not want to take antibiotics may be assured that if they do not have risk factors, risk of disease in the newborn is 1 in 1000 greater than the risk if they were to take antibiotics. This is the only set of guidelines to give this option.

The recommended IPC is Penicillin G (5 million units intravenously [IV] for the initial dose, then 2.5 million units IV every 4 hours until delivery) or Ampicillin (2 g IV for the initial dose, then 1 g IV every 4 hours until delivery). If a patient has a history of a penicillin allergy then Cefazolin, Clindamycin, or Erythromycin is the antibiotic of choice.

Currently there is no universal approach to the management of the neonate born to a GBS-positive mother. The treatment can range from observation of the neonate for 48 hours, to limited evaluation (including pediatric consult, CBC with differential, blood culture, and 48 hours observation in hospital), to a full diagnostic evaluation and empiric therapy. Variations in approaches will depend on individual circumstances and institutional preferences.[3]

◤ REFERENCES ◢

1. *Pediatric Child Health* 7(6):July/Aug, 2002.
2. Prevention of perinatal group B streptococcal disease, *MMWR* Revised Guidelines from CDC, No. RR-11, 51:August 16, 2002.
3. Prevention of group B streptococcal infection in newborns. Recommendation statement from the Canadian Task Force on Preventative Health Care, *CMAJ* 166(7), 2002.

Hypertensive Disorders of Pregnancy

(See also hypertension)

Classification

The hypertensive disorders of pregnancy may be divided into four main categories. In the list below, traditional terms are followed in parentheses by terms recommended by the Canadian Hypertension Society.[1,2]

Chronic hypertension (pre-existing hypertension)
Gestational hypertension (gestational hypertension without proteinuria)
Pre-eclampsia (gestational hypertension with proteinuria)
Chronic hypertension with superimposed pre-eclampsia (pre-existing hypertension plus superimposed gestational hypertension with proteinuria)

Definition

Hypertension in pregnancy has been traditionally defined as any reading over 140/90 mm Hg.[1,2] In addition, several guidelines have recommended that the diagnosis be made if there is an increase of the systolic level by 30 mm Hg or of the diastolic level by 15 mm Hg compared with average readings before 20 weeks gestation.[3,4] The Canadian Hypertension Society rejects changing blood pressure levels during pregnancy as a criterion for hypertension because rises above these levels occur commonly and do not result in the detection of more true cases of hypertension than are found by using absolute figures alone.[2,5] Blood pressure in pregnant women should be measured when they are sitting up. The women should not use tobacco or caffeine 30 minutes prior to measurement.[6]

Prevention

A Cochrane review showed a reduction in the incidence of high blood pressure with and without proteinuria with calcium supplementation (at least 1 gm daily).[7] In both cases, the effect was greater among women at high risk of developing hypertension and those with low baseline dietary calcium. This did not translate into any significant effect on risk of stillbirth or death before discharge from the hospital. A decreased risk of preterm delivery was shown only in those women at high risk of hypertension. The optimal dose of calcium is not known.

Laboratory investigations

Standard investigations for patients with hypertensive disorders of pregnancy include a complete blood count and platelet count, urinalysis, and measurements of serum uric acid, serum creatinine, and liver enzymes.[2] Proteinuria should be quantified with 24-hour urine collection.

Non-pharmacological management

At present this consists primarily of watchful waiting; the traditional therapeutic modalities of strict bedrest and salt restriction have no value.[5]

Pharmacological management

Antihypertensive drug treatment for mild to moderate hypertension (systolic BP 140 to169 mm Hg, diastolic BP 90 to 109 mm Hg) halves the risk of developing severe hypertension.[8] It does not reduce the risk of developing hypertension with proteinuria, nor does it have any clinical effect on the risks for the fetus such as death, small for gestational age, or preterm birth. Overall, it is not clear whether drug therapy for this group has any significant benefits.[9] Medications are required for all women with systolic pressures above 169 mm Hg or diastolic pressures above 109 mm Hg to reduce the risk of maternal mortality and morbidity.[1,10] Decisions about pharmacotherapy have to take into account the gestational age, the presence or absence of proteinuria, and perhaps evidence of end organ damage.[11]

Many antihypertensive drugs are inadequately studied in pregnancy. Methyldopa (Aldomet) is the drug of first choice in non-severe hypertension. Second-line drugs include labetalol (Trandate), pindolol (Visken), oxprenolol (Trasicor), and sustained release nifedipine (Adalat, Procardia). A 2004 Cochrane review showed a trend toward small for gestational age infants in users of β-blockers, a finding that needs to be further evaluated.[12] For severe hypertension in pregnancy the first-line drug is hydralazine (Apresoline); second-line drugs are labetalol and long-acting nifedipine. ACE inhibitors and angiotensin II receptor antagonists are contraindicated in pregnancy.[1,11]

Chronic hypertension (pre-existing hypertension)

Diagnosis of chronic hypertension is made when patients have a history of hypertension before pregnancy or when the blood pressure is 140/90 mm Hg or higher before 20 weeks of gestation. Use of the latter criterion results in many missed cases because blood pressure normally drops during the second trimester. Most women with chronic hypertension who have systolic levels below 170 mm Hg or diastolic levels below 110 mm Hg do not require pharmacotherapy.[1]

Gestational hypertension (gestational hypertension without proteinuria)

Gestational hypertension is the new onset of hypertension after 20 weeks gestation without associated symptoms or signs of pre-eclampsia. In general, drug treatment is not required and pregnancy outcome is good.[1]

Pre-eclampsia (gestational hypertension with proteinuria)

A working clinical definition of pre-eclampsia is hypertension plus hyperuricemia or proteinuria. Proteinuria is defined as 1+ on a dipstick on two or more occasions, or 300 mg [0.3 g] or higher in a 24-hour urine collection. The severity of pre-eclampsia is measured by the degree of hypertension and proteinuria. Edema is common but not necessary for the diagnosis.[1,3] The problem with this or any other clinical definition is that patients may have the disorder without hypertension or proteinuria. For example, 20% of women in whom seizures (eclampsia) later develop have diastolic blood pressure readings below 90 mm Hg or no proteinuria.[1]

A probable explanation for the lack of hypertension or proteinuria in some women who later have serious disease is that one of the basic pathophysiological abnormalities is reduced vascular perfusion, which is often localized. If decreased perfusion does not involve the glomeruli, proteinuria will not occur. Another basic abnormality in pre-eclampsia is endothelial cell dysfunction, which can cause increased vascular permeability with edema, thromboses, and low platelet counts.[1,3]

Severe pre-eclampsia is diagnosed by the following:
- Systolic BP of 160 mm Hg or diastolic BP of 110 mm Hg or greater on two separate occasions more than 6 hours apart
- Proteinuria of more than 5 g in 24 hours or more than 3+ protein on two urine samples longer than 4 hours apart
- Oliguria
- Pulmonary edema or cyanosis
- Impairment of liver function

- Visual or cerebral dysfunction
- Pain in the epigastric area
- Decreased platelet count

Eclampsia is a new onset of grand mal seizures in a woman with pre-eclampsia.[6]

Risk factors for pre-eclampsia include first pregnancy, family history of pre-eclampsia, previous personal history of pre-eclampsia, older age, pre-existing hypertension, diabetes, multiple pregnancies, hydatidiform mole, and hydrops fetalis.[3] Women with pre-eclampsia are at greater risk for seizures, cerebral hemorrhage, liver and renal failure, disseminated intravascular coagulation, and placental abruption.[1] Fetal complications include intrauterine growth restriction (IUGR), placental abruption, prematurity, oligohydramnios, and fetal loss.

A meta-analysis of randomized control trials involving pregnant women with historical risk factors for pre-eclampsia and prophylaxis with aspirin showed decrease in perinatal death, pre-eclampsia, rate of spontaneous preterm birth, and small for gestation age births. There was no increase in placental abruption.[13]

Studies involving supplementation of vitamin C (1000 mg/d) and vitamin E (400 mg/d) for prevention of pre-eclampsia have shown improvement in biochemical indices of disease (placental function and oxidative stress) for women at high risk of pre-eclampsia.[1,14] Management of mild pre-eclampsia is controversial. Whether bedrest, hospitalization, antihypertensive therapy, or prophylactic anticonvulsants are beneficial is unknown, but it is generally agreed that if the woman is at 34 weeks or more and the cervix is favourable for induction, immediate delivery should be undertaken. In all cases, close monitoring (weight, fetal status, blood pressure, proteinuria, and platelet count) is needed because the pre-eclampsia may progress rapidly.[1]

Women with severe pre-eclampsia who are at 34 or more weeks of gestation require immediate delivery, as do many who are at earlier stages. For those with a diastolic pressure of 110 mm Hg or more, the usual medical treatment is intravenous hydralazine (Apresoline) or, if contraindicated, intravenous labetalol or oral nifedipine.[1,12]

Prophylactic anticonvulsants are given to patients with severe pre-eclampsia. In North America, magnesium sulfate is the drug most frequently used, whereas in Europe the more common practice has been antihypertensive therapy with or without phenytoin (Dilantin).[1] Magnesium sulphate more than halves the risk of pre-eclampsia and probably reduces maternal mortality. In the short term, it does not affect the outcome for the baby.[15] One trial comparing the prophylactic use of magnesium sulfate with phenytoin in women with pre-eclampsia demonstrated a small benefit for the magnesium sulfate-treated group.[10,16] Magnesium sulfate is the anticonvulsant of choice for women with eclampsia.[16,17] It is

At very high doses can cause hypocalcemia and tetany

the drug recommended by the Canadian Hypertension Society.[11]

HELLP syndrome

The acronym HELLP stands for *h*emolysis, *e*levated *l*iver enzymes, and *l*ow *p*latelet counts. It most frequently occurs as a complication of severe pre-eclampsia, but it can develop in pregnant women who are normotensive and have no proteinuria, as well as in postpartum women. Ninety percent of patients with the HELLP syndrome have right upper quadrant pain secondary to focal hepatic necrosis. At the slightest suspicion of this condition a complete blood count and blood smear should be obtained. The blood smear may reveal the presence of fragmented red cells (schistocytes), which are usually seen in microangiopathic conditions such as this.[18]

◁ REFERENCES ▷

1. Sibai BM: Treatment of hypertension in pregnant women, *N Engl J Med* 335:257-265, 1996.
2. Helewa ME, Burrows RF, Smith J, et al: Report of the Canadian Hypertension Society Consensus Conference. 1. Definitions, evaluation and classification of hypertensive disorders in pregnancy, *CMAJ* 157:715-725, 1997.
3. Zamorski MA, Green LA: Preeclampsia and hypertensive disorders of pregnancy, *Am Fam Physician* 53:1595-1604, 1996.
4. National High Blood Pressure Education Program Working Group report on high blood pressure in pregnancy, *Am J Obstet Gynecol* 163(5 Pt 1):1691-1712, 1990.
5. Moutquin J-M, Garner PR, Burrows RF: Report of the Canadian Hypertension Society Consensus Conference. 2. Nonpharmacologic management and prevention of hypertensive disorders in pregnancy, *CMAJ* 157:907-919, 1997.
6. Schroeder BM: ACOG Practice Bulletin on Diagnosing and managing preeclampsia and eclampsia, *Am Fam Physician* 66(2):July 15, 2002
7. Atallah AN, Hofmeyr GJ, Duley L: Calcium supplementation during pregnancy for preventing hypertensive disorders and related problems (Cochrane Review), In *The Cochrane Library*, Issue 2, 2004, Chichester, 2004, Wiley & Sons.
8. Abalos E, Duley L, Steyn DW, et al: Antihypertensive drug therapy for mild to moderate hypertension during pregnancy (Cochrane Review). In *The Cochrane Library*, Issue 2, 2004, Chichester, 2004, John Wiley & Sons.
9. Afifi Y, Churchill D: Pharmacological treatment of hypertension in pregnancy, *Curr Pharm Des* 9(21):1745-53, 2003.
10. Duley L, Henderson-Smart DJ: Drugs for the treatment of very high blood pressure during pregnancy (Cochrane Review). In *The Cochrane Library*, Issue 2, 2004, Chichester, 2004, John Wiley & Sons.
11. Rey é: Report of the Canadian Hypertension Society Consensus Conference. 3. Pharmacologic treatment of hypertensive disorders in pregnancy, *CMAJ* 157:1245-1254, 1997.
12. Magee LA, Duley L: Oral beta blockers for mild to moderate hypertension during pregnancy (Cochrane Review). In *The Cochrane Library*, Issue 2, 2004, Chichester, 2004. Wiley & Sons.
13. Coomarasamy A: Aspirin for prevention of preeclampsia in women with historical risk factors: a systematic review, *Obstet Gynecol* 101(6):1319-32, 2003.
14. Chappell LC: Vitamin C and E supplementation in women at risk of preeclampsia is associated with changes in indices of oxidative stress and placental function, *Am J Obstet Gynecol* 187(3)777-84, 2002.
15. Duley L, Glumezoglu AM, Henderson-Smart DJ: Magnesium sulfate and other anticonvulsants for women with pre-eclampsia (Cochrane Review). In *The Cochrane Library*, Issue 2, 2004, Chichester, 2004, John Wiley & Sons.
16. Lucas MJ, Leveno KJ, Cunningham FG: A comparison of magnesium sulfate with phenytoin for the prevention of preeclampsia, *N Engl J Med* 333:201-205, 1995.
17. Eclampsia Trial Collaborative Group: Which anticonvulsant for women with eclampsia? Evidence from the Collaborative Eclampsia Trial, *Lancet* 242:1455-1463, 1995.
18. Stone JH: HELLP syndrome: hemolysis, elevated liver enzymes, and low platelets, *JAMA* 280:559-562, 1998.

Infectious Diseases in Pregnancy

(See also erythema infectiosum; HIV and AIDS)

Erythema infectiosum

Erythema infectiosum is caused by parvovirus B19 and usually affects children between the ages of 5 and 14 years. It is contagious for 5 to 10 days before the onset of the rash, but not once the rash has appeared. The mode of transmission is respiratory secretions or from hand to mouth contact. Fifty to sixty-five percent of adults have acquired immunity. Among infants carried by women who became infected with parvovirus B19 during the first 20 weeks of pregnancy, 20% develop a non-immune form of hydrops fetalis because of transient red blood cell aplasia. Although a few cases of fetal loss result from this infection, spontaneous recovery without sequelae is the usual outcome.[1] The spontaneous loss rate of fetuses affected with parvovirus B19 before 20 weeks gestation is 14.8% and 2.3% after 20 weeks gestation.[2]

Pregnant women who have been exposed to erythema infectiosum should be tested for specific IgG and IgM antibodies. If IgG antibody is present, the patient is immune, and if neither antibody is present, she is not infected but remains at risk. If IgM antibodies develop, the woman should be carefully monitored with serial ultrasounds to detect the presence of hydrops. In a very few cases fetal blood transfusions are indicated, but in most instances the condition resolves spontaneously.[1]

Herpes simplex

The risk of transmitting herpes simplex virus (HSV) to the neonate is up to 50% in cases of primary herpes, whereas for women with recurrent episodes it is only 2%

to 3% with vaginal birth even in the presence of lesions. The lesser risk with recurrent herpes is due in part to a lesser quantity of virus and in part to the presence of protective IgG in the baby. Serial cultures of HSV during the last weeks of pregnancy are no longer advised. The current recommendation of both the Society of Obstetricians and Gynecologists of Canada and the American College of Obstetricians and Gynecologists is to examine the vulva, buttocks, and thighs for lesions and offer Cesarean section if they are present.[3] New recommendations suggest that women with known recurrent genital HSV infection can be offered acyclovir suppression (acyclovir 400 mg twice a day) near term (36 weeks gestation to delivery.) For clinical suspicion or culture evidence of neonatal infection, antiviral therapy should be initiated as soon as possible.[4]

HIV and AIDS

The risks of vertical transmission of HIV and methods of management of the infection in pregnant women are discussed in the section on HIV and AIDS.

Mumps

Mumps is very rare in pregnancy. It is not known to be teratogenic. Women who have the disease in the first trimester have a higher incidence of spontaneous abortions.[5]

Rubella

Rubella is contagious from a few days before the appearance of the rash until 5 to 7 days after its development. About half of those who acquire the disease are asymptomatic. In North America, lack of immunity is most common in recent immigrants and refugees.[6]

Major features of the congenital rubella syndrome (CRS) are cataracts, sensorineural hearing loss, and congenital heart disease, especially patent ductus arteriosus, and pulmonary stenosis. Other features that may be seen are microphthalmia, retinopathy, and intrauterine growth retardation. The congenital rubella syndrome occurs only when the mother is infected with rubella in the first 20 weeks of gestation, and the earlier the infection occurs, the greater the risk. Between one fifth and one third of infants born to mothers infected during the first 20 weeks of pregnancy are affected. Up to 90% of infants born to mothers infected during the first 11 weeks of gestation will develop CRS. Infection late in the first half of pregnancy is more likely to result in hearing impairment and less likely to be associated with other defects.[7] Although rubella vaccine is contraindicated in pregnancy, no cases of congenital rubella syndrome have been reported in women who accidentally received such vaccinations in early pregnancy.[6]

Pregnant women should be screened for rubella immunity (rubella IgG) at the earliest prenatal visit. A positive rubella IgG antibody test indicates rubella immunity.[7] If a woman whose immune status to rubella is unknown is exposed to the disease, she should be tested for rubella IgG within 7 days. If the test is positive, the patient is immune, but if it is negative, she should be tested for rubella IgG and IgM after 3 weeks. Recent infection is indicated by either the new development of IgM or a fourfold or greater increase in IgG. If serological tests are positive, infection of the fetus can be diagnosed prenatally by testing fetal blood for rubella-specific IgM or by chorionic villus biopsy and polymerase chain reaction assessment.[6]

Rubeola

Rubeola is very rare in pregnancy. No evidence of teratogenesis or spontaneous abortion in infected women has been reported. The risk of premature labour, spontaneous abortion, and neonatal mortality is slightly increased.[8]

Toxoplasmosis

Toxoplasmosis acquired by the mother during pregnancy, even if asymptomatic, may infect the fetus and cause a variety of disorders such as chorioretinitis, developmental delay, and hearing loss.[9] The risk of vertical transmission is much greater in late pregnancy than in early pregnancy, but the risk of clinical disease in the infant is much greater when maternal infection is acquired early in pregnancy.[10]

About two thirds of women in Canada have no protective immunity. Measures for preventing infection include avoiding undercooked meat and unpasteurized milk; carefully washing raw foods, utensils, counters, and hands during the preparation of food; wearing gloves while gardening; and washing hands after contact with soil or sand. Cats, particularly kittens, can transmit the infection through their feces. Cats should not be fed undercooked meat, and kitty litter should be changed daily because the toxoplasmosis oocysts take 2 to 3 days to become infectious. If possible the litter change should be done by a non-pregnant person. However, it can safely be done by the pregnant woman if she wears gloves, washes her hands afterward, and disinfects the litter box with boiling water (see also discussion of HIV and AIDS).[9]

Screening pregnant women for toxoplasmosis is a routine practice in some European countries such as Austria and France. A systematic literature review concluded that the value of screening pregnant women for toxoplasmosis or treating those who are infected is uncertain.[11]

Varicella

The risk of acquiring varicella in pregnancy is low (1 to 7 per 10,000 pregnancies). The disease is infectious from 2 days before the onset of the eruption until all the vesicles have crusted, which usually takes about 5 days.[12] The most feared complication of varicella in pregnancy is congenital varicella embryopathy (limb hypoplasia, skin scarring, eye defects, and neurological abnormalities). When mothers are infected in the first 20 weeks of pregnancy, 2.2% of infants are affected by the syndrome.[13] Pregnancies complicated by maternal primary varicella infection should have a detailed anatomical ultrasound performed between 20 and 22 weeks of gestation to evaluate fetal growth, limbs, and the anatomy of the cerebral and ocular systems.[14] Treatment of the mother with antiviral medications does not alter that risk.[12]

Varicella in pregnancy puts the mother at increased risk because the mortality of varicella pneumonia during pregnancy is high.

Twenty four percent to sixty percent of infants born to mothers who develop varicella between 2.5 weeks before and 1 week after delivery contract varicella. The Centers for Disease Control and Prevention (CDC) recommends the administration of varicella zoster immunoglobulin (VZIG) to any infant born to a mother who develops varicella between 5 days before and 2 days after delivery. The infant should also be treated with intravenous acyclovir at 30 mg/kg divided 3 times per day for 10 days.[14] If a pregnant woman with no history of chickenpox is exposed to an infected person, her antibody status should be determined (over 85% of women who do not know if they have had chickenpox are found to be immune). If she is antibody negative, or if serological results are unavailable within 96 hours of exposure, she should be given passive immunization with VZIG[12]; the usual dose is four vials, each containing 125 units. If given within 96 hours of exposure, VZIG is likely to abort the disease; if given later, it may modify the disease.[12]

────────── ❧ **REFERENCES** ❧ ──────────

1. Mankuta D, Bar-Oz B, Koren G: Erythema infectiosum (fifth disease) and pregnancy, *Can Fam Physician* 45:603-605, 1999.
2. Parvovirus B19 infection in pregnancy, Sept 2002, Society of Obstetricians and Gynecologists of Canada.
3. Sanderson F: Perinatal viral infections: 5 scenarios to manage, *Patient Care Can* 7(1):43-60, 1996.
4. Guidelines for perinatal care: Obstetric guideline 3. Herpes in the perinatal period, July 2003, British Columbia Reproductive Care Program.
5. Boucher M: Les maladies virales de l'enfance et de la grossesse: petit guide pratico-pratique, *Clin Mar* 10:55-70, 1995.
6. Bar-Oz B, Ford-Jones L, Koren G: Congenital rubella syndrome, *Can Fam Physician* 45:1865-1867, 1999.
7. Control and prevention of rubella: evaluation and management of suspected outbreaks, rubella in pregnant women, and surveillance for congenital rubella syndrome, *MMWR Morb Mortal Wkly Rep* 50(RR-12):1, 2001.
8. Stein SJ, Greenspoon JS: Rubeola during pregnancy, *Obstet Gynecol* 78:925-929, 1991.
9. Phillips E: Toxoplasmosis, *Can Fam Physician* 44:1823-1825, 1998.
10. Dunn D, Wallon M, Peyron F, et al: Mother- to child transmission of toxoplasmosis: risk estimates for clinical counselling, *Lancet* 353:1829-1833, 1999.
11. Wallon M, Liou C, Garner P, et al: Congenital toxoplasmosis: systematic review of evidence of efficacy of treatment in pregnancy, *BMJ* 318:1511-1514, 1999.
12. Hudson SP: Selected viral infections in pregnancy, *J SOGC* 16:1245-1251, 1994.
13. Inocencion G, Loebstein R, Lalkin A, et al: Managing exposure to chickenpox during pregnancy, *Can Fam Physician* 44:745-747, 1998.
14. Herpesviridae infections in newborns: varicella zoster virus, herpes simplex virus, and cytomegalovirus. *Pediatr Clin North Am* 51(4):889, 2004.

Nausea and Vomiting in Pregnancy

Nausea and vomiting in pregnancy (NVP) is the most common medical condition in pregnancy, affecting 50% to 90% of women. The most severe form of NVP is referred to as hyperemesis gravidarum (HG). Defined as persistent vomiting that leads to weight loss greater than 5% of prepregnancy weight with associated electrolyte imbalance and ketonuria, HG occurs in about 1% of pregnancies.

The physical and emotional impact of NVP has a negative effect on family relationships and has major consequences on women's working abilities. It leads to anxiety and worry about the effect of the symptoms on the fetus. In Canada, as many as 14 hospitalizations per 1000 live births are attributable to NVP. Therefore, early recognition and management of NVP can have significant effects on health and quality of life during pregnancy as well as financial impact on the health care system.

The pathogenesis of NVP is poorly understood and the etiology is multifactorial. Other causes of nausea and vomiting must be ruled out, including gastrointestinal, genitourinary, CNS, and toxic or metabolic problems. In addition idiopathic NVP must be distinguished from that caused by hydatidiform mole or multiple gestation.

Pharmacological antiemetic therapy is still viewed with caution due to thalidomide (causing limb reduction defects) and Bendectin (voluntarily withdrawn from the market in 1983 due to legal actions resulting from false claims of teratogenicity). Hence, primary care providers play a major role in counselling and reassuring patients on safe and effective treatments available for NVP.

Dietary and lifestyle changes

Because RCTs are difficult to perform, there has been no evidence to prove the effectiveness of dietary changes in relieving NVP symptoms. Neither is there evidence that short-term dietary deficiencies during the early weeks of pregnancy will have long-term consequences on pregnancy outcome. Women should be counselled to eat whatever appeals to them. Since fatigue seems to exacerbate NVP, and sleep requirements increase in early pregnancy, women should be encouraged to have extra rest. Short-term leave from work may be appropriate (Level "C" recommendation).

Non-pharmacological therapies

Ginger. Ginger is a spice present in foods and beverages. It is also available in teas and tablet extracts. There is one RCT which examines the efficacy of 1000 mg per day of ginger. Safety at higher doses has not yet been determined. Hence, ginger can be recommended at any time as an oral dose of 250 mg every 6 hours.

Acupuncture and Acupressure. Acupuncturists have used stimulation of the P6 (Neiguan) point, located three fingers' breadth proximal to the wrist for thousands of years, to treat nausea and vomiting. Non-blinded RCTs have demonstrated a decrease in persisting nausea by at least 50%. Bands worn on the wrist (Sea Bands) to apply acupressure may also be helpful (Level "A" recommendation).

Vitamins

Pyridoxine Monotherapy. Pyridoxine, vitamin B_6, has been shown to be effective in two RCTs (75 mg/day and 30 mg/day orally). A retrospective cohort study concluded that its use conferred no risk for major malformations. It may be considered at any time as an adjuvant measure (Level "A" recommendation).

Pharmacological therapies

Pharmacological therapies should be initiated when conservative measures are not effective and should be initiated, when appropriate, as soon as possible after the diagnosis of NVP. Primary care physicians should be familiar with the most commonly used drugs (see following review). Assuming non-NVP causes have been ruled out, a more detailed algorithm is available in the SOGC guidelines for more refractory cases.

Antihistamines

Doxylamine Combinations. Doxylamine is an H1 receptor antagonist that has been shown to be effective in the treatment of NVP. It is currently marketed in Canada as a fixed combination, delayed-release formulation containing 10 mg doxylamine with 10 mg pyridoxine (vitamin B6). The standard dose is up to 4 tablets per day, taken in two doses (one in the morning and one in the evening). Recent reviews of safety and efficacy of this product have not shown risk to the fetus; hence, it is currently considered to be standard of care (Level "A" recommendation).

Other Antihistamines. The most commonly used alternative antihistamine is dimenhydrinate (Gravol). A wide body of evidence suggests that this drug is effective, carries no human teratogenic potential, and may in fact confer a slightly decreased risk of malformations with use in the first trimester. It is a good choice for acute and breakthrough episodes of NVP. The usual dose is 50 to 100 mg by mouth or as a suppository every 4 to 6 hours (Level "A" recommendation).

Other pharmacotherapies

Please refer to the SOGC guidelines.[1]

Refractory NVP

When NVP is refractory to initial pharmacotherapy, other causes or exacerbating factors should be sought. Investigations should include electrolytes, TSH, renal function, liver function, drug levels, ultrasound, and possibly *Helicobacter pylori* testing (Level "A" recommendation).

_____ ≈ REFERENCES ≈ _____

1. Arsenault M, Lane C: SOGC Clinical practice guidelines; The management of nausea and vomiting of pregnancy, *JOGC* 24(10):817-823, 2002. Accessed at www.sogc.org on May 23, 2005.

Classification of recommendations

Recommendations included in these guidelines have been adapted from the ranking method found in the Report of the Canadian Task Force on Preventive Health Care, accessible at http://www.ctfphc.org (accessed May 23, 2005).

EPISIOTOMY

Historically, episiotomies have been thought to reduce the mechanical and metabolic morbidity of the infant, prevent pelvic floor relaxation, and decrease the incidence of perineal pain, urinary incontinence, and sexual dysfunction.[1,2] Well-designed randomized controlled trials have since proven these hypotheses wrong.[2-4] When compared with restrictive episiotomy (i.e. only when condition of mother or fetus necessitates urgent delivery), patients who had routine episiotomies not only had more pain and sexual dysfunction, but also had a much higher incidence of third- and fourth-degree tears.[3] Labrecque and co-workers[5] in a retrospective cohort study involving over 4000 women also found a much higher rate of third- and fourth-degree tears in patients who had episiotomies. A review of trials by the Cochrane Collaboration demonstrated that a policy of restrictive episiotomy had many benefits compared with routine, including less posterior perineal trauma, less suturing and fewer healing complications. There was no difference between the groups with respect to rates of severe vaginal or perineal trauma, dyspareunia, incontinence or pain. The only benefit to routine episiotomy was increased rates of anterior perineal trauma in the restrictive group.

❧ REFERENCES ❧

1. Helewa ME: Episiotomy and severe perineal trauma: of science and fiction (editorial), *Can Med Assoc J* 156:811-813, 1997.

2. Klein M, Gauthier R, Robbins JM, et al: Relation of episiotomy to perineal trauma and morbidity, sexual dysfunction, and pelvic floor relaxation, *Am J Obstet Gynecol* 171:591-598, 1994.

3. lein MC, Gauthier RC, Jorgensen SH, et al: Does episiotomy prevent perineal trauma and pelvic floor relaxation? *Online J Curr Clin Trials* [serial online], Jul 1, 2 (Doc No 10), 1992.

4. Carroli G, Belizan J. Episiotomy for vaginal birth (Cochrane Review). In The Cocrane Library, Issue 3, 2004, updated May 4, 1999. Chichester, UK, John Wiley and Sons, Ltd.

5. Labrecque M, Baillargeon L, Dallaire M, et al: Association between median episiotomy and severe perineal lacerations in primiparous women, *Can Med Assoc J* 156:797-802, 1997.

POSTPARTUM DEPRESSION

Postpartum depression (PPD) occurs within 6 to 12 weeks of delivery in about 10% of pregnancies. It should be distinguished from postnatal blues, which are experienced by 50% to 80% of women and are mild and self-limited, and postpartum or puerperal psychosis, which affects about 0.2% of pregnant women[1]. The "blues" appear 2 to 7 days after delivery and usually resolve within 2 weeks. Deficiency or imbalance of sex hormones has been suggested as a cause of PPD.[2] However, a recent Cochrane review found that treatment of women with progestins made them worse, and treatment with estrogen produced only modest improvement in symptoms.[3] Psychoses complicate about one in 1000 deliveries. The most common is related to manic depression, in which neuroleptic drugs should be used with caution. Post-traumatic stress disorder, obsessions of child harm, and a range of anxiety disorders all require specific psychological treatments. Postpartum depression necessitates thorough exploration. Cessation of breastfeeding is not necessary, because most antidepressant drugs seem not to affect the infant. Controlled trials have shown the benefit of involving the child's father in therapy and of interventions promoting interaction between mother and infant. Owing to its complexity, multidisciplinary specialist teams have an important place in postpartum psychiatry[1]. There is evidence that the use of a screening tool, the Edinburg Postpartum Depression Scale, during well-child visits in the first year of life, can effectively identify those at risk[4].

The duration of untreated PPD is usually 2 to 6 months, which is similar to depression occurring at any other time[5]. Women whose initial manifestation of an affective disorder is PPD are at increased risk for subsequent postpartum depressions. Also, women with a first-degree relative who has bipolar disorder are at higher risk of PPD. Women with PPD who have had a past history of depressions unrelated to pregnancy are not at increased risk for subsequent PPD.[6] A previous stillbirth is also a risk factor for PPD, particularly if the subsequent pregnancy occurs within 12 months of that event.[7]

Children of women with PPD have been found to have some degree of cognitive impairment and emotional and behavioral problems when evaluated at ages 18 months and 4 to 5 years. Whether treatment of PPD alters this outcome is uncertain, but preliminary studies are encouraging. One explanation for this finding is that associative learning in young infants is related to the quality of the "child-directed speech" to which they are exposed. Among other characteristics, child-directed speech is distinguished by exaggerated modulation of tone, increased amplitude, longer pauses, and more repetitions. Depressed mothers are less capable of generating child-directed speech than are non-depressed mothers.[8] Therefore detection and treatment of PPD are priorities because treatment improves the quality of life of both mother and infant.

Although a number of studies have shown counselling and psychotherapy to be beneficial,[1,5,6] most workers advocate pharmacotherapy (even for nursing mothers) because withholding drugs has serious consequences for mother, baby, and other family members. First-choice drugs are SSRIs.[9] Tricyclics are also effective, and ECT leads to rapid improvement in refractory cases.[1]

An open clinical trial in a small group of women with a past history of postpartum depression compared the effects of antidepressants given immediately after delivery against clinical monitoring only. The rate of recurrent postpartum depression was much higher in the group not receiving antidepressants.[10]

(handwritten annotation: — onset up to 6m P.P.)

❧ REFERENCES ❧

1. Brockington I. Postpartum psychiatric disorders. *Lancet* 363(9405);303-310:2004

2. Murray D: Oestrogen and postnatal depression (editorial), *Lancet* 347:918-919, 1996.

3. Lawrie TA, Herxheimer A, Dalton K: Oestrogens and progestins in preventing and treating postnatal depression (Cochrane review). In: The Cochrane Library, Issue 4, 2004. Chichester, UK. John Wiley & Sons Ltd.

4. Chaudron LH, Szilagyi PG, Kitzman HJ, Wadkins HI, Conwell Y. Detection of postpartum depressive symptoms by screening at well-child visits. *Pediatrics* 2004 Mar;113(3 Pt 1):551-8.

5. Epperson CN: Postpartum major depression: detection and treatment, *Am Fam Physician* 59:2247-2254, 1999.

6. Cooper PJ, Murray L: Postnatal depression, *BMJ* 316:1884-1886, 1998.

7. Hughes PM, Turton P, Evans CD: Stillbirth as risk factor for depression and anxiety in the subsequent pregnancy: cohort study, *BMJ* 318:1721-1724, 1999.

8. Kaplan PS, Bachorowski J-A, Zarlengo-Strouse P: Child-directed speech produced by mothers with symptoms of depression fails to promote associative learning in 4-month-old infants, *Child Dev* 70:560-570, 1999.

9. Kulinn NA, Pastuszak A, Sage SR, et al: Pregnancy outcome following maternal use of the new selective serotonin reuptake inhibitors: a prospective controlled multicenter study, *JAMA* 279:609-610, 1998.

10. Wisner KL, Wheeler S: Prevention of recurrent postpartum major depression, *Hosp Commun Psychiatry* 45:1191-1196, 1994.

Migraines in pregnancy → tend to improve
- estrogen drop can cause HA
- Postpartum may worsen
- first Trimester worst
- MRI choice

acute
Tylenol 650mg
Mod-severe
   Acet 650-1000
   Maxeran 10mg
   Codeine 30-60mg
Ø NSAIDs, ASA, triptans,
Ø prophylaxis